Vascular
Manifestations
of
Systemic
Autoimmune
Diseases

Vascular Manifestations
of
Systemic Autoimmune Diseases

Edited by

Ronald A. Asherson, M.D.
Ricard Cervera, M.D.

Associate Editors

Steven B. Abramson, M.D.
Jean-Charles Piette, M.D.
Douglas A. Triplett, M.D.

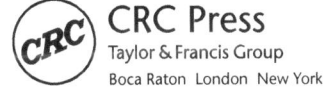
CRC Press
Taylor & Francis Group
Boca Raton London New York

CRC Press is an imprint of the
Taylor & Francis Group, an **informa** business

CRC Press
Taylor & Francis Group
6000 Broken Sound Parkway NW, Suite 300
Boca Raton, FL 33487-2742

First issued in paperback 2019

© 2001 by Taylor & Francis Group, LLC
CRC Press is an imprint of Taylor & Francis Group, an Informa business

No claim to original U.S. Government works

ISBN-13: 978-0-8493-1335-6 (hbk)
ISBN-13: 978-0-367-39761-6 (pbk)

Library of Congress Card Number 00-060809

Library of Congress Cataloging-in-Publication Data

Vascular manifestations of systemic autoimmune disease / edited by Ronald A. Asherson, Ricard Cervera, Douglas A. Triplett.
  p. cm.
  Includes bibliographical references and index.
  ISBN 0-8493-1335-X (alk. paper)
  1. Vasculitis. 2. Autoimmune diseases—Complications. 3. Blood-vessels—Diseases—Immunological aspects. I. Asherson, Ronald A. II. Cervera, Ricard. III. Triplett, Douglas A.
  [DNLM: 1. Autoimmune Disease—complications. 2. Vascular Diseases—etiology. WD 305 V331 2000]
  RC694.5.I53 V365 2000
  616.1'3—dc21

                       00-060809
                           CIP

Visit the Taylor & Francis Web site at
http://www.taylorandfrancis.com

and the CRC Press Web site at
http://www.crcpress.com

Dedication

Dr. Asherson dedicates this book to the research fellows with whom he has worked at the Royal Postmedical School of London and the St. Thomas' Hospital in London, and to Professors Robert Lahita of New York, Jean-Charles Piette of Paris, and Yehuda Schoenfeld of Israel.

Dr. Cervera dedicates this book to his wife Carme and his daughters Marta and Laura.

Foreword

In the beginning, we thought inflammation of blood vessels was the sole manifestation of systemic autoimmune diseases. Now, by this new millennium, we have learned that disorders of coagulation, autoantibodies to phospholipids, vasospasm, both injury to and antibodies to neutrophils and endothelial cells, and certain lipids and amino acids are all intricately involved in the development of vascular disease in these patients. How are all these processes linked? What strategies can we employ or develop to halt the progression of vascular damage? What are the best ways to control acute vasculitis and vasospasm therapeutically? What are the risks and benefits of various strategies to prevent clotting? How soon should we initiate preventive strategies that protect blood vessels from arteriosclerosis in people with acute rheumatic diseases? What should those strategies be?

The biology of these attacks on blood vessels, the clinical consequences, therapeutic approaches, and preventive strategies are all addressed in this book. International experts in the vascular diseases associated with autoimmunity, Drs. Ronald Asherson, Ricard Cervera, Douglas Triplett, Jean-Charles Piette, and Steven Abramson, have gathered other experts who lead the thinking in such studies — experts of great international standing. Together they have assembled a comprehensive look at this ever-increasing problem. Now that most individuals survive the onset of severe acute systemic autoimmune diseases and live for decades more, halting the long-term attack on the vasculature is increasingly important.

Welcome to you, the reader. Whether you use this volume to look up a particular aspect of vascular disease in autoimmune settings or whether you read it from cover to cover, you are sure to have your thinking stimulated and your knowledge increased. Perhaps you will pursue some of these questions further and will be the first to solve some of these most puzzling problems.

Bevra H. Hahn, M.D., FACR
Professor of Medicine, Chief of Rheumatology
University of California, Los Angeles
Immediate Past President, American College of Rheumatology

The Editors

Ronald A. Asherson, M.D., FACP, FRCP (London), FCP (SA), FACR, is Honorary Consultant Physician and Principal Scientific Officer at the Rheumatic Disease Unit, Department of Medicine, Groote Schuur Hospital, University of Cape Town, South Africa.

Dr. Asherson qualified in Medicine at the University of Cape Town in 1957 and, after completing his internship, became H/P at the Hammersmith Hospital, London, in 1960. In 1961, he accepted a fellowship at the Columbia Presbyterian and Francis Delafield Hospitals in New York, returning to become Senior Registrar at the Groote Schuur Hospital in Cape Town from 1961 to 1964. After 10 years as a Clinical Tutor in the Department of Medicine, he returned to the U.S. and was appointed as Assistant Clinical Professor of Medicine at the New York Hospital–Cornell Medical Center. From 1981 to 1986, he was associated with the Rheumatology Department at the Royal Postgraduate Medical School of London. It was at that time that he developed his interest in systemic autoimmune diseases and antiphospholipid antibodies. In 1986 he moved to the Rayne Institute and St. Thomas' Hospital in London, where he was appointed Honorary Consultant Physician and Senior Research Fellow. In 1991 he took a year's sabbatical at St. Luke's Roosevelt Hospital Center in New York before returning to South Africa.

He is a Fellow of the American College of Physicians (FACP), a Founding Fellow of the American College of Rheumatology (FACR), and a Fellow of the Royal College of Physicians (FRCP) of London. From 1988 to 1991 he was on the Council of the Royal Society of Medicine in London. In 1992 he was the co-winner of the European League Against Rheumatism (EULAR) Prize and in 1993 was the co-recipient of the International League Against Rheumatism (ILAR) Prize, both for research on antiphospholipid antibodies.

Dr. Asherson has been an invited speaker at many universities and international conferences. He is the author of more than 200 papers on systemic autoimmune diseases and has contributed to more than 40 leading textbooks of medicine, rheumatology, and surgery as well as having co-edited the books *Phospholipid-Binding Antibodies,* CRC Press (1991), and *The Antiphospholipd Syndrome,* CRC Press (1996). Dr. Asherson is on the editorial boards of several international journals and is a member of the "Rheume 21st" group of international experts on rheumatology. He is currently engaged in research on systemic autoimmune diseases, particularly on the antiphospholipd syndrome, and is involved in clinical practice in South Africa.

Ricard Cervera, M.D., Ph.D., is Senior Specialist Physician at the Systemic Autoimmune Diseases Unit, Hospital Clinic of Barcelona, and Associate Professor of Medicine at the University of Barcelona School of Medicine, Barcelona, Catalonia, Spain.

Dr. Cervera qualified in Medicine in 1983 from the University of Barcelona and from 1984 until 1988 trained in Internal Medicine at the Hospital Clinic of Barcelona. He obtained his Ph.D. degree from the University of Barcelona in 1988 for his thesis on anticardiolipin antibodies. His postdoctoral experience included 2 years at the Lupus Research Unit, The Rayne Institute, St. Thomas' Hospital, London, working with Drs. Graham R. V. Hughes and Ronald A. Asherson.

Among other awards, he has received the Spanish Society of Internal Medicine Award for research on antibodies to endothelial cells, the Fernández-Cruz Award from the Rhône-Poulenc Farma Foundation, and the Juan Vivancos Award from the Consorci d'Hospitals de Barcelona. He has been the recipient of research grants from the Spanish Departments of Health and Education and Science, the British Council, and the European Commission.

Dr. Cervera is a member of the Catalan, Spanish, and International Societies of Internal Medicine, Spanish Society of Rheumatology, and honorary member of the Argentinian and Slovak Societies of Rheumatology. He is coordinator of the "Euro-lupus" and "Euro Phospholipid" projects, and of the European Working Party on Systemic Lupus Erythematosus, and has organized eight international workshops in several cities in Europe. He is on the editorial boards of several journals, including *Clinical Rheumatology, Clinical Application of Immunological Investigations,* and *Medicina Clinica* (Barcelona).

Dr. Cervera has presented over 100 invited lectures and has published more than 300 scientific papers. He is co-editor of several books, including *Antibodies to Endothelial Cells and Vascular Damage,* CRC Press (1994), *The Antiphospholipid Syndrome,* CRC Press (1996), and *Enfermedades Autoimmunes Sistémicas,* MRA (1998). His current major research interest includes clinical and immunological aspects of systemic autoimmune diseases, particularly the pathogenesis of vascular damage in systemic lupus erythematosus, primary Sjögren's syndrome and the antiphospholipid syndrome.

Associate Editors

Douglas A. Triplett, M.D., FACP, FCAP, FASCP, Vice President for Medical Education, Ball Memorial Hospital; Professor of Pathology and Assistant Dean, Indiana University School of Medicine; and Director of Midwest Hemostasis and Thrombosis Laboratories, Muncie, Indiana.

Dr. Triplett received his M.D. in 1968 from Indiana University School of Medicine and completed his pathology residency training at Methodist Hospital, Indianapolis, and Ball Memorial Hospital, Muncie. Following completion of his residency program, he assumed the responsibility of Director of Hematology, Ball Memorial Hospital/Pathologists Associated. In 1997 he became Laboratory Director for Midwest Hemostasis and Thrombosis Laboratories.

He was Valedictorian of his medical school class, and was the recipient of the prestigious Roy Reinhardt Award. He was elected Fellow of the American College of Physicians (FACP) in 1986, and served as Chairman of the Coagulation Resource Committee for the College of American Pathologists 1980—1992. In 2000 he assumed the position of Chairman, Council in Clinical Pathology (CCP), College of American Pathologists.

Dr. Triplett has been an invited speaker at many universities and international conferences. He has written more than 124 papers dealing with various aspects of hematopathology, and hemostasis and thrombosis, is the author or co-author of 7 books, and has written 45 book chapters.

Steven Abramson, M.D., is Professor of Medicine and Pathology at the New York University School of Medicine, where he is also Vice Dean for Medical Education. He was recently appointed as Chief, Division of Rheumatology, and is also Physician-in-Chief and Chairman of the Department of Rheumatology and Medicine at the Hospital for Joint Diseases. He graduated from Dartmouth College and earned his medical degree from Harvard Medical School. He completed his internship and residency at the New York University Medical Center-Bellevue Hospital, where he also pursued a fellowship in rheumatology.

Currently a member of the Board of Trustees of the National Arthritis Foundation, Dr. Abramson is a former Chairman of the Arthritis Advisory Committee, Center for Drug Evaluation and Research, of the Food and Drug Administration (FDA), and continues as an active consultant to the Committee. He has served on several committees and has organized many symposia at the American College of Rheumatology. He is also on the Board of Directors of Osteoarthritis Research Society International (OARSI).

Dr. Abramson is known internationally for his research contributions to the basic understanding of inflammation and immunologically induced tissue injury. He has published numerous reports in refereed journals and books, has served on the editorial boards of several journals, and is currently Associate Editor of *Arthritis and Rheumatism.*

Contributors

Steven B. Abramson
Department of Rheumatology
Hospital for Joint Diseases
New York, NY

Ronald A. Asherson
Rheumatic Diseases Unit
Department of Medicine
University of Cape Town School of Medicine
Cape Town, South Africa

A. Olcay Aydintug
Department of Clinical Immunology –
  Rheumatology
Division of Internal Medicine
Medical School of Ankara University
Ankara, Turkey

Paul A. Bacon
Department of Rheumatology
Division of Immunology and Infection
University of Birmingham
Birmingham, U.K.

Pierre-André Bécherel
Department of Internal Medicine
Pitié-Salpêtrière University Hospital
Paris, France

H. Michael Belmont
Department of Rheumatology
Hospital for Joint Diseases
New York, NY

Carol M. Black
Center for Rheumatology (Royal Free Campus)
Royal Free and University College
  Medical School
London, U.K.

Miri Blank
Research Unit for Autoimmune Diseases
Chaim Sheba Medical Center
Sackler Faculty of Medicine
Tel-Aviv University
Tel-Aviv, Israel

Xavier Bosch
Systemic Autoimmune Diseases Unit
Hospital Clinic
Barcelona, Catalonia, Spain

Kevin G. Burnand
Academic Department of Surgery
St. Thomas' Hospital
London, U.K.

Mario García-Carrasco
Rheumatic Disease Unit
School of Medicine
Universidad Autónoma de Puebla
Puebla, México

David M. Carruthers
Department of Rheumatology
Division of Immunity and Infection
University of Birmingham
Birmingham, U.K.

Manuel Ramos-Casals
Systemic Autoimmune Diseases Unit
Hospital Clinic
Barcelona, Catalonia, Spain

Marco Matucci-Cerinic
Department of Medicine
Division of Rheumatology
University of Florence
Florence, Italy

Ricard Cervera
Systemic Autoimmune Diseases Unit
Hospital Clinic
Barcelona, Catalonia, Spain

Maria C. Cid
Department of Internal Medicine
Hospital Clinic
Barcelona, Catalonia, Spain

H. Terence Cook
Department of Histopathology
Imperial College School of Medicine
Hammersmith Hospital
London, U.K.

Kevin A. Davies
Rheumatology Section
Imperial College School of Medicine
Hammersmith Hospital
London, U.K.

David P. D'Cruz
The Lupus Research Unit
The Rayne Institute
St. Thomas' Hospital
London, U.K.

Nicoletta Del Pappa
Department of Internal Medicine
University of Milan
Milan, Italy

Christopher P. Denton
Center for Rheumatology (Royal Free Campus)
Royal Free and University College Medical
  School
London, U.K.

Gerard Espinosa
Systemic Autoimmune Diseases Unit
Hospital Clinic
Barcelona, Catalonia, Spain

Pan Sheng Fan
Department of Medicine
Division of Rheumatology
Medical College of Ohio
Toledo, OH

Josep Font
Systemic Autoimmune Diseases Unit
Hospital Clinic
Barcelona, Catalonia, Spain

Camille Francès
Department of Internal Medicine
Pitié-Salpêtrière University Hospital
Paris, France

Sergio Generini
Department of Medicine
Division of Rheumatology
University of Florence
Florence, Italy

Anne Gompel
Service de Gynécologie
Hotel-Dieu de Paris
Paris, France

Scott Goodnight
Division of Laboratory Medicine
The Oregon Health Sciences University
Portland, OR

Josep M. Grau
Department of Internal Medicine
Hospital Clinic
Barcelona, Catalonia, Spain

Tim W. Higenbottam
Department of Respiratory Medicine
Royal Hallamshire Hospital
Sheffield, U.K.

Miguel Ingelmo
Systemic Autoimmune Diseases Unit
Hospital Clinic
Barcelona, Catalonia, Spain

M. Bashar Kahaleh
Department of Medicine
Division of Rheumatology
Medical College of Ohio
Toledo, OH

Cees G.M. Kallenberg
Department of Clinical Immunology
University Hospital Groningen
Groningen, The Netherlands

Ilan Krause
Research Unit of Autoimmune Diseases
Chaim Sheba Medical Center
Sackler Faculty of Medicine
Tel-Aviv University
Tel-Aviv, Israel

Robert G. Lahita
Department of Rheumatology
New York Medical College
St. Vincent's Hospital
New York, NY

Thomas J.A. Lehman
Division of Pediatric Rheumatology,
Hospital for Special Surgery
Stanford Weill Medical College
  of Cornell University
New York, NY

Sozos Loizou
Rheumatology Section
Imperial College School of Medicine
Hammersmith Hospital
London, U.K.

Gale A. McCarty
Indiana University
Rheumatology Division
Indianapolis, IN

Pier Luigi Meroni
Department of Internal Medicine
University of Milan
Milan, Italy

Joan T. Merrill
St. Lukes Roosevelt Hospital
Columbia University
New York, NY

Fujio Numano
Department of Internal Medicine
Tokyo Medical and Dental University
Tokyo, Japan

Ann L. Parke
Division of Rheumatic Diseases
University of Connecticut Health
  Science Centre
Farmington, CT

Michelle Petri
Division of Rheumatology
Johns Hopkins University School of Medicine
Baltimore, MD

Jean-Charles Piette
Department of Internal Medicine
Pitié-Salpêtrière University Hospital
Paris, France

Charles D. Pusey
Department of Medicine
Imperial College School of Medicine
Hammersmith Hospital
London, U.K.

Elena Raschi
Department of Internal Medicine
University of Milan
Milan, Italy

Karim Raza
Department of Rheumatology
City Hospital
Birmingham, U.K.

Joan-Carles Reverter
Hemotherapy and Hemostasis Department
Hospital Clinic
Barcelona, Catalonia, Spain

José Hernández-Rodríguez
Department of Internal Medicine
Hospital Clinic
Barcelona, Catalonia, Spain

Robert A.S. Roubey
Associate Professor of Medicine
Division of Rheumatology and Immunology
University of North Carolina
Chapel Hill, NC

Michael Samarkos
Rheumatology Section
Imperial College School of Medicine
Hammersmith Hospital
London, U.K.

James R. Seibold
Robert Wood Johnson Medical School,
Scleroderma Program
University of Medicine and Dentistry
  of New Jersey
New Brunswick, NJ

Yehuda Shoenfeld
Department of Medicine "B"
Research Unit of Autoimmune Diseases
Chaim Sheba Medical Center
Tel-Aviv University
Tel-Aviv, Israel

Ronit Simantov
Division of Hematology/Oncology
Stanford Weill Medical College
 of Cornell University
New York, NY

Dolors Tàssies
Hemotherapy and Hemostasis Department
Hospital Clinic
Barcelona, Catalonia, Spain

Jan Willem Cohen Tervaert
Department of Clinical Immunology
University Hospital Groningen
Groningen, The Netherlands

Douglas A. Triplett
Indiana University School of Medicine
Midwest Hemostasis
 and Thrombosis Laboratories
Muncie, IN

Outi Vaarala
Department of Biochemistry
Mannerheimintie
Helsinki, Finland

Phillippe Vinceneux
Department of Internal Medicine
Pitié-Salpêtrière University Hospital
Paris, France

Matthew Waltham
Academic Department of Surgery
St. Thomas' Hospital
London, U.K.

Babette B. Weksler
Division of Hematology/Oncology
Stanford Weill Medical College
 of Cornell University
New York, NY

Simon P. Wharton
Department of Respiratory Medicine
Royal Hallamshire Hospital
Sheffield, U.K.

Table of Contents

Section I: Mechanisms of Vascular Disease

Ronald A. Asherson and Ricard Cervera, Editors
Douglas A. Triplett, Associate Editor

Section II: Clinical Manifestations

Ronald A. Asherson and Ricard Cervera, Editors
Jean-Charles Piette, Associate Editor

Section III: Treatment

Ronald A. Asherson and Ricard Cervera, Editors
Steven B. Abramson, Associate Editor

Section I

Mechanisms of Vascular Disease

1 Pathology of Vascular Disease

H. Terence Cook and Charles D. Pusey

CONTENTS

I. SYSTEMIC VASCULITIS

Vasculitis is inflammation in blood vessels. It may be divided into inflammation-involving arteries (arteritis), arterioles (arteriolitis), capillaries (capillaritis), or veins (venulitis). Localized vasculitis may be seen at sites of infection or of inflammation secondary to other causes such as trauma, damage due to chemicals or toxins, or irradiation. Systemic vasculitis may arise in infections from the dissemination of organisms through the circulation, as is seen, for example, in meningococcal septicemia. However, the majority of cases of systemic vasculitis arise through noninfectious mechanisms and these forms of noninfectious systemic vasculitis are the subject of this section. These vasculitides form a number of relatively clear cut, although overlapping, clinical and patho-

---

TABLE 1.1
Classification of Systemic Vasculitis

Large Vessel Vasculitis
Giant-cell (temporal) arteritis
Takayusu's arteritis

Medium-Sized Vessel Arteritis
Classical polyarteritis nodosa
Kawasaki's disease

Small Vessel Vasculitis
Associated with immune deposits
Henoch-Schonlein purpura
Cryoglobulinemia
Goodpasture's (anti-GBM) disease
Other immune complex vasculitis (e.g., serum sickness, SLE)

Without conspicuous immune deposits
Microscopic polyangiitis
Wegener's granulomatosis
Churg-Strauss syndrome

---

logical entities. Since, in most cases, the etiology and pathogenesis are still obscure, they are classified mainly on the tissue morphology and more specifically on the basis of the size of vessel involved, the type of inflammatory response, and any associated pathological features (Table 1.1).[1-3]

A. GIANT CELL (TEMPORAL) ARTERITIS

Temporal arteritis is the most common form of systemic arteritis, with an incidence of up to 20 to 30 cases per 100,000 per year for those over 50 years old.[4] It is uncommon below the age of 50. It is a focal inflammation of arteries of medium and small size that mainly affects extracranial branches of the carotid arteries, particularly the temporal arteries. However, in severe cases, lesions may be found in arteries throughout the body and in the arch of the aorta. The major clinical manifestations are of headache, tenderness over the temporal artery, visual loss, and facial pain. It is frequently associated with the syndrome of polymyalgia rheumatica in which there is nonspecific malaise, anorexia, weight loss, and aching around the shoulders and hips. In cases with involvement of visceral vessels, there may be myocardial ischemia, gastrointestinal symptoms, or neurological disturbances. If the aortic arch is involved, the presentation may be identical to that of Takayusu's arteritis.

Histologically, the most common appearance is of granulomatous inflammation which is closely related to fragmented internal elastic lamina. In these areas the inflammatory infiltrate is composed of epithelioid macrophages with frequent macrophage giant cells. However, in one third of cases giant cells are absent or very scanty and many sections may have to be examined to find them. Adjacent to the areas of granulomatous inflammation there is typically a nonspecific inflammatory infiltrate of neutrophils, lymphocytes, and eosinophils which may involve the full thickness of the arterial wall. The majority of the lymphocytes are T helper cells.[5] There is often prominent intimal fibrosis (Figure 1.1) and superimposed thrombosis. The lesions heal with fibrous tissue replacing the damaged internal elastic lamina or with fibrous obliteration of the lumen. The disease often only involves short segments of the arterial wall, with the important practical implication that temporal artery biopsies should be of adequate size and examined histologically at several levels. Ideally at least 1 cm and preferably 2 to 3 cm of artery should be biopsied.[6] We routinely cut biopsies into 2 mm-long segments which are then embedded on end and each cut at 3 levels, with

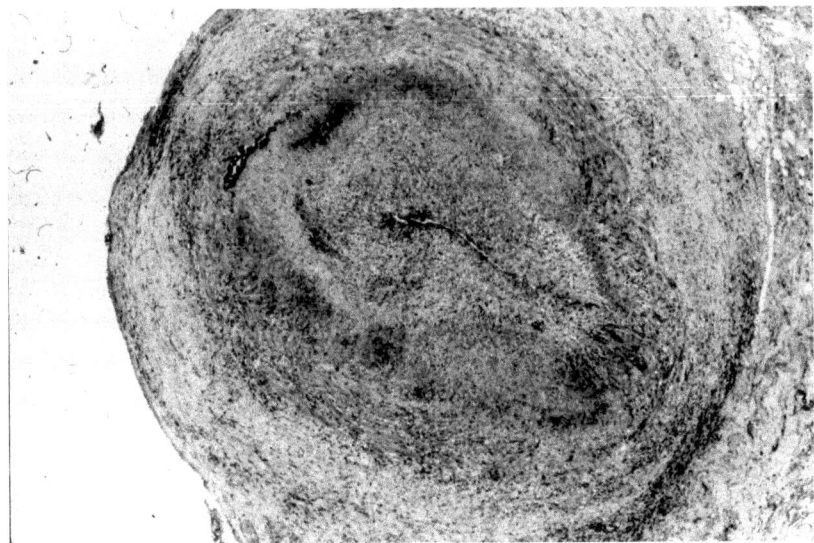

FIGURE 1.1 Temporal arteritis. The temporal artery shows transmural inflammation which is most marked in the inner media, together with marked intimal thickening almost obliterating the lumen (H&E, × 10).

hematoxylin and eosin and elastic van Gieson staining. Histological changes may be present in clinically normal vessels. Even in cases in which the clinical features are classical only about 60% of temporal artery biopsies will show disease.

The etiology and pathogenesis of this relatively common disease are still unknown. The presence of granulomatous inflammation has led to the suspicion that an infectious agent may be involved, but none has been identified. The morphological features suggest an immunologic reaction against a component of the arterial wall, such as elastin.

B. TAKAYASU'S ARTERITIS

This condition, named after the Japanese ophthalmologist who described its ocular manifestations in 1908, is an arteritis of large vessels, principally involving the thoracic or abdominal aorta, or both, and their major branches.[7] It is a rare disease that is found worldwide, but most of the patients are young women from Asia, India, Africa, and South America. However, it is increasingly reported in Europe and in the U.S. It is seven times more common in women than men. It is seen predominantly between the ages of 10 to 50 years, and 90% of patients are under the age of 30. Almost all patients with the disease have multiple sites of arterial involvement. It classically involves the aortic arch, but in 30% of cases it also affects the remainder of the aorta and its branches. In 12% it is limited to the descending thoracic and abdominal aorta. The coronary arteries are involved in about 10% of cases and the pulmonary artery in about 50%. The symptoms depend on the location and severity of the process and include weakening of the pulses of the upper extremities sometimes with increased blood pressure in the lower extremities, ocular disturbances, and various neurological defects. Involvement of the root of the aorta may lead to dilatation and aortic valve regurgitation. The most common cause of death is heart failure or sudden death due to aortic rupture.

The gross morphological changes are irregular thickening of the aortic wall with intimal wrinkling. The orifices of the major arteries to the upper extremities may be markedly narrowed or obliterated accounting for the clinical designation of "pulseless disease." Histologically there is an inflammatory infiltrate which is most prominent in the media. It is predominantly lymphoplasmacytic with variable numbers of eosinophils and macrophages. There may be focal granulomatous inflammation with scattered macrophage giant cells, but the number of giant cells is quite variable. In some cases the granulomas show central necrosis resembling tuberculosis. The inflammation in the media eventually leads to intimal hyperplasia and fibrosis. The histological appearances may be indistinguishable from those of giant cell (temporal) arteritis and the distinction is made mainly on the clinical presentation including the age of the patient. The cause is unknown.

C. Classical Polyarteritis Nodosa (Classical PAN)

This is a necrotizing inflammation which may affect medium- or small-sized arteries in any organ or system of the body. The more usual sites of involvement found in autopsy series are the kidneys (85%), heart (75%), liver (65%), and gastrointestinal tract (50%), with less common involvement of the pancreas, testes, skeletal muscle, nervous system, and skin. As defined here, cases in which there is glomerulonephritis or involvement of arterioles, capillaries, or venules are excluded. Classical PAN is a disease of young adults although it may be seen in children and older individuals. It affects two to three times as many men as women. The symptoms and signs may vary depending on the particular organ system affected, but result from the effects of ischemia and infarction in the involved organs.[8]

Grossly, the lesions in the arteries involve sharply localized segments often at branching points and bifurcations. Macroscopically, they may be apparent as nodular grey or red swellings of the vessel and rarely small aneurysmal dilatations or perivascular hematomas may result from weakening or rupture of the wall. Ulceration, infarction, ischemic atrophy or hemorrhage may be found in the areas supplied by these vessels.

Microscopically the acute lesions are characterized by necrosis which may involve the intima alone or the full thickness of the arterial wall. The necrotic area has a characteristic eosinophilic staining pattern resembling that of fibrin, hence the designation "fibrinoid" necrosis (Figure 1.2). Numerous leukocytes, including neutrophils, may be present within the vessel wall and extending into the perivascular tissue; in some cases eosinophils are prominent. The necrosis may involve the entire circumference of the vessel wall, but is often localized to one segment. There may be luminal thrombosis overlying the inflamed area. As the lesions heal the inflammatory infiltrate becomes rich in macrophages and plasma cells and concentrically arranged fibroblasts are seen. The fibroblastic response may extend into the surrounding tissue. Thrombus may also become organized leading to fibrous obliteration of the lumen. In healed lesions there is fibrous replacement of part of the vessel wall and, in elastic stains, the internal elastic lamina is seen to be replaced by fibrous

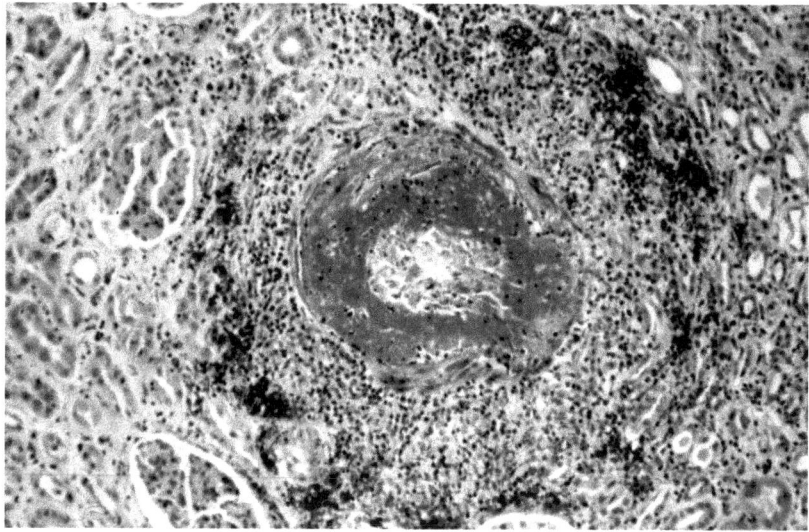

FIGURE 1.2 Classical polyarteritis nodosa. An arcuate artery in the kidney shows circumferential fibrinoid necrosis with surrounding inflammation and hemorrhage (H&E, × 25).

tissue. At any particular time, both active necrotizing inflammation and healed lesions may be seen in different vessels or even in different parts of the same vessel.

The cause is unknown. An association with hepatitis B infection has been reported raising the possibility of an immune complex pathogenesis, but immunofluorescence and electron microscopy provide little support for this. The presence of antibodies to neutrophil cytoplasmic antigens (ANCA) is rare in patients with classical polyarteritis, indicating that they do not play a role in pathogenesis.

D. KAWASAKI'S DISEASE

This condition, also called mucocutaneous lymph node syndrome of childhood, is characterized by lymphadenopathy, an exfoliative cutaneous eruption and arteritis involving medium-sized arteries, particularly the coronary arteries. It is a disease of young children with a peak incidence in the first year of life. It is not found in neonates and is rarely seen for the first time after 5 years of age. The onset is abrupt, with high fever, malaise, and a nonspecific rash. A striking feature is plantar and palmar erythema with edema and subsequent desquamation.

Histologically, the arteritis resembles that of classical PAN, with necrosis and inflammation affecting the entire thickness of the vessel wall. There may be superimposed thrombosis. Aneurysm formation may occur at the site of inflammation. Coronary artery aneurysms are reported in up to a quarter of those affected. Two thirds of these occur in the left coronary artery, mainly in its proximal part. Death in Kawasaki's disease, due to superimposed thrombosis in a coronary artery or to rupture of a coronary artery aneurysm, occurs in 1 to 2.8% of patients in the first 3 months of the illness, and sudden death has been reported months to years after the initial illness. The kidney is the second most commonly affected organ after the heart, with lesions usually affecting interlobar or arcuate arteries

The cause is unknown. The disease may occur in an epidemic form and shows a seasonal incidence with more cases in the spring months in the Northern Hemisphere. It is common in Japan and in persons of Japanese ancestry in other countries. A variety of infectious agents have been suggested as etiological factors, but there is no firm evidence for their involvement. In some patients cytotoxic antibodies which react with cytokine-activated endothelial cells have been found.[9]

E. VASCULITIS INVOLVING SMALL VESSELS

Many forms of vasculitis involve arterioles, capillaries, or venules. Glomerulonephritis is also common in these forms. They may be classified into those in which there are easily detected immune deposits in the vessel wall and those in which immune deposits are not found. The latter group is further subclassified on the basis of the type of vessel involved and other associated features, such as the presence of circulating ANCA. Morphologically, the features of these diseases overlap and, in particular, any of them may give rise to inflammation of small vessels in the skin to produce the histological picture of leukocytoclastic vasculitis. This is a vasculitis involving the capillaries and venules of the dermis. The major findings are neutrophils, nuclear dust from fragmented neutrophils, and fibrin both within and around capillaries and venules (Figure 1.3). The amount of nuclear dust and fibrin is very variable. In addition, there may be a mixed inflammatory infiltrate surrounding the venules of the superficial and/or deep dermal plexuses and sometimes those in the subcutis.

1. Small Vessel Vasculitis with Immune Deposits

a. Henoch-Schonlein purpura

In this syndrome there is necrotizing inflammation of small vessels with deposition of IgA in vessel walls. It typically involves the skin, gut, and glomeruli and is associated with arthralgia or arthritis. It is predominantly an illness of children, but may be seen at any age. The peak incidence is 4 to 5 years of age. The skin lesions characteristically affect the extensor surfaces of the lower legs,

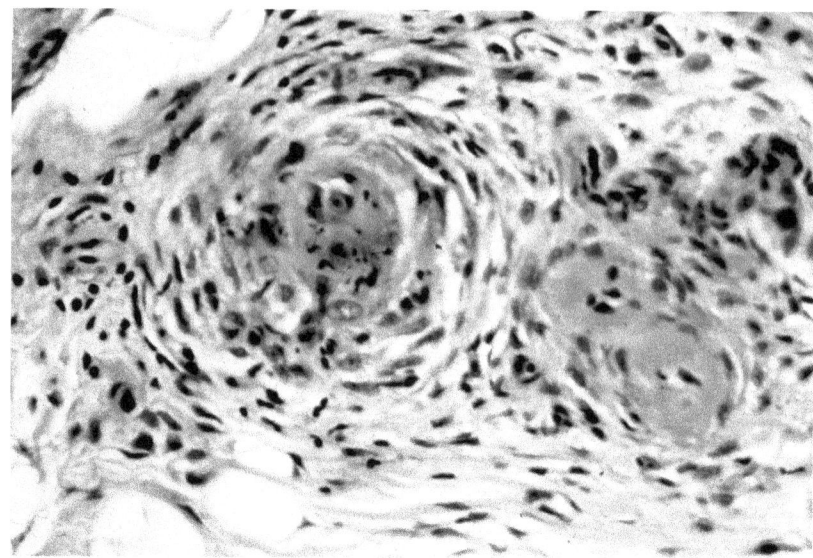

FIGURE 1.3 Leukocytoclastic vasculitis. Small vessels show fibrinoid necrosis of their walls associated with inflammatory cells and nuclear debris (H&E, × 100).

the buttocks, and the forearms. Histologically, the changes in the skin are those of a leukocytoclastic vasculitis (see above). IgA and C3 can be demonstrated by immunohistochemistry in the vasculitic lesions and may also be present in apparently uninvolved vessels. Similar changes to those in the skin may be found in other organs, particularly in the gastrointestinal tract. The incidence of renal involvement is estimated to be 40 to 60%.

The typical lesion in the kidney is a focal and segmental proliferative glomerulonephritis (Figure 1.4). Glomeruli show segmental areas of increased cellularity, including increased numbers of cells in capillary lumens, often on a background of slight generalized mesangial hypercellularity. The increase in intraluminal cells is, in part, due to the presence of infiltrating neutrophils or mononu-

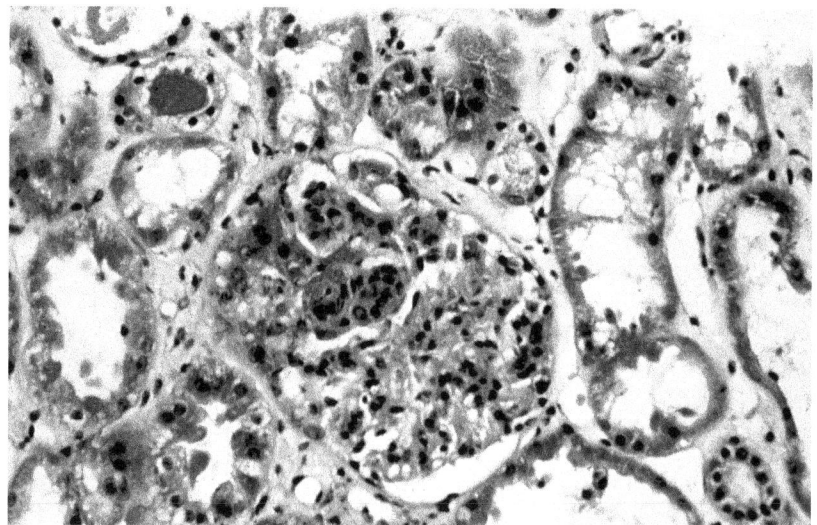

FIGURE 1.4 Henoch-Schonlein purpura. The glomerulus shows a segmental area of fibrinoid necrosis with a small cellular crescent in Bowman's space. The rest of the tuft shows mild mesangial hypercellularity (H&E, × 60).

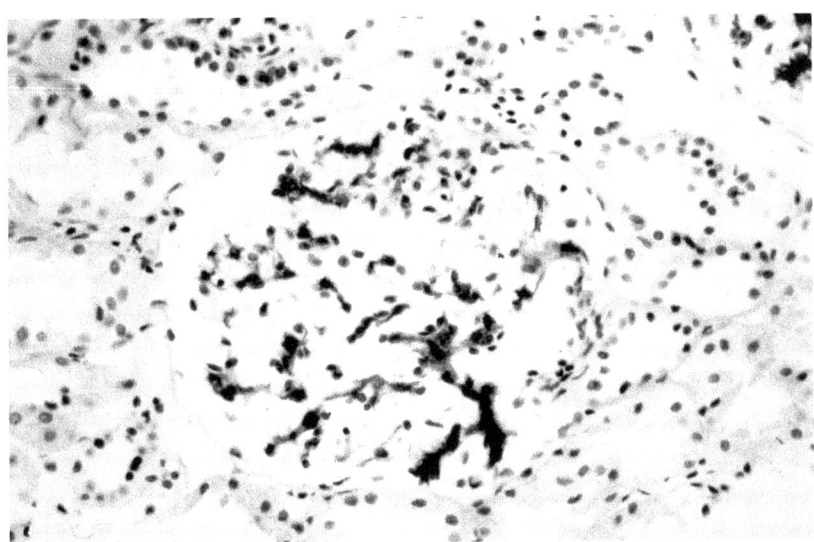

FIGURE 1.5 Henoch-Schonlein purpura. The glomerulus shows IgA deposition in the mesangium (peroxidase counterstained with hematoxylin, × 60).

clear cells. There may be segmental areas of fibrinoid necrosis with disruption of the glomerular architecture and the presence of eosinophilic amorphous material which stains immunohistochemically for fibrin. In more severe cases, crescents are present in Bowman's space. Following the acute phase, crescents become progressively less cellular and more fibrous, and areas of segmental glomerular necrosis heal with obliteration of capillary lumens and the development of segmental scars with adhesion of the glomerular tuft to Bowman's capsule. Tubulointerstitial changes are thought to be secondary to the glomerular changes and reflect their severity. There is often tubular dedifferentiation and red cell casts may be present. The interstitium shows edema and a nonspecific mononuclear cell inflammatory infiltrate. The blood vessels in the kidney only rarely show evidence of necrotizing inflammation. By immunohistochemistry, IgA is found within the glomeruli (Figure 1.5) and may be accompanied by C3 and IgG. The deposits are found in all glomeruli, most prominently in the mesangium, but there may also be deposits in a granular pattern on capillary walls. Electron microscopy demonstrates the presence of immune complexes as electron dense deposits in the mesangium. The capillary wall deposits may be seen in both subendothelial and subepithelial locations. In many cases the glomerular appearances are indistinguishable from those seen in IgA nephropathy (Berger's disease), and some have suggested that IgA nephropathy represents a localized form of HSP.

Although HSP is immunologically mediated, its cause is unknown. It sometimes follows infections, particularly of the upper respiratory tract, or drug administration.

b. Vasculitis in cryoglobulinemia

Cryoglobulins are circulating immunoglobulins which form insoluble precipitates in the cold. They may be classified into three types: (1) type I consists of a single monoclonal immunoglobulin, (2) type II is a mixed cyoglobulinemia consisting of a monoclonal immunoglobulin (usually IgM) directed against a polyclonal immunoglobulin (usually IgG), and (3) type III is a mixed cryoglobulin consisting of two polyclonal immunoglobulins. Type I cryoglobulins are usually found in lymphoproliferative disorders such as multiple myeloma or other malignancies of B cells. Mixed cryglobulinemias have been described in a number of settings such as lymphoproliferative disorders, autoimmune diseases such as SLE, and in chronic infections including those due to hepatitis B, hepatitis C, and Epstein-Barr virus. Recent evidence suggests that many cases, previously termed essential cryoglobulinemia because the etiology was unknown, are due to hepatitis C infection.

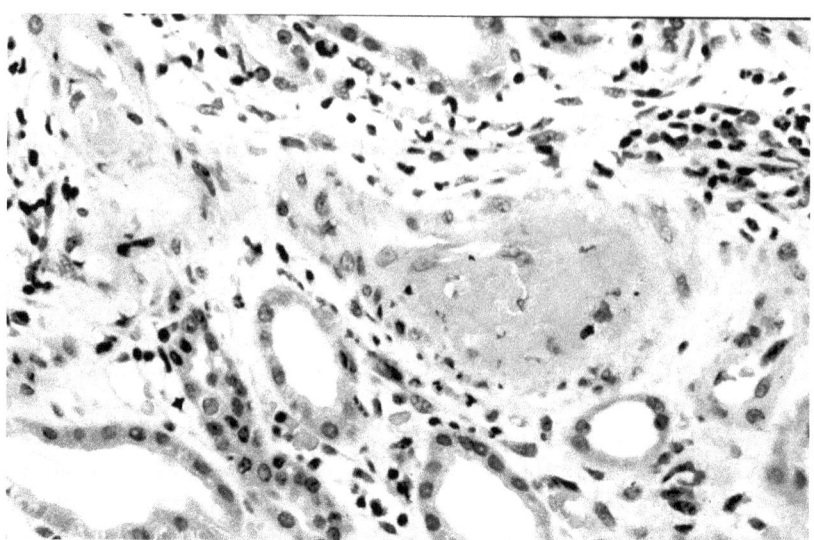

FIGURE 1.6 Cryoglobulinemia. An intrarenal arteriole with a large deposit of eosinophilic cryoglobulin bulging into the lumen (H&E, × 100).

Hepatitis C antigens have been detected in circulating cryoglobulins and many of the cryoglobulins have been shown to bind hepatitis C nucleocapsid core antigen.

Cryoglobulins may cause vasculitis and glomerulonephritis. The most common site of vascular involvement is the skin although many other organs may be affected. The most common manifestation is purpura on the skin of the lower extremities, trunk, or face. There may also be arthralgia, hepatosplenomegaly, and peripheral neuropathy. Histologically, the skin lesions resemble those of a typical leukocytoclastic vasculitis, but a distinct and characteristic feature is that deposits of the cryoglobulin itself may be seen as eosinophilic material within the lumen of the affected small vessels (Figure 1.6). As well as involvement of capillaries and post-capillary venules there may be inflammation in arterioles and small arteries. The cryoglobulin deposits can be stained immuno-histochemically to show their component immunoglobulins.

The acute changes in the glomeruli are of a diffuse endocapillary proliferative glomerulone-phritis which may have mesangiocapillary features. Typically the glomeruli show marked hyper-cellularity with increased cells in capillary lumens, although there may be marked variation between glomeruli. There is often prominent infiltration by both neutrophils and macrophages. Cryoglobulins are seen as homogeneous eosinophilic material lying either beneath the capillary loop endothelium or within capillary lumens and sometimes referred to as *thrombi* (Figure 1.7). The presence of subendothelial immune deposits may lead to the laying down of new basement membrane material on the luminal side of the deposit giving rise to a double contour appearance to the capillary wall, so called mesangiocapillary change. Areas of segmental necrosis or crescents are only rarely seen. The composition of the glomerular deposits as detected by immunohistochemistry corresponds to that of the circulating cryoglobulins. Thus, in type II cryoglobulinemia the deposits characteristically stain for IgG and IgM. In addition, C1q, C3, and C4 are also found in mixed cryoglobulinemia since there is activation of complement via the classical pathway. This is also reflected in the reduced circulating levels of these complement components. By electron microscopy, most of the cryoglobulin deposits are seen to be located beneath the glomerular endothelium. These deposits often have a characteristic substructure. In type II cryoglobulinemia, the typical appearance is of curved annular-tubular structures approximately 30 nm in diameter. Type I cryoglobulins are more typically straight fibrils with cross hatching. Other ultrastructural findings include the presence of numerous intracapillary macrophages and of mesangiocapillary change with mesangial cell inter-position between the layers of basement membrane in the capillary wall. Vasculitic lesions affect

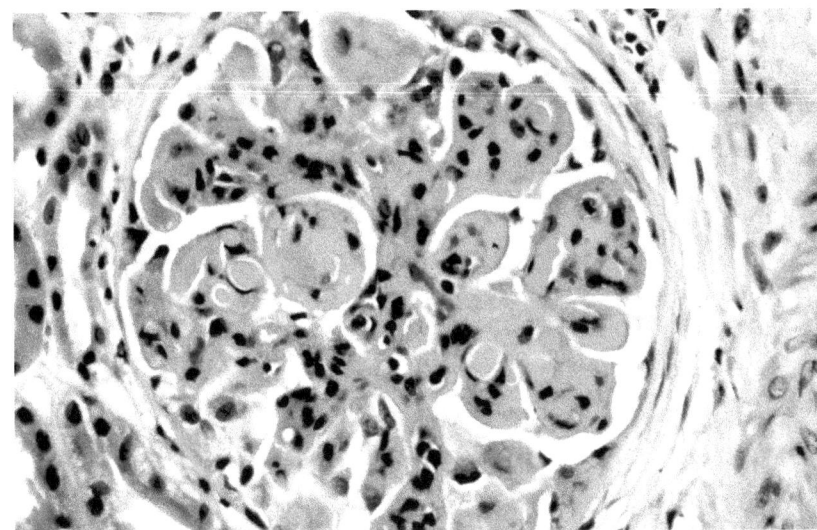

FIGURE 1.7 Cryoglobulinemia. The glomerulus shows accentuated lobulation and hypercellularity. Cryoglobulin is seen as hyaline eosinophilic material which, in some loops, appears as intraluminal "thrombi" (H&E, × 100).

arterioles and interlobular arteries in about one third of renal biopsies. They range from obvious necrotizing arteritis to more subtle intraluminal deposition of eosinophilic material resembling that in the glomeruli, without significant inflammatory reaction.

c. Goodpasture's (anti-GBM) disease

This may be regarded as a form of small vessel vasculitis caused by antibodies directed against the Goodpasture antigen, located in the noncollagenous domain of the α3 chain of type IV collagen. Type IV collagen is a major component of all basement membranes, but the α3 chain has a limited distribution, being co-expressed with the α4 chain in the glomerular basement membrane and distal tubular basement membrane in the kidney, and in the alveolus of the lung, the choroid plexus, the cochlea, and the eye. The major clinical manifestations of anti-GBM disease are rapidly progressive glomerulonephritis and/or alveolar hemorrhage. In a cohort of 71 patients from the U.K., 65% had glomerulonephritis without lung hemorrhage and 35% had both glomerulonephritis and lung hemorrhage (Goodpasture's syndrome).[10]

The characteristic features of renal involvement are focal and segmental glomerular fibrinoid necrosis with crescent formation (Figure 1.8). The uninvolved glomerular segments typically show only mild hypercellularity which may help in the distinction from cases of crescentic glomerulonephritis due to immune complex deposition, in which there is usually more hypercellularity and thickening of glomerular capillary walls. Macrophages are more prominent in crescents associated with anti-GBM disease than in immune complex mediated crescentic glomerulonephritis.[11] The crescents may disrupt Bowman's capsule and there may be prominent periglomerular inflammatory infiltrates. A useful clue to the diagnosis of anti-GBM disease is that the crescents are typically all of the same age, in contrast to the varying ages often seen in crescentic glomerulonephritis associated with ANCA. The crescents progressively evolve into fibrocellular and then fibrous crescents as the lesions age. There may be interstitial inflammation which parallels the severity of the glomerular disease. The characteristic immunofluorescence finding is linear capillary wall staining for IgG which may be accompanied by C3. Linear staining for IgA and/or IgM is less commonly present.

In the lungs, alveolar hemorrhage is the major histological finding (Figure 1.9). Infiltration of alveolar septa by neutrophils, with some showing nuclear fragmentation, may be present but is

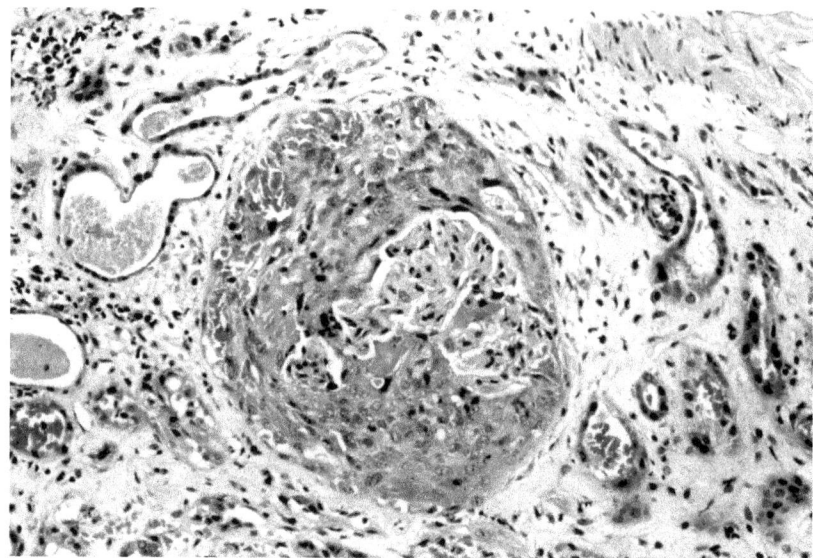

FIGURE 1.8 Goodpasture's (anti-GBM) disease. The glomerulus shows a large cellular crescent with fibrinoid necrosis in the underlying tuft (H&E, × 60).

usually inconspicuous. Immunofluorescence microscopy may show linear staining of alveolar wall for IgG and lesser amounts of C3. During resolution of the intra-alveolar hemorrhage there is a progressive increase in hemosiderin-laden macrophages and there may be mild septal fibrosis.

2. Small Vessel Vasculitis without Immune Deposits

The best characterized diseases in this category are those associated with ANCA.[12] They can be classified on the basis of organ involvement and other clinical features into microscopic polyangiitis, Wegener's granulomatosis, and Churg-Strauss syndrome. The overall incidence of this type of small vessel vasculitis has been estimated at about 20 per million per year. It appears to be increasing in

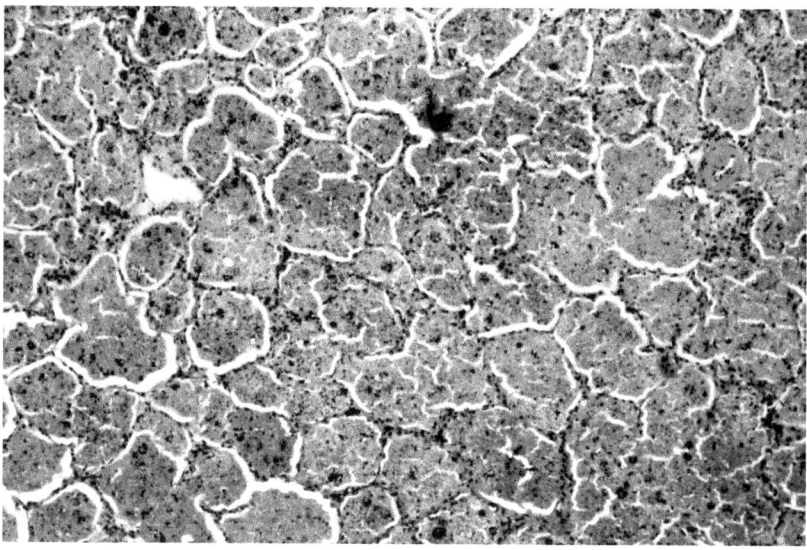

FIGURE 1.9 Goodpasture's (anti-GBM) disease. Lung showing extensive intra-alveolar hemorrhage (H&E, × 60).

frequency, but this may, in part, reflect better diagnosis following the discovery of ANCA. The role of ANCA in pathogenesis remains unproven, although their close association with active disease and various biological effects *in vitro*, suggest they are important. These conditions have in common the fact that they may cause small vessel vasculitis and necrotizing glomerulonephritis, but it should be emphasized that the inflammation may not be confined to small vessels and can also involve larger arteries. The renal changes seen are similar in all three diseases and will be described first.

a.   Renal lesions in ANCA-associated vasculitis

The typical pattern of glomerular involvement is a focal and segmental necrotizing glomerulonephritis. The characteristic lesion is a segmental area of glomerular fibrinoid necrosis — that is an area of the glomerulus in which there is disruption of the basement membrane, often with nuclear fragmentation, and associated with the deposition of intensely eosinophilic material which stains immunohistochemically for fibrin-related antigens. There is often associated crescent formation in Bowman's space. There may be a few inflammatory cells associated with the lesion itself, but the uninvolved glomerular segments appear normal, in contrast to segmental glomerulonephritis associated with immune complexes where there is usually more prominent glomerular hypercellularity. In severe cases, there may be disruption of Bowman's capsule with extension of fibrin into the renal parenchyma and this may give rise to a granulomatous response (Figure 1.10). It should be emphasized that the presence of such granulomatous periglomerular inflammation is not specific for Wegener's granulomatosis. Immunohistochemistry reveals the presence of fibrin in the acute lesions, but there is absent, or only scanty, staining for immunoglobulins or complement — hence, the description of these lesions as *pauci-immune*. Electron microscopy may demonstrate breaks in the glomerular basement membrane in areas of necrosis and shows electron-dense accumulations of fibrin, but typical electron-dense immune deposits are absent. There are usually associated inflammatory changes in the interstitium, the severity of which is proportional to the glomerular involvement. The tubules appear dedifferentiated and the interstitium is edematous with an infiltrate of mononuclear leukocytes. The renal vessels may show necrotizing vasculitis with segmental fibrinoid necrosis accompanied by infiltration of leukocytes. Neutrophils are prominent in early lesions, while mononuclear leukocytes predominate in older lesions. Necrotizing inflammation may also be seen in the medullary vasa recta with infiltration by neutrophils, neutrophil fragmentation, and hemorrhage.

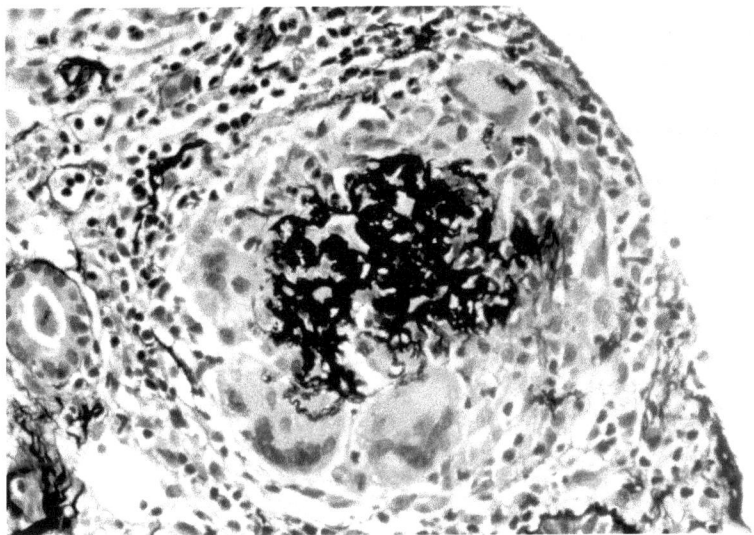

FIGURE 1.10 ANCA-associated vasculitis in the kidney. The glomerulus shows rupture of Bowman's capsule with surrounding granulomatous infiltrate in which giant cells are prominent (Jone's silver methenamine, × 60).

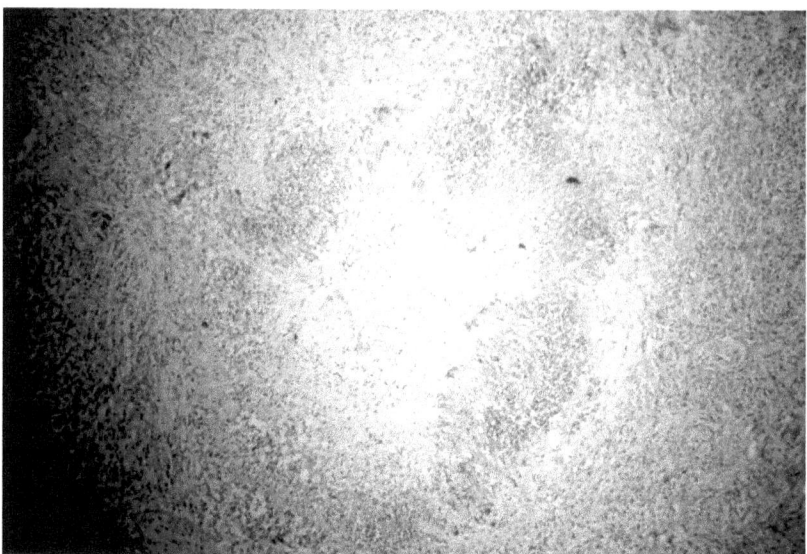

FIGURE 1.11 Wegener's granulomatosis. Lung biopsy showing an area of necrosis surrounded by a poorly defined granulomatous infiltrate containing occasional macrophages (H&E, × 10).

The glomerular lesions of fibrinoid necrosis heal with the development of areas of segmental glomerular sclerosis. Cellular crescents undergo progressive fibrosis to become fibrocellular and finally fibrous crescents. In renal biopsies, glomerular lesions of different ages may be seen, so that cellular crescents and fibrous crescents both may be present in contrast to anti-GBM disease where the lesions are usually of similar ages.

b. Wegener's granulomatosis

Wegener's granulomatosis is a necrotizing vasculitis characterized by the triad of (1) acute necrotizing granulomas of the upper respiratory tract, the lower respiratory tract, or both; (2) focal necrotizing or granulomatous vasculitis affecting small- to medium-sized vessels (capillaries, venules, arterioles, and arteries) most prominent in the lungs and upper airways, but affecting other sites as well; and (3) focal and segmental necrotizing glomerulonephritis. The respiratory tract granulomas may involve the ears, nose, sinuses, throat, or the lungs. Some patients may not show the full triad but have involvement limited to the respiratory tract. Wegener's granulomatosis is associated with ANCA in over 90% of cases with active systemic disease. The peak incidence is in the fourth and fifth decades of life with a slight male predominance.

A granuloma is defined as an accumulation of macrophages some of which have acquired an epithelioid phenotype, i.e., the macrophages have come to resemble epithelial cells in that, in hematoxylin- and eosin-stained sections, they have moderate amounts of pale pink cytoplasm with indistinct cell boundaries. Frequently, but not invariably, epithelioid cells fuse to form giant cells which are multinucleated and may have diameters of up to 50 μm. Granulomas may occur as very clearly defined discrete lesions, as in sarcoidosis, or may be very ill-defined lesions, as is often the case in Wegener's granulomatosis (Figure 1.11). In many cases it is only the presence of scattered multinucleate giant cells that allows the inflammation to be identified as granulomatous. The lesions of Wegener's granulomatosis in the upper respiratory tract usually show areas of ulceration in which there is necrosis and an inflammatory infiltrate of neutrophils, mononuclear leukocytes, and a variable number of giant cells. Definitive diagnosis in biopsies may be difficult both because of the nonspecific nature of the inflammatory infiltrate and because such lesions in the upper respiratory tract often show secondary changes due to superimposed infection.

The gross appearance of the granulomatous lesions in the lung parenchyma is variable. They are nodules which may be solid but may show central necrosis or cavitation. Microscopically, the predominant finding is of necrosis with a prominent neutrophil infiltrate. As emphasised above the granulomatous component of the inflammation may be difficult to identify, but when present it consists of palisading of epithelioid macrophages around the necrotic foci. If compact, easily identifiable granulomas are present, this suggests another diagnosis such as infection or sarcoidosis. Similar granulomatous foci may, less commonly, be found in virtually any other organ in the body.

Vasculitis in Wegener's granulomatosis may affect both small- and medium-to-large-sized vessels. Small vessel vasculitis in the skin gives rise to the typical pattern of leukocytoclastic vasculitis as described above. Microvasculitis can also be found in the lung, where it consists of infiltration of capillaries, venules, and arterioles by neutrophils with resulting alveolar hemorrhage. The second type of vasculitis is a granulomatous arteritis which involves medium- and larger-sized arteries. The granulomas may be seen within the vessel wall, but in some lesions may be clearly separate from it.

The glomerular changes seen in Wegener's granulomatosis have been described separately above. Approximately 80% of patients with Wegener's granulomatosis will go on to have glomerulonephritis, but less than 20% have nephritis at the time of presentation.[13]

c. Microscopic polyangiitis

This is a systemic vasculitis which characteristically affects arterioles, capillaries, and venules. Over 80% of patients with microscopic polyangiitis have ANCA. It may, in some cases, also cause inflammation of arteries indistinguishable from that seen in classical polyarteritis nodosa. The approach to classification suggested by the Chapel Hill Consensus Conference[1] is that classical polyarteritis nodosa and microscopic polyangiitis should be distinguished pathologically by the absence of vasculitis in vessels other than arteries in classical PAN and the presence of vasculitis in vessels smaller than arteries in microscopic polyangiitis. The lesions in microscopic polyangiitis may be found in skin, mucous membranes, lungs, brain, heart, gastrointestinal tract, kidneys, and muscle. Approximately 90% of patients have glomerulonephritis.

Histologically, the typical lesions in small vessels resemble those of leukocytoclastic vasculitis discussed above. The vessels show segmental foci of fibrinoid necrosis of the vessel wall with an influx of neutrophils (Figure 1.12). As the lesions age, the neutrophils are replaced by mononuclear leukocytes and fibrosis replaces the fibrinoid necrosis. If lesions in arteries are found, they are similar to those seen in classical PAN. In general, immunoglobulin and complement deposition is absent or scanty.

d. Churg-Strauss syndrome

Churg-Strauss syndrome, or *allergic granulomatosis and angiitis,* is a syndrome in which necrotizing vasculitis occurs in association with eosinophilia and asthma.[14] The classical description by Churg and Strauss[15] described three major histological features: necrotizing vasculitis, tissue infiltration by eosinophils, and extravascular granulomas. Clinically, allergic rhinitis is usually the first manifestation of disease with asthma developing later. The vasculitic phase mainly affects the skin, heart, lungs, nervous system, and gastrointestinal tract. Renal involvement is less frequent and less severe than in microscopic polyangiitis or Wegener's granulomatosis. Vasculitis usually develops within 3 years of the onset of asthma. Approximately 70% of patients have ANCA.

Histologically, the lesions are similar to those that may be found in Wegener's granulomatosis and microscopic polyangiitis, but show, in addition, prominent eosinophilic infiltration and may have other associated features. The granulomatous lesions found in the respiratory tract show necrosis with eosinophils and poorly defined granulomas with occasional giant cells. In the upper respiratory tract, the granulomatous lesions may be accompanied by polyp formation, a manifestation of long-standing allergic rhinitis. The skin may show a typical leukocytoclastic vasculitis, but there may also be granulomas in the dermis or subdermis. Renal involvement takes the form

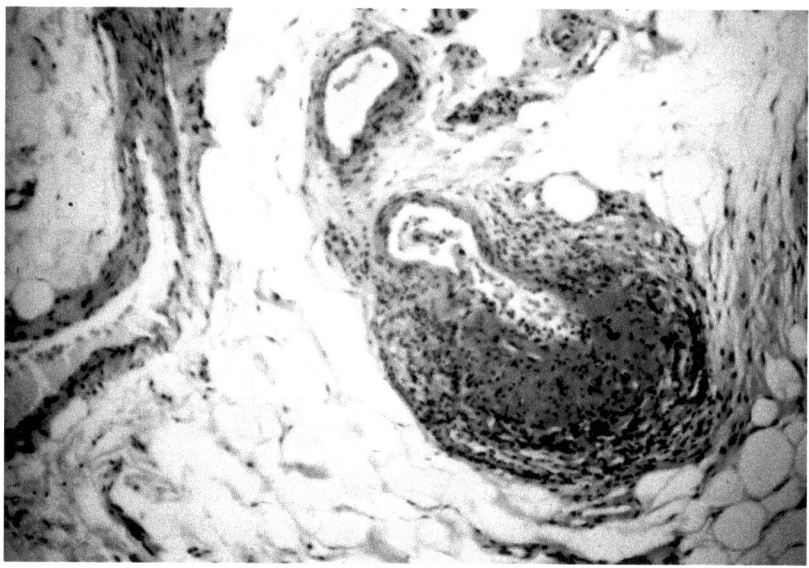

FIGURE 1.12 Microscopic polyangiitis. A small vessel in the wall of the gut showing segmental fibrinoid necrosis with adjacent inflammatory infiltrate (H&E, × 60).

of focal and segmental necrotizing glomerulonephritis which may be accompanied by necrotizing vasculitis as described above. The renal lesions are indistinguishable from those found in microscopic polyangiitis and Wegener's granulomatosis. Eosinophils may be seen in perivascular and interstitial infiltrates in all three diseases and are not specific for Churg-Strauss syndrome, although their presence should raise the suspicion of this diagnosis.

F. VASCULITIS IN OTHER DISEASES

1. Vascular Lesions in Systemic Lupus Erythematosus

Systemic Lupus Erythematosus (SLE) may give rise to a number of vascular lesions, including immune deposition without inflammation, thrombotic microangiopathy, necrotizing vasculitis, and accelerated atherosclerosis.

The most common vascular lesion of SLE seen in renal biopsies is immune complex deposition in the walls of small arteries and arterioles without an inflammatory response. In mild cases the vessels appear normal by light microscopy or show only slight deposition of eosinophilic glassy material in vessel walls. With more severe involvement the vessels show changes of noninflammatory necrotizing vasculopathy in which affected vessels are markedly narrowed by abundant intimal deposits that may extend into the media. The endothelium may be swollen or denuded and there may be loss of medial myocytes. The lesions predominantly affect preglomerular arterioles, but may also be seen in interlobular arteries. Immunofluorescence shows variable staining of the intima for immunoglobulins (IgA, IgG, and IgM in various combinations) and complement components (C1q and C3). The finding of IgM or C3 alone is insufficient to diagnose this condition, since these may be frequently found in areas of arteriolar hyalinosis associated with aging or hypertension. Some authors have used the term *lupus vasculitis* to refer to these changes, but, in view of the absence of inflammation, lupus vasculopathy is probably a better term.

True inflammatory vasculitis may also be seen in SLE. Involvement of the skin gives rise to a leukocytoclastic vasculitis. In the kidney, true inflammatory arteritis is the least common vascular lesion encountered in renal biopsies from lupus patients. Morphologically, there is infiltration of the intima and media by neutrophils and mononuclear leukocytes, often accompanied by fibrinoid necrosis and rupture of the elastic laminae. Immunofluorescence demonstrates strong staining for fibrin-related antigens, but staining for immunoglobulin and complement may be weak and variable. The presence of true inflammatory vasculitis in the kidney is associated with an extremely poor prognosis.

Thrombotic microangiopathy may occur in patients with SLE and the morphological features are discussed below. It may be associated with antiphospholipid antibodies. In some patients it gives rise to systemic manifestations, but in a significant number of patients thrombotic lesions are found in the renal biopsies in the absence of systemic manifestations.

Accelerated atherosclerosis is common in patients with SLE, particularly in young patients who have been treated with corticosteroids, and leads to presentation with complications of coronary artery atherosclerosis including angina and myocardial infarction. The pathogenesis is multifactorial and may reflect the fact that the traditional risk factors including hypertension, obesity, and hyperlipidemia are more common in patients with SLE. In addition, immune complexes may cause endothelial damage and promote atherosclerosis.

2. Vascular Involvement in Rheumatoid Arthritis

Patients with rheumatoid arthritis may develop inflammation in medium- to small-sized arteries similar to that seen in classical PAN, although, in contrast to that disease, there is rarely renal involvement. Vasculitis may involve nerves (with the development of mononeuritis multiplex), mesenteric arteries, and coronary arteries. Involvement of the skin usually takes the form of a leukocytoclastic vasculitis.

3. Vascular Involvement in Behçet's Disease

Behçet's disease is a symptom complex of oral and genital ulceration and uveitis. It may also cause arthritis, neurological manifestations, and gastrointestinal ulceration. The histological features are best described in the skin where the most common vascular involvement is a "lymphocytic vasculitis" characterized by mononuclear cell infiltration around small vessels with variable mural and luminal fibrin deposition. There may be thrombosis in small vessels in the skin without significant inflammation resembling a thrombotic microangiopathy. A typical leukocytoclastic vasculitis may also be seen.

4. Hypocomplementemic Urticarial Vasculitis

This is a syndrome characterized by an erythematous urticaria-like skin rash, arthralgia or arthritis, and variable renal involvement.[16,17] It is most common in young and middle-aged women. It is associated with autoantibodies to the collagen-like region of complement component C1q and reduced levels of circulating C1q. The characteristic skin lesion is a leukocytoclastic vasculitis with immune deposits of IgG, IgA, and IgM. Kidneys have been reported as showing mesangial proliferative or mesangiocapillary glomerulonephritis.

II. THROMBOTIC MICROANGIOPATHY

Thrombotic microangiopathy describes a set of histological appearances, including glomerular thrombosis, arteriolar thrombosis, and loose intimal thickening of small arteries. In hemolytic uremic syndrome, these changes are predominantly in the kidney, while in thrombotic thrombocytopenic purpura widespread systemic manifestations occur. The features overlap with those found in systemic sclerosis and malignant hypertension.

A. Hemolytic Uremic Syndrome (HUS)

Clinically this is characterized by renal failure with thrombocytopenia and hemolytic anemia with red blood cell fragmentation (microangiopathic hemolytic anemia). Histologically, changes are seen in glomeruli, arterioles, and interlobular arteries. Early in the course of the disease, the glomeruli

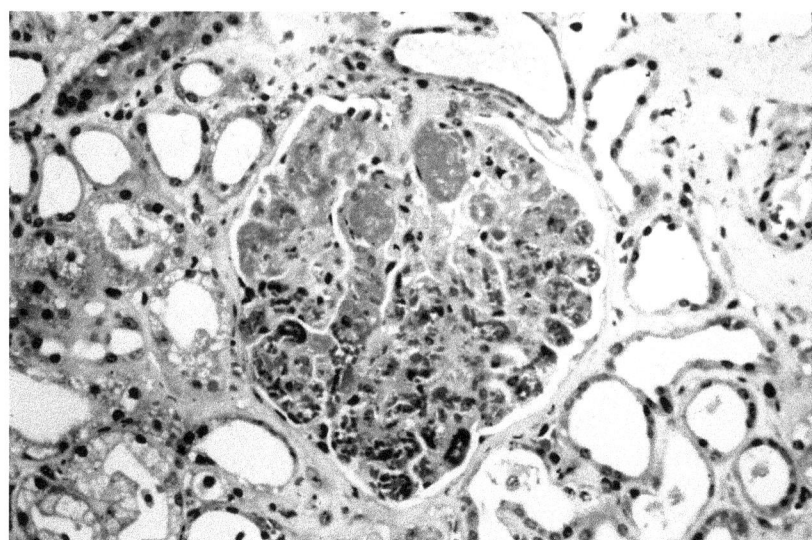

FIGURE 1.13 Hemolytic uremic syndrome. The glomerulus shows granular, platelet-rich thrombi in capillary loops together with many trapped red blood cells. The adjacent tubules show acute ischemic damage (H&E, × 60).

show intraluminal capillary thrombi in which platelets are often prominent (Figure 1.13). Although capillary loops anywhere in the glomerular tuft may be involved, thrombosis is often particularly apparent at the glomerular hilum where it may be continuous with thrombus in the afferent arteriole. At this stage, electron microscopy demonstrates fibrin within glomerular capillary loops and may also show swelling of the glomerular endothelium and a separation of the endothelium from the underlying basement membrane. The intervening space is filled with relatively electron-lucent flocculant material. Glomerular capillary loops are often distended and contain trapped red blood cells, many of which may appear fragmented. A change which may occur in more florid cases is mesangiolysis with microaneurysm formation. As the lesion ages, the lucent layer seen ultrastructurally beneath the glomerular endothelium becomes more prominent and then new basement membrane material is laid down beneath the endothelial cell. By light microscopy this is seen as a thickened capillary wall with a typical double contour appearance on silver staining. The mesangium may show irregular expansion with a foamy appearance. Scattered crescents may be present in severe disease. Eventually the lesions heal with sclerosis of the glomerular tuft.

The changes in the afferent arterioles include insudation of fibrin in the arteriolar wall often with trapped, fragmented red blood cells and intraluminal thrombosis. Interlobular arteries show a striking expansion of the intima by material which is almost translucent in H&E stains and which contains only scattered elongated cell nuclei. This is referred to a myxoid or mucoid intimal hyperplasia. In time collagen is deposited within the thickened intima. In severe cases the vascular changes may lead to focal or extensive cortical necrosis.

Hemolytic uremic syndrome with these typical pathological appearances may be seen in several clinical settings.

1. Secondary to infection, particularly infection with verocytotoxin producing *Escherichia coli.*
2. Complicating pregnancy, the post-partum period and the use of estrogen preparation.
3. Associated with drugs, particularly cytotoxic drugs, including mitomycin, cisplatin, and 5-flurouracil, and the immunosuppressive drugs cyclosporine and tacrolimus.
4. Renal transplant rejection may have identical histological appearances.

It seems likely that in all these settings the primary injury is to the endothelium and the evidence for this is strongest in *E. coli* infection where the toxin produced has been shown *in vitro* to be directly toxic to endothelial cells. HUS may occur with none of these precipitating factors or prodromal illnesses and can be sporadic or familial (in some cases related to factor H deficiency). Microangiopathic hemolysis is thought to arise from mechanical damage to red blood cells as they pass through the developing thrombi in the renal microcirculation.

B. THROMBOTIC THROMBOCYTOPENIC PURPURA (TTP)

This is a form of disseminated thrombotic microangiopathy characterized by thrombocytopenia, hemolytic anemia, fever, renal abnormalities, and neurological disturbances. There are widespread thrombi within arterioles throughout the body particularly in the central nervous system. The renal changes are similar to those of HUS, but usually less severe. The disease is associated with a defect in the processing of the von Willebrand factor which accumulates as unusually large multimers that facilitate the adhesion of platelets to endothelium.[18] Normally the multimers are degraded by a metalloprotease, but in TTP there is a deficiency of this protease which may be constitutive, in patients with relapsing disease, or due to the presence of an autoantibody against components of the enzyme. In contrast, patients with HUS have normal levels of this enzyme, showing a clear difference in the pathogenesis of the two diseases.

C. MALIGNANT HYPERTENSION

In malignant hypertension the vascular changes in the kidney are similar to those of HUS. Thus, there is fibrin insudation in the walls of arterioles, sometimes accompanied by thrombosis, and myxoid expansion of the intima of interlobular arteries (Figure 1.14). Glomeruli typically show ischemic tuft collapse, but there may be segmental fibrinoid necrosis or thrombosis. These features are commonly seen on a background of changes of long-standing hypertension, including arteriolar hyalinosis and arterial intimal thickening with reduplication of the internal elastic lamina. Fibrin within arteriolar walls may also be seen in other organs, particularly the brain.

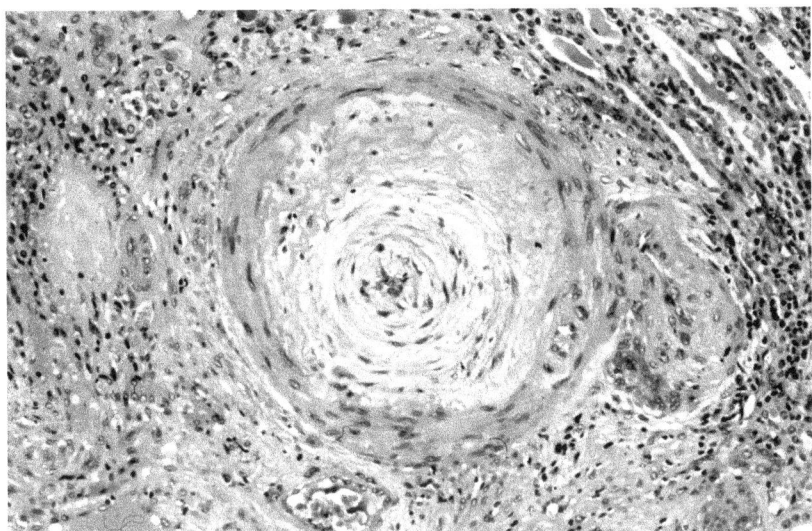

FIGURE 1.14 Malignant hypertension. A renal interlobular artery showing severe myxoid intimal thickening (onion skin) (H&E, × 60).

D. SYSTEMIC SCLEROSIS

Patients with systemic sclerosis may develop acute deterioration in renal function usually accompanied by severe hypertension and with changes in the kidney indistinguishable to those seen in HUS or malignant hypertension. It is difficult to be sure whether the morphological changes are a cause or a consequence of hypertension.

E. ANTIPHOSPHOLIPID SYNDROME

This syndrome occurs in patients with circulating antibodies directed against various phospholipids.[19] These antibodies may be seen as an isolated phenomenon, or may arise in association with a known connective tissue disease, particularly SLE. Autoantibodies to phospholipids may also arise in the context of viral infections or cancers. They may be detected in laboratory tests by their activity against cardiolipin, leading to false-positive tests for syphilis, and by their interference with phospholipid-dependent coagulation tests such that they act as *in vitro* anticoagulants — "the lupus anticoagulant." However, *in vivo* their effect is to produce a thrombophilic state. They may lead to a typical acute thrombotic microangiopathy resembling acute HUS, but more commonly the patients have a protracted illness. Common manifestations include recurrent arterial and venous thrombosis, recurrent miscarriages, thrombocytopenia, livido reticularis, and neurological manifestations.

Histologically, the changes may resemble those described above for HUS, but in chronic cases the kidney may show a mesangiocapillary pattern of injury. There is duplication of the glomerular basement membrane best revealed by PAS or silver staining. Differentiation from immune complex mediated mesangiocapillary glomerulonephritis (MCGN) is on the basis of immunohistochemistry and electron microscopy. In MCGN, there is typically deposition of immune complexes which stain for IgG and C3 and are seen as subendothelial electron-dense deposits by electron microscopy. In chronic thrombotic microangiopathy, immune deposits are not found and the subendothelial space is expanded by lucent material which may contain platelets and fibrin.

REFERENCES

1. Jennette JC, Falk RJ, Andrassy K, Bacon PA, Churg J, Gross WL, Hagen EC, Hoffman GS, Hunder GG, Kallenberg CGM, McCluskey RT, Sinico RA, Rees AJ, Van Es LA, Waldherr R, and Wiik A: Nomenclature of systemic vasculitis. Proposal of an international consensus conference. *Arthritis Rheum* 1994;37:187–192.
2. Jennette JC and Falk RJ: Small-vessel vasculitis. *N Engl J Med* 1997;337:1512–1523.
3. Gaskin G and Pusey CD: Systemic vasculitis; in Davison AM, Cameron JS, Grunfeld J-P, Kerr DNS, Ritz E, and Winearls CG (Eds): *Oxford Textbook of Clinical Nephrology.* Oxford: Oxford University Press, 1998, 877–910.
4. Bengtsson B-A: Epidemiology of giant cell arteritis; in Hazleman B and Bengtsson B-A (Eds.), *Bailliere's Clinical Rheumatology.* Vol. 5/No. 3, *Giant Cell Arteritis and Polymyalgia Rheumatica.* London: Balliere Tindall, 1991, pp 379–386.
5. Banks PM, Cohen MD, Ginsburg WW, and Hunder GG: Immunohistologic and cytochemical studies of temporal arteritis. *Arthritis Rheum* 1983;26:1201–1207.
6. Temporal artery biopsy. *Lancet* 1983;i:396–397.
7. Hall S, Barr W, Lie JT, Stanson AW, Kazmier FJ, and Hunder GG: Takaysu's arteritis: a study of 32 North American patients. *Medicine* 1985;64:89–99.
8. Travers RL, Allison DJ, Brettle RP, and Hughes GRV: Polyarteritis nodosa: a clinical and angiographic analysis of 17 cases. *Sem Arthritis Rheum* 1979;8:184–199.
9. Leung DY, Geha RS, Newburger JW, Burns JC, Fiers WX, Lapierre LA, and Pober JS: Two monokines, interleukin 1 and tumor necrosis factor, render cultured vascular endothelial cells susceptible to lysis by antibodies circulating during Kawasaki syndrome. *J Exp Med* 1986;164:1958.

10. Savage CO, Pusey CD, Bowman C, Rees AJ, and Lockwood CM: Antiglomerular basement membrane antibody mediated disease in the British Isles 1980–4. *Br Med J Clin Res Educ* 1986;292:301–304.

11. Magil AB and Wadsworth LD: Monocyte involvement in glomerular crescents. *Lab Invest* 1982;47:160–166.

12. Jennette JC: Antineutrophil cytoplasmic autoantibody-associated diseases: a pathologist's perspective. *Am J Kidney Dis* 1991;18:164–170.

13. Duna GF, Galperin C, and Hoffman GS: Wegener's granulomatosis. *Rheum Dis Clin N Am* 1995;21:949–986.

14. Lanham JG, Elkon KB, Pusey CD, and Hughes GR: Systemic vasculitis with asthma and eosinophilia: a clinical approach to the Churg-Strauss syndrome. *Medicine* 1984;63:65–81.

15. Churg J and Strauss L: Allergic granulomatosis, allergic angiitis and periarteritis nodosa. *Am J Pathol* 1951;27:277–301.

16. Grishman E and Spiera H: Vasculitis in connective tissue diseases, including hypocomplementemic vasculitis; in Churg A and Churg J (Eds.): *Systemic Vasculitides.* New York: Igaku-Shoin, 1991, 273–292.

17. Wisnieski JJ, Baer AN, Christensen J, Cupps TR, Flagg DN, Jones JV, Katzenstein PL, McFadden ER, McMillen JJ, and Pick MA: Hypocomplementaemic urticarial vasculitis syndrome. Clinical and serologic findings in 18 patients. *Medicine-Baltimore* 1995;74:24–41.

18. Moake JL: Moschcowitz, multimers and metallprotease. *N Engl J Med* 1998;339:1629–1631.

19. Greaves M: Antiphospholipid antibodies and thrombosis. *Lancet* 1999;353:1348–1353.

2 Coagulation Abnormalities

Douglas A. Triplett

CONTENTS

I. INTRODUCTION

The hemostatic response is designed to generate a fibrin/platelet plug at the site of vascular injury. In order to have a normal hemostatic response, platelets, coagulation proteins, and the vascular wall must interact in an orchestrated interactive sequence of events. Perturbation of any component may result in clinical bleeding or thrombosis.[1]

In addition to the procoagulant response, there are a number of plasma proteins which function as "physiologic inhibitors of the coagulation cascade." Among these proteins are antithrombin (previously referred to as antithrombin III), protein C, protein S, and tissue factor pathway inhibitor (TFPI).[1] (Table 2.1) Hereditary or acquired abnormalities of antithrombin, protein C, and protein S are associated with thromboembolic complications.[2]

Autoantibodies have been implicated in the pathogenesis of both acquired hemorrhagic disorders and acquired thrombotic complications.[3] The concept of antibody mediated thrombosis was originally proposed by Vermylen and colleagues in 1997.[3,4] This review will focus on the role of antiphospholipid antibodies (APA) and their association with acquired bleeding disorders and thrombosis.

II. ANTIPHOSPHOLIPID ANTIBODIES

APA were originally thought to be antibodies that recognized phospholipids (PLs). However, recent studies have clearly demonstrated APA, which are identified in the setting of autoimmune disease, recognize a variety of plasma proteins that bind to activated PL membranes (e.g., activated platelets, endothelium, monocytes, tumor cells).[5] Among the proteins which have been identified as antigenic targets are β_2 Glycoprotein I (β_2 GPI), prothrombin, protein C, protein S, factor XI, and high and low molecular weight kininogens.[6] (Table 2.2)

A second group of APA react only with phospholipids (do not require protein binding to PLs). These antibodies are typically seen in response to infections (e.g., syphilis, hepatitis C, etc.). Biologic false-positive serologic tests for syphilis are often seen following various infections and autoimmune diseases.[7-9] It is important to differentiate infection-related APA from APA requiring

TABLE 2.1
Down-Regulation of Coagulation

Regulatory Proteins	Procoagulant Proteins
Antithrombin	Serine Proteases (e.g., Xa, Thrombin)
PC, PS	Va, VIIIa
TFPI	Extrinsic Pathways (VIIa-TF)
Plasmin	Fibrin Clot

Note: PC = Protein C, PS = Protein S, TFPI = Tissue factor pathway inhibitor, Factors Xa, Va, VIIIa, VIIa = Activated forms of clotting factors.

TABLE 2.2
APA: Antigenic Targets

β_2 Glycoprotein I (β_2 GPI)	Prothrombin
Annexin V	Protein C
Complement factor H	Protein S
High mol. wt. kininogen	Factor XI
Low mol. wt. kininogen	C4b-BP
Lipopolysaccharide binding protein	Thrombin modified antithrombin

TABLE 2.3
β_2 GPI: Physiologic Functions

Anticoagulant	Procoagulant
Inhibit contact system	Inhibit APC[b]
Inhibit prothrombinase	
Inhibit ADP plt. aggreg.[a]	

[a] Platelet aggregation.
[b] Activated protein C.

"protein cofactors." Infection-related APA are not associated with thromboembolic complications, while protein cofactor dependent APA are linked to thrombosis.[5,10-12]

III. β_2 GLYCOPROTEIN I (GPI)

β_2 GPI is a 50 kD protein present in human plasma in a concentration of approximately 200 µg/ml.[13] β_2 GPI also has been designated apolipoprotein H. β_2 GPI is lipophilic and will bind to negatively charged surfaces (e.g., activated cellular membranes, heparan sulfate on the surface of endothelium, and lipoproteins).[5,13] β_2 GPI has a number of anticoagulant properties, including inhibition of contact system of coagulation, inhibition of prothrombinase reaction, and decreased ADP-induced platelet aggregation.[4,15-17] (Table 2.3) Although these anticoagulant properties have been demonstrated *in vitro*, hereditary deficiency of β_2 GPI is **not** associated with clinical thrombophilia. *In vitro* studies have demonstrated antibodies to β_2 GPI may inhibit activated protein C (APC) resulting in a potential prothrombotic condition.[8,19-21]

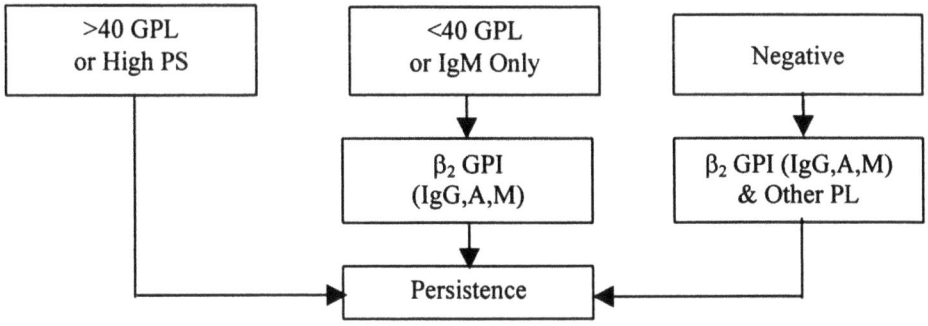

GPL = IgG Anticardiolipin Units
PS = Phosphatidylserine
PL = Phospholipid

FIGURE 2.1 ACA algorithm.

β_2 GPI and prothrombin are the major proteins involved in the binding of APA to PL surfaces.[22-25] The majority of patients who have lupus anticoagulants (LA) or positive anticardiolipin antibodies (ACA) have antibodies to **both** β_2 GPI and prothrombin. In ACA assay systems using "high sensitivity microtiter plates," β_2 GPI is an absolute requirement for the binding of ACA to the cardiolipin-coated surfaces of the microtiter plate.[16,22] With the recognition of β_2 GPI as an essential cofactor in the ACA assay, enzyme-linked immunosorbent assay (ELISA) for β_2 GPI have become available.[26,27] β_2 GPI ELISAs are less sensitive than the standard ACA assay (i.e., they do not identify infection-related ACA positive patients). However, the anti-β_2 GPI assay is much more specific than the standard ACA assay.[28] There is a higher correlation with clinical thrombosis when one uses the anti-β_2 GPI assay. As a part of the evaluation of patients with antibody-mediated thrombosis, a specific β_2 GPI ELISA is essential (Figure 2.1).

A recent report described immunolocalization of β_2 Glycoprotein I in human atherosclerotic plaques.[29] In the study by George et al., β_2 GPI was identified within the subendothelial region, intimal-medial borders of human atherosclerotic plaques, and β_2 GPI colocalized with CD4-positive lymphocytes. The authors concluded that colocalization of CD4-positive lymphocytes with β_2 GPI suggested β_2 GPI is the antigenic target in an immune-mediated reaction which could potentially influence progression of atherosclerotic plaques.

IV. ANTIBODIES TO PROTHROMBIN

Loeliger was the first to describe a case of a patient with LA and hypoprothrombinemia.[30] The addition of normal plasma to the patient's plasma resulted in enhanced LA activity (lupus cofactor effect). Subsequent to this observation, several additional investigators reported patients with hypoprothrombinemia and clinical bleeding.[31,32]

Using various configurations of microtiter plates (e.g., gamma irradiated plates, "high activated" PVC plates, and microtiter plates coated with phosphatidylserine), antibodies to prothrombin can be demonstrated in 50 to 90% of cases with demonstrable LA/ACA positivity.[11,33] Thus, the frequency of antibodies to prothrombin is greater than antibodies to β_2 GPI in patients with the APA syndrome. In most cases, antiprothrombin antibodies recognize human and bovine prothrombin. Typically, the patient's antibody population is diverse with varying affinities for prothrombin. These antibodies bind to prothrombin fragment 1 as well as prethrombin 1.[34]

TABLE 2.4
LA and Clinical Bleeding[37-39]
(Associated Predisposing Factors)

Specific factor inhibition
  Factor VIII inhibitors
  Factor II inhibitors
Thrombocytopenia
Platelet dysfunction
Uremia
Concomitant drug administration (e.g., aspirin)

The vast majority of patients with antiprothrombin antibodies will have normal circulating plasma levels of prothrombin. The unusual patient with high titer/high avidity antibodies to prothrombin may present with prolonged screening coagulation studies (activated partial thromboplastin time (APTT), prothrombin time (PT)). In these patients, complexes of immunoglobulins and prothrombin are presumably cleared from the circulation resulting in prolonged clotting times and, in some cases, significant/severe clinical bleeding.[11,35,36] These cases are relatively rare and have been reported in all age groups although pediatric patients represent a disproportionate number of the cases. In most cases, the hypoprothrombinemia will respond to the use of prednisone. Hemorrhagic complications may also be seen in LA-positive patients due to a variety of associated conditions.[37-39] (Table 2.4)

Galli and colleagues have emphasized the differences between LAs due to prothrombin antibodies and those due to β_2 GPI antibodies.[40-42] In the former case, the kaolin clotting time (KCT) is disproportionately prolonged when compared to the dilute Russell viper venom time (dRVVT).[42] Patients with LA due to anti-β_2 GPI will have a greater prolongation of the dRVVT when compared to the KCT.[41,42] (Table 2.5) In the majority of patients with demonstrable LA, patient plasmas will contain antibodies to both prothrombin and β_2 GPI. Thus, the relative titers and affinities of antibodies to these two proteins determines the coagulation profile (dRVVT/KCT).

The association of antiprothrombin antibodies as a cause of thromboembolic events remains a matter of some controversy. In a study by Horbach and colleagues, patients with systemic lupus erythematosus (SLE) were evaluated for IgG and IgM antiprothrombin antibodies.[23] In their study, antiprothrombin antibodies appeared to be a risk factor (odds ratio 2.53 and 2.72 for IgG and IgM antibodies, respectively). When the study was analyzed using multivariant analysis, antiprothrombin antibodies did not appear to be a risk factor. Funke and colleagues reported IgG and IgM antibodies

TABLE 2.5
Antiprothrombin and Anticardiolipin Antibodies

	Antiprothrombin	Anticardiolipin
Antigen	Prothrombin	β_2 GPI
Epitopes	Fragment 1, prethrombin 1	Domains 1 and 4
Species specificity	Yes	No
Affinity	Mainly low	Low
LA	Yes	Yes
	(KCT > dRVVT)	(dRVVT > KCT)
Thrombosis	+	+++

Source: Adapted from Galli, M. and Barbui, T., *Blood,* 93, 2149–2157, 1999.

to prothrombin/PL complexes gave an odds ratios of 2.8 for venous thrombosis and 4.1 for arterial thrombosis in SLE patients.[44] Vaarala and colleagues reported antibodies to prothrombin result in an increased risk of myocardial infarction in middle-aged men.[45]

Further studies of antibodies to prothrombin are necessary to clarify their role in thrombosis (both venous and arterial). In some experimental studies, antibodies to prothrombin have resulted in increased generation of thrombin. The prothrombotic nature of these antibodies may be due to their affinity, antigenic target(s) within the prothrombin molecule, titer as well as antigenic "clustering" on phospholipid surfaces allowing for bivalent binding.

Bivalent antibody binding results in an increased localized concentration of prothrombin on the cellular membranes.[10] As a result, there is "transmembrane signaling" resulting in a prothrombotic cellular surface.

V. ANTIBODIES TO PROTEIN S AND ANNEXIN V

There are a number of reports documenting reduced concentrations of protein S in patients with LA.[18,20,46] One hypothesis to explain the reduced protein S concentration involves LA/β_2 GPI-induced binding of free protein S to C4b-BP (complement 4-binding protein).[18,20,46] Physiologically, approximately 40% of protein S circulates in the free state and 60% bound to C4-BP. Free protein S is required as a cofactor for the activated protein C downregulation of factors Va and VIIIa (Figure 2.2). The redistribution of free protein S to the bound state may result in an acquired prothrombotic condition.

Other components of the protein C/protein S pathway also have been suggested as potential targets of APA.[47] There are several reports of antibodies to protein C and also thrombomodulin. However, the most important potential antigenic target is protein S.[18,20,46]

Annexins are a family of proteins that may be antigenic "targets" for APA.[48,49] Over 20 members of the Annexin family have been identified.[50] These proteins bind calcium and phospholipids. Annexin V has recently been reported as an important protein found in trophoblasts as well as endothelial cells.[51] The role of Annexin V is presumably to block the participation of anionic phospholipids in phospholipid-dependent coagulation reactions. Based on studies by Rand et al., patients with APS lose the Annexin V protective activity resulting in exposure of phospholipids

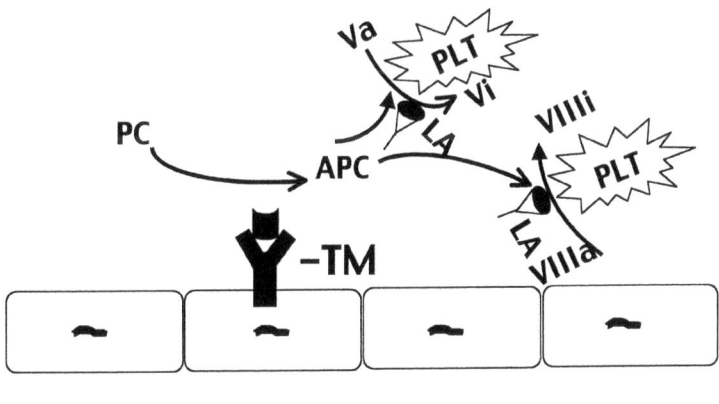

TM = Thrombomodulin
= Thrombin
= PL Binding Protein (e.g., β_2 Glycoprotein I and Prothrombin)

FIGURE 2.2 Activated protein C downregulation of factors Va and VIIIa.

and resulting coagulation reactions.[51] Antibodies to Annexin V have been described in SLE patients with antipaspholipid syndrome (APS).[52]

VI. ANTIBODIES TO PROTEINS OF THE CONTACT SYSTEM OF COAGULATION

The initiation of the hemostatic response involves activation of the "contact system." Activation of the contact system requires loss of endothelial cells resulting in exposure of subendothelial matrix. Hageman factor (factor XII) will bind to the site of vascular injury initiating the subsequent assembly of the contact system. High molecular weight kininogen (also known as the Fitzgerald factor) circulates in plasma as a carrier protein binding either factor XI or prekallikrein (Fletcher factor). The activation of factor XII and, subsequently, factor XI leads to the amplification of the coagulation cascade. However, there remains some controversy regarding the overall role of the "contact system." Hereditary deficiencies of factor XII, and Fletcher and Fitzgerald factors do not result in clinical bleeding. Although these patients have markedly prolonged APTTs, they are clinically asymptomatic with respect to bleeding.

Recently, there have been reports of low levels of factor XII and factor XI in APA positive patients.[53-55] In some cases, both functional activity and antigen levels of these proteins have been decreased. In the case of factor XI, it appears the functional assay (conventional factor assays) is critical in identifying the situation.[56] If one uses human factor XI deficient substrate plasma, often the apparent factor XI activity is decreased.[57] However, if bovine factor XI deficient substrate plasma is used in the assay, the resulting factor XI activity is normal.[57] This emphasizes the "species specificity" of patients with LA positivity. Presumably, one would expect to see the same results in factor XII deficient plasmas; however, these studies have not, as yet, been reported.

In APA-positive patients, antibodies to high molecular weight kininogen (HMWK) have been identified.[58] HMWK is a cofactor for the binding of APA to phosphatidylethanolamine (PE).[59] Antibodies to PE have been linked to thromboembolic complications. Currently, ELISA assays for antibodies to PE are not commercially available.

VII. SUMMARY

APA react with many of the coagulation proteins essential for normal hemostasis. In the vast majority of cases, APA-positive patients have antibodies to either β_2 GPI or prothrombin. These antibodies result in a predisposition to thrombosis involving both the venous and arterial circulation. Commercially available ELISAs for antibodies to β_2 GPI are now available. In the near future, ELISAs for detection of antibodies to prothrombin should become available. Antibodies to these two plasma proteins are by far the most commonly encountered APAs. Nevertheless, there are a number of other plasma proteins which are antigenic targets for APAs. Among these proteins, Annexin V has attracted the greatest attention. Antibodies to Annexin have been associated with recurrent spontaneous abortion due to loss of the protective activity of Annexin V in the placenta.[60-62] The loss of Annexin V anticoagulant properties from endothelial cells may also represent another mechanism accounting for venous thrombosis.

Although significant advances have been made over the past several years in understanding APA-induced thrombosis, there is still much which remains unknown. Ideally, a functional assay system to identify the procoagulant APAs would greatly enhance our diagnostic/management capabilities. Acquired activated protein C-resistance (APC-R) appears to be the most common pathophysiologic mechanism for venous thromboembolic events. On the arterial side of the circulation, activation of platelets is the most common pathophysiologic mechanism. The use of flow cytometry may prove to be the best approach to identifying patients at risk for APA-related arterial thromboembolic events.

REFERENCES

1. Hathaway, W.E. and Goodnight, S.H., *Disorders of Hemostasis and Thrombosis. A Clinical Guide,* McGraw-Hill, New York, 1993.
2. Rosendaal, F.R., Venous thrombosis: a multicausal disease, *Lancet,* 353, 1167–1173, 1999.
3. Vermylen, J., Hoylaerts, M.F., and Arnout, J., Antibody mediated thrombosis, *Thromb. Haemost.,* 78, 420–423, 1997.
4. Hoylaerts, M.F., Thys, C., Arnout, J., and Vermylen, J, Recurrent arterial thrombosis linked to auto-immune antibodies enhancing von Willebrand factor binding to platelets and inducing FcγRII receptor-mediated platelet activation, *Blood,* 91, 2810–2817, 1998.
5. Triplett, D.A., Antiphospholipid protein antibodies: laboratory detection and clinical relevance, *Thromb. Res.,* 78, 1–31, 1995.
6. Arvieux, J., Pernod, G., Regnault, V., Darnige, L., and Garin, J., Some anticardiolipin antibodies recognize a combination of phospholipids with thrombin-modified antithrombin complement C4b-binding protein and lipopolysaccharide binding protein, *Blood,* 93, 4248–4255, 1999.
7. Davis, B., Biologic false-positive serologic tests for syphilis, *Medicine,* 23, 359–365, 1944.
8. Moore, J.E. and Mohr, C.F., Biologically false-positive serologic tests for syphilis, *JAMA,* 150, 467–473, 1952.
9. Harvey, A.M. amd Shulman, L.E., Connective tissue disease and chronic biologic false-positive test for syphilis (BFP reaction), *Med. Clin. N. Am.,* 50, 1271–1279, 1966.
10. Roubey, R.A.S. and Hoffman, M., From antiphospholipid syndrome to antibody-mediated thrombosis, *Lancet,* 350, 1491–1493, 1997.
11. Galli, M. and Barbui, T., Antiphospholipid antibodies: detection and clinical significance in the antiphospholipid syndrome, *Blood,* 93, 2149–2157, 1999.
12. Oosting, J.D., Derksen, R.H.W.M., Bobbink, I.W.G., Hackeng, T.M., Bouma, B.N., and deGroot, P.G., Antiphospholipid antibodies directed against a combination of phospholipid with prothrombin, protein C, or protein S: an explanation for their pathogenic mechanism, *Blood,* 81, 2618–2625, 1993.
13. Kamboh, M.I. and Mehdi, H., Genetics of apolipoprotein H (β_2 Glycoprotein I) and anionic phospholipid binding, *Lupus,* 7, S10–S13, 1998.
14. Schousboe, I., β_2 Glycoprotein I: a plasma inhibitor of the contact activation of the intrinsic blood coagulation pathway, *Blood,* 66, 1086–1091, 1985.
15. Nimpf, J., Wurm, H., and Kostner, G.M., β_2 Glycoprotein I (apo-H) inhibits release reaction of human platelets during APA induced aggregation, *Atherosclerosis,* 63, 109–114, 1987.
16. McNeil, H.P., Simpson, R.J., Chesterman, C.N., and Krilis, S.A., Antiphospholipid antibodies are directed to a complex antigen that includes a lipid-binding inhibitor of coagulation: β_2 Glycoprotein I (apolipoprotein H), *Proc. Natl. Acad. Sci. USA,* 87, 4120–4124, 1990.
17. Nimpf, J., Bevers, E.M., Bomans, P.H.H., Till, U., Wurm, H., Kostner, G.M., and Zwaal, R.F.A., Prothrombinase activity of human platelets is inhibited by β_2 Glycoprotein I, *Biochim. Biophys. Acta,* 884, 142–149, 1986.
18. Ginsberg, J.S., Demers, C., Brill-Edwards, P., Bona, R., Johnston, M., Wong, A., and Denburg, J.A., Acquired free protein S deficiency is associated with antiphospholipid antibodies and increased thrombin generation in patients with systemic lupus erythematosus, *Am. J. Med.,* 98, 379–383, 1995.
19. Galli, M., Ruggeri, L., and Barbui, T., Differential effects of anti-β_2 Glycoprotein I and anti-prothrombin antibodies on the anticoagulant activity of activated protein C, *Blood,* 91, 1999–2004, 1998.
20. Merrill, J.T., Zhang, H.W., Shen, C., Butman, B.T., Jeffries, E.P., Lahita, R.G., and Myones, B.L., Enhancement of protein S anticoagulant function by β_2 Glycoprotein I, a major target antigen of antiphospholipid antibodies: β_2 Glycoprotein I interferes with binding of protein S to its plasma inhibitor, C4b-binding protein, *Thromb. Haemost.,* 81, 748–757, 1999.
21. Sheng, Y., Kandiah, D.A., and Krilis, S.A., β_2 Glycoprotein I: target antigen for "antiphospholipid" antibodies. Immunological and molecular aspects, *Lupus,* 7, S5–S9, 1998.
22. Roubey, R.A.S., Ersenberg, R.A., Harper, M.F., and Winfield, J.B., Anticardiolipin autoantibodies recognize β_2 Glycoprotein I in the absence of phospholipid: importance of Ag density and bivalent binding, *J. Immunol.,* 154, 954–960, 1995.
23. Horbach, D.A., Van Oort, E., Derksen, R.H.W.M., and deGroot, P.G., The contribution of antiprothrombin antibodies to lupus anticoagulant activity, *Thromb. Haemost.,* 79, 790–795, 1998.

24. Funke, A., Bertolaccini, M.L., Atsumi, T., Amerngual, O., Khamashta, M.A., and Hughes, G.R.V., Autoantibodies to prothrombin-phosphatidylserine complex: clinical significance in systemic lupus erythematosus, *Lupus*, 7, S221, 1998.

25. Biasiolo, A., Rampazzo, P., Brocca, T., Barbero, F., Rosato, A., and Pengo, V., [anti-β_2 Glycoprotein I-β_2 Glycoprotein I] immune complexes in patients with antiphospholipid syndrome and other autoimmune diseases, *Lupus*, 8, 121–125, 1999.

26. Arvieux, J., Roussel, B., Jacob, M.C., and Colomb, M.G., Measurements of antiphospholipid antibodies by ELISA using β_2 Glycoprotein I as an antigen, *J. Immunol. Methods*, 143, 223–229, 1991.

27. Koike, T., Ichikawa, K., Kasahara, H., Atsumi, T., Tsutsumi, A., and Matsuura, E., Epitopes on β_2 GPI recognized by anticardiolipin antibodies, *Lupus*, 7, S14–S17, 1998.

28. Sanmarco, M., Soler, C., Christides, C., Raoult, D., and Weiller, P.J., Gerolami, V., Bernard, D., Prevalence and clinical significance of IgG isotype anti-β_2 Glycoprotein I antibodies in antiphospholipid syndrome: a comparative study with anticardiolipin antibodies, *J. Lab. Clin. Med.*, 129, 499–506, 1997.

29. George, J., Harats, D., Gilburd, B., Afek, A., Levy, Y., Schneiderman, J., Barshack, I., Ropolovic, J., and Shoenfeld, Y., Immunolocalization of β_2 Glycoprotein I (apolipoprotein H) to human atherosclerotic plaque, *Circulation*, 99, 2227–2230, 1999.

30. Loeliger, A., Prothrombin as cofactor of the circulating anticoagulant in systemic lupus erythematosus, *Thromb. Diath. Haemost.*, 3, 237, 1959.

31. Rapaport, S.I., Ames, S.B., and Duval, B.J., A plasma coagulation defect in systemic lupus erythematosus arising from hypoprothrombinemia combined with antiprothrombinase activity, *Blood*, 15, 212, 1960.

32. Corrigan, J.J., Patterson, J.H., and May, N.E., Incoagulability of the blood in systemic lupus erythematosus. A case due to hypoprothrombinemia and a circulating anticoagulant, *Am. J. Dis. Child.*, 119, 365–369, 1970.

33. Fleck, R.A., Rapaport, S.I., and Rao, L.V.M., Anti-prothrombin antibodies and the lupus anticoagulant, *Blood*, 72, 512–519, 1988.

34. Rao, V.M., Hoang, A.D., and Rapaport, S.I., Mechanism and effects of the binding of lupus anticoagulant IgG and prothrombin to surface phospholipid, *Blood*, 88, 4173–4182, 1996.

35. Triplett, D.A. and Brandt, J.T., Lupus anticoagulants: misnomer, paradox, riddle, epiphenomenon, *Hematol. Pathol.*, 2, 121–143, 1988.

36. Edson, J.R., Vogt, J.M., and Hasegawa, D.K., Abnormal prothrombin crossed-immunoelectrophoresis in patients with lupus inhibitors, *Blood*, 64, 807–816, 1984.

37. Triplett, D.A., Simultaneous occurrence of lupus anticoagulant and factor VIII inhibitors. *Am. J. Hematol.*, 56, 195–196, 1997.

38. Biron, C., Durand, L., Lemkecher, T., Dauverchain, J., Meunier, L., Meynadier, J., and Schved, J.F., Simultaneous occurrence of lupus anticoagulant, factor VIII inhibitors and localized pemphigoid, *Am. J. Hematol.*, 51, 250–251, 1996.

39. Ballard, H.S. and Nyamush, A.G., Life threatening haemorrhage in a patient with rheumatoid arthritis and a lupus anticoagulant coexisting with acquired autoantibodies against factor VIII, *Br. J. Rheumatol.*, 32, 515–517, 1993.

40. Galli, M., Finazzi, G., Bevers, E.M., and Barbui, T., Kaolin clotting time and dilute Russell's viper venom time distinguish between prothrombin and β_2 Glycoprotein I-dependent antiphospholipid antibodies, *Blood*, 86, 617–623, 1995.

41. Norbis, F., Barbui, T., and Galli, M., Dilute Russell's viper venom time and colloidal silica clotting time for the identification of the phospholipid-dependent inhibitors of coagulation, *Thromb. Res.*, 85, 427–431, 1997.

42. Galli, M., Finazzi, G., and Barbui, T., Antiphospholipid antibodies: predictive value of laboratory tests, *Thromb. Haemost.*, 78, 75–78, 1997.

43. Vaarala, O., Puurunen, M., Manttari, M., Manninen, V., Aho, K., and Palosuo, T., Antibodies to prothrombin imply a risk of myocardial infarction in middle-aged men, *Thromb. Haemost.*, 75, 456–459, 1996.

44. Parke, A.L., Weinstein, R.E., Bona, R.D., Maier, D.B., and Walker, J.F., The thrombotic diathesis associated with the presence of phospholipid antibodies may be due to low levels of free protein S, *Am. J. Med.*, 93, 49–56, 1992.

45. Oosting, J.D., Derksen, R.H.W.M., Bobbink, I.W.G., Hackeng, T.M., Bouma, B.N., and deGroot, P.G., Antiphospholipid antibodies directed against a combination of phospholipid binding with prothrombin, protein C, or protein S: an explanation of their pathogenic mechanism, *Blood*, 81, 2618–2625, 1993.

46. Pigault, C., Follenius-Wund, A., Schmutz, M., Freyssinet, J.M., and Brisson, A., Formation of two-dimensional assays of annexin V on phosphatidylserine containing liposomes, *J. Mol. Biol.*, 236, 199–208, 1994.

47. Nakamura, N., Ban, T., Yamaji, K., Yoneda, Y., and Wada, Y., Localization of the apoptosis-inducing activity of lupus anticoagulants in an annexin V-binding antibody subset, *J. Clin. Invest.*, 101, 1951–1959, 1998.

48. Rand, J.H., "Annexinopathies" — a new class of diseases, *N. Engl. J. Med.*, 340, 1035–1036, 1999.

49. Rand, J.H., Wu, X.X., Andree, H.A.M., Ross, A., Rusinova, E., Gascon-Lema, M.E., Calandri, C., and Harpel, P.C., Antiphospholipid antibodies accelerate plasma coagulation by inhibiting annexin V binding to phospholipids: a "lupus procoagulant" effect, *Blood*, 92, 1652–1660, 1998.

50. Kaburaki, J., Kuwawa, M., Yamamoto, M., Kawai, S., and Ikeda, Y., Clinical significance of anti-annexin V antibodies in patients with systemic lupus erythematosus, *Am. J. Hematol.*, 54, 209–213, 1997.

51. Jaeger, U., Kapiotis, S., Pabinger, I., Puchhammer, E., Kryle, P., and Lechner, K., Transient lupus anticoagulant associated with hypoprothrombinemia and factor XII deficiency following adenovirus infection, *Ann. Haematol.*, 67, 95–99, 1993.

52. Habmayer, W.M., Haushofer, A., Angerer, V., and Fischer, M., The discrimination of factor XII deficiency and lupus anticoagulant, *Thromb. Haemost.*, 75, 698–699, 1996.

53. Jones, D.W., Gallimore, M.J., and Winter, M., Pseudo factor XII deficiency and phospholipid antibodies, *Thromb. Haemost.*, 75, 696–697, 1996.

54. Dolan, G., Kirby, R., Vong, S.T., Horn, E.H., and Westby, J., Interference on factor XI: measurement by antiphospholipid antibodies: potential source of error in diagnosis of factor XI deficiency, *Br. J. Haemost.*, 97, 85, 1997.

55. Triplett, D.A. and Barna, L.K., Use of a factor XI assay to screen for β_2 GPI dependent or prothrombin dependent lupus anticoagulants, *Lupus*, 3, 354, 1994.

56. Boffa, M.C., Berard, M., Toshitaka, S., and McIntyre, J.A., Antiphosphatidylethanolamine antibodies as the only antiphospholipid antibodies detected by ELISA II kininogen reactivity, *J. Rheumatol.*, 23, 1375–1379, 1996.

57. Sugi, T. and McIntyre, J.A., Autoantibodies to phosphatidylethanolamine (PE) recognize a kininogen-PE complex, *Blood*, 86, 3083–3089, 1995.

58. Rand, J.H., Wu, X.X., Guller, S., Gil, G., Schet, J., and Lockwood, C.J., Reduction of annexin V (placental anticoagulant protein-1) on placental villi of women with antiphospholipid antibodies and recurrent spontaneous abortion, *Am. J. Obstet. Gynecol.*, 171, 1566–1572, 1994.

59. Vogt, E., Ng, A., and Rote, N.S., Antiphosphatidylserine antibody removes annexin V and facilitates the binding of prothrombin at the surface of a chomocarcinoma model of trophoblast differentiation, *Am. J. Obstet. Gynecol.*, 177, 964–972, 1997.

60. Rand, J.H., Wu, X.X., Guller, S., Scher, J., Andree, H.A., and Lockwood, C.J., Antiphospholipid immunoglobulin G antibodies reduce annexin V levels on syncytiotrophoblasts apical membranes and in culture media of placental villi, *Am. J. Obstet. Gynecol.*, 177, 918–923, 1997.

3 Antiphospholipid Antibodies

Robert A. S. Roubey

CONTENTS

I. INTRODUCTION

The antiphospholipid syndrome (APS) is the association of antibodies with an apparent specificity for anionic phospholipids with arterial and venous thrombosis, recurrent fetal loss, thrombocytopenia, a form of valvular heart disease, livedo reticularis, cutaneous ulceration, chorea, and certain other neurological manifestations. There is increasing evidence that the autoantibodies associated with APS are not only serological markers of the syndrome, but play a direct role in hypercoagulability and other clinical manifestations. This chapter will review the autoimmune response and spectrum of autoantibodies associated with APS and the possible contribution of autoantibodies in the pathophysiology of APS-associated thrombosis. The clinical features of APS, as well as its diagnosis and treatment, are discussed in detail by R. Asherson and R. Cervera in Chapter 20.

II. AUTOANTIBODIES AND ANTIGENS

The antibodies associated with APS are traditionally detected in two types of laboratory assays. So-called anticardiolipin antibodies are detected in enzyme-linked immunosorbent assays (ELISAs) in which cardiolipin, a negatively-charged phospholipid, dried onto wells of a microtiter plate is the putative antigen. In contrast, lupus anticoagulant assays detect antibodies based on their ability to inhibit certain phospholipid-dependent coagulation reactions. The antibodies detected in anticardiolipin ELISAs and/or lupus anticoagulant tests were originally thought to be directed against anionic phospholipids. Over the past decade, however, data from many laboratories have shown that this is not generally the case.[1] For the most part, the antibodies in APS patient sera that are detected in anticardiolipin ELISAs do not recognize cardiolipin, but rather bind to β_2-Glycoprotein I (β_2GPI), a phospholipid-binding plasma protein. Most autoantibodies with lupus anticoagulant activity in APS patients are directed against either β_2GPI or prothrombin. These key observations have led to a reevaluation of the nature of "antiphospholipid" antibodies (APA) and may provide important clues into the nature of the autoimmune response and potential mechanisms of autoantibody-mediated thrombosis in APS.

A. β_2-GLYCOPROTEIN I

Approximately a decade ago three independent laboratories reported that affinity-purified "anticardiolipin" antibodies did not bind to cardiolipin in the absence of serum or plasma.[2-4] The plasma component required for antibody-binding was β_2GPI (also termed *apolipoprotein* H). The major source of β_2GPI in most anticardiolipin ELISAs is bovine serum, which is used in the blocking buffer and sample diluent of these assays. A small amount of human β_2GPI is also present in the diluted serum sample itself.

1. β_2GPI Structure and Function

β_2GPI was first identified by Schultze in 1961.[5] It is a 50 kD glycoprotein present in normal plasma at a concentration of approximately 200 μg/ml (4 μM). β_2GPI belongs to the complement control protein family of molecules, containing five characteristic consensus repeats or "sushi" domains.[6] β_2GPI binds to anionic phospholipids;[7] hence, its interaction with cardiolipin-coated plates in the anticardiolipin ELISA. Lysine-rich segments in the fifth "sushi" domain have been implicated as major phospholipid-binding regions.[8-10] The physiological function of β_2GPI is not known. *In vitro* data demonstrate that β_2GPI can inhibit prothrombinase activity,[11-13] contact pathway activation,[14] ADP-induced platelet aggregation,[15] and factor Xa generation by platelets,[16] suggesting that the protein may function as a natural anticoagulant. Evidence against such a role, however, includes the fact that many of the *in vitro* activities require supraphysiological concentrations of β_2GPI and/or nonphysiological buffers. Recent data demonstrate that the binding of β_2GPI to membranes containing physiological concentrations of anionic phospholipids is actually weak compared to coagulation factors and other phospholipid-binding proteins involved in hemostasis. Normal plasma levels of β_2GPI would not effectively compete with these proteins for membrane binding sites *in vivo*.[17,18] Further, inherited deficiency of β_2GPI, either heterozygous or homozygous, is not clearly associated with an increased risk of thrombosis.[19]

β_2GPI may interact with other plasma proteins or molecules on cell surfaces. A fraction of plasma β_2GPI circulates in association with lipoproteins[20] and a specific interaction with apolipoprotein (a) has recently been reported.[21] There is also evidence of relatively tight binding of β_2GPI to calmodulin[22] and annexin II,[23] although the physiological importance of these interactions is unknown. "Anticardiolipin" antibodies bind to vascular endothelial cells and platelets in a β_2GPI-dependent fashion and, in some instances, trigger intracellular events.[24-26] The mechanism of signal transduction is not known, but appears to be independent of Fc receptors.[25] These observations suggest the existence of one or more β_2GPI transmembrane receptor proteins. β_2GPI also binds to cells undergoing apoptosis, presumably through an interaction with phosphatidylserine that is exposed on the outer membrane leaflet of such cells.[27] This observation and *in vivo* clearance experiments suggest that β_2GPI might serve as an opsonin for the recognition and clearance of apoptotic cells.[28,29]

2. Characterization of Anti-β_2GPI Autoantibodies

In APS patient sera, most anticardiolipin antibodies bind to epitopes expressed on β_2GPI, and antibody binding to β_2GPI in the absence of phospholipid has been observed by most groups.[30-36] Autoantibody binding to native β_2GPI has been demonstrated in fluid-phase inhibition experiments and by the immunoaffinity purification of these antibodies using β_2GPI immobilized on agarose beads. These data do not exclude the possibility that certain anti-β_2GPI antibodies may be directed against conformational epitopes on phospholipid-bound β_2GPI.[31] Most autoantibodies to β_2GPI in patient sera are of low intrinsic affinity ($K_d \sim 10^{-5}$ M for fluid-phase binding),[32,37] which may have important implications for pathophysiology. Anti-β_2GPI antibodies appear to circulate free from β_2GPI and do not decrease plasma β_2GPI levels via the formation and clearance of circulating immune complexes. *In vivo*, high avidity binding to β_2GPI may occur through multivalent attachment to β_2GPI that is clustered and/or immobilized on cell surfaces. Recent studies of polyclonal anti-β_2GPI antibodies indicate that immunodominant epitopes reside in the first domain of β_2GPI.[38,39] In contrast, several patient-derived monoclonal antibodies recognize epitopes located in the fourth domain.[40]

Certain autoantibodies to β_2GPI have lupus anticoagulant activity[12,13] and anti-β_2GPI antibodies account for one third to one half of lupus anticoagulants in APS patients.[41] The probable mechanism by which anti-β_2GPI antibodies express lupus anticoagulant activity has recently been elucidated. Although β_2GPI binding to physiological membranes is weak, in the presence of anti-β_2GPI antibodies, complexes of antibody cross-linked β_2GPI may bind to membranes with extraordinarily high avidity.[17,42,43] This high avidity is due to the fact that antibody cross-linked β_2GPI complexes contain two or more β_2GPI molecules and bind bivalently or multivalently to the phospholipid membrane. Whereas physiological concentrations of monomeric β_2GPI do not effectively compete with coagulation factors for anionic membrane sites, antibody-β_2GPI complexes may compete very effectively. These complexes reduce the number of anionic phospholipid sites available to the prothrombinase complex and inhibit coagulation reactions in lupus anticoagulant assays. It is not known why certain anti-β_2GPI antibodies have lupus anticoagulant (LA) activity but others do not. It is likely that both fine specificity and average affinity are important factors.

B. PROTHROMBIN

The other major specificity of autoantibodies with lupus anticoagulant activity is prothrombin.[44] Antiprothrombin autoantibodies may account for one half to two thirds of LA in APS patients. The mechanism of LA activity is probably similar to that of anti-β_2GPI autoantibodies. Complexes of antibody cross-linked prothrombin bind anionic phospholipid membranes with high avidity, displacing other coagulation factors.[45] Antiprothrombin autoantibodies also may interfere with assembly of the prothrombinase complex or directly retard activation of prothrombin by factor Xa.

Most antiprothrombin autoantibodies are probably of relatively low affinity; however, a small subset of patients have higher affinity antiprothrombin antibodies. These patients are hypoprothrombinemic due to the clearance of prothrombin antigen-antibody complexes and, unlike APS patients, have a bleeding tendency rather than an increased risk of thrombosis. Antiprothrombin autoantibodies associated with APS are commonly species specific, i.e., they recognize human prothrombin but not prothrombin of other species. The observation that most antiprothrombin autoantibodies fail to bind to bovine prothrombin was important in identifying these antibodies as lupus anticoagulants.[44]

For technical reasons, antiprothrombin antibodies are not usually detectable in anticardiolipin ELISAs. These include the low concentration of prothrombin in serum, species specificity, and low calcium ion concentration. Antiprothrombin ELISAs have been developed recently; however, optimization, standardization, and key methodological issues have not been resolved.[41,46,47] Calcium has a major influence on the conformation of prothrombin and differences in calcium ion concentration may profoundly affect antiprothrombin immunoassays.

C. OTHER AUTOANTIBODIES

A number of other autoantibodies may be associated with APS. These include certain antibodies that are detected in anticardiolipin and/or lupus anticoagulant assays, and antibodies that are not detectable in standard antiphospholipid antibody tests. In theory, anticardiolipin ELISAs may detect antibodies to any cardiolipin-binding protein in bovine serum or to cardiolipin itself. Examples of the former include complement factor H and C4b-binding protein. The relevance of antibodies to these proteins to APS is not known. Antibodies that bind directly to cardiolipin occur in patients with syphilis and certain other infectious diseases, as well as certain normal individuals. These antibodies do not appear to be associated with APS.

One group of investigators has recently emphasized the fact that the fatty acid chains of cardiolipin derived from natural sources are readily oxidizable, and that some degree of oxidation is likely under the conditions used in most anticardiolipin ELISAs.[48] Anticardiolipin assays may therefore detect antibodies directed against these oxidized lipids. It is also possible that β_2GPI or certain other serum proteins may bind covalently to oxidized cardiolipin. The presence of oxidized lipids in anticardiolipin assays is intriguing in light of some reports suggesting the cross-reactivity of anticardiolipin antibodies and antibodies to oxidized lipoproteins.[49] It is unclear whether there is true cross-reactivity between antibodies to oxidized lipids or if this observation is due to detection of antibodies to β_2GPI or other proteins in both assays.

The protein C pathway is a clinically important physiological anticoagulant mechanism,[50] and inhibition of this pathway may be an important mechanism of hypercoagulability in APS. Autoantibodies to components of this pathway have been reported in association with APS, although they are not detectable in anticardiolipin or lupus anticoagulant assays. Autoantibodies to thrombomodulin,[51-53] protein C, and protein S[54,55] have been reported.

Autoantibodies to annexin V (placental anticoagulant protein-1) have been reported by some groups.[56] Annexins are a family of calcium-dependent phospholipid-binding, intracellular proteins thought to have an important function in membrane processes, such as exocytosis.[57] It is postulated that annexin V may be involved in hemostasis.[58]

Heparan sulfate proteoglycan (HSPG) is expressed on vascular endothelium and plays an important role in vascular structure and function. Vascular HSPG is required for the activation and optimal anticoagulant activity of antithrombin III. Autoantibodies to both the heparan sulfate moiety and the core protein of vascular HSPG have been detected in certain lupus sera.[59,60]

Analogous to the role of β_2GPI in anticardiolipin ELISAs, high and/or low molecular weight kininogens are required for the binding of certain antibodies in antiphosphatidylethanolamine assays.[61]

III. AUTOIMMUNITY IN APS

Although our knowledge of the autoantibodies associated with APS has increased considerably in recent years, very little is known about the autoimmune disorder leading to their production. As a primary syndrome, APS may be viewed as an "organ-specific" autoimmune disease with autoantibodies directed against a small number of phospholipid-binding plasma proteins and related antigens. On the other hand, APS and the same autoantibodies also occur as a secondary syndrome in the setting of systemic lupus erythematosus and more generalized autoimmunity.

A. ANIMAL MODELS

Appropriate animal models are important tools for studying several aspects of APS, i.e., the cellular basis of the autoimmune response, the contribution of genetic factors, and mechanisms by which autoantibodies may contribute to thrombosis and fetal loss. To date, most attention has focused on the pathogenic effects of antibodies with relatively little attention to the nature of the autoimmune response.

1. Spontaneous Models

Putative spontaneous models of APS include the MRL/lpr and NZW × BXSB F1 strains of mice.[62,63] Although MRL/lpr mice have antibodies detectable in anticardiolipin assays, the exact nature of these anticardiolipin antibodies is controversial. NZW × BXSB F1 mice develop true anti-β_2GPI autoantibodies (autoantibodies to murine β_2GPI).[64] In addition to features of lupus, these mice develop a degenerative coronary vasculopathy with myocardial infarction. Two BXSB alleles contributing to the production of anticardiolipin (anti-β_2GPI) antibodies have recently been identified.[65] The genetics of this model are complex, however, in that different alleles were associated with antiplatelet antibodies/thrombocytopenia and with myocardial infarction. Other genes involved include those in the major histocompatibility complex[65,66] and genes encoded on the BXSB Y-linked autoimmune accelerator (Yaa) gene.[67] A recent study suggests that CD4+ cells play an important role in the NZW × BXSB F1 model.[68] Treatment of mice with an anti-CD4 monoclonal antibody ameliorated the autoimmune disease, whereas an anti-CD8 monoclonal antibody worsened it.

2. Induced Models

There are two general types of induced animal models of APS: (1) those involving passive transfer of antibodies from patients to animals, and (2) those involving various forms of active immunization. Passive transfer models evaluate the short-term effects of antibodies on coagulation and/or pregnancy in recipient animals, but are not designed to investigate the immune abnormalities underlying APS. Active immunization models include those in which animals are immunized with APS-associated antigens and an idiotype/antiidiotype model in which mice are immunized with APS-associated antibodies. Experiments in which normal mice are immunized with APS-associated antigens generally confirm the observation that phospholipids themselves are poor antigens. In contrast, immunization of mice with heterologous (human) β_2GPI and an adjuvant induces an initial antibody response to the foreign protein. Over time tolerance is broken with the development of antimurine β_2GPI autoantibodies.[69] Interestingly, mice immunized with human β_2GPI appear to develop clinical features of APS in temporal association with the appearance of autoreactive antimurine β_2GPI antibodies. Immunization of mice with heterologous β_2GPI bound to apoptotic cells, in the absence of adjuvant, also breaks tolerance.[70] In the idiotype/antiidiotype model of APS developed by Shoenfeld and colleagues,[71] mice immunized with an anticardiolipin (anti-β_2GPI) antibody produce antibodies of the same specificity. The disease can be transferred by bone marrow T cells suggesting an important role for these cells.[72] While this model may be useful for studying antibody effects, it's relevance to the immunopathogenesis of human APS is not known.

B. HUMAN STUDIES

1. Cellular Immune Response

Visvanathan and McNeil have recently identified and characterized the cellular immune response to β_2GPI in patients with APS.[73] Peripheral blood mononuclear cells from 8 of 18 patients with APS proliferated in response to β_2GPI, whereas no response was observed with cells from healthy controls, patients with other autoimmune diseases, or anticardiolipin antibody-positive patients without clinical manifestations of APS. The response to β_2GPI was antigen-specific and required HLA class II molecules, CD4+ T cells, and antigen-presenting cells. The proliferating cells were CD4+ T cells producing interferon-γ, but not IL-4, suggesting a predominantly T_H1 response.

2. Immunogenetics

The HLA associations of APS have been studied by several groups. Arnett et al. observed a strong association with DQw7 (DQB1*0301) linked to HLA-DR5 and -DR4 haplotypes.[74] Among the patients who were DQw7 (DQB1*0301) negative, all possessed DQw8 (DQB1*0302) and/or DQw6 (DQB1*0602 or DQB1*0603) alleles. These molecules and DQw7 (DQB1*0301) all contain an identical seven amino acid sequence in the third hypervariable region of the HLA-DQ molecule, suggesting a possible "epitope" associated with APS. Other investigators have reported associations with DR4, DR7, and DRw53.[75]

There are several studies of the familial occurrence of APS. In the largest study to date, seven families were identified, in which 30 of 101 family members met diagnostic criteria for APS.[76] Segregation analysis strongly supported a genetic basis for the disease that was best explained by a dominant or codominant model. Interestingly, in these families APS was not linked with HLA, Fas, or other candidate genes.

IV. PATHOPHYSIOLOGY

A. Autoantibody–Antigen Interactions

There are a limited number of mechanisms by which autoantibodies to phospholipid-binding plasma proteins, such as β_2GPI and prothrombin, could interact with their respective antigens. First, high affinity, neutralizing autoantibodies may directly inhibit an antigen's function and/or decrease plasma antigen levels via clearance of antigen–antibody complexes. This type of interaction typically occurs with acquired inhibitors to coagulation factors. With the exception of the small subset of patients with lupus anticoagulants and hypoprothrombinemia, antibodies associated with APS tend to be of relatively low affinity and do not decrease plasma antigen levels. A second possibility is that autoantibodies and antigens may form immune complexes that deposit in vessel walls, leading to inflammation and tissue injury. This occurs in serum sickness and many vasculitides, but does not appear to occur with either acquired factor inhibitors or autoantibodies associated with APS.

Two other possibilities may be particularly relevant to APS. As discussed above, although relatively low affinity autoantibodies to phospholipid-binding plasma proteins may not bind to their antigens in the fluid phase, high avidity bivalent or multivalent antibody–antigen reactions may occur when the antigens are bound to membranes. Autoantibody cross-linking of membrane bound antigens will markedly decrease the rate at which the antigens dissociate from the membrane, causing dysregulation of phospholipid-dependent reactions. This is the likely mechanism by which certain anti-β_2GPI autoantibodies exhibit lupus anticoagulant activity, as previously discussed. If the antigens are bound to receptor proteins on the cell surface, cross-linking by antibodies may trigger signal transduction and certain cellular responses. This may well be the mechanism by which β_2GPI and anti-β_2GPI autoantibodies cause the upregulation of adhesion molecules on endothelial cells.[24,25]

B. Mechanisms of Autoantibody-Mediated Thrombosis

The literature implicates a confusing variety of mechanisms by which autoantibodies contribute to a hypercoagulable state in APS. Most of these studies were performed prior to our current understanding of autoantibody specificities, which may explain many of the apparent discrepancies. The diversity of mechanisms may be due to the likelihood that different autoantibodies have different pathophysiological activities. The spectrum of autoantibodies and their characteristics (specificity, fine specificity, valency, affinity/avidity, titer) may explain the spectrum of clinical manifestations in APS, e.g., why some patients experience only arterial thrombosis and others have exclusively venous events. Based on the antibody–antigen interactions discussed above, potential mechanisms of thrombosis will be grouped as those involving antibody interference with hemostatic reactions (physiological anticoagulant reactions, fibrinolysis) and those involving cell-mediated events.

1. Interference with Hemostatic Reactions

a. Inhibition of physiological anticoagulants

Inhibition of the protein C pathway has been one of the most common mechanisms of thrombosis observed in experimental studies of APS associated autoantibodies. The clinical importance of the protein C system in normal hemostasis is evidenced by the association of inherited deficiencies of protein C or protein S with thrombosis, and by the recent identification of resistance to activated protein C as one of the most common inherited cause of thrombosis.[77]

Inhibition of both protein C activation by thrombin and thrombomodulin and of the proteolytic cleavage of factor Va and factor VIIIa by activated protein C have been observed in association with APS.[54,78-82] Anti-β_2GPI autoantibodies may be involved, although data are equivocal.[83-85] There is also evidence that autoantibodies directed against protein C pathway components, i.e., thrombo-modulin, protein C, and protein S, may be involved.[53,54]

Antithrombin III is the major plasma inhibitor of factor IXa, factor Xa, and thrombin. In order to optimally inhibit these factors, antithrombin III must bind to heparan sulfate expressed on vascular endothelium. Autoantibodies to vascular heparan sulfate proteoglycan (HSPG) and/or heparin could contribute to a thrombotic tendency by blocking the activation of antithrombin III.[86-88] In view of the fact that β_2GPI binds to heparin, anti-β_2GPI antibodies could have a similar effect.

It has been proposed that both annexin V and β_2GPI may act as physiological anticoagulants, although data supporting such roles are quite limited. Rand and colleagues have proposed that displacement of annexin from cell surfaces by certain antiphospholipid antibodies (perhaps in the presence of β_2GPI) may be a pathophysiological mechanism in APS.[89] One study suggests that β_2GPI acts as inhibitor of factor Xa generation on the surface of platelets and that autoantibodies to β_2GPI may block this activity.[16]

b. Inhibition of fibrinolysis

Studies of fibrinolytic activity in patients with APS have generally been inconclusive, although increased levels of plasminogen activator inhibitor-1 (PAI-1) have been reported.[90-92] The possible effects of autoantibodies on factor XII-dependent fibrinolysis[93] has received less attention. Two studies reported inhibition of this pathway in a significant number of patients with lupus antico-agulants.[94,95]

2. Cellular Interactions

a. Monocytes

There is increasing evidence that increased expression of tissue factor (TF) on circulating blood monocytes is an important mechanism of hypercoagulability in APS.[96-99] Anticardiolipin (anti-β_2GPI) antibodies from patient sera as well as patient-derived monoclonal anti-β_2GPI autoantibodies induced TF expression on normal blood monocytes.

b. Endothelial cells

There are several mechanisms by which autoantibodies may enhance the procoagulant activity of vascular endothelial cells. Sera and IgG fractions from certain patients increase the expression of TF,[100,101] the production of endothelin 1,[102] and the expression of the adhesion molecules E-selectin, VCAM-1, and ICAM-1.[24,25] The latter activities have been shown to be dependent on β_2GPI and anti-β_2GPI autoantibodies.

Another mechanism involves dysregulation of eicosanoid metabolism. There is some evidence that autoantibodies in APS may inhibit production of endothelial cell prostacyclin (PGI_2), a potent vasodilator and platelet inhibitor.[103] Autoantibody effects on platelet eicosanoids may be more important, however, as discussed below.

c. Platelets

Some studies suggest that APS antibodies induce platelet aggregation,[104] whereas others have observed inhibition,[105] perhaps due to differences in antibody subsets. Monoclonal anti-β_2GPI antibodies bind to platelets in a β_2GPI-dependent fashion and lead to platelet activation in the presence of subthreshold concentrations of weak agonists.[106]

There is consistent evidence that APS autoantibodies enhance platelet thromboxane A_2 production.[107-109]

V. SUMMARY

There have been significant advances in our understanding of the autoantibodies and antigens involved in APS. These findings are contributing to more specific studies of the autoimmune responses in the syndrome and to the development of appropriate animal models. Increased knowledge of the relevant autoantibodies and antigens is helping to explain the clinical diversity of APS and the variety of proposed pathophysiological mechanisms.

REFERENCES

1. Roubey, R. A. S., Immunology of the antiphospholipid antibody syndrome, *Arthritis Rheum.*, 39, 1444–1454, 1996.
2. Galli, M., P. Comfurius, C. Maassen, H. C. Hemker, M. H. De Baets, P. J. C. van Breda-Vriesman, T. Barbui, R. F. A. Zwaal, and E. M. Bevers, Anticardiolipin antibodies directed not to cardiolipin but to a plasma protein cofactor, *Lancet*, 335, 1544–1547, 1990.
3. McNeil, H. P., R. J. Simpson, C. N. Chesterman, and S. A. Krilis, Anti-phospholipid antibodies are directed against a complex antigen that includes a lipid-binding inhibitor of coagulation: β_2-glycoprotein I (apolipoprotein H), *Proc. Natl. Acad. Sci. USA*, 87, 4120–4124, 1990.
4. Matsuura, E., Y. Igarashi, M. Fujimoto, K. Ichikawa, and T. Koike, Anticardiolipin cofactor(s) and differential diagnosis of autoimmune disease, *Lancet*, 336, 177–178, 1990.
5. Schultze, H. E., K. Heide, and H. Haupt, Über ein bisher unbekanntes niedermolekilares β_2-globulin der humanserums, *Naturwissenschaften*, 23, 719–719, 1961.
6. Reid, K. B. M., D. R. Bentley, R. D. Campbell, L. P. Chung, R. B. Sim, T. Kristensen, and B. F. Tack, Complement system proteins which interact with C3b or C4b: a superfamily of structurally related proteins, *Immunol. Today*, 7, 230–234, 1986.
7. Wurm, H., β_2-glycoprotein I (apolipoprotein H) interactions with phospholipid vesicles, *Int. J. Biochem.*, 16, 511–515, 1984.
8. Hunt, J. E., R. J. Simpson, and S. A. Krilis, Identification of a region of β_2-glycoprotein I critical for lipid binding and anti-cardiolipin cofactor activity, *Proc. Natl. Acad. Sci. USA*, 90, 2141–2145, 1993.
9. Steinkasserer, A., P. N. Barlow, A. C. Willis, Z. Kertesz, I. D. Campbell, R. B. Sim, and D. G. Norman, Activity, disulphide mapping and structural modelling of the fifth domain of human β_2-glycoprotein I, *FEBS Lett.*, 313, 193–197, 1992.
10. Kertesz, Z., B. Yu, A. Steinkasserer, H. Haupt, A. Benham, and R. B. Sim, Characterization of binding of human β_2-glycoprotein I to cardiolipin, *Biochem. J.*, 310, 315–321, 1995.
11. Nimpf, J., E. M. Bevers, P. H. H. Bomans, U. Till, H. Wurm, G. M. Kostner, and R. F. A. Zwaal, Prothrombinase activity of human platelets is inhibited by β_2-glycoprotein I, *Biochim. Biophys. Acta*, 884, 142–149, 1986.
12. Galli, M., P. Comfurius, T. Barbui, R. F. A. Zwaal, and E. M. Bevers, Anticoagulant activity of β_2-glycoprotien I is potentiated by a distinct subgroup of anticardiolipin antibodies, *Thromb. Haemost.*, 68, 297–300, 1992.

13. Roubey, R. A. S., C. W. Pratt, J. P. Buyon, and J. B. Winfield, Lupus anticoagulant activity of autoimmune antiphospholipid antibodies is dependent upon β_2-glycoprotein I, *J. Clin. Invest.*, 90, 1100–1104, 1992.

14. Schousboe, I., β_2-glycoprotein I: a plasma inhibitor of the contact activation of the intrinsic blood coagulation pathway, *Blood*, 66, 1086–1091, 1985.

15. Nimpf, J., H. Wurm, and G. M. Kostner, β_2-glycoprotein-I (apo H) inhibits the release reaction of human platelets during ADP-induced aggregation, *Atherosclerosis*, 63, 109–114, 1987.

16. Shi, W., B. H. Chong, P. J. Hogg, and C. N. Chesterman, Anticardiolipin antibodies block the inhibition by β_2-glycoprotein I of the factor Xa generating activity of platelets, *Thromb. Haemost.*, 70, 342–345, 1993.

17. Willems, G. M., M. P. Janssen, M. M. A. L. Pelsers, P. Comfurius, M. Galli, R. F. A. Zwaal, and E. M. Bevers, Role of divalency in the high-affinity binding of anticardiolipin antibody-β_2-glycoprotein I complexes to lipid membranes, *Biochemistry*, 35, 13833–13842, 1996.

18. Roubey, R. A. S., M. F. Harper, and B. R. Lentz, The interaction of β_2-glycoprotein I with phospholipid membranes (abstract), *Arthritis Rheum.*, 38, S211–S211, 1995.

19. Bancsi, L. F., I. K. van der Linden, and R. M. Bertina, β_2-glycoprotein I deficiency and the risk of thrombosis, *Thromb. Haemost.*, 67, 649–653, 1992.

20. Polz, E., H. Wurm, and G. M. Kostner, Investigations on β_2-glycoprotein-I in the rat: isolation from serum and demonstration in lipoprotein density fractions, *J. Biochem.*, 11, 265–270, 1980.

21. Kochl, S., F. Fresser, E. Lobentanz, G. Baier, and G. Utermann, Novel interaction of apolipoprotein(a) with β_2-glycoprotein I mediated by the kringle IV domain, *Blood*, 90, 1482–1489, 1997.

22. Rojkjaer, R., D. A. Klaerke, and I. Schousboe, Characterization of the interaction between β_2-glycoprotein I and calmodulin, and identification of a binding sequence in β_2-glycoprotein I, *Biochim. Biophys. Acta Protein Struct. Mol. Enzymol.*, 1339, 217–225, 1997.

23. Ma, K., J. -C. Zhang, K. Wan, M. Poncz, K. A. Hajjar, and K. R. McCrae, The binding of β_2-glycoprotein I (β_2GPI) to endothelial cells is mediated through a high affinity interaction with annexin II (abstract), *Blood*, 92, 172A, 1998.

24. Del Papa, N., L. Guidali, L. Spatola, P. Bonara, M. O. Borghi, A. Tincani, G. Balestrieri, and P. L. Meroni, Relationship between anti-phospholipid and anti-endothelial cell antibodies III: β_2-glycoprotein I mediates the antibody binding to endothelial membranes and induces the expression of adhesion molecules, *Clin. Exp. Rheumatol.*, 13, 179–185, 1995.

25. Simantov, R., J. M. LaSala, S. K. Lo, A. E. Gharavi, L. R. Sammaritano, J. E. Salmon, and R. L. Silverstein, Activation of cultured vascular endothelial cells by antiphospholipid antibodies, *J. Clin. Invest.*, 96, 2211–2219, 1995.

26. Shi, W., B. H. Chong, and C. N. Chesterman, β_2-Glycoprotein I is a requirement for anticardiolipin antibodies binding to activated platelets: differences with lupus anticoagulants, *Blood*, 81, 1255–1262, 1993.

27. Price, B. E., J. Rauch, M. A. Shia, M. T. Walsh, W. Lieberthal, H. M. Gilligan, T. O'Laughlin, J. S. Koh, and J. S. Levine, Anti-phospholipid autoantibodies bind to apoptotic, but not viable, thymocytes in a β_2-glycoprotein I-dependent manner, *J. Immunol.*, 157, 2201–2208, 1996.

28. Chonn, A., S. C. Semple, and P. R. Cullis, β_2-glycoprotein I is a major protein associated with very rapidly cleared liposomes *in vivo*, suggesting a significant role in the immune clearance of "non-self" particles, *J. Biol. Chem.*, 270, 25845–25849, 1995.

29. Balasubramanian, K., J. Chandra, and A. J. Schroit, Immune clearance of phosphatidylserine-expressing cells by phagocytes. The role of β_2-glycoprotein I in macrophage recognition, *J. Biol. Chem.*, 272, 31113–31117, 1997.

30. Hunt, J. and S. Krilis, The fifth domain of β_2-glycoprotein I contains a phospholipid binding site (cys281-cys288), and a region recognised by anticardiolipin antibodies, *J. Immunol.*, 152, 653–659, 1994.

31. Matsuura, E., Y. Igarashi, T. Yasuda, T. Koike, and D. A. Triplett, Anticardiolipin antibodies recognize β_2-glycoprotein I structure altered by interacting with an oxygen modified solid phase surface, *J. Exp. Med.*, 179, 457–462, 1994.

32. Roubey, R. A. S., R. A. Eisenberg, M. F. Harper, and J. B. Winfield, "Anticardiolipin" autoantibodies recognize β_2-glycoprotein I in the absence of phospholipid. Importance of antigen density and bivalent binding, *J. Immunol.*, 154, 954–960, 1995.

33. Pengo, V., A. Biasiolo, and M. G. Fior, Autoimmune antiphospholipid antibodies are directed against a cryptic epitope expressed when β_2-glycoprotein I is bound to a suitable surface, *Thromb. Haemost.*, 73, 29–34, 1995.

34. Keeling, D. M., A. J. G. Wilson, I. J. Mackie, S. J. Machin, and D. A. Isenberg, Some "antiphospholipid antibodies" bind to β_2-glycoprotein I in the absence of phospholipid, *Br. J. Haematol.*, 82, 571–574, 1992.

35. Arvieux, J., B. Roussel, M. C. Jacob, and M. G. Colomb, Measurement of anti-phospholipid antibodies by ELISA using β_2-glycoprotein I as an antigen, *J. Immunol. Methods*, 143, 223–229, 1991.

36. Viard, J. -P., Z. Amoura, and J. -F. Bach, Association of anti-β_2 glycoprotein I antibodies with lupus-type circulating anticoagulant and thrombosis in systemic lupus erythematosus, *Am. J. Med.*, 93, 181–186, 1992.

37. Tincani, A., L. Spatola, E. Prati, F. Allegri, P. Ferremi, R. Cattaneo, P. Meroni, and G. Balestrieri, The anti-β_2-glycoprotein I activity in human anti-phospholipid syndrome sera is due to monoreactive low-affinity autoantibodies directed to epitopes located on native β_2-glycoprotein I and preserved during species evolution, *J. Immunol.*, 157, 5732–5738, 1996.

38. Marquis, D., E. Victoria, and G. M. Iverson, β_2GPI-dependent anticardiolipin autoantibodies recognize an epitope on the first domain of β_2GPI (abstract), *Lupus*, 7, S176–S176, 1998.

39. McNeeley, P. A., E. J. Victoria, D. Marquis, J. F. Crisologo, D. C. Tuyay, and M. D. Linnik, APS patient sera preferentially recognize the first domain of β_2-glycoprotein I (abstract), *Lupus*, 7, S176–S176, 1998.

40. Igarashi, M., E. Matsuura, Y. Igarashi, H. Nagae, K. Ichikawa, D. A. Triplett, and T. Koike, Human β_2-glycoprotein I as an anticardiolipin cofactor determined using deleted mutants expressed by a baculovirus system, *Blood*, 87, 3262–3270, 1996.

41. Arvieux, J., L. Darnige, C. Caron, G. Reber, J. C. Bensa, and M. G. Colomb, Development of an ELISA for autoantibodies to prothrombin showing their prevalence in patients with lupus anticoagulants, *Thromb. Haemost.*, 74, 1120–1125, 1995.

42. Arnout, J., C. Wittevrongel, M. Vanrusselt, M. Hoylaerts, and J. Vermylen, β_2-glycoprotein I-dependent lupus anticoagulants form stable bivalent antibody β_2-glycoprotein I complexes on phospholipid surfaces, *Thromb. Haemost.*, 79, 79–86, 1998.

43. Takeya, H., T. Mori, E. C. Gabazza, K. Kuroda, H. Deguchi, E. Matsuura, K. Ichikawa, T. Koike, and K. Suzuki, Anti-β_2-glycoprotein I (β_2GPI) monoclonal antibodies with lupus anticoagulant-like activity enhance the β_2GPI binding to phospholipids, *J. Clin. Invest.*, 99, 2260–2268, 1997.

44. Bevers, E. M., M. Galli, T. Barbui, P. Comfurius, and R. F. A. Zwaal, Lupus anticoagulant IgG's (LA) are not directed to phospholipids only, but to a complex of lipid-bound human prothrombin, *Thromb. Haemost.*, 66, 629–632, 1991.

45. Rao, L. V. M., A. D. Hoang, and S. I. Rapaport, Mechanisms and effects of the binding of lupus anticoagulant IgG and prothrombin to surface phospholipid, *Blood*, 88, 4173–4182, 1996.

46. Galli, M., G. Beretta, M. Daldossi, E. M. Bevers, and T. Barbui, Different anticoagulant and immunological properties of anti-prothrombin antibodies in patients with antiphospholipid antibodies, *Thromb. Haemost.*, 77, 486–491, 1997.

47. Horbach, D. A., E. van Oort, R. H. Derksen, and P. G. De Groot, The contribution of anti-prothrombin-antibodies to lupus anticoagulant activity — discrimination between functional and non-functional anti-prothrombin-antibodies, *Thromb. Haemost.*, 79, 790–795, 1998.

48. Hörkkö, S., E. Miller, D. W. Branch, W. Palinski, and J. L. Witztum, The epitopes for some antiphospholipid antibodies are adducts of oxidized phospholipid and β_2-glycoprotein I (and other proteins), *Proc. Natl. Acad. Sci. USA*, 94, 10356–10361, 1997.

49. Hörkkö, S., E. Miller, E. Dudl, P. Reaven, L. K. Curtiss, N. J. Zvaifler, R. Terkeltaub, S. S. Pierangeli, D. W. Branch, W. Palinski, and J. L. Witztum, Antiphospholipid antibodies are directed against epitopes of oxidized phospholipids, *J. Clin. Invest.*, 98, 815–825, 1996.

50. Esmon, C. T., The protein C anticoagulant pathway, *Arterioscler. Thromb.*, 12, 135–145, 1992.

51. Ruiz-Argüelles, G. J., A. Ruiz-Argüelles, M. Deleze, and D. Alarcón-Segovia, Acquired protein C deficiency in a patient with primary antiphospholipid syndrome. Relationship to reactivity of anticardiolipin antibody with thrombomodulin, *J. Rheumatol.*, 16, 381–383, 1989.

52. Oosting, J. D., K. T. Preissner, R. H. W. M. Derksen, and P. G. De Groot, Autoantibodies directed against the epidermal growth factor-like domains of thrombomodulin inhibit protein C activation *in vitro*, *Br. J. Haematol.*, 85, 761–768, 1993.

53. Carson, C. W., P. C. Comp, N. L. Esmon, A. R. Rezaie, and C. T. Esmon, Thrombomodulin antibodies inhibit protein C activation and are found in patients with lupus anticoagulant and unexplained thrombosis (abstract), *Arthritis Rheum.*, 37, S296–S296, 1994.

54. Oosting, J. D., R. H. W. M. Derksen, I. W. G. Bobbink, T. M. Hackeng, B. N. Bouma, and P. G. De Groot, Antiphospholipid antibodies directed against a combination of phospholipids with pro-thrombin, protein C, or protein S: an explanation for their pathogenic mechanism? *Blood*, 81, 2618–2625, 1993.

55. Pengo, V., A. Biasiolo, T. Brocco, S. Tonetto, and A. Ruffatti, Autoantibodies to phospholipid-binding plasma proteins in patients with thrombosis and phospholipid-reactive antibodies, *Thromb. Haemost.*, 75, 721–724, 1996.

56. Matsuda, J., N. Saitoh, K. Gohchi, M. Gotoh, and M. Tsukamoto, Anti-annexin V antibody in systemic lupus erythematosus patients with lupus anticoagulant and/or anticardiolipin antibody, *Am. J. Hematol.*, 47, 56–58, 1994.

57. Creutz, C. E., The annexins and exocytosis, *Science*, 258, 924–931, 1992.

58. van Heerde, W. L., P. G. De Groot, and C. P. M. Reutelingsperger, The complexity of the phospholipid binding protein annexin V, *Thromb. Haemost.*, 73, 172–179, 1995.

59. Fillit, H. and R. Lahita, Antibodies to vascular heparan sulfate proteoglycan in patients with systemic lupus erythematosus, *Autoimmunity*, 9, 159–164, 1991.

60. Fillit, H., S. Shibata, T. Sasaki, H. Speira, L. D. Kerr, and M. Blake, Autoantibodies to the protein core of vascular basement membrane heparan sulfate proteoglycan in systemic lupus erythematosus, *Autoimmunity*, 14, 243–249, 1993.

61. Sugi, T. and J. A. McIntyre, Autoantibodies to phosphatidylethanolamine (PE) recognize a kininogen-PE complex, *Blood*, 86, 3083–3089, 1995.

62. Smith, H. R., C. L. Hansen, R. Rose, and R. T. Canoso, Autoimmune MRL-lpr/lpr mice are an animal model for the secondary APS, *J. Rheumatol.*, 17, 911–915, 1990.

63. Hashimoto, Y., M. Kawamura, K. Ichikawa, T. Suzuki, T. Sumida, S. Yoshida, E. Matsuura, S. Ikehara, and T. Koike, Anticardiolipin antibodies in NZW × BXSB F1 mice: a model of antiphospholipid antibody syndrome, *J. Immunol.*, 149, 1063–1068, 1992.

64. Monestier, M., D. A. Kandiah, S. Kouts, K. E. Novick, G. L. Ong, M. Z. Radic, and S. A. Krilis, Monoclonal antibodies from NZW × BXSB F_1 mice to β_2-glycoprotein I and cardiolipin, *J. Immunol.*, 2631–2641, 1996.

65. Ida, A., S. Hirose, Y. Hamano, S. Kodera, Y. Jiang, M. Abe, D. Zhang, H. Nishimura, and T. Shirai, Multigenic control of lupus-associated antiphospholipid syndrome in a model of (NZW × BXSB) F_1 mice, *Eur. J. Immunol.*, 28, 2694–2703, 1998.

66. Ibnou-Zekri, N., M. Iwamoto, L. Fossati, P. J. McConahey, and S. Izui, Role of the major histocompatibility complex class II Ea gene in lupus susceptibility in mice, *Proc. Natl. Acad. Sci. USA*, 94, 14654–14659, 1997.

67. Fossati, L., M. Iwamoto, R. Merino, and S. Izui, Selective enhancing effect of the Yaa gene on immune responses against self and foreign antigens, *Eur. J. Immunol.*, 25, 166–173, 1995.

68. Adachi, Y., M. Inaba, A. Sugihara, M. Koshiji, K. Sugiura, Y. Amoh, S. Mori, T. Kamiya, H. Genba, and S. Ikehara, Effects of administration of monoclonal antibodies (anti-CD4 or anti-CD8) on the development of autoimmune diseases in (NZW × BXSB)F_1 mice, *Immunobiology*, 198, 451–464, 1998.

69. Tincani, A., B. Beltrami, P. L. Meroni, F. Allegri, L. Spatola, M. Cinquini, Y. Shoenfeld, and G. Balestrieri, Immunization of naive BALB/c mice with human β_2-glycoprotein I (β_2GPI) breaks tolerance against the murine molecule (abstract), *Lupus*, 7, S173–S173, 1998.

70. Levine, J. S., R. Subang, J. S. Koh, and J. Rauch, Induction of anti-phospholipid autoantibodies by β_2-glycoprotein I bound to apoptotic thymocytes, *J. Autoimmun.*, 11, 413–424, 1998.

71. Blank, M., J. Cohen, V. Toder, and Y. Shoenfeld, Induction of anti-phospholipid syndrome in naive mice with mouse lupus monoclonal and human polyclonal anti-cardiolipin antibodies, *Proc. Natl. Acad. Sci. USA*, 88, 3069–3073, 1991.

72. Blank, M., I. Krause, N. Lanir, P. Vardi, B. Gilburd, A. Tincani, Y. Tomer, and Y. Shoenfeld, Transfer of experimental antiphospholipid-syndrome by bone marrow cell transplantation: the importance of the T cell, *Arthritis Rheum.*, 38, 115–122, 1995.

73. Visvanathan, S. and H. P. McNeil, Cellular immunity to β_2-glycoprotein I in patients with the antiphospholipid syndrome, *J. Immunol.*, 162, 6919–6925, 1999.

74. Arnett, F. C., M. L. Olsen, K. L. Anderson, and J. D. Reveille, Molecular analysis of major histo-compatibility complex alleles associated with the lupus anticoagulant, *J. Clin. Invest.,* 87, 1490–1495, 1991.

75. Sebastiani, G. D., M. Galeazzi, G. Morozzi, and R. Marcolongo, The immunogenetics of the antiphos-pholipid syndrome, anticardiolipin antibodies, and lupus anticoagulant, *Semin. Arthritis Rheum.,* 25, 414–420, 1996.

76. Goel, N., T. L. Ortel, D. Bali, J. Anderson, I. S. Gourley, H. Smith, C. Morris, D. W. Branch, P. Ford, D. Berdeaux, R. A. S. Roubey, S. F. Kingsmore, T. Thiel, C. Amos, and M. F. Seldin, Familial antiphospholipid antibody syndrome: criteria for disease and evidence for autosomal dominant inher-itance, *Arthritis Rheum.,* 42, 318–327, 1999.

77. Dahlbäck, B., Physiological anticoagulation: resistance to activated protein C and venous thromboem-bolism, *J. Clin. Invest.,* 94, 923–927, 1994.

78. Borrell, M., N. Sala, C. de Castellarnau, S. Lopez, M. Gari, and J. Fontcuberta, Immunoglobulin fractions isolated from patients with antiphospholipid antibodies prevent the inactivation of factor Va by activated protein C on human endothelial cells, *Thromb. Haemost.,* 68, 268–272, 1992.

79. Cariou, R., G. Tobelem, S. Bellucci, J. Soria, C. Soria, J. Maclouf, and J. Caen, Effect of lupus anticoagulant on antithrombogenic properties of endothelial cells — inhibition of thrombomodulin-dependent protein C activation, *Thromb. Haemost.,* 60, 54–58, 1988.

80. Comp, P. C., L. E. DeBault, N. L. Esmon, and C. T. Esmon, Human thrombomodulin is inhibited by IgG from two patients with non-specific anticoagulants (abstract), *Blood,* 62 (Suppl. 1), 299a, 1983.

81. Malia, R. G., S. Kitchen, M. Greaves, and F. E. Preston, Inhibition of activated protein C and its cofactor protein S by antiphospholipid antibodies, *Br. J. Haematol.,* 76, 101–107, 1990.

82. Marciniak, E. and E. H. Romond, Impaired catalytic function of activated protein C: a new *in vitro* manifestation of lupus anticoagulant, *Blood,* 74, 2426–2432, 1989.

83. Keeling, D. M., A. J. G. Wilson, I. M. Mackie, D. A. Isenberg, and S. J. Machin, β_2-glycoprotein I inhibits the thrombin/thrombomodulin dependent activation of protein C (abstract), *Blood,* 78, 184a, 1991.

84. Oosting, J. D., R. H. W. M. Derksen, T. M. Hackeng, M. Van Vliet, K. T. Preissner, B. N. Bouma, and P. G. De Groot, *In vitro* studies of antiphospholipid antibodies and its cofactor, beta-2-glycoprotein I, show negligible effects on endothelial cell mediated protein C activation, *Thromb. Haemost.,* 66, 666–671, 1991.

85. Matsuda, J., K. Gohchi, K. Kawasugi, M. Gotoh, N. Saitoh, and M. Tsukamoto, Inhibitory activity of anti-β_2-glycoprotein I antibody on factor Va degradation by activated-protein C and its cofactor protein S, *Am. J. Hematol.,* 49, 89–91, 1995.

86. Shibata, S., T. Sasaki, P. Harpel, and H. Fillit, Autoantibodies to vascular heparan sulfate proteoglycan in systemic lupus erythematosus react with endothelial cells and inhibit the formation of thrombin-antithrombin III complexes, *Clin. Immunol. Immunopathol.,* 70, 114–123, 1994.

87. Chamley, L. W., E. J. McKay, and N. S. Pattison, Inhibition of heparin/antithrombin III cofactor activity by anticardiolipin antibodies: a mechanism for thrombosis, *Thromb. Res.,* 71, 103–111, 1993.

88. Shibata, S., P. C. Harpel, A. Gharavi, J. Rand, and H. Fillit, Autoantibodies to heparin from patients with antiphospholipid antibody syndrome inhibit formation of antithrombin III-thrombin complexes, *Blood,* 83, 2532–2540, 1994.

89. Rand, J. H., X. X. Wu, H. A. M. Andree, C. J. Lockwood, S. Guller, J. Scher, and P. C. Harpel, Pregnancy loss in the antiphospholipid-antibody syndrome — a possible thrombogenic mechanism, *N. Engl. J. Med.,* 337, 154–160, 1997.

90. Matsuda, J., K. Kawasugi, K. Gohchi, N. Saitoh, M. Tsukamoto, M. Kazama, and T. Kinoshita, Clinical significance of the venous occlusion test on systemic lupus erythematosus patients with a focus on changes in blood levels of tissue plasminogen activator, von Willebrand factor antigen, and thrombomodulin, *Acta Haemmatol.,* 88, 22–26, 1992.

91. Nilsson, T. K. and E. Lofvenberg, Decreased fibrinolytic capacity and increased von Willebrand factor levels as indicators of endothelial cell dysfunction in patients with lupus anticoagulant, *Clin. Rheu-matol.,* 8, 58–63, 1989.

92. Violi, F., D. Ferro, G. Valesini, C. Quintarelli, M. Saliola, M. A. Grandilli, and F. Balsano, Tissue plasminogen activator inhibitor in patients with systemic lupus erythematosus and thrombosis, *Br. Med. J.,* 300, 1099–1102, 1990.

93. Wachtfogel, Y. T., R. A. DeLa Cadena, and R. W. Colman, Structural biology, cellular interactions and pathophysiology of the contact system, *Thromb. Res.*, 72, 1–21, 1993.

94. Sanfelippo, M. J. and C. J. Drayna, Prekallikrein inhibition associated with the lupus anticoagulant: a mechanism of thrombosis, *Am. J. Clin. Pathol.*, 77, 275–279, 1982.

95. Killeen, A. A., K. C. Meyer, J. M. Vogt, and J. R. Edson, Kallikrein inhibition and C_1-esterase inhibitor levels in patients with lupus inhibitor, *Am. J. Clin. Pathol.*, 88, 223–228, 1987.

96. Amengual, O., T. Atsumi, M. A. Khamashta, and G. R. V. Hughes, The role of the tissue factor pathway in the hypercoagulable state in patients with the antiphospholipid syndrome, *Thromb. Haemost.*, 79, 276–281, 1998.

97. Cuadrado, M. J., C. López-Pedrera, M. A. Khamashta, M. T. Camps, F. Tinahones, A. Torres, G. R. V. Hughes, and F. Velasco, Thrombosis in primary antiphospholipid syndrome: a pivotal role for monocyte tissue factor expression, *Arthritis Rheum.*, 40, 834–841, 1997.

98. Kornberg, A., M. Blank, S. Kaufman, and Y. Shoenfeld, Induction of tissue factor-like activity in monocytes by anti-cardiolipin antibodies, *J. Immunol.*, 153, 1328–1332, 1994.

99. Reverter, J. C., D. Tassies, J. Font, M. A. Khamashta, K. Ichikawa, R. Cervera, G. Escolar, G. R. Hughes, M. Ingelmo, and A. Ordinas, Effects of human monoclonal anticardiolipin antibodies on platelet function and on tissue factor expression on monocytes, *Arthritis Rheum.*, 41, 1420–1427, 1998.

100. Oosting, J. D., R. H. W. M. Derksen, L. Blokzijl, J. J. Sixma, and P. G. De Groot, Antiphospholipid antibody positive sera enhance endothelial cell procoagulant activity — studies in a thrombosis model, *Thromb. Haemost.*, 68, 278–284, 1992.

101. Tannenbaum, S. H., R. Finko, and D. B. Cines, Antibody and immune complexes induce tissue factor production by human endothelial cells, *J. Immunol.*, 137, 1532–1537, 1986.

102. Atsumi, T., M. A. Khamashta, R. S. Haworth, G. Brooks, O. Amengual, K. Ichikawa, T. Koike, and G. R. V. Hughes, Arterial disease and thrombosis in the antiphospholipid syndrome: a pathogenic role for endothelin 1, *Arthritis Rheum.*, 41, 800–807, 1998.

103. Carreras, L. O. and J. Maclouf, The lupus anticoagulant and eicosanoids, *Prostaglandins Leukot. Essent. Fatty Acids*, 49, 483–488, 1993.

104. Escolar, G., J. Font, J. C. Referter, A. Lopez-Soto, M. Garrido, R. Cervera, M. Inglemo, R. Castillo, and A. Ordinas, Plasma from systemic lupus erythematosus patients with antiphospholipid antibodies promotes platelet aggregation, *Arterioscler. Thromb.*, 12, 196–200, 1992.

105. Ostfeld, I., N. Dadosh-Goffer, S. Borokowski, J. Talmon, A. Mani, U. Zor, and J. Lahav, Lupus anticoagulant antibodies inhibit collagen-induced adhesion and aggregation of human platelets *in vitro*, *J. Clin. Immunol.*, 12, 415–423, 1992.

106. Arvieux, J., B. Roussel, P. Pouzol, and M. G. Colomb, Platelet activating properties of murine monoclonal antibodies to β_2-glycoprotein I, *Thromb. Haemost.*, 70, 336–341, 1993.

107. Hasselaar, P., R. H. W. M. Derksen, L. Blokzijl, and P. G. De Groot, Thrombosis associated with antiphospholipid antibodies cannot be explained by effects on endothelial and platelet prostanoid synthesis, *Thromb. Haemost.*, 59, 80–85, 1988.

108. Maclouf, J., F. Lellouche, M. Martinuzzo, P. Said, and L. O. Carreras, Increased production of platelet-derived thromboxane in patients with lupus anticoagulants, *Agents Actions Suppl.*, 37, 27–33, 1992.

109. Martinuzzo, M. E., J. Maclouf, L. O. Carreras, and S. Lévy-Toledano, Antiphospholipid antibodies enhance thrombin-induced platelet activation and thromboxane formation, *Thromb. Haemost.*, 70, 667–671, 1993.

4 Platelet Disorders in Autoimmune Diseases

Ronit Simantov and Babette B. Weksler

CONTENTS

I. INTRODUCTION

Platelets are essential for normal hemostasis, acting in the initial phase (primary hemostasis) to form an occlusive platelet plug at the site of injury and to accelerate the localized activation of circulating plasma procoagulants. Normal platelet counts range from 150,000 to 450,000/µl and the normal lifespan of circulating platelets is 7 to 10 days, with younger platelets displaying greater hemostatic efficacy than older ones. A level of >50,000/µl is generally needed for normal hemostasis. The spleen sequesters about one third of circulating platelets which can be released by stress or increased plasma catecholamines. The bone marrow can increase platelet production about sevenfold in the face of increased peripheral destruction or external loss, both by expanding the megakaryocyte population and by inducing earlier release of platelets from megakaryocytes. Such "stress platelets" are large in size and often have enhanced functional capacity. The rate of platelet production is governed by the hormone thrombopoietin, which rises if circulating platelet mass falls; thrombopoietin receptors (c-mpl) on the platelet surface control plasma thrombopoietin levels. Platelet removal from the circulation is stochastic, independent of platelet age. Early platelet removal can reflect ongoing intravascular thrombosis, mechanical trauma, or reticuloendothelial endocytosis of platelets coated with antibodies, as in immune thrombocytopenias. In the latter instance, platelets may circulate for only a few hours.

Both defective platelet function and thrombocytopenia are characterized by similar bleeding diatheses. Bruising, petechiae, and mucosal bleeding are typical manifestations, in contrast to joint and deep organ bleeds that characterize deficiencies of soluble procoagulant factors, such as hemophilia. However, intracerebral bleeds occur with severe thrombocytopenia and constitute an unusual but severe complication of thrombocytopenia.

Acquired disorders of platelets are much more common than inherited defects, and are caused by many factors, including drugs, autoimmune diseases, malignancy, or mechanical damage. Drug-induced platelet dysfunctions are the most frequent platelet disorders, and impaired platelet aggregation due to aspirin is by far the most common platelet dysfunction. Drug-related immune thrombocytopenias are also relatively common, and hundreds of different medications have been implicated as causes of immune thrombocytopenia. Different drugs have different mechanisms of action in producing immune thrombocytopenia, ranging from specific antiplatelet antibodies against membrane receptors or against drugs bound to platelet surfaces, to abnormal activation of platelets by immune complexes involving drugs bound to platelet proteins. All of these mechanisms cause early removal of circulating platelets. Idiopathic autoimmune thrombocytopenias represent another important category of immunologically mediated thrombocytopenias in which antibodies arise that are directed against specific platelet membrane components; these are common in children after viral infections and in adults in the absence of known causes.

In the autoimmune disorders, the increased tendency to form autoantibodies or antidrug antibodies, as well as disturbed T-cell function, results in an increased incidence of immune thrombocytopenias as well as immunologically mediated platelet dysfunctions. Conversely, during immunosuppression with long-acting T-cell directed medications, such as fludarabine, or after bone marrow transplantation, disturbance in T-cell regulation of B-cell function is associated with an increased incidence of autoimmune cytopenias, including thrombocytopenias.

II. NORMAL PLATELET FUNCTION

Platelets circulate as nonreactive discs that neither stick to one another, nor to other types of blood cells, nor to the vascular endothelium. However, at sites of vascular injury, individual platelets alter membrane receptors to rapidly adhere to sites of injury, display receptors for binding of fibrinogen and other coagulant factors, aggregate together to form a hemostatic plug, and catalyze the rapid, localized production of thrombin. Within seconds, activated platelets release preformed vasoactive substances that contract vessels and accelerate blood clotting. They rapidly synthesize and release lipid mediators, such as thromboxane A2 (TXA2), a potent vasoconstrictor and platelet activator. At least three major types of activation (via ADP, via TXA2, and via thrombin) can initiate these steps which interact in a final common pathway centered on activation of GPIIb/IIIa, the glycoprotein membrane receptor for fibrinogen.

In addition, platelets augment the adhesion of neutrophils and monocytes to the vessel wall, increase leukocyte activation, secrete inhibitors of fibrinolysis, and release multiple growth factors that initiate wound healing. Insufficient platelet activation, or low platelet numbers increases bleeding risk, whereas excessive platelet activation is associated with thrombosis. Either bleeding or thrombosis, or sometimes bleeding and thrombosis together, can be seen in platelet disorders associated with autoimmune disease.

III. ABNORMALITIES OF PLATELET FUNCTION

Abnormal platelet function resulting in poor hemostasis can result from a variety of defects:

- Impaired platelet adhesion to the injured blood vessel wall
- Decreased platelet aggregation
- Lack of release from platelets of vasoactive substances
- Decreased synthesis of lipid mediators

Conversely, excessive platelet adhesion, aggregation, or release may promote thrombosis. Immune mechanisms may be responsible for both hyporeactivity and hyperreactivity of platelets. Aspirin use is the most common cause of platelet dysfunction in normal individuals as well as in patients treated with this antiinflammatory drug, as is frequently done in autoimmune disorders. Aspirin specifically blocks TXA2 formation by platelets by irreversibly inactivating platelet cyclooxygenase, a key enzyme in synthesis of TXA2. The thromboxane pathway is important for normal platelet function. One "baby" (81 mg) aspirin tablet suffices to inhibit normal platelet aggregation for several days in almost all persons, so that aspirin-impaired platelet dysfunction clearly outnumbers any other type of platelet disorder, given the enormous usage of aspirin throughout the world. Indeed, the sensitivity of platelet cyclooxygenase to inhibition by aspirin is therapeutically used to prevent heart attacks and strokes in atherosclerotic patients, and in prothrombotic states associated with autoimmune disease. The bleeding time is usually doubled by aspirin, but not further increased by higher doses. Platelets do not contain the inducible enzyme, cyclooxygenase-2, but only the constitutive form, cyclooxygenase-1, so that the new specific inhibitors of COX-2 recently developed for antiinflammatory effects do not inhibit platelet function and thus do not induce a bleeding tendency. Because the TXA2 pathway is only one of several independent mechanisms for platelet activation, hemostasis is generally maintained even when TXA2 generation is inhibited. This is why aspirin use produces only a rather mild hemorrhagic tendency unless other aspects of hemostasis are also abnormal, as in anticoagulated patients or in hemophilia.

IV. ADENOSINE DIPHOSPHATE (ADP) AND
THROMBIN PATHWAYS

Adenosine diphosphate (released from platelet-dense granules upon platelet activation) causes a change in platelet shape and induces activation of the GPIIb/IIIa receptors on platelet membranes, permitting the binding of plasma fibrinogen. This is a central mechanism of platelet activation and allows bridging among individual, activated platelets resulting in formation of platelet aggregates and acceleration of thrombin formation. If ADP release is decreased (after aspirin, for example, or in storage-pool disease, a deficiency of platelet dense granules), platelet aggregation may be impaired. Specific drugs can interfere with this pathway. The thienopyridines (ticlopidine and clopidogrel) block ADP binding to its receptors on platelets and, therefore, decrease platelet activation without blocking the TXA2 pathway. Clopidogrel, which is related to but safer than ticlopidine, is gaining widespread use in prevention of thrombosis in vascular stents and for prevention of TIA, stroke, and myocardial infarction. ADP-blocking drugs prolong the bleeding time, but do so in relation to dose. Thrombin, acting on thrombin receptors at the platelet surface, independently activates platelets by a PKC-dependent pathway, leading to activation of GPIIb/IIIa, full aggregation, and release of platelet vasoactive contents even in the absence of TXA2 production. Specific antithrombins, such as lepirudin (a hirudin analog) or antithrombin peptides, and peptidomimetic drugs block only thrombin-mediated activation, while GPIIb/IIIa antagonists, such as the monoclonal antibody, abciximab (ReoPro), block all platelet activation, since the final activation pathway for platelet activation requires this fibrinogen receptor.

V. IMMUNOLOGICALLY MEDIATED PLATELET DYSFUNCTION

As demonstrated by abciximab, antibodies that interact with GPIIb/IIIa on the platelet surface can inhibit platelet function directly or can nonspecifically block activation of these receptors that require rearrangement of component receptor units for activation. Outside the therapeutic arena, immunologically mediated platelet dysfunction is rare, but occurs in diseases where immune function is disturbed, such as systemic lupus erythematosus (SLE), lymphomas, multiple myeloma, and chronic myeloproliferative syndromes. Antibodies directed against GPIIb/IIIa have been reported in SLE and can induce a thrombasthenia-like syndrome if they interact with or block functional sites on the GPIIb/IIIa complex.

Platelet adhesion requires interaction of membrane GPIb receptors with collagen or von Willebrand's factor (vWF) present in vascular subendothelium; it is not altered by aspirin nor dependent on cyclooxygenase integrity. Normal platelet adhesion, required for normal hemostasis, is defective in a rare congenital condition, Bernard-Soulier disease, in which the GPIb receptors are deficient. In congenital von Willebrand's disease, a common bleeding disorder, vWF is diminished or dysfunctional and platelet adhesion is impaired. Acquired von Willebrand's disease is uncommon, but almost always represents an autoimmune process and is associated with states of disturbed immunity such as SLE.[1] In acquired von Willebrand's disease, the pathogenic mechanisms responsible include (1) binding of anti-vWF IgG antibodies to vWF on endothelial cells and platelets leading to early removal of the vWF and a diminished level of large multimeric vWF, and (2) the inactivation of vWF function in adhesion by circulating anti-vWF antibodies, producing abnormal vWF molecules with poor function and thus impairing platelet adhesion.[2] One of the differences between inherited and acquired vWD is that in the acquired form, platelet vWF is normal; laboratory and clinical abnormalities relate to decreased levels or decreased function of plasma vWF. Treatment of congenital and acquired vWD is similar, with replacement of factor or use of desmopressin to augment release of vWF.[3]

VI. IDIOPATHIC THROMBOCYTOPENIC PURPURA

A. PATHOGENESIS

Idiopathic thrombocytopenic purpura (ITP) is defined as decreased numbers of circulating platelets without any known cause, and normal or increased numbers of megakaryocytes in the bone marrow. Clinical features include petechiae, ecchymoses, and mucosal bleeding. The peripheral blood smear in ITP reveals a decrease in the number of platelets and an increase in megathrombocytes, and the bone marrow contains an increased number of megakaryocytes. In general, the thrombopoietin level is normal.[4]

The pathogenesis of ITP involves the binding of IgG autoantibodies to platelets, with subsequent Fc receptor-mediated phagocytosis by splenic macrophages. Therefore, platelet survival is markedly decreased. The platelet autoantibodies may be directed toward glycoprotein IIb/IIIa or GPIb/IX, the major adhesive protein receptors on the platelet surface. In chronic ITP, GPIb antibodies may be associated with activation of complement (Table 4.1). Circulating immune complexes are

---

TABLE 4.1
Antiplatelet Antibodies Characteristic of Autoimmune Thrombocytopenia

Disease Category	Antibodies Reactive with:
Idiopathic thrombocytopenic purpura	GP IIb/IIIa, GPIb/IX, GPIa/IIa, GPIV
Antiphospholipid syndrome	GP IIb/IIIa, GPIb/IX, β_2GP1, prothrombin, other proteins
Heparin-induced thrombocytopenia	Heparin-PF4 complex, other heparin-like molecules complexed with PF4
HIV-associated ITP	GPIIIa-(44-69) peptide

TABLE 4.2
Evaluation of Thrombocytopenia of Possible Immune Etiology

Platelet count	Less than 100,000
Size of platelets	Large
History	
Hemorrhagic Diathesis	+
Drug history	May increase risk
Autoimmune disorder	Increases risk
Ongoing infection	Children: +, especially viral
	Adults: infection associated with decreased production
Malignancy	Increases risk, possible DIC
Physical Examination	
Petechiae and purpura	If platelets < 50,000
Splenomegaly	Not associated with ITP
Bone marrow cellularity	Usually normal
Bone marrow megakaryocytes	Usually increased
Platelet kinetics	Short platelet lifespan

observed in some patients. In patients with chronic ITP, T-cells reactive with altered GPIIb/IIIa complexes or with peptide fragments of GPIIb/IIIa have been detected. These reactive T-cells were CD4+ and HLA-DR restricted, and were involved in production of anti-GPIIb/IIIa antibodies in peripheral blood mixed lymphocyte cultures from ITP patients.[5] Circulating immune complexes are observed in some patients, particularly those with HIV and ITP. Indeed, in patients with HIV who have ITP, antibodies that are cross-reactive with GPIIIa and HIV GP120 have been detected.[6,7]

B. Diagnosis

The diagnosis of ITP remains one of exclusion despite many attempts to develop specific diagnostic tests (Table 4.2). Although the pathogenesis clearly involves peripheral destruction of platelets sensitized by autoantibodies, assays of platelet-associated IgG (PAIgG) have a low specificity, partly because immunoglobulins are normally present in platelet alpha granules and nonspecifically on the platelet membrane. Protein-specific assays that measure autoantibodies against the complexes GPIIb/IIIa or GPIb/IX have a higher specificity for ITP (>90%) but sensitivity is moderate (about 30%).[8] Platelet counts have not correlated with the likelihood of a positive result nor with its extent.[9] The difficult task of distinguishing ITP from immune-complex-associated thrombocytopenias that are encountered in SLE, chronic liver disease/hepatitis or HIV has been studied by using a battery of tests that measure platelet-associated IgG, complement C3C4, and IgM.[10] High levels of C3C4 and immune complexes were associated with these secondary immune-complex-associated thrombocytopenias, but not with ITP. In the face of the difficulty in establishing a clear laboratory diagnosis of ITP, illustrated even in these recent sophisticated approaches, the American Society of Hematology has suggested practice guidelines for establishing the diagnosis of ITP based principally on history, physical examination (absence of splenomegaly), and blood counts together with examination of the peripheral blood smear.[11] If the picture is not typical — thrombocytopenia with large platelets, CBC otherwise normal, no hepatosplenomegaly, absence of other underlying hematologic or systemic disease — then a test for HIV antibodies in patients at risk of HIV and a bone marrow examination in patients >60 years old to exclude myelodysplasia, have been recommended by the American Society of Hematology.

C. Presentation and Clinical Features

Clinically, ITP can be classified into childhood and adult types. ITP in children is often preceded by a viral illness, and is characterized by an acute course. Eighty to 90% of children with ITP recover spontaneously in 2 weeks to 6 months. Once remission is achieved in children, recurrence is rare. The disease course differs in adults, however. Spontaneous remissions are rare (about 10%); most adults with ITP will require therapy.

D. Management

The management differs between children and adults with ITP. In children, where the disease is often self-limited in duration, an asymptomatic child with platelet count >20,000/µl is often observed without treatment. Relative indications for corticosteroid therapy in children include platelet counts less than 10,000/µl, significant mucosal hemorrhage, and increased risk of traumatic bleeding. In symptomatic children and adults, corticosteroids are the conventional initial therapy of ITP, using a dose of 1 mg/kg. The mechanism of corticosteroid effect is decreased Fc receptor-mediated clearance of antibody-coated platelets, and, to a lesser degree, decreased immunoglobulin production.[12] In addition, corticosteroids will often reverse the bleeding diathesis prior to a rise in platelet count, by inhibition of vascular endothelial cell activation with resultant decrease in vascular permeability and vasoconstriction of the capillary bed.[13] The platelet count will often rise within a week of starting this therapy. Approximately 60% of adults with ITP will have a response within 4 weeks. After achievement of normal platelet levels, the steroids are gently tapered off over a number of weeks in a stepwise manner. Up to 40% of adults and the majority of children may achieve a sustained remission. Patients who do not maintain a sustained complete remission generally undergo splenectomy to remove the major site of destruction of opsonized platelets. Seventy percent of patients who undergo a splenectomy will have a sustained remission. In one recent series, the patient outcome following splenectomy showed a probability of disease-free survival at 10 years of 83% and overall survival of 93%.[14]

Chronic ITP is characterized by exacerbations and remissions over long periods of time.[15] Patients who have persistent platelet counts below 40,000/ml and spontaneous bleeding can be treated with corticosteroids.[16] Intravenous gamma globulin (IVIgG) is used in patients whose platelet counts are dangerously low or who are refractory to corticosteroids. The mechanism of action of IVIgG is likely the binding and blockade of Fc receptors on fixed macrophages, preventing the recognition and phagocytosis of autoantibody-coated platelets. Anti-D has been used with some success in Rh(D)-positive patients with ITP, particularly in nonsplenectomized patients.[17] The proposed mechanism of action is blockade of the reticuloendothelial system with antibody-red cell antigen complexes. An advantage over IVIgG is the lower cost. Reversal of thrombocytopenia by IVIgG or anti-D occurs in the majority of patients but is usually temporary in effect. In emergency situations, IVIgG is preferred because it acts more rapidly, whereas for maintenance prior to splenectomy, anti-D is easier to administer and less expensive.[18] Anti-D is not effective post-splenectomy nor in patients who are Rh-negative. Hemolysis may be seen, although it is generally moderate and self-limited.

E. Platelet Kinetics in ITP

Since ITP is associated with increased platelet destruction, it has been assumed that platelet production is increased, and that the resulting level of thrombocytopenia represents the balance between destruction and enhanced production of platelets. Direct assessment of this premise in a large series of untreated patients with ITP using indium-labeled, autologous platelets to determine platelet lifespan has shown that platelet kinetics may be variable in ITP.[19] In this series, 58% of patients had normal or increased platelet production and increased peripheral destruction characterized by a reduced platelet survival time of 1.6 ± 1.4 days. Eighty-eight percent of these patients who underwent splenectomy had remission of the thrombocytopenia. However, a large second group (42%) had decreased platelet production that was correlated with a longer platelet survival (3.6 ± 2 days) and a lesser response to splenectomy (62%). These latter patients displayed ineffective thrombopoiesis, despite seemingly normal numbers of megakaryocytes on bone marrow examination.[20]

VII. THROMBOCYTOPENIA IN PATIENTS WITH UNDERLYING IMMUNE DISEASE

Immune-mediated thrombocytopenias can occur in association with other immune disorders, including systemic lupus erythematosus, systemic sclerosis, lymphoma, and infectious mononucleosis. The mechanism in these settings, as in classic ITP, involves the coating of platelets with IgG and clearance from the circulation by the phagocytic cells of the reticuloendothelial system. Evan's syndrome is characterized by autoimmune hemolytic anemia in association with ITP. The disease is often relapsing, with alternating exacerbations of thrombocytopenia and hemolytic anemia. Therapy includes corticosteroids, splenectomy, and other immunosuppressive modalities in refractory patients.

A. PLATELET DISORDERS IN SYSTEMIC LUPUS ERYTHEMATOSUS

Thrombocytopenia is often an initial manifestation of SLE, and may be important in prognosis of the disease.[21,22] Thrombocytopenia was found to be the only independent risk factor of poor prognosis in a study of 389 patients with SLE.[23] Interestingly, however, hemorrhagic complications of thrombocytopenia are a rare cause of death in SLE. Acute thrombocytopenia occurring during SLE flares are particularly associated with complications and increased mortality.[24] In addition, the presence of a circulating lupus anticoagulant or anticardiolipin antibody is increased in incidence in patients with SLE. Patients with SLE have also been shown to have qualitative platelet defects, including absent collagen-induced platelet aggregation and impaired ADP- and epinephrine-induced platelet response. In some SLE patients observation of decreased platelet serotonin levels (serotonin being a normal component of platelet-dense granules and platelets are the major site of blood serotonin) and increased urinary serotonin levels suggests that these abnormalities may reflect ongoing intravascular blood coagulation and platelet activation, resulting in release of platelet serotonin.[25]

B. PLATELETS AND THE ANTIPHOSPHOLIPID ANTIBODY SYNDROME

The presence of circulating antibodies to anionic phospholipids is associated with a syndrome of venous and arterial thrombosis, fetal loss, and thrombocytopenia, particularly in young individuals. Antiphospholipid antibodies (aPL) are observed in patients with SLE, but can also occur in the absence of specific autoimmune disease (primary antiphospholipid syndrome). The aPL includes the lupus anticoagulant (LA) and anticardiolipin antibodies (aCL). LA is associated with more severe thrombocytopenia in patients with SLE, but incurs a greater risk of thrombosis rather than of clinical bleeding.[26] Thrombocytopenia has also been described in patients with the primary antiphospholipid antibody syndrome.[27] The frequency of thrombocytopenia in SLE patients with antiphospholipid antibodies has been shown to be 13 to 40% according to several series.[28,29] Conversely, a study of 109 patients with ITP showed that 69 (46%) had a positive LA or aCL antibody.[30]

The aPL autoantibodies were originally described as reactive with negatively charged phospholipids, but recent evidence suggests that they are directed towards neo-epitopes on plasma proteins such as β_2-glycoprotein 1 and prothrombin when those are complexed with phospholipid.[31] In the laboratory, aPL antibodies tend to inhibit clotting in tests such as the activated partial thromboplastin time or the dilute Russell's viper venom time. The pathogenic mechanism by which the aPL antibodies lead to clinical thrombosis likely involves the interaction of aPL with the vascular endothelium. The aPLs activate endothelial cells, inducing the expression of adhesion molecules associated with a thrombogenic phenotype, or possibly enhancing tissue factor expression.[32] Specific impairment of the natural anticoagulant protein C/protein S system, or enhanced binding of prothrombin to endothelium, or direct activation of platelets by the aPL antibodies, do not appear to be responsible for the prothrombotic effects of aPL antibodies.[33] Neither could thrombocytopenia in primary antiphospholipid syndrome be correlated with presence of platelet autoantibodies.[34] Different types of aPL may have quite different biologic effects.[35] The presence of the lupus anticoagulant also has been correlated with increased urinary excretion of a TXA2 metabolite characteristically produced by platelets (11-dehydroxythromboxane B2), indicative of systemic platelet activation without accompanying signs of compensatory increase in vascular prostacyclin formation.[36] Moreover, the F(ab)2 fragments of these antibodies induced serotonin release and increased TXA2 generation by normal platelets, further suggesting that presence of the LA correlated with increased risk for intravascular thrombosis and suggesting a rationale for using antiplatelet therapy as prophylaxis in patients with LA and antiphospholipid syndrome.[37] Presence of anticardiolipin, in contrast, was not associated with increased excretion of thromboxane metabolites.

Numerous studies have not provided conclusive evidence that platelets are directly activated by aPL. However, aPL has been shown to bind to previously activated platelets, which display a rich array of anionic phospholipids on their surface.[38,39] Recent studies have confirmed these findings and also have shown that plasma from patients with both LA and aCL did not induce platelet activation, but augmented the platelet activation response to ADP, as measured by surface expression of CD62P.[40]

VIII. PLATELET DISORDERS IN HIV DISEASE

Thrombocytopenia commonly occurs in individuals with HIV disease.[41] In a large, longitudinal survey of HIV-infected patients, the 1-year incidence of thrombocytopenia was 8.7% in persons with one or more AIDS-defining opportunistic illnesses and 3.1% in patients with a CD4 count < 200 cells/mm^3, and was associated with decreased survival.[42] The mechanisms of thrombocytopenia appear to be multifactorial and include thrombocytopenia in HIV disease related to an immune destruction by antiplatelet antibodies (Table 4.1) as well as HIV infection of megakaryocytes that express CD4, the receptor for HIV.[43] A study of patients with patients with HIV and thrombocytopenia showed that although the endogenous thrombopoietin level was increased along with the marrow megakaryocyte number, peripheral platelet mass turnover and splenic sequestration were also increased, suggesting that thrombocytopenia in these patients was due to impairment in platelet formation by HIV-infected marrow megakaryocytes, as well as increased peripheral destruction.[44] Other causes of thrombocytopenia in these patients include adverse effects of drug therapy, opportunistic infections, and malignancies. There is an increased incidence of throbmotic thrombocytopenic purpura (TTP) in HIV-infected patients, associated with a severe course and poor prognosis.

Treatment is directed towards optimal management of the underlying HIV infection; antiretroviral therapy has been shown to be particularly effective in increasing platelet counts. Corticosteroids and intravenous gamma globulin, as well as splenectomy, have been used effectively in patients with HIV-related immune thrombocytopenia. In one series, 19 of the 21 patients treated with splenectomy maintained platelet counts greater than 98,000/mm^3. In addition, splenectomies did not accelerate the progression of the AIDS in these patients.[45] Platelet transfusions are sometimes needed for the treatment of thrombocytopenia caused by decreased production.

IX. IMMUNE THROMBOCYTOPENIA IN CHRONIC LYMPHOCYTIC LEUKEMIA

Chronic lymphocytic leukemia (CLL), the most common adult leukemia, is characterized by the expression of CD5 and low expression of surface membrane immunoglobulin on B lymphocytes. ITP occurs in 2 to 3% of CLL patients, often in early stages of the disease. Platelet-associated immunoglobulins may be detected in the absence of ITP as well. Initial therapy for ITP in CLL, as in primary ITP, is corticosteroids. ITP in CLL will generally respond to therapy for the underlying disease with alkylating agents, steroids, or purine analogs. Seventy percent of patients respond. Splenectomy is sometimes used. CLL is also associated with other autoimmune manifestations such as AIHA. The mechanism of these autoimmune phenomena is related to T cell dysregulation with loss of tolerance to self antigens, leading to increased autoantibody production and destruction of platelets.[46] In addition, it has been proposed that autoreactive CLL B lymphocytes are being constantly challenged by self-antigens, leading to proliferation and potential malignant transformation in the disease.[47]

X. ALLOIMMUNE THROMBOCYTOPENIAS

A. ALLOIMMUNE NEONATAL PURPURA

The Pl^{A1} (HPA-1a) antigen is present on the surface of platelets in 98% of the population, while $\leq 2\%$ of the population have the Pl^{A2} (HPA-1b) antigen. Other platelet antigens include HPA-5 and HPA-4 (Yuk), which is found in the Japanese population. If a fetus has inherited a paternal antigen that induces alloantibody formation in an antigen-negative mother, alloimmune neonatal purpura may occur. Clinically, infants present with markedly low platelet counts and hemorrhage, which may be devastating. Laboratory evaluation includes the demonstration of platelet alloantibodies in maternal and fetal plasma. Maternal plasma is tested for reactivity against neonatal or paternal platelets. Treatment includes steroids and exchange transfusion. Therapeutic options also include intravenous gamma globulin as well as transfusion of antigen-negative platelets. Approximately 50% of cases of alloimmune neonatal purpura occur in first-born infants. Recurrence of neonatal thrombocytopenia in subsequent pregnancies should be prevented with monitoring of fetal platelet counts with percutaneous umbilical blood sampling at 20 to 24 weeks gestation. Frequent ultrasound examinations are necessary to monitor the condition of the fetus. Treatments include antepartum treatment with steroids and/or immune globulin, as well as fetal platelet transfusions with antigen-negative platelets in selected cases. Cesarean section is often performed in the setting of neonatal thrombocytopenia due to the risk of intracranial hemorrhage in vaginal delivery.

B. POST-TRANSFUSION PURPURA

Post-transfusion purpura (PTP) occurs 7 to 10 days after blood transfusion in patients who lack the platelet antigen Pl^{A1}. This rare condition occurs in multiparous women sensitized to the Pl^{A1} antigen through pregnancy or in patients who have had previous exposures to transfusions. The thrombocytopenia is usually severe, with platelet counts in the 1000 to 10,000 range, and may be accompanied by clinically significant hemorrhage. Treatment involves supportive care with management of hemorrhagic complications and intravenous gamma globulin. All other nonessential medications should be discontinued, as many have been implicated in thrombocytopenia; captopril, in particular, may exacerbate the binding of antibodies in PTP.[48] Other treatment modalities include corticosteroids, plasmapharesis, and rarely, exchange transfusion. Patients who require subsequent transfusions should receive washed erythrocytes or Pl^{A1}-negative blood. The pathophysiology of PTP is not clear. Patients will develop alloantibodies to Pl^{A1}, yet will paradoxically destroy their own platelets which lack the antigen. Proposed mechanisms include immune complex formation leading to nonspecific platelet destruction, broad specificity of the alloantibody to platelet antigens leading to destruction of Pl^{A1}-negative platelets, and production of concurrent autoantibodies with platelet reactivity.

C. DRUG-INDUCED IMMUNE THROMBOCYTOPENIA

Many drugs are capable of causing antibody-mediated thrombocytopenia by a variety of mechanisms (Table 4.3). Drugs that bind to platelet membrane glycoproteins may stimulate the production

TABLE 4.3
Mechanisms of Immune Thrombocytopenia Related to Drugs

Mechanism	Example
Drug covalently bind platelet membrane glycoprotein and acts as hapten	Penicillin
Drug binds platelet membrane glycoprotein and produces novel compound epitopes or changes conformation	Quinidine
	Qunine
	Sulfas
Drug induces antiplatelet antibodies without itself being bound to platelet	Procainamide
	Quinidine
	Quinine
Drug binds to normal platelet component forming immunogenic complexes; immune complexes with drug activate platelets via Fc receptors	Heparin
	Low molecular weight heparin
Drug binds to fibrinogen receptor changing conformation	Abciximab
	Other GPIIb/IIIa blockers

of hapten-dependent antibodies that recognize drug-membrane glycoprotein targets. Quinidine, quinine, and sulfonamides induce the formation of antibodies that bind to membrane glycoproteins only when soluble drug or metabolite is present. Drugs may also trigger the production of autoantibodies that bind directly to cell membrane proteins.[49] A recent study to determine the strength of clinical evidence for individual drugs as a cause of thrombocytopenia reviewed 515 case reports on patients with drug-induced thrombocytopenia (excluding heparin). In 247 patient case reports (48%), the drug appeared to be the causal agent of thrombocytopenia. The reports included 98 drugs, most frequently quinidine, trimethoprim-sulfamethoxazole, and gold. However, many of the reports reviewed in this study did not provide evidence for drug-related thrombocytopenia.[50]

Acute profound thrombocytopenia has been reported following therapy with abciximab, a chimeric monoclonal antibody Fab fragment directed against platelet GPIIb/IIIa. This medication is used in the setting of percutaneous coronary procedures to reduce early closure and other adverse events. In one series, of three cases (0.7%) of severe thrombocytopenia (range 1000 to 16,000) were found among 452 patients who underwent percutaneous coronary revascularization procedures within 2 to 31 hours after treatment with abciximab.[51] Platelet transfusion can be used to treat hemorrhage associated with abciximab-induced thrombocytopenia.

D. HEPARIN-INDUCED THROMBOCYTOPENIA

Immune thrombocytopenia related to heparin use is becoming more and more common among hospitalized patients and among those with recurrent cardiovascular episodes, because heparin is increasing as prophylaxis against perioperative thromboembolism during many invasive procedures, or to flush indwelling vascular devices or intravenous lines. Estimates suggest that from 5 to 30% of patients receiving heparin may have this complication, depending on the length of time the drug is given, whether there has been previous administration of heparin, and which type of heparin is used. Two types of heparin-associated thrombocytopenia have been identified. In HIT I, heparin binding to the platelet surface nonspecifically causes a mild, progressive thrombocytopenia, usually asymptomatic, which resolves when heparin is discontinued. In HIT II, rapid development of severe thrombocytopenia is associated with life-threatening thromboses. The pathogenesis of HIT II is unusual but clearly explains the combination of thrombocytopenia and thrombosis.[52] In HIT II, heparin binds to platelet factor 4, a positively charged α granule protein released during platelet activation (e.g., during a thrombotic episode for which the heparin therapy was first given). This complex antigen elicits the synthesis of antibodies that then bind to the complex of heparin and

PF4 on the surface of platelets and on the vascular endothelium, to which PF4 also binds.[53] The bound antibodies interact with Fcγ RII-A receptors causing rapid clearance of circulating sensitized platelets and activation of endothelium, which leads to both arterial and venous thrombosis. Expression of Fcγ RII-A receptors increases during inflammation and during platelet activation, and there is some evidence that polymorphisms of this receptor are also associated with increased risk of HIT thrombosis. In addition, the release of procoagulant platelet microparticles during HIT II thrombocytopenia further increases the risk of thrombosis. In HIT II, thrombocytopenia usually appears between 5 to 10 days after initiation of heparin therapy, although this interval may be shorter if the patient has had previous exposure to heparin. Immediate cessation of heparin administration is crucial, but usually the original thrombotic or risk condition necessitates continuing anticoagulation. Low molecular weight heparins are to be avoided because of their high rate of cross reactivity for binding to PF4, participation in complex formation, and elicitation of antibodies. Other anticoagulants, such as the nonheparin glycosaminoglycan danaparoid sodium; direct thrombin inhibitors, such as recombinant hirudin or argatroban; or the defibrinating agent ancrod can be substituted until oral anticoagulants can become effective.[54] Risk of morbidity or death in HIT II has been >60% and >20%, respectively, but with early recognition (following the platelet count daily of patients on heparin), immediately stopping heparin and using platelet inhibitors, the morbidity recently decreased to 7% and mortality to 1% in one large study of 100 consecutive patients with heparin-associated antiplatelet antibodies measured by platelet aggregation testing.[55]

XI. THROMBOTIC THROMBOCYTOPENIA PURPURA (TTP)

TTP is a syndrome defined by a pentad of symptoms: thrombocytopenia, microangiopathic hemolytic anemia, fever, renal failure, and neurologic disease. The process is characterized by the formation of small vessel microthrombi with consumption of platelets and erythrocyte damage, leading to the characteristic peripheral blood smear showing schistocytes and thrombocytopenia. Treatment of TTP includes emergent plasma infusion, plasmapharesis, and steroids, although mortality remains high. HIV infection has been found to be a predisposing factor. In addition, TTP has been reported to be associated with the antiplatelet medication ticlopidine.[56]

Although TTP is not generally classified as an autoimmune disease, its increased incidence in the HIV population and its often fatal course in SLE suggest that immune modulation may be important in its pathophysiology. A number of autoantibodies have been reported in TTP patients, including anti-CD36 antibodies and anti-vWF-cleaving metalloprotease.[57] Further indirect evidence for an autoimmune component includes the response to therapy with administration of corticosteroids and other immunosuppressant agents, and of plasma-exchange therapy.

Recent work has shown that pathophysiology of TTP may be related to the effect of plasma factors in TTP patients on microvascular endothelial cells. Exposure of microvascular EC to plasma from patients with TTP induces apoptosis of EC.[58] Other studies have focused on the presence of large von Willebrand factor multimers in the circulation, possibly due to a defect in cleavage of vWF by the EC.[59] Identification of plasma factors mediating apoptosis of EC in this disorder and experimental approaches to therapy are subjects of intense investigation.[60]

REFERENCES

1. Mohri, H., Motomura, S., Kanamori, H., Matsuzaki, M., Watanabe, S., Maruta, A., Kodama, F., and Okubo, T., Clinical significance of inhibitors in acquired von Willebrand syndrome, *Blood*, 91, 3623, 1998.
2. Viallard, J.F., Pellegrin, J.L., Vergnes, C., Borel-Derlon, A., Clofent-Sanchez, G., Nurdan, A.T., Leng, B., and Nurden, P., Three cases of acquired von Willebrand disease associated with systemic lupus erythematosus, *Br. J. Haematol.*, 105, 532, 1997.

3. Rodeghiero, F., Castaman, G., and Mannucci, P. M., Clinical indications for desmopressin (DDAVP) in congenital and acquired von Willebrand disease, *Blood Rev.*, 5, 155, 1991.

4. Karpatkin, S., Autoimmune (idiopathic) thrombocytopenic purpura, *Lancet*, 349, 1531, 1997.

5. Kuwana, M., Kaburaki, J., and Ikeda, Y., Autoreactive T cells to platelet GPIIb:GPIX in immune thrombocytopenic purpura. Role in productions of antiplatelet autoantibody, *J. Clin. Invest.*, 102, 1393, 1998.

6. Bettareb, A., Oksenhendler, E., Duedari, N., and Bierling, P., Cross-reactive antibodies between HIV-GP120 and platelet gpIIIa (CD61) in HIV-related immune thrombocytopenic purpura, *Clin. Exp. Immunol.*, 103, 19, 1996.

7. Nardi, M.A., Liu, L.X., and Karpatkin, S., GPIIIa-(49-66) is a major pathophysiologically relevant antigenic determinant for antiplatelet GPIIIa of HIV-1-related immunologic thrombocytopenia, *Proc. Natl. Acad. Sci. USA*, 94,7589, 1997.

8. Berchtold, P., Muller, D., Beardsley, D., Fujisawa, K., Kaplan, C., Kekomaki, R., Lipp, E., Morell-Kopp, M.C., Kiefel, V., McMillan, R., von dem Borne, A.E., and Imbach, P., International study to compare antigen-specific methods used for the measurement of antiplatelet autoantibodies, *Br. J. Haematol.*, 96, 477, 1997.

9. Warner, M.N., Moore, J.C., Warkentin, T.E., Santos, A.V., and Kelton, J.G., A prospective study of protein-specific assays used to investigate idiopathic thrombocytopenic purpura, *Br. J. Haematol.*, 104, 447, 1999.

10. Samuel, H., Nardi, M., Karpatkin, M., Hart, D., Belmont, M., and Karpatkin, S., Differentiation of autoimmune thrombocytopenia from thrombocytopenia associated with immune complex disease, systemic lupus erythematosus, hepatitis-cirrhosis and HIV-infection by platelet and serum immunologic measurement, *Br. J. Haematol.*, 105, 1086, 1999.

11. George, J.N., Woolf, S.H., Raskob, G.E., Wasser, J.S., Aledort, L.M., Ballem, P.J., Blanchette, V.S., Bussel, J.B., Cines, D.B., Kelton, J.G., Lichtin, A.E., McMillan, R., Okerbloom, J.A., Regan, D.H., and Warner, I., Idiopathic thrombocytopenic purpura: a practice guideline developed by explicit methods for the American Society of Hematology, *Blood*, 88, 3, 1996.

12. Fries, L.F., Brickman, C.M., and Frank, M.M., Monocyte receptors for the Fc portion of IgG increase in number of autoimmune hemolytic anemia and other hemolytic states and are decreased by glucocorticoid therapy, *J. Immunol.*, 131, 1240, 1983.

13. Boumpas, D.T., Chrousos, G.P., Wilder, R.L., Cupps, T.R., and Balow, J.E., Glucocorticoid therapy for immune-mediated diseases: basic and clinical correlates, *Ann. Int. Med.*, 119, 1198, 1993.

14. Mazzucconi, M.G., Arista, M.C., Pernaino, M., Chistolini, A., Felici, C., Francavilla, V., Macale, E., Conti, L., and Gandolfo, G.M., Long-term follow-up of autoimmune thrombocytopenic purpura (ATP) patients submitted to splenectomy, *Eur. J. Haematol.*, 62, 219, 1999.

15. McMillan, R., Therapy for adults with refractory chronic immune thrombocytopenic purpura, *Ann. Intern. Med.*, 126, 307, 1997.

16. George, J.N., El-Harake, M.A., and Raskob, G.E., Chronic idiopathic thrombocytopenic purpura, *N. Eng. J. Med.*, 331, 1207, 1994.

17. Scaradavou, A., Woo, B., and Woloski, B.M., et al., Intravenous anti-D treatment of immune thrombocytopenic purpura: experience in 272 patients, *Blood*, 89, 2689, 1997.

18. Blanchette, V. and Carcao, M., Intravenous immunoglobulin G and anti-D as therapeutic interventions in immune thrombocytopenic purpura, *Transfu. Sci.*, 19, 231, 1998.

19. Louwes, H., Zeinali Lathori, O.A., Vellenga, E., and deWolf, J.T., Platelet kinetic studies in patients with idiopathic thrombocytopenic purpura, *Am. J. Med.*, 106, 430, 1999.

20. Rand, M.L. and Dean, J.A., Platelet function in autoimmune (idiopathic) thrombocytopenic purpura, *Acta Paediatr. Supp.*, 424, 57, 1998.

21. Pistiner, M., Wallace, D.J., Nessim, S., Metzger, A.L., and Klinenberg, J.R., Lupus erythematosus in the 1980s. A survey of 570 patients, *Semin. Arthr. Rheum.* 21, 55, 1991.

22. Abu-Shakra, M., Urowitz, M.B., Gladman, D.D., and Gough, J., Mortality studies in systemic lupus erythematosus: results from a single center. II. Predictor variables for mortality, *J. Rheum.*, 22, 1265, 1997.

23. Reveille, J.D., Bartolucci, A., and Alarcon, G.S., Prognosis in systemic lupus erythematosus. Negative impact of increasing age at onset, black race, and thrombocytopenia, as well as causes of death, *Arthr. Rheum.*, 33, 37, 1990.

24. Miller, M.H., Urowitz, M.B., and Gladman, D.D., The significance of thrombocytopenia in systemic lupus erythematosus, *Arthr. Rheum.*, 26, 1181, 1983.

25. Kanai, H., Tsuchida, A., Yano, S., and Naruse, T., Intraplatelet and urinary serotonic concentrations in systemic lupus erythematosus with reference to its clinical manifestations, *J. Med.*, 20, 371, 1989.

26. Alarcon-Segovia, D., Deleze, M., Oria, C.V., Sanchez-Guerrero, J., Gomez-Pacheco, L., Cabiedes, J., Fernandez, L., and Ponce de Leon, S., Antiphospholipid antibodies and the antiphospholipid syndrome in systemic lupus erythematosus: a prosepective analysis of 500 consecutive patients, *Medicine,* 68, 353, 1989.

27. Out, H.J., de Groot, P.G., van Vilet, M., de Gast, G.C., Nieuwenhaus, H.K., and Derksen, R.H.W.M., Antibodies to platelets in patients with antiphospholipid antibodies, *Blood,* 77, 2655, 1991.

28. Averbuch, M., Koifman, B., and Levo, Y., Lupus anticoagulant, thrombosis, and thrombocytopenia in systemic lupus erythematosus, *Am. J. Med. Sci.,* 293, 2, 1987.

29. Sturfelt, G., Nived, O., Norberg, R., Thorstensson, R., and Krook, K., Anticardiolipin antibodies in patients with systemic lupus erythematosus, *Arth. Rheum.,* 30, 382, 1987.

30. Stasi, R., Stipa, E., Masi, M., Cecconi, M., Scimo, M.T., Oliva, F., Sciarra, A., Perrotti, A.P., Adomo, G., and Amadori, S., et al., Prevalence and clinical significance of elevated antiphospholipid antibodies in patients with idiopathic thrombocytopenic purpura, *Blood,* 88, 3354, 1996.

31. Roubey, R.A., Autoantibodies to phospholipid-binding plasma proteins: a new view of lupus antico-agulants and other "antiphospholipid" autoantibodies, *Blood,* 84, 2854, 1994.

32. Simantov, R., LaSala, J.M., Lo, S.K., Gharavi, A., Sammaritano, L.R., Salmon, J.E., and Silverstein, R.L., Activation of cultured vascular endothelial cells by antiphospholipid antibodies, *J. Clin. Invest.,* 96, 2211, 1995.

33. Rao, L.V.M., Mechanisms of activity of lupus anticoagulants, *Curr. Opin. Hematol.,* 4, 344, 1997.

34. Shechter, Y., Tal, Y., Greenberg, A., and Brenner, B., Platelet activation in patients with antiphospho-lipid syndrome, *Blood Coagul. Fibrinol.,* 9, 653, 1998.

35. Joseph, J.E., Donohoe, S., Harrison, P., Mackie, I.J., and Machin, S.J., Platelet activation and turnover in the primary antiphospholipid syndrome, *Lupus,* 7, 333, 1998.

36. Lellouche, F., Martinuzzo, M., Said, P., Maclouf, J., and Carreras, L.O., Imbalance of thrombox-ane/prostacyclin biosynthesis in patients with lupus anticoagulant, *Blood,* 78, 2894, 1991.

37. Leung, S., Zoboh, V.A., Miller-Blair, D.J., and Robbins, D.L., Isolation and purification of anticardi-olipin antibody from plasma of a patient with antiphospholipid syndrome: induced generation of platelet thromboxane A2 synthesis, *Prostagland. Leuko. Essent. Fatty Acids,* 55, 385, 1996.

38. Shih, W., Chong, B.H., and Chesterman, L.N., Beta-2-glycoprotein 1 is a requirement for anticardi-olipin antibody to activated platelets: differences with lupus anticoagulants, *Blood,* 81, 1255, 1993.

39. Khamashta, M.A., Harris, E.N., Gharavi, A.E. Derue, G., Gil, A., Vasquez, J.J., and Hughes, G.R.V., Immune mediated mechanism for thrombosis: antiphospholipid antibody binding to platelet mem-branes, *Ann. Rheumatol. Dis.,* 47, 849, 1988.

40. Nojimo, J., Suehisa, E., Kuratsune, H., Machii, T., Koike, T., Kitani, T., Kanakura, Y., and Amino, N., Platelet activation induced by combined effects of anticardiolipin and lupus anticoagulant IgG antibodies in patients with systemic lupus erythematosus, *Thromb. Haematol.,* 41, 436, 1999.

41. Louache, F. and Vainchenker, W., Thrombocytopenia in HIV infection, *Curr. Opin. Hematol.,* 1, 369, 1994.

42. Sullivan, P.S., Hanson, D.L, Chu, S.Y., Jones, J.L., and Ciesielski, C.A., *AIDS Hum. Retrovirol.,* 14, 374, 1997.

43. Chelucci, C., Federico, M., Guerriero, R., Mattia, G., Casella, I., Pelosi, E., Testa, U., Mariani, G., Hassan, H.J., and Peschle, C., Productive human immunodeficiency virus-1 infection of purified megakaryocytic progenitors/precursors and maturing megakaryocytes, *Blood,* 91, 1225, 1998.

44. Cole, J.L., Marzec, U.M., Gunthel, C.J., Karpatkin, S., Worford, L., Sundell, I.B., Lennox, J.L., Nichol, J.L., and Harker, L.A., Ineffective platelet production in thrombocytopenic human immunodeficiency virus-infected patients, *Blood,* 91, 3239, 1998.

45. Aboolian, A., Ricci, M., Shapiro, K., Connors, A., and LaRaja, R.D., Surgical treatment of HIV-related immune thrombocytopenia, *Int. Surg.,* 84, 81, 1999.

46. Diehl, L.F. and Ketchum, L.H., Autoimmune disease and chronic lymphocytic leukemia: autoimmune hemolytic anemia, pure red cell aplasia, and autoimmune thrombocytopenia, *Semin. Oncol.,* 80, 1998.

47. Pritsch, O., Maloum, K., and Dighiero, G., Basic biology of autoimmune phenomena in chronic lymphocytic leukemia, *Semin. Oncol.*, 25, 34, 1998.
48. Bepler, G., Hoffman, S.E., Thompson, B.P., Telem, M.J., and Rosse, W.F., Captopril-enhanced binding of PlA1 antibodies in post-transfusion purpura, *Transfusion*, 31, 752, 1991.
49. Aster, R.A., Drug-induced immune thrombocytopenia: an overview of pathogenesis, *Sem. Hematol.*, 36 (suppl 1), 2, 1999.
50. George, J.N., Raskob, G.E., Shah, S.R., Rizvi, M.A., Hamilton, S.A., Osborne, S., and Vondracek, T., Drug-induced thrombocytopenia: a systematic review of published case reports, *Ann. Intern. Med.*, 129, 886, 1998.
51. Jubelirer, S.J., Koenig, B.A., and Bates, M.C., *Am. J. Hematol.*, 61, 205, 1999.
52. Vermylen, J., Hoylaerts, M.F., and Arnout, J., Antibody mediated thrombosis, *Thromb. Haemost.*, 78, 420, 1997.
53. Warkentin, T.E., Clinical presentation of heparin-induced thrombocytopenia, *Semin. Hematol.*, 35 (Suppl 5), 9, 1998.
54. Greinacher, A., Volpel, H., Janssens, U., Hac Wunderle, V., Kemkes-Matthes, B., Eichler, P., Mueller-Velten, H.G., and Potzsch, B., Recombinant hirudin (lepirudin) provides safe and effective anticoagulation in patients with heparin-induced thrombocytopenia: a prospective study, *Circulation*, 99, 73, 1999.
55. Almeida, J.I., Coats, R., Liem, T.K., and Silver, D., Reduced morbidity and mortality rates of the heparin-induced thrombocytopenia syndrome, *J. Vasc. Surg.*, 27, 309, 1998.
56. Mukamal, K.J., Wu, B., and McPhedran, P., Ticlopidine-associated thrombotic thrombocytopenic purpura, *Ann. Intern. Med.*, 129, 837, 1998.
57. Tsai, H.-M. and Lian, E.C.-Y., Antibodies to von Willebrand factor-cleaving protease in acute thrombotic thrombocytopenic purpura, *N. Eng. J. Med.*, 339, 1585, 1998.
58. Mitra, D., Jaffe, E.A., Weksler, B., Hajjar, K.A., Soderland, C., and Laurence, J., Thrombotic thrombocytopenic purpura and sporadic hemolytic-uremic syndrome plasma induce apoptosis in restricted lineages of human microvascular endothelial cells, *Blood*, 89, 1224, 1997.
59. Furlan, M., von Willebrand factor-cleaving protease in thrombotic thrombocytopenic purpura and hemolytic-uremic syndrome, *N. Eng. J. Med.*, 339, 1578, 1998.
60. Laurence, J. and Mitra, D., Apoptosis of microvascular endothelial cells in the pathophysiology of thrombotic thrombocytopenic purpura/sporadic hemolytic uremic syndrome, *Sem. Hematol.*, 34, 98, 1997.

5 Immunology of Atherosclerosis

Outi Vaarala, M.D., Ph.D.

CONTENTS

I. AUTOIMMUNE MECHANISMS IN ATHEROSCLEROSIS

A. IMMUNE ACTIVATION IN ATHERSCLEROSIS

The basic characteristic of the atherosclerotic vessel is the accumulation of lipids, lipoproteins, and inflammatory cells, such as T-lymphocytes and macrophages, in the arterial intima and the proliferation of the smooth muscle cells.[1] Atherosclerosis is a systemic disease characterized by narrowing arteries with endothelial dysfunction, impaired vasodilatation, and the hemostatic imbalance. Formation of atheroma is considered as a chronic inflammatory process in the arterial wall. Atherosclerosis is converted to an acute clinical event by the induction of plaque rupture which leads to the development of thrombosis and occlusion of the vessel. The risk of plaque rupture depends more on the structural type of the plaque than on the size of the plaque (i.e., the degree of stenosis). Accordingly, atherosclerotic plaques can be divided into "vulnerable" and "stable" plaques, the latter showing often luminal narrowing in angiography but being less prone to rupture. The "vulnerable" plaques may have a well-preserved lumen without angiographically evident flow-limiting stenosis, but the arteries with "vulnerable" plaques seem to be the most infarct-prone arteries.

Enhanced inflammation response in the "vulnerable" plaques, characterized by accumulation of macrophages and activated T lymphocytes, seems to be a crucial factor predisposing to plaque rupture and development of thrombosis. Genetic factors regulating, e.g., the cytokine secretion and plasma lipoprotein profile as well as environmental factors, like infections and dietary factors, are important determinants of the inflammatory reaction in the atherosclerotic vessel. Recently, nonspecific inflam-

TABLE 5.1
Evidence for the Role of Autoimmunity in the Pathogenesis of Atherosclerosis

Expression of autoantigens including modified LDL, HSP60/65, and β_2-glycoprotein I is demonstrated in human atherosclerotic plaques.[5,14,15,47]

Antibodies to oxidized LDL predict clinical progression of atherosclerosis.[16,18,19]

Autoreactive T cells against oxidized LDL can be derived from human atherosclerotic plaques.[4]

Antibodies binding to cardiolipin and prothrombin predict myocardial infarction.[19,35,48]

Antibodies to cardiolipin/β_2-glycoprotein I increase the uptake of oxidized LDL by macrophages.[44]

Immunization with β_2-glycoprotein I resulted in accelerated atherosclerosis in LDL receptor-deficient mice and apoE-knockout mice.[45,46]

Immunization with HSP65 induces atherosclerosis in normocholesterolemic rabbits.[57]

matory markers such as elevated levels of serum C-reactive protein[2] and activation of peripheral blood lymphocytes[3] have been associated with the risk of coronary atherosclerosis. Besides nonspecific inflammatory reactions, antigen-specific autoimmune reactivity occurs in atherosclerosis.

T lymphocyte clones derived from the target organ, i.e., atherosclerotic plaques, have been shown to possess autoreactivity against oxidatively modified, low-density lipoprotein (LDL), the major autoantigen in atheroma.[4] T-cell clones recognizing oxidized LDL secreted IFN-γ and represented, thus, Th1-type reactivity which means help for cytotoxic immune function. Also, expression of heat shock protein 65, which is a stress protein expressed in response to stress and injury, has been demonstrated in atheroma.[5] Circulating autoantibodies to these self-proteins, such as oxidized LDL and heat shock protein 65, occur in the patients with atherosclerosis.[6,7] The role of autoimmunity in the atherosclerotic process may include nonspecific inflammatory factors, which maintain the vascular inflammation, and antigen-specific autoimmunity, which potentiates atherosclerosis by specific mechanisms involved with atherogenesis and development of atherothrombosis. The evidence on the involvement of autoimmune reactivity in atherosclerosis is shown in Table 5.1.

B. Systemic Lupus Erythematosus as a Model of Autoimmune-Mediated Atherosclerosis

Vascular inflammation accompanying multiple immunological abnormalities is a basic feature of systemic autoimmune diseases with vascular manifestations, such as systemic lupus erythematosus (SLE). In the patients with SLE, premature atherosclerosis is a considerable clinical problem.[8-10] According to the epidemiological studies by Manzi and coworkers, women with SLE in the 35- to 44-year-old age group had over 50 times higher rate ratio of cardiovascular events than healthy women of similar age.[9]

In the Hopkins Lupus Cohort, the majority of the prospectively followed thrombotic events were arterial thrombosis, such as myocardial infarction and stroke.[11] Venous thrombosis was clustered early in the history of the disease and arterial events occurred late pointing to the poor therapeutic efficacy in prevention of atherothrombosis in SLE. Several studies clearly indicate that accelerated atherosclerosis is a clinical challenge in the treatment of patients with SLE.[8-10,12] Classical risk factors of atherosclerosis, such as the prolonged treatment with prednisone, high blood pressure, and high levels of LDL cholesterol contribute to the atherosclerosis also in SLE. but do not wholly explain this clinical peculiarity. The possible atherogenic role of autoimmune responses associated with systemic autoimmune diseases including SLE and antiphospholipid syndrome are discussed in this review. The studies showing an association of antiphospholipid antibodies with clinical manifestations of atherosclerosis suggest that patients with antiphospholipid syndrome are at an increased risk of atherosclerosis (Figure 5.1).

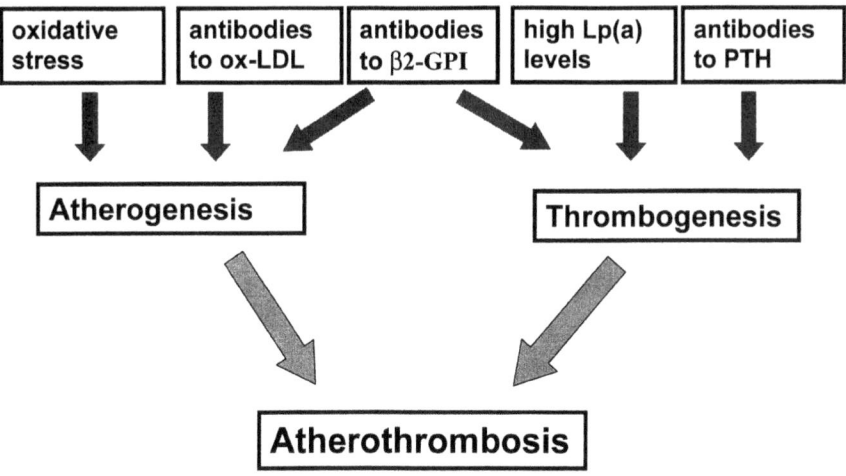

Atherogenic and thrombogenic factors common in atherosclerosis and antiphospholipid syndrome

FIGURE 5.1 Atherogenic and thrombogenic factors.

II. AUTOIMMUNE RESPONSE TO OXIDIZED LDL

A. The Role of Oxidized LDL as an Autoantigen in Atherosclerosis

The "oxidative-modification hypothesis" in the pathogenesis of atherosclerosis is based on the oxidative modification of LDL leading to lipid accumulation due to the enhanced uptake of oxidized LDL by scavenger receptors of macrophages.[13] Increasing evidence indicates that the accumulation of the lipids on the arterial wall is dependent on the modification of LDL by oxidation, although the molecular changes in LDL molecule induced by oxidation are not well characterized. Inflammation in the atherosclerotic vessel wall leads to increased oxidative capacity that causes peroxidation of lipids. The end products of lipid peroxidation further propagate changes in the proteins, such as production of malondialdehyde-conjugated LDL. The modifications of LDL by other mechanisms than oxidation also may potentiate its atherogenic nature. Generation of enzymatically modified LDL molecules may be important in the atherogenesis, especially hypochlorite-conjugated LDL produced by myeloperoxidase present in the atherosclerotic vessel wall.[14]

Modified LDL molecules have been identified in the atherosclerotic vessels indicating their accumulation in the atherosclerotic plaques.[14,15] The modified LDL molecules induce chemotactic agents and increased expression of endothelial adhesion molecules for monocytes and lymphocytes potentiating the vascular inflammatory reaction.[16,17] The modified self-proteins also induce autoimmune responses. As mentioned before, T-cell clones reactive with oxidized LDL have been derived from the human atherosclerotic plaques[4] and elevated levels of autoantibodies to oxidized LDL are associated with atherosclerosis and have been reported to imply an active atherosclerotic process.[6,18,19]

The pathogenic role of antibodies to oxidized LDL have been suggested by studies showing that *in vitro* these antibodies enhance the accumulation of LDL into macrophages.[20] However, *in vivo* immunization with oxidized LDL has been shown to protect from atherosclerosis in ApoE-deficient mice[21] and in LDL-receptor deficient mice.[22] This protective effect seems not to be dependent on the generation of antibodies to oxidized LDL and has been suggested to be related to T-cell-dependent mechanisms.[22] It must be pointed out that due to the absence of LDL receptor in these mice the mechanisms and the effect of immunization may differ from those observed in normal animal or in humans. In apo E-knockout mice, severe hypercholesterolemia modified the production subtypes of IgG autoantibodies to oxidized LDL and induced a switch from Th1 to Th2-type reactivity, whereas moderate hypercholesterolemia was associated with Th1-type reactivity.[23a] These kinds of changes in the functional profile of immune responses may influence the development of atherosclerosis and the effect of the modifying factors may be dependent on the experimental model used.

In humans the elevated levels of autoantibodies to oxidized LDL have been found to be markers or predictors of accelerated atherosclerotic process suggesting their importance in the pathogenesis of atherosclerosis. Two prospective studies in non-SLE subjects have shown that antibodies to oxidized LDL are predictive for myocardial infarction[18,19] and progression of carotid atherosclerosis.[6] In addition, the levels of antibodies to oxidized LDL represented an independent determinant of impaired endothelium-dependent and endothelium-independent vasodilatation, which was detected in the forearm vasculature with a strain-gauge plethysmography in a series of patients with coronary heart disease.[23b] These findings suggest that increased levels of antibodies to oxidized LDL in humans are closely associated with the atherosclerotic process in the vessel wall.

B. ANTIBODIES TO OXIDIZED LDL AS MEMBERS OF ANTIPHOSPHOLIPID ANTIBODIES

Antibodies to oxidized LDL occur frequently also in the patients with SLE[24] and are associated with arterial thrombosis in these patients.[25,26] Antibodies to oxidized LDL comprise heterogenous groups of antibodies with respect to their specificity. A subpopulation of these antibodies bind to oxidized lipids in the LDL molecule and are likely responsible for cross-reactivity with phospholipids such as cardiolipin.[27,28]

Another subpopulation of antibodies to oxidized LDL recognizes oxidized apolipoprotein B of LDL which is modified during oxidation.[29] Since a small amount of plasma β_2-glycoprotein I (GPI), an antigenic target of antiphospholipid antibodies, is bound to LDL molecules in circulation, antibodies to β_2-GPI may show binding to oxidized LDL.[30] However, studies on SLE sera-derived autoantibodies have not been able to demonstrate a true cross reactivity between the antibodies to oxidized LDL and β_2-GPI.[31,32] Since antibodies to oxidized LDL cross react with antiphospholipid antibodies, they are considered as members of the family of antiphospholipid antibodies.[24,27,28,33] The major population of the cross-reactive antibodies react likely with oxidized phospholipids (e.g., cardiolipin). Despite the overlapping specificities, a separate population of antibodies to oxidized LDL with no cross-reactivity to cardiolipin can be eluted from SLE sera.[27]

Also, clinical associations of the antibodies to oxidized LDL differ from those of antibodies binding to the cardiolipin-β_2-GPI complex.[25,26,34] The antibodies to cardiolipin-β_2-GPI complex are associated with both arterial and venous thrombosis in SLE, but antibodies to oxidized LDL do not show association with venous thrombosis. Instead, these antibodies are associated with arterial thrombosis in antiphospholipid syndrome.[25,26] The question of the direct involvement of antibodies to oxidized LDL in the development of atherothrombosis is open, but several studies indicate that these antibodies serve as markers of pathogenic determinants of atherosclerosis, such as oxidation of LDL, endothelial dysfunction, and arterial inflammation. The frequent occurrence of antibodies to oxidized LDL in SLE and antiphospholipid syndrome may be associated with enhanced oxidative stress which activates the atherosclerotic process.

III. ANTICARDIOLIPIN ANTIBODIES IN ATHEROSCLEROSIS

Elevated levels of antibodies binding to cardiolipin have been associated with myocardial infarction. Also, prospective studies have shown that elevated levels of cardiolipin-binding antibodies in non-SLE population imply an increased risk for the development of myocardial infarction.[19,35-37] Some evidence supports the view that cardiolipin-binding antibodies are a risk for myocardial infarction especially in young individuals.[36,37] Prospective studies have not confirmed the association of cardiolipin-binding antibodies with myocardial infarction.[38,39]

Studies on the clinical importance of cardiolipin-binding antibodies have several problems due to the methodological differences between laboratories. The antibodies binding to cardiolipin on solid-phase immunoassay may be directed against several different antigenic structures available in the assay. Some recognize phospholipids, some bind to plasma-phospholipid proteins such as β_2-GPI or protrombin, and some of these antibodies may be directed against cross-reactive epitopes common with oxidized LDL. The heterogeneity of cardiolipin-binding antibodies makes it difficult to compare the results from separate studies. Some anticardiolipin assays may detect more specific antibodies directed against phospholipid-binding plasma proteins and be less sensitive for antibodies showing cross-reactivity with oxidized LDL.

As discussed above, some of the cardiolipin-binding antibodies may cross react with oxidatively modified LDL due to cross-reactivity between oxidized lipids[27,28] and act in the same way as antibodies to oxidized LDL in atherosclerosis. Immunization with anticardiolipin antibodies has been reported to result in accelerated atherosclerosis in LDL-receptor knockout mice without changing the plasma lipid profile.[40] However, the fine specificity of these antibodies remained unclear in this study (i.e., cross-reactivity with oxidized LDL or affinity to β_2-GPI). Interestingly, elevated levels of cardiolipin-binding antibodies have been reported in smokers in whom the levels of these antibodies correlated inversely with the plasma vitamin C concentration.[41] Smoking induces oxidative stress, production of free radicals, and consumption of antioxidants. Also, the recent studies showing that markers of enhanced lipid peroxidation are associated with antiphospholipid antibodies indicate that increased oxidative stress may contribute to the development of cardiolipin-binding antibodies.[42,43] It is of interest whether the use of antioxidants in the patients with anticardiolipin antibodies would decrease the risk of atherothrombosis.

IV. ANTIBODIES BINDING TO β_2-GLYCOPROTEIN I AND PROTHROMBIN

The role of antibodies to β_2-GPI has been suggested in human atherosclerosis. β_2-GPI-binding antibodies represent the major population of antiphospholipid antibodies in the patients with antiphospholipid syndrome. These autoantibodies are associated with arterial and venous thrombosis in SLE and antiphospholipid syndrome.

In vitro studies suggest that antiphospholipid antibodies may contribute to the development of atherosclerotic process in antiphospholipid syndrome by enhancing of the lipid accumulation and inflammation in the arterial vessel wall. Antibodies to β_2-GPI have been shown to enhance the accumulation of oxidized LDL into macrophages.[44] The binding to β_2-GPI-LDL complex may be the mechanism with which these antibodies increase LDL uptake by Fc-receptors and contribute to the development of premature atherosclerosis in patients with antiphospholipid syndrome. Also, animal studies indicate that immunity to β_2-GPI plays a role in the development of atherosclerosis. When LDL receptor-deficient or apolipoprotein E-deficient mice were immunized with human β_2-GPI, acceleration of early atherosclerosis was observed.[45,46] Although the mechanisms are not known, these studies suggest an involvement of β_2-GPI in the atherosclerotic process. The recent finding of the presence of β_2-GPI in the atherosclerotic plaque is of great interest and emphasizes the role of β_2-GPI in atherosclerosis.[47] In a prospective study including dyslipidemic middle-aged men without autoimmune diseases antibodies to β_2-GPI however, were not associated with the development of myocardial infarction.[48]

Prothrombin is an antigenic target of antiphospholipid antibodies and a subgroup of these antibodies possess lupus anticoagulant activity.[49] Antibodies to prothrombin have been associated with myocardial infarction in a prospective followup of healthy dyslipidemic men.[48] A twofold risk of myocardial infarction was found in middle-aged men with antibody levels to prothrombin in the highest tertile when compared to men with antibody levels in the lowest tertile. This risk was multiplied by an additive manner when the joint effect with other risk factors for myocardial infarction was taken into account, such as high levels of antibodies to oxidized LDL, smoking, and high lipoprotein(a) (Lp(a)) levels. These findings suggest that autoimmunity to prothrombin may be associated with atherothrombosis, but this issue needs further studies. The mechanisms involved with the development of atherothrombosis may be related to the procoagulant activity of these antibodies *in vivo* as we have already suggested.[50]

Antibody responses to other plasma proteins than LDL may develop in atherosclerosis due to the modification of the plasma proteins in the inflamed arterial wall. The production of autoantibodies to β_2-GPI or prothrombin may reflect the focal inflammatory reaction and, thus, be a marker for thrombotic risk in atherosclerosis. However, generation of antiphospholipid antibodies directed against β_2-GPI may independently influence the development of atherothrombosis by changing the hemostatic balance towards hypercoagulation. In antiphospholipid syndrome (also known as Hughes syndrome), the antiphospholipid antibodies may interfere with blood coagulation and essentially increase the risk for clinical manifestation of atherosclerosis as thrombosis.[51] Besides the possible effect of antiphospholipid antibodies on blood coagulation, their occurrence is associated with high Lp(a) levels which is a hemostatic risk factor for atherothrombosis.[52,53] The prothrombotic stage in antiphospholipid syndrome may result in high risk of thrombosis even in association with early atherosclerotic changes in the arterial wall.

V. AUTOIMMUNITY TO HEAT SHOCK PROTEINS IN ATHEROSCLEROSIS

Immune response against heat shock proteins (HSP) has been suggested to be involved in atherogenesis. Increased levels of antibodies to HSP60/65 have been shown to associate with carotid atherosclerosis and coronary heart disease.[7,54] Antibodies to HSP60/65 are not uncommon in healthy subjects probably due to their cross-reactivity with bacterial HSPs encountered by humans. Increased levels of antibodies to HSP60/65 have been reported in patients with systemic vasculitis, in SLE, and other autoimmune diseases without vascular complications, such as rheumatoid arthritis and type 1 diabetes.[55] Although HSP60/65 is known to be expressed in human atherosclerotic lesions the wide spectrum of antibodies to HSP60/65 in different diseases and also in healthy subjects causes problems in the evaluation the role of these antibodies in atherosclerosis. In normocholesterolemic rabbits, immunization with HSP65 has been shown to induce atherosclerosis,[56] and human autoantibodies to HSP60/65 have been demonstrated to mediate endothelial cytotoxicity,[57] which favors the role of HSP60/65-specific immunity in atherogenesis. However, further studies are needed to justify the importance of HSP65 as an autoantigen in atherosclerosis.

VI. CONCLUSIONS

The inflammatory risk factors of atherothrombosis identified in common atherosclerosis without underlying autoimmune diseases seem to have importance also in the vascular manifestations of certain systemic autoimmune diseases, such as SLE and antiphospholipid syndrome. The autoimmunity associated with these diseases may enhance atherogenesis and the development of atherosclerotic thrombotic occlusion in these diseases. Autoimmune responses to autoantigens involved with the atherosclerotic process, such as oxidized LDL and HSP65, are common in patients with SLE who show accelerated atherosclerosis. In addition, a role for autoantibodies against the antigenic targets of antiphospholipid antibodies, such as β_2-glycoprotein I and prothrombin, has been suggested in atherosclerosis. The importance of the intensive treatment of the classical risk factors of atherosclerosis, i.e., high blood pressure and plasma LDL cholesterol, is emphasized by the current knowledge on the pathogenesis of atherosclerosis. Based on the evidence on the involvement of immune mechanisms in the atherosclerotic process several experimental studies have suggested that immunosuppressive treatments may protect from atherosclerosis.[58-60] In the future, the studies on the immunological proatherogenic factors in patients with SLE and antiphospholipid syndrome may lead to the development of more specific treatments for atherosclerotic complications, not only in these autoimmune diseases but also in common atherosclerosis.

REFERENCES

1. Libby, P., Molecular bases of the acute coronary syndromes, *Circulation*, 91, 2844, 1995.
2. Mendall, M.A., Patel, P., Ballam, L., Strachan, D., and Northfield, T.C., C reactive protein and its relation to cardiovascular risk factors: a population based cross sectional study, *B. M. J.*, 312, 1061, 1996.
3. Neri, G., Prisco, D., Martini, F., Gori, A.M., Brunelli, T., Poggesi, L., Rostagno, C., Gensini, G.F., and Abbate, R., Acute T-cell activation is detectable in unstable angina, *Circulation*, 95, 1806, 1997.
4. Stemme, S., Faber, B., Holm, J., Wiklund, O., Witztum, J.L., and Hansson, G.K., T lymphocytes from human atherosclerotic plaques recognize oxidized low density lipoprotein, *Proc. Natl. Acad. Sci. USA*, 92, 3893, 1995.
5. Kleindienst, R., Xu, Q., Willeit, J., Waldenberger, F.R., Weimann, S., and Wick, G., Immunology of atherosclerosis: demonstration of heat shock protein 60 expression and T lymphocytes bearing alpha/beta or gamma/delta receptor in human atherosclerotic lesions, *Am. J. Pathology*, 142, 1927, 1993.
6. Salonen, J.T., Ylä-Herttuala, S., Yamamoto, R., Butler, S., Korpela, H., Salonen, R., Nyyssönen, K., Palinski, W., and Witztum, J.L., Autoantibody against oxidized LDL and progression of carotid atherosclerosis, *Lancet*, 339, 883, 1992.
7. Xu, Q., Willeit, J., Marosi, M., Kleindienst, R., Oberhollenzer, F., Kiechl, S., Slutnig, T., Luef, G., and Wick, G., Association of serum antibodies to heat-shock protein 65 with carotid atherosclerosis, *Lancet*, 341, 255, 1993.
8. Urowitz, M.B., Bookman, A.A.M., Koehler, B.E., Gordon, D.A., Smythe, H.A., and Ogryzlo, M.A., The bimodal mortality pattern of systemic lupus eryhtematosus, *Am. J. Med.*, 69, 221, 1976.
9. Manzi, S., Meilahn, E.N., Rairie, J.E., Conte, C.G., Medsger, T.A., Jansen-McWilliams, L., D'Agostino, R.B., and Kuller, L.H., Age-specific incidence rates of myocardial infarction and angina in women with systemic lupus erythematosus: comparison with the Framingham study, *Am. J. Epidemiol.*, 145, 408, 1997.
10. Ward, M.M., Premature morbidity from cardiovascular and cerebrovascular diseases in women with systemic lupus erythematosus, *Arth. Rheum.*, 42, 338, 1999.
11. Petri, M., Thrombosis and systemic lupus erythematosus: the Hopkins Lupus Cohort perspective, *Scand. J. Rheumatol.*, 25, 191, 1995.
12. Manzi, S., Selzer, F., Sutton-Tyrrell, K., Fitzgerald, S.G., Rairie, J.E., Tracy, R.P., and Kuller, L.H., Prevalence and risk factors of carotid plaque in women with systemic lupus erythematosus, *Arth. Rheum.*, 42, 51, 1999.
13. Witztum, J.L., The oxidation hypothesis of atherosclerosis, *Lancet,* 344, 793, 1994.
14. Hazell, L.J., Arnold, L., Flowers, D., Waeg, G., Malle, E., and Stocker, R., Presence of hypochlorite-modified proteins in human atherosclerotic lesions, *J. Clin. Inv.,* 97, 1535, 1996.
15. Yla-Herttuala, S., Palinski, W., Rosenfeld, M.E., Parthasarathy, S., Carew, T.E., Butler, S., Witztum, J.L., and Steinberg, D., Evidence for the presence of oxidatively modified low density lipoprotein in atherosclerotic lesions of rabbit and man, *J. Clin. Inv.,* 84, 1086, 1989.
16. Shih, P.T., Elices, M.J., Fang, Z.T., Ugarova, T.P., Strahl, D., Territo, M.C., Frank, J.S., Kovach, N.L., Cabanas, C., Berliner, J.A., and Vora, D.K., Minimally modified low-density lipoprotein induces monocyte adhesion to endothelial connecting segment-1 by activating beta1 integrin, *J. Clin. Inv.,* 103, 613, 1999.
17. Klouche, M., May, A.E., Hemmes, M., Messner, M., Kanse, S.M., Preissner, K.T., and Bhakdi, S., Enzymatically modified, nonoxidized LDL induces selective adhesion and transmigration of monocytes and T-lymphocytes through human endothelial cell monolayers, *Arterioscler. Thromb. Vasc. Biol.,* 19, 784, 1999.
18. Puurunen, M., Mänttäri, M., Manninen, V., Tenkanen, L., Alfthan, G., Ehnholm, C., Vaarala, O., Aho, K., and Palosuo, T., Antibody against oxidized low-density lipoprotein predicting myocardial infarction, *Arch. Intern. Med.,* 154, 2605, 1994.

19. Wu, R., Nityanand, S., Berglund, L., Lithell, H., Holm, G., and Lefvert, A.K., Antibodies against cardiolipin and oxidatively modified LDL in 50-year-old men predict myocardial infarction, *Arterioscler. Tromb. Vasc. Biol.*, 17, 3159, 1997.

20. Lopes-Virella, M.F., Binzafar, N., Rackley, S., Takei, A., La Via, M., and Virella, G., The uptake of LDL-IC by human macrophages: predominant involvement of the Fc gamma RI receptor, *Atherosclerosis*, 135, 161, 1997.

21. George, J., Afek, A., Gilburd, B., Levkovitz, H., Shaish, A., Goldberg, I., Kopolovic, Y., Wick, G., Shoenfeld, Y., and Harats, D., Hyperimmunization of apo-E-deficient mice with homologous malondialdehyde low-density lipoprotein suppresses early atherogenesis, *Atherosclerosis*, 138, 147, 1998.

22. Freigang, S., Hörkkö, S., Miller, E., Witztum, J.L., and Palinski, W., Immunization of LDL receptor-deficient mice with homologous malondialdehyde-modified and native LDL reduces progression of atherosclerosis by mechanisms other than induction of high titers of antibodies to oxidative neoepitopes, *Arterioscler. Thromb. Vasc. Biol.*, 18, 1972, 1998.

23a. Zhou, X., Paulsson, G., Stemme, S., and Hansson, G.K., Hypercholesterolemia is associated with a T helper (Th) 1/Th2 switch of the autoimmune response in atherosclerotic apo E-knockout mice, *J. Clin. Inv.*, 101, 1717, 1998.

23b. Sinisalo, J., et al., unpublished data, 1999.

24. Vaarala, O., Alfthan, G., Jauhiainen, M., Leirisalo-Repo, M., Aho, K., and Palosuo, T., Crossreaction between antibodies to oxidized lipoprotein and to cardiolipin in systemic lupus erythematosus, *Lancet*, 341, 923, 1993.

25. Amengual, O., Atsumi, T., Khamashta, M.A., Tinahones, F., and Hughes, G.R., Autoantibodies against oxidized low-density lipoprotein in antiphospholipid syndrome, *Br. J. Rheumatol.*, 36, 964, 1997.

26. Cuadrado, M.J., Tinahones, F., Camps, M.T., de Ramon, E., Gomez-Zumaquero, J.M., Mujic, F., Khamashta, M.A., and Hughes, G.R. Antiphospholipid, anti-β_2-glycoprotein I and antioxidized low-density antibodies in antiphospholipid syndrome, *Q. J. Med.*, 91, 619, 1998.

27. Vaarala, O., Puurunen, M., Lukka, M., Alfthan, G., Leirisalo-Repo, M., Aho, K., and Palosuo, T., Affinity-purified cardiolipin-binding antibodies show heterogeneity in their binding to oxidized low-density lipoprotein, *Clin. Exp. Immunol.*, 104, 269, 1986.

28. Hörkkö, S., Miller, E., Dudl, E., Reaven, P., Curtiss, L.K., Zvaifler, N.J., Terkeltaub, R., Pierangeli, S.S., Branch, D.W., Palinski, W., and Witztum, J.L., Antiphospholipid antibodies are directed against epitopes of oxidized phospholipids, *J. Clin. Invest.*, 98, 815, 1996.

29. Palinski, W., Yla-Herttuala, S., Rosenfeld, M.E., Butler, S.W., Socher, S.A., Parthasarathy, S., Curtiss, L.K., and Witztum, J.L., Antisera and monoclonal antibodies specific for epitopes generated during oxidative modification of low-density lipoprotein, *Arteriosclerosis*, 10, 325, 1990.

30. Matsuura, E., Katahira, T., Igarashi, Y., and Koike. T., β_2-glycoprotein I bound to oxidatively modified lipoproteins could be targeted by anticardiolipin antibodies, *Lupus*, 3, 314, 1994.

31. Matsuda, J., Gotoh, M., Kawasugi, K., Gohchi, K., Tsukamoto, M., and Saitoh, N., Negligible synergistic effect of β_2-glycoprotein I on the reactivity of antioxidized low-density lipoprotein antibody to oxidized low-density lipoprotein, *Am. J. Hematol.*, 52, 114, 1996.

32. Tinahones, F.J., Cuadrado, M.J., Khamashta, M.A., Mujic, F., Gomez-Zumaquero, J.M., Collantes, E., and Hughes, G.R., Lack of cross-reaction between antibodies to β_2-glycoprotein-I and oxidized low-density lipoprotein in patients with antiphospholipid syndrome, *Br. J. Rheumatol.*, 37, 746, 1998.

33. Mizutani, H., Kurata, Y., Kosugi, S., Shiraga, M., Kashiwagi, H., Tomiyama, Y., Kanakura, Y., Good, R.A., and Matsuzawa, Y., Monoclonal anticardiolipin autoantibodies established from the (New Zealand White x BXSB)F1 mouse model of antiphospholipid syndrome cross react with oxidized low-density lipoprotein, *Arth. Rheum.*, 38, 1382, 1995.

34. Aho, K., Vaarala, O., Tenkanen, L., Julkunen, H., Jouhikainen, T., Alfthan, G., and Palosuo, T., Antibodies binding to anionic phospholipids but not to oxidized low-density lipoprotein are associated with thrombosis in patients with systemic lupus erythematosus, *Clin. Exp. Rheumatol.*, 14, 499, 1996.

35. Vaarala, O., Mänttäri, M., Manninen, V., Tenkanen, L., Puurunen, M., Aho, K., and Palosuo, T., Anticardiolipin antibodies and risk of myocardial infarction in a prospective cohort of middle-aged men, *Circulation*, 91, 23, 1995.

36. Zuckerman, E., Toubi, E., Shiran, A., Sabo, E., Shmuel, Z., Golan, T.D., Abinader, E., and Yeshurun, D., Anticardiolipin antibodies and acute myocardial infarction in nonsystemic lupus erythematosus: a controlled prospective study, *Am. J. Med.*, 101, 381, 1996.

37. Levine, S.R., Salowich-Palm, L., Sawaya, K.L., Perry, M., Spencer, H.J., Winkler, H.J., Alam, Z., and Carey, J.L., IgG anticardiolipin antibody titer > 40 GPL and the risk of subsequent thrombo-occlusive events and death: a prospective cohort study, *Stroke,* 28, 1660, 1997.

38. Sletnes, K.E., Smith, P., Abdelnoor, M., Arnesen, H., and Wisloff, F., Antiphospholipid antibodies after myocardial infarction and their relation to mortality, reinfarction, and nonhemorrhagic stroke, *Lancet,* 339, 451, 1992.

39. Zsakiris, D.A., Marbet, G.A., Burkat, F., and Duckert, F., Anticardiolipin antibodies and coronary heart disease, *Eur. Heart. J.,* 13, 1645, 1992.

40. George, J., Afek, A., Gilburd, B., Levy, Y., Blank, M., Kopolovic, J., Harats, D., and Shoenfeld, Y., Atherosclerosis in LDL-receptor knockout mice is accelerated by immunization with anticardiolipin antibodies, *Lupus,* 6, 723, 1997.

41. Fickl, H., Van Antwerpen, V.L., Richards, G.A., Van der Westhuyzen, D.R., Davies, N., Van der Walt, R., Van der Merwe, C.A., and Anderson, R., Increased levels of autoantibodies to cardiolipin and oxidized low density lipoprotein are inversely associated with plasma vitamin C status in cigarette smokers, *Atherosclerosis,* 24, 5, 1996.

42. Iuliano, L., Pratico, D., Ferro, D., Pittoni, V., Valesini, G., Lawson, J., FitzGerald, G.A., and Violi, F., Enhanced lipid peroxidation in patients positive for antiphospholipid antibodies, *Blood,* 90, 3931, 1997.

43. Ames, P.R., Nourooz-Zadeh, J., Tommasino, C., Alves, J., Brancaccio, V., and Anggard, E.E., Oxidative stress in primary antiphospholipid syndrome, *Thromb. Haemost.,* 79, 447, 1998.

44. Hasunuma, Y., Matsuura, E., Makita, Z., Katahira, T., Nishi, S., and Koike, T., Involvement of β_2-glycoprotein I and anticardiolipin antibodies in oxidatively modified low-density lipoprotein uptake by macrophages, *Clin. Exp. Immunol.,* 107, 569, 1997.

45. George, J., Afek, A., Gilburd, B., Blank, M., Levy, Y., Aron-Maor, A., Levkovitz, H., Shaish, A., Goldberg, I., Kopolovic, J., Harats, D., and Shoenfeld, Y., Induction of early atherosclerosis in LDL-receptor-deficient mice immunized with β_2-glycoprotein I, *Circulation,* 98, 1108, 1998.

46. Afek, A., George, J., Shoenfeld, Y., Gilburd, B., Levy, Y., Shaish, A., Keren, P., Janackovic, Z., Goldberg, I., Kopolovic, J., and Harats, D., Enhancement of atherosclerosis in β_2-glycoprotein I-immunized apolipoprotein E-deficient mice, *Pathobiology,* 67, 19, 1999.

47. George, J., Harats, D., Gilburd, B., Afek, A., Levy, Y., Schneiderman, J., Barshak, I., Kopolovic, J., and Shoenfeld, Y., Immunolocalization of β_2-glycoprotein I (Apolipoprotein H) to human atherosclerotic plaques: potential implications for lesion progression, *Circulation,* 99, 2227, 1999.

48. Vaarala, O., Puurunen, M., Mänttäri, M., Manninen, V., Aho, K., and Palosuo, T., Antibodies to prothrombin imply a risk of myocardial infarction in middle-aged men, *Thromb. Haemost.,* 75, 456, 1996.

49. Galli, M. and Barbui, T., Antiprothrombin antibodies: detection and clinical significance in the antiphospholipid syndrome, *Blood,* 93, 2149, 1999.

50. Puurunen, M., Mänttäri, M., Manninen, V., Palosuo, T., and Vaarala, O., Antibodies to prothrombin cross react with plasminogen in patients developing myocardial infarction, *Br. J. Haematol.,* 100, 374, 1998.

51. Vaarala, O., Atherosclerosis in SLE and Hughes syndrome (editorial), *Lupus,* 6, 489, 1997.

52. Yamazaki, M., Asakura, H., Jokaji, H., Saito, M., Uotani, C., Kumabashiri, I., Morishita, E., Aoshima, K., Ikeda, T., and Matsuda, T., Plasma levels of lipoprotein(a) are elevated in patients with the antiphospholipid antibody syndrome, *Thromb. Haemost.,* 71, 424, 1994.

53. Atsumi, R., Khamashta, M.A., Andujar, C., Leandro, M.J., Amengual, O., Ames, P.R., and Hughes, G.R. Elevated plasma lipoprotein(a) level and its association with impaired fibrinolysis in patients with antiphospholipid syndrome, *J. Rheumatol.,* 25, 69, 1998.

54. Hoppichler, F., Lechleitner, M., Traweger, C., Schett, G., Dzien, A., Sturm, W., and Xu, Q., Changes of serum antibodies to heat-shock protein 65 in coronary heart disease and acute myocardial infarction, *Atherosclerosis,* 126, 333, 1996.

55. Kaufmann, S.H., Heat shock proteins and autoimmunity: a critical appraisal, *Int. Arch. Allergy Immunol.,* 103, 317, 1994.

56. Schett, G., Xu, Q., Amberger, A., Van der Zee, R., Recheis, H., Willeit, J., and Wick, G., Autoantibodies against heat shockprotein 60 mediate endothelial cytotoxicity, *J. Clin. Inv.,* 96, 2569, 1995.

57. Xu, Q., Dietrich, H., Steiner, H.J., Gown, A.M., Schoel, B., Mikuz, G., Kaufmann, S.H., and Wick, G., Induction of arteriosclerosis in normocholesterolemic rabbits by immunization with heat shock protein 65, *Arterioscl. Thromb.,* 12, 789, 1992.

58. Drew, A.F. and Tipping, P.G., Cyclosporine treatment reduces early atherogenesis in the cholesterol-fed rabbit, *Atherosclerosis*, 116, 181, 1995.
59. Matsumoto, T., Saito, E., Watanabre, H., Fujioka, T., Yamada, T., Takahashi, Y., Ueno, T., Tochihara, T., and Kanmatsuse, K., Influence of FK 506 on experimental atherosclerosis in cholesterol-fed rabbits, *Atherosclerosis*, 139, 95, 1998.
60. Nicoletti, A., Kaveri, S., Caligiuri, G., Bariety, J., and Hansson, G.K., Immunoglobulin treatment reduces atherosclerosis in apo E knockout mice, *J. Clin. Inv.*, 102, 910, 1998.

6 Homocysteine and Vascular Disease in the Autoimmune Connective Tissue Diseases

Michelle Petri

CONTENTS

I. INTRODUCTION

Premature, or accelerated, atherosclerosis has become recognized as a major determinant of both morbidity and mortality in chronic autoimmune diseases, especially systemic lupus erythematosus (SLE) and rheumatoid arthritis (RA). The pathogenesis of accelerated atherosclerosis is almost certainly multifactorial. The initial insult is likely a direct attack on the endothelial surface of blood vessels, due to immune complex deposition, cytokines, or other immune-derived factors. The chronic phase, however, is more complicated, and is less likely to involve factors related to active autoimmune disease, and more likely to involve so-called "traditional" cardiovascular risk factors (Figure 6.1). It is now recognized that the levels of some "traditional" risk factors can be increased by common treatments of autoimmune disease, including prednisone and methotrexate, and by organ system involvement in specific autoimmune diseases, such as renal involvement in SLE leading to hypertension and hyperlipidemia. This chapter will review the role of homocysteine, a newly recognized, but important "traditional" cardiovascular risk factor, and its importance in both systemic lupus erythematosus and rheumatoid arthritis.

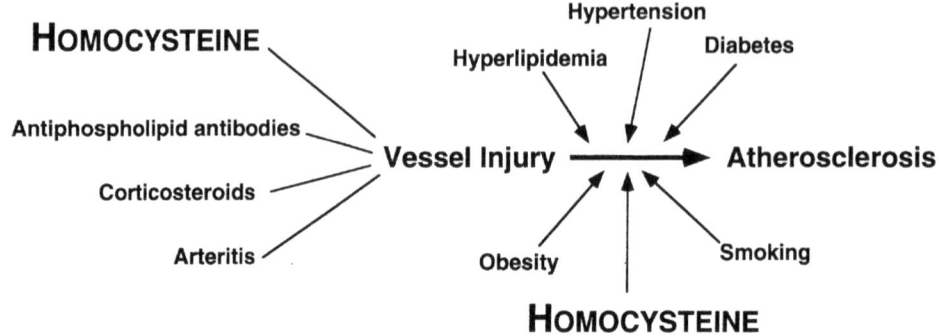

FIGURE 6.1 Role of homocysteine in atherosclerosis in SLE.

II. HOMOCYSTEINE: A NEWLY IDENTIFIED RISK FACTOR FOR ATHEROTHROMBOSIS

McCully was the first to describe the association of hyperhomocysteinemia and atherosclerosis.[1] Even mild increases in plasma homocysteine (HC) are now recognized to increase the risk of both atherosclerosis and thrombosis. Homocysteinemia is usually detected through fasting levels in plasma, but only 50% of hyperhomocysteinemic subjects can be identified in this way. Methionine loading can be used to further identify those at risk.

Homocysteine potentiates atherosclerosis and thrombosis through multiple mechanisms, including direct injury of endothelial surfaces, activating coagulation and blocking fibrinolysis, activating platelets, and reducing vascular reactivity. The major effect of homocysteine appears to be mediated by endothelial dysfunction on both the arterial and venous side of the circulation, decreasing the release or the action of nitric oxide in response to blood flow. Endothelial-modulated vasoconstriction in coronary vessels,[2] endothelium-dependent flow-mediated dilation,[3] and decreased flow-mediated endothelium-dependent (NO-mediated) vasodilation[4] have all been demonstrated with homocysteine. A threshold concentration of homocysteine may be necessary to induce endothelial lesions.[5]

Homocysteine has multiple additional effects that contribute to atherosclerosis, including smooth muscle proliferation, extracellular matrix modification, and lipoprotein oxidation. There is increased growth and collagen in arterial smooth muscle cells.[6] Serine elastase is increased in arterial smooth muscle.[7]

The effects of hyperhomocysteinemia go beyond its atherogenic potential because it is also thrombogenic. It inhibits thrombomodulin, inhibits antithrombin III-binding activity, inhibits ADPase activity by HUVECS (ADP is a potent platelet aggregatory agent), and inhibits binding of t-PA (thereby interfering with fibrinolysis[8,9]). The effect of homocysteine has been likened to a permanent hemostatic system activation, documented by increased levels of prothrombin fragment F1.2.[10]

III. GENETIC CAUSES OF HYPERHOMOCYTEINEMIA

Hyperhomocysteinemia is usually due to an autosomal recessive disorder, whereby deficiency of cystathione β-synthase results in plasma HC levels as high as 400 μmol/l. This syndrome, homocystinuria, was classically described as resulting in mental retardation, ectopic lens, and skeletal abnormalities. It also leads to premature atherosclerosis in the coronary and carotid distributions and to thrombosis, both arterial and venous. Heterozygous homocystinuria due to heterozygous cystathione β-synthase deficiency occurs in about one out of 300 people, but can also lead to atherothrombotic risk. Thermolabile mutations in a second enzyme, methylene tetrahydrofolate reductase (MTHFR), which remethylates homocysteine into methionine, also lead to increased levels of homocysteine. Up to 50% of people are heterozygous for one of seven mutations in MTHFR, the most common genetic cause of mildly increased homocysteine levels.

IV. DEMOGRAPHIC AND DIETARY CAUSES OF ELEVATED HOMOCYSTEINE LEVELS

Demographic factors also determine homocysteine levels. Males have higher levels than females.[11] Postmenopausal women have higher levels than premenopausal women. Homocysteine levels increase with age in both sexes.[11] Means and percentiles for homocysteine are now available by race and sex.[12] Homocysteine is a risk factor for cardiovascular disease in both blacks and whites.[13] Elevated levels of homocysteine in black stroke victims may be partially explained by renal insufficiency.[14] Premenopausal black women have higher homocysteine levels than whites.[15]

Homocysteine levels may be independently related to isolated systolic hypertension in the elderly.[16] Hypertensive subjects have higher homocysteine than normotensive subjects.[17] Homocysteine increases with smoking.[11] Interaction effects were noted in one study between homocysteine and smoking or hypertension,[18] such that homocysteine powerfully increased the cardiovascular risk associated with smoking and hypertension.[19]

Diet appears to be another important determinant of homocysteine levels, especially in the elderly. Depressed levels of several B vitamins, including folic acid, B_6, and B_{12} (all of which are cofactors in homocysteine metabolic pathways) can lead to increased homocysteine levels. Dietary supplementation with these B vitamins can lower homocysteine levels. There is an inverse dose-response relation between dietary protein and homocysteine levels. Increased coffee consumption increases homocysteine levels.[20]

Estrogen and similar drugs affect homocysteine levels. Estrogen reduces homocysteine in elderly men.[21] Hormone replacement reduced homocysteine 12.3% in women with higher baseline levels.[22] Tamoxifen reduces homocysteine levels, especially the higher baseline levels.[23,24]

V. RISK ESTIMATES OF CARDIOVASCULAR DISEASE WITH ELEVATED HOMOCYSTEINE

Meta-analyses have shown that elevated fasting HC levels are associated with at least a twofold increase in risk of coronary artery disease and stroke, and perhaps even a higher risk of peripheral arterial disease.

A. RISK ESTIMATES FOR CORONARY ARTERY DISEASE

In the Physicians Health Study, elevated levels of HC increased the risk of myocardial infarction threefold. Young women with homocysteine = 15.6 µmol/l had twice the risk of myocardial infarction as those with homocysteine = 10.0 µmol/l (OR 2.3, 95% CI 0.94 to 5.64).[25] A homocysteine level of 14 µmol/l conferred an odds ratio of cornary artery disease of 4.8 (p < 0.001) in a case-control study.[26] In a meta-analysis, a 5 µmol/l increment in homocysteine led to an odds ratio for CAD of 1.6 in men and 1.8 in women. A total of 10% of the population had CAD risk attributable to homocysteine.[27]

B. RISK ESTIMATES FOR CAROTID ATHEROSCLEROSIS AND STROKE

Homocysteine levels are associated with increased common carotid artery wall thickness in men: the adjusted intima-media thickness was 1.12 mm vs. 1.02 mm with homocysteine concentration above and below 11.5 µmol/l (p = 0.029).[28] For carotid artery stenosis, an odds ratio of 2.0 was found for the highest homocysteine quartile.[29] The relative risk of stroke increases with the second, third, and fourth quartiles of homocysteine, with odds ratios of 1.3, 1.9, and 2.8, respectively.[30] In a meta-analysis, the odds ratio for cerebrovascular disease (for a 5 μmol/l homocysteine increment) was 1.5.[27]

C. Risk Estimates of Peripheral Arterial Disease

Using transesophageal echocardiography to evaluate the thoracic aorta, a correlation of homocysteine with atherosclerotic plaque was found (r = 0.63, p < 0.0001).[31] Homocysteine has been found to be an independent risk factor for peripheral vascular disease with a fourfold increase in risk.[32]

D. Risk Estimates of Venous Thrombosis with Elevated Homocysteine

Several recent meta-analyses have examined the relationship between hyperhomocysteinemia and venous thrombosis. In one meta-analysis of 10 case-control studies, a pooled estimate of the odds ratio was 2.5 (95% CI 1.8 to 3.5) for fasting plasma HC above the 95th percentile or above the mean + 2 SD, and 2.6 (95% CI 1.6 to 4.4) for a postmethionine increase in homocysteine level.[33] In a second meta-analysis of nine studies, a pooled odds ratio of 2.95 (95% CI 2.08 to 4.17, p < 0.001) was found and, for postmethionine levels, an odds ratio 2.15 (95% CI 1.20 to 3.85) was determined. If patients older than 60 were excluded, the odds ratio for venous thrombosis rose to 4.37 (95% CI 1.94 to 9.84).[34]

Elevated homocysteine levels are a risk factor for recurrent venous thromboembolism as well. In one study, 264 patients with venous thrombosis were followed prospectively after discontinuing warfarin. Recurrent venous thromboembolism occurred in 12 of 66 (18%) with homocysteine levels above the 95th percentile vs. 8% with normal homocysteine levels. The cumulative probability of recurrent venous thromboembolism 24 months after stopping warfarin was 19.2% in the hyperhomocysteinemia group vs. 6.3% in those with normal levels (p = 0.0001). The relative risk of recurrent thrombosis with hyperhomocysteinemia was 2.7 (95% CI 1.3 to 5.8, p = 0.009).[35]

Case-control studies have demonstrated that homocysteinemia is associated with venous thrombosis even when other causes of venous hypercoagulability are excluded. In contrast to the meta-analysis,[34] however, in one case-control study the association was increased with age and was stronger among women.[36]

VI. INTERVENTION TRIALS

Intervention trials to lower homocysteine need to address multiple issues, including the B vitamins needed, the doses needed, and whether certain subgroups (i.e., renal failure) are resistant to treatment. True outcome studies (i.e., reduction of cardiovascular events) have not been done.

Three B vitamins (folic acid, B_6, and B_{12}) are involved in homocysteine metabolism. In a trial using 1 mg folic acid, B_6, and B_{12}, a 27.9% reduction in homocysteine occurred; antioxidants had no effect.[37] In a trial of folic acid and B_6 supplementation, B_6 had no added effect.[38] Similarly, in a trial of folic acid, B_{12}, and B_6, the effect of folic acid alone was similar to the multiple vitamin effect.[39]

Several doses of folic acid have been examined. In a study that used folic acid at 400 mcg, 1 mg, or 5 mg (along with vitamin B_{12} and B_6), 400 mcg of folic acid appeared to be equivalent to higher doses, with reduction in total plasma homocysteine from 13.8 ± 8.8 to 9.6 ± 2 μmol/l (p = 0.001).[40] Even low-dose folic acid is beneficial, such as 250 mcg of folic acid, which reduced homocysteine in healthy young women.[41] The usual amount of folic acid in breakfast cereal, 127 mcg of folic acid, only decreased homocysteine by 3.7% (p = NS), but cereals with higher folic acid content (499 and 665 mcg) reduced homocysteine by 11% and 14% (p = 0.001).[42] Similarly, 100 mcg of folic acid was not effective, but doses as low as 200 mcg were effective, in lowering homocysteine in normals.[43]

In renal failure patients, folic acid supplementation (2.5 or 5 mg folic acid) does not normalize homocysteine, but a 35% reduction was achieved.[44] Even a standard multiple vitamin, Nephro-Vite, which contains B vitamins and 1 mg of folic acid, reduced plasma homocysteine by 23.7%, from 27.8 ± 5.9 to 21.2 ± 6.6 µmol/l ($p = 0.007$), in hemodialysis patients.[45] Reduction of homocysteine in diabetic nephropathy patients is of special interest because homocysteine elevation is associated with increased albumin excretion rate.[46]

Outcome studies to determine if homocysteine reduction protects against cardiovascular and thrombotic complications should be done. However, it should not be assumed that results will be positive. Long-term reduction in plasma homocysteine did not result in improvement of endothelial function in peritoneal dialysis patients.[47] Similarly, in atherosclerotic monkeys, *in vivo* responses of resistance vessels to endothelium-dependent vasodilators (acetylcholine or ADP) did not improve after vitamin supplementation.[48]

VII. PREMATURE ATHEROSCLEROSIS IN SYSTEMIC LUPUS ERYTHEMATOSUS

Improved survival in systemic lupus erythematosus (SLE) has led to recognition that the major long-term threat in SLE is not active SLE, but atherosclerosis.[49] Autopsy studies have shown that atherosclerosis is a frequent problem in the poststeroid era.[50,51] Clinically recognized atherosclerosis, presenting as angina pectoris or myocardial infarction, occurs in about 8% of most lupus cohorts, worldwide.[52]

Noninvasive screening tests for atherosclerosis, including exercise stress tests and carotid duplex, suggest that the true prevalence of atherosclerosis in SLE is much higher.[53,54] Although the initiating factor in atherosclerosis in SLE is autoimmune, potentiating factors include multiple traditional cardiovascular risk factors that are amenable to intervention strategies, both lifestyle and pharmacologic.

Chronic treatment with prednisone increases the levels of some of the traditional cardiovascular risk factors in SLE patients. Using longitudinal regression analysis, we have shown that an increase in daily prednisone dose increases cholesterol, blood pressure, and weight.[55] Thus, "prednisone sparing" strategies are likely to reduce the atherosclerotic burden. For example, the antimalarial drugs, such as hydroxychloroquine, lower lipid levels, in addition to favorable rheologic properties.[56]

Some of the cardiovascular risk factors — such as hypertension and hyperlipidemia — can also represent chronic renal damage from lupus nephritis and nephrotic syndrome. Aggressive control of these risk factors, with both lifestyle modification and drug therapy, needs to be instituted in even the young SLE patients.

Antiphospholipid antibodies, specifically the lupus anticoagulant and anticardiolipin antibody, are a known risk factor for thromboembolic disease. In the author's Hopkins Lupus Cohort, the lupus anticoagulant also is a prospective risk factor for coronary artery disease and for asymptomatic atherosclerosis on carotid duplex scan.[53] The mechanisms by which antiphospholipid antibodies potentiate atherosclerosis are now better understood. The plasma protein target of most antiphospholipid antibodies, β_2-glycoprotein I (GPI), serves as a natural protection against atherosclerosis by retarding uptake of oxidized low-density lipoprotein (LDL), one of the initiating steps. In contrast, in the presence of antiphospholipid antibodies, a conformational change occurs, and β_2-GPI then accelerates the uptake of oxidized LDL.[57] Antiphospholipid antibodies represent a cardiovascular risk factor that could be important throughout the course of SLE, even at times when disease activity appears to be well-controlled.

A. Homocysteine in SLE

Using the prospective Hopkins Lupus Cohort database, the author performed a nested case-control study to determine if homocysteine levels at baseline (entry into the cohort) were predictive of later cardiovascular events. It was found that 15% of the patients had homocysteine levels greater than 14.1 µmol/l. In univariate analyses, SLE male patients who had renal insufficiency, took prednisone, or had the lupus anticoagulant had higher plasma homocysteine levels. One of the most important determinants of homocysteine levels in the SLE patients turned out to be B vitamin levels, folic acid and B_6, even though the SLE patients were young and not thought to have limited diets.[58] After adjustment for established risk factors, plasma homocysteine levels remained an independent risk factor for stroke (OR 2.44, 95% CI 1.04 to 5.75, p = 0.04) and arterial thrombosis (OR 3.49, 95% CI 0.97 to 12.54, p = 0.05). In a multiple regression model, a one standard deviation change in homocysteine led to a twofold increase in the odds ratio for stroke.

We proceeded to do a B vitamin intervention trial to determine if homocysteine levels could be decreased in SLE. An initial concern was that the HC levels, which were associated with prednisone use and with renal insufficiency, might not be modifiable. However, in preliminary analyses, the mean level of homocysteine decreased significantly with supplementation with folic acid, B_6, and B_{12}.[59]

A second group has now confirmed that SLE patients have increased levels of homocysteine.[60] SLE patients with arterial thrombosis had higher levels of homocysteine (20.6 ± 10 vs. 13.2 ± 6.8 μmol/l, p < 0.001). The crude odds ratio for arterial thrombosis for the highest vs. lowest quartile of homocysteine was 4.4 (95% CI 1.3 to 14.9). Similar to the results in the Hopkins Lupus Cohort, no association was found with venous thrombosis. Homocysteine levels were higher in patients on prednisone and lower in those on oral contraceptives. The increased levels do not appear to be genetic, i.e., due to thermolabile mutations in MTHFR. Thus, homocysteine should be considered an acquired cardiovascular risk factor in SLE, present throughout the disease course, but modifiable by a simple, safe, and inexpensive intervention, B vitamin supplementation.

VIII. ATHEROSCLEROSIS IN RHEUMATOID ARTHRITIS

Rheumatoid arthritis is well recognized as a disabling polyarthritis, and most recognize that it is associated with increased mortality. It is less recognized that atherosclerosis and thrombosis have become increasing problems in rheumatoid arthritis over the past few decades. In a study using dipyridamole-thallium scintiography, 27 of 54 patients with rheumatoid arthritis had perfusion defects. At autopsy, 7 of 12 cases had microvasculitis and microthrombosis.[61] In a Holter monitoring study, silent myocardial ischemic episodes were more frequent in rheumatoid arthritis than in controls.[62] Early deaths with thrombolytic therapy for myocardial infarction have occurred in seropositive, corticosteroid-treated patients.[63]

A. HOMOCYSTEINE IN RHEUMATOID ARTHRITIS

The immunosuppressive regimen of choice for rheumatoid arthritis in the U.S. is methotrexate.[64] Methotrexate acts as both an antiinflammatory and antierosive therapy in rheumatoid arthritis. Its toxicity includes mouth ulcers, nausea, elevated liver function tests, and, rarely, cirrhosis and pulmonary alveolitis. A landmark clinical trial demonstrated that folic acid supplementation decreased most methotrexate toxicity, especially elevated liver function tests and mouth ulcers.[65]

A potentially hidden toxicity of methotrexate has been elevated levels of homocysteine. Whether homocysteine has played a role in atherosclerosis in rheumatoid arthritis can only be inferred indirectly. However, supplementation with folic acid reduced homocysteine levels in rheumatoid arthritis patients[66] who participated in a trial of placebo vs. 5 mg or 27.5 mg folic acid supplementation.

IX. CONCLUSION

Although atherosclerosis and thrombosis are multifactorial in SLE and in rheumatoid arthritis, with immune-mediated mechanisms playing a major role in initiation, traditional cardiovascular and thrombotic risk factors play an increasing role in the chronic phase. To this end, the recognition that homocysteine is elevated in both SLE and in rheumatoid arthritis, and is potentially modifiable by B vitamin supplementation, has been an important therapeutic advance.

REFERENCES

1. McCully, K. S., Vascular pathology of homocysteinemia: implications for pathogenesis of arteriosclerosis, *Am. J. Pathol.*, 56, 111, 1969.
2. Tyagi, S. C., Smiley, L. M., Mujumdar, V. S., Clonts, B., and Parker, J. L., Reduction-oxidation (Redox) and vascular tissue level of homocyst(e)ine in human coronary atherosclerotic lesions and role in extracellular matrix remodeling and vascular tone, *Mol. Cell. Biochem.*, 181, 107, 1998.
3. Woo, K. S., Chook, P., Lolin, Y. I., Cheung, A. S., Chan, L. T., Sun, Y. Y., Sanderson, J. E., Metreweli, C., and Celermajer, D. S., Hyperhomocyst(e)inemia is a risk factor for arterial endothelial dysfunction in humans, *Circulation*, 96, 2542, 1997.
4. Tawakol, A., Omland, T., Gerhard, M., Wu, J. T., and Creager, M. A., Hyperhomocyst(e)inemia is associated with impaired endothelium-dependent vasodilation in humans, *Circulation*, 95, 1119, 1997.
5. Hladovec, J., Sommerova, Z., and Pisarikova, A., Homocysteinemia and endothelial damage after methionine load, *Thromb. Res.*, 88, 361, 1997.
6. Majors, A., Ehrhart, L. A., and Pezacka, E. H., Homocysteine as a risk factor for vascular disease: enhanced collagen production and accumulation by smooth muscle cells, *Arterioscler. Thromb. Vasc. Biol.*, 17, 2074, 1997.
7. Jourdheuil-Rahmani, D., Rolland, P. H., Rosset, E., Branchereau, A., and Garcon, D., Homocysteine induces synthesis of a serine elastase in arterial smooth muscle cells from multiorgan donors, *Cardiovasc. Res.*, 34, 597, 1997.
8. Harpel, P. C., Zhang, X., and Borth, W., Homocysteine and hemostasis: pathogenic mechanisms predisposing to thrombosis, *J. Nutr.*, 126, 1285S, 1996.
9. Hajjar, K. A. and Jacovina, A. T., Modulation of annexin II by homocysteine: implications for atherothrombosis, *J. Investig. Med.*, 46, 364, 1998.
10. Kyrle, P. A., Stumpflen, A., Hirschl, M., Bialonczyk, C., Herkner, K., Speiser, W., Weltermann, A., Kaider, A., Pabinger, I., Lechner, K., and Eichinger, S., Levels of prothrombin fragment F1+2 in patients with hyperhomocysteinemia and a history of venous thromboembolism, *Thromb. Haemost.*, 78, 1327, 1997.
11. Nygard, O., Vollset, S. E., Refsum, H., Stensvold, I., Tverdal, A., Nordrehaug, J. E., Ueland, M., and Kvale, G., Total plasma homocysteine and cardiovascular risk profile: the Hordaland Homocysteine study, *J.A.M.A.*, 274, 1526, 1995.
12. Jacques, P. F., Rosenberg, I. H., Rogers, G., Selhub, J., Bowman, B. A., Gunter, E. W., Wright, J. D., and Johnson, C. L., Serum total homocysteine concentrations in adolescent and adult Americans: results from the third National Health and Nutrition Examination Survey, *Am. J. Clin. Nutr.*, 69, 482, 1999.
13. Giles, W. H., Kittner, S. J., Ou, C. Y., Croft, J. B., Brown, V., Buchholz, D. W., Earley, C. J., Feeser, B. R., Johnson, C. J., Macko, R. F., McCarter, R. J., Price, T. R., Sloan, M. A., Stern, B. J., Wityk, R. J., Wozniak, M. A., and Stolley, P. D., Thermolabile methylenetetrahydrofolate reductase polymorphism (C677T) and total homocysteine concentration among African-American and white women, *Ethn. Dis.*, 8, 149, 1998.
14. Delport, R., Ubbink, J. B., Vermaak, W. J., Rossouw, H., Becker, P. J., and Joubert, J., Hyperhomocysteinaemia in black patients with cerebral thrombosis, *Q. J. Med.*, 90, 635, 1997.
15. Gerhard, G. T., Sexton, G., Malinow, M. R., Wander, R. C., Connor, S. L., Pappu, A. S., and Connor, W. E., Premenopausal black women have more risk factors for coronary heart disease than white women, *Am. J. Cardiol.*, 82, 1040, 1998.
16. Sutton-Tyrrell, K., Bostom, A., Selhub, J., and Zeigler-Johnson, C., High homocysteine levels are independently related to isolated systolic hypertension in older adults, *Circulation*, 96, 1745, 1997.
17. Malinow, M. R., Levenson, J., Giral, P., Nieto, F. J., Razavian, M., Segond, P., and Simon, A., Role of blood pressure, uric acid, and hemorrheological parameters on plasma homocyst(e)ine concentration, *Atherosclerosis*, 114, 175, 1995.

18. Graham, I. M., Daly, L. E., Refsum, H. M., Robinson, K., Brattstrom, L. E., Ueland, P. M., Palma-Reis, R. J., Boers, G. H., Sheahan, R. G., Israelsson, B., Uiterwaal, C. S., Meleady, R., McMaster, D., Verhoef, P., Witteman, J., Rubba, P., Bellet, H., Wautrecht, J. C., de Valk, H. W., Sales Luis, A. C., Parrot-Rouland, F. M., Tan, K. S., Higgins, I., Garcon, D., and Andria, G., et al., Plasma homocysteine as a risk factor for vascular disease: the European Concerted Action Project, *J.A.M.A.*, 277, 1775, 1997.

19. Boers, G. H., The case for mild hyperhomocysteinaemia as a risk factor, *J. Inherit. Metab. Dis.*, 20, 301, 1997.

20. Stolzenberg-Solomon, R. Z., Miller, E. R., III, Maguire, M. G., Selhub, J., and Appel, L. J., Association of dietary protein intake and coffee consumption with serum homocysteine concentrations in an older population, *Am. J. Clin. Nutr.*, 69, 467, 1999.

21. Giri, S., Thompson, P. D., Taxel, P., Contois, J. H., Otvos, J., Allen, R., Ens, G., Wu, A. H., and Waters, D. D., Oral estrogen improves serum lipids, homocysteine and fibrinolysis in elderly men, *Atherosclerosis*, 137, 359, 1998.

22. van der Mooren, M. J., Demacker, P. N., Blom, H. J., de Rijke, Y. B., and Rolland, R., The effect of sequential three-monthly hormone replacement therapy on several cardiovascular risk estimators in postmenopausal women, *Fertil. Steril.*, 67, 67, 1997.

23. Cattaneo, M., Baglietto, L., Zighetti, M. L., Bettega, D., Robertson, C., Costa, A., Mannucci, P. M., and Decensi, A., Tamoxifen reduces plasma homocysteine levels in healthy women, *Br. J. Cancer*, 77, 2264, 1998.

24. Anker, G., Lonning, P. E., Ueland, P. M., Refsum, H., and Lien, E. A., Plasma levels of the atherogenic amino acid homocysteine in postmenopausal women with breast cancer treated with tamoxifen, *Int. J. Cancer*, 60, 365, 1995.

25. Schwartz, S. M., Siscovick, D. S., Malinow, M. R., Rosendaal, F. R., Beverly, R. K., Hess, D. L., Psaty, B. M., Longstreth, W. T., Jr., Koepsell, T. D., Raghunathan, T. E., and Reitsma, P. H., Myocardial infarction in young women in relation to plasma total homocysteine, folate, and a common variant in the methylenetetrahydrofolate reductase gene, *Circulation*, 96, 412, 1997.

26. Robinson, K., Mayer, E. L., Miller, D. P., Green, R., van Lente, F., Gupta, A., Kottke-Marchant, K., Savon, S. R., Selhub, J., and Nissen, S. E., et al., Hyperhomocysteinemia and low pyridoxal phosphate: common and independent reversible risk factors for coronary artery disease, *Circulation*, 92, 2825, 1995.

27. Boushey, C. J., Beresford, S. A., Omenn, G. S., and Motulsky, A. G., A quantitative assessment of plasma homocysteine as a risk factor for vascular disease: probable benefits of increasing folic acid intakes, *J.A.M.A.*, 274, 1049, 1995.

28. Voutilainen, S., Alfthan, G., Nyyssonen, K., Salonen, R., and Salonen, J. T., Association between elevated plasma total homocysteine and increased common carotid artery wall thickness, *Ann. Med.*, 30, 300, 1998.

29. Selhub, J., Jacques, P. F., Bostom, A. G., D'Agostino, R. B., Wilson, P. W. F., Belanger, A. J., O'Leary, D. H., Wolf, P. A., Schaefer, E. J., and Rosenberg, I. H., Association between plasma homocysteine concentrations and extracranial carotid-artery stenosis, *N. Engl. J. Med.*, 332, 286, 1995.

30. Perry, I. J., Refsum, H., Morris, R. W., Ebrahim, S. B., Ueland, P. M., and Shaper, A. G., Prospective study of serum total homocysteine concentration and risk of stroke in middle-aged British men, *Lancet*, 346, 1395, 1995.

31. Konecky, N., Malinow, M. R., Tunick, P. A., Freedberg, R. S., Rosenzweig, B. P., Katz, E. S., Hess, D. L., Upson, B., Leung, B., Perez, J., and Kronzon, I., Correlation between plasma homocyst(e)ine and aortic atherosclerosis, *Am. Heart J.*, 133, 534, 1997.

32. Cheng, S. W., Ting, A. C., and Wong, J., Fasting total plasma homocysteine and atherosclerotic peripheral vascular disease, *Ann. Vasc. Surg.*, 11, 217, 1997.

33. den Heijer, M., Rosendaal, F. R., Blom, H. J., Gerrits, W. B., and Bos, G. M., Hyperhomocysteinemia and venous thrombosis: a meta-analysis, *Thromb. Haemost.*, 80, 874, 1998.

34. Ray, J. G., Meta-analysis of hyperhomocysteinemia as a risk factor for venous thromboembolic disease, *Arch. Intern. Med.*, 158, 2101, 1998.

35. Eichinger, S., Stumpflen, A., Hirschl, M., Bialonczyk, C., Herkner, K., Stain, M., Schneider, B., Pabinger, I., Lechner, K., and Kyrle, P. A., Hyperhomocysteinemia is a risk factor of recurrent venous thromboembolism, *Thromb. Haemost.*, 80, 566, 1998.

36. den Heijer, M., Koster, T., Blom, H. J., Bos, G. M., Briet, E., Reitsma, P. H., Vandenbroucke, J. P., and Rosendaal, F. R., Hyperhomocysteinemia as a risk factor for deep-vein thrombosis, *N. Engl. J. Med.*, 334, 759, 1996.

37. Woodside, J. V., Yarnell, J. W., McMaster, D., Young, I. S., Harmon, D. L., McCrum, E. E., Patterson, C. C., Gey, K. F., Whitehead, A. S., and Evans, A., Effect of B-group vitamins and antioxidant vitamins on hyperhomocysteinemia: a double-blind, randomized, factorial-design, controlled trial, *Am. J. Clin. Nutr.*, 67, 858, 1998.

38. Dierkes, J., Kroesen, M., and Pietrzik, K., Folic acid and Vitamin B_6 supplementation and plasma homocysteine concentrations in healthy young women, *Int. J. Vitam. Nutr. Res.*, 68, 98, 1998.

39. den Heijer, M., Brouwer, I. A., Bos, G. M., Blom, H. J., van der Put, N. M., Spaans, A. P., Rosendaal, F. R., Thomas, C. M., Haak, H. L., Wijermans, P. W., and Gerrits, W. B., Vitamin supplementation reduces blood homocysteine levels: a controlled trial in patients with venous thrombosis and healthy volunteers, *Arterioscler. Thromb. Vasc. Biol.*, 18, 356, 1998.

40. Lobo, A., Naso, A., Arheart, K., Kruger, W. D., Abou-Ghazala, T., Alsous, F., Nahlawi, M., Gupta, A., Moustapha, A., van Lente, F., Jacobsen, D. W., and Robinson, K., Reduction of homocysteine levels in coronary artery disease by low-dose folic acid combined with vitamins B_6 and B_{12}, *Am. J. Cardiol.*, 83, 821, 1999.

41. Brouwer, I. A., van Dusseldorp, M., Thomas, C. M., Duran, M., Hautvast, J. G., Eskes, T. K., and Steegers-Theunissen, R. P., Low-dose folic acid supplementation decreases plasma homocysteine concentrations: a randomized trial, *Am. J. Clin. Nutr.*, 69, 99, 1999.

42. Malinow, M. R., Duell, P. B., Hess, D. L., Anderson, P. H., Kruger, W. D., Phillipson, B. E., Gluckman, R. A., Block, P. C., and Upson, B. M., Reduction of plasma homocyst(e)ine levels by breakfast cereal fortified with folic acid in patients with coronary heart disease, *N. Engl. J. Med.*, 338, 1009, 1998.

43. Ward, M., McNulty, H., McPartlin, J., Strain, J. J., Weir, D. G., and Scott, J. M., Plasma homocysteine, a risk factor for cardiovascular disease, is lowered by physiological doses of folic acid, *Q. J. Med.*, 90, 519, 1997.

44. Dierkes, J., Domrose, U., Ambrosch, A., Bosselmann, H. P., Neumann, K. H., and Luley, C., Response of hyperhomocysteinemia to folic acid supplementation in patients with end-stage renal disease, *Clin. Nephrol.*, 51, 108, 1999.

45. House, A. A. and Donnelly, J. G., Effect of multivitamins on plasma homocysteine and folate levels in patients on hemodialysis, *ASAIO J.*, 45, 94, 1999.

46. Chico, A., Perez, A., Cordoba, A., Arcelus, R., Carreras, G., de Leiva, A., Gonzalez-Sastre, F., and Blanco-Vaca, F., Plasma homocysteine is related to albumin excretion rate in patients with diabetes mellitus: a new link between diabetic nephropathy and cardiovascular disease? *Diabetologia*, 41, 684, 1998.

47. van Guldener, C., Janssen, M. J., Lambert, J., ter Wee, P. M., Donker, A. J., and Stehouwer, C. D., Folic acid treatment of hyperhomocysteinemia in peritoneal dialysis patients: no change in endothelial function after long-term therapy, *Perit. Dial. Int.*, 18, 282, 1998.

48. Lentz, S. R., Malinow, M. R., Piegors, D. J., Bhopatkar-Teredesai, M., Faraci, F. M., and Heistad, D. D., Consequences of hyperhomocyst(e)inemia on vascular function in atherosclerotic monkeys, *Arterioscler. Thromb. Vasc. Biol.*, 17, 2930, 1997.

49. Urowitz, M. B., Bookman, A. A. M., Koehler, B. E., Gordon, D. A., Smythe, H. A., and Ogryzlo, M. A., The bimodal mortality pattern of systemic lupus erythematosus, *Am. J. Med.*, 60, 221, 1976.

50. Bulkley, B. H. and Roberts, W. C., The heart in systemic lupus erythematosus and the changes induced in it by corticosteroid therapy: a study of 36 necropsy patients, *Am. J. Med.*, 58, 243, 1975.

51. Abu-Shakra, M., Urowitz, M. B., Gladman, D. D., and Gough, J., Mortality studies in systemic lupus erythematosus: results from a single center. I. Causes of death, *J. Rheumatol.*, 22, 1259, 1995.

52. Petri, M., Perez-Gutthann, S., Spence, D., and Hochberg, M. C., Risk factors for coronary artery disease in patients with systemic lupus erythematosus, *Am. J. Med.*, 93, 513, 1992.

53. Petri, M. and Hamper, U., Frequency of atherosclerosis detected by carotid duplex in SLE [abstract], *Arthritis Rheum.*, 40, 9(Suppl.), S219, 1997.

54. Manzi, S., Selzer, F., Sutton-Tyrrell, K., Fitzgerald, S. G., Rairie, J. E., Tracy, R. P., and Kuller, L. H., Prevalence and risk factors of carotid plaque in women with systemic lupus erythematosus, *Arthritis Rheum.*, 42, 51, 1999.

55. Petri, M., Lakatta, C., Magder, L., and Goldman, D. W., Effect of prednisone and hydroxychloroquine on coronary artery disease risk factors in systemic lupus erythematosus: a longitudinal data analysis, *Am. J. Med.*, 96, 254, 1994.

56. Petri, M., Hydroxychloroquine use in the Baltimore Lupus Cohort: effects on lipids, glucose and thrombosis, *Lupus*, 5, S16, 1996.

57. Matsuura, E., Hasunuma, Y., Makita, Z., Nishi, S., and Koike, T., Oxidatively modified LDL as a target for β_2-glycoprotein I antibodies [abstract], *Lupus*, 5, 517, 1996.

58. Petri, M., Roubenoff, R., Dallal, G. E., Nadeau, M. R., Selhub, J., and Rosenberg, I. H., Plasma homocysteine as a risk factor for atherothrombotic events in systemic lupus erythematosus, *Lancet*, 348, 1120, 1996.

59. Petri, M., Vu, D., Omura, A., Yuen, J., Selhub, J., Rosenberg, I., and Roubenoff, R., Effectiveness of B-vitamin therapy in reducing plasma total homocysteine in patients with systemic lupus [abstract], *Arthritis Rheum*, 41, S241, 1998.

60. Fijnheer, R., Roest, M., Haas, F. J., De Groot, P. G., and Derksen, R. H., Homocysteine, methylene-tetrahydrofolate reductase polymorphism, antiphospholipid antibodies, and thromboembolic events in systemic lupus erythematosus: a retrospective cohort study, *J. Rheumatol.*, 25, 1737, 1998.

61. Momose, S., Detection of myocardial lesions by dipyridamole thallium-201 scintigraphy in patients with rheumatoid arthritis, *Ryumachi*, 35, 559, 1995.

62. Wislowska, M., Sypula, S., and Kowalik, I., Echocardiographic findings, 24-hour electrocardiographic Holter monitoring in patients with rheumatoid arthritis according to Steinbrocker's criteria, functional index, value of Waaler-Rose titre and duration of disease, *Clin. Rheumatol.*, 17, 369, 1998.

63. Kotha, P., McGreevy, M. J., Kotha, A., Look, M., and Weisman, M. H., Early deaths with thrombolytic therapy for acute myocardial infarction in corticosteroid-dependent rheumatoid arthritis, *Clin. Cardiol.*, 21, 853, 1998.

64. Weinblatt, M. E., Coblyn, J. S., Fox, D. A., Fraser, P. A., Holdsworth, D. E., Glass, D. N., and Trentham, D. E., Efficacy of low-dose methotrexate in rheumatoid arthritis, *N. Engl. J. Med.*, 312, 818, 1985.

65. Morgan, S. L., Baggott, J. E., Vaughn, W. H., Austin, J. S., Veitch, T. A., Lee, J. Y., Koopman, W. J., Krumdieck, C. L., and Alarcon, G. S., Supplementation with folic acid during methotrexate therapy for rheumatoid arthritis: a double-blind, placebo-controlled trial, *Ann. Intern. Med.*, 121, 833, 1994.

66. Morgan, S. L., Baggott, J. E., Lee, J. Y., and Alarcon, G. S., Folic acid supplementation prevents deficient blood folate levels and hyperhomocysteinemia during long-term, low-dose methotrexate therapy for rheumatoid arthritis: implications for cardiovascular disease prevention, *J. Rheumatol.*, 25, 441, 1998.

7 Vascular Tone Control and Raynaud's Phenomenon

Marco Matucci-Cerinic, Sergio Generini, Pan Sheng Fan, and M. Bashar Kahaleh

CONTENTS

I. INTRODUCTION

It is now clear that the endothelium is not a passive barrier but is the largest organ in the body that exerts striking control over several fundamental functions essential for life. One of the main functions of the endothelium is its contribution to the control of vascular tone. This is achieved by the continuous release of vasoactive mediators that oppose the vasodepressive effect of atmospheric and interstitial pressures. Thus, the regulation of vascular tone control is a fundamental function of the endothelium that allows organ function and survival through the maintenance of physiologic blood perfusion to tissues.

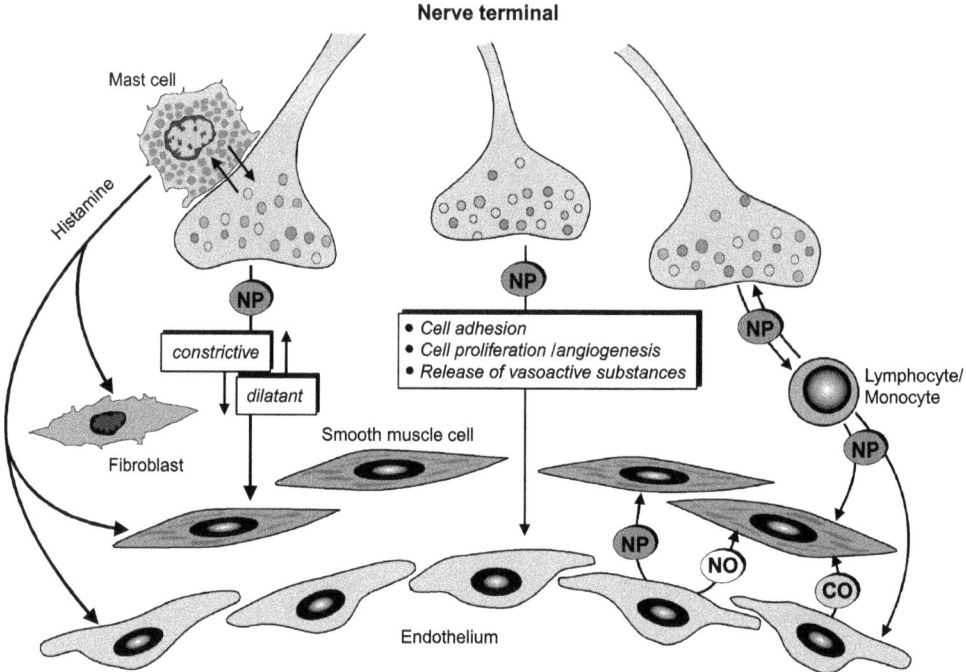

FIGURE 7.1 The effects of neuropeptides (NP) on smooth muscle cells and endothelial cells are reported. Neuropeptides may not only exert a vasodilating/constricting action but they may start mast cell and lymphocyte activation, thus, indirectly mediating immune and fibroblast activity.

In the past two decades, a great deal of knowledge has been achieved following the demonstration by Furchgott and Zawadski that the endothelium was one of the mediators and controllers of the vascular tone.[1] The statement, "obligatory role of endothelial cells to relax smooth muscle cells," that was used in their work to describe the function of the endothelium[1] is now believed to be an essential part of a larger interactive network which includes the nervous system. This network is multifaceted and operates in a complex fashion to maintain delicate balance between different cellular systems and mediators.

Several mediators, derived from the endothelium itself or present in the circulatory system, stimulate the endothelium to produce relaxing or constricting factors (Figure 7.1). This network is further refined by recent discoveries that will have an immense impact on our understanding and management of the regulation of vascular tone both in physiology and pathology. In humans, Raynaud's phenomenon (RP) is the best clinical example of defective vascular tone control that results from diverse sources. In this chapter we will examine the contributions of the two controlling systems — nervous and endothelial — of the vascular tone and discuss potential mechanisms that may lead to defective control of vascular tone in RP.

II. THE NERVOUS SYSTEM

The nervous system is one of the main contributors to the control of vascular tone. In the past, vascular tone was considered the domain of α1-adrenergic control and vasodilatation only a reflex event. The impressive advancement in the understanding of the function of the peripheral nervous system (PNS) and in particular of its perivascular nerve terminals (once considered noradrenergic or cholinergic) has allowed a wider awareness of the complexity of vascular tone control.

The capacity of neurotransmitters, released from different sets of nerve terminals (sensory and autonomic), to influence and control the functional performance of the vascular endothelium and of numerous other cells (mast cells, lymphocytes, macrophages, fibroblasts, and smooth muscle cells), suggests a dominant role for the PNS in the microenvironment (Figure 7.1). PNS does not only "sense" the surrounding events (immune, inflammatory, etc.) and inform the corresponding specialized nervous centers, but it also exerts a pivotal local control on these events, in particular on the vascular tone.[2] Thus, PNS and the vascular endothelium can be viewed as preferential partners in the maintenance of the desired blood flow in any given circumstance.

Nerve terminals release different neuropeptides that contribute to vascular tone control through their interaction with endothelial cells and smooth muscle cells. Sensory motor nerves release the neuropeptides substance P and calcitonin gene-related peptide (CGRP) which share an endothelial-dependent relaxing action by inducing the production and release of nitric oxide (NO). CGRP has also direct endothelium independent relaxing action on smooth muscle cells. The parasympathetic system, both through acethylcholine and the vasoactive intestinal peptide, relaxes smooth muscle cells that are contracted by the sympathetic system through the release of adrenaline, ATP, that act as cotransmitters, and neuropeptide Y.

A. SUBSTANCE P

Substance P (SP) is an undecapeptide of the tachykinins family, present in the central and peripheral nervous system. It is released by unmyelinated C type and small myelinated A-δ fibers of capsaicin-sensitive sensory neurons, which innervate the skin, mucous membranes, lungs, gastrointestinal system, and joints. SP contributes to vascular tone control by its potent vasodilating properties, and mediates nociceptive and neurogenic vasodilatation.[3] It also contributes to plasma extravasation[4] and induces mast cells to produce histamine, leukotrienes C_4 and B_4.[5] SP exerts important immune-modulating activities by enhancing chemotaxis, modulating neutrophil function, activation of macrophages (with consequent thromboxane release), monocytes (with cytokines release), platelets and leukocytes, and by the induction of the endothelial leukocyte adhesion molecule (ELAM) expression in microvascular endothelial cells.[6] SP is a mitogen to endothelial cells (stimulates neovascularization *in vivo* and the proliferation of endothelial cells *in vitro*), to fibroblasts and smooth muscle cells.[6] SP may also modulate lymphocyte function, stimulating T-cell proliferation and immunoglobulin synthesis *in vitro*, B-lymphocytes differentiation, and IL-2 expression in activated human T cells.[6]

At the peripheral level, SP directly stimulates nociceptors, partly acting via histamine release and partly via activation of neurokinin NK1 receptors on the postcapillary venular endothelial cells. This action results in increase local production of pain-producing substances, such as kinins and prostaglandins.

The several linked effects for SP on the vascular, immune, and connective tissue systems promote this peptide as an important mediator of inflammatory events with a peculiar proinflammatory activity. In particular, SP might be a protagonist of "neurogenic inflammation" that has a role in different phases in the pathogenesis of connective tissue and articular disorders.[7]

B. NEUROKININ A

Neurokinin A (NK-A) also belongs to the family of tachykinins and is as potent as SP in increasing vascular permeability.[8] NK-A acts through the interaction with several neurokinins receptors (NK1, NK2, and NK3) on the endothelial surface. In general, NK-A causes an endothelium-dependent vasorelaxation via activation of the NK2 receptor; still, the final effect can vary widely in different organs due to the engagement of different receptor subtypes and their density. For instance, in the skin microvasculature, NK-A induces vasodilation and extravasation of blood that are not related to NO release,[9] while in the stomach, it induces vasoconstriction that is mediated via an unusual NK2-like receptor.[10] In the intrapulmonary vessels, NK-A exerts an endothelium-independent constrictive effect[11] and, in cultured endothelial cells, it induces prostacyclin release by activation of the NK1 receptor subtype.[12]

C. Calcitonin Gene-Related Peptide

Calcitonin gene-related peptide (CGRP) is a 37 amino acid peptide, a product of an alternative processing of the calcitonin gene that is localized in the same capsaicin-sensitive sensory neurons that release SP. CGRP is a very potent vasodilator, relaxing vascular smooth muscle through an endothelium independent mechanism,[3] but, unlike SP, it exerts little effects on microvascular permeability. Moreover, CGRP potentates the edematous effect of IL-1,[13] promotes the activation of leukocytes and their adhesion to endothelial cells, and is a chemotactic to human T cells.[6]

CGRP's role in inflammation is controversial because, beside the proinflammatory action synergistic with SP, it also acts as a potent antiinflammatory substance by inhibiting edema and the inflammatory actions induced by histamine, leukotriene B_4, and serotonin.[14] CGRP also has immunomodulating action. The greatest component of its immunoregulatory activities is the modulation or antagonism of SP actions on immune cells. CGRP is able to reduce T-cell proliferation and IL-2 production and to inhibit natural killer (NK) activity, IFN-γ-induced H_2O_2 production, and antigen presentation by macrophages.[6]

The intradermal injection of CGRP in picomolar doses induces local erythema, which lasts for several hours. This effect is due to increase in cutaneous blood flow. Higher doses of CGRP can cause a painful sensation; this may be of relevance in pathological conditions. The intravenous administration of CGRP leads to facial flushing that highlights the potent microvascular vasodilating activity of CGRP.

D. Somatostatin

Somatostatin (SOM) is a tetradecapeptide released from the hypothalamus. It inhibits the release of growth hormone, thyrotropin-releasing hormone, and prolactine. It is also present in peripheral sensory fibers and in several organs, in particular the gastrointestinal tract. SOM has a wide range of biologic effects mediated by specific cell surface receptors. It acts as a neurotransmitter that affects glandular secretion, smooth muscle contractility, cell proliferation, immune and inflammatory cells.[6] SOM participates with other neuropeptides in nociception, employing different pathways than SP. SOM exhibits a potent analgesic activity and is utilized in the treatment of pain of diverse origin.[15] SOM induces marked vasoconstriction, particularly of the splanchnic circulatory system. For this reason, SOM is successfully used in esophageal bleeding and in gastrointestinal hemorrhagic disorders.

SOM inhibits the proliferation of human T lymphocytes and reduces γ-IFN production by monocytes.[6] SOM inhibits the release of histamine and leukotriene D_4 from immunologically stimulated human basophils, but fails to inhibit the release of histamine from mast cells.[6] SOM seems to be a selective antagonist of SP, inhibiting neutrophils chemotaxis and GTPase activity induced by SP.[16]

E. Acetylcholine

Acetylcholine (Ach) is localized in the neuromuscular junctions and, in the central nervous system (CNS), it is found in the basal forebrain cholinergic complex and the pontomesencephalotegmental cholinergic complex. It represents the neurotransmitter of all preganglionic vegetative nervous system fibers (both sympathetic and parasympathetic) acting by nicotinic receptors; the neurotransmitter of all postganglionic effector parasympathetic fibers, acting by muscarinic receptors; and the neurotransmitter of postganglionic sympathetic fibers innervating sudoripar glands. Certain data suggest that Ach may participate in circuits involved in nociception (e.g., Ach applied to a blister produced a brief but severe pain). Ach may act as a sensory neurotransmitter in thermal receptors, taste fiber endings, and chemoreceptors. The main effect of Ach, through specific muscarinic membrane receptors, is a negative dromotropic effect. In the blood vessels, Ach is a vasodilator that induces the release of NO from endothelial cells leading to smooth muscle cells relaxation.

F. Vasoactive Intestinal Polypeptide

Vasoactive intestinal polypeptide (VIP) is a 29 amino acids peptide, originally isolated from porcine intestine and named for its ability to alter enteric blood flow. It shares amino acid sequences similarity to other neuropeptides, like the VIP-related family, comprising glucagon, secretin, gastric inhibiting peptide, and growth-releasing hormone.

VIP is colocalized in postganglionic effector fibers of parasympathetic nervous system, together with Ach. Its action is synergistic with Ach (e.g., in salivary glands it increases vasodilatation and enhances the secretory effects of Ach). VIP induces endothelium-dependent relaxation in human uterine arteries, acting as a partial agonist on this vascular bed. It appears that endothelium-dependent relaxation, induced by VIP, can be entirely explained by the release of NO from endothelial cells.

G. Norepinephrine

Norepinephrine (NE) is concentrated in the CNS and is the main neurotransmitter of postganglionic nerves in the sympathetic PNS. NE is stored in vesicles inside the nerve terminals and released into the synaptic space together with dopamine in response to appropriate nervous stimulation. It activates pre- and post-synaptic receptors generating different effects depending on the characteristics and location of the receptors (α1, α2, β1, β2). NE has a generalized, potent, constrictive effect on peripheral vasculature. The constrictive effect of NE may be potentiated by endothelin that, with an endothelium-dependent mechanism, is able to increase locally the vascular sensitivity to NE.[17] This effect is counterbalanced by NO which may be released through stimulation of α1 and α2-adrenoceptors on the endothelium leading to and dampened NE-induced contractions of smooth muscle.[18] In specific vascular beds, such as the cerebral and coronary arteries, NE induces an endothelium-dependent relaxation.

H. Neuropeptide Y

Neuropeptide Y (NPY) is a peptide widely distributed throughout the central and peripheral nervous system, in the gastrointestinal tract, in the skin, and in several other organ systems. In many nerves, NPY is colocalized with noradrenergic transmitters in postganglionic sympathetic fibers, although in some parasympathetic ganglia, it is found in nerves containing acetylcholine.[19] In the sympathetic nerve terminals, NPY is also frequently colocalized with dynorphin, an opiate peptide. NPY is not unique to NE fibers, since it may also be found in megakaryocytes and platelets. It is released during nerve activation and ischemia and causes vasoconstriction and smooth muscle cell proliferation. It also has an angiogenic effect. NPY potentiates vasoconstriction produced by sympathetic nerve stimulation acting at the postjunctional level, primarily on endothelial cells.[19] Moreover, NPY may induce the release of cyclooxigenase metabolites, particularly TXA2; it also may have a synergistic effect on the vasoconstriction induced by the noradrenergic mediator in systemic venous and arterial circulation.[20] Thus, NPY, together with NE and dynorphin, may interact to regulate vascular smooth muscle contractility and, in particular, in the maintenance of the sympathetic tone.

III. THE ENDOTHELIUM

The endothelium has autocrine, paracrine, and endocrine activities[21] that are partially controlled by the PNS. Endothelial cells have the unusual duty of a twofold sensory-effector function. They sense the changes on both cellular poles, the circulatory and the interstitial, and respond by synthesizing factors that affect circulating elements (i.e. von Willebrand factor, adhesion molecules, tissue plasminogen activator, endothelin, etc.), but also acquaint the PNS terminals of the changes in order to work in concert in controlling smooth muscle cells leading to relaxation or contraction (Figure 7.1). The balance between the actions of the endothelium and that of the PNS is very

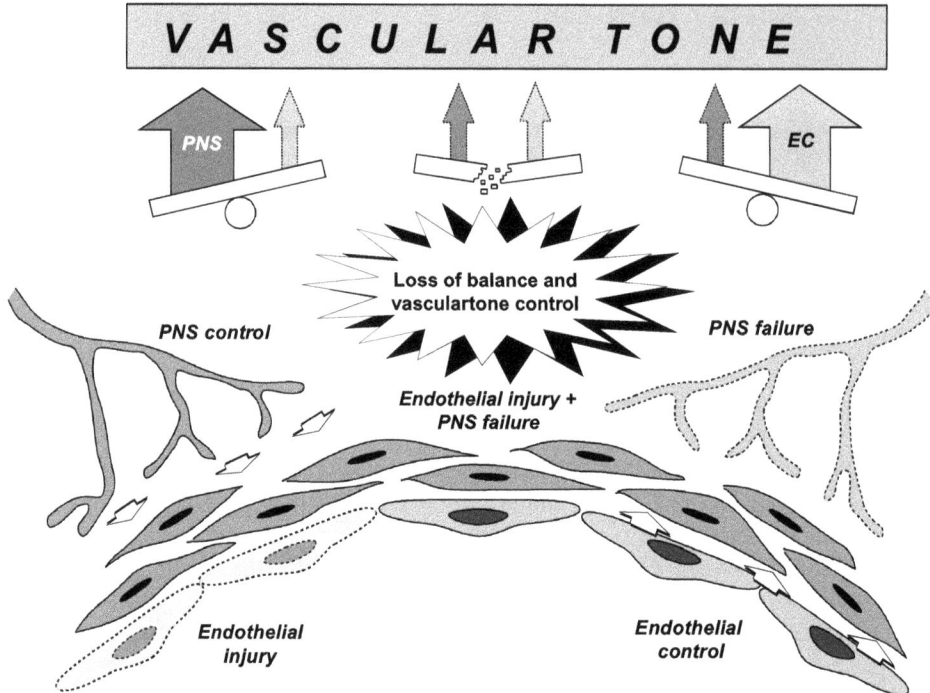

FIGURE 7.2 The balance of the endothelial and nervous control of the vascular tone is presented. The injury of both systems leads to the collapse of the vascular tone.

delicate and includes the concept of "dual" regulation of vascular tone (Figure 7.2). Around this duet, other circulating elements and other cells as platelets, mast cells, fibroblasts, and smooth muscle cells, contribute to the control of the vascular tone.

The endothelium modulates the vascular tone through the release of substances that relax or contract smooth muscle cells. Endothelium-derived vasoconstricting (endothelin, angiotensin II, and superoxide anions) and vasodilating (nitric oxide, carbon monoxide, prostacyclin, bradykinin, endothelium-derived hyperpolarizing factor) factors interact through binding to specific receptors on vascular cells and constitute an endocrine, paracrine, and autocrine system that integrates the mutual regulation of vascular factors production and action. This endothelial network modulates the vascular tone and, in a broader fashion, controls the trafficking of cells and fluid through the vessel wall. Moreover, these factors have an important impact on platelet activation, the function of the coagulation-fibrinolysis cascade and the proliferation of the endothelium itself and of smooth muscle cells, thus affecting vessel wall growth.

A. NITRIC OXIDE

The labile substance nitric oxide (NO) has a very short half-life of 5 to 6 sec. It is synthesized from L-arginine and oxygen through a NO synthase enzyme. The oxydoreduction reaction progresses through many passages, needs several cofactors (calcium, calmodulin, NADPH, FAD, and others), and the terminal products are NO and citrulline. In smooth muscle cells, NO-dependent relaxation is achieved through the activation of cyclic 3′-5′-guanosine monophosphate and, independently, by the hyperpolarizing effect of NO. Two types of NOS are present in the cells, constitutive (c-NOS) and an inducible (iNOS) form.

The first one, cNOS (also termed eNOS, for endothelium), is present in endothelial cells, but has been found also in platelets and in the CNS and PNS. Physiologic stimuli, like shear stress, stimulate the surface chemoreceptors of the endothelium that in turn activate c-NOS leading to an immediate NO production in picomolar quantities. This basal activity, linked to the pulsatility of the blood flow, is fundamental for the maintenance of the vascular tone.[22] Other factors may stimulate cNOS to promptly release NO, like acetylcholine, histamine, vasopressin, oxytocin, substance P, as well as thrombin, ADP, and serotonin. In particular, bradykinin stimulates its receptors on endothelial surfaces, increases calcium concentration, and activates cNOS, and, therefore, NO production.

The activation of the second enzyme system, iNOS, is slower (hours), but is associated with a release of nanomolar quantities of NO; in fact, NO synthesis in this system continues until the substrate is exhausted. iNOS is expressed not only in endothelial cells but also in immune cells, smooth muscle cells, hepatocytes, and astrocytes. The activation of iNOS is achieved mainly by bacterial lipopolysaccharides and/or the proinflammatory cytokines (IL-1, g IFN, TNF a).

The other important effect for NO includes inhibition of smooth muscle cells proliferation and platelet aggregation and adhesion. It is interesting here to note that NO can regulate eicosanoid synthesis,[23] inhibit the formation of endothelial-derived hyperpolarizing factor,[24] and modulate endothelin production.[25] Moreover, NO may guard against excessive vasoconstriction during maximal sympathetic stimulation.[26] These actions position NO as a principal regulator of vasorelaxation and the inflammatory response.

B. CARBON MONOXIDE

Carbon monoxide (CO) has been recently shown to be produced by endothelial cells and to induce vasorelaxation. Convincing evidence supports the presence of heme-oxygenase 2, which synthesizes carbon monoxides in endothelial cells and the adventitial nerves of blood vessels. The inhibition of heme-oxygenase 2 blocks endothelial dependent relaxation independent of the NO pathway. This suggests that CO, like NO, may have a role in endothelial derived relaxation properties.[27]

C. PROSTACYCLIN AND OTHER EICOSANOIDS

Prostaglandins are derived primarily from arachidonic acid stored in the cellular membrane of all cells. Arachidonic acid is released from membrane phospholipids primarily via the enzyme phospholipase A2. Release of arachidonic acid is a key rate-limiting step in prostaglandin synthesis. Once released, arachidonic acid can be either directly oxidized or converted via a number of biochemical pathways to prostaglandins, thromboxanes, leukotrienes, and hydroperoxides. Mechanical or chemical stimulation of the EC membrane activates prostaglandin biosynthetic pathways, in which cycloxygenase is the initial enzyme, inducing the production and release of biologically active prostaglandins (prostacyclin (PGI_2), PGE_2, PGD_2, $PGF_{2\alpha}$, and thromboxane A_2 (TXA_2)).

The biologic effects of prostaglandins depend on their interactions with their receptors and the relative amounts of the types of prostaglandins produced.[28] Thus, three different PGE_2 receptors have been isolated; moreover, receptors for PGD_2, PGI_2, $PGF_{2\alpha}$, and TXA_2 have also been characterized. All these receptors are expressed on smooth muscle cells, although the type of receptor expressed varies in different organs. Stimulation of the primary PGE_2 receptor, the PGI_2 receptor, and the PGD_2 receptor leads to smooth muscle relaxation through the release of intracellular cAMP. The other two PGE_2 receptors, the PGF_2 receptor, and the TXA_2 receptor initiate smooth muscle contraction through the release of intracellular calcium.

Two receptors expressed on platelets also have opposing actions — PGI_2 inhibits platelet aggregation, whereas TXA_2 induces platelet aggregation. PGE_2 receptor (EP_2) which is expressed on PMNs and lymphocytes, modulates many of the prostaglandins effect on immune functions. A confounding factor is that most receptors can be stimulated by most prostaglandins; the receptors merely differ in the relative amounts of individual prostaglandins needed for stimulation. Thus, if PGI_2 is present in large amounts in a tissue with PGE_2 receptors, a PGE_2-like response will occur.

Overall, PGE_2 and PGI_2 are proinflammatory, leading to vasodilatation and increased vascular permeability and, together with NO, have a synergic effect on vasodilatation and inhibition of platelet aggregation. In fact, PGI_2 is the most potent endogenous inhibitor of platelet aggregation yet discovered. PGE_2 also induces T-cell migration and production of metalloproteinases. In contrast, the direct effects of PGE_2 and PGI_2 on cellular immune functions are inhibitory; thus, PGE_2 inhibits T-cell responses and IL-2 production *in vitro,* and blocks B-cell maturation.

The upregulation of PGI_2 production by shear stress is mediated by increased arachidonic acid release and by a combined increase in the expression of COX and PGI_2 synthases[29] assuring a continuous production of prostanoids.[30] Bradykinin, adenosine, and thrombin are potent endothelial stimulators of the production and release of PGI_2 as well.

The physiological role of PGI_2 has been difficult to define. It has been suggested that the endothelium responds to vasoconstriction by the release of PGI_2 to restrain an aggressive vasoconstrictive process. Thus, in the lungs, "pulses" of PGI_2 reverse the sustained vasoconstriction initiated by PGF_2 or TXA_2.[31] Moreover, ET-1 mediated venoconstriction in humans is attenuated by the local generation of PGI_2.[32] Similar to NO, PGI_2 prevents the release of growth factors by the vascular wall and prevents vascular wall thickness. In contrast, potent vasoconstriction is regularly achieved by TXA_2, leucotrienes, and hydroperoxides.[33] Thus, stimulation of TXA_2 receptors not only results in smooth muscle contraction, but also in platelet aggregation, increased intestinal secretion, and increased glomerular filtration.

D. ENDOTHELIAL-DERIVED HYPERPOLARIZING FACTOR

Endothelial cells produce an endothelial-derived hyperpolarizing factor (EDHF) that induces smooth muscle cell hyperpolarization. This factor is neither NO nor PGI_2.[34] Still, it is similar to these vasoactive mediators since it mediates a vasorelaxing effect after endothelial stimulation by bradykinin and substance P.[35] EDHF has been characterized as an epoxyeicosatrienoic acid or a cannabinoid agonist such as anandamide, but its true nature remains unknown.[34] The hyperpolarizing effects are believed to be mediated through the opening of potassium channels in cell membranes.[36]

E. ANGIOTENSIN II

An intensely potent constrictive effect by angiotensin II (AT-II) on smooth muscle cells is mediated by activation of two distinct receptors, AT-I and AT-II. AT-II-induced vasodepression is associated with increased intracellular calcium levels and activation of protein kinase C. Norepinephrine is a potent stimulator of the production and release of AT-II, which in turn activates the sympathetic terminals, in a feed-back loop that links the endothelium with the PNS. AT-II stimulates the production of NO and peroxynitrite from endothelial cells[37] by activation of Ca^{2+}/calmodulin-dependent cNOS via AT-1 receptor.[38] Indeed, AT-II stimulates the proliferation of smooth muscle cells and angiogenesis. Thus, AT-II may be considered as a fundamental element in the integrated regulation of vascular tone.[39]

F. ENDOTHELIN

Endothelin (ET) is a 21 aminoacid peptide[40] that features 3 isoforms (ET1, 2, 3) with corresponding receptors on endothelial and smooth muscle cells membrane.[41] The release of ET from endothelial cells is a shear-sensitive process. Moreover, other substances like norepinephrine and thrombin stimulate the endothelial release of ET that in turn stimulate phospolipase C; consequently, accumulation of intracellular calcium activates a prolonged smooth muscle cell contraction. ET has a potent mitogenic effect on smooth muscle cells.[42] ET's role in vascular tone control is a modulatory one since it stimulates the production of TXA_2[43] leading to constriction and also it has the capacity to induce the release of NO, PGI_2, and PGE_2 that, in turn, induce a reactive vasorelaxation. On the other hand, PGE_2 and PGI_2 inhibit the production and secretion of ET from cultured endothelial cells. These interactive mechanisms illustrate the complexity of the balance between relaxation and constriction that assures the control of vascular tone and physiologic vessel patency.

G. Purinoreceptor

New insight in the functional multitude of the vascular endothelium is the description of the purinergic system[44] and the discovery of purinergic receptors on smooth muscle cells and endothelial cells.[45] Purines are thought to be involved in the tolerance of endothelial cells to acute and chronic hypoxia.[46] Thus, during reactive hyperemia following episodes of ischemia, ATP is released in conspicuous quantity from endothelial cells to activated platelets and interact with the P2Y-purinoceptor leading to NO releases that induces smooth muscle cell relaxation. It has been demonstrated that the preservation of guanine and adenine nucleotides may contribute the hypoxic tolerance of the endothelium.

H. The Endothelium as Producer of Neurotransmitters

Endothelial cells are shown recently to produce neurotransmitters, such as substance P, CGRP, and acetylcholine in rats[47] and humans.[48] Substance P, produced by endothelial cells, inhibits basal release of endothelin via a mechanism that requires the production of NO, and both substance P and CGRP suppress thrombin-stimulated endothelin release.[49] These findings enforce the unique capacity of the vascular endothelium in the control of vascular tone and demonstrate a new potential for therapeutic intervention in situations associated with defective control vascular tone.

A new important hypothesis is that endocannabinoids (anandamide) may be produced by endothelial cells and that may be involved in the regulation of the microvascular environment.[50] In particular, anandamide has been shown to stimulate NO release from endothelial cells[51] and to stimulate intracellular endothelial calcium transients.[52] This shows that new systems of signaling may play a role in the dynamic net that regulates the vascular tone in humans.

IV. THE LOSS OF VASCULAR TONE CONTROL IN RAYNAUD'S PHENOMENON

The pathophysiologic pathways that lead to RP are profoundly different in view of the diverse conditions associated with this phenomenon. Still, and in view of the preceding discussion, the PNS and the endothelium are inevitably involved in the genesis of all forms of RP. In general, it can be argued that in conditions where the endothelium is affected, the PNS will compensate and command the control of vascular tone, while if the PNS is affected by a disease process, then the endothelium will likely guide vascular tone. However, when both are affected, then the vascular tone control will definitively be compromised (Figure 7.2). For instance, in vasculitis, involvement of the endothelium may lead to a vascular instability; here if the disease process does not affect the PNS then it can offset and mask endothelial breakdown by rescuing the physiologic control of vascular tone. While, in carpal tunnel syndrome, where the insult involves the PNS, endothelial related mechanisms could counterbalance neuronal dysfunction. Unfortunately in disorders like systemic sclerosis, both systems are profoundly affected equally and early in the disease that a significant disintegration of the major mechanisms of vascular tone control ensues leading to the emergence of an aggressive RP and consequent vascular complications.

A. Endothelial Dysfunction

Endothelial dysfunction is the main event associated with the development of RP, particularly in the connective tissue disorders. Discussions concerning mechanisms of endothelial injury/dysfunction are beyond the scope of this chapter. Still, antiendothelial antibodies, products of cytotoxic T

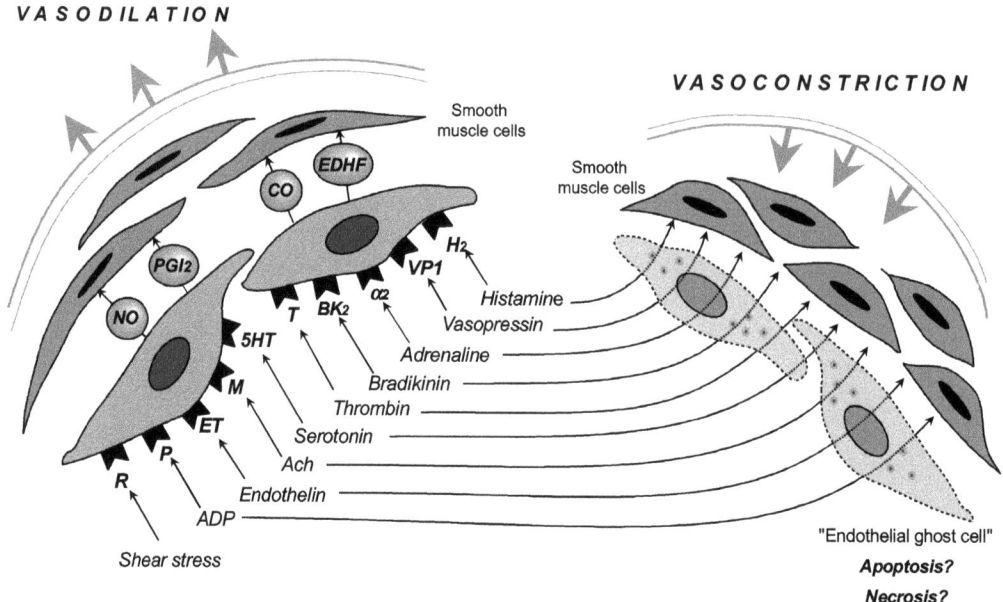

FIGURE 7.3 Several substances interact with specific receptors and induce an endothelial mediated vasorelaxation. When the endothelial cell is injured or apoptotic, the substances interact directly with smooth muscle cells inducing vasoconstriction (NO = nitric oxide, PGI_2 = prostacyclin, CO = carbon monoxide, EDHF = endothelial-derived hyperpolarizing factor).

cells, endothelial apoptosis and ischemia-reperfusion injury are some of the proposed mechanisms for endothelial dysfunction. The net effect of endothelial damage is a coordinated shift in the expression of endothelial genes leading to the appearance of proinflammatory, proconstrictive and proproliferative endothelial phenotype. Indeed, this leads to a cascade of events beginning with the reduction of intracellular G proteins,[53] activation of vascular cytokines (IL1, TNFα)[54] and expression of vascular adhesion molecules[55] which attract monocytes and leukocytes to adhere to the vessel wall. Thus, endothelial damage immensely affect the endothelial input in the control of vascular tone and eventually contributes to the proliferative vasculopathy that characterized these disorders. The enhanced platelet aggregation and the release of vasoconstrictor substances such as thrombin, serotonin, and thromboxane A_2 further accentuate this. The absence of functional endothelium may also lead to exposure of the interstitium and the vascular wall to the harmful effects of circulating elements and mediators. This may be critical since it allows a switch in the function of some substances from vasodilatation to vasoconstriction. Thus, substances that interact usually with the intact endothelium to induce vasodilatation, may in the absence of functional endothelium, act directly on smooth muscle cells inducing vasoconstriction and proliferation (i.e. bradykinin, serotonin etc.)[53] (Figure 7.3). This mechanism is deleterious because it may provoke not only profound vasoconstriction but also may contribute to the pathogenesis of occlusive vascular disease.

In the vasculature, the major source of oxidative stress is the superoxide anion, produced in endothelial cells in physiological conditions. Overwhelming evidence indicates that increased oxygen free radicals levels are the prime underlying mechanism for endothelial dysfunction in RP. The occurrence of daily episodes of RP and thus ischemia reperfusion-injury (I/R) leads to enhanced production of reactive oxygen species and oxidative modifications of low-density lipoproteins. However, it should be stressed that the endothelium possesses a cellular mechanism to adapt rapidly to the changing local environment. This important phenomenon is known as endothelial adaptation. I/R derived from RP stress endothelial cells inducing a process of adaptation that enables the cells to overcome stressful events.[56] The development of cell adaptation to oxygen radicals is related to increase in certain enzyme activities (catalase, superoxide dismutase, glutathione peroxidase etc), endothelial cells thus will promptly response to oxidative stress by synthesis of stress inducible proteins and scavenging enzymes. Still, in the phase of recurrent and sustained I/R, exhaustion of endothelial capacity for adaptation may finally evolve. Deficient endothelial adaptation to I/R may facilitate the development of vascular injury, and a cascade of events leading to the progression from benign RP to occlusive vascular disease.[57]

I/R injury may initiate or perpetuate the vascular disease since I/R is an inflammatory process that results from interplay of humoral and cellular components including the complement, cytokines and the contact activated cascades.[58] Platelets and neutrophils are routinely seen adhering to the endothelium following reperfusion injury. In general, soon after the start of reperfusion, endothelial dysfunction of ischemic vascular bed ensues. The initial endothelial dysfunction appears to be related to adhesion molecule expression and the recruitment of neutrophils and platelets. Indeed, EC dependent vascular responses are preserved after I/R in adhesion molecules deficient mice (ICAM and P-selectin); moreover, ICAM-1 deficient mice are resistant to cerebral I/R injury.[59,60] Both TNF-α and IL1 are released during I/R and contribute to upregulation of adhesion molecules expression. Moreover, TNF-α release in post-ischemic extremities is implicated in the genesis of the no-reflow since anti-TNF-α antibodies prevent the no-flow phenomenon.[61] Other cytokines released in the process of reperfusion includes IL-8 that further help recruit neutrophils, IL-1 convertase that may induce EC apoptosis, and endothelin-1 that enhances vasospasm and vascular injury.[62] Mast cell involvement in this process is mediated by adenosine that induces mast cells degranulation and subsequent arteriolar vasoconstriction.[63]

EC injury is believed to be mediated by superoxide radicals formed by endothelial cells and by neutrophils. Superoxide inhibits the release of NO, PGI_2, TPA, protein S, and heparin sulfate from EC leading to impairment of the vascular tone control and the thrombo-resistance within the microvasculature. Increased vascular permeability and loss of endothelial dependent vasodilatation[64] characterize EC dysfunction. Reduction in NO production by injured EC is suggested by prevention of EC dysfunction by direct NO donors. Moreover, inhaled NO can reduce the adhesive properties, vasoconstriction, and permeability of injured blood vessels in NO depleted tissue, suggesting a blood borne molecules that have an NO carrying capacity.[65] Complement activation may also play a decisive role in EC injury after I/R since the soluble complement receptor CR1 significantly reduces tissue injury by blocking complement deposition.[66] Moreover, intracellular oxygen derived free radicals activate NF-kappa B mediated complement C3b deposition on MVEC membrane.[67]

It is intriguing here to note that localized I/R vascular insult may lead to generalized vascular dysfunction as noted in the pulmonary vascular beds after mesenteric I/R.[68]

B. Peripheral Nervous System Dysfunction

Damage to the PNS in different physiological and pathophysiological circumstances may alter the balance between relaxing and constricting factors. In carpal tunnel syndrome, prolonged compression of the median nerve provokes failure of the sensory system and therefore may initiate RP. In systemic sclerosis the dysregulation of the neural control of vascular tone in RP is suggested by deficiency of the vasodilatory neuropeptides, possibly due to sensory system damage.[69] The possibility that selective dysfunction in CGRP nerve fibers may be implicated in the pathophysiology of RP and consistent with a local fault in the digital vasculature has been suggested. In the skin of RP, scleroderma and vibration white fingers, a consistent deficiency of CGRP fibers has been detected.[70,71] Indeed, the sensitivity of the digital cutaneous microvasculature to intradermal injection of endothelin 1 (that elicits the erythematous flare that is propagated by CGRP-ergic fibers) and CGRP is strongly diminished suggesting that a deficiency of CGRP containing nerves is present in the digital skin of RP.[72] An interesting finding here is the reported tendency toward higher density of neuropeptide Y positive fibers in the forearm skin of RP patients.[73,74] The tight correlation between the dysfunction of the peripheral nervous system and RP has been recently confirmed in a study where the involvement of the peripheral nervous system has been found to overlap topographically with surface areas involved in dysregulated vascular tone control.[75] Suggesting again the intricate interplay between the vascular and neurologic system in disease pathogenesis. Better understanding of this interplay will undoubtedly improve our understanding of the disease itself and will result in more effective therapeutic interventions.

REFERENCES

1. Furchgott RF and Zawadski JV: The obligatory role of endothelial cells in the relaxation of arterial smooth muscle by acethylcholine. *Nature* 1980; 288: 373–6.
2. Ralevic V and Burnstock G: *Neural Endothelial Interactions in the Control of Vascular Tone.* Texas: Landes Publishing Co., 1993.
3. Mione MC, Ralevic V, and Burnstock G: Peptides and vasomotor mechanisms. *Pharmacol Ther* 1990; 46: 429–468.
4. Lembeck F and Holzer P: Substance P as a neurogenic mediator of antidromic vasodilation and neurogenic plasma extravasation. *Naunyn Schmiedebergs Arch Pharmacol* 1979; 310: 175–183.
5. Bienenstock J et al.: Evidence for mast cells nerve interactions. In E. Goetz (Ed): *Neuroimmune Networks: Physiology and Diseases,* New York: Alan R. Liss, 1989; 275–310.
6. Matucci-Cerinic M: Sensory neuropeptides and rheumatic diseases. *Rheum Dis Clinics N Am* 1993; 19, 975.
7. Matucci-Cerinic M, Cutolo M, Generini S, and Konttinen Y: Neuropeptides and hormones in arthritis. *Curr Op Rheumatol* 1998;
8. Couture R and Kerouac R: Plasma extravasation induced by mammalian tachykinins in rat skin: influence of anaesthetic agents and an acetylcholine antagonist. *Br J Pharmacol* 1987; 91: 265–273.
9. Ralevic V, Khalil Z, Helme RD, and Dusting GJ: Role of nitric oxide in the actions of substance P and other mediators of inflammation in rat skin microvasculature. *Eur J Pharmacol* 1995; 25: 231–9.
10. Lippe I, Wachter CH, and Holzer P: Neurokinin A-induced vasoconstriction and muscular contraction in the rat isolated stomach: mediation by distinct and unusual neurokinin 2 receptors. *J Pharmacol Exp Ther* 1997; 28: 1294–302.
11. Shirahase H, Kanda M, Kurahashi K, Nakamura S, Usui H, and Shimizu Y: Endothelium-dependent contraction in intrapulmonary arteries: mediation by endothelial NK1 receptors and TXA2. *Br J Pharmacol* 1995; 115: 1215–20.
12. Marceau F, Tremblay B, Couture R, and Regoli D: Prostacyclin release induced by neurokinins in cultured human endothelial cells. *Can J Physiol Pharmacol* 1989; 67: 159–62.
13. Buckley TL, Brain SD, Collins PD, and Williams TJ: Inflammatory edema induced by interactions between Il-1 and the neuropeptide calcitonin gene related peptide. *J Immunol* 1991; 146: 3424–3430.
14. Raud J, Lundeberg T, Brodda-Jansen G, Theodorsson E, and Hedqvist P: Potent anti-inflammatory action of calcitonin gene related peptide. *Biochem Biophys Res Comun* 1991; 180: 1429–1435.
15. Chrubasik J, Meynadier J, Blond S, Scherpereel P, Ackerman E, Weinstock M, Bonath K, Cramer H, and Wunsch E: Somatostatin, a potent analgesic. *Lancet* 1984, 2: 1208–1209.
16. Kolasinski SL, Haines KA, Siegel EL, Cronstein BN, and Abramson SB: Neuropeptides and inflammation: a somatostatin analog as a selective antagonist of neutrophil activation by substance P. *Arthritis Rheum* 1992, 35: 369–375.
17. Zerrouk A, Champeroux P, Safar M, and Brisac AM: Role of endothelium in the endothelin-1-mediated potentiation of the norepinephrine response in the aorta of hypertensive rats. *J Hypertens* 1997; 15: 1101–11.
18. Kaneko K and Sunano S: Involvement of alpha-adrenoceptors in the endothelium-dependent depression of noradrenaline-induced contraction in rat aorta. *Eur J Pharmacol* 1993; 24: 195–200.
19. McDonald JK: NPY and related substances. *CRC Crit Rev Neurobiol* 1988; 4: 97–107.
20. Fabi F, Argiolas L, Ruvolo G, and del Basso P: Neuropeptide Y-induced potentiation of noradrenergic vasoconstriction in the human saphenous vein: involvement of endothelium generated thromboxane. *Br J Pharmacol* 1998; 124: 101–10.
21. Luscher TF and Barton M: Biology of the endothelium. *Clin Cardiol* 1997; 34: 425–35.

22. Busse R and Fleming I: Pulsatile stretch and shear stress: physical stimuli determining the production of endothelium derived relaxing factors. *J Vasc Res* 1998; 35: 73–84.
23. Kosonen O, Kankaanranta H, Malo-Ranta U, and Ristimaki A: Moilanen: inhibition by nitric oxide-releasing compounds of prostacyclin production in human endothelial cells. *Br J Pharmacol* 1998; 125: 247–54.
24. Bauersachs J, Popp R, Fleming I, and Busse R: Nitric oxide and endothelium-derived hyperpolarizing factor: formation and interactions. *Prostaglan Leukot Essent Fatty Acids* 1997; 57: 439–46.
25. Rizvi MA and Myers PR: Nitric oxide modulates basal and endothelin induced coronary artery vascular smooth muscle cell proliferation and collagen levels. *J Mol Cell Cardiol* 1997; 29: 1779–89.
26. King-van Vlack CE, Curtis SE, Mewburn JD, Cain SM, and Chapelr CK: Endothelial modulation of neural sympathetic vascular tone in canine skeletal muscle. *J Appl Physiol* 1998; 85: 1362–7.
27. Zakhary R, Gaine SP, Dinerman JL, Ruat M, and Flavahan NA: Heme oxygenase 2: endothelial and neuronal localisation and role in endothelium dependent relaxation. *PNAS* 1996; 93: 795–798.
28. Salvati P, Lamberti E, Ferrario R, et al: Long-term thromboxane-synthase inhibition prolongs survival in murine lupus nephritis. *Kidney Int* 1995; 47: 1169–1175.
29. Okahara K, Sun B, and Kambayashi J: Upregulation of prostacyclin synthesis-related gene expression by shear stress in vascular endothelial cells. *Arthrerioscler Thromb Vasc Biol* 1998; 18: 1922–6.
30. Duffy SJ, Tran BT, New G, Tudball RN, Esler MD, Harper RW, and Meredith IT: Continuous release of vasodilator prostanoids contributes to regulation of resting forearm bloof flow in humans. *Am J Physiol* 1998; 274: H1174–83.
31. Higenbottam T: Pathophysiology of pulmonary hypertension: a role for endothelial dysfunction. *Chest* 1994; 105 (Suppl. 2): 7s–12s.
32. Webb DJ and Haynes WG: Venoconstriction to endothelin-1 in humans is attenuated by local generation of prostacyclin but not nitric oxide. *J Cardiovasc Pharmacol* 1993; 22 (Suppl. 8): s317–20.
33. Camacho M, Lopez-Belmonte J, and Vila L: Rate of vasoconstrictor prostanoids released by endothelial cells depends on cyclooxygenase 2 expression and prostaglandin I synthase activity. *Circ Res* 1998; 83: 353–65.
34. Edwards G and Weston AH: Endothelium-derived hyperpolarizing factor: a critical appraisal. *Prog Drug Res* 1998; 50: 107–33.
35. Urakami-Harasawa L, Shimokawa H, Nakashima M, Egashira K, and Takeshita A: Importance of endothelium-derived hyperpolarizing factor in human arteries. *J Clin Invest* 1997; 100: 2793–9.
36. Vanhoutte PM: Other endothelial derived vasoactive factors. *Circulation* 1993; 87: V9–V17.
37. Pueyo ME, Arnal JF, Rami J, and Michel JB: Angiotensin II stimulates the production of NO and peroxynitrite in endothelial cells. *Am J Physiol* 1998; 274: C2414–20.
38. Saito S, Hirata Y, Emori T, Imai T, and Marumo F: Angiotensin II activates endothelial constitutive nitric oxide synthase via AT1 receptors. *Hypertens Res* 1996; 19: 201–206.
39. Cody RJ: The integrated effects of angiotensin II. *Am J Cardiol* 1997; 79: 9–11.
40. Ortega Mateo A and de Artinano AA: Highlights on endothelins-a review. *Pharmacol Res* 1997; 36: 339–51.
41. Lipa JE, Neligan PC, Perreault TM, Baribeau J, Levine RH, Knowlon RJ, and Pang CY: Vasoconstrictor effect of endothelin 1 in human skin: role of ETA and ETB receptors. *Am J Physiol* 1999; 276: H359–67.
42. Kahaleh BM and Fan PS: Effect of cytokines on the production of endothelin by endothelial cells. *Clin Exp Rheumatol* 1997; 15: 163–167.
43. Miura K, Yukumura T, Yamashita Y, et al: Renal and femoral vascular responses to endothelin-1 in dogs: role of prostaglandins. *J Pharmacol Exp Ther* 1991; 256: 11–17.
44. Burnstock G: Purinergic nerves. *Pharmacol Rev* 1972; 24: 509–581.
45. Burnstock G: Development and perspectives of the purinoceptor concept. *J Autonom Pharmacol* 1996; 16: 295–302.
46. Tretyakov AV and Farber HW: Endothelial cell tolerance to hypoxia: potential role of purine nucleotide phosphates. *J Clin Invest* 1995; 95: 738–744.
47. Milner P, Ralevic V, Hopwood AM, Fehér E, Lincoln J, Kirpatrick KA, and Burnstock G: Ultrastructural localisation of substance P and choline acetyltransferase in endothelial cells of rat coronary artery and release of substance P and acethycholine during hypoxia. *Experientia* 1989; 45: 121–125.

48. Milner P, Kirpatrick K, Ralevic V, Toothill V, Pearson J, and Burnstock G: Endothelial cells cultured from human umbilical vein release ATP substance P and acetylcholine in response to increased flow. *Proc R Soc London B,* 1990, 241: 245–248.

49. Spencer SP, Milner P, Bodin P, and Burnstock G: Modulation of endothelin release by vasoactive peptides localised in human umbilical vein endothelial cells. *Endothelium* 1996; 4: 309–317.

50. Bilfinger TV, Salzet M, Fimiani C, Deutsch D, and Stefano GB: Pharmacological evidence for anandamide amidase in human cardiac and vascular tissues. *Int J Cardiol* 1998; 30 (Suppl. 1): S3–13.

51. Stefano GB, Salzet M, Magazine HI, et al: Antagonist of LPS and IFN-γ induction of iNOS in human saphenous vein endothelium by morphine and anandamide by nitric oxide inhibition of adenylate cyclase. *J Cardiovasc Pharmacol* 1998; 31: 813–820.

52. Fimiani C, Mattocks D, Cavani F, et al: Morphine and anandamide stimulate intracellular calcium transients in human arterial endothelial cells: coupling to nitric oxide release. *Cell Signaling* 1999; (in press).

53. Boulanger CM and Vanhoutte PM: G proteins and endothelium-dependent relaxations. *J Vascu Res* 1997; 34: 175–85.

54. Matucci-Cerinic M, Kahaleh BM, and LeRoy EC: The vascular involvement in systemic sclerosis. In *Systemic Sclerosis.* D Furst and P Clements, Eds. Lea and Febiger, Philadelphia, 153–173, 1995.

55. Kahaleh BM and Matucci-Cerinic M: Endothelial injury and its implication. In: G Neri Serneri, GF Gensini, R Abbate, D Prisco, Eds. *Thrombosis: An Update.* Scientific Press, Firenze, Italy, 649–658, 1992.

56. Briner VA, Tsai P, and Schrier RW: Bradykinin: potential for vascular constriction in the presence of endothelial injury. *Am J Physiol* 1993; 264: F322–327.

57. Matucci-Cerinic M, Generini S, Pignone A, and Cagnoni M: From Raynaud's phenomenon to systemic sclerosis: lack or exhaustion of adaptation? *Adv Org Biol* 1998; 6: 241–253.

58. Miller BE and Levy JH: The inflammatory response to cardiopulmonary bypass. *J Cardiothor Vasc Anest* 1997; 11: 355–66.

59. Banda MA, Lefer DJ, and Granger DN: Postischemic endothelium-dependent vascular reactivity is preserved in adhesion molecule-deficient mice. *Am J Physiol* 1997; 273: H2721–5.

60. Connelly ES Jr, Winfree CJ, Springer TA, Naka Y, Liao H, Yan SD, Stern DM, Soloman RA, Gutierrez-Ramos JC, and Pinksy DJ: Cerebral protection in homozygous null ICAM-1 mice after middle cerebral artery occlusion: role of neutrophil adhesion in the pathogenesis of stroke. *J Clin Invest* 1996; 97: 209–216.

61. Sternbergh WC III, Tuttle TM, Makhoul RG, Bear HD, Sobel M, and Fowler AA III: Postischemic extremities exhibit immediate release of tumor necrosis factor. *J Vasc Surg* 1994; 20: 474–481.

62. Hofman FM, Chen P, Jayaseelan R, Incardona F, Fisher M, and Zidovetzki R: Endothelin-1 induces production of the neutrophil chemotactic factor interleukin-8 by human brain-derived endothelial cells. *Blood* 1998; 92: 3064–3072.

63. Keller MW: Arteriolar constriction in skeletal muscle during vascular stunning: role of mast cells. *Am J Physiol* 1997; 272: H 2154–2163.

64. Fullerton DA, Eisenach JH, Friese RS, Agrafojo J, Sheridan BC, and McIntyre RC Jr: Impairment of endothelial-dependent pulmonary vasorelaxation after mesenteric ischemia/reperfusion. *Surgery* 1996; 120: 979–984.

65. Fox-Robichaud A, Payne D, Hasan SU, Ostrovsky L, Fairhead T, Reinhardt P, and Kubes P: Inhaled NO as a viable antiadhesive therapy for ishcemia/reperfusion injury of distal mircrovascular beds. *J Clin Invest* 1998; 101: 2497–2505.

66. Lehmann TG, Koeppel TA, Kirschfink M, Gebhard MM, Herfarth C, Otto G, and Post S: Complement inhibition by soluble complement receptor type 1 improves microcirculation after rat liver transplantation. *Transplantation* 1998; 66: 717–722.

67. Collard CD, Agah A, and Stahl GL: Complement activation following reoxygenation of hypoxic human endothelial cells: role of intracellular reactive oxygen species, NF-kappaB and new protein synthesis. *Immunopharmacology* 1998; 39: 39–50.

68. Fullerton DA, Eisenach JH, Friese RS, Agrafojo J, Sheridan BC, and McIntyre RC Jr: Impairment of endothelial-dependent pulmonary vasorelaxation after mesenteric ischemia/reperfusion. *Surgery* 1996; 120: 879–884.

69. Kahaleh BM and Matucci-Cerinic M: Raynaud's phenomenon and scleroderma: dysregulated neuroendothelial control of vascular tone. *Arth Rheum* 1995; 38: 1–4.

70. Bunker CB, Terenghi G, Springall DR, Polak JM, and Dowd PMl: Deficiency of calcitonin gene related peptide in RP. *Lancet* 1990; 336: 1530–1535.

71. Goldsmith PC, Molina FA, Bunker CB, and Dowd P: Cutaneous nerve fibre depletion in vibration white finger. *J R Soc Med* 1994; 87: 77–381.

72. Bunker CB, Goldsmith PC, Leslie TA, Hayes N, Foreman JC, and Dowd PM: Calcitonin gene related peptide, endothelin 1, the cutaneous microvasculature and RP. *Br J Dermatol* 1996; 134: 399–406.

73. Wallengren A, Akesson A, Scheja A, and Sundler F: Occurrence and distribution of peptidergic fibers in skin biopsies from patients with systemic sclerosis. *Acta Derm Venereol* 1996; 76: 126–128.

74. Akesson A and Ekman R: Gastrointestinal regulatory peptides in systemic sclerosis. *Arth Rheum* 1993; 36: 698–703.

75. Lori S, Matucci-Cerinic M, Casale R, Generini S, Lombardi A, Pignone A, Scaletti C, Gangemi PF, and Cagnoni M: Peripheral nervous system involvement in systemic sclerosis: the median nerve as target structure. *Clin Exp Rheumatol* 1996; 14: 601–605.

8 Antineutrophil Cytoplasmic Antibodies

Xavier Bosch and Josep Font

CONTENTS

I. INTRODUCTION

Antibodies against neutrophils were described as early as 1974 in patients with rheumatoid arthritis[1] and shortly thereafter in patients with renal disease.[2] The association of antineutrophil cytoplasmic autoantibodies (ANCA) with Wegener's granulomatosis (WG) was first reported in 1985 in a Dutch-Danish collaborative study.[3] Detection of ANCA is now an established tool in the clinical workup of patients with suspected systemic vasculitis, acute renal failure, or other signs of glomerular disease. Since the first reports on ANCA, the number of scientific papers investigating their clinical significance as well as their causative role in the development of systemic vasculitis has increased yearly.

II. ANCA TERMINOLOGY

The standard method for ANCA measurement is an indirect immunofluorescence (IIF) test in which ethanol-fixed neutrophils from healthy donors are incubated with patients' sera.[4,5] The IIF test is the most widely used screening test for ANCA, and it provides a means to divide ANCA into three groups according to the staining pattern of the granulocytes:

Cytoplasmic ANCA (C-ANCA): coarse granular staining of the cytoplasm, often with accentuated staining of the central part of the cell (between the nuclear lobes) (Figure 8.1).

Perinuclear ANCA (P-ANCA): staining of the nucleus, perinuclear area, or both, leaving the cytoplasm unstained (Figure 8.2).

Atypical staining (atypical ANCA): any positive staining of the cells other than the C-ANCA or P-ANCA pattern[6]

Various efforts have been made to subclassify atypical ANCA using allusive names such as "xANCA" or "snowdrift ANCA," but because these patterns have not been unequivocally described,

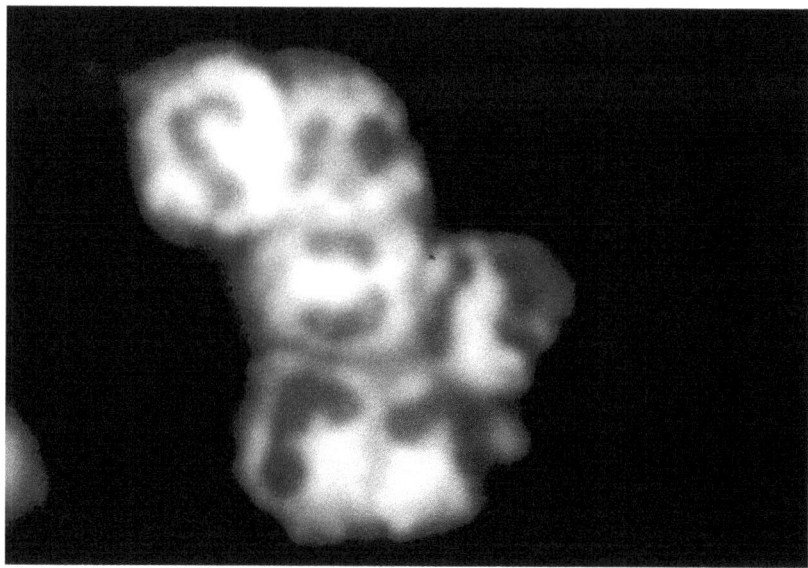

FIGURE 8.1 Cytoplasmic immunofluorescence staining pattern of ANCA on ethanol-fixed neutrophils.

their clinical meaning is unclear, and the antigenic targets not uniformly recognized, the preferred name for these staining patterns should be "atypical" until further research provides a better understanding of their significance.

The notation of the IIF patterns and the full form of the abbreviation ANCA tend to differ among authors. At the last meeting of the European Vasculitis Study Group in April 1998, its members agreed that ANCA stands for "antineutrophil cytoplasmic autoantibodies" and should be used as a clinical term, excluding, for instance, antibodies generated in animal models. References to ANCA patterns in immunofluorescence tests should be written with a capital letter followed by a hyphen, for instance, "C-ANCA," and the antibody specificity should be put in front, for instance,

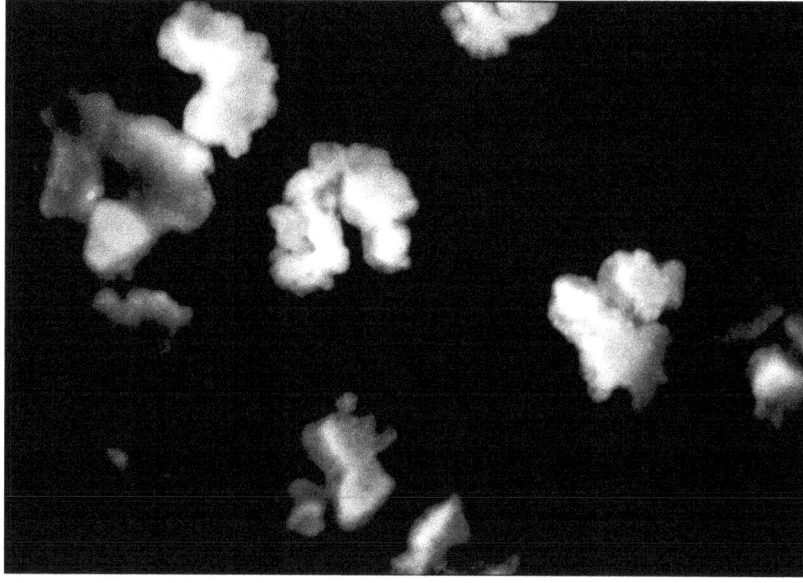

FIGURE 8.2 Perinuclear immunofluorescence staining pattern of ANCA on ethanol-fixed neutrophils.

"PR3-ANCA" (proteinase-3 ANCA). To indicate a combination of the immunofluorescence pattern and the antigen, the following format was suggested: "C-ANCA+/PR3-ANCA+."

III. ANCA-RELATED ANTIGENS AND TESTING METHODOLOGY

The number of antigens described as targets for ANCA is still increasing. The C-ANCA pattern is most strongly associated with PR3, whereas the P-ANCA pattern can be caused by antibodies against a number of different target antigens (Table 8.1). Examples of recently described antigens include catalase and alpha-enolase,[7] actin,[8] and high-mobility group nonhistone chromosomal proteins (HMG-1 and HMG-2).[9,10] Most of these specificities were found in atypical ANCA or P-ANCA sera.

The standard IIF test is still the most widely used screening test for ANCA, but only by the addition of solid phase assays can the antigenic specificity of ANCA be established. Especially in P-ANCA-positive sera, antigenic specificity determination of the antibodies is mandatory because several antigens with different clinical impacts are known to generate nuclear or perinuclear staining patterns (Table 8.1). Moreover, antinuclear antibodies (ANA) may give rise to nuclear reactivity that cannot be distinguished from that caused by other antibodies with the IIF test. ANCA enzyme-linked immunosorbent assays (ELISAs) may help overcome the diagnostic uncertainty of an unexpected P-ANCA positivity. In patients with systemic vasculitis, P-ANCA are most strongly associated with anti-myeloperoxidase (anti-MPO) antibodies. Other P-ANCA sera or atypical ANCA sera may react with lactoferrin, elastase, or bactericidal/permeability-increasing protein (BPI). ELISAs to detect these antigens are available in research settings.

Standardization of assay methodology and a number of antigens have been accomplished in a multicenter European study in which it was shown that PR3 and MPO, isolated from neutrophils by various methods, are good antigenic substrates for ELISAs.[11] With standardized assay methodology, reproducible results could be obtained between laboratories.[11] Results from a recent prospective study involving about 170 patients with new-onset systemic vasculitis[12] indicated that, for diagnostic purposes, the IIF test is an appropriate screening test for ANCA; that a positive IIF

TABLE 8.1
Target Antigens for ANCA

Azurophilic Granules	Specific Granules	Other	IIF Pattern
Proteinase-3			C-ANCA
Myeloperoxidase			P-ANCA
Elastase			
Cathepsin-G			P-ANCA
Beta-glucuronidase			P-ANCA
Lysozyme	Lysozyme		P-ANCA
Azurocidin			C-ANCA
BPI			C-ANCA
	Lactoferrin		P/Atypical
		Catalase	P/Atypical
		Alpha-enolase	P/Atypical
		HMG-1, HMG-2	P/Atypical
		Actin	Unknown

Note: BPI = bactericidal/permeability-increasing protein; HMG = high-mobility group non-histone chromosomal proteins; P/Atypical = P-ANCA pattern or atypical pattern.

test result should always be confirmed by an antigen-specific ELISA, at least for anti-PR3 and for anti-MPO; and that especially P-ANCA without an ELISA result has a low specificity for systemic vasculitis.

In conclusion, ANCA testing methodology should consist of screening by the IIF test, with confirmation of a positive test by ELISAs for the detection of anti-PR3 and anti-MPO antibodies. The value of refining assay technology (e.g., catching ELISAs, recombinant antigens) needs further investigation.

IV. DISEASES ASSOCIATED WITH ANCA

Since the first descriptions of ANCA, the number of diseases in which ANCA may be encountered has continued to increase. In addition to small-vessel vasculitis (i.e., WG, microscopic polyangiitis, and Churg-Strauss syndrome), the list now includes various rheumatic autoimmune diseases, inflammatory bowel disease, autoimmune liver diseases, infections, malignancies, myelodysplastic processes, and many others, even diabetes mellitus. The interpretation of many reports is, however, compromised by limited information about the methods utilized for ANCA detection.

ANCA-associated small-vessel vasculitis affects people of all ages but is most common in older adults in their 50s and 60s, and it affects men and women equally. In the U.S. the disease is more frequent among whites than blacks. Its incidence is approximately 2 in 100,000 people in the United Kingdom, and approximately 1 in 100,000 in Sweden. Although WG, microscopic polyangiitis, and Churg-Strauss syndrome are categorized as ANCA-associated small-vessel vasculitis, it is important to realize that a minority of patients with typical clinical and pathological features of these diseases are ANCA-negative.[13] Of importance, massive pulmonary hemorrhage caused by capillaritis (Figures 8.3 and 8.4) is the most life-threatening manifestation of ANCA-associated small-vessel vasculitis and warrants rapid institution of aggressive immunosuppressive therapy.

The most clear-cut association of a disease with ANCA directed against a specific target antigen remains the association between WG and PR3-ANCA. Between 80 and 95% of all ANCA found in WG are C-ANCA. The use of more sensitive PR3-ANCA-specific methods of detection has

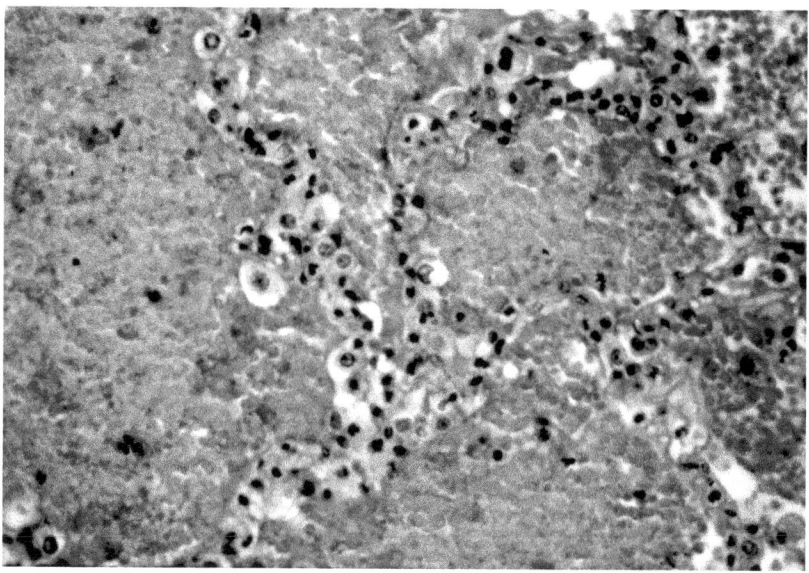

FIGURE 8.3 Necrotizing alveolar capillaritis. Massive alveolar hemorrhage with enlargement of interalveolar septa.

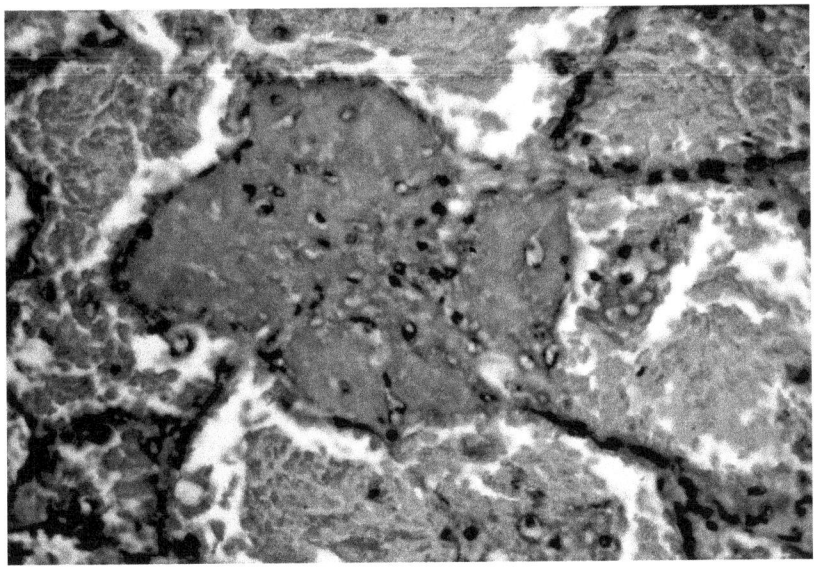

FIGURE 8.4 Necrotizing alveolar capillaritis. Fibrin clot projecting into adjacent alveoli.

confirmed that the C-ANCA phenomenon in WG is almost always associated with anti-PR3. It is estimated that 5 to 20% of ANCA in WG may be P-ANCA, which are mostly directed against MPO.[14]

More than 80% of patients with microscopic polyangiitis have ANCA, most often P-ANCA or anti-MPO. This helps distinguish microscopic polyangiitis from ANCA-negative small-vessel vasculitis, but does not distinguish microscopic polyangiitis from other types of disease associated with ANCA. Positive ANCA and negative serologic test for hepatitis B help differentiate microscopic polyangiitis from polyarteritis nodosa.[13] Finally, approximately 70% of patients with Churg-Strauss syndrome have ANCA, usually P-ANCA or anti-MPO.[13]

V. THE USEFULNESS OF ANCA FOR CLINICAL PRACTICE AND PREDICTIVE VALUE

The ANCA test can be negative even in active generalized disease, and a negative ANCA test does not rule out the diagnosis of systemic vasculitis. This is one of the main reasons why the ANCA test should not be used in place of a biopsy. ANCA may also be used to monitor disease activity. The predictive value of an ANCA rise for subsequent disease activity is disputed, however, and further studies are needed to confirm earlier reports about ANCA titer-guided therapy changes.[15]

As with any diagnostic test, the predictive value of ANCA depends on the pretest probability of the disease. In light of the wide variety of disease manifestations in patients with systemic vasculitis, the positive predictive value (PPV) and negative predictive value (NPV) can be calculated only for well-defined patient subgroups. If the sensitivity and specificity figures from the above-mentioned European study[12] are used for patients with renal disease, the PPV for pauci-immune necrotizing glomerulonephritis can be calculated to be 98% in patients with hematuria, proteinuria, and rapidly progressive renal insufficiency (NPV, 80%). In patients with hematuria and proteinuria but with normal renal function, the PPV drops to 47% (NPV, 99%).[15]

Because of the variation in presentation of WG and microscopic polyangiitis, with limited forms of disease and often an incomplete clinical picture, prevalence figures are not available and predictive values cannot be calculated. Thus, even with well-performing assays for ANCA testing, the value of the test is determined by the indication of ordering the test.[15]

VI. THE POTENTIAL PATHOGENETIC ROLE OF ANCA

Starting with the early publications on ANCAs, hypotheses have been raised about their role in the development of the necrotizing vasculitic lesion, but until today little has been known about their causative functions. In inflammatory conditions, leukocytes transmigrate across the endothelial wall, which involves a complex process of loose adhesion, rolling, integrin activation, firm adhesion, and the final arrival at the site of inflammation, possibly through a chemotactic gradient.[15] This process, in general, is not accompanied by lytic necrosis of the vessel wall. In systemic vasculits, however, it is believed that instead of migrating through the vessel wall, neutrophils degranulate onto the endothelium, causing direct vessel wall injury. Experimental research concentrating on how necrotizing vasculitis develops is therefore concentrated on deviations in the various components involved in the process of inflammatory cell activation and transmigration, and it is generally believed that ANCA may influence some if not all of these components.

What causes ANCA? No answer can be provided as yet. Prolonged or unusual presentation of ANCA antigens to the immune system in the context of infections or specific genetic background could lead to the formation of theses autoantibodies, but the process is not fully understood. Experimentally, the immune response toward ANCA antigens can now be studied by means of recombinant antigens. Recombinant proteinase-2, which is enzymatically active and recognized by ANCA sera, has been successfully expressed in a hematopoietic cell line.[16]

Data indicate that ANCA interfere with the effector pathway of the immune response relevant for vasculitic inflammation. Accessibility of ANCA antigens as targets for circulating antibodies appears to be a prerequisite for such an interaction. The ANCA antigens are stored in granules of cells of myelomonocytic lineages, and they can be translocated from the cytoplasm to the cell surface after stimulation by cytokines (e.g., TNF-alpha priming). The current concept implies that priming occurs at sites of infection whereby ANCA antigens are made accessible on circulating polymorphonuclear cells and monocytes. In contrast to viable polymorphonuclear cells, ANCA can interact with their antigens on the surface of apoptotic polymorphonuclear cells in the absence of priming.[17]

What is the consequence when ANCA bind to their cell-surface exposed antigens? *In vitro* primed polymorphonuclear cells are activated to produce reactive oxygen species, release lysosomal enzymes, and upregulate adhesion molecules to adhere to the endothelium.[18,19] On monocytes, ANCA have recently been shown to induce the release of interleukine-8.[20]

ANCA-mediated adherence of polymorphonuclear cells to the endothelium and release of toxic components from the granules could finally lead to endothelial damage. The presence of ANCA antigens in target tissue itself would help to explain the effect of ANCA binding even more directly. However, experiments so far have provided conflicting evidence for their presence in other tissue, such as the endothelium or renal tubular epithelium.[21,22] At present it should be assumed that the interaction of ANCA with their antigens occurs on the surface of polymorphonuclear cells or monocytes, or after they have been released and deposited on the target tissue. It is known from various animal models that proteolytic enzymes from neutrophil granules such as myeloperoxidase or elastases, which are at the same time ANCA antigens, can lead to damage of capillary walls, apoptosis of endothelial cells, loss of heparan sulfate in glomerular basement membranes, glomerulonephritis, and proteinuria when perfused to kidneys.[23,24] Table 8.2 lists the potential biologic functions of most ANCA target antigens. ANCA might facilitate proteolytic damage indirectly through interference of ANCA with the tight control of the proteolytic action by the enzyme's natural inhibitors (e.g., alpha-1 antitrypsin for proteinase-3 or ceruloplasmin for MPO). That the net effect of such interference would be increased tissue damage due to proteolysis has not been proved; indeed, the recent finding that anti-proteinase-3 ANCA inhibit the enzyme's proteolytic activity[25] does not support this view.

To date, no unequivocal animal models of ANCA-induced vasculitis have been reported, although there are several models that suggest a pathogenic role for ANCA. Brouwer et al.[24] immunized rats with human myeloperoxidase and then perfused the renal artery with hydrogen peroxide and human neutrophil extracts that included myeloperoxidase. The rats developed glom-

---

TABLE 8.2
Some Potential Biologic Functions of ANCA Antigens

Target Antigen	Biologic Functions
Proteinase-3	Favors migration of neutrophils to inflammatory tissue sites
	Platelet activation enhancement
	Modulation of the biologic activity of some inflammation mediators
	Bactericidal against Escherichia coli
	IL-8 release stimulation from endothelial cells
Myeloperoxidase	Macrophage function modulation
	Microbicidal activity against bacteria, viruses, and fungi
Cathepsin-G	Facilitates migration to inflammation sites
	Platelet activation
	Bactericidal activity
	Stimulation of lymphocytes
Elastase	Bactericidal against Escherichia coli
	Favors migration to inflammatory tissues
Lactoferrin	Bactericidal and bacteriostatic activities
	Immune response modulation

---

erulonephritis with crescent formation and had only transient low-level glomerular immune complexes. The authors concluded that the lesion resembled ANCA-associated glomerulonephritis in humans. However, Yang et al.[26] tried to reproduce these experiments but found extensive glomerular immune complexes by immunohistology. They concluded that this was a model of glomerulonephritis caused by *in situ* immune complex formation and did not resemble ANCA-glomerulonephritis, which is characterized by few or no immune deposits.

Several animal models with vasculitis and polyclonal B-cell activation have been found to have circulating ANCA, especially anti-MPO, including rats treated with mercury chloride and MRL-lpr/lpr mice. The importance of ANCA in these models, if any, is obscured by the many other potentially pathogenic autoantibodies that are also present.

Kobayashi et al.[27] reported in 1995 the interesting observation that rats injected with subnephritogenic doses of rabbit antiglomerular basement membrane as well as rabbit anti-rat MPO developed glomerular inflammation, but rats receiving anti-MPO alone or anti-glomerular basement membrane alone did not. They proposed that the dose of antiglomerular basement membrane antibodies was too low to cause nephritogenic activation of neutrophils, but was high enough to cause priming of neutrophils in glomeruli, which then allowed nephritogenic activation of neutrophils by the anti-MPO antibodies.

Herringa et al.[28] observed similar but more dramatic effects in a rat model with circulating anti-rat MPO antibodies induced by immunization with human MPO. When rats with circulating anti-rat MPO were injected with subnephritogenic doses of antiglomerular basement membrane antibodies, a severe glomerulonephritis with crescents developed. Normal rats given the same dose of antiglomerular basement membrane antibodies developed only minor glomerular injury.

Shoenfeld and associates[29,30] have induced ANCA production in mice by initiating an anti-idiotypic network response to intradermal immunization with human C-ANCA. Anti-anti-idiotypic antibodies were detected that had specificity for proteinase-3. The mice did not develop overt vasculitis, but they did develop perivascular mononuclear leukocyte infiltrates in the lungs.

VII. CONCLUSIONS

There is no doubt that ANCA are quite heterogeneous. There continues to be substantial progress in refining and standardizing techniques to detect and classify ANCA. Certainly, the diagnostic associations of these antibodies have been most consistent with WG and microscopic polyangiitis. There remains the possibility that certain ANCA may play a significant role, perhaps in enhancing disease expression in WG, microscopic polyangiitis, and other diseases; however, data at present are controversial and incomplete. The determination of ANCA status can be a very useful diagnostic aid to the evaluation of patients with WG or microscopic polyangiitis, but it cannot substitute for clinical expertise and, when feasible, histopathologic data, in the course of providing patient care. New developments in detection and characterization of ANCA will probably influence the diagnostic performance of these antibodies and concepts about their pathogenesis. On the basis of these conclusions, some authors consider it prudent at present to delay decisions to revise classification systems for vasculitis based principally on the presence and type of ANCA.[14]

REFERENCES

1. Wiik A and Munthe E. Complement fixing granulocyte-specific antinuclear factors in neutropenic cases of rheumatoid arthritis. *Immunology* 1974; 26: 1127–1134.
2. Davies DJ, Moran JE, and Niall JF. Segmental necrotising glomerulonephritis with antineutrophil antibody: possible arbovirus aetiology?. *BMJ* 1982; 285: 606.
3. Van der Woude FJ, Rasmussen N, Lobatto S, Wiik A, Permin H, van Es LA, et al. Autoantibodies against neutrophils and monocytes: tool for diagnosis and marker of disease activity in Wegener's granulomatosis. *Lancet* 1985; II: 425–429.
4. Wiik A. Delineation of a standard procedure for indirect immunofluorescence detection of ANCA. *APMIS* 1989; 6 (Suppl): 12–13.
5. Wiik A, Rasmussen N, and Wieslander J. Methods to detect autoantibodies to neutrophilic granulocytes. *Manual of Biological Markers of Disease* 1993; A9: 1–14.
6. Wiik A and van der Woude FJ. The new ACPA/ANCA nomenclature. *Neth J Med* 1990; 36: 107–108.
7. Roozendaal C, Zhao MH, Horst G, Lockwood CM, Kleibeuker JH, Limburg PC, et al. Catalase and alpha-enolase: two novel granulocyte autoantigens in inflammatory bowel disease (IBD). *Clin Exp Immunol* 1998; 112: 10–16.
8. Orth T, Gerken G, Kellner R, Meyer zum Buschenfelde KH, and Mayet WJ. Actin is a target antigen of anti-neutrophil cytoplasmic antibodies (ANCA) in autoimmune hepatitis type-1. *J Hepatol* 1997; 26: 37–47.
9. Uesugi H, Ozaki S, Sobajima J, Osakada F, Shirakawa H, Yoshida M, and Nakao K. Prevalence and characterization of novel pANCA, antibodies to the high mobility group non-histone chromosomal proteins HMG1 and HMG2, in systemic rheumatic diseases. *J Rheumatol* 1998; 25: 703–709.
10. Orth T, Kellner R, Diekmann O, Faust J, Meyer zum Buschenfelde KH, and Mayet WJ. Identification and characterization of autoantibodies against catalase and alpha-enolase in patients with primary sclerosing cholangitis. *Clin Exp Immunol* 1998; 112: 507–515.
11. Hagen EC, Andrassy K, Csernok E, Daha MR, Gaskin G, Gross W, et al. Development and standardization of solid phase assays for the detection of anti-neutrophil cytoplasmic antibodies (ANCA): a report on the second phase of an international cooperative study on the standardization of ANCA assays. *J Immunol Methods* 1996; 196: 1–15.
12. Hagen EC, Daha MR, Hermans J, Andrassy K, Csernok E, Gaskin G, et al. The diagnostic value of standardized assays for anti-neutrophil cytoplasmic antibodies (ANCA) in idiopathic systemic vasculitis: results of an international collaborative study. *Kidney Int* 1998; 53: 743–753.
13. Jennette JC and Falk RJ. Small-vessel vasculitis. *N Engl J Med* 1997; 337: 1512–1523.
14. Hoffman GS and Specks U. Antineutrophil cytoplasmic antibodies. *Arthritis Rheum* 1998; 41: 1521–1537.
15. Bajema IM and Hagen EC. Evolving concepts about the role of antineutrophil cytoplasm autoantibodies in systemic vasculitides. *Curr Opin Rheumatol* 1999; 11: 34–40.
16. Specks U, Fass DN, Fautsch MP, Hummel AM, and Viss M. Recombinant human proteinase 3, the Wegener's autoantigen, expressed in HMC-1 cells is enzymatically active and recognized by c-ANCA. *FEBS Lett* 1996; 390: 265–270.

17. Gilligan HM, Bredy B, Brady HR, Hebert MJ, Slayter HS, Xu Y, et al. Antineutrophil cytoplasmic autoantibodies interact with primary granule constituents on the surface of apoptotic neutrophils in the absence of neutrophil priming. *J Exp Med* 1996; 184: 2231–2241.

18. Falk RJ, Terrell RS, Charles LA, and Jennette JC. Anti-neutrophil cytoplasmic autoantibodies induce neutrophils to degranulate and produce oxygen radicals *in vitro. Proc Natl Acad Sci USA* 1990; 87: 4115–4119.

19. Keogan MT, Rifkin I, Ronda N, Lockwood CM, and Brown DL. Antineutrophil cytoplasm antibodies increase neutrophil adhesion to cultured human endothelium. *Adv Exp Med Biol* 1993; 336: 115–119.

20. Ralston DR, Marsh CB, Lowe MP, and Wewers MD. Antineutrophil cytoplasmic antibodies induce monocyte IL-8 release. Role of surface proteinase-3, alpha-1-antitrypsin, and fc-gamma receptors. *J Clin Invest* 1997; 100: 1416–1424.

21. Mayet WJ, Csernok E, Szymkowiak C, Gross WL, and Meyer zum Büschenfelde KH. Human endothelial cells express proteinase 3, the target antigen of anticytoplasmic antibodies in Wegener's granulomatosis. *Blood* 1993; 82: 1221–1229.

22. King WJ, Adu D, Daha MR, Brooks CJ, Radford DJ, Pall AA, et al. Endothelial cells and renal epithelial cells do not express the Wegener's autoantigen, proteinase 3. *Clin Exp Immunol* 1995; 102: 98–105.

23. Herringa P, van den Born J, Brouwer E, Dolman KM, Klok PA, Huitema MG, et al. Elastase, but not proteinase 3 (PR3), induces proteinuria associated with loss of glomerular basement membrane heparan sulphate after *in vivo* renal perfusion in rats. *Clin Exp Immunol* 1996; 105; 321–329.

24. Brouwer E, Huitema MG, Klok PA, de Weerd H, Cohen Tervaert JW, Weening JJ, et al. Anti-myeloperoxidase associated proliferative glomerulonephritis: an animal model. *J Exp Med* 1993; 177: 905–914.

25. Daouk GH, Palsson R, and Arnaout MA. Inhibition of proteinase 3 by ANCA and its correlation with disease activity in Wegener's granulomatosis. *Kidney Int* 1995; 47: 1528–1536.

26. Yang JJ, Jennette JC, and Falk RJ. Immune complex glomerulonephritis is induced in rats immunized with heterologous myeloperoxidase. *Clin Exp Immunol* 1994; 97: 466–473.

27. Kobayashi K, Shibata T, and Sugisaki T. Aggravation of rat nephrotoxic serum nephritis by anti-myeloperoxidase antibodies. *Kidney Int* 1995; 47: 454–463.

28. Herringa P, Brouwer E, Klok PA, Huitema MG, van dem Born J, Weening JJ, et al. Autoantibodies to myeloperoxidase aggravate mild anti-glomerular-basement-membrane-mediated glomerular injury in the rat. *Am J Pathol* 1996; 149: 1695–1706.

29. Blank M, Stein TM, Kopolovic J, Wiik A, Meroni PL, Conforti G, et al. Immunization with anti-neutrophil cytoplasmic antibody (ANCA) induces the production of mouse ANCA and perivascular lymphocyte infiltration. *Clin Exp Immunol* 1995; 102: 120–130.

30. Tomer Y, Gilburd B, Blank M, Lider O, Hershkoviz R, Fishman P, et al. Characterization of biologically active antineutrophil cytoplasmic antibodies in mice. *Arthritis Rheum* 1995; 38: 1375–1381.

9 Anti-Endothelial Cell Antibodies

Pier Luigi Meroni, Nicoletta Del Papa, and Elena Raschi

CONTENTS

I. INTRODUCTION

The endothelial cell (EC) surface is now considered a dynamic, heterogeneous organ that possesses synthetic, secretory, metabolic, and immunologic functions. Endothelial cells directly and indirectly play key roles in the development of vessel inflammatory injury associated with several vascular disorders.[1] In addition, EC surface molecules carry epitopes which may be targeted by anti-endothelial cell antibodies (AECA).[2]

Anti-endothelial cell antibodies were identified more than 20 years ago by using an indirect immunofluorescence (IIF) technique with mouse kidney sections as substrate.[3,4] Then, the availability of techniques for EC culture led to the development of sensitive and reproducible assays with the formal demonstration of AECA in a wide variety of disorders. Most of them have in common an immune-mediated damage to the vessel wall.[5] More recently, an extensive experimental literature has emerged supporting the possible pathogenetic role for AECA in human vasculitis. Several AECA-mediated effects on EC functions, including cytotoxic effects, release of endothelial mediators (vWF, prostacyclin), and the induction of an endothelial pro-inflammatory phenotype have been reported.[5]

II. AECA IN PRIMARY VASCULITIS

There is a general consensus in literature on the presence and high prevalence of AECA in primary autoimmune vasculitis (see Table 9.1).[2,5] Positivities for AECA have been found in more than 50% of Wegener's granulomatosis (WG) and micropolyarteritis (MPA) patients.[2,5] It is noteworthy that AECA coexist with anti-neutrophil cytoplasmic antigen antibody (ANCA), the other serological marker present in the majority of these patients.[6] However, both epidemiological and cross-inhibition studies clearly demonstrated that AECA is an antibody population distinct from ANCA.[7-10] Titration of AECA has been used in the follow-up of patients with WG, and it has been shown that titres fluctuate and correlate with other clinical or laboratory parameters of disease activity and of

TABLE 9.1
AECA in Systemic Autoimmune Vasculitis

Disease	Prevalence	Correlation with Disease Activity
WG/MPA	up to 50%	Yes, predictive for relapses
KS	up to 70% on resting EC	detected during acute disease
HUS	93% (13/14)	detected during acute disease
TTP	100% (3/3)	
SLE	up to 80%; higher prevalence in pts with renal involvement	Yes, renal involvement
APS	up to 60%	
RA with vasculitis	up to 60%; higher prevalence in pts with vasculitis	Yes, vasculitis
MCTD	45% (20/44)	
PSS/CREST	20–60%	Yes, vascular involvement
Polymyositis/dermatomyositis	44% (8/18)	
Behcet	25–50%; up to 80% in active disease	Yes
Idiopatic retinal vasculitis	35% (7/20)	
Takayasu Arteritis	up to 94% (17/18)	
Giant cell arteritis	up to 50%,with or without polymyalgia rheumatica	

endothelial damage.[7,8,10,11] Prospective analysis showed that the AECA titre rise preceded the development of relapses in ANCA-negative WG patients, and the persistence of AECA positivity after remission was associated with a highly increased risk for relapse in WG ANCA-negative patients.[10,11] As a whole, these findings suggest that AECA detection might also represent a useful serologic tool for monitoring primary small vessel vasculitis.

Kawasaki Disease (KD) is an immunologically mediated systemic vasculitis which affects almost exclusively the early childhood.[12] The etiology of the disease is still unknown, but it seems to be triggered, in a susceptible host, by a variety of infectious agents, resulting in a marked generalized immune activation. High levels of circulating pro-inflammatory cytokines have been described in the acute phase of KD.[13,14] These findings, together with the demonstration of com-plement-dependent cytotoxic AECA on cytokine-activated EC, suggested the hypothesis that endot-helial activation and neo-antigen expression or antigen up-regulation could represent a key patho-genetic mechanism.[15] In addition, several groups found a significantly increased prevalence of AECA in acute KD, even with resting EC. Increased IgM and IgG AECA (up to 72% and 42% of patients, respectively) were originally reported in KD children, as compared with both febrile and non-febrile controls.[16-19] Interestingly, a strong relationship has been shown between autoantibody levels and disease activity,[16,17] and in one study a switch from IgM to IgG AECA positivity was described during the follow-up.[18] However, no significant correlation between the presence of AECA and the development of cardiac aneurysms was observed in those studies.

III. AECA IN SECONDARY VASCULITIS

As reported in Table 9.1, AECA were found to be associated with vasculitis in several systemic autoimmune diseases.[2] In this chapter the main clinical association with the widest literature support will be addressed.

Systemic Lupus Erythematosus (SLE): several groups described AECA in sera of patients with SLE.[20-33] Endothelial binding was reported to be unrelated to the presence of other circulating autoantibodies (including anti-nuclear and anti-extractable nuclear antigen autoantibodies) and of immunocomplexes.[23,24,27-33] The prevalence of AECA in SLE patients was up to 88% depending on the different populations studied and the detection methods used. Several groups also showed a correlation between AECA levels and disease activity, and an association with lupus nephritis was reported.[27,28,30,31] Correlations between AECA and cutaneous vasculitis, pulmonary hypertension, serositis, and joint involvement were also anedoctically described.[2]

Systemic Sclerosis (SSc): AECA have been found in SSc sera with a prevalence ranging from 20 to 44%.[22,23,34-40] Recently, a significant tendency for AECA titres to increase with disease severity was described.[36-40] Interestingly, another group reported an association between AECA and other parameters of vessel damage such as increased pulmonary pressure values, digital ulcers, capillaroscopic abnormalities, and alveolo-capillary dysfunction.[40]

Rheumatoid Arthritis (RA): AECA prevalence was found higher (up to 67%) in patients with RA complicated by vasculitis compared to RA patients without vascular complications (up to 16%).[41,42] In the same studies a correlation between AECA levels and disease activity was also described.

Sjogren Syndrome (SS): a higher prevalence of AECA has been described in SS in comparison with normal controls. However, although the high levels of vWF in sera from SS patients suggested endothelial damage, no correlation was found between the AECA titres and any other clinical or serological features of the disease.[38,43]

Antiphospholipid Syndrome (APS): although APS cannot be regarded as a true vasculitis,[44] it is important to mention that a significant association between aPL and AECA has been reported by different groups, suggesting that AECA might represent another autoantibody present in APS sera.[21,24,45-48] *In vitro* and *ex-vivo* studies showed that antibodies against beta 2 glycoprotein I (β2GPI) — one of the anti-phospholipid antibody plasma cofactors — can recognize β2GPI adhered to endothelial surfaces and can be responsible for most of the whole anti-endothelial activity.[49-56] However, in addition to antibodies against adhered β2GPI, aPL sera contain true AECA since they are also able to immunoprecipitate constitutive endothelial cell membrane proteins.[47,51,57]

IV. ASSAYS FOR AECA DETECTION

Circulating antibodies directed against EC have been described independently by Lindqvist and Osterland and by Tan and Pearson using indirect immunofluorescence on tissue sections.[3,4] Recently, the availability of human EC cultures facilitated the development of more sensitive and specific techniques to detect antibodies reacting with surface endothelial antigens. Live or lightly fixed whole cells are now widely used in cell-surface radioimmunoassays or enzyme-linked immunosorbent (ELISA) assays.[5] However, the heterogenicity in AECA assays makes it difficult to compare results.[58] Nevertheless, it is now generally accepted that AECA might be of IgG, IgM, and IgA isotypes, IgG being the most common, and that the binding is mediated by F(ab)$_2$ fragments.[5] AECA have also been detected by standard complement-dependent microcytotoxicity assay[25] or by cytofluorimetry.[59,60] The presence of circulating autoantibodies against endothelial proteins has been confirmed by immunoblotting (IB) against crude EC preparations as well as membrane-enriched preparations.[42,62-64] Furthermore, two groups independently showed that selectively radio-labeled EC surface proteins can be immunoprecipitated by AECA-positive sera.[47,57] In WG and SLE sera the analysis of the immunoprecipitated proteins identified proteins with a molecular weight ranging from 200 to 25 kDa. The number of the immunoprecipitated bands was smaller (9 bands) than previously reported by using an immunoblotting against crude cell-membrane extract (19 bands).[62] Such a difference is likely related to the selective involvement of surface proteins in the immunoprecipitation assay with no contamination by endothelial intracellular structures.

TABLE 9.2
Characteristics of AECA in Systemic Autoimmune Vasculitis

Disease	Endothelial Ag	Methods of Detection	Cross-Reactivity	Pathogenetic Mechanisms
WG/MPA	Constitutive EC surface Proteins 120 KDa molecule Specifically recognized	Cell-ELISA, IB, IP	Fibroblasts and partially with mononuclear cells	C-fixation ADCC EC activation
KS	Non-immuno-precipitable IL-1, TNF-α, IFNγ-inducible	C'-cytotoxicity, cell-ELISA		C'-cytotoxicity
HUS	Non-immuno-precipitable Downregulated by IFNγ	C'-cytotoxicity	Non cross-reactivity with dermal fibroblasts or VSMC	C'-dependent cytoxicity
TTP	Immunoprecipitates a 43KDa cytosolic and nuclear protein	C'-cytotoxicity, IFF		C'-dependent cytotoxicity in large part due to IC
SLE	Directed against a group of constitutive and adhered proteins (15 to 200 KDa) or nucleosomal components	C'-cytotoxicity, cell-ELISA, IB, IP cytofluorimetry	Fibroblasts and partially with mononuclear cells	C'-fixation, ADCC
APS	In part directed against anti-β2GPI	Cell-ELISA, IB, IP	Dermal Fibroblasts	EC activation
RA Vasculitis	Directed against a group of molecules (16 to 68 KDa)	Cell-ELISA, IB, cytofluorimetry	Fibroblasts, PBMC, erythrocytes	
PSS/CREST	Constitutive EC Ag molecules ranging in size from 16–68 KDa	C'-cytotoxicity cell-ELISA, IB	Dermal Fibroblasts T-lymphoma cell line	C'-fixation, ADCC, EC activation
Behçet	Higher reactivity with microvascular EC	Cell-ELISA		
Takayasu Arteritis		cytofluorimetry		

V. CELL AND ANTIGEN SPECIFICITY

Despite their identification 25 years ago, little is known about the antigen specificities recognized by these antibodies. AECA-positive sera react with EC obtained from different human anatomical sources (large arterial as well as venous vessels, or small vessels, such as omental and renal microvasculature), with endothelial cell lines, or with EC of different animal origin.[2,5] Altogether these data support the presence of non-species-specific autoantibodies to endothelial antigens commonly expressed on the majority of vascular tissues. Higher reactivity of AECA-positive sera from Behçet patients with human omental microvascular EC in comparison with EC from umbilical cord vein (HUVEC) suggested the expression of antigens strictly related to the anatomical origin of cells.[65] However, no differential reactivity was found between HUVEC and brain endothelial cells when sera from SLE patients with central nervous system involvement were tested.[66] Antigenic epitopes for AECA are likely a heterogeneous family of molecules, some of them are specific for EC only, but the majority are apparently shared by human fibroblasts and, at least partially, by platelets and peripheral mononuclear cells. The anti-endothelial binding is unrelated to blood group antigens or HLA Class I or II molecules.[2,5,67]

Our own group clearly showed that AECA-positive WG and SLE sera immunoprecipitate several constitutive endothelial proteins exposed on the cell surface. In addition to the bands shared in common, some antigens were recognized only by WG or SLE sera, respectively. These findings suggest a selective endothelial antigen involvement in primary and secondary vasculitis.[29] Using immunoblotting analysis, two groups independently noted that SLE nephritis sera frequently recognized 38, 41, and 150 kDa antigens.[43,63] Sera from patients with diffuse or localized cutaneous SSc displayed antibodies reacting with proteins of enriched membranes or cytosol fractions ranging in size from 18 to 120 kDa.[68] Analysis of cellular proteins derived from human microvascular renal EC showed antibodies to 43 kDa cytosolic and nuclear proteins in sera from patients with thrombotic thrombocytopenic purpura (TTP) and hemolytic uremic syndrome (HUS); comparable reactivity was occasionally also found in sera from SLE, anti-glomerular basement nephropathy, and heparin-associated immune-thrombocytopenic purpura.[63]

Other specific AECA target antigens include sulphate proteoglycan or heparin-like molecules constitutively expressed on EC. Heparan sulphate shares sequences and functions with heparin and humoral autoimmunity to HS, and heparin has also been documented in human and murine SLE.[69,70] In SLE and other autoimmune diseases, antibodies to HS were shown to react with EC.[71,72] Furthermore, Shibata demonstrated that heparin inhibits AECA binding in a dose-dependent manner.[72] Studies demonstrated that part of the antigens recognized by AECA are expressed in the subendothelial matrix, and that anti-collagen antibodies can be part of the whole anti-endothelial reactivity in sera of primary and secondary autoimmune vasculitis.[43,73]

Endothelial antigens recognized by AECA can be modulated by cytokines. In fact, AECA in KS sera were cytotoxic only for IL-1β-, TNFα-, or IFNγ-treated, but not for resting EC. In contrast, the complement-cytotoxicity, found in HUS and in some TTP patients, was down-regulated by EC treatment with IFNγ.[15] Increased anti-endothelial binding to cytokine-activated EC was also reported in SLE sera.[59,74] These latter findings were not confirmed by other authors and AECA-positive sera from primary vasculitis recognized determinants constitutively present on EC surfaces that were not up-regulated (or only partially upregulated) by cytokine treatment.[9,75]

Specific targets for AECA also include molecules that adhere to EC ("planted" antigens). In line is the demonstration that part of the endothelial proteins immunoprecipitated by SLE sera were removed by extensive washes with high-molar buffers.[29] In addition, both polyclonal and monoclonal anti-DNA antibodies bind to EC *in vitro* by reacting with DNA or DNA/histone molecules adhered to the cell membranes through electric charges.[76,77] Similarly, the anti-endothelial activity described in sera from patients with anti-phospholipid syndrome has been shown to be largely mediated by antibodies specific for β2GPI, the anionic phospholipid binding plasma protein able to adhere to the EC surface membranes.[52,56] Antibodies reacting with platelet factor 4 (PF4) complexed to glycosaminoglycan molecules on the surface of EC may be part of the AECA detectable in heparin-associated thrombocytopenia.[78]

VI. THE PATHOGENETIC ROLE OF AECA

Immuno-mediated inflammatory damage of vessel walls is a feature common to several autoimmune vascular diseases. Endothelium is available for circulating autoantibodies and AECA were shown to react with surface EC membrane proteins. Altogether these findings suggest a possible pathogenetic role for these autoantibodies. Moreover, the clear correlation between AECA and an active vascular damage in autoimmune vasculitis supports their direct involvement.

In vitro studies showed that AECA are able to fix complement in primary and secondary vasculitis, raising the possibility that such a mechanism might participate in the vessel inflammation.[20,25,26] However, other studies have been unable to confirm these findings.[23,27,75,79] On the other hand, when endothelial monolayers, sensitized with WG AECA-positive sera or their IgG fractions, were incubated with Fcγ receptor positive mononuclear cells, an antibody-dependent cellular cytotoxicity (ADCC) could be found.[75] Interestingly, not all the sera displayed such an activity despite the presence of AECA, and there was no correlation with the antibody titres. It has been suggested that a peculiar immunoglobulin isotype might be a limiting factor in the ADCC phenomenon. These findings, together with the fact that ADCC requires a huge effector/target ratio, raise the possibility that an AECA-mediated endothelial cytotoxicity does not represent the main *in vivo* mechanism of vascular damage. On the contrary, AECA in KS and HUS display a complement-dependent cytotoxicity on cytokine-activated (IFNγ, IL1α/β, and TNFα) EC, suggesting that these patients generate an immune response directed to their abnormally stimulated vascular structures.[15]

Recently, AECA have been found to have functional effects on the endothelium. It has been reported that both polyclonal as well as monoclonal AECA induce an endothelial cell activation *in vitro* studies.[32,33,52,54,55,80-83] Actually, polyclonal IgG from primary vasculitis and from SSc and SLE patients were found to affect endothelial-leukocyte interactions as shown by cytokine and chemokine secretion, and E-Selectin, ICAM-1, and VCAM-1 expression on HUVEC monolayers.[32,33,80-83] Similarly, the incubation of EC with antibodies reacting with β2GPI, the plasma cofactor for anti-phospholipid antibodies, has been shown to induce EC activation with up-regulation of adhesion molecules, IL-6 production, and alteration in prostacyclin metabolism.[52,54,55,82,84] Experiments performed with specific antagonists for IL-1β and TNFα showed that activation occurs in part through autocrine cytokines secreted by the EC themselves.[32,55,80] Moreover, a murine AECA monoclonal antibody (mAb) generated by idiotypic manipulation immunoprecipitated a 70 kDa endothelial cell protein and displayed comparable EC activation effects *in vitro*.[83] Altogether these findings provide strong evidence of a pathogenetic role for AECA in autoimmune vasculitis.

More recently, Bordron et al. showed that AECA from SSc sera and a murine AECA mAb can induce phosphatidylserine (PS) exposure and DNA fragmentation in EC, raising the possibility of the induction of endothelial apoptosis by AECA.[85,86] The authors hypothesized that the AECA-induced EC apoptosis could explain, at least in part, the association between AECA and aPL since the latter could be produced after the exposure of PS (or PS/phospholipid-binding protein complexes) on EC undergoing apoptosis.[86]

Finally, AECA from APS sera have been shown to affect endothelial cell migration *in vitro*, providing an additional pathogenetic mechanism.[87]

Several *in vivo* experimental models support a role for AECA in endothelial damage. Goat anti-rabbit angiotensin converting enzyme (ACE) antibodies repeatedly injected intravenously in rabbits induce granular deposits of goat IgG on the glomerular endothelium, followed by the development of sub-epithelial granular deposits.[88] Preformed xeno- or allo-antibodies reactive with endothelial transplantation antigens were shown to lead to severe endothelial damage in animal models of xeno- or allo-grafts.[89]

Antibodies reactive with EC have been found to occur spontaneously in MLR *lpr/lpr*, a murine strain that develops a disease resembling human SLE.[53] It is not known whether anti-β2GPI and/or anti-HS antibodies, also detectable in the same mice, are involved in the whole anti-endothelial activity.

Naive mice can be induced to develop autoimmune disorders (such as SLE-, APS-, and WG-like diseases) when actively immunized with human autoantibodies carrying peculiar pathogenetic idiotypes. A disregulation of the physiological idiotypic network caused by the injected autoantibody was claimed to be responsible for the appearance of murine autoantibodies with the same antigen specificity, and for the demonstration of pathological findings resembling the respective human autoimmune disease characterized by a given autoantibody.[90] Accordingly, the injection of WG IgG fractions, displaying both anti-proteinase 3 (PR3) and AECA activity, was found to induce the appearance of murine anti-PR3 and anti-endothelial antibodies together with histopathological signs of renal and pulmonary vasculitis.[91] Interestingly, mice sera immunoprecipitated radiolabeled cell surface endothelial proteins with a molecular weight quite comparable to that recognized by human AECA positive WG sera.[91] In addition, when the same experimental design was performed by immunizing naive mice with human WG IgG depleted of anti-PR3 antibodies but still with anti-endothelial activity, the appearance of murine AECA and glomerular vascular inflammation was found once again.[92] The last findings strongly support the hypothesis of the direct *in vivo* pathogenetic activity of AECA.

An IgG mAb was obtained from these mice and it was shown (1) to bind to both human and murine EC, (2) to immunoprecipitate an EC membrane protein of 70 kDa quite comparable to that precipitated either by the WG IgG used for the immunization and by the whole mice sera, (3) to mediate an ADCC towards EC monolayers, and (4) to activate EC as demonstrated by the up-regulation of IL-6 secretion by HUVEC incubated in its presence.[83] The murine mAb is likely to be representative of the antibodies experimentally induced in naive mice and bears structural and relevant functional similarities with the AECA WG IgG spontaneously occurring in human pathology.

REFERENCES

1. Cines, D. B., Pollak, E. S., Buck, C. A., Loscalzo J., Zimmerman, G. A., McEver, R. P., Pober, J. S., Wick, T. M., Konkle, B. A., Schwartz, B. S., Barnathan, E. S., McCrae, K. R., Hug, B. A., Schmidt, A., and Stern, D. M., Endothelial cells in physiology and in the pathophysiology of vascular disorders, *Blood,* 91, 3527, 1998.
2. Meroni, P. L., Del Papa, N., Raschi, E., Tincani, A., Balestrieri, G., and Youinou, P., Antiendothelial cell antibodies (AECA): from a laboratory curiosity to another useful autoantibody, *The Decade of Autoimmunity,* Shoenfeld,Y., ed., Elsevier Science, Amsterdam, 1998.
3. Lindquist, K. J. and Osterland, C. K., Human antibodies to vascular endothelium, *Clin Exp Immunol,* 9, 753, 1971.
4. Tan, E. M. and Pearson, C. N., Rheumatic disease sera reactive with capillaries in the mouse kidney, *Arthritis Rheum,* 15, 23, 1972.
5. Meroni, P. L. and Youinou, P., Endothelial cell autoantibodies, *Autoantibodies,* Peter, J., Shoenfeld, Y. eds., Elsevier Science, Amsterdam, 1996.
6. Bajema, I. M. and Hagen, E. C., Evolving concepts about the role of antineutrophil cytoplasm autoantibodies in systemic vasculitides, *Curr Opin Rheumatol,* 11, 34, 1999.
7. Ferraro, G., Meroni, P. L., Tincani, A., Sinico, A., Barcellini, W., Radice, A., Gregorini, G., Froldi, M., Borghi, M. O., and Balestrieri, G., Anti-endothelial cell antibodies in patients with Wegener's granulomatosis and micropolyartheritis, *Clin Exp Immunol,* 79, 47, 1990.
8. Frampton, G., Jayne, D. R., Perry, G. J., Lockwood, C. M., and Cameron, J. S., Autoantibodies to endothelial cells and neutrophil cytoplasmic antigens in systemic vasculitis, *Clin Exp Immunol,* 82, 227, 1990.
9. Savage, C. O. S., Pottinger, B. E., Gaskin, G., Lockwood, C. M., Pusey, C. D., and Pearson, J. D., Vascular damage in Wegener's granulomatosis and microscopic polyartheritis: presence of antiendothelial cell antibodies and their relation to anti-neutrophil cytoplasmic antibodies, *Clin Exp Immunol,* 85, 14, 1991.
10. Chan, T. M., Frampton, G., Staines, N. A., Hobby, P., Perry, G. J., and Cameron, J. S., Clinical significance anti-endothelial cell antibodies in systemic vasculitis: a longitudinal study comparing anti-endothelial cell antibodies and anti-neutrophil cytoplasm antibodies, *Am J Kidney Dis,* 86, 727, 1993.
11. Del Papa, N., Guidali, L., Radice, A., Sinico, R. A., Moroni, G., Ponticelli, C., Domeneghetti, M. P., Farsi, A., Emmi, L., Tincani, A., Gregorini, G., Rizzi, R., Pasaleva, A., Dammacco, F., and Meroni, P. L., Antiendothelial cell antibodies in Wegener's granulomatosis and mycropolyarteritis, *Sarcoidosis,* 13, 260, 1996 (abstr).
12. Kawasaki, T., Acute febrile mucocutaneous syndrome with lymphoid involvement with specific desquamation of the fingers and the toes in children, *Jap J Allergy,* 16, 21, 1967.
13. Leung, D. Y. M., New developments in Kawasaki's disease, *Curr Opin Rheumatol,* 3, 46, 1990.
14. Barron, K. S., Immune abnormalities in Kawasaki disease: prognostic implications and insight into pathogenesis, *Cardiol Young,* 1, 206, 1991.
15. Leung, D. Y. M., Kawasaki's disease, *Curr Opin Rheumatol,* 5, 41, 1993.
16. Tizard, E. J., Baguley, E., Hughes, G. R. V., and Dillon, M. J., Anti-endothelial cell antibodies detected by a cellular based ELISA in Kawasaki disease, *Arch Dis Child,* 66, 189, 1991.
17. Kaneko, K., Savage, C. O. S., Pottinger, B. E., Shah, V., and Pearson, J. D., Antiendothelial cell antibodies can be cytotoxic to endothelial cells without cytokine pre-stimulation and correlate with ELISA antibody measurement in Kawasaki disease, *Clin Exp Immunol,* 98, 264, 1994.

18. Del Papa, N., Guidali, L., Salice, P., Pietrogrande, M. C., Cattaneo, E., De Gasperi, G. C., Bardare, M., Grazioli, S., Cattaneo, R., and Meroni, P. L., Anti-endothelial cell antibodies and anti-neutrophil cytoplasmic antibodies in Kawasaki disease, *Sarcoidosis*, 13, 276, 1996 (abstr).

19. Fujieda, M., Oishi, N., and Kurashige, T., Antibodies to endothelial cells in Kawasaki disease lyse endothelial cells without cytokine pretreatment, *Clin Exp Immunol*, 107, 120, 1997.

20. Cines, D. B., Lyss, A. P., Reeber, M., Bina, M., and De Horatius, R. J., Presence of complement-fixing anti-endothelial cell antibodies in systemic lupus erythematosus, *J Clin Invest*, 73, 611, 1984.

21. Le Roux, G., Wautier, M. P., Guillevin, L., and Wautier, J. L., IgG binding to endothelial cells in systemic lupus erythematosus, *Thromb Haemost*, 56, 144, 1986.

22. Hashemi, S., Smith, C. D., and Izaguite, C. A., Antiendothelial cell antibodies: detection and characterization using a cellular enzyme-linked immunosorbent assay, *J Lab Clin Med*, 109, 434, 1987.

23. Rosenbaum, J., Pottinger, B. E., Woo, P., Black, C. M., Louzou, S., Byron, M. A., and Pearson, J. D., Measurement and characterization of circulating anti-endothelial cell IgG in connective tissue diseases, *Clin Exp Immunol*, 72, 450, 1988.

24. Vismara, A., Meroni P. L., Tincani, A., Harris, E. N., Barcellini, W., Brucato, A., Khamashta, M. A., Hughes, G. R. V., Zanussi, C., and Balestrieri, G., Antiphospholipid antibodies and endothelial cells, *Clin Exp Immunol*, 74, 247, 1988.

25. Brasile, L., Kremer, J. M., Clarke, J. L, and Cerilli, J., Identification of an autoantibody to vascular endothelial cell-specific antigens in patients with systemic vasculitis, *Am J Med*, 87, 74, 1989.

26. Quadros, N. P., Roberts-Thompson, P. J., and Gallus, A. S., IgG and IgM antiendothelial cell antibodies in patients with collagen-vascular disorders, *Rheum Int,* 10, 113, 1990.

27. D'Cruz, D. P., Houssiau, F. A., Ramirez, G., Baguley, E., McCutcheon, J., Vianna, J., Haga, H. J., Swana, G. T., Khamashta, M. A., Taylor, J. C., Davies, D. R., and Hughes, G. R. V., Antibodies to endothelial cells in systemic lupus erythematosus: a potential marker for nephritis and vasculitis, *Clin Exp Immunol*, 85, 254, 1991.

28. Perry, G. J., Elston, T., Khouri, N. A., Chan, T. M., Cameron, J. S., and Frampton, G., Antiendothelial cell antibodies in lupus: correlations with renal injury and circulating markers of endothelial damage, *Quarterly J Med*, 86, 727, 1993.

29. Del Papa, N., Conforti, G., Gambini, D., La Rosa, L., Tincani, A., D'Cruz, D., Khamashta, M. A., Hughes, G. R. V., Balestrieri, G., and Meroni, P. L., Characterization of the endothelial surface proteins recognized by anti-endothelial antibodies in primary and secondary autoimmune vasculitis, *Clin Immunol Immunopath,* 70, 211, 1994.

30. Chan, E. M. and Chenk, I. H. P., Prospective study of antiendothelial cell antibodies in patients with systemic lupus erythematosus, *Clin Immunol Immunopath,* 78, 41, 1996.

31. Navarro, M., Cervera, R., Font, J., Reverter, J. C., Monteagudo, J., Escolar, G., Lopez-Soto, A., Ordinas, A., and Ingelmo, M., Antiendothelial cell antibodies in systemic autoimmune diseases: prevalence and clinical significance, *Lupus,* 6, 521, 1997.

32. Carvalho, D., Savage, C. O. S., Isenberg, D., and Pearson, J. D., IgG Anti-endothelial cell autoantibodies from patients with systemic lupus erythematosus or systemic vasculitis stimulate the release of two endothelial cell-derived mediators, which enhance adhesion molecule expression and leukocyte adhesion in an autocrine manner, *Arthritis Rheum,* 42, 631,1999.

33. Del Papa, N., Raschi, E., Moroni, G., Panzeri, P., Borghi, M. O., Ponticelli, C., Tincani, A., Balestrieri, G., and Meroni, P. L., Anti-endothelial cell IgG fractions from systemic lupus erythematosus patients bind to human endothelial cells and induce a pro-adhesive and a pro-inflammatory phenotype *in vitro, Lupus* (in press).

34. Holt, C. M., Lindsey, N., Moult, J., Malia, R. G., Greaves, M., Hume, A., Nowell, N. R., and Hughes, P., Antibody-dependent cellular cytotoxicity of vascular endothelium: characterization and pathogenic associations in systemic sclerosis, *Clin Exp Immunol*, 78, 359,1989.

35. Lima, J., Fonollosa, V., Fernandez-Cortijo, J., Ordi, J., Cuenca, R., Khamastha, M. A., Vilarderll, M., Simeon, C. P., and Pico, M., Platelet activation, endothelial cell dysfunction in the absence of anticardiolipin antibodies in systemic sclerosis, *J Rheumatol*, 18, 1833, 1991.

36. Salozhin, K. V., Shcherbakov, A. B., Nasonov, E. L., Kolesova, N. V., Romanov, I. A., and Guseva, N. G., Antiendothelial antibodies in systemic scleroderma and Raynaud's disease, *Terapevticheskii Arkhiv*, 67, 54, 1995.

37. Salojin, K. V., Le Tonqueze, M., Saraux, A., Nassonov, E. L., Dueymes, M., Piette, J. C., and Youinou, P., Antiendothelial cell antibodies: useful markers of systemic sclerosis, *Am J Med,* 102, 178, 1997.

38. Hebbar, M., Lassalle, P., Delneste, Y., Haltron, P. Y., Devulder, B., Tonnel, A. B., and Janin, A., Assessment of anti-endothelial cell antibodies in systemic sclerosis and Sjogren's syndrome, *Ann Rheum Dis,* 56, 230,1997.

39. Negi, V. S., Tripathy, N. K., Misra, R., and Nityanand, S., Antiendothelial cell antibodies in scleroderma correlate with severe digital ischemia and pulmonary arterial hypertension, *J Rheumatol*, 25, 462, 1998.

40. Pignone, A., Scaletti, C., Matucci-Cerinic, M., Generini, S., Cagnoni, M., Del Papa, N., Meroni, P. L., Falcini, F., Vazquez Abad, D., and Rothfield, N., Anti-endothelial cell antibodies in systemic sclerosis, *Clin Exp Rheumatol,* 16, 528, 1998.

41. Heurkens, A. H. M., Hiemstra, P. S., Lafeder, G. J. M., Daha, M. R., and Breedveld, F. C., Antiendothelial cell antibodies in patients with rheumatoid arthritis complicated by vasculitis, *Clin Exp Immunol,* 78, 7, 1989.

42. Van der Zee, J. M., Heurkens, A. H., van de Voort, E. A., Daha, M. R., and Breedveld, F. C., Characterization of anti-endothelial antibodies in patients with rheumatoid arthritis complicated by vasculitis, *Clin Exp Rheumatol,* 9, 589, 1991.

43. D'Cruz, D., Jedryka-Goral, A., and Hughes, G. R. V., Antibodies to endothelial cells in systemic lupus erythematosus and Sjogren's syndrome, *Endothelial Cell Autoantibodies,* Peter, J. and Shoenfeld, Y. Eds., Elsevier Science, Amsterdam, 1996.

44. Lie, J. T., Vasculopathy of the anti-phospholipid syndromes revisited: thrombosis is the culprit and vasculitis the consort, *Lupus,* 5, 368, 1996.

45. Hasselaar, P., Derksen, R. H. W., Blokzjil, L., and De Groot, P. G., Cross-reactivity of antibodies directed against cardiolipin, DNA, endothelial cells and blood platelets, *Thromb Haemost,* 63, 169, 1990.

46. Cervera, R., Khamashta, M. A., Font, J., Ramirez, G., D'Cruz, D., Montalban, J., Ingelmo, M., and Hughes, G. R. V., Antiendothelial cell antibodies in patients with the anti-phospholipid syndrome, *Autoimmunity,* 11, 1, 1991.

47. McCrae, K. R., DeMichele, A., Samuels P., Roth, D., Kuo A., Meng, K. H., Rauch, J., and Cines, D. B., Detection of endothelial cell reactive immunoglobulin in patients with antiphospholipid antibodies, *Br J Haemathol,* 79, 595, 1991.

48. Del Papa, N., Meroni, P. L., Tincani, A., Harris, E. N., Pierangeli, S. S., Barcellini, W., Borghi, M. O., Balestrieri, G., and Zanussi, C., Relationship between anti-phospholipid and anti-endothelial cell antibodies: further characterization of the reactivity on resting and cytokine-activated endothelial cells, *Clin Exp Rheumatol,* 10, 37, 1992.

49. McIntyre J. A., Immune recognition at the maternal-fetal interface: overview, *Am J Reprod Immunol,* 28, 127, 1992.

50. La Rosa, L., Meroni, P. L., Tincani, A., Balestrieri, G., Faden, A., Lojacono, A., Morassi, L., Brocchi, E., Del Papa, N., Gharavi, A. E., Sammaritano, L., and Lockshin, M. D., β2-glycoprotein I and placental anti-coagulant protein I in placentae from patients with anti-phospholipid syndrome, *J Rheumatol,* 21, 1684, 1994.

51. Del Papa, N., Conforti, G., Gambini, D., Barcellini, W., Borghi, M. O., Fain, C., Tincani, A., Balestrieri, G., Tedesco, F., and Meroni, P. L., Characterization of anti-endothelial cell antibodies in anti-phospholipid syndrome, *Molecular Basis of Human Diseases,* Polli, E. E. Ed., Amsterdam, London, New York, Tokyo, Excerpta Medica, 1994.

52. Del Papa, N., Guidali, L., Spatola, L., Bonara, P., Borghi, M. O., Tincani, A., Balestrieri, G., and Meroni, P. L., Relationship between anti-phospholipid and anti-endothelial antibodies III: β2-glycoprotein I mediates the antibody binding to endothelial membranes and induces the expression of adhesion molecules, *Clin Exp Rheumatol,* 13, 179, 1995.

53. Le Tonqueze, M., Salozhin, K., Dueymes, M., Piette, J. C., Lovalev, V., Shoenfeld, Y., Nassonov, E., and Youinou, P., Role of β2-glycoprotein I in the anti-phospholipid antibody binding to endothelial cells, *Lupus,* 4, 179, 1995.

54. Del Papa, N., Guidali, L., Sala, A., Buccellati, C., Khamashta, M. A., Ichikawa, K., Koike, T., Balestrieri, G., Tincani, A., Hughes, G. R. V., and Meroni, P. L., Endothelial cell as target for antiphospholipid antibodies, *Arthritis Rheum*, 40, 551, 1997.

55. Del Papa, N., Raschi, E., Catelli, L., Khamashta, M. A., Ichikawa, K., Tincani, A., Balestrieri, G., and Meroni, P. L., Endothelial cells as a target for antiphospholipid antibodies: role of anti-beta2 glycoprotein I antibodies, *Am J Reproduct Immunol*, 38, 212, 1997.

56. Del Papa, N., Sheng, Y. H., Raschi, E., Kandiah, D. A., Tincani, A., Khamashta, M. A., Atsumi, T., Hughes, G. R. V., Ichikawa, K., Koike, T., Balestrieri, G., Krilis, S. A., and Meroni P. L., Human β2-glycoprotein I binds to endothelial cells through a cluster of lysine residues that are critical for anionic phospholipid binding and offers epitopes for anti-β2-glycoprotein I antibodies, *J Immunol*, 1998.

57. Del Papa, N., Conforti, G., Gambini, D., La Rosa, L., Tincani, A., D'Cruz, D., Khamashta, M. A., Hughes, G. R. V., Balestrieri, G., and Meroni, P. L., Characterization of the endothelial surface proteins recognized by anti-endothelial antibodies in primary and secondary autoimmune vasculitis, *Clin Immunol Immunopath*, 70, 211, 1994.

58. Youinou, P., Meroni, P. L., Khamashta, M. A., and Shoenfeld, Y. A., Need for standardization of the anti-endothelial-cell antibody test, *Immunology Today*, 16, 363, 1995.

59. Quadros, N. P., Roberts-Thomson, P. J., and Gallus, A. S., Sera from patients with systemic lupus erythematosus demonstrate enhanced IgG binding to endothelial cells pretreated with tumour necrosis factor alpha, *Rheumatol Intern*, 153, 99, 1995.

60. Westphal, R., Boerbooms, A. M. T. H., Schalkwijk, C. J. M., Kwast, H., De Weijert, M., Jacobs, C., Vierwinden, G., Ruiter, D. J., Van de Putte, L. B. A., and De Waal, R. M. W., Antiendothelial cell antibodies in sera of patients with autoimmune diseases: comparison between ELISA and FACS analysis, *Clin Exp Immunol*, 96, 444, 1994.

61. Heurkens, A. H. M., Gorter, A., de Vreede, T. M., Edgell, C. S., Breedveld, F. C., and Daha, M. R., Methods for the detection of anti-endothelial antibodies by enzyme-linked immunosorbent assay, *J Immunol Methods*, 141, 33, 1991.

62. van der Zee, J. M., Siegert, C. E. H., de Vreede, T. A., Daha, M. R., and Breedveld, F. C., Characterization of anti-endothelial antibodies in systemic lupus erythematosus (SLE), *Clin Exp Immunol*, 84, 238, 1991.

63. Koenig, D. W., Barley-Maloney, L., and Daniel, T. O., A Western blot assay to detect autoantibodies to criptic endothelial antigens in thrombotic microangiopathies, *J Clin Immunol*, 13, 204, 1993.

64. Jiann Shyong, L., Ming-Fei, L., and Huan-Yao, L., Characterization of antiendothelial cell antibodies in the patients with systemic lupus erythematosus: a potential marker for disease activity, *Clin Immunol Immunopath*, 79, 211, 1996.

65. Cervera, R., Navarro, M., Lopez-Soto, A., Cid, M. C., Font, J., Esparza, J., Reverter, J. C., Monteagudo, J., Ingelmo, M., and Urbano-Marquez, A., Antibodies to endothelial cells in Behçet's disease: cell-binding heterogeneity and association with clinical activity, *Ann Rheum Dis*, 53, 265, 1994.

66. Hess, D. C., Shepard, J. C., and Adams, R. J., Increased immunoglobulin binding to cerebral endothelium in patients with aPL, *Stroke*, 24, 994, 1993.

67. Meroni, P. L., D'Cruz, D., Khamastha, M. A., and Hughes, G. R. V., Antiendothelial cell antibodies: for scientists or for clinicians too?, *Clin Exp Immunol*, 104, 1992, 1996.

68. Hill, M. B., Phipps, J. L., Milford-Ward, A., Greaves, M., and Hughes, P., Further characterization of antiendothelial cell antibodies in systemic lupus erythematosus by controlled immunoblotting, *Br J Rheumatol*, 35, 1231, 1996.

69. Fillit, H. and Lahita, R., Antibodies to vascular heparan sulphate proteoglycan in patients with systemic lupus erythematosus, *Autoimmunity*, 9, 159, 1991.

70. Fillit, H., Edstrom, W., Yang, C. P., Moran, T., and Dimitriu-Bona, A., Autoimmune MRL mice express high-affinity IgG2b monoclonal autoantibodies to heparin, *Clin Immunol Immunopathol*, 81, 62, 1996.

71. Renaudineau, Y., Revelen, R., Bordron, A., Mottier, D., Youinou P., and Le Corre, R., Two populations of endothelial cell antibodies cross-react with heparin, *Lupus*, 7, 86, 1998.

72. Shibata, S., Sasaki, T., Harpel, P., and Fillit, H., Autoantibodies to heparin sulphate proteoglycan in systemic lupus erythematosus react with endothelial cells and inhibit the formation of thrombin-anti-thrombin III complexes, *Clin Immunol Immunopathol*, 70, 114, 1994.

73. Direkeseli, H., D'Cruz, D., Khamashta, M. A., and Hughes, G. R. V., Autoantibody against endothelial cells, extracellular matrix, and human collagen type IV in patients with systemic vasculitis, *Clin Immunol Immunopathol*, 70, 206, 1994.

74. van der Zee, J. M., Miltenburg, A. M., Siegert, C. E., Daha, M. R., and Breedveld, F. C., Antiendothelial cell antibodies in systemic lupus erythematosus: enhanced antibody binding to interleukin-1-stimulated endothelium, *Int Arch Allergy & Immunol*, 104, 131, 1994.

75. Del Papa, N., Meroni, P. L., Barcellini, W., Sinico, A., Radice, A., Tincani, A., D'Cruz, D., Nicoletti, F., Borghi, M. O., Khamashta, M. A., Hughes, G. R. V., and Balestrieri, G., Antibodies to endothelial cells in primary vasculitides mediate *in vitro* endothelial cytotoxicity in the presence of normal peripheral blood mononuclear cells, *Clin Immunol Immunopathol*, 63, 267, 1992.
76. Chan, T. M., Frampton, G., Staines, N. A., Hobby, P., Perry, G. J., and Cameron, J. S., Different mechanisms by which anti-DNA moabs bind to human endothelial cells and glomerular mesangial cells, *Clin Exp Immunol*, 88, 65, 1992.
77. Chan, T. M., Yu, P. M., Tsang, K. L. C., and Cheng, I. K. P., Endothelial cell binding by human polyclonal anti-DNA antibodies: relationship to disease activity and endothelial functional alterations, *Clin Exp Immunol,* 100, 506, 1995.
78. Visentin, G., Ford, S., Scott, J., and Aster, R., Antibodies from patients with heparin-induced thrombocytopenia/thrombosis are specific for platelet factor 4 complexed with heparin or bound to endothelial cells, *J Clin Invest*, 93, 81, 1994.
79. Penning, C. A., French, M. A., Rowell, N. R., and Hughes, P. J., Antibody-dependent cellular cytotoxicity of human vascular endothelium in systemic lupus erythematosus, *J Clin Lab Immunol,* 17, 125, 1985.
80. Carvalho, D., Savage, C. O. S., Black, C. M., and Pearson, J. D., IgG antiendothelial cell autoantibodies from scleroderma patients induce leukocyte adhesion to human vascular endothelial cells *in vitro, J Clin Invest,* 97, 111, 1996.
81. Del Papa, N., Guidali, L., Sironi, M., Shoenfeld, Y., Mantovani, A., Tincani, A., Balestrieri, G., Radice, A., Sinico, R. A., and Meroni, P. L., Antiendothelial IgG antibodies from Wegener's granulomatosis bind to human endothelial cells *in vitro* and induce adhesion molecule expression and cytokine secretion, *Arthritis Rheum*, 39, 758, 1996.
82. Simantov, R., La Sala, J. M., Lo, S. K., Gharavi, A. E., Sammaritano, L. R., Salmon, J. E., and Silverstein, R. L., Activation of cultured vascular endothelial cells by antiphospholipid antibodies, *J Clin Invest,* 96, 2211, 1995.
83. Levy, Y., Gilburd, B., George, J., Del Papa, N., Mallone, R., Damianovich, M., Blank, M., Radice, A., Renaudineau, Y., Youinou, P., Wiik, A., Malavasi, F., Meroni, P. L., and Shoenfeld, Y., Characterization of murine monoclonal anti-endothelial cell antibodies (AECA) produced by idiotypic manipulation with human AECA, *Intern Immunol*, 10, 861, 1998.
84. George, J., Blank, M., Levy, Y., Meroni, P. L., Damianovich, M., Tincani, A., and Shoenfeld, Y., Differential effects of anti-beta 2 glycoprotein I antibodies on endothelial cells and on the manifestations of experimental antiphospholipid syndrome, *Circulation,* 97, 900, 1998.
85. Bordron, A., Dueymes, M., Levy, Y., Jamin, C., Leroy, J .P., Piette, J. C., Shoenfeld, Y., and Youinou, P., The binding of some human antiendothelial cell antibodies induces endothelial cell apoptosis, *J Clin Invest,* 101, 2029, 1998.
86. Bordron, A., Dueymes, M., Levy, Y., Jamin, C., Ziporen, L., Piette, J. C., Shoenfeld, Y., and Youinou, P., Anti-endothelial cell antibody binding makes nevatively charged phospholipids accessible to antiphospholipid antibodies, *Arthritis Rheum,* 41, 1738, 1998.
87. Lanir, N., Zilberman, M., Yron, I., Tennenbaum, G., Shechter, Y., and Brenner, B., Reactivity patterns of anti-phospholipid antibodies and endothelial cells: effect of anti-endothelial antibodies on cell migration, *J Lab Clin Med*, 131, 548, 1998.
88. Matsuo, M., Fukatsu, A., Taub, M. L., Caidwell, P. R., Brentjens, J. R., and Andres, C., Glomerulonephritis induced in the rabbit by anti-endothelial antibodies, *J Clin Invest*, 79, 1798, 1987.
89. Platt, J. L. and Back, F. H., Discordant xenografting: challenges and controversies, *Curr Opin Immunol*, 3, 735, 1991.
90. Shoenfeld, Y., Idiotypic induction of autoimmunity: a new aspect of the idiotypic network, *FASEB J*, 8, 1296, 1994.
91. Blank, M., Tomer, Y., Stein, M., Kopolovic, A., Wiik, A., Meroni, P. L., Conforti, G., and Shoenfeld, Y., Induction of Wegener's granulomatosis in mice by active immunization with anti-neutrophil cytoplasmic antibody (ANCA): a new aspect of Jerne's idiotypic network, *Clin Exp Immunol*, 102, 120, 1995.
92. Damianovich, M., Gilburd, B., George, J., Del Papa, N., Afek, A., Goldberg, I., Kopolovic, Y., Roth, D., Barkai, G., Meroni, P. L., and Shoenfeld, Y., Pathogenic role of anti-endothelial cell antibodies in vasculitis, *J Immunol*, 156, 4946, 1996.

10 Cryoglobulins

*Mario García-Carrasco, Manuel Ramos-Casals,
Ricard Cervera, and Josep Font*

CONTENTS

I. DEFINITION

A cryoglobulin is an immunoglobulin (Ig) that precipitates when serum is incubated at a temperature of less than 37°C. Although cold-induced precipitation of serum proteins was first described in 1933,[1] the term "cryoglobulinemia" was introduced by Lerner et al. in 1947.[2] In 1966, Meltzer et al.[3] described the typical clinical symptoms associated with cryoglobulinemia, particularly the triad of purpura, arthralgia, and weakness. The existence of circulating cryoglobulins (cryoglobulinemia) is not always related to the presence of symptomatology, and we use the term "cryoglobulinemic syndrome" when patients with cryoglobulinemia have clinical manifestations.

Cryoglobulinemia leads to systemic vasculitis due to a direct obstruction of the vessels, or to inflammation induced by the deposition of the Ig aggregate mediated to a large extent through complement activation. Most frequently small arteries and veins are involved. The deposition of rheumatoid factor (RF), IgG, and complement in the vessel wall suggests that it is triggered by the (cryo)precipitation of RF-IgG and subsequent complement activation. The main histological findings include endothelial swelling, blood extravasates, perivascular infiltrates of monocytes and neutrophils, and impairment of the interstice.

II. CLASSIFICATION

Classification of cryoglobulins into three types on the basis of their immunochemical properties, as proposed by Brouet et al.[4] in 1974, is still used since it offers correlations with associated diseases and clinical manifestations. Type I cryoglobulins are composed of single monoclonal immunoglobulins, while type II and III cryoglobulins are composed of immunocomplexes formed by monoclonal (in type II) or polyclonal (in type III) IgM with RF activity and the corresponding antigen (usually polyclonal IgG). For this reason, these last two types are referred to as mixed cryoglobulinemia (MC).

Finally, the existence of cryoglobulins that do not fit well into any of the categories described above should be noted. Some authors have described the presence of oligoclonal IgM with trace amounts of polyclonal immunoglobulins and have proposed the existence of a new cryoglobulin type, the type II-III variant.[5,6] The microheterogeneity of the IgM in these cases probably represents a transition from type III to type II, and may indicate the natural evolution of cryoglobulinemia in some patients. The transformation from polyclonal (type III) to oligoclonal (microheterogeneity or type II-III) and finally to monoclonal RF (type II) may somehow be induced by the continous B cell stimulation caused by infectious or other exogenous agents. Recently, Musset et al.[7] reported that 25 (12%) of 210 cases of mixed cryoglobulinemia exhibited a monoclonal IgG on immunoblot. It is noteworthy that all of these monoclonal IgG were IgG1 (37%) or IgG3 (63%) isotypes. It has been reported that murine IgG3 plays a major role in the generation of cryoglobulins due to their unique physicochemical properties (including self-association resulting from Fc-Fc interaction), and because IgM RF with the specificity of anti-IgG3 activity are more potent for the generation of cryoglobulins than those lacking this anti-IgG3 activity.[8] Despite several functional and structural differences, human and mouse IgG3 seem to have the same tendency to self-aggregate, and this could play a role in the nucleation of the cryoprecipitate.

III. ETIOPATHOGENIC FACTORS

A. GENETIC FACTORS

Cryoglobulinemic syndrome may be a consequence of the interaction of an exogenous agent with a host characterized by a particular genetic background. Thus, the main etiopathogenic factor in cryoglobulin production is probably the individual genetic background which regulates the response to infections. Polymorphism of HLA molecules may be responsible for the different repertoires of immune responses against antigens through the recognition of viral peptides in the context of MHC molecules. HLA expression has beeen investigated in patients with cryoglobulinemia with controversial results. Some studies have failed to demonstrate an association between MC and HLA,[9-11] and others have found significant association. Ossi et al.[12] reported that HLA-B35 and B51 were highly expressed in MC patients. In another study, Lenzi et al.[13] found a significant association with class I HLA-B8 and class II HLA-DR3 alleles. Although the association was stronger with HLA-B8 than with DR3, it is remarkable that 8 of 25 (32%) MC patients were positive for HLA-B8 and DR3, and that the calculated odds ratio (8.2) was higher for the haplotype B8-DR3 than

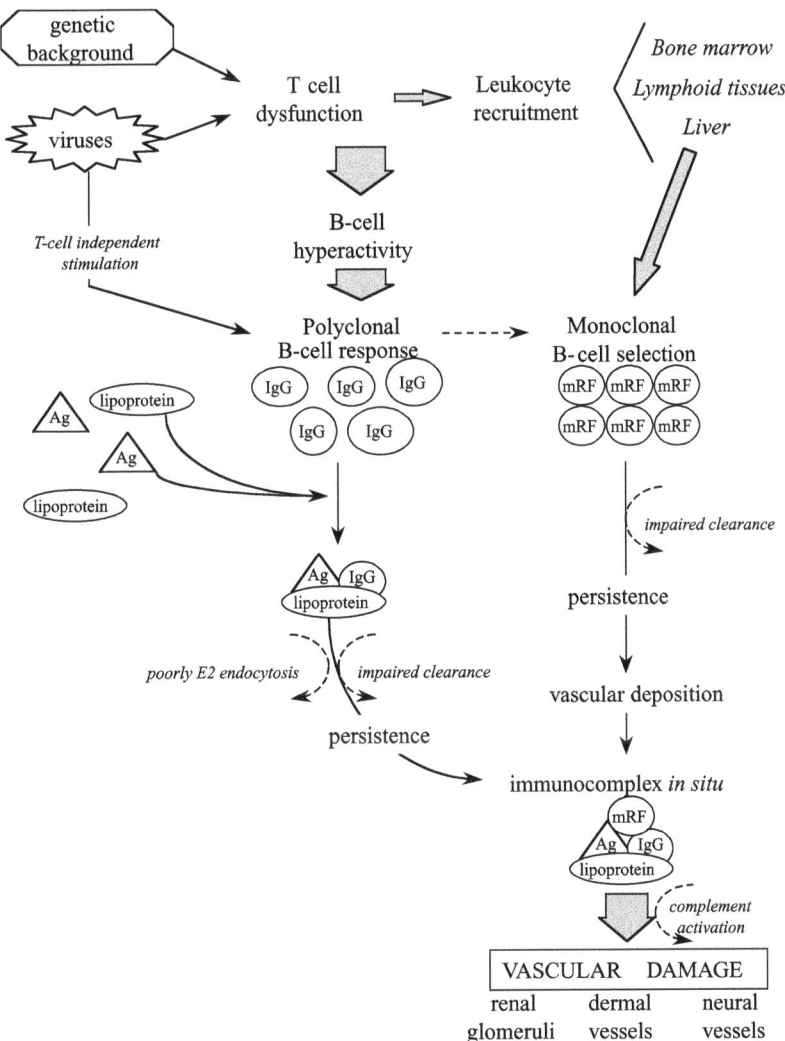

FIGURE 10.1 Etiopathogenic mechanisms in mixed cryoglobulinemia.

for each single specificity. The authors concluded that HLA-B8 and DR3 may be considered risk factors for HCV-related MC in addition to cirrhosis,[14] and suggested that patients exhibiting the B8-DR3 phenotype may carry a deletion in the C4A locus. Finally, Amoroso et al.[11] studied Ig heavy chain polymorphism and found that patients with MC showed different frequencies of polymorphic markers within the IGHG1 locus than did those of a control population.

B. Infectious Agents

Over the last 20 years a possible association between several infectious diseases and cryoglobulins has been proposed[15] and different types of acute and chronic infections associated with production of circulating cryoglobulins have been reported.[16] These observations strongly suggest the possibility that cryoglobulin production is a consequence of antigen stimulation directly or indirectly caused by infectious agents. In the majority of cases circulating cryoglobulins disappear from the circulation when the antigenic stimuli vanish,[16] but in some chronic infections small amounts of cryoglobulins may be detectable in the sera for a long time.[17-19] The infectious agents associated most frequently with cryoglobulinemia are viruses, mainly hepatotropic viruses.

1. Hepatotropic Viruses

a. Hepatitis C virus

Since the development in 1989 of a test for the detection of antibodies to hepatitis C virus (HCV), it has been established that almost all cases of MC previously called essential are related to chronic HCV infection.[4,20] At present, several findings suggest a close association between HCV and MC, including the presence of anti-HCV antibodies in sera from a high proportion of MC patients,[21,22] the presence of HCV-RNA sequence in serum and plasma samples,[22,23] bone marrow cells[24] and peripheral blood mononuclear cells (PBMC)[24-26] from cryoglobulinemic patients and, the presence of anti-HCV antibodies and specific HCV-RNA sequences in cryoprecipitates.[14,27,28]

Most patients with chronic HCV infection do not develop MC, with percentages ranging from 13 to 54%.[29-32] It is not yet clear why HCV induces the production of MC in some patients but not in others, and this indicates that other factors in addition to HCV infection are needed for the development of cryoglobulinemia. The presence of several HCV genotypes that coexist over a wide geographical distribution suggests that MC-HCV may be caused by a specific HCV genotype. At least five genotypes of HCV have been identified which differ from each other in more than 21% of about 9,400 nucleotides.[33] All of the common genotypes have been found in patients with MC-HCV,[34-35] and none of these studies has demonstrated an increased prevalence of specific genotypes among patients with MC compared with control groups. In contrast to these studies, an increased prevalence of genotype 2 in Italian patients with MC-HCV has recently been reported,[36] but it is possible that the prevalence of genotype 2 may be higher than that of genotype 1 in the HCV-infected population of Northern Italy. However, some authors have found that HCV genotype 1b is associated with monoclonal or oligoclonal cryoglobulin types, whereas genotype 3a is associated with type III cryoglobulins.[37] Finally, the existence of mutations in the HCV hypervariable region (HVR) of the E2/NS1 region may be responsible for the establishment of persistent viral infection by providing an escape route from the host immune system.[38,39] Aiyama et al.[40] studied two patients with MC and found that both HCV RNA and anti-HVR antibodies were concentrated in cryoglobulins compared with serum and supernatant. Thus, circulating HCV may be captured by anti-HVR antibody, resulting in the formation of cryoglobulins. Other mechanisms may be postulated in cryoglobulin formation, such as a cross-reactivity to IgG, since a motif inside the core protein (EGLGWAGWL, conserved in HCV genotypes) was identified as homologous to a sequence of IgG heavy chains.[41]

The detection of HCV-RNA in the PBMC of MC patients[26] may suggest a correlation between this phenomenon and the pathogenesis of cryoglobulinemia. The HCV infection of the circulating lymphocytes could trigger the mono- or polyclonal B-cell proliferation which is responsible for the production of CIC, including mixed cryoglobulins, and the consequent vasculitis.[42] However, De Maddalena et al.[43] did not observe any difference in positivity between the PBMC collected from MC patients and those from non-cryoglobulinemic HCV infection. This suggests a tropism of HCV for PBMC, regardless of the presence of a cryoglobulinemic syndrome.

Finally, more recent studies have provided evidence for a new hypothesis on the etiology and pathophysiology of MC-HCV.[4,22] HCV/IgG complexes and HCV/lipoprotein (very low density lipoprotein, VLDL) complexes have been detected in sera of HCV-infected patients,[44] and these complexes might serve as a B-cell superantigen, inducing the synthesis of non-HCV-reactive IgM with RF-like activity, thus leading to immunocomplex formation by means of a direct chronic stimulation of a specific population of B cells in the liver. The main findings supporting this hypothesis are the selective concentration of HCV with monoclonal RF (mRF) and VLDL in the cryoglobulins, the low density lipoprotein (LDL) receptor (LDLR) mediation of HCV endocytoses, the tripled risk of developing MC among HCV-infected patients who carry the apolipoprotein (apo) E2 allele, and the finding that hepatic lymphoid follicles in patients with MC consist predominantly of monoclonal IgMk B cells that are CD5+, strongly Bcl-2+, and weakly Ki-67+. Several observations suggest that the LDLR mediates endocytosis of HCV: the specific concentration of HCV in type II cryoglobulins with mRF of the WA idiotype[45] and VLDL,[46] the apparent endocytosis of HCV in skin lesions by keratinocytes known to have LDLR,[47] and the precipitation of HCV from infected serum by anti-beta lipoprotein.[48] Furthermore, endocytosis of HCV by the LDLR has been demonstrated *in vitro* in cultured cell lines.[49] Inhibition experiments using antisera to apoB and apoE, which are known to bind to LDLR, have demonstrated that most but not all of the endocytosis of HCV is blocked. These *in vitro* studies suggest that LDLR may be a major receptor for infection of hepatocytes by HCV and also indicate that LDLR may mediate the HCV infection of cells that may or may not be permissive to HCV replication. It also seems that HCV complexed to VLDL containing apo E2 may persist in the circulation and stimulate WA mRF production. Agnello et al.[50] compared the prevalence of the apoE alleles in HCV-infected patients with and without MC and found that the prevalence of the apo E2 allele was significantly higher in the MC-HCV population and that the risk factor for developing MC in the HCV-infected population was three times greatest in individuals carrying the apoE2 allele. These results support the hypothesis that HCV complexes containing apo E2 are poorly endocytosed by the LDLR and may persist in the circulation, thereby stimulating WA mRF production.

b. Other hepatotropic viruses

Acute type A hepatitis is clearly associated with a large increase in circulating IgMs and cryoglobulin production.[45,51] The cryoprecipitates contain type III cryoglobulins, and IgM anti-hepatitis A virus (HAV) has been detected in virtually all cases,[16] although some cryoprecipitates have only contained polyclonal IgM. The reduction in serum cryoglobulin concentrations generally occurs with the remission of symptoms.

Before the isolation of HCV in 1989, the possibility that hepatitis B virus (HBV) might play a predominant role in causing "essential" MC was supported by some authors[52] who reported the existence of HBsAg and/or HBsAb in a substantial number of patients with MC.[19,52] Subsequent studies failed to confirm these findings[53,54] and showed that the prevalence of HBV-related markers in large series of cryoglobulinemic patients was not significantly different from the prevalence observed in blood donors.[55] It is possible that HBV exerts a primary role in causing cryoglobulinemia in a small number of patients with chronic liver disease in whom no other causes of cryoglobulin induction can be found since some reports concerning the replication of HBV in lymphocytes[56,57] support the possibility of this virus as an inducer of cryoglobulin production.

The role of hepatitis G virus (HGV) in cryoglobulin production has been recently analyzed. Misiani et al.[58] detected GBV-C RNA in 40% of cryoglobulinemic patients, usually associated with HCV infection, and those patients with GBV-C infection alone had no detectable GBV-C RNA in cryoprecipitate. On the other hand, Cassan et al.[59] and Cacoub et al.[60] found a lower prevalence of HGV/HCV coinfection as a cause of cryoglobulinemia.

2. Lymphotropic Viruses

Cryoglobulin production has been described during the course of some lymphotropic viral infections. There has been a single report of cryoglobulins in association with adenovirus infection,[61] but greater attention has been reserved for other viruses such as the Epstein-Barr virus and, more recently, human retroviruses such as HIV-1 and the HTLV-I. Dimitrakopoulos et al.[62] found a high prevalence of cryoglobulins in HIV-1-infected patients (27%), with a higher prevalence in anti-HCV-positive patients (55%) than in anti-HCV-negative (23%). Additionally, the authors showed that the formation of cryoglobulins is strongly associated with high serum titers of HIV-1 RNA, which is a direct marker of HIV-1 viremia, active HIV-1 replication, and continous antigenic stimulation of B lymphocytes.[63] Of the 24 cryoglobulinemic HIV patients, 9 (38%) had clinical manifestations of cryoglobulinemia.

IV. PATHOGENIC MECHANISMS

A. Alteration of Immune Response

1. Leukocyte Recruitment

Recent studies indicate that specific leukocyte subpopulations are differentially recruited to the site of inflammation depending on specific pathogenetic stimuli.[64] In chronic HCV infection, Sansonno et al.[65] suggest that lymphocytes are recruited in the liver, and in a fraction of cases they are also expanded and activated to secrete molecules with RF activity. It is interesting to consider that, like the synovial membrane in patients with rheumatoid arthritis,[66] the liver may represent a microenvironment apart from lymphoid tissue in which a germinal center-like reaction is induced by HCV infection that probably stimulates B cells to produce IgM molecules bearing the 17.109 XId. It seems that clonal V-D-J products can be amplified from foci of liver B cells, and different foci may derive from different B cells within the polyclonal repertoire of liver-infiltrating B cells. The frequent detection of oligoclonal B cell expansion may indeed represent a key pathobiologic feature of HCV-associated, nonmalignant B cell lymphoproliferation, but the preferential expansion of one of these clones would in turn lead to a monoclonal pattern. Thus, it seems reasonable to speculate that infection of B lymphocytes, clonal B cell expansion, and RF production are closely related events in the natural history of chronic hepatitis C.[65]

2. B-Cell Activation and Monoclonal Rheumatoid Factor Production

The persistence of HCV or other viruses in the host may cause continous B cell stimulation with the hyperproduction of polyclonal Ig and polyclonal RF, thus inducing the formation of type III cryoglobulins. Continuous HCV viral replication may be representative of enhanced and/or long-duration immune pressure in response to chronic HCV infection with subsequent selection of oligoclonal or monoclonal RF secreting B cells.[67] This IgM results from the chronic stimulation of the immune system, either by complexes consisting of IgG bound to HCV or by the infectious agent directly, and leads to the monoclonal expansion of B cells expressing the corresponding RF in peripheral blood and in bone marrow biopsies.[68]

A major question about the pathogenesis of MC is whether it occurs in subgroups of patients with HCV infection, and it seems likely that MC is restricted to a subgroup of patients predisposed to the formation of RF. RF B cells are part of the normal immune repertoire, and significant titers of RF are induced during normal antiviral or antibacterial immune responses. RF also plays an important role in immunocomplex formation, being the antibody of circulating mixed cryoglobulins.[20,69] The antigens involved can be autologous denatured Ig,[20,69] HCV genomic sequences,[45] or other unknown factors. Under the pressure of chronic antigen stimulation, the RF repertoire is remodeled and progressively includes monospecific, somatically mutated RF similar to those observed in chronic autoimmune diseases such as RA.[67]

Previous studies using polyclonal anti-idiotypes have shown that monoclonal RF share cross-reactive idiotypes (XId)[70-71] that have been originally classified into three XId groups: WA and PO, which include 60% and 20% of monoclonal RF, respectively, and the BLA group, which defines a minor subgroup. The recent demonstration of the specific concentration of HCV in type II cryoglobulins in association with WA mRF[68] has suggested that HCV is involved in the production of the WA mRF. The WA mRF are encoded by VKIIIb and V_H1 or V_H3 germline genes.[20,69] The WA XId appears to be highly conserved and unaltered by the limited number of somatic mutations manifested by WA mRF, suggesting an antigen selection process for WA XId-positive B cells with survival benefits from this process.[73] The association of HCV with WA mRF suggests that HCV may be the pathogen that stimulates the proliferation of WA XId-positive B cells. The type of germline genes that encode the WA mRF are usually produced by CD5+ B cells. The monoclonal IgMK cells infiltrating the liver and bone marrow of patients with type II cryoglobulinemia have been reported to be CD5+,[45] whereas the IgMK monoclonal cell in the peripheral blood have been reported to be CD5–.[67,76] The significance of these observations remains to be determined since the role of the CD5 antigen as a marker of cell linage is at present controversial. In mouse studies there is evidence that the CD5 antigen is a linage marker for primordial B cells arising predominantly in the peritoneal cavity. In humans there is no such evidence, and CD5 may be a marker for a T cell-independent B cell developmental pathway.

Finally, the demonstration of WA XId + RF-IgM,[73] the lack of HCV-IgG complexes in cryoglobulin,[13] the association of serum lipoproteins with HCV, and the known characteristics of the CD5+ cells[77] have led to the recently proposed hypothesis that mixed cryoglobulins result from the chronic stimulation by HCV-lipoprotein of a specific population of WA-XId-CD5+ cells in the liver, and that these cells modulate WA-XId-CD5-cells (B-1 b) that produce the WA mRF by continued stimulation in the peripheral blood. In conclusion, the chronicity and low morbidity of HCV infection suggest that the long-term evolution of chronic HCV infection stimulates the production of a monoclonal population of B cells.

3. Cryoglobulins and Lymphoproliferation

The demonstration of HCV genoma in circulating lymphocytes[26] suggests a direct involvement of the immune system in the pathogenesis of the clinico-serological features of MC. It has long been known that lymphomas may develop in some patients with MC, usually after a long-term follow-up period.[72,78] In patients with type II MC, the appearance of non-Hodgkin's B cell lymphoma has been recorded after a mean period of six years from disease onset.[79,80] In all cases, circulating HCV markers were present, and viral RNA was detectable in both fresh and cultured PBMC from cryoglobulinemic patients.[79,80] Thus, HCV-related proteins, genomic HCV sequences, and ongoing viral replication have been identified in PBMC and lymph node cells from patients with type II MC and neoplastic lymphoproliferation.[81,82] The lymphotropism of HCV[83] could explain the appearance of a "benign" B-cell expansion in MC, which at some point may switch to evident B-cell malignancy. Since HCV cannot be integrated into the host genome, it may be hypothesized that HCV is involved in the oncogenesis through indirect mechanisms.[26,79,84] The lymphoproliferation and its evolution from benign to malignant neoplasia is probably a multifactorial and multistep process in which one or more infectious agents and genetic and environmental factors may be involved.

Lymphoma also complicates many cases of cryoglobulinemia secondary to Sjögren's syndrome (SS). In primary SS, cryoglobulinemia is detected in 16% of patients.[85] Recently, Tzioufas et al.[86] reported that MC and mRF can be used as laboratory predictive factors for lymphoma development in SS. The frequent association of HCV infection and SS,[87] lymphoproliferation and SS,[88] and MC and SS suggests a close relationship between HCV infection, MC, and lymphoproliferation in SS patients.[89]

B. PERSISTENCE OF CIRCULATING CRYOGLOBULINS

The mononuclear phagocitic system plays an important role in removing immunocomplexes (IC) from the circulation. Clearance of circulating immune complexes (CIC) is carried out by the liver and spleen mononuclear phagocytic system, in particular the Kupffer cells, whose activation can promote parenchymal inflammation and fibrosis.[69,96] The importance of the splenic reticuloendothelial function has been suggested in a study that examined splenic extraction of antibody-coated erythrocytes in autoimmune diseases.[91]

In patients with MC, a defective clearance of cryoglobulins and immune complexes has been postulated to be due to hypocomplementemia, inability of cryoglobulins to bind activated C3, low erythrocyte complement receptor (CR1), and impaired binding of cryoglobulins to erythrocytes for transport and uptake by the reticuloendothelial system.[92,93] Roccatello et al.[94] have shown that the liver and spleen mononuclear phagocytic system plays a major role in the handling of cryoglobulins in the blood. The relative lack of cryoglobulin binding to erythrocytes may lead to their persistence in the plasma phase, a condition that enhances the potential for cryoglobulin deposition in different tissues.[92] Furthermore, the high prevalence of liver involvement in patients with MC and HCV infection suggests that the removal of cryoglobulins by the liver mononuclear phagocytic system may be also impaired.

C. PATHOGENICITY OF CRYOGLOBULINS

1. Local Factors

Cryoprecipitation can be regarded as the result of the temperature-dependent association and dissociation of cryoglobulinemic components, although the molecular mechanism of cryoprecipitation, particularly the contribution of low temperature, is unclear. Low temperature may favor formation of cryo-IgM/IgG complexes. Multivalent cryo-IgM may have high functional affinity at a low temperature, but it is interesting that physicochemical characterization of purified monoclonal cryoglobulins revealed no evidence of low-temperature-dependent conformational changes. On the other hand, Ferri et al.[95] have demonstrated in MC patients a high frequency of hemorrheological alterations such as abnormally increased blood viscosity and/or reduced blood filtration. Hemorrheological alterations may contribute, at least in part, to the pathogenesis of neurological and cutaneous lesions. This is particularly important for the lower limbs, where both clinical manifestations typically appear more frequently. In these areas, a lower temperature and a slower blood flow can induce rheological alterations that could enhance the formation of IC.

2. Cryoglobulin Deposition

The cryoglobulinemic syndrome represents one of the best examples of IC disease. The vascular deposition of cryoglobulins and complement, with the possible contribution of other factors such as rheological alterations,[95] is responsible for the organ damage observed in MC patients. The vasculitic process affecting the small vessels, capillaries, and postcapillary venules consists of a neutrophilic infiltrate indicative of leukocytoclastic vasculitis. The extent of cryoglobulin deposition and possibly a critical antigen:antibody ratio in the CIC are important factors in triggering vasculitis, and it is also speculated that intravascular deposition of cryoproteins may cause luminal narrowing and obliteration of the microvascular space, leading to ischemic injury. However, cryocrit levels do not correlate with the presence and the degree of clinical and histological signs of vasculitis, suggesting that there is no direct relation between the amount of circulating cryoglobulins and vascular damage.[96]

The pathogenicity of cryoglobulins is related to the pathogenicity of the IC and, specifically, to the presence of an IgM RF which depletes complement proteins and reduces adherence to erythrocyte receptors, leading to the abnormal processing of IC.[97] The pathogenic effects of IC are especially related to their thermosolubility, their antibody affinity, the antigen/antibody ratio, the nature and type of the proteins involved, and the efficiency of the system that should prevent the deposition of IC in the tissue. It should be remarked that all these variables have been shown to be totally unrelated to the *in vitro* reaction of IgM RF with IgG during a three-day incubation of sera at 4°C to isolate the cryoprecipitate. Under such conditions, low-affinity RF can easily react with IgG, resulting in the enhanced formation of cryoprecipitate. At 37°C, mixed cryoglobulins circulate dissociated into monomeric IgG and monomeric IgM RF with little or no evidence of high molecular weight complexes of IgG and IgM RF. The finding that circulating cryoglobulins dissociate almost completely to their monomeric components at 37°C is consistent with the known low-affinity binding of RF bound to IgG crosslinked to antigen at corporal temperature. Other studies[98] have confirmed that the complexes precipitated at 4°C as cryoglobulins are present in the serum as dissociated components and not as IC. Hence, some physiological or pathological events on the site of inflammation may promote the IC formation of these low-avidity antibodies with their antigens.

3. Complement Activation

It has previously been claimed that IC leading to *in vivo* activation of the complement system may be a physiological component of the immune system in controlling infectious disease.[99] However, the *in vitro* activation of the classical complement pathway at a low temperature is known as cold activation of complement, and has been frequently observed among patients with liver disease.[100,101] Ueda et al.[102] found that some epitopes of HCV stimulate the synthesis of an antibody that preferentially reacts with antigen at lower temperatures, and that the HCV or HCV-antibody complex stimulates the synthesis of RF, which also binds to the IC with higher affinity at lower temperatures. Other clues to the pathophysiology of the disease may be gleaned from the unusual pattern of complement activation present in the serum of patients with MC, which involves only early components C1, C4, and C2, possibly related to action of the C4 binding protein.[103] However, C3 has been shown to be present in glomerular deposits in membranoproliferative glomerulone-phritis lesions in type II MC, and C3 serum levels have been reported to correlate inversely with the severity of nephritis.[104] In addition, cryoglobulins from these patients have been shown to activate C3.[103]

D. Tissue Damage

1. Cutaneous Vasculitis

The main clinical hallmark of MC is palpable purpura, a cutaneous vasculitis caused by the deposition of the components of cryoglobulins, polyclonal IgG, and monoclonal RF in the vessel walls.[3] Purpura, with sometimes severe ulcerations of the legs, is described in almost 100% of patients. Other skin manifestations include urticaria and Raynaud's phenomenon, sometimes with acral necrosis.

Several studies have investigated the presence of HCV or its components in the cutaneous lesions of MC patients with chronic HCV infection. In skin biopsy samples taken near the vasculitic lesion, the HCV antigens have been localized in the vessel walls and perivascular spaces, and the presence of HCV has been demonstrated in both the dermis and epidermis in the palpable purpuric lesions of patients with type II cryoglobulinemia. Although no replication of the virus appeared in the dermis, the presence of HCV predominantly in the basal cell layer and the predominant staining in suprabasal cells are consistent with the spread of HCV from the dermis to the epidermis.[47] The presence of HCV has also been detected in several cutaneous cell types such as keratinocytes, glandular, or endothelial cells. The most likely explanation for the presence of HCV in keratinocytes and endothelial cells is the recently described mechanism of endocytosis of HCV via the LDLR.[105] LDLR are present on keratinocytes[106] and, as in most other cells, the LDLR increase in number when activated during inflammation. A surprising finding in these studies was that positive-strand HCV could be detected in keratinocytes, glandular ductal epithelial cells, and vascular endothelial cells in the lesions, but not in normal skin of the same patient. Furthermore, evidence of replication could not be detected. The likely explanation for this observation was that up-regulation of the LDLR on these cells in the setting of inflammation mediated endocytosis of HCV by these cells, which are not apparently permissive to replication of the virus.[47] The HCV detected in vascular endothelial cells also appeared to be associated to the inflammatory process because HCV was not evident in endothelial cells in the absence of inflammation.

Using immunofluorescence analysis, the cutaneous deposits have been shown to contain IgG and IgM. Two pieces of evidence suggests the *in situ* formation of complexes of IgG, mRF, and HCV. First, in all cases the serum cryoglobulins circulate dissociated into IgG, monomeric mRF, and HCV with no evidence of HCV-IgG complexes or high molecular weight complexes containing HCV, IgG, and mRF. This suggests that the components of the cryoglobulins were present in the serum as monomeric components. Second, when resolving lesions were analyzed and vessel walls showed only evidence of edema with minimal perivascular inflammatory cell infiltrate, HCV was the only component detected in the vessel wall (presumably, HCV was trapped in the vessel wall due to its large size). The demonstration of HCV within the vessel wall in the absence of inflammatory reactions sustains the hypothesis that the virus is responsible for vasculitis by targeting cryoglobulin deposition and other circulating factors capable of initiating vessel damage.[107] The infected endothelial cells could help to maintain the viremic phase, and their damage or destruction might result in the loss of the barrier function, with spread of the virus into the tissues. However, it seems unlikely that endothelial cells may represent an active site of HCV replication in MC. Sansonno et al.[65] failed to demonstrate endothelial HCV reactivity in patients with HCV infection without circulating cryoglobulins, suggesting that the peculiar characteristics of IC and local factors play a crucial role in endothelial HCV deposition in MC. The presence of HCV-related material within and between endothelial cells up to the basement membrane could reflect the possible mechanism by which serum-derived HCV reaches the basal membrane as the result of an enhanced phagocytosis process occurring in both damaged and undamaged vessels in MC.[108] Another possible mechanism for the development of cutaneous vasculitis is that complexes activate endothelial cells and alter vascular permeability, leading to neutrophil infiltration and vessel wall damage which permit *in situ* IC formation. It is known that *in vitro* cryoprecipitation is enhanced by decreasing the temperature and increasing the concentration of the IgG and IgM components, and these particular conditions may be mimicked in the superficial vascular plexus of the dermis.

2. Renal Vasculitis

Cryoglobulinemia is a systemic vasculitis characterized in 20 to 30% of cases by renal involvement.[109] Typical glomerular lesions are found especially in type II cryoglobulinemia and represent a peculiar type of membranoproliferative exudative glomerulonephritis characterized by a particular monocyte infiltration and, in some cases, by the presence of massive endoluminal occlusion of capillary lumina by the same Ig classes seen in the cryoprecipitating Ig (the so-called "hyaline thrombi"), along with subendothelial deposits. Milder focal or mesangial proliferative glomerulonephritis can also occur.[110-111] Using immunofluorescence analysis, the glomerular deposits have been shown to contain IgG, IgM, and the C3 component of complement.[110] By idiotype analysis, the IgM in the glomerular deposits corresponds to the mRF in the serum.[112] By electron microscopy, the glomerular deposits have been shown to have crystalloid structures that occur in tubular and annular shapes.[113] These structures are thought to be IgG-mRF complexes since similar structures have been seen in the serum cryoglobulins, and recombination studies of mRF and IgG have reproduced these structures.[114]

Concentration of cryoglobulins in glomerular capillaries induced by the filtration process has been proposed as the mechanism for deposition of the immune complexes which mediate the glomerulonephritis.[110] According to Lockwood,[115] the glomerular localization of cryoglobulins can be favored by a high endocapillary concentration of cryoglobulin complexes occurring as a result of the glomerular filtration process, which increases the viscosity of the capillary contents through fluid loss. The results of studies on IgG3 cryoglobulins in MRL/lpr/lpr mice are consistent with this mechanism since deposition of the IgG3 in the glomeruli was sufficient to induce the nephritis.[116] However, Fornasieri et al.[117] demonstrated that human IgMk RF-IgG cryoglobulin from a patient in the acute phase of cryoglobulinemic glomerulonephritis was able to induce massive deposition of hyaline material in 100% of capillary loops in mice after an early phase of pure mesangial deposits. The deposits identified by immunofluorescence were composed of human IgMk and human IgG with concomitant mouse C3 activation. Thus, the continued circulation and the *in situ* formation of complexes in the renal tissue, aided by the special renal environment of increased protein concentration in the glomerular capillary loops, may contribute to the evolution of renal injury in MC.

Recently, Fornasieri et al.[118] demonstrated the affinity of cryoglobulin IgMk RFs for immobilized cellular fibronectin, an adhesive glycoprotein that connects adjacent cells and mediates cell anchorage to the extracellular matrix, and suggested a possible etiopathogenic mechanism for induction of *in situ* complex glomerulonephritis (GN).[118] The nephritogenicity of type II cryoglobulins could be due to the capacity of their IgMk RF to bind to cellular fibronectin, which is strongly represented in human mesangium, leading to growth *in situ* of mesangial, paramesangial, and subendothelial deposits.[118]

Other studies have focused on the possible role of the monocyte-macrophage system in the renal involvement of MC. Monocyte-macrophage infiltration into the glomerulus, and the periglomerular and perivascular areas, is a common histopathological feature of this form of glomerular disease.[109,119] MCP-1 is a chemokine with a highly specific chemotactic effect on monocytes,[120] produced *in vitro* by mesangial, endothelial, and proximal tubular cells, and its production is induced by different cytokines as well as by IgG aggregates.[121,122] Gesualdo et al.[123] have shown that MCP-1 is expressed at both the gene and protein levels *in vivo* during cryoglobulinemic membranoproliferative GN. Although monocyte infiltration is a common histopathological feature of several primary and secondary glomerulonephritis, the mechanisms involved in monocyte recruitment in renal tissue are still under debate. The strong corrrelation, found by Gesualdo et al.,[123] between MCP-1 expression and monocyte/macrophage infiltration supports the hypothesis that MCP-1 may play an important role in the recruitment of these cells into the renal glomerulus. The deposition of cryoglobulins at a renal level may cause the monocyte/macrophage influx through an induction of MCP-1 expression by resident cells. In addition, since monocytes themselves produce the chemokine, once these cells reach the mesangial or the interstitial areas they could generate a positive loop maintaining the inflammatory process.

Finally, some authors[124] have observed specific antibodies to alpha-enolase in patients with MC and renal involvement, and have concluded that the antibodies against alpha-enolase, which are highly expressed in renal tissues, are suggestive of the *in situ* formation of IC in patients with MC and glomerulonephritis.

3. Peripheral Neuropathy

The frequency of peripheral nervous system (PNS) disorders in MC ranges from 7 to 60%[125,126] and, clinically, patients may present mononeuropathy, multiple mononeuropathy, or polyneuropathy. Nerve biopsies from affected patients disclose axonal pathology, in accordance with electrophysiological findings.[127,128] The severity of PNS involvement and its course are unpredictable and variable even in patients sharing the same cryoglobulin type or with identical underlying disorders. This can be partly explained by the role played by extrinsic factors in inducing exacerbation that characterize the course of the disease, in addition to intrinsic cellular and humoral immune factors responsible for tissue damage. The pathogenesis of cryoglobulinemic neuropathy is not yet completely understood, and several observations suggest three possible mechanisms: vasculitis,[108,129,130] occlusion of vasa nervorum by cryoglobulin deposition, or immunologically mediated demyelinization.[108]

Histologic studies have shown, in the majority of cases, inflammatory vessel damage with axonal degeneration,[129,130] supporting the vascular origin of nerve lesions. The clearcut correlation between serum cryoglobulin levels and various neurologic findings (presence of objective symptoms, conduction velocity, and F wave alterations) suggests that an IC-mediated vasculitis may be responsible for nerve injury. A similar pathogenetic mechanism has been demonstrated for other frequent complications of MC, such as purpura and renal involvement.[20] Epineurial vasculitis is also currently viewed as a consequence of vascular IC deposition.[131,132] However, transmural neutrophilic infiltration with leukocytoclastic changes, the distinctive pathological picture of IC-mediated vasculitis, has rarely been observed in cryoglobulinemic neuropathy, and perivascular lympho-histiocytic infiltrates suggest a disorder mediated by T-cells.[64] Cryoglobulins and/or IC seem to contribute to the generation of microvascular, but not vasculitic, changes in epineurial inflammation. On the other hand, necrotizing vasculitis with transmural inflammatory infiltration of small epineurial arterioles was found in the biopsies of some patients.[77]

The second mechanism postulated in nerve injury due to cryoglobulins is the occlusion of the vasa nervorum by cryoglobulin precipitation. Previous studies have suggested that axonal degeneration is produced by acute and chronic ischemia as a consequence of multifocal epineurial arteriopathy and/or diffuse endoneurial microangiopathy.[77,134] The presence of Ig in endoneurial capillaries suggests that the microangiopathy could be the consequence of IC entrapment along vascular basement membranes or the result of microvessel occlusion by cryoprecipitates.[128]

Finally, demyelination is found in a minority of cases with cryoglobulinemic neuropathy, with mixed features of demyelination and axonal alterations.[135]

V. CONCLUSION

Since the initial report in 1990 of the association between MC and HCV infection, it has become clear that most of the so-called "essential" cryoglobulinemias are in fact associated with HCV infection. A necessary step for their development seems to be long-standing infection with liver disease and hypergammaglobulinemia. It seems reasonable to remark that infection of B lymphocytes, clonal B cell expansion, and RF production are closely related events in the natural history of chronic hepatitis C, and that the formation of RF(anti-IgG)/IgG immune complexes is a major step preceding cryoprecipitation. Finally, recent studies have focused on the close relationship between MC and a higher risk of evolution to lymphoid malignancies.

REFERENCES

1. Wintrobe MM, Buell MV. Hypertroteinemia associated with multiple myeloma. *Bull Johns Hopkins Hosp* 1933; 52:156–65.
2. Lerner AB, Watson CJ. Studies of cryoglobulins. I. Unusual purpura associated with the presence of a high concentration of cryoglobulin (cold precipitable serum globulin). *Am J Med Sci* 1947; 214:410–15.
3. Meltzer M, Franklin EC. Cryoglobulinemia: a study of 29 patients. I. IgG and IgM cryoglobulins and factors effecting cryoprecipitability. *Am J Med* 1966; 40:828–36.
4. Brouet JC, Clauvel JP, Danon F et al. Biological and clinical significance of cryoglobulins: a report of 86 cases. *Am J Med* 1974; 57:775–88.
5. Musset L, Diemert MC, Taibi F et al. Characterization of cryoglobulins by immunoblotting. *Clin Chem* 1992; 38:798–802.
6. Tissot JD, Schifferli JA, Hochstrasser DF et al. Two-dimensional polyacrylamide gel electrophoresis analysis of cryoglobulins and identification of an IgM-associated peptide. *J Immunol Meth* 1994; 173:63–75.
7. Musset L, Duarte F, Gaillard O et al. Immunochemical characterization of monoclonal IgG containing mixed cryoglobulins. *Clin Immunol Immunopathol* 1994; 70:166–70.
8. Abelmoula M, Spertini F, Shibata T et al. IgG3 is the major source of cryoglobulins in mice. *J Immunol* 1989; 143:526–32.
9. Nightingale SD, Pelley RP, Delaney NL et al. Inheritance of mixed cryoglobulinemia. *Am J Hum Genet* 1981; 33:735–44.
10. Migliorini P, Bombardieri S, Castellani A, Ferrara GB. HLA antigens in essential mixed cryoglobulinemia. *Arthritis Rheum* 1981; 24:932–6.

11. Amoroso A, Berrino M, Canale L et al. Are HLA class II and immunoglobulin constant region genes involved in the pathogenesis of mixed cryoglobulinemia type II after hepatitis C virus infection? *J Hepatol* 1998; 29:36–44.

12. Ossi E, Bordin MA, Businaro MA et al. HLA expression in type II mixed cryoglobulinemia and chronic hepatitis C virus. *Clin Exp Rheumatol* 1995; 13(Suppl 13):S91–S93.

13. Lenzi M, Frisoni M, Mantovani V et al. Haplotype HLA-B8-DR3 confers susceptibility to hepatitis C virus-related mixed cryoglobulinemia. *Blood* 1998; 91:2062–6.

14. Lunel F, Musset L, Cacoub P et al. Cryoglobulinemia in chronic liver disease: role of hepatitis C virus and liver damage. *Gastroenterology* 1994; 106:1291.

15. Levo Y. Nature of cryoglobulinemia. *Lancet* 1980; i:285–7.

16. Galli M, Invernizzi F, Chemotti M et al. Cryoglobulins and infectious diseases. *La Ricerca Clin Lab* 1986; 16:301–13.

17. Lassus A. Development of rheumatoid factor activity and cryoglobulins in primary and secondary syphilis. *Int Arch Allergy* 1970; 36:515–8.

18. Mcintosh RM, Koss MN, Gocke DJ. The nature and incidence of cryoproteins in hepatitis B antigen (HBsAg)-positive patients. *Q J Med* 1976; 45:23–38.

19. Realdi G, Alberti A, Rigoli A, Tremolada F. Immune complexes and Australia antigen in cryoglobulinemic sera. *Z Immunitats-Forsch* 1974; 147:114–26.

20. Gorevic PD, Kassab HJ, Levo Y et al. Mixed cryoglobulinemia: clinical aspects and long term follow up of 40 patients. *Am J Med* 1980; 69:287–309.

21. Casato M, Taliani G, Pucillo LP, Goffredo F, Lagana B, Bonomo L. Cryoglobulinemia and hepatitis C virus. *Lancet* 1991; 337:1047–8.

22. Misiani R, Bellavita P, Fenili D et al. Hepatitis C virus infection in patients with essential mixed cryoglobulinemia. *Ann Intern Med* 1992; 117:573–7.

23. Pascual M, Perrin L, Giostra E, Schifferli JA. Hepatitis C virus in patients with cryoglobulinemia type II. *J Infect Dis* 1990; 162:569–70.

24. Gabrielli A, Manzin A, Candela M et al. Active hepatitis C virus infection in bone marrow and peripheral blood mononuclear cells from patients with mixed cryoglobulinemia. *Clin Exp Immunol* 1994; 97:97:87–93.

25. Bouffard P, Hayasshi PH, Acevedo R, Levy N, Zeldis JB. Hepatitis C virus infection is detected in a monocyte/macrophage subpopulation of peripheral blood mononuclear cells. *J Infect Dis* 1992; 166:1276–80.

26. Ferri C, Monti M, La Civita L et al. Infection of peripheral blood mononuclear cells by hepatitis C virus in mixed cryoglobulinemia. *Blood* 1993; 82:3701–5.

27. Muñoz-Fernández S, Barnado FJ, Martin-Mola E et al. Evidence of hepatitis C virus antibodies in the cryoprecipitate of patients with mixed cryoglobulinemia. *J Rheumatol* 1994; 21:229–33.

28. Cacoub P, Lunel F, Fabiani F et al. Mixed cryoglobulinemia and hepatitis C virus. *Am J Med* 1994; 40:124–32.

29. Werner C, Joller-Jemelka HI, Fontana A. Hepatitis C virus and cryoglobulinemia. *N Engl J Med* 1993; 328:1122–3.

30. Galli M, Monti G, Monteverde A, Invernizzi F, Pietrogrande M. Hepatitis C virus and mixed cryoglobulinemia. *Lancet* 1992; 339:989.

31. Cacoub P, Lunel F, Musset L, Opolon P, Piette JC. Hepatitis C virus and cryoglobulinemia. *N Engl J Med* 1993; 328:1121–2.

32. Levey M, Bjornsson B, Banner B et al. Mixed cryoglobulinemia in chronic hepatitis C infection: a clinicopathologic analysis of 10 cases and review of recent literature. *Medicine* 1994; 73:53–67.

33. Choo QL, Richman KH, Han JH et al. Genetic organization and diversity of the hepatitis C virus. *Proc Natl Acad Sci USA* 1991; 88:2451–5.

34. Crovatto M, Ceselli S, Mazzaro C et al. HCV genotypes and cryoglobulinemia. *Clin Exp Rheumatol* 1995; 13:S79.

35. Pawlotsky JM, Roudot-Thoraval F, Simmonds P et al. Extrahepatic immunologic manifestations in chronic hepatitis C virus serotypes. *Ann Intern Med* 1995; 122:169.

36. Zignego AL, Ferri C, Giannini C et al. Hepatitis C virus genotype analysis in patients with type I cryoglobulinemia. *Ann Intern Med* 1996; 124:31.

37. Antonescu C, Mayerat C, Mantegani A, Frei PC, Spertini F, Tissot JD. Hepatitis C virus (HCV) infection: serum rheumatoid factor activity and HCV genotype correlate with cryoglobulin clonality. *Blood* 1998; 92:3486–7.

38. Weiner AJ, Geysen HM, Cristopherson C et al. Evidence for immune selection of hepatitis C virus (HCV) putative envelope glycoprotein variants: potential role in chronic HCV infections. *Proc Natl Acad Sci USA* 1992; 89:3468–72.

39. Higashi Y, Kakumu S, Yoshioka K et al. Dynamics of genome change in the E2/NS1 region of hepatitis C virus *in vivo. Virology* 1993; 197:659–668.

40. Aiyama T, Yoshioka K, Okumura A et al. Hypervariable region sequence in cryoglobulin-associated hepatitis C virus in sera of patients with chronic hepatitis C: relationship to antibody response against hypervariable region genome. *Hepatology* 1996; 24:1346–50.

41. Hartmann H, Schott P, Polzien F et al. Cryoglobulinemia in chronic hepatitis C virus infection: prevalence, clinical manifestations, response to interferon treatment and analysis of cryoprecipitates. *Z Gastroenterol* 1995; 33:643–50.

42. Ferri C, Zignego AL, Bombardieri S et al. Etiopathogenetic role of hepatitis C virus in mixed cryoglobulinemia, chronic liver diseases and lymphomas. *Clin Exp Rheumatol* 1995; 13 (Suppl 13):S135–140.

43. De Maddalena C, Zehender G, Bianchi A et al. HCV-RNA detection using different PCR methods in sera, cryoglobulins and peripheral blood mononuclear cells of patients with mixed cryoglobulinemia. *Clin Exp Rheumatol* 1995; 13 (Suppl 13):S119–122.

44. Thomssen R, Bonk S, Thiele A. Density heterogeneities of hepatitis C virus in human sera due to the binding of beta-lipoproteins and immunoglobulins. *Med Microbiol Immunol* 1993; 74:669–76.

45. Agnello V, Chung RT, Kaplan LM. A role for hepatitis C virus infection in type II cryoglobulinemia. *N Engl J Med* 1992; 327:1490–5.

46. Agnello V, Zhang QX, Elfahal M, Abel G, Knight GB. Association of hepatitis C virus with VLDL in type II cryoglobulinemia. 3rd International Meeting on Hepatitis C Virus and Related Viruses, 1995 (abstract).

47. Agnello V, Abel G. Localization of hepatitis C virus in cutaneous vasculitic lesions in patients with type II cryoglobulinemia. *Arthritis Rheum* 1997; 40:2007–15.

48. Thomssen R, Monazahian M, Bonk S et al. The binding of HCV to lipoproteins. Keystone Symposium on Hepatitis C and Beyond, 1996, abstract.

49. Agnello V, Barnes JL. Human rheumatoid factor cross-idiotype. I. Wa and BLA are heat labile conformational antigens requiring both heavy and light chains. *J Exp Med* 1986; 164:1809.

50. Agnello V, Abel G, Zhang QX, Elfahal M, Knight GB. The etiology of mixed cryoglobulinemia: the role of the LDL receptor and apolipoprotein E2. *Arthritis Rheum* 1997; 39:5315.

51. Galli M, Invernizzi F, Fiorenza AM et al. Crioglobuline ed immunocomplesi circolanti in epatite A. *Acta Medit Patol Infett Trop* 1982; 1:93–103.

52. Levo Y, Gorevic PD, Kassab HJ, Zucker-Franklin D, Franklin EC. Association between hepatitis B virus and essential mixed cryoglobulinemia. *N Engl J Med* 1977; 297:946–7.

53. Montagnino G. Reappraisal of the clinical expression of mixed cryoglobulinemia. *Springer Semin Immunopathol* 1988; 10:1–19.

54. Popp JW Jr, Dienstag JL, Wands JR, Bloch KJ. Essential mixed cryoglobulinemia without evidence for hepatitis B virus infection. *Ann Intern Med* 1980; 92:379–83.

55. Galli M, Monti G, Invernizzi F et al. Hepatitis B virus-related markers in secondary and in essential mixed cryoglobulinemias: a multicentric study of 596 cases. *Ann Ital Med Int* 1992; 7:209–14.

56. Rommet-Lemmone JL, McLane MF, Elfassi E, Haseltine WA, Azocar J, Essex M. Hepatitis B virus infection in cultured human lymphoblastoid cells. *Science* 1983; 221:667–9.

57. Pontisso P, Poon HC, Tiollais P, Brechot C. Detection of hepatitis B virus in mononuclear blood cells. *Br Med J* 1984; 288:1561–6.

58. Misiani R, Mantero G, Bellavita P et al. GB virus C infection in patients with type II mixed cryoglobulinemia. *Ann Intern Med* 1997; 127:891–4.

59. Casan M, Lilli D, Rivanera D et al. HCV/HGV coinfection and cryoglobulinemia. *J Hepatol* 1998; 28:355–7.

60. Cacoub P, Frangeul L, Musset L. Hepatitis G and mixed cryoglobulinemia. *Ann Intern Med* 1997; 126:1002.

61. Utsinger PD. Immunologic studies of arthritis associated with adenoviral infection. *Arthritis Rheum* 1977; 3:188 (abstr).
62. Dimitrakopoulos A, Kordossis T, Hatzakis A, Moutsopoulos HM. Mixed cryoglobulinemia in HIV-1 infection: the role of HIV-1. *Ann Intern Med* 1999; 130:226–230.
63. Mellors JW, Kingsley LA, Rinaldo CR Jr et al. Quantitation of HIV-1 RNA in plasma predicts outcome after seroconversion. *Ann Intern Med* 1995; 122:573–9.
64. Moore PM. Immune mechanisms in the primary and secondary vasculitides. *J Neurol Sci* 1989; 93:129–145.
65. Sansonno D, De Vita S, Iacobelli AR, Cornacchiulo V, Boiocchi M, Dammacco F. Clonal analysis of intrahepatic B cells from HCV-infected patients with and without mixed cryoglobulinemia. *J Immunol* 1998; 160:3594–601.
66. Schroder AE, Greiner C, Seyfert C, Berek C. Differentiation of B cells in the nonlymphoid tissue of the synovial membrane of patients with rheumatoid arthritis. *Proc Natl Acad Sci USA* 1996; 93:221.
67. Djavad N, Bas S, Shi SW et al. Comparison of rheumatoid factors of rheumatoid arthritis patients, of individuals with mycobacterial infections and of normal controls: evidence for maturation in the absence of an autoimmune response. *Eur J Immunol* 1996; 26:2480.
68. Perl A, Gorevic PD, Ryan DH et al. Clonal B cell expansions in patients with essential mixed cryoglobulinemia. *Clin Exp Immunol* 1989; 76:54–60.
69. Bombardieri S, Ferri C, Migliorini P et al. Cryoglobulins and immune complexes in essential mixed cryoglobulinemia. *La Ricerca Clin Lab* 1986; 16:281.
70. Kunkel HG, Agnello V, Joslin FG et al. Cross idiotypic specificity among monoclonal IgM proteins with anti-gamma-globulin activity. *J Exp Med* 1973; 137:331–7.
71. Agnello V, Arbetter A, DeKasep GI et al. Evidence for a subset of rheumatoid factor that cross-react with DNS-histone and have a distinct cross-idiotype. *J Exp Med* 1980; 151:1514–19.
72. Gorevic PD, Frangione B. Mixed cryoglobulinemia cross-reactive idiotypes: implications for the relationship of MC to rheumatic and lymphoproliferative diseases. *Semin Hematol* 1991; 28:79–94.
73. Knight GB, Agnello V, Bonagura V, Barnes JL, Panka DJ, Zhang QX. Human rheumatoid factor cross-idiotypes. IV. Studies on WA Xid-positive IgM without rheumatoid factor activity provide evidence that the WA Xid is not unique to rheumatoid factors and is distinct from the 17109 and G6 Xids. *J Exp Med* 1993; 178:1903–11.
74. Monteverde A, Ballara M, Bertoncelli MC et al. Lymphoproliferation in type II mixed cryoglobulinemia. *Clin Exp Rheumatol* 1995; 13:141–7 (Suppl 13).
75. Pasquali JL, Walkinger C, Kunk L, Knapp AM, Levallois H. The majority of peripheral blood monoclonal IgM rheumatoid factor secreting cells are CD5 negative in three patients with mixed cryoglobulinemia. *Blood* 1991; 77:1761.
76. Crouzier R, Martin T, Pasquali JL. Monoclonal IgM rheumatoid factor secreted by CD5-negative B cells during mixed cryoglobulinemia. *J Immunol* 1995; 41:3421.
77. Bonetti B, Invernizzi F, Rizzuto N et al. T-cell-mediated epineurial vasculitis and humoral-mediated microangiopathy in cryoglobulinemic neuropathy. *J Neuroimmunol* 1997; 73:145–54.
78. Monteverde A, Rivano MT, Allegra GC et al. Essential mixed cryoglobulinemia, type II: a manifestation of low-grade malignant lymphoma? Clinical morphological study of 12 cases with special reference to immunohistochemical findings. *Acta Haematol* 1988; 79:20–5.
79. Ferri C, Monti M, La Civita L et al. Hepatitis C virus infection in non-Hodgkin's B cell lymphoma complicating mixed cryoglobulinemia. *Eur J Clin Invest* 1994; 24:781–4.
80. La Civita L, Zignego AL, Monti M, Longombardo G, Pasero G, Ferri C. Mixed cryoglobulinemia as a possible preneoplastic disorder. *Arthritis Rheum* 1995; 38:1859–60.
81. Zignego AL, Decarli M, Monti M et al. Hepatitis C virus infection of mononuclear cells from peripheral blood and liver infiltrates in chronically infected patients. *J Med Virol* 1995; 47:58.
82. Sansonno D, De Vita S, Cornacchiulo V, Carbone A, Boiocchi M, Dammaco F. Detection and distribution of hepatitis C virus-related proteins in lymph nodes of patients with type II mixed cryoglobulinemia and neoplastic or non-neoplastic lymphoproliferation. *Blood* 1996; 88:4296.
83. Ferri C, Marzo E, Longombardo G et al. Alpha-interferon in mixed cryoglobulinemia patients: a randomized crossover controlled trial. *Blood* 1993; 81:1132–6.
84. Ferri C, Caracciolo F, Zignego AL et al. Hepatitis C virus infection in patients with non-Hodgkin's lymphoma. *Br J Haematol* 1994; 88:392–4.

85. Ramos-Casals M, Cervera R, Yagüe J, García-Carrasco M, Trejo O, Jiménez S, Morlá RM, Font J, Ingelmo M. Cryoglobulinemia in primary Sjögren's syndrome: prevalence and clinical characteristics in a series of 115 patients. *Semin Arthritis Rheum* 1998; 28:200–205.

86. Tzioufas AG, Boumba DS, Skopouli FN, Moutsopoulos HM. Mixed monoclonal cryoglobulinemia and monoclonal rheumatoid factor cross-reactive idiotypes as predictive factors for the development of lymphoma in primary Sjögren's syndrome. *Arthritis Rheum* 1996; 39:767–72.

87. García-Carrasco M, Ramos-Casals M, Cervera R, Font J, Vidal J, Muñoz FJ, Miret C, Espinosa G, Ingelmo M. Hepatitis C virus infection in "primary" Sjögren's syndrome: prevalence and clinical significance in a series of 90 patients. *Ann Rheum Dis* 1997; 56:173–175.

88. Ramos-Casals M, García-Carrasco M, Cervera R, Font J, Sjögren's syndrome and lymphoproliferative disease, In: *Cancer and Autoimmunity,* Shoenfeld, Yehuda and Gershwin, M Eric, Eds., Elsevier Science, Amsterdam, 2000, 55–80.

89. Ramos-Casals M, García-Carrasco M, Cervera R, Font J. Sjögren's syndrome and hepatitis C virus (review). *Clin Rheumatol* 1999; 18:93–100.

90. Bradfield JW. Control of spillover. The importance of Kupffer-cell function in clinical medicine. *Lancet* 1974; 2:883–7.

91. Walport MJ, Peters AM, Elkon KB, Puset CD, Lavender JP, Hughes GRV. The splenic extraction ratio of antibody-coated erythrocytes and its response to plasma exchange and pulse methylprednisolone. *Clin Exp Immunol* 1985; 60:465–73.

92. Ng YC, Schifferli JA. Clearance of cryoglobulins in man. *Springer Semin Immunopathol* 1988; 10:75–89.

93. Madi N, Steiger G, Estreicher J et al. Effective immune adherence and elimination of hepatitis surface antigen/antibody complexes in patients with mixed essential cryoglobulinemia type II. *J Immunol* 1991; 147:495–502.

94. Roccatello D, Morsica G, Picciotto G et al. Impaired hepatosplenic elimination of circulating cryoglobulins in patients with essential mixed cryoglobulinaemia and hepatitis C virus (HCV) infection. *Clin Exp Immunol* 1997; 110:9–14.

95. Ferri C, Mannini L, Bartoli V et al. Blood viscosity and filtration abnormalities in mixed cryoglobulinemia patients. *Clin Exp Rheumatol* 1990; 8:271–81.

96. Sansonno D, Cornacchiulo V, Iacobelli AR, Di Stefano R, Lospalluti M, Dammacco F. Localization of hepatitis C virus antigens in liver and skin tissues of chronic hepatitis C virus-infected patients with mixed cryoglobulinemia. *Hepatology* 1995; 21:305–12.

97. Invernizzi F, Pietrogrande M, Sangramoso B. Classification of the cryoglobulinemic syndrome. *Clin Exp Rheumatol* 1995; 13(Suppl 13):S123–8.

98. Agnello V. The etiology and pathophysiology of mixed cryoglobulinemia secondary to hepatitis C virus infection. *Springer Semin Immunopathol* 1997; 19:111–29.

99. Chen PP, Fong S, Goni F et al. Cross-reacting idiotypes on cryoprecipitating rheumatoid factor. *Springer Semin Immunopathol* 1988; 10:35–55.

100. Kitamura H, Nagaki K, Inoshita K et al. The cold activation of the classical complement pathway, the cause of the differences between plasma and serum complement in liver cirrhosis. *Clin Exp Immunol* 1977; 27:34–7.

101. Inai S, Kitamura H, Fujita T et al. Differences between plasma and serum complement in patients with chronic liver disease. *Clin Exp Immunol* 1976; 25:403–9.

102. Ueda K, Nakajima H, Nakagawa T, Shimizu A. The association of complement activation at a low temperature with hepatitis C virus infection in comparison with cryoglobulin. *Clin Exp Immunol* 1995; 101:284–7.

103. Gigli I. Complement activation in patients with mixed cryoglobulinemia. In: Ponticelli C, Minetti L, D'Amico G (eds). *Antiglobulins, Cryoglobulins and Glomerulonephritis.* Martinus Nijhoff, Dordrecht, pp 135–146.

104. Maggiore Q, Bartolomeo F, L'Abate A et al. Glomerular localization of circulating antiglobulin activity in essential mixed cryoglobulinemia with glomerulonephritis. *Kidney Int* 1982; 21:387.

105. Agnello V, Abel G, Zhang QX, Elfahal M, Knight GB. Low density lipoprotein receptor (LDLR) mediated endocytosis of HCV: a potential mechanism for infection of hepatocytes. IX Triennal International Symposium on Viral Hepatitis and Liver Disease. Rome, April 1996.

106. Ponec M, te Pas MF, Havekes L, Boonstra J, Mommaas AM, Vermeer BJ. LDL receptors in kerati-nocytes. *J Invest Dermatol* 1992 (suppl 6); 98:50S–56S.

107. Hundt M, Zielinska-Skowronel M, Schmidt RE. Fcgamma receptor activation of neutrophils in cryoglobulin-induced leukocytoclastic vasculitis. *Arthritis Rheum* 1993; 36:974–82.

108. Feiner HD. Relationship of tissue deposits of cryoglobulin to clinical features of mixed cryoglobu-linemia. *Hum Pathol* 1983; 14:710–5.

109. Ben-Bassat M, Boner G, Rosenfeld J et al. The clinicopathologic features of cryoglobulinemic nephropathy. *Am J Clin Pathol* 1983; 79:147–156.

110. D'Amico G, Colasanti G, Ferrario F, Sinico RA. Renal involvement in essential mixed cryoglobu-linemia. *Kidney Int* 1989; 35:1004–14.

111. Monga A, Mazzuco G, Barbiano DI, Belgioioso G, Busnach G. The presence and possible role of monocyte infiltration in human chronic proliferative glomerulonephritis. *Am J Pathol* 1979; 94:271–84.

112. Sinico RA, Winearls CG, Sabadini E, Fornasieri A, Castiglione A, D'Amico G. Identification of glomerular immune deposits in cryoglobulinemia glomerulonephritis. *Kidney Int* 1988; 34:109.

113. Cordonnier D, Martin H, Groslambert P et al. Mixed IgG-IgM cryoglobulinemia with glomerulone-phritis: immunochemical, fluorescent and ultrastructural study of kidney and *in vitro* cryoprecipitate. *Am J Med* 1975; 59:867.

114. Stoebner P, Renversez JC, Groulade J, Vialtel P, Cordonner D. Ultrastructural study of IgG and IgG-IgM crystal cryoglobulins. *Am Soc Clin Pathol* 1978; 4:404.

115. Lockwood CM. Lymphoma, cryoglobulinemia and renal disease. *Kidney Int* 1979; 16:522–30.

116. Reininger L, Berney T, Shibata T, Spertini F, Merino R, Izui S. Cryoglobulinemia induced by a murine IgG3 rheumatoid factor: skin vasculitis and glomerulonephritis arise from distinct pathogenic mech-anisms. *Proc Natl Acad Sci USA* 1990; 87:10038.

117. Fornasieri A, Tazzari S, Li M et al. Electron microscopy study of genesis and dynamics of immunodepo-sition in IgMk-IgG cryoglobulin-induced glomerulonephritis in mice. *Am J Kidney Dis* 1998; 31:435–42.

118. Fornasieri A, Armelloni S, Bernasconi P et al. High binding of immunoglobulin M kappa rheumatoid factor from type II cryoglobulins to cellular fibronectin: a mechanism for induction of *in situ* immune complex glomerulonephritis? *Am J Kidney Dis* 1996; 27:476–83.

119. Van Goor H, Ding G, Kees-Folts D et al. Macrophages and renal disease. *Lab Invest* 1994; 71:456–64.

120. Leonard EJ, Yoshimura T. Human monocyte chemoattractant protein-1 (MCP-1). *Immunol Today* 1993; 11:97–101.

121. Rovin BH, Yoshimura T, Tan L. Cytokine-induced production of monocyte chemoattractant protein-1 by cultured human mesangial cells. *J Immunol* 1992; 148:2148–53.

122. Schmouder RL, Strieter RM, Kunkel SL. Interferon gamma regulation of human cortical epithelial cell-derived monocyte chemotactic peptide-1. *Kidney Int* 1993; 44:43–9.

123. Gesualdo L, Grandaliano G, Ranieri E et al. Monocyte recruitment in cryoglobulinemic membrano-proliferative glomerulonephritis: a pathogenetic role for monocyte chemotactic peptide-1. *Kidney Int* 1997; 51:155–63.

124. Sabbatini A, Dolcher MP, Marchini B. Alpha-enolase is a renal-specific antigen associated with kidney involvement in mixed cryoglobulinemia. *Clin Exp Rheumatol* 1997; 15:655–8.

125. Logothetis J, Kennedy WR, Ellington A, Williams RC. Cryoglobulinemic neuropathy: incidence and clinical characteristics. *Arch Neurol* 1968; 19:389–97.

126. Gemignani F, Pavesi G, Fiocchi A, Manganelli P, Ferraccioli G, Marbibi A. Peripheral neuropathy in essential mixed cryoglobulinemia. *J Neurol Neurosurg Psych* 1992; 55:116–120.

127. García-Bragado F, Fernández JM, Navarro C. Peripheral neuropathy in essential mixed cryoglobu-linemia. *Arch Neurol* 1988; 45:1210–14.

128. Nemni R, Corbo M, Fazio R, Quattrini A, Comi G, Canal N. Cryoglobulinemic neuropathy. A clinical, morphological and immunohistochemical study of 8 cases. *Brain* 1988; 111:541–2.

129. Chad D, Pariser K, Bradley WG, Adelman LS, Pinn VW. Pathogenesis of cryoglobulinemic neurop-athy. *Neurology* 1982; 32:725–9.

130. Cream JJ, Hern JEC, Hughes RAC, Mackenzie ICK. Mixed or immune complex cryoglobulinemia and neuropathy. *J Neurol Neurosurg Psychiatry* 1974; 37:82–7.

131. Bruyn GW. Angiopathic Neuropathy in Collagen Vascular Diseases. In: PJ Vinken, GW Bruyn and HL Klawans (Eds). *Handbook of Clinical Neurology*. Vol 51. WB Matthews, Amsterdam, p 446.

132. Conn DL, Hunder GG, O'Duffy JD. Vasculitis and Related Disorders. In: WN Kelley, DE Harris, S Ruddy and CB Sledge (Eds). *Textbook of Rheumatology,* 4th Edn. WB Saunders, Philadelphia, pp 1077–1102.

133. Chalk CH, Dick PJ, Conn DL, Vasculitic Neuropathy. In: PJ Dick, PK Thomas, JW Griffin, PA Low and JF Poduslo (Eds). *Peripheral Neuropathy,* Vol 2, 3rd. De WB Saunders, Philadelphia, pp 1424–36.

134. Vital C, Deminière C, Lagueny A et al. Peripheral neuropathy with essential mixed cryoglobulinemia: biopsies from 5 cases. *Acta Neuropathol* 1988; 75:605–610.

135. Thomas FP, Lovelace RE, Ding XS et al. Vasculitic neuropathy in a patient with cryoglobulinemia and anti-MAG IGM monoclonal gammopathy. *Muscle Nerve* 1992; 15:891–8.

11 Markers of Endothelial Damage

David P. D'Cruz

CONTENTS

I. INTRODUCTION

Vascular endothelial involvement is a characteristic feature of the systemic autoimmune diseases. The major manifestations of diseases such as systemic lupus erythematosus (SLE) include thrombosis, vasculitis, glomerulonephritis, synovitis, and central nervous system disease. In each of these manifestations the vascular endothelium is involved in different ways and may result in transient or permanent damage. The aim of this chapter is to review some of the mechanisms of vascular damage and serological markers that may be surrogate markers of endothelial damage, and to review the correlation of these values with clinical features.

II. MECHANISMS OF VASCULAR DAMAGE

The pathology of vascular disease was reviewed in detail in Chapter 1. However, it is worth summarizing the basic mechanisms by which the endothelium may be involved in vascular inflammation in autoimmune rheumatic diseases. While the precise mechanisms that initiate vascular inflammation remain poorly understood, the main processes are summarized in Table 11.1.

These pathological processes may result in endothelial activation, damage, or complete destruction of the endothelial layer as well as disruption of the subendothelial basement membrane and its related matrices. These processes may result in the release of various molecules into the circulation that could be useful markers of vascular damage.

III. ADHESION MOLECULES AND ENDOTHELIAL ACTIVATION

Endothelial cells express a large number of molecules on their surfaces either constitutively, or through signal transduction and protein synthesis that regulate the adhesion and transmigration of

---

TABLE 11.1
Putative Mechanisms of Vascular Damage in Autoimmune Disease

Immune complex-mediated disease with complement activation
Direct antibody-mediated endothelial cytotoxicity
Indirect antibody-dependent cell-mediated endothelial cytotoxicity
Phagocyte-mediated endothelial damage
T-cell reactivity against endothelium
Loss of protective antiinflammatory processes at the endothelium
Thrombosis and vascular occlusion

---

cells through the endothelial monolayer. These cell adhesion molecules are membrane-bound proteins that fall into three broad families: the integrins, the immunoglobulin superfamily, and the selectins.[1] The integrins may be divided into three subfamilies based on a common β chain: the very late antigen (VLA) proteins, the leucocyte integrins, and the cytoadhesins. The immunoglobulin superfamily of receptors generally bind to integrin receptors found on leucocytes and include the intercellular and vascular cell adhesion molecules (ICAM-1 and VCAM-1). The selectins include three members: E-, P-, and L-selectin, which are important in interactions between vascular endothelium and leucocytes, platelets, and lymphocytes.

Endothelial adhesion molecules are central to the recruitment of inflammatory cells to sites of infection and inflammation and may be upregulated by mediators such as IL-1, TNF-α, histamine, and bacterial lipopolysaccharide (LPS). The expression of these molecules may be measured by several means. For example, leucocyte adhesion molecule expression may be assessed *ex-vivo* using FACS analysis of peripheral blood samples. Vascular endothelial cell adhesion molecule expression can only be directly assessed by staining tissue sections from patients with vasculitis with specific monoclonal antibodies, and this does not allow a dynamic picture of adhesion molecule expression to be gained.[1] Conveniently, however, these adhesion molecules may be shed from the surface of endothelial cells and leucocytes, and these soluble forms may be detected in peripheral blood and other body fluids relatively easily.[2]

E-selectin is a good example to illustrate what may be achieved by monitoring circulating levels of soluble adhesion molecules. E-selectin is only expressed on activated endothlium and is released into the circulation. Thus measurements of soluble E-selectin may indicate the extent of endothelial activation in a given disease process. For example, soluble E-selectin levels are elevated in rheumatoid arthritis, the systemic vasculitides, polyarteritis nodosa and giant cell arteritis, systemic sclerosis and SLE.[3-7] In systemic sclerosis, soluble E-selectin levels are significantly elevated in patients with renal crisis but do not correlate with pulmonary hypertension,[3] and serial measurements correlate with changes in disease severity including changes in skin score and pulmonary and renal function.[4] A further study confirmed that E-selectin levels are elevated in systemic sclerosis and correlated with pulmonary fibrosis.[5] In SLE and the sytemic vasculitides, however, E-selectin is either not elevated or does not correlate with clinical features of active disease.[7-12] Similarly, E-selectin levels do not correlate with vasculitic complications in rheumatoid arthritis.[13]

Measurements of circulating cell adhesion molecules have shown good correlations with disease severity/activity in most of the autoimmune connective tissue diseases. For example, soluble intercellular adhesion molecule 1 (sICAM-1) levels correlate with disease relapse in patients with idiopathic retinal vasculitis.[14] Elevated levels of sICAM-1 and sVCAM-1 and correlations with disease activity have been shown in Wegener's granulomatosis and other systemic vasculitides, SLE, scleroderma, and rheumatoid arthritis.[4-6,8-11,13,15] In renal biopsies from patients with a variety of glomerulonephritides including lupus nephritis, ICAM-1 was found in the glomerular lesion and correlated with endocapillary proliferation with exudative lesions, hematuria, and circulating sICAM-1 levels.[16] Furthermore, elevated urinary excretion of sVCAM-1 as well as proinflammatory cytokines such as TNF-α, IL-6, and increased fractional excretion of IL-8 were observed in patients with ANCA-positive glomerulonephritis and lupus nephritis.[17] Thus measurement of circulating adhesion molecules may be a useful tool to monitor disease activity, and may be useful in the early detection of glomerulonephritis.

IV. PROCOAGULANT MOLECULES AS MARKERS OF ENDOTHELIAL DAMAGE

The vascular endothelium has a central physiological role in maintaining the patency of vessels and regulating thrombosis via procoagulant, antithrombotic, and fibrinolytic actions. Procoagulant molecules synthesized by endothelial cells include von Willebrand factor antigen (vWF), tissue factor, plasminogen activator-inhibitor-1 and 2 (PAI-1, PAI-2), factor V, and platelet activating factor. Many of these molecules have been measured in the autoimmune connective tissue diseases but are not all are endothelial specific.

A. VON WILLEBRAND FACTOR ANTIGEN

vWF is synthesized by the endothelium, stored as vWF multimers in the Weibel-Palade bodies, and released as multimeric molecules. vWF is important in platelet adhesion and aggregation, and its release from endothelium is enhanced by thrombin. vWF release from platelets is induced by ADP, collagen, and thrombin in vitro.[18] vWF has the advantage that it is easily measured by ELISA, though it should be remembered that vWF levels also rise with the acute phase response to infective episodes, rather like C-reactive protein.

Increased levels of vWF have been observed in a wide variety of autoimmune connective tissue diseases and correlate with clinical features such as vasculitis and glomerulonephritis. There is a consensus that raised vWF levels are broadly reflective of endothelial damage rather than being a non-specific acute phase reactant, though in the context of infection this may not be true.[18] In the systemic vasculitides, a large number of studies have shown that vWF levels are raised, but not all studies show a correlation with disease activity. An example is the study of Hergesell et al.,[19] who found high vWF levels in Wegener's granulomatosis and microscopic polyangiitis compared to healthy controls, but found that levels were not significantly different between patients with active disease and those in remission. Our own studies in Wegener's granulomatosis showed that vWF levels were elevated in patients and correlated with disease activity, ESR, CRP, ANCA titers, and serum creatinine levels.[20] vWF levels were particularly elevated in patients with active renal disease, and in the patients as a whole, vWF levels correlated weakly with soluble levels of IL-2 receptor, an indirect marker of lymphocyte activation (Figure 11.1).[20]

Elevated vWF levels were first noted in scleroderma in 1981,[21] and since then many studies have confirmed this and have observed correlations with major organ involvement.[22] Prospective studies of vWF levels in patients with scleroderma suggest that persistently elevated levels are associated with a higher risk of mortality.[23] Elevated vWF levels are seen in patients with rheumatoid vasculitis, and are also associated with cardiovascular events such as myocardial infarction in RA patients.[24,25]

In the 1970s vWF was studied as a marker of endothelial damage in adults and children with a variety of renal diseases and chronic renal failure. Several authors noted elevated levels of vWF in patients with early glomerulonephritis associated with a variety of diseases, chronic renal impairment, and renal diseases in children, respectively.[26-28] Ekberg et al.[26] suggested that elevated vWF levels were associated with a poor outlook in terms of deteriorating renal function, although this did not seem to be the case in Ambruso's study.[28] We showed that patients with lupus nephritis have significantly elevated vWF levels and vWF levels correlated with the presence of cutaneous and digital vasculitis and with nephrotic syndrome, but not with renal impairment.[29]

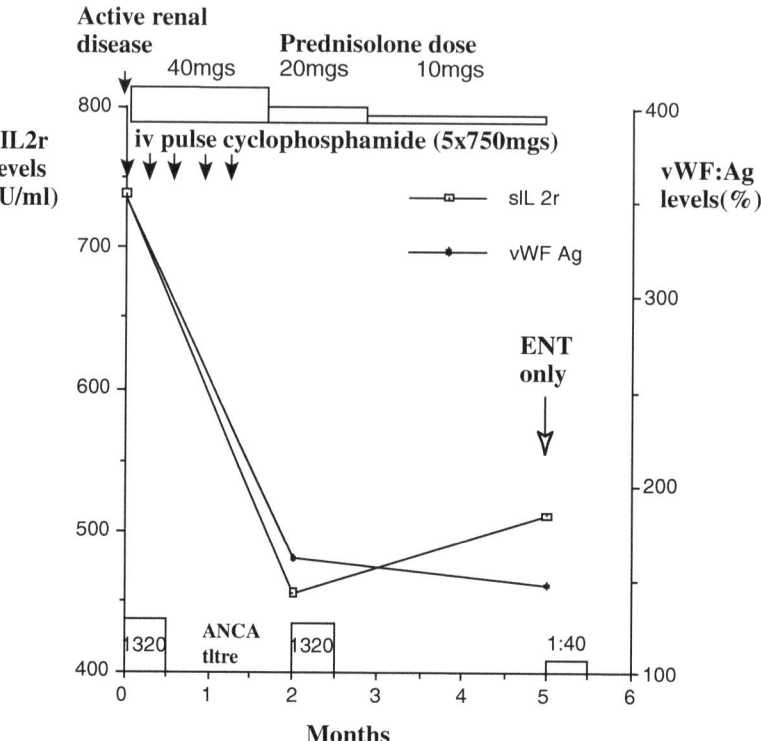

FIGURE 11.1 Serological profile of a patient treated with intravenous cyclophosphamide and prednisolone showing falls in sIL2r and vWF:Ag levels. (ENT = Ear, nose, and throat disease.) (Reprinted with permission).

VWF levels are elevated in patients with Behçet's disease although the proportion of patients with elevated levels varies between studies. For example, Yazici et al.[30] found elevated levels of vWF in 13 patients with Behçet's disease and vascular involvement compared to 17 patients without vascular disease. Direskeneli et al.[31] found elevated vWF levels in Behçet's disease patients compared to controls, but there were no specific correlations either with vascular complications or with disease activity. Thus, vWF levels may be useful markers of endothelial damage in some connective tissue diseases, and in a few diseases these levels may correlate with disease severity and prognosis. Although the vWF assay has been available for many years, the monitoring of vWF levels in connective tissue diseases has not been widely utilized.

V. THROMBOMODULIN

Thrombomodulin (Tm) is a transmembrane endothelial glycoprotein receptor that binds thrombin and catalyzes Protein C activation. It has powerful antithrombotic properties on the vascular surface, and measurement of Tm levels may be a useful marker of endothelial damage.[32,33] Tm is present on all vascular endothelia, is especially rich in the lung and placental vascular beds, and may be detected in a soluble form in most body fluids. Tm is excreted by the kidneys, so renal failure may result in elevated plasma Tm levels — the plasma Tm/creatinine ratio may be more useful in distinguishing Tm that has been released from damaged endothelia from Tm that has accumulated simply through renal impairment.[33] Tm is a more specific marker of endothelial damage than vWF and is not an acute phase reactant.

Plasma Tm levels are measured with an ELISA using two monoclonals recognizing different epitopes on the Tm molecule though the assay has not been internationally standardized.[32,33] There is wide variation in Tm levels between healthy individuals and according to age, sex, and blood group, though within individuals Tm levels remain relatively constant.[33]

Soluble Tm levels have been measured in a wide variety of vascular diseases. In the systemic vasculitides, for example, Tm levels were markedly elevated in both Wegener's granulomatosis and microscopic polyangiitis, and correlated with clinical disease activity.[12,34,35] In SLE, Tm levels correlated with active disease[36,37] and lupus nephritis but not with other measures of disease activity.[38] Since Tm is so closely related to mechanisms of thrombosis, there has been some interest in measuring Tm levels in the antiphospholipid syndrome. Takaya et al. did not find any correlation with antiphospholipid antibodies (aPL),[38] whereas Karmochkine et al. noted that Tm correlated with aPL but not with disease activity.[39] Further studies by Ohdama suggested that Tm levels may be a predictor of thrombotic complications in SLE although Tm levels did not correlate with antiphospholipid antibodies.[40] In Behçet's disease there have been conflicting studies of Tm levels,[34,41] with one study showing elevated levels and the other showing lower levels compared to healthy controls.

There have been a number of studies examining Tm levels in systemic sclerosis, and some studies demonstrated elevated Tm levels which correlated with the clinical extent of the disease. For example, Salojin et al.[42] found elevated Tm levels in patients with primary Raynaud's phenomenon, and even higher levels in limited systemic sclerosis patients compared to healthy controls. Mizutani et al. also noted high Tm levels in both the plasma and skin biopsies from patients with systemic sclerosis — Tm levels also correlated with anti-Scl-70 antibodies.[43] However, Herrick et al.[44] found no differences in Tm levels between patients with primary Raynaud's and those with limited or diffuse systemic sclerosis.

Decreased Tm levels may also be significant and result from microthrombosis and hypoxia that downregulates endothelial Tm synthesis. An example of this is severe primary pulmonary hypertension where hypoxia is severe and prolonged.[45]

VI. ENDOTHELINS

The endothelins (ET-1, ET-2, and ET-3) are a family of 21-aminoacid peptides. They are potent vasoconstrictor peptides produced by endothelial cells and are important in maintaining vascular tone. Elevated ET-1 levels have been described in a variety of conditions including SLE, Raynaud's phenomenon, systemic sclerosis, pulmonary hypertension, Buerger's disease, Kawasaki's disease, and Takayasu's disease. In these conditions ET-1 levels may contribute to the pathogenesis of the disease and be markers of endothelial involvement.

In SLE, Shen et al. found that ET levels were elevated particularly in patients with pulmonary hypertension, which was seen in 11% of their patients.[46] Elevated ET levels also correlated with active disease, Raynaud's phenomenon, and rheumatoid factors.

Systemic sclerosis is characterized by fibrosis, and vascular disease, particularly vasoconstriction, is a hallmark of the disease. The majority of ET is produced from the vascular endothelium but a recent study demonstrated that cultured fibroblasts from patients with systemic sclerosis are also able to produce excessive amounts of ET which is further enhanced by IL-1β.[47] Furthermore, alveolar macrophages from patients with lung involvement in systemic sclerosis produced more ET in response to LPS than macrophages from control subjects.[48] Thus ET production is not endothelial specific.

There have been a number of studies examining serum ET levels in systemic sclerosis, and the consensus is that ET-1 levels are markedly elevated.[49-55] These studies differ, however, in the correlation between elevated ET levels and clinical features. For example, Vancheeswaran et al.[52] noted that patients with diffuse systemic sclerosis had elevated ET levels irrespective of fibrotic skin or lung disease or hypertensive lung or renal disease. However, they found that only patients with limited systemic sclerosis and hypertensive lung or renal disease had elevated ET levels. In contrast, two studies by Morelli et al. demonstrated elevated ET levels but failed to find correlations with fibrotic or hypertensive lung disease.[53,54]

There have been very few studies in the systemic vasculitides. Elevated ET levels were found in patients with Kawasaki's disease compared to age-matched healthy and febrile controls.[56] In an unpublished pilot study, elevated ET levels were found in bronchoalveolar lavage fluid from patients with Wegener's granulomatosis.[57] The paucity of studies in this area is perhaps not surprising since neither vasoconstriction nor fibrosis are characteristic of the systemic vasculitides.

VII. LAMININ

The subendothelial basement membrane contains collagen type IV, laminin, and heparan sulphate proteoglycans together with the smaller molecules nidogen and BM-40. Basement membranes are important in such processes as the control of cell phenotype, tissue invasion by cells, and the filtration of macromolecules through glomeruli.

Laminin, with a molecular weight of 900 kDa, has a cruciate structure consisting of three polypeptide chains B1, B2, and A.[58] Laminin has been demonstrated in all renal and placental basement membranes, has fundamental structural and functional roles within basement membranes, and is produced by a variety of cells including endothelial cells. Laminin has well-defined domains that are responsible for cell binding, and binds calcium and collagen type IV within the matrix.

A pepsin digest of laminin obtained from human placenta produces up to eight fragments, including the antigenic P1 fragment. Using this fragment in inhibition radioimmunoassays, elevated laminin P1 (LP1) levels have been shown in conditions where there are increased turnovers or degradations of basement membranes, such as diabetic microangiopathy with renal involvement, pregnancy, and alcoholic liver disease.

In the autoimmune connective tissue diseases, Schneider et al.[59] showed that LP1 levels are elevated in patients with SLE, particularly during a flare of lupus. LP1 levels have also been described in systemic sclerosis, though without any correlation with clinical features[60] and cryo-globulinemic vasculitis where levels correlated with disease activity and visceral involvement.[61] Circulating levels of laminin fragments may therefore be surrogate markers of vascular damage in the autoimmune connective tissue diseases.

VIII. SUMMARY AND CONCLUSIONS

Vascular endothelial involvement is characteristic of the autoimmune connective tissue diseases, though the precise mechanisms of etiology and pathophysiology remain to be elucidated. A number of surrogate markers of endothelial damage have been described and some of these have proved to be useful clinical and prognostic markers. The description of novel markers such as endothelial adhesion molecules and endothelins may give further insights into the pathology of these diseases, and may add to the growing list of surrogate markers of endothelial dysfunction.

REFERENCES

1. Bradley JR, Lockwood CM, Thiru S. Endothelial cell activation in patients with systemic vasculitis. *QJM* 1994; 87:741–5.
2. Gearing AJH, Newman W. Circulating adhesion molecules in disease. *Immunol Today* 1993; 14:506–12.
3. Stratton RJ, Coghlan JG, Pearson JD, Burns A, Sweny P, Abraham DJ, Black CM. Different patterns of endothelial cell activation in renal and pulmonary vascular disease in scleroderma. *QJM* 1998; 91:561–6.

4. Denton CP, Bickerstaff MC, Shiwen X, Carulli MT, Haskard DO, Dubois RM, Black CM. Serial circulating adhesion molecule levels reflect disease severity in systemic sclerosis. *Br J Rheum* 1995; 34:1048–54.

5. Ihn H, Sato S, Fujimoto K, Takehara K, Tamaki K. Increased serum levels of soluble vascular cell adhesion molecule-1 and E-selectin in patients with systemic sclerosis. *Br J Rheum* 1998: 37; 1188–1192.

6. Salih AM, Nixon NB, Dawes PT, Mattey DL. Soluble adhesion molecules and anti-endothelial cell antibodies in patients with rheumatoid arthritis complicated by peripheral neuropathy. *J Rheumatol* 1999; 26:551–5.

7. Janssen BA, Luqmani RA, Gordon C, Hemingway IH, Bacon PA, Gearing AJ, Emery P. Correlation of blood levels of soluble vascular cell adhesion molecule-1 with disease activity in systemic lupus erythematosus and vasculitis. *Br J Rheum* 1994; 33:1112–6.

8. Mrowka C, Sieberth HG. Detection of circulating adhesion molecules ICAM-1, VCAM-1 and E-selectin in Wegener's granulomatosis, systemic lupus erythematosus and chronic renal failure. *Clinical Nephrol* 1995; 43:288–96.

9. Nyberg F, Acevedo F, Stephansson E. Different patterns of soluble adhesion molecules in systemic and cutaneous lupus erythematosus. *Exp Dermatol* 1997; 6:230–5.

10. Pall AA, Adu D, Drayson M, Taylor CM, Richards NT, Michael J. Circulating soluble adhesion molecules in systemic vasculitis. *Nephrol Dialysis Transplant* 1994; 9:770–4.

11. Stegeman CA, Tervaert JW, Huitema MG, de Jong PE, Kallenberg CG. Serum levels of soluble adhesion molecules intercellular adhesion molecule 1, vascular cell adhesion molecule 1, and E-selectin in patients with Wegener's granulomatosis. Relationship to disease activity and relevance during follow-up. *Arthritis Rheum* 1994; 37:1228–35.

12. Boehme MW, Schmitt WH, Youinou P, Stremmel WR, Gross WL. Clinical relevance of elevated serum thrombomodulin and soluble E-selectin in patients with Wegener's granulomatosis and other systemic vasculitides. *Am J Med* 1996; 101:387–94.

13. Voskuyl AE, Martin S, Melchers L, Zwinderman AH, Weichselbraun I, Breedveld FC. Levels of circulating intercellular adhesion molecule-1 and -3 but not circulating endothelial leucocyte adhesion molecule are increased in patients with rheumatoid vasculitis. *Br J Rheum* 1995; 34:311–5.

14. Palmer HE, Zaman AG, Ellis BA, Stanford MR, Graham EM, Wallace GR. Longitudinal analysis of soluble intercellular adhesion molecule 1 in retinal vasculitis patients. *Eur J Clin Inves* 1996; 26:686–91.

15. Kuryliszyn-Moskal A, Bernacka K, Klimiuk PA. Circulating intercellular adhesion molecule 1 in rheumatoid arthritis — relationship to systemic vasculitis and microvascular injury in nailfold capillary microscopy. *Clin Rheumatol* 1996; 15:367–73.

16. Yokoyama H, Takaeda M, Wada T, Ohta S, Hisada Y, Segawa C, Furuichi K, Kobayashi K. Glomerular ICAM-1 expression related to circulating TNF-alpha in human glomerulonephritis. *Nephron* 1997; 76(4):425–33.

17. Tesar V, Masek Z, Rychlik I, Merta M, Bartunkova J, Stejskalova A, Zabka J, Janatkova I, Fucikova T, Dostal C, Becvar R. Cytokines and adhesion molecules in renal vasculitis and lupus nephritis. *Nephrol Dialysis Transplant* 1998; 13:1662–7.

18. Blann AD. von Willebrand factor as a marker of injury to the endothelium in inflammatory vascular disease. *J Rheumatol* 1993; 20:1469–71.

19. Hergesell O, Andrassy K, Nawroth P. Elevated levels of markers of endothelial cell damage and markers of activated coagulation in patients with systemic necrotizing vasculitis. *Thromb Haemostas* 1996; 75:892–8.

20. D'Cruz D, Direskeneli H, Khamashta M, Hughes GR. Lymphocyte activation markers and von Willebrand factor antigen in Wegener's granulomatosis: potential markers for disease activity. *J Rheumatol* 1999; 26:103–9.

21. Kahaleh MB, Osborn I, LeRoy EC. Increased factor VIII/von Willebrand factor antigen and von Willebrand factor activity in scleroderma and in Raynaud's phenomenon. *Ann Intern Med* 1981; 94:482–4.

22. Greaves M, Malia RG, Milford Ward A, Moult J, Holt CM, Lindsey N, Hughes P, Goodfield M, Rowell NR. Elevated von Willebrand factor antigen in systemic sclerosis: relationship to visceral disease. *Br J Rheum* 1988; 27:281–5.

23. Blann AD, Sheeran TP, Emery P. von Willebrand factor: increased levels are related to poor prognosis in systemic sclerosis and not to tissue autoantibodies. *Br J Biomed Science* 1997; 54:5–9.

24. Belch JJF, Zoma AA, Richards IM, McLaughlin K, Forbes CD, Sturrock RD. Vascular damage and factor VIII related antigen in rheumatic diseases. *Rheumatology Int* 1987; 7:107–11.

25. Nilsson TK, Norberg B, Wallberg-Jonnson S, Dahlqvist SR. von Willebrand factor in plasma as risk indicator for cardiovascular events. *J Intern Med* 1991; 229:557–8.

26. Ekberg MR, Nilsson IM, Linell F. Significance of increased Factor VIII in early glomerulonephritis. *Ann Int Med* 1975; 83:337–341.

27. Warrell RP, Hultin M, Coller BS. Increased Factor VIII/von Willebrand factor antigen and von Willebrand factor activity in renal failure. *Am J Med* 1979; 66:226–228.

28. Ambruso DR, Durante DP, McIntosh RM, Hathway WE. Factor VIII and renal disease. *Ann Int Med* 1977; 87:636–637.

29. D'Cruz D, Jedryka-Goral A, Khamashta MA, Hughes GRV. von Willebrand factor antigen in lupus nephritis. *Arthritis Rheum* 1991; 34 (Supplement 9):130.

30. Yazici H, Hekim N, Ozbakir F, Yurdakul S, Tuzun Y, Pazarli H, Muftuoglu A. Von Willebrand factor in Behçet's syndrome. *J Rheumatol* 1987; 14:305–6.

31. Direskeneli H, Keser G, D'Cruz D, Khamashta MA, Akoglu T, Yazici H, Yurdakul S, Hamuryudan V, Ozgun S, Hughes GRV. Antiendothelial cell antibodies, endothelial proliferation and von Willebrand factor antigen in Behçet's disease. *Clin Rheumatol* 1995; 14:55–61.

32. Ishii H, Uchiyama H, Kazama M. Soluble thrombomodulin antigen in conditioned medium is increased by damage of endothelial cells. *Thromb Haemostas* 1991; 65:618–23.

33. Boffa MC, Karmochkine M. Thrombomodulin: an overview and potential implications in vascular disorders. *Lupus* 1998; 7 (Suppl 2):S120–5.

34. Ohdama S, Takano S, Miyake S, Kubota T, Sato K, Aoki N. Plasma thrombomodulin as a marker of vascular injuries in collagen vascular diseases. *Am J Clin Path* 1994; 101(1):109–13.

35. Ohdama S, Matsubara O, Aoki N. Plasma thrombomodulin in Wegener's granulomatosis as an indicator of vascular injuries. *Chest* 1994; 106:666–71.

36. Kawakami M, Kitani A, Hara M, Harigai M, Suzuki K, Kawaguchi Y, Ishii H, Kazama M, Kawagoe M, Nakamura H. Plasma thrombomodulin and alpha 2-plasmin inhibitor-plasmin complex are elevated in active systemic lupus erythematosus. *J Rheumatol* 1992; 19:1704–9.

37. Boehme MW, Nawroth PP, Kling E, Lin J, Amiral J, Riedesel J, Raeth U, Scherbaum WA. Serum thrombomodulin. A novel marker of disease activity in systemic lupus erythematosus. *Arthritis Rheum* 1994; 37:572–7.

38. Takaya M, Ichikawa Y, Kobayashi N, Kawada T, Shimizu H, Uchiyama M, Moriuchi J, Watanabe K, Arimori S. Serum thrombomodulin and anticardiolipin antibodies in patients with systemic lupus erythematosus. *Clin Exp Rheumatol* 1991; 9:495–9.

39. Karmochkine M, Boffa MC, Piette JC, Cacoub P, Wechsler B, Godeau P, Juhan I, Weiller PJ. Increase in plasma thrombomodulin in lupus erythematosus with antiphospholipid antibodies [letter]. *Blood* 1992; 79:837–8.

40. Ohdama S, Yoshizawa Y, Kubota T, Aoki N. Plasma thrombomodulin as an indicator of thromboembolic disease in systemic lupus erythematosus. *Int J Cardiol* 1994; 47(1 Suppl):S1–6.

41. Tribout B, Huong-Du LT, Gozin D et al. Low levels of circulating thrombomodulin in patients with Behçet's disease. *Rev Med Int* 1993; 14 (Suppl 1): 27 abstract CO9.

42. Salojin KV, Le Tonqueze M, Saraux A, Nassonov EL, Dueymes M, Piette JC, Youinou PY. Antiendothelial cell antibodies: useful markers of systemic sclerosis. *Am J Med* 1997; 102:178–85.

43. Mizutani H, Hayashi T, Nouchi N, Inachi S, Suzuki K, Shimizu M. Increased endothelial and epidermal thrombomodulin expression and plasma thrombomodulin level in progressive systemic sclerosis. *Acta Medica Okayama* 1996; 50:293–7.

44. Herrick AL, Illingworth K, Blann A, Hay CR, Hollis S, Jayson MI. von Willebrand factor, thrombomodulin, thromboxane, beta-thromboglobulin and markers of fibrinolysis in primary Raynaud's phenomenon and systemic sclerosis. *Ann Rheum Dis* 1996; 55:122–7.

45. Cacoub P, Karmochkine M, Dorent R, Nataf P, Piette JC, Godeau P, Gandjbakhch I, Boffa MC. Plasma levels of thrombomodulin in pulmonary hypertension. *Am J Med* 1996; 101:160–4.

46. Shen JY, Chen SL, Wu YX, Tao RQ, Gu YY, Bao CD, Wang Q. Pulmonary hypertension in systemic lupus erythematosus. *Rheum International* 1999; 18:147–51.

47. Kawaguchi Y, Suzuki K, Hara M, Hidaka T, Ishizuka T, Kawagoe M, Nakamura H. Increased endothelin-1 production in fibroblasts derived from patients with systemic sclerosis. *Ann Rheum Dis* 1994; 53:506–10.

48. Odoux C, Crestani B, Lebrun G, Rolland C, Aubin P, Seta N, Kahn MF, Fiet J, Aubier M. Endothelin-1 secretion by alveolar macrophages in systemic sclerosis. *Am J Resp & Critical Care Med* 1997; 156:1429–3.

49. Kadono T, Kikuchi K, Sato S, Soma Y, Tamaki K, Takehara K. Elevated plasma endothelin levels in systemic sclerosis. *Arch Dermatol Res* 1995; 287:439–42.

50. Kahaleh MB. Endothelin, an endothelial-dependent vasoconstrictor in scleroderma. Enhanced production and profibrotic action. *Arthritis Rheum* 1991; 34:978–83.

51. Zachariae H, Heickendorff L, Bjerring P, Halkier-Sorensen L, Sondergaard K. Plasma endothelin and the aminoterminal propeptide of type III procollagen (PIIINP) in systemic sclerosis. *Acta Dermato-Venereol* 1994; 74:368–70.

52. Vancheeswaran R, Magoulas T, Efrat G, Wheeler-Jones C, Olsen I, Penny R, Black CM. Circulating endothelin-1 levels in systemic sclerosis subsets — a marker of fibrosis or vascular dysfunction? *J Rheumatol* 1994; 21:1838–44.

53. Morelli S, Ferri C, Polettini E, Bellini C, Gualdi GF, Pittoni V, Valesini G, Santucci A. Plasma endothelin-1 levels, pulmonary hypertension, and lung fibrosis in patients with systemic sclerosis. *Am J Med* 1995; 99:255–60.

54. Morelli S, Ferri C, Di Francesco L, Baldoncini R, Carlesimo M, Bottoni U, Properzi G, Santucci A. Plasma endothelin-1 levels in patients with systemic sclerosis: influence of pulmonary or systemic arterial hypertension. *Ann Rheum Dis* 1995; 54:730–4.

55. Matsuda J, Tsukamoto M, Gohchi K, Saitoh N, Miyajima Y, Kazama M. Effect of total-body cold exposure on plasma concentrations of von Willebrand factor, endothelin-1 and thrombomodulin in systemic lupus erythematosus patients with or without Raynaud's phenomenon. *Acta Haematologica* 1992; 88:189–93.

56. Morise T, Takeuchi Y, Takeda R, Karayalcin U, Yachie A, Miyawaki T. Increased plasma endothelin levels in Kawasaki disease: a possible marker for Kawasaki disease. *Angiology* 1993; 44:719–23.

57. Ehrenreich H, Anderson RW, Fox CH, Rieckmann P, Hoffman GS, Travis WD, Coligan JE, Kehrl JH, Fauci AS. Endothelins, peptides with potent vasoactive properties, are produced by human macrophages. *J Exp Med* 1990; 172:1741–8.

58. Timpl R. Review: Structure and biological activity of basement membrane proteins. *Eur J Biochem* 1989; 180:487–502.

59. Schneider M, Hengst K, Waldendorf M, Högeman B, Gerlach U. The value of serum laminin P1 in monitoring disease activity in patients with systemic lupus erythematosus. *Scan J Rheumatol* 1988; 17:417–22.

60. Gerstmeier H, Gabrielli A, Meurer M, Brocks D, Braun-Falco O, Krieg T. Levels of type IV collagen and laminin fragments in serum from patients with progressive systemic sclerosis. *J Rheumatol* 1988; 15:969–72.

61. Gabrielli A, Marchegiani G, Rupoli S, Ansuini G, Brocks DG, Danieli G, Timpl R. Assessment of disease activity in essential cryoglobulinemia by serum levels of a basement membrane antigen, laminin. *Arthritis Rheum* 1988; 31:1558–62.

12 Systemic Inflammatory Response Syndrome, Systemic Lupus Erythematosus, and Thrombosis

H. Michael Belmont and Steven B. Abramson

CONTENTS

I. INTRODUCTION

The systemic inflammatory response syndrome (SIRS) is a reaction characterized by widespread inflammation primarily affecting the vascular endothelium. A consequence of SIRS is multiorgan failure or dysfunction syndrome, with manifestations that include catecholamine unresponsive hypotension, decreased myocardial contractility, cerebral dysfunction, and ARDS.[1-3] It is now recognized that SIRS may arise from both sepsis and noninfectious causes such as immune-mediated organ injury.[1] Serious exacerbations of systemic lupus erythematosus (SLE) can produce a syndrome that is indistinguishable from SIRS and can be accompanied by similar organ failure. Severe flares of SLE share many features with endotoxemia and SIRS, and are best modeled experimentally by the Shwartzman phenomenon.[4-6] Among the features common to both SIRS and active SLE are uncontrolled activation of the complement and clotting cascades, production of inflammatory cytokines, leukocyte-platelet activation within the microvasculature, and upregulation of adhesion molecules. Therefore, the Shwartzman phenomenon may serve as both a model for SIRS and the multiorgan dysfunction that can accompany acute lupus crisis. Additionally, the circulating mediators and endothelial cell activation that are the hallmarks of SIRS can provide the substrate permissive for the widespread, diffuse thrombosis that defines the catastrophic antiphospholipid antibody syndrome (CAPS).

This chapter will review the relationship between the Shwartzman phenomenon, SIRS, and mediators that act on inflammatory and endothelial cells promoting vascular injury in autoimmune disorders such as SLE and CAPS.

II. SIRS: SHWARTZMAN-LIKE INFLAMMATORY VASCULAR INJURY

Some patients with SLE have small vessel disease and inflammatory vasculopathy in the absence of local immune complex deposition, particularly those patients with central nervous system involvement.[7-9] Several lines of investigation now suggest a mechanism for this complement-mediated vascular injury in SLE, one not dependent on immune complex deposition.[10-15] This mechanism is best modeled experimentally by the Shwartzman phenomenon. The local Shwartzman lesion requires a preparatory intradermal injection of endotoxin, which is followed in 4–18 hours by the intravenous injection of endotoxin.[16,17] This results in the intravascular activation of complement triggering the release of anaphylatoxins such as C3a and C5a into the circulation.[18] The split products attract and activate inflammatory cells such as neutrophils and platelets, causing them to aggregate, to adhere to the vascular endothelium, to occlude small vessels, and to release toxic mediators. Activation of complement thus leads to an occlusive vasculopathy that may also result in widespread ischemic injury.[18]

The Shwartzman phenomenon was originally described as a model of meningococcal sepsis, but it is now recognized that cytokines such as IL-1β and TNF-α can substitute for endotoxin.[19] Such agents stimulate the up-regulation on the endothelial cell surface of intercellular adhesion molecule 1 (ICAM-1) and E-selectin, which are the counterreceptors for the neutrophil adhesion molecule CD11b/CD18 and Sialyl-Lewis X, respectively.[20] It has long been established that complement activation in plasma stimulates circulating neutrophils to produce the local Shwartzman lesion, but it was only recently recognized that the preparatory phase represents a time of ICAM-1 and E-selectin up-regulation.[17] The importance of this local endothelial cell activation is supported by the capacity of antibodies to ICAM-1, administered intravenously, to prevent the development of the experimental lesion.[17]

III. ACTIVATION OF THE COMPLEMENT SYSTEM

In most instances, inflammatory disease of blood vessels and tissues in SLE involves complement activation in the presence or absence of immune complex deposition. Complement cleavage products, particularly C3a, C5a, and C5b-9, are key mediators in the promotion of local tissue injury.

A. THE COMPLEMENT SYSTEM

The complement system is comprised of at least 20 plasma proteins which participate in a variety of host defense and immunological reactions. Each complement component is cleaved via a limited proteolytic reaction which proceeds by either the classical or alternative pathway. The alternative pathway is more primitive and may be activated by contact with a variety of substances including polysaccharides (such as endotoxin) found in the cell walls of microorganisms. The activation of the classical pathway by immune complexes requires binding of the first complement component, C1, to sites on the Fc portions of immunoglobulins, particularly of the IgG-1, IgG-3, and IgM isotypes.

1. Activation of C3

Activation of the third component of complement is central to both the classical and alternative pathways. C3 is cleaved by convertases to two active products, C3a and C3b. C3a, released into the fluid phase, provokes the release of histamine from mast cells and basophils, causes smooth muscle contraction, and induces platelet aggregation. C3b has two functions: it is part of the C5 convertase which continues the complement cascade, and is also the major opsonin of the complement system. It binds to immune complexes and to a variety of activators such as microbial organisms. The binding of C3b to these particles facilitates the attachment of the particle to the C3b receptor on cells, and on complement receptor 1 (CR1), which is present on erythrocytes, neutrophils, monocytes, B lymphocytes, and glomerular podocytes. CR1 on phagocytes potentiates phagocytosis. CR1 on erythrocytes, which accounts for approximately 90% of CR1 in blood, facilitates the clearance of immune complexes from the circulation by transporting erythrocyte-bound complexes to the liver and spleen for removal. Recently, a new biologic role for C3a and C3a desArg was described in the regulation of TNF-α and IL-1β synthesis in nonadherent peripheral blood mononuclear cells (PBMC).[21] C3a and C3a desArg suppressed endotoxin-induced synthesis of TNF-α and IL-1β. In contrast, in adherent PBMC, C3a and C3a desArg enhanced endotoxin-induced production of these cytokines. Thus, both C3a and C3a desArg may enhance cytokine synthesis by adherent monocytes at local inflammatory sites while inhibiting the systemic synthesis of proinflammatory cytokines by circulating cells.

2. Activation of C5

In addition to its role as an opsonin, C3b forms part of the C5 convertase which leads to the generation of C5a and C5b. C5a, like C3a, is an anaphylatoxin capable of activating basophils and mast cells. C5a is also among the most potent biological chemoattractants for neutrophils. C5b, which will attach to the surface of cells and microorganisms, is the first component in the assembly of C5b-9, the membrane attack complex.

3. Membrane Attack Complex

The Membrane Attack Complex (MAC), or the terminal complement assembly of C5b-9, has long been known to lytic bacteria. However, assembly of MAC on homologous leukocytes is not a cytotoxic event. After insertion of MAC into a leukocyte membrane, the cell sheds a small membrane vesicle containing the MAC complex. What is less appreciated is that insertion of MAC into the cell membrane triggers cell activation before it is shed.[22,23] MAC acts as an ionophore, provoking increases in cytosolic calcium and consequently triggering cell functions.[24] These include generation of toxic oxygen products as well as activation of both the cyclooxygenase (platelets, monocyte/macrophages, synoviocytes) and lipoxygenase pathways of arachidonate metabolism. Furthermore, the deposition of MAC increases the surface expression of P-selectin on the endothelial cell surface, promoting adhesion to circulating neutrophils.[25] *In vivo* evidence that vascular endothelium represents a site of C5b-9 deposition has been demonstrated in immune vasculitis[26-28] and infarcted myocardium.[29]

B. COMPLEMENT ACTIVATION DURING EXACERBATIONS OF SLE

A major consequence of immune complex deposition in SLE is the activation of complement. The consumption of complement components and their deposition in tissue is reflected by a decrease

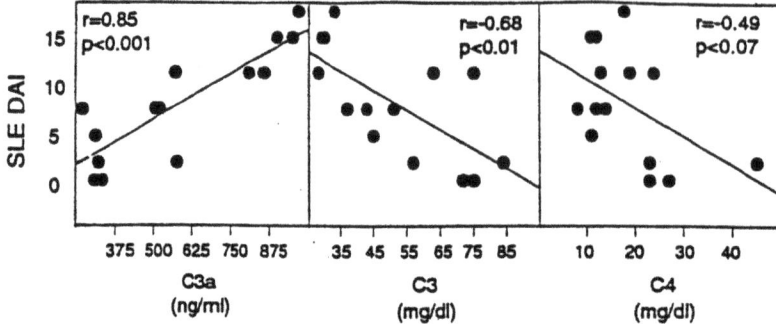

FIGURE 12.1 Correlation between complement levels (C3a desArg, C3, and C4) and the Systemic Lupus Erythematosus Activity Index (SLEDAI) score. There is a positive correlation between the SLEDAI and C3a and a negative correlation of a lesser magnitude between SLEDAI and C3 and C4.

in serum levels of C3 and C4 in most patients with active disease.[30] However, since the synthesis of both C3 and C4 increases during periods of disease activity, the serum levels of these proteins may be normal despite accelerated consumption.[31] Conversely, chronically depressed levels of individual complement components due to decreased synthesis, hereditary deficiencies, or increased extravascular distribution of complement proteins has been reported in SLE.[32] The decreased serum complement levels in these patients may lead to the mistaken conclusion that excessive complement activation is ongoing. To define more precisely the role of complement activation with respect to clinical disease, activity of SLE circulating levels of complement degradation products during periods of active and inactive disease have been measured.[7,33-37] Levels of plasma C3a, Ba, and the serum complement attack complex SC5b-9 were each shown to be more sensitive indicators of disease activity than either total C3 or C4 level.[7,33-35,37] Elevations of plasma C3a levels may precede other serologic or clinical evidence of an impending disease flare.[37]

The episodic, uncontrolled activation of complement proteins is a characteristic feature of SLE. Disease exacerbations are typically accompanied by decreases in total C3 and C4 values in association with elevations in plasma of the biologically active complement split products C3a desArg and C5a desArg.[7,35,38,39] During periods of disease flare, circulating neutrophils are activated to increase their adhesiveness to vascular endothelium, as indicated by the upregulation of the surface B2-integrin CD11b/CD18 (Complement receptor 3).[40,41] A recent study demonstrated that the surface expression of three distinct endothelial cell adhesion molecules, E-selectin, VCAM-1, and ICAM-1, is also upregulated in patients with SLE (Figures 12.1, 12.2).[9] Endothelial cell activation was most marked in patients with disease exacerbations characterized by significant elevations of plasma C3a desArg, and the activation reversed with improvement in disease activity.[9] In these studies, endothelial cell adhesion molecule up-regulation was observed in otherwise histologically normal skin, and was notable for the absence of local immune complex deposition.[9] These data suggest that excessive complement activation in association with primed endothelial cells can induce neutrophil-endothelial cell adhesion and predispose to leukoocclusive vasculopathy during SLE disease flares. This pathogenic mechanism may be of particular relevance to vascular beds which lack the fenestrations that permit the trapping of circulating immune complexes. Such an example is the central nervous system (CNS) where the blood-brain barrier can prevent the access of circulating immune complexes to the perivascular tissues. But in the setting of widespread endothelial cell activation, exuberant systemic complement activation can promote diffuse microvascular injury in the absence of immune complex deposition and produce the most common pathologic finding of CNS lupus, microinfarction.[38,42-45] Similar pathologic events may also be present in the mesenteric circulation and produce features of SLE enteritis,[8] or produce pulmonary leukosequestration and acute, reversible hypoxemia during disease exacerbations.[46]

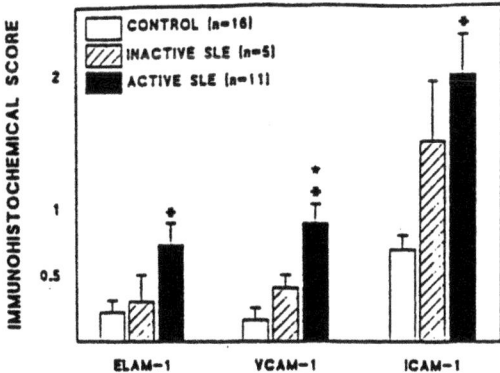

FIGURE 12.2 Endothelial cell adhesion molecule expression in patients with active vs. inactive SLE, and in healthy control subjects. The mean expression of all three adhesion molecules was significantly greater in patients with active SLE vs. controls. Adhesion molecule expression was also greater in patients with active vs. those with inactive SLE. Bars show the mean and SEM. (Note: ELAM-1 is now designated as E-selectin.)

IV. THE ROLE OF ENDOTHELIAL CELL ACTIVATION

A. Upregulation of Endothelial Adhesion Molecules

Recent *in vitro* and *in vivo* investigations have indicated that the perturbation of endothelial cells in SLE is an important accompaniment of active disease. It is increasingly clear that the endothelium is not just a passive target of injury, but plays an active role in accounting for the localization and propagation of the leucocyte and autoantibody-mediated inflammation.[47] The potential importance of endothelial adhesion molecule expression in SLE was recently illustrated by a report from Elkon and co-workers. These investigators demonstrated in MRL/MpJ-Faslpr (Faslpr) mice that ICAM-1 deficiency resulted in a striking improvement in survival.[48] Histological examination of ICAM-1-deficient mice revealed a significant reduction in glomerulonephritis and vasculitis of kidney, lung, and skin.

In human disease, Jones et al.[49] examined lesional skin in patients with SLE and scored the intensity of adhesion molecule expression immunohistochemically. They demonstrated increased expression of ICAM-1, VCAM-1, and E-selectin in lesional skin versus normal controls. We have examined endothelial cell adhesion molecule expression immunohistochemically in biopsy specimens from nonlesional, non-sun-exposed skin from SLE patients. Our findings demonstrated upregulation of the surface expression of all three adhesion molecules, E-selectin, VCAM-1, and ICAM-1, in patients with active SLE.[9,20] The abnormal expression of these endothelial cell adhesion molecules in histologically normal-appearing skin was most marked in patients with active disease characterized by significant elevations of the complement split product C3a desArg. In related studies we could also demonstrate that endothelial cells in these same biopsy specimens overexpressed the inducible form of nitric oxide synthase (NOS-2).[50] The activation of endothelial cells of nonlesional skin is a striking reminder of the systemic nature of immune stimulation in SLE, and is likely due to the circulation of a variety of stimuli capable activating endothelium.

Consistent with activation and perturbation of vascular endothelium, elevations of soluble adhesion molecules (E-selectin, sICAM-1, sVCAM-1) have been reported in active SLE.[47,51] While levels of soluble adhesion molecules reflect immune stimulation and tend to correlate with disease activity, their utility as monitors of disease activity remains to be established.

V. RECEPTORS FOR COMPLEMENT AND
INTERCELLULAR ADHESION IN SIRS

A. COMPLEMENT RECEPTORS AND SURFACE INTEGRINS

1. Neutrophils

The first event in an inflammatory process initiated by complement activation and the generation of potent chemoattractants, such as C5a, requires the margination, attachment, and egress of activated neutrophils from the circulation. Neutrophils express receptors for the complement fragment C3b (receptor designated CR1) and its inactivated cleavage product iC3b (receptor designated CR3 or CD11b/CD18).[52] On the surface of phagocytes, both CR1 and CD11b/CD18 play important roles in the clearance of particles, such as opsonized bacteria, to which C3b or iC3b are bound. This clearance mechanism is also essential for the removal of immune complexes containing C3b and iC3b.[53] In addition to its role as a receptor for iC3b, CD11b/CD18 is the major neutrophil adhesion molecule responsible for the capacity of the neutrophil to adhere to vascular endothelium and to other neutrophils.[41] CD11b/CD18 is a member of a family of surface glycoproteins known as beta2 integrins, which are heterodimers consisting of a common beta subunit (CD18) and distinct alpha subunits (CD11a, CD11b, CD11c). In the neutrophil the most important beta2 integrin appears to be CD11b/CD18, required for normal phagocytosis, aggregation, adhesion, and chemotaxis. Intercellular adhesion molecule-1 (ICAM-1), expressed on resting and activated endothelial cells, has been identified as a ligand for the CD18 integrins.[54] Interaction between CD18 and ICAM-1 modulates both the adhesion of neutrophils to vascular endothelium and their egress to the extravascular space. The initial rolling of activated neutrophils on endothelium, a prerequisite for CD18-dependent adhesion under conditions of flow, is mediated by a separate molecular interaction: that between the selectins, E-selectin, and P-selectin on the endothelial cell, and a carbohydrate ligand, sialyl-Lex, on the neutrophil.[54-56] In addition, the neutrophil expresses L-selectin on its surface, which also promotes rolling and is shed from the plasma membrane upon cell activation. The redundancy with regard to selectin function may be explained in part by the different kinetics of their participation in the events of intracellular adhesion: L-selectin is shed within seconds of neutrophil activation; P-selectin is stored in the Weibel-Palade bodies in endothelial cells and expressed on the surface within minutes following exposure of the cells to acute stimuli such as thrombin; and E-selectin is upregulated over several hours following cytokine exposure in a process which requires transcription and translation of new protein.

2. Macrophages/Monocytes

Macrophages/monocytes play an important role in immune-mediated tissue injury, particularly in nephritis.[57] These cells express the three major classes of Fc receptors as well as beta1, beta2, and beta3 integrins which facilitate phagocytosis of opsonized particles, intercellular adhesion, and adhesion to extracellular matrix proteins. Monocytes are recruited into tissues from the circulation in response to chemotactic factors (e.g., C5a, IL-8, TGF-beta, fragments of collagen, and fibronectin) produced at inflammatory sites. Recruitment requires the expression of adhesion molecules on activated vascular endothelium (e.g., ICAM-1, VCAM-1) which are recognized by counterligands of the circulating monocyte (e.g., LFA-1, VLA-4). When monocytes emigrate into tissues they can be transformed into activated macrophages following exposure to cytokines such as interferon-gamma, IL-1, and TNF. Macrophage activation results in an increase in cell size, increased synthesis of proteolytic enzymes, and the secretion of a variety of inflammatory products (Table 12.1).

3. Platelets

Platelets express two surface adhesion promoting molecules: gpIIb/IIIa (activated by ADP) which binds fibrinogen, fibronectin, vitronectin, and von Willebrand Factor,[58] and P-selectin (GMP-140,

TABLE 12.1
Local Mediators Released by Neutrophils, Macrophages, and Platelets

I.   Secretory products produced by neutrophils and macrophages
    1. Reactive oxygen intermediates (e.g., superoxide anion)
    2. Proteolytic enzymes
    3. Reactive nitrogen intermediates (e.g., nitric oxide)
    4. Bioactive lipids
      a. COX products: prostaglandin E_2 (PGE$_2$), PG F$_{2\alpha}$, prostacyclin, thromboxane (TX)
      b. LO products: monohydroxyeicosatetraenoic acids, dihydroxyeicosatetraenoic acids, leukotrienes, lipoxins
      c. PAFs (1 *O*-alkyl-2-acetyl-*sn*-glyceryl-3-phosphorylcholine)
    5. Chemokines (e.g., IL-8)
II. Secretory products produced by macrophages
    1. Polypeptide hormones
      a. IL-1α and IL-1β (collectively, IL-1)
      b. TNF-α (cachectin, TNF)
      c. IFN-α
      d. IFN-γ (confirmation needed)
      e. Platelet-derived growth factor(s) (PDGF)
      f. TGF-β
      g. b-Endorphin
    2. Complement (C) components
      a. Classical path: C1, C4, C2, C3, C5
      b. Alternative path: factor B, factor D, properdin
    3. Coagulation factors
      a. Intrinsic path: IX, X, V, prothrombin
      b. Extrinsic path: VII
      c. Surface activities: tissue factor, prothrombinase
      d. Prothrombolytic activity: plasminogen activator inhibitors, plasmin inhibitors
III. Secretory products produced by platelets
    1. Plasminogen
    2. α2-Plasmin inhibitor
    3. PDGF
    4. Platelet factor 4
    5. TGF-α and TGF-β
    6. Serotonin
    7. Adenosine diphosphate
    8. Thromboxane A_2
    9. 12-hydroxytetraenoic acid

PADGEM), a membrane glycoprotein located in the alpha granules of platelets and Weibel-Palade bodies of endothelium. When these cells are activated by agents such as thrombin, P-selectin is rapidly translocated to the plasma membrane where it functions as a receptor for neutrophils and monocytes. Expression of P-selectin on activated platelets may therefore facilitate recruitment of neutrophils and monocytes to sites of thrombosis or inflammation.[55]

Platelets have been identified in the glomeruli of patients with SLE nephritis, where they are believed to play a particularly important role.[59] Urinary thromboxane levels are elevated in patients with active lupus nephritis, a finding with several implications: first, it is a sign of abnormal platelet aggregation in the microvasculature with the potential for thrombosis and endothelial injury; second, the vasoconstrictive properties of TXA2 would be expected to decrease glomerular filtration rate (GFR) and renal blood flow (RBF); and, third, the release of growth factors and other mediators by activated platelets could aggravate the proliferative glomerular lesion. Recent studies of the administration of specific TXA2 antagonists have shown promise in the improvement of both GFR and RBF in SLE nephritis.[60]

Platelet activation in lupus glomerulonephritis has been attributed to a variety of substances, including immune complexes, activated complement components (including C3a and the membrane attack complex, C5b-9), PAF, and vasopressin. Neutrophils may also be able to activate platelets via the release of oxidants and proteases. Platelets may aggravate immune injury in glomerulonephritis via several mechanisms, which include: promoting thrombosis; reducing glomerular filtration rate (GFR) through the production of thromboxane and other vasoactive substances; and release of products which activate macrophages, neutrophils, and glomerular mesangial cells.[61]

VI. SIRS AND CAPS

SIRS, as modeled by the Shwartzman phenomenon, is characterized by inflammatory vascular injury and leukothrombosis. However, SIRS is not only accompanied by activation of complement, neutrophils, and platelets, but also by the triggering of the serine protease cascades of the coagulant and fibrinolytic systems.[62] Therefore, SIRS associated with endotoxemia can produce a consumptive coagulopathy and DIC. However, immune-mediated SIRS, with its emphasis on endothelial cell activation, may be a model for the thrombosis that accompanies the antiphospholipid antibody syndrome, especially catastrophic APS.

Catastrophic APS occurs in a minority of patients with aPL; is characterized by acute, vascular occlusions involving multiple organs; and is an example of a noninflammatory thrombotic microvasculopathy.[63] The pathogenesis of microvasculopathy in autoimmune disease includes classic leukocytoclastic vasculitis secondary to subendothelial immune complex deposition in vessel walls; leukothrombosis secondary to intravascular activation of complement, neutrophils, and endothelium in the absence of local immune complex deposition as modeled by the Shwartzman phemomenon; or thrombosis of vessels secondary to a noninflammatory vasculopathy.[4-6]

Besides APS, thrombotic microangiopathic syndromes include thrombotic thrombocytopenia purpura (TTP), hemolytic uremic syndrome (HUS), disseminated intravascular coagulation (DIC), and HELLP (hemolysis, elevated liver enzymes, and low platelets associated with preeclampsia) syndrome. The latter is an uncommon complication of pregnancy and, interestingly, Neuwelt described a woman who developed catastrophic APS 31 years after a pregnancy accompanied by HELLP, suggesting a unifying pathophysiologic mechanism.[64] On the other hand, evidence suggests that an immunoglobulin inhibitor of von Willebrand factor-cleaving protease causes the thrombotic microangiopathic hemolytic anemia that characterizes autoimmune-associated TTP.[65] The uncatabolized von Willebrand multimers promote disseminated intravascular platelet aggregation.

The diffuse and multiorgan yet episodic nature of catastrophic APS occurring in only a minority of patients with likely longstanding circulating aPL is consistent with the hypothesis that additional biological factors are required for the widespread microvasculopathy. A candidate target for activation that would then be permissive for the development of APS is endothelial cells. The common pathophysiologic substrate in SIRS and CAPS is activation of vascular endothelium to express proinflammatory surface adhesion molecules that interact with circulating inflammatory cells (e.g. neutrophils), elements of the phospholipid-dependent coagulation factors, and platelets.[4,66] The endogenous mediators of SIRS include immune stimuli that activate endothelial cells and likely contribute to providing preparatory signals for catastrophic APS. These stimuli include cytokines, complement components, and autoantibodies.

A. IMMUNE STIMULI THAT ACTIVATE ENDOTHELIAL CELLS

1. Cytokines

Cytokines are likely to be important mediators of endothelial cell activation and injury in SLE vasculitides. TNF-α INF-γ and IL-1 each stimulate adhesion molecule expression. Different studies have variably reported increased levels of TNF-α, IL-1β, IL-6, IFN-γ, and IL-8 in the circulation during vasculitis,[47] but the specific role of a specific cytokine remains to be determined. It should be noted that while endothelial cells may be acted upon by cytokines produced by other inflammatory cells, they also can be stimulated to produce cytokines such as IL-1, IL-6, IL-8, and TNF-α which can act as autacoids to upregulate adhesion molecule expression.[67]

2. Complement Components

Several products of the activated complement system (e.g., C3b, iC3b, and C5a) are known to activate endothelial cells *in vitro*. More recently, the role of the membrane attack complex (MAC) in endothelial cell activation has emerged. Kilgore et al. demonstrated, using human umbilical vein endothelial cells (HUVECs), that assembly of the MAC resulted in a marked increase in neutrophil binding as compared with that observed in cells treated with TNF-α alone.[68] Enhanced neutrophil binding was attributable to upregulation of E-selectin and ICAM-1.

The MAC has also recently been shown, in a study by Saadi et al., to participate in the upregulation of endothelial cell tissue factor activity.[69] The expression of tissue factor by the endothelium promotes a procoagulant state that is likely to be of major importance in the pathogenesis of the vascular injury. Using the interaction of antiendothelial cell (EC) antibodies and complement with cultured endothelium as a model, the authors studied the expression and function of tissue factor, a cofactor for factor VIIa-mediated conversion of factor X to factor Xa. Cell surface expression of tissue factor activity required activation of complement and assembly of the membrane attack complex. Expression of tissue factor was not a direct consequence of the action of the MAC on the endothelial cell, but was a secondary response that required as an intermediate step the release of IL-1α, an early product of the endothelial cell response to complement activation.

Finally, there is recent evidence that C1q is a cofactor required for immune complexes to stimulate endothelial expression of E-selectin, ICAM-1 and VCAM-1.[70] In these studies, immune complexes caused the upregulation of HUVEC adhesion molecules and stimulated endothelial cell adhesiveness for added leukocytes in the presence of complement-sufficient normal human serum. The dependency on serum could be shown to be due to a requirement for complement activation and the generation of C1q. HUVECs expressed a 100- to 126-kDa C1q-binding protein. However, soluble C1q alone, unbound to immune complexes, did not induce adhesion molecule upregulation.

3. Autoantibodies

Autoantibodies to phospholipids, endothelial cells, and DNA have each been demonstrated to react with endothelial cells *in vitro* and promote the upregulation of adhesion molecules or tissue factor. The capacity of antiendothelial cell antibodies, for example, to increase tissue factor expression in the presence of complement was noted above.[69] Neng et al. reported that anti-DNA autoantibodies stimulate the release of interleukin-1 and interleukin-6 from human endothelial cells.[71] In these studies, the incubation of endothelial cells with purified IgG containing anti-ds-DNA (compared with those incubated with anti-ds-DNA-depleted IgG) caused a significant increase of supernatant IL-1 and IL-6 in association with increased mRNA expression for these cytokines. The investigators, using a similar strategy, also demonstrated the upregulation of adhesion molecule expression on endothelial cells by anti-DNA autoantibodies in patients with SLE.[72] In these studies, the expression of ICAM-1 and VCAM-1 on HUVECs cultured with either control IgG or anti-ds-DNA were compared by flow cytometry. Compared with either control IgG or anti-ds-DNA-depleted-IgG, HUVEC incubated with anti-ds-DNA expressed a significantly higher mean fluorescence intensity of ICAM-1 and VCAM-1. At the same time, ICAM-1 mRNA was also raised.

Simanitov et al. showed that IgG from patients with aPL was able to enhance endothelial cell adhesion molecule expression and monocyte adherence.[73] This capacity of aPL to activate endothelial cells may be required in catastrophic APS before aPL interacts with platelets or coagulation proteins to mediate diffuse thrombotic microvasculopathy.

The activation of endothelial cells and accompanying upregulation of adhesion molecules and tissue factor typical of SIRS is likely pivotal to the development of catastrophic APS. It is the collaboration of cytokines, activated complement components, and autoantibodies that act on endothelial cells to increase adhesiveness, and procoagulant activity that provides the preparatory signals for aPL in catastrophic APS. This interaction between activated endothelial cells, neutrophils, and platelets in the presence of aPL generates the diffuse microvasculopathy that characterizes catastrophic APS. This diffuse thrombotic microvasculopathy is responsible for the clinical features of catastrophic APS by producing tissue injury, which can include pulmonary capillary leak or ARDS, brain capillary leak or "acute cerebral distress syndrome," myocardial dysfunction, and, potentially, systemic inflammatory response syndrome (SIRS) with multiorgan failure.

VII. CONCLUSION

Based on the shared pathogenesis and clinical features, severe SLE exacerbations may be viewed as immune-mediated SIRS, while CAPS as SIRS occurs in the setting of high titer antiphospholipid antibodies. Vascular injury results in each of these syndromes due to a collaboration of cytokines, activated complement components, and autoantibodies acting on endothelial cells to increase adhesiveness and procoagulant activity. These same mediators act locally on leukocytes and platelets to increase their adhesion to vascular endothelium and to stimulate the local release of toxic inflammatory mediators, including proteases and oxygen-derived free radicals. SIRS occurring in the setting of autoimmune disorders can generate either leukothrombosis in the presence of complement, neutrophil and endothelial cell activation, or noninflammatory thrombotic vasculopathy in the presence of aPL. The precise trigger for endothelial cell activation, the reason that clinical exacerbations and remissions are episodic and separated in time, and the ameliorative effects of immunosuppressive and anticoagulation therapy require further clarification. Blockade of the interactions between inflammatory cells, adhesion molecules, and endothelial cells could provide useful therapeutic strategy in the future.

REFERENCES

1. Bone RC. Why new definitions of sepsis and organ failure are needed. *Am J Med* 1993; 95:348.
2. Nogare D. Septic shock. *Am J Med Sci* 1991; 302:50–65.
3. Waage A, Brandtzaeg P, Espevik T, Halstensen A. Current understanding of the pathogenesis of gram-negative shock. *Infect Dis Clin North Am* 1991; 5:781–789.
4. Belmont HM, Abramson SB, Lie JT. Pathology and pathogenesis of vascular injury in systemic lupus erythermatosus: Interactions of inflammatory cells and activated endothelium. *Arthritis Rheum* 1996; 39:9–22.
5. Golden BD, Belmont HM. The role of microvasculopathy in the catastrophic antiphospholipid syndrome: comment on the article by Neuwelt et al (letter). *Arth Rheum* 1997; 40 (8):1534–1539.
6. Abramson SA, Belmont HM. SLE: Mechanisms of vascular injury. *Hosp Prac* 1998; 33 (4):107–127.
7. Belmont HM, Hopkins P, Edelson HS, et al. Complement Activation during systemic lupus erythematosus. C3a and C5a anaphylatoxins circulate during exacerbations of disease. *Arth Rheum* 1986; 29:1085–1089.
8. Hopkins P, Belmont M, Buyon J, Philips MR, Weissmann G, Abramson SB. Increased plasma anaphylotoxins in systemic lupus erythematosus predict flares of the disease and may elicit the adult cerebral distress syndrome. *Arth Rheum* 1988; 31:632–641.
9. Belmont HM, Buyon J, Giorno R, Abramson SB. Upregulation of endothelial cell adhesion molecules characterizes disease activity in systemic lupus erythematosus: The Shwartzman Phenomenon revisited. *Arth Rheum* 1994; 37:376–383.
10. Jacob HS, Craddock PR, Hammerschmidt DE, Moldow CF. Complement-induced granulocyte aggregation: an unsuspected mechanism of disease. *N Eng J Med* 1980; 302:789–794.

11. Hammerschmidt DE, Weaver LJ, Hudson LD, Craddock PR, Jacob HS. Association of complement activation and elevated plasma-C5a with adult respiratory distress syndrome. *Lancet* 1980; 1:947–949.

12. Hakim R, Breillatt J, Lazarus M, Prt K. Complement activation and hypersensitivity reactions to hemodialysis membranes. *N Eng J Med* 1984; 311:878–882.

13. Craddock P, Fehr J, Dalmasso A, Brigham K, Jacob H. Hemodialysis leukopenia. *J Clin Invest* 1977; 59:879–888.

14. Chenoweth DE, Cooper SW, Hugli TE, Stewart RW, Balckstone EH, Kirklin SW. Complement activation during cardiopulmonary bypass. *N Eng J Med* 1981; 304:497–505.

15. Perez HD, Horn JK, Ong R, Goldstein I. Complement (C5)-derived chemotactic activity in serum from patients with pancreatitis. *J Lab Clin Med* 1983; 101:123–129.

16. Shwartzman G. *Phenomenon of Local Tissue Reactivity.* New York: Paul Hoeber, 1937.

17. Argenbright L, Barton R. Interactions of leukocyte integrins with intercellular adhesion molecule 1 in the production of inflammatory vascular injury *in vivo.* The Shwartzman phenomenon revisited. *J Clin Invest* 1992; 89:259–273.

18. Abramson SB, Weissmann G. Complement split products and the pathogenesis of SLE. *Hosp Prac* 1988; 23(12):45–55.

19. Pohlman TM, Stanness KA, Beatty PG, Ochs HD, and Harlan JM. *J Immunol* 1986; 136:4548–4553.

20. Pober JS, Gimbrone M, Lapierre D, et al. Overlapping patterns of activation of human endothelial cells by interleukin-1, tumor necrosis factor and immune interferon. *J Immunol* 1986; 137:1893–1896.

21. Takabayashi T, Vannier E, Clark BD, et al. A new biologic role for C3a and C3a desArg: regulation of TNF-alpha and IL-1 beta synthesis. *J Immunol* 1996; 156:3455–3460.

22. Stein JM, Luzio JP. Membrane sorting during vesicle shedding from neutrophils during sublytic complement attack. *Biochem Soc Trans* 1989; 16:1082–1083.

23. Morgan BP, Dankert JR, Esser AF. Recovery of human neutrophils from complement attack: Removal of the membrane attack complex by endocytosis and exocytosis. *J Immunol* 1987; 138:246–253.

24. Morgan BP. Complement membrane attack on nucleated cells: resistance, recovery and non-lethal effects. *Biochem J* 1989; 264:1–14.

25. Hattori R, Hamilton KK, McEver RP, Sims PJ. Complement proteins C5b-9 induce secretion of high molecular weight multimers of endothelial von Willebrand Factor and translocation of granule membrane. *J Biol Chem* 1989; 264:9053–9060.

26. Biesecker G, Katz S, Koffler D. Renal localization of the membrane attack complex in systemic lupus erythematosus nephritis. *J Exp Med* 1981; 154:1779–1794.

27. Biesecker G, Lavin L, Zisking M, Koffler D. Cutaneous localization of the membrane attack complex in discoid and systemic lupus erythematosus. *N Eng J Med* 1982; 306:264–270.

28. Kissel JT, Mendell JR, Rammohan KW. Microvascular deposition of complement membrane attack complex in dermatomyositis. *N Eng J Med* 1986; 314:329–334.

29. Schafer H, Mathey D, Hugo F, Bhakdi S. Deposition of the terminal C5b-9 complement complex in infarcted areas of human myocardium. *J Immunol* 1986; 137:1945–1949.

30. Ruddy S, Carpenter CB, Chin KW, et al. Human complement metabolism: an analysis of 144 studies. *Medicine* (Baltimore) 1975; 54:165–178.

31. Charlesworth JA, Williams DG, Sherington E, Lachmann PJ, Peters DK. Metabolic studies of the third component of complement and the glycine rich glycoprotein in patients with hypocomplementemia. *J Clin Invest* 1974; 53:1578–1587.

32. Sliwinski AJ, Zvaifler NJ. Decreased synthesis of the third component (C3) in hypocomplementemic systemic lupus erythematosus. *Clin Exp Immunol* 1972; 11:21–29.

33. Kerr L, Adelsberg BR, Schulman P, Spiera H. Factor B activation products in patients with systemic lupus erythematosus: A marker of severe disease activity. *Arth Rheum* 1989; 32:1406–1413.

34. Falk RJ, Dalmasso AP, Kim Y, Lam S, Michael A. Radioimmunoassay of the attack complex of complement in serum from patients with systemic lupus erythematosus. *N Eng J Med* 1985; 312:1594–1599.

35. Buyon J, Tamerius J, Belmont HM, Abramson S. Assessment of disease activity and impending flare in patients with systemic lupus erythematosus: comparison of the use of complement split products and conventional measurements of complement. *Arth Rheum* 1992; 35:1028–1037.

36. Buyon J, Tamerius J, Ordica S, Young B, Abramson S. Activation of the alternative complement pathway accompanies disease flares in systemic lupus erythematosus during pregnancy. *Arth Rheum* 1992; 35:55–61.
37. Hopkins PT, Belmont HM, Buyon J, Philips MR, Weissmann G, Abramson SB. Increased levels of plasma anaphylatoxins in systemic lupus erythematosus predict flares of the disease and may elicit vascular injury in lupus cerebritis. *Arth Rheum* 1988; 31:632–641.
38. Fletcher MP, Seligmann BE, Gallin JI. Correlation of human neutrophil secretion, chemoattractant receptor mobilization and enhanced functional capacity. *J Immunol* 1982; 128:941.
39. Schur PH, Sandson J. Immunologic factors and clinical activity in systemic lupus erythematosus. *N Eng J Med* 1968; 278:533–538.
40. Buyon JP, Shadick N, Berkman R, et al. Surface expression of gp165/95, the complement receptor CR3, as a marker of disease activity in systemic lupus erythematosus. *Clin Immunol Immunopath* 1988; 46:141–149.
41. Philips MR, Abramson SB, Weissmann G. Neutrophil adhesion and autoimmune vascular injury. *Clin Aspects Autoimmun* 1989; 3:6–15.
42. Johnson RT, Richardson EP. The neurological manifestations of systemic lupus erythematosus: a clinical pathological study of 24 cases and a review of the literature. *Medicine* (Baltimore) 1968; 47:337–369.
43. Ellis SG, Verity MA. Central nervous system involvement in systemic lupus erythematosus: a review of the neuropathologic findings in 57 cases, 1955–1977. *Semin Arth Rheum* 1979; 8:212–233.
44. Hammad A, Tsukada Y, Torre N. Cerebral occlusive vasculopathy in systemic lupus erythematosus and speculation on the part played by complement. *Ann Rheum Dis* 1992; 51:550–552.
45. Devinsky O, Petito CK, Alonso DR. Clinical and neuropathological findings in systemic lupus erythematosus: The role of vasculitis heart emboli and thrombotic thrombocytopenic purpura. *Ann Neurol* 1988; 23:380.
46. Abramson SB, Dobro J, Eberle MA, et al. The syndrome of acute reversible hypoxemia of systemic lupus erythematosus. *Ann Int Med* 1991; 114:941–947.
47. Arnaout MA, Colten HR. Complement C3 receptors: Structure and function. *Molec Immun* 1984; 21:1191–1199.
48. Wright SD, Rao PE, VanVoorhis WC, et al. Identification of the C3bi receptor of human monocytes and macrophages by using monoclonal antibodies. *Proc Natl Acad Sci USA* 1983; 80:5699–5705.
49. Springer TZ, Teplow DB, Dreyer WJ. Sequence homology of the LFA-1 and Mac-1 leukocyte adhesion glycoprotein and unexpected relation to leukocyte interferon. *Nature* 1985; 314:540–542.
50. Belmont HM, Levartovsky D, Goel A, et al. Increased nitric oxide production accompanied by the upregulation of inducible nitric oxide synthase in vascular endothelium from patients with systemic lupus erythematosus. *Arth Rheum* 1997; 40:1810–1816.
51. Fearon DT, Collins LA. Increased expression of C3b receptors on polymorphonumclear leukocytes induced by chemotactic factors and by purification procedures. *J Immunol* 1983; 130:370–375.
52. Ross GD, Medof ME. Membrane complement receptors specific for bound fragments of C3. *Adv Immunol* 1985; 37:217–267.
53. Schifferli JA, Ng YC, Peters DK. The role of complement and its receptor in the elimination of immune complexes. *N Eng J Med* 1986; 315:488–495.
54. Yong K, Khwaja A. Leukocyte cellular adhesion molecules. *Blood Rev* 1990; 4:211–225.
55. McEver RP, Roder P. Selectins: Novel receptors that mediate leukocyte adhesion during inflammation. *Thromb & Haemostasis* 1991; 65:223–228.
56. Lawrence MB, Springer TA. Leukocytes role on a selection of physiologic flow rates: Distinction from and prerequisite for adhesion through integrins. *Cell* 1991; 65:859–873.
57. Nikolic–Paterson DJ, Lan HY, Hill PA, Atkins RC. Macrophages in renal injury. *Kidney Int* 1994; 45:S79-S82.
58. Pytela R, Pierschbacher M, Ginsberg M, Plow E, Rouslahti E. Platelet membrane glycoprotein IIb/IIIa: member of a family of Arg-Gly-Asp-specific adhesion receptors. *Science* 1986; 231:1559–1562.
59. Johnson RJ. Platelets in inflammatory glomerular injury. *Sem Nephrol* 1991; 11:276–284.
60. Pierucci A, Simonetti BM, Pecci G. Improvement in renal function with selective thromboxane antagonism in lupus nephritis. *N Eng J Med* 1989; 320:421–425.

61. Johnson RJ, Lovett D, Lehrer RI, Couser WG, Klebanoff SJ. Role of oxidants and proteases in glomerular injury. *Kidney Int* 1994; 45:352–359.

62. Van Deventer SJH, Buller HR, Ten Cate JW, et al. Experimental endotoxemia in humans: Analysis of cytokine release and coagulation, fibrinolytic, and complement pathways. *Blood* 1990; 76:2520–2526.

63. Asherson RA. The catastrophic antiphospholipid syndrome. *J Rheumatol* 1992; 19:508–512.

64. Neuwelt CM, Daikh DI, Linfoot JA, et al. Catastrophic antiphospholipid syndrome. Response to repeated plasmapheresis over three years. *Arth Rheum* 1997; 40:1534–1539.

65. Tsai H-M, Lian EC-Y. Antibodies to von Willebrand factor-cleaving protease in acute thrombotic thrombocytopenic purpura. *N Engl J Med* 1998; 339:1585–1594.

66. Cockwell P, Tse WY, Savage CO. Activation of endothelial cells in thrombosis and vasculitis. *Scan J of Rheum* 1997; 26:145–150.

67. Berger MD, Birx L, Wetzler EM, O'Shea JJ, Brown EJ, Cross AS. *J Immunol* 1985; 135:1342–1348.

68. Kilgore KS, Shen JP, Miller BF, Ward PA, Warren JS. Enhancement by the complement membrane attack complex of tumor necrosis factor-alpha-induced endothelial cell expression of E-selectin and ICAM-1. *J Immunol* 1995; 155:1434–1441.

69. Saadi S, Holzknecht RA, Patte CP, Stern DM, Platt JL. Complement-mediated regulation of tissue factor activity in endothelium. *Lupus* 1995; 4:104–108.

70. Lozada C, Levin RI, Huie M, et al. Identification of C1q as the heat-labile serum cofactor required for immune complexes to stimulate endothelial expression of the adhesion molecules E-selectin and intercellular and vascular cell adhesion molecules. *Proc Natl Acad Sci USA* 1995; 92:8378–8382.

71. Neng Lai LK, Leung JC, Bil Lai K, Li PK, Lai CK. Anti-DNA autoantibodies stimulate the release of interleukin-1 and interleukin-6 from human endothelial cells. *J Pathol* 1996; 178:451–458.

72. Lai KN, Leung JC, Lai KB, Wong KC, Lai CK. Upregulation of adhesion molecule expression on endothelial cells by anti-DNA autoantibodies in systemic lupus erythematosus. *Clin Immunol Immunopath* 1996; 81:229–238.

73. Simantov R, LaSala J, Lo SK, et al. Activation of cultured vascular endothelial cells by antiphospholipid antibodies. *J Clin Invest* 1995; 96:2211–2219.

13 Leukocyte Cell Adhesion Molecules in Vasculitis

Jan Willem Cohen Tervaert and Cees G.M. Kallenberg

CONTENTS

I. INTRODUCTION

The vascular endothelium forms the biologic interface between circulating blood and all other tissues and organs. Endothelial cells respond to various stimuli by initiating a series of molecular events (endothelial cell activation) that culminate in adhesion and emigration of leukocytes from the bloodstream. Activation of the vascular endothelium by several different stimuli plays a crucial role in the initiation, localization, and propagation of vascular injury.[1] *In vitro* studies have demonstrated that activation of cultured vascular endothelial cells (EC) renders them hyperadhesive for leukocytes. Coincubation of activated EC with unstimulated polymorphonuclear neutrophils (PMNs) results in EC injury, a process that is dependent upon direct neutrophil-endothelial cell contact and is mainly due to serine proteases.[2] Furthermore, *in vitro* studies have shown that neutrophil-mediated injury of activated EC in culture is more severe when those EC are coincubated

TABLE 13.1
Adhesion Molecules Potentially Involved in Vasculitis

Molecule	CD Name	Expression	Ligands
		Selectins Important for Tethering and Rolling	
L-selectin	CD62L	Leukocytes	Carbohydrate linked to CD34, GlyCAM-1 and/or MAdCAM-1
P-selectin	CD62P	Endothelium, Platelets	Sialyl Lewis a,x linked to PSGL-1
E-selectin	CD62E	Endothelium	Sialyl Lewis a,x
		Immunoglobulin Superfamily Important for Adhesion and Transmigration	
ICAM-1	CD54	Endothelium, Leukocytes, Other	CD11a/CD18, CD11b/CD18
ICAM-2	CD102	Endothelium, Subpopulation leukocytes	CD11a/CD18
ICAM-3	CD50	Leukocytes	CD11a/CD18
VCAM-1*	CD106	Endothelium, Macrophages, Vascular SMC	$\alpha 4\beta 1$ (VLA-4), $\alpha 4\beta 7$
PECAM-1	CD31	Endothelium, Platelets, Leukocytes	PECAM-1

* GlyCAM-1 = glycosylation-dependent cell adhesion molecule-1; the interaction between VCAM-1 and $\alpha 4\beta 1$ (VLA-4) is also important for tethering and rolling MAdCAM-1 = mucosal addressin cell adhesion molecule-1; PSGL-1 = P-selectin glycoprotein ligand-1; ICAM = intercellular cell adhesion molecule; VCAM-1 = vascular cell adhesion molecule-1; PECAM-1 = platelet-endothelial cell adhesion molecule-1; VLA-4 = very late activation antigen-4; SMC = smooth muscle cell.

with primed PMN in the presence of anti-neutrophil cytoplasmic autoantibodies (ANCA) than when incubated with primed PMN in the presence of normal IgG.[3] Those ANCA are found in patients with systemic necrotizing vasculitis and are capable of stimulating primed neutrophils *in vitro* to produce radical oxygen species and to degranulate resulting in the release of serine proteases and other potentially damaging products.[4]

Activated endothelial cells and cytokine-primed leukocytes play a pivotal role in the pathophysiology of vasculitis.[1,4-7] During the last two decades it has become evident which cell adhesion molecules play a critical role in the interaction between the vascular endothelium and leukocytes (Table 13.1).[8-11] In this review, we focus on the demonstration of (soluble) adhesion molecules in vasculitis, and on the use of adhesion molecules as targets for treatment of vasculitis.

II. DEMONSTRATION OF ADHESION MOLECULES IN VASCULITIS

Several studies have investigated the expression of adhesion molecules on circulating leukocytes and the *in situ* expression of adhesion molecules in vasculitic lesions.

A. DEMONSTRATION OF ADHESION MOLECULES ON CIRCULATING LEUKOCYTES

1. β1 Integrins

In 1993, Takeuchi et al.[12] reported increased expression of the β1 integrin VLA-4 (CD49d/CD29) on purified peripheral blood lymphocytes (PBL) from six patients with vasculitis secondary to systemic lupus erythematosus (SLE) as compared to patients with SLE without vasculitis and/or normal controls. VLA-4 on these cells is important for tethering and rolling on, firm adhesion to, and transmigration through endothelial cells that express VCAM-1.[9] In addition, VLA-4 is important for T-cell costimulation and cell-matrix adhesion via binding to the CS-1 domain of fibronectin. During follow-up studies performed in two patients with SLE vasculitis, VLA-4 expression returned to normal during treatment, but increased again during relapse.[12] Functional studies further showed that T-cells from SLE patients with vasculitis, in comparison with T-cells from SLE patients without vasculitis, demonstrated increased adhesion to cultured endothelial cells and/or CS-1 peptide.[12]

This suggests that lymphocytes in SLE vasculitis not only exhibit upregulated expression of VLA-4, but also functional upregulation of VLA-4.

Gutfleisch et al.[13] reported increased expression of the β1 integrin subunit (CD29) on CD4 positive cells in patients with Wegener's granulomatosis (WG) compared to normal controls. Furthermore, Haller et al.[14] found increased expression of the β1 integrin subunit (CD29) on granulocytes and monocytes of patients with either active or inactive WG. Expression of the alpha 4 integrin subunit (CD49d), however, was not increased on these cells as confirmed by Muller Kobold et al.[15,16]

2. β2 Integrins

Takeuchi et al.[12] found increased CD11a and CD18 expression on purified PBL from SLE patients with and without vasculitis. CD11a/CD18 on these cells plays an important role in adhesion and transendothelial migration via binding to either ICAM-1 and/or ICAM-2 on endothelial cells. In addition, CD11a/CD18 is involved in the adhesion of lymphocytes to other cells via binding to either ICAM-1, ICAM-2, and/or ICAM-3.

Haller et al.[14] reported increased expression of CD11a on lymphocytes and monocytes of patients with active WG when compared with healthy controls. In addition, increased expression of CD18 on granulocytes, monocytes, and lymphocytes, and increased expression of CD11b on granulocytes and monocytes, was found in patients with active WG. CD11b/CD18 (CR3 receptor, MAC-1) binds to ICAM-1, iC3b, fibrinogen, factor X, lipo-polysaccharide (LPS), and β-glucan. CD11b/CD18 on neutrophils is involved in phagocytosis and adhesion of neutrophils to EC. Patients with WG and inactive disease had persistently elevated CD18 expression on granulocytes and/or monocytes, whereas CD11a and Cd11b expression was not higher in these patients when compared with healthy controls.[14] Recently, Muller Kobold et al. also reported increased expression of CD11b on monocytes.[16] CD11b expression on granulocytes, however, was only increased in patients with newly diagnosed vasculitis, but not in patients with relapsing disease.[15]

3. L-Selectin

Riecken et al. analyzed L-selectin expression on neutrophils from patients with WG[17] and found decreased levels of L-selectin on purified neutrophils in six out of seven patients with active disease, and in four out of thirteen patients with partial or complete remission. L-selectin is important for tethering and rolling of leukocytes on EC. After activation by chemoattractants, adhesiveness of leukocytes increases and migration of leukocytes starts. Soon after activation, L-selectin is shed from neutrophils. Whether this process also takes place in the circulation in patients with WG is questionable. The observed decrease of L-selectin expression in this study may be due to the isolation procedure of neutrophils, which may have activated the neutrophils *in vitro*. Indeed, Muller Kobold et al. did not find a decrease of L-selectin expression on neutrophils in WG by using a whole blood method in which neutrophils were not isolated.[15]

4. ICAM-1

On purified PBL (both T- and B-cells), ICAM-1 expression was found to be increased in patients with WG and/or microscopic polyangiitis compared to normals.[13] We studied ICAM-1 expression on circulating neutrophils in patients with ANCA-associated vasculitis (Wegener's granulomatosis, microscopic polyangiitis, or Churg-Strauss syndrome), patients with sepsis, and healthy controls and found increased ICAM-1 expression on neutrophils of patients with sepsis but not in patients with vasculitis as compared to normal controls.[15]

From these studies it can be concluded that circulating lymphocytes in SLE vasculitis and active WG demonstrate upregulated expression of different adhesion molecules, i.e., VLA-4, CD11a, and ICAM-1. Studies regarding adhesion molecule expression on neutrophils are, however, inconclusive, probably because of technical differences resulting in different levels of activation of neutrophils *in vitro*. Upregulation of CD11b on neutrophils can only be found in patients with ANCA-associated vasculitis who have very active disease. Finally, circulating monocytes in active WG demonstrate upregulation of CD11a and CD11b. Taken together, these studies point to activation of granulocytes, lymphocytes, and monocytes in SLE-associated and ANCA-associated vasculitis. The full extent of this activation may, however, be underestimated since activated circulating leukocytes may adhere to the endothelium and, therefore, may be missed during analysis.

B. *In Situ* Expression of Adhesion Molecules in Biopsies

Several investigators have studied the *in situ* expression of adhesion molecules in vasculitic lesions. These studies mainly focused on the endothelial expression of the selectins, ICAM-1, VCAM-1, and PECAM.

E-selectin (CD62E), a member of the selectin family, is an endothelial-specific adhesion molecule and is only expressed upon activation by inflammatory mediators such as LPS and/or cytokines. P-selectin (CD62P), also a member of the selectin family, is stored in the alpha granules of platelets and Weibel-Palade bodies of endothelial cells. In response to mediators such as thrombin, histamine, the membrane attack complex of complement, and C5a, P-selectin is mobilized to the plasma membrane to bind neutrophils and monocytes.[18,19]

ICAM-1 (CD54), VCAM-1 (CD106), and PECAM-1 (CD31) belong to the immunoglobulin superfamily.[9] ICAM-1 has a very broad distribution, being constitutively expressed on endothelial cells and lymphoid cells. In addition, ICAM-1 can be induced on a wide variety of cells by inflammatory mediators. VCAM-1 is expressed on endothelial cells, macrophages, follicular dendritic cells, and vascular smooth muscle cells.[20] PECAM-1 is expressed on leukocytes, platelets, and at cell-cell junctions on the endothelium. PECAM-1 can bind homophilically to itself and heterophilically to a counter-receptor that is not yet characterized. The constitutive expression of both ICAM-1 and VCAM-1 on EC is increased by stimulation with inflammatory mediators; the upregulated expression of these adhesion molecules may increase leukocyte extravasation at inflammatory sites. PECAM-1 is found constitutively on endothelial cells and plays a pivotal role in leukocyte transmigration.

1. Skin Biopsies

In 1989, Leung et al.[21] reported E-selectin expression in lesional tissues obtained from five children with Kawasaki's disease before intravenous gammaglobulin treatment was started. E-selectin expression was particularly observed in venules in the papillary and superficial dermis. In contrast, E-selectin expression was not found on endothelial cells of normal skin and, in addition, little or no E-selectin expression was found in four of six biopsies from lesional skin obtained after intravenous gammaglobulin treatment.[21] Patients with decrease of endothelial activation had a marked clinical improvement during treatment, whereas in the two patients with persistent endothelial activation, persistence of disease activity despite gammaglobulin treatment was noted. Endothelial staining for ICAM-1 correlated with expression of E-selectin and was upregulated in pretreatment samples, reduced in those patients with good clinical response, but persistently upregulated in the two patients with more protracted clinical courses. The reversal of EC activation in patients during clinical improvement, as was found in this study, supports a pathogenic role for EC activation in Kawasaki disease.

In skin biopsies from normal subjects and nonlesional skin specimens from patients with vasculitis, no endothelial expression of E-selectin and/or VCAM-1 is detected.[22] In contrast, post-capillary venules in skin lesions of patients with vasculitis showed endothelial E-selectin expression in 15 of 24 biopsies (63% of the patients) and endothelial VCAM-1 expression in 8 of 24 biopsies

(33% of the patients).[22] In addition, keratinocyte ICAM-1 expression was significantly increased in skin biopsies from patients with lymphocytic vasculitis, suggesting an active role for gamma interferon-producing T-cells in the pathogenesis of this form of vasculitis. Bradley et al.[23] examined skin biopsies from patients with leukocytoclastic angiitis of the skin (LCA), either idiopathic or secondary to a systemic illness. E-selectin expression was observed in 75% of the specimens and was associated with neutrophil infiltration. Neutrophil infiltrates were not observed in the absence of E-selectin, and the most intense neutrophil infiltration occurred in biopsies that had the most intense staining for E-selectin. In contrast, endothelial ICAM-1 expression (100% of the cases) and endothelial VCAM-1 expression (85% of the cases) was associated with a mononuclear cell inflammatory infiltrate. Expression of ICAM-1 and VCAM-1 was also found on perivascular inflammatory cells. A sequential analysis of adhesion molecules in 42 patients with LCA was performed by Sais et al.[24] The most pronounced E-selectin expression was found in lesions of less than 48 hours' duration. Furthermore, an inverse relation between the staining intensity of E-selectin and the duration of the lesion was found. In addition, E-selectin expression was correlated with (CD11b positive) neutrophils in the inflammatory infiltrate and with deposition of IgG, IgA, IgM, and/or C3 in the vessel walls. Endothelial VCAM-1 expression was only infrequently observed, and only in lesions of more than 24 hours' duration. In addition, in vasculitis that also involved medium-sized vessels, perivascular cells demonstrated a significant increase of VCAM-1 immunoreactivity, which was associated with a higher amount of infiltrating inflammatory cells. Endothelial expression of ICAM-1 was moderately upregulated, but endothelial expression of P-selectin was not observed in skin biopsies from patients with LCA.

These data demonstrate that endothelial activation occurs early during development of vasculitic lesions in the skin. Furthermore, they suggest that the nature of leukocyte infiltration at sites of cutaneous inflammation is determined by the pattern of endothelial adhesion molecule expression.

2. Kidney Biopsies

In normal kidneys, E-selectin is not found, whereas VCAM-1 is found on epithelial cells of Bowman's capsule, on occasional tubular epithelial cells, and on endothelial cells of small interstitial vessels, but not on glomerular endothelial cells.[7,26,29,30] ICAM-1 in normal kidneys is found on Bowman's capsule epithelium and on glomerular endothelial cells, peritubular capillaries, and small-sized and medium-sized vessels in the interstitium.[7,25,27-30] In addition, the brush border of proximal tubules and some interstitial cells are occasionally ICAM-1-positive. In renal biopsies of patients with pauci-immune necrotizing and/or crescentic glomerulonephritis (either idiopathic or in association with Wegener's granulomatosis or microscopic polyangiitis), we and others[25-34] found that all cells forming crescents are positive for VCAM-1 and ICAM-1. When crescents become fibrous with no or only a few cells, decreased expression of ICAM-1 and VCAM-1 is observed.[33] Furthermore, in many cases extraglomerular vessels demonstrate positive VCAM-1 staining.[33] Expression of E-selectin has been found on extraglomerular vessels by some[33] but not by others.[32] In addition, about 20% of the inflammatory cells of periglomerular granulomatous lesions and/or interstitial infiltrates are positive for ICAM-1 and/or VCAM-1.[34] Finally, upregulation of VCAM-1 and ICAM-1 expression is found on tubular epithelial cells. Interestingly, Rastaldi et al.[34] reported that marked expression of VCAM-1 corresponding exactly with the necrotizing lesions and upregulated glomerular expression of VCAM-1 was associated with intraglomerular infiltration of macrophages. These data suggest that intraglomerular expression of VCAM-1 might be a useful marker of disease activity in biopsies that demonstrate ANCA-associated renal vasculitis.

The expression of adhesion molecules in other forms of renal vasculitis has been studied incidentally. In Henoch-Schönlein purpura and cryoglobulinemia, Bruyn and Dinklo[29] reported upregulation of VCAM-1 on the glomerular capillary wall, interstitial vessels, and mesangial cells, whereas ICAM-1 was upregulated on the glomerular mesangium, and on parietal and tubular epithelial cells.

From these studies it can be concluded that glomerular expression of VCAM-1 is associated with areas of necrosis and crescent formation, whereas both ICAM-1 and VCAM-1 are strongly upregulated in peritubular regions and on tubular epithelial cells in different forms of renal vasculitis. These findings suggest that ICAM-1 and VCAM-1 are involved in the recruitment of intraglomerular leukocytes. In contrast, E-selectin is not detected in glomerular lesions, and at present it is not clear what adhesion molecules leukocytes use to tether and roll during lesion development in renal vasculitis.

3. Other Lesional Tissues

Panegyres[35] reported endothelial ICAM-1 upregulation in muscle and nerve vessels from seven patients with various forms of vasculitis involving small and/or medium-sized blood vessels. Induction of endothelial expression of E-selectin was only found in one of the biopsies. A detailed study of muscle and/or nerve biopsies of 30 patients with polyarteritis nodosa was reported by Coll-Vinent et al.[36] They found intense upregulation of E-selectin in early lesions and, in 10 of 30 patients, also in noninflamed vessels.[36] In well-established lesions, E-selectin was only occasionally found, and VCAM-1 was found on vessels that were still preserved. Luminal expression of ICAM-1, PECAM-1, and P-selectin, adhesion molecules that are constituvely expressed in muscle biopsies, was decreased and had completely disappeared in vessels that were occluded. Since a similar pattern was observed with an endothelial cell marker (i.e., ulex europeus), the authors conclude that luminal endothelium disappears after damage. In biopsies from patients with PAN with well-established lesions, many microvessels were found that were probably derived from inflammation-induced angiogenesis. The microvessels in PAN were positive for ICAM-1, PECAM-1, and P-selectin. In addition, microvessels stained positive for E-selectin and VCAM-1, but these adhesion molecules were no longer present on microvessels of healed lesions. From this study, the authors hypothesize that luminal endothelium probably participates only in early phases of leukocyte adhesion, whereas angiogenesis plays an important role in leukocyte recruitment later on, and contributes to the persistence of inflammation in PAN.[36]

Wawryk et al.[37] reported regional induction of ICAM-1 on intimal myofibroblasts and vascular smooth muscle cells adjacent to granulomatous arteritis lesions in biopsies from patients with temporal arteritis. Flipo et al.[38] studied the expression of adhesion molecules in labial salivary glands from six patients with rheumatoid vasculitis and found E-selectin and ICAM-1 expression, but not VCAM-1 expression in areas of microvascular damage. The expression of these adhesion molecules was only occasionally found in control biopsies from salivary glands obtained from patients with rheumatoid arthritis without vasculitis and/or patients with Sjögren's syndrome.[38]

In summary, increased endothelial expression of adhesion molecules has been consistently reported in studies on biopsies of patients with different forms of vasculitis. In vasculitis involving the skin, muscle, and/or nerve, early lesions show strong upregulation of E-selectin, which is associated with a predominantly neutrophilic infiltrate. During lesion development the pattern changes, E-selectin disappears and VCAM-1 staining associated with an infiltrate consisting of lymphocytes and monocytes/macrophages is present. Finally, when blood vessels are severely damaged, endothelial cells disappear and staining for adhesion molecules that are constitutively expressed on the endothelium of normal, medium-, and/or small-sized vessels, e.g., ICAM-1, PECAM-1, and P-selectin, disappears. In biopsies of patients with renal vasculitis, E-selectin is only occasionally found on interstitial vessels, but is notoriously absent in glomeruli. During the early phase of crescent formation, there is strong expression of VCAM-1 and ICAM-1 on cells that form crescents, whereas the staining of these adhesion molecules decreases during later stages when crescents become fibrous.

Upregulation of endothelial-leukocyte adhesion molecules in vasculitis may reflect a complex interplay of various stimuli at the level of transcriptional regulation.[39,40] Such stimuli may include cytokines (e.g., interleukin-1 and tumor necrosis factor-α), oxidant stresses,[41,42] angiogenic factors,[43]

TABLE 13.2
Soluble Leukocyte Adhesion Molecules in Vasculitis

	sICAM-1	sVCAM-1	sE-selectin
Takayasu arteritis	–	+/–	+/–
Temporal arteritis	+	nt.	+/–
PAN	++	+	++
Kawasaki	++	+	++
Wegener granulomatosis			
-generalized	++	++	++
-limited	–	++	+/–
MPA	++	++	++
Churg-Strauss	nt.	nt.	nt.
Henoch-Schönlein	–	nt.	+/–
LCA	–	nt.	nt.

Note: ++ = highly elevated; + = moderately elevated; +/– = elevated in some studies, but not in others; – = not different from healthy controls; nt. = not tested. sICAM-1 = soluble intercellular adhesion molecule-1; sVCAM-1 = soluble vascular cell adhesion molecule-1. PAN = classic polyarteritis nodosa; MPA = microscopic polyangiitis; LCA = leukocytoclastic angiitis of the skin.

and biochemical forces.[44] In addition, autoantibodies such as anti-endothelial cell antibodies (AECA) and ANCA may be such stimuli.[45-50] Mayet et al.[45,46] reported that incubation of cultured EC with affinity-purified ANCA (i.e., anti-PR3) resulted in an increased membrane expression of E-selectin and VCAM-1. The mechanism of ANCA-stimulated induction of adhesion molecules is not known. Mayet et al. suggest that anti-PR3 antibodies bind to membrane expressed PR3 on cultured endothelial cells and subsequently induce activation of endothelial cells.[51] This latter viewpoint, however, is challenged by others[52] who could not detect membrane expression of PR3 on cultured endothelial cells.

III. SOLUBLE ADHESION MOLECULES AS CLINICAL MARKERS

Many adhesion molecules are released from cell surfaces.[53-55] Serum levels of soluble adhesion molecules can be measured and can be regarded as an index of endothelial cell activation. In addition, there is some evidence that soluble adhesion molecules may have biological functions.[56-58] Finally, it has been hypothesized that levels of soluble adhesion molecules can be used as markers of disease activity in different diseases. Several studies have focused on the measurement of soluble adhesion molecules in patients with vasculitis. These studies will be discussed (Table 13.2).

A. Takayasu's Arteritis

Hoffman and Ahmed measured soluble E-selectin, ICAM-1, VCAM-1, and PECAM-1 levels in a small cohort of patients with active (n = 6) and inactive (n = 20) Takayasu's arteritis.[59] Levels of soluble VCAM-1 and ICAM-1 did not differ from levels found in healthy controls. Levels of soluble PECAM-1 were significantly higher in patients with inactive (2x higher) than in active disease or healthy controls.[59] Soluble E-selectin levels were higher (21%) in patients compared with healthy controls, but no differences were found between active and inactive patients. Boehme et al.[60] could not detect differences in sE-selectin levels between patients with active Takayasu's arteritis (n = 12) and healthy controls. In another study,[61] levels of sVCAM-1 were found to be higher (44%)

in patients with Takayasu's arteritis (n = 73) than in healthy controls. No relation between sVCAM-1 and fibrinogen levels were found, suggesting that sVCAM-1 is not a marker of activity in this disease. No difference in sICAM-1 levels was found between patients and controls.[61]

B. Temporal Arteritis

Elevated levels of sE-selectin (2.2 × higher than in controls) were also reported in patients with temporal arteritis (n = 34).[62] sE-selectin levels in patients with active temporal arteritis were not different from levels in patients in which the disease was inactive. A trend towards higher E-selectin levels was found in patients in whom the disease was complicated by polymyalgia rheumatica. sICAM-1 levels were also found to be significantly higher than in controls (1.7 × higher) in patients with polymyalgia rheumatica with or without temporal arteritis (n = 16), and, in a prospective study, it was demonstrated that elevated levels returned to normal after one week of steroid therapy.[63]

C. Classic Polyarteritis Nodosa (PAN)

Carson et al.[62] studied 56 patients with polyarteritis. Patients were classified according to the 1990 American College of Rheumatology criteria as having PAN. Hence, most of these patients, when classified according to the Chapel Hill Consensus Conference classification criteria, are probably having microscopic polyangiitis.[64,65] In these patients, elevated sE-selectin levels were found (2.3 × higher than healthy controls). No clear relation with disease activity was found, although a trend towards higher levels was observed in those patients who had liver involvement.

More recently, Coll-Vinent et al. measured soluble ICAM-1, VCAM-1, E-selectin, L-selectin, and P-selectin in 22 patients with classic PAN who were classified according to the Chapel Hill Consensus Conference criteria.[66] At the time of diagnosis, sICAM-1 levels (2.0 × higher), sVCAM-1 levels (1.6 × higher), and sE-selectin levels (1.8 × higher) were significantly higher than in controls. At diagnosis, sP-selectin levels were not different from those in controls, and sL-selectin levels were only slightly lower than in controls, possibly because circulating L-selectin binds to activated endothelium. Shortly after the start of treatment with prednisolone and cyclophosphamide, a significant increase of sICAM-1 and sP-selectin was observed (Figure 13.1). The authors hypothesize that this phenomenon might be explained by a release of bound soluble adhesion molecules since treatment might have modulated receptor/ligand affinity. Subsequently, during further follow-up, levels of sVCAM-1 and sP-selectin normalized, whereas levels of sICAM-1 and sE-selectin decreased but remained significantly elevated when compared to levels in normal controls. Finally, sL-selectin levels that were already slightly lower at diagnosis further decreased during follow-up and became significantly lower than levels of normal controls when measured during remission. In summary, in PAN, highly elevated levels for sE-selectin, sICAM-1, and s-VCAM-1 are found that decrease but do not normalize during follow-up. Whether this latter finding reflects low-grade subclinical activity in these patients has to be further investigated in a long-term follow-up study.

D. Kawasaki Disease

Furukawa et al.[67] measured soluble ICAM-1 levels in 29 patients with acute Kawasaki disease (KD). The mean sICAM-1 level at admission was 2.0 × higher in acute KD than in healthy young children and/or children suffering from measles. Patients who developed coronary artery lesions (n = 7) during follow-up had higher levels of sICAM-1 at onset. Levels of sICAM-1 correlated with serum TNFα levels. During treatment with intravenous infusions of gamma globulin and aspirin, sICAM-1 levels decreased to normal ranges.

Soluble sE-selectin levels were also found to be markedly (8.9 ×) increased in patients with acute KD (n = 24) compared to age-matched control children.[68] The highest levels of sE-selectin were found in three children who developed coronary artery lesions. sE-selectin levels correlated with serum TNF-α and IL-6 levels, but not with CRP or ESR. Three weeks after the start of

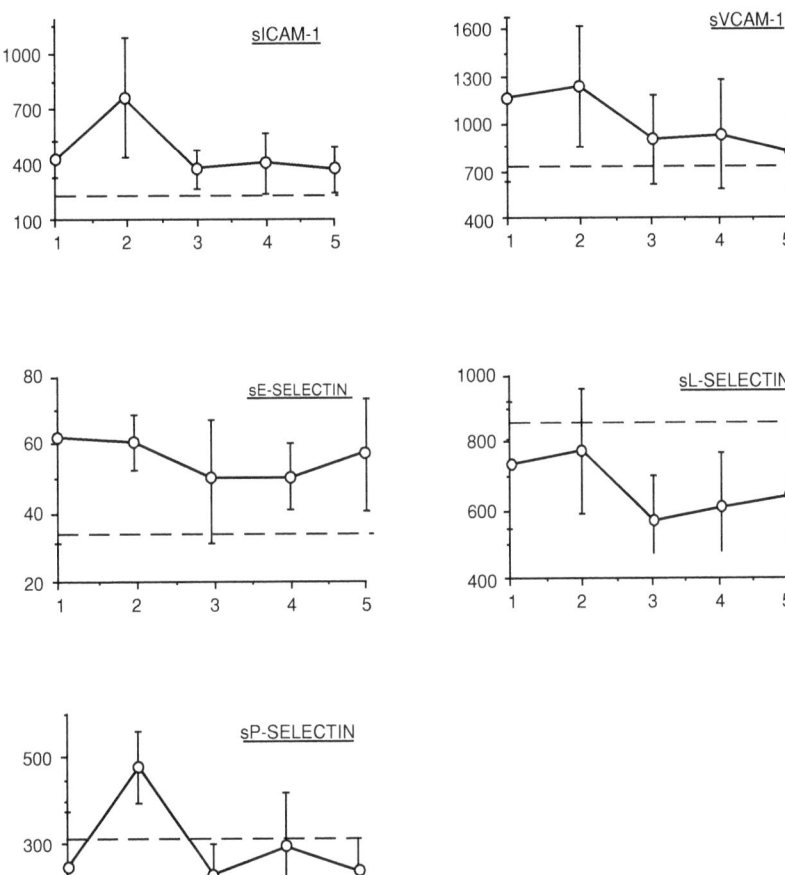

FIGURE 13.1 Serum levels of soluble ICAM-1, soluble VCAM-1, soluble E-selectin, sL-selectin and sP-selectin (mean levels and s.d.) were measured in patients with classic polyarteritis nodosa (n = 22). Numbers on the horizontal axis represent different groups: group 1 = active untreated patients, group 2 = patients within the first 7 days of treatment; group 3 = patients with partial remission btween the first week and the first 3 months of treatment; group 4 = patients in remission still receiving immunosuppressive treatment; group 5 = patients in remission no longer receiving therapy. The broken line stands for the mean level found in the controls. (From Coll-Vinent et al.[66] With permission.)

treatment with intravenous infusions of gammaglobulin and aspirin, sE-selectin levels were lower than in acute KD, but still higher than in controls.[68]

Nash et al.,[69] studying 59 acute KD patients, confirmed that median levels of sE-selectin (2.7 × controls) and sICAM-1 (1.5 × controls) are elevated in KD. In addition, sVCAM-1 levels were also significantly higher (1.2 × controls) in acute KD than in afebrile controls. In 35 children with fever, levels of sICAM-1 and sE-selectin were also elevated, but were significantly lower than in acute KD. In contrast, sVCAM-1 levels in febrile controls were even higher than in acute KD. In acute KD, levels of sE-selectin, sICAM-1, and sVCAM-1 correlated with each other. In addition, sE-selectin levels correlated with CRP. Levels of soluble adhesion molecules decreased during treatment. Although no data were shown, the authors state that levels of soluble adhesion molecules do not predict the development of coronary artery lesions. Spertini et al. studied sL-selectin levels in 55 KD patients and found that these were lower than sL-selectin levels in normal blood donors.[70] Kanekura measured sL-selectin in nine patients with acute KD, of which three developed coronary artery lesions.[71] The patients who developed coronary artery lesions had significantly lower sL-selectin levels compared to patients with acute KD without coronary lesions and/or healthy controls (2.0 lower). Also, during the convalescent stage, sL-selectin levels were consistently lower in patients who developed coronary artery lesions compared to patients with acute KD without coronary lesions and/or healthy controls.

In summary, in patients with acute KD, the levels of sE-selectin, sVCAM-1, and sICAM-1 are elevated compared to age-matched children. It remains to be studied in a prospective study whether the measurement of soluble adhesion molecules is a good predictor of the development of coronary artery aneurysms.

E. WEGENER'S GRANULOMATOSIS

Hauschild et al.[72] studied sICAM-1 levels in 23 patients with generalized WG and 8 patients with limited WG. sICAM-1 levels were significantly elevated (1.6 × controls) in patients with active generalized WG compared with controls, whereas patients with active locoregional WG had sICAM-1 levels that were only slightly higher than in controls (1.2 × controls). During remission, sICAM-1 levels fell. Stegeman et al.[73] studied sE-selectin, sVCAM-1, and sICAM-1 levels in patients with newly diagnosed active WG (n = 22) before and at the time of a relapse (n = 12), and during the occurrence of an upper respiratory tract infection without signs of disease reactivation (n = 18). In patients with newly diagnosed, untreated, active, generalized WG (i.e., with renal involvement) sICAM-1 levels (1.9 × higher), sVCAM-1 levels (2.9 ×) and sE-selectin (1.5 ×) were higher than in healthy controls (Figure 13.2). In patients with "limited" WG (i.e., without renal involvement), sVCAM-1 levels were also significantly higher compared to controls; however, sE-selectin and sICAM-1 levels in these patients were not different from controls (Figure 13.2). At the time of diagnosis, levels of sE-selectin, sICAM-1, and sVCAM-1 correlated with CRP and disease activity, but not with ANCA titer. At the time of relapse, only a minority of the patients had elevated levels of either sVCAM-1, sICAM-1, and/or sE-selectin levels. Levels of sVCAM-1, but not of sICAM-1 and sE-selectin, were higher than in controls. Compared with levels obtained six months prior to relapse, levels of sE-selectin, sVCAM-1, and sICAM-1 were, however, significantly higher at

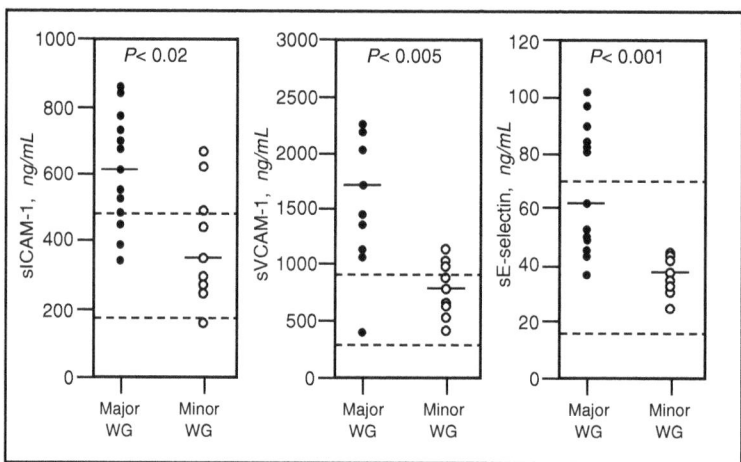

FIGURE 13.2 Serum levels of soluble ICAM-1, soluble VCAM-1, and soluble E-selectin were measured at the time of diagnosis in 22 consecutive patients with Wegener's granulomatosis ('WG') with either disease activity in the upper or lower airways without evidence of vasculitic activity in other organs ('Minor') or with disease activity involving the kidneys and/or with pulmonary involvement with impending respiratory failure and/or cerebral or abdominal vasculitis ('Major'). Short horizontal bars indicate median values; broken lines indicate the upper and lower limits of the normal range. (From Stegeman et al.[52] With permission.)

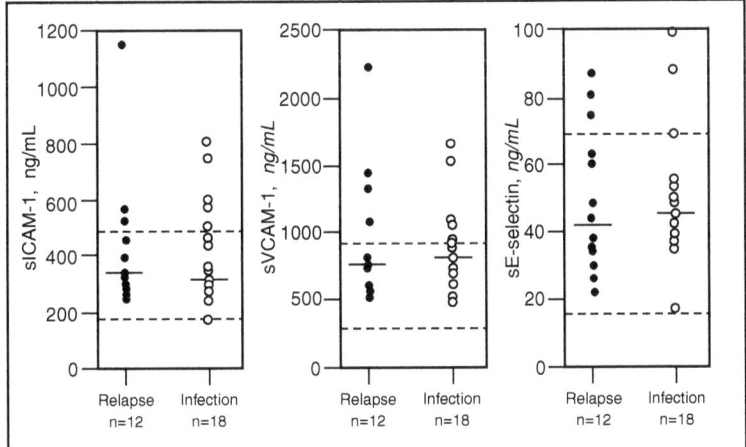

FIGURE 13.3 Serum levels of soluble ICAM-1, soluble VCAM-1, and soluble E-selectin were measured at the time of relapse in 12 patients with Wegener's granulomatosis ('Relapse') and during 18 episodes of documented upper airways infection in 17 patients with inactive Wegener's granulomatosis ('Infection'). Short horizontal bars indicate median values; broken lines indicate the upper and lower limits of the normal range; n = number of subjects. (From Stegeman et al.[52] With permission.)

the time of relapse. During an upper respiratory tract infection without disease reactivation, levels of sVCAM-1 were also elevated compared to normal controls. No differences were found in serum levels of sVCAM-1, sICAM-1, and sE-selectin between relapse and upper airway infection (Figure 13.3), so measurement of soluble adhesion molecules cannot discriminate between immune activation during infection and during activity of WG.

Elevated levels of sVCAM-1 (1.9 × higher than in controls), sICAM-1 (2.0 × higher), and sE-selectin (1.5 × higher) were found in another study in patients with active generalized WG (n = 19).[74] Patients with active WG and a need for renal replacement therapy had higher levels of sVCAM-1 and sICAM-1 than WG patients not requiring dialysis. In this study, elevated levels of sVCAM-1 and sICAM-1, however, were also found in ten patients on chronic hemodialysis but without WG. The authors suggested that elevated levels of soluble adhesion molecules in these patients may be due to a retention of adhesion molecules as a consequence of impaired renal function.[74] In patients with chronic renal failure, levels of soluble adhesion molecules, however, do not correlate with serum creatinine,[74,75] suggesting that elevated levels in patients on dialysis might reflect increased endothelial injury rather than impaired clearance. Finally, Boehme et al.[60] reported elevated sE-selectin levels in both locoregional WG (3.6 × higher) and patients with WG who had more extensive disease (1.9 × higher), despite the fact that most samples were obtained during treatment. No correlations were found in this study between sE-selectin levels, CRP, ANCA, and/or disease activity.[60]

In summary, elevated levels of sVCAM-1 are found in patients with WG. sE-selectin and sICAM-1 levels, however, are elevated in patients with renal involvement, but not in all patients with a more limited form. The clinical relevance of measuring these soluble adhesion molecules in WG is limited as they do not discriminate between disease activity and upper respiratory tract infection without disease reactivation.

F. MICROSCOPIC POLYANGIITIS

Patients with ANCA-associated pauci-immune necrotizing and/or crescentic glomerulonephritis (NCGN) have either (generalized) WG, microscopic polyarteriitis, or idiopathic NCGN. Since the therapeutic approach of these patients is not influenced by the diagnosis, these patients are often grouped together as "ANCA-associated glomerulonephritis/vasculitis." Yaqoob et al. measured sE-selectin levels in nine patients with ANCA-associated glomerulonephritis and found elevated levels at presentation (n = 7) and during relapse (n = 2) that fell within normal limits after one week of treatment, before other disease activity markers such as C-reactive protein and von Willebrand factor normalized.[76] Elevated plasma levels of sVCAM-1 and s-ICAM-1 were also found in patients with ANCA-associated glomerulonephritis (n = 14).[77] Urinary levels of sVCAM-1 but not of sICAM-1 were also elevated in these patients.[77]

Finally, Tesar et al.[78] reported highly elevated sICAM-1 (3.9 × healthy controls) and sVCAM-1 (1.9 ×) levels, in ten patients with ANCA-associated glomerulonephritis, that decreased during treatment with steroids, cyclophosphamide, and plasma exchange. Interestingly, each single plasma exchange was accompanied by a decrease in serum levels of sICAM-1 and s-VCAM-1, but not of cytokines such as IL-1β, IL-6, or IL-8. Furthermore, concentrations of sICAM-1 and sVCAM-1 in plasma filtrate were significantly lower than in serum obtained before plasma exchange, but significantly higher than in serum taken at the end of the procedure, suggesting effective filtration of both molecules.[78]

G. HENOCH-SCHÖNLEIN PURPURA

In children with Henoch-Schönlein purpura, sICAM-1 levels are not elevated when compared with healthy controls.[67,79,80] Contradictory results are available with respect to levels of sE-selectin in this disease. In one study, high sE-selectin levels were reported in patients with Henoch-Schönlein purpura compared to age-matched controls (4.2 × higher),[68] whereas in two other studies, sE-selectin levels were not different from age-matched controls.[79,80] Willis, however, found raised sE-selectin levels in a small subgroup of patients and suggested that these patients had more severe systemic and renal vasculitis.[80]

H. OTHER FORMS OF VASCULITIS

In patients with isolated cutaneous leukocytoclastic angiitis (without systemic vasculitis), Wang et al.[81] found normal sICAM-1 levels. Finally, Voskuyl et al.[82] found elevated sICAM-1 (1.7 × higher) and only slightly elevated sE-selectin (1.2 × higher) levels in patients with rheumatoid vasculitis. In addition, in this study sICAM-3 levels were measured and found to be markedly elevated in patients with rheumatoid vasculitis (2.2 × higher than controls). During follow-up, when vasculitis was inactive sICAM-3 levels fell significantly, whereas sE-selectin and sICAM-1 levels revealed no significant change. Whether measurement of sICAM-3 is also useful as a marker of disease activity in other forms of vasculitis, has not yet been studied.

In summary, levels of sICAM-1, sVCAM-1, and sE-selectin are elevated in patients with systemic necrotizing vasculitis with involvement of medium-sized and/or small vessels. In more limited forms of small-vessel vasculitis and/or vasculitis involving large-sized vessels, measurement of soluble adhesion molecule levels gives rise to more variable results: in some studies elevated levels are reported, in other studies they are not. During treatment with corticosteroids and cyclo-phosphamide with or without plasma exchange, levels of these adhesion molecules decrease, but during remission of the disease, levels are not always completely normal. Finally, during a relapse, levels rise again. The value of these markers as predictors of disease activity, however, is limited since elevated levels are also found during other conditions in which endothelial cells are activated, e.g., infections,[69,73,83] atherosclerosis,[84] hypertension,[85] and/or dyslipidemia.[86] The clinical value of measurement of other soluble adhesion molecules such as sL-selectin, sP-selectin, sPECAM, and sICAM-3 in vasculitis patients is at present unknown. Interestingly, sL-selectin levels in patients with vasculitis are lower compared to healthy controls.[66,70,71,87] Since sL-selectin retains functional binding activity,[58] low levels may promote leukocyte-endothelial adhesion, and may point to a state of less protection against endothelial injury.

IV. THERAPY

Many antiinflammatory agents influence the adhesion of leukocytes to endothelial cells. For instance, it has been suggested that inhibition of endothelial cell activation by inhibition of NFκB activity is a major component of the antiinflammatory activity of steroids.[88,89] NFκB is a key transcription factor in inflammation. In quiescent cells, NFκB is present in the cytosol bound to its inhibitor IkappaB. Stimulation of cells with various stimuli, such as IL-1β, TNF-a, and LPS, leads to proteolytic degradation of IkappaB and, hence, activation of latent NFκB.[90] It is postulated that all stimuli ultimately converge to enhance intracellular reactive oxygen metabolism.[39] Once NFκB is activated, it translocates into the nucleus and stimulates transcription of a variety of target genes such as those coding for cell adhesion molecules, cytokines, and chemoattractants. Thus, antiinflammatory agents that inhibit NFκB are good candidates to use in the treatment of vasculitis.[7] Different possibilities are currently under study: antisense oligonucleotides that block transcription factors,[9] anti-oxidant inhibitors of NFκB,[92] and inhibitors of the proteasome pathway.[93,94]

During the last several years other strategies have been developed to directly inhibit mechanisms of endothelial-leukocyte adhesion. For this purpose, a fast-growing amount of modalities are being developed such as monoclonal antibodies to leukocyte-adhesion molecules,[95] carbohydrates that inhibit selectin function,[96] antisense oligonucleotides that block adhesion molecules,[97] flavonoids,[98] and synthetic peptides that block integrin-mediated adhesion.[99] These modalities have been exhaustively tested in multiple animal models, especially experimental models of immune-complex-mediated glomerulonephritis, dermal vasculitis, or lung injury. In addition, the role of endothelial-leukocyte adhesion molecules has been studied in animal models that may be relevant for human vasculitides. The first model is a rat model of antimyeloperoxidase-associated renal vasculitis,[100] in which rats develop pauci-immune necrotizing crescentic glomerulonephritis, vasculitis, and periglomerular granulomatous inflammation. By studying this animal model, Coers et al. found increased expression of ICAM-1 during lesion development in the glomerulus, the proximal tubules, and the interstitium.[101] Intervention with blocking monoclonal antibodies to ICAM-1, however, did not mitigate renal damage in this model.[102] Another animal model is pulmonary granulomatous vasculitis induced by injection of β-glucan. During lesion development in this model, upregulation of P-selectin, VCAM-1, and ICAM-1, but not of E-selectin, is found on the endothelial lining of pulmonary vessels.[103-105] Therapy with anti-VLA4 antibodies, anti-oxidant inhibitors of NFκB, anti-ICAM-1 antibodies, and GM2941, a sulfated carbohydrate that inhibits P-selectin-mediated neutrophil-endothelial cell interactions, all caused a significant reduction of lesion development in this model.[104-106] Finally, Li et al.[107] demonstrated reduction of lesions when β-glucan was injected in mice deficient for the Ig-like domain 4 of VCAM-1, resulting in alternatively spliced forms of VCAM-1 with only a single a4 integrin binding site.

In summary, many different, new therapeutic antiadhesive strategies are being tested *in vitro* and *in vivo* in animal models of vasculitis. Trials with these new antiadhesive modalities in patients have recently started, and the first results are promising.[108]

V. CONCLUSIONS

Increasing evidence has been found that induction and/or upregulation of endothelial-leukocyte adhesion molecules plays a major role in the pathogenesis of vasculitis. Increased expression of adhesion molecules on circulating leukocytes has been mainly reported in patients with active Wegener's granulomatosis, but endothelial expression of adhesion molecules has been consistently observed in skin and/or renal biopsies of patients with different forms of vasculitis. Furthermore, levels of soluble adhesion molecules, i.e., sICAM-1, sVCAM-1, and sE-selectin, are highly elevated in patients with systemic necrotizing vasculitis.

Many different, new therapeutic antiadhesive strategies have been tested *in vitro* and *in vivo* in animal models of vasculitis, and experimental antiadhesive therapy has just recently been introduced in patients with forms of vasculitis that are refractory to standard treatment.

REFERENCES

1. Cohen Tervaert JW, Kallenberg CGM: The Role of Autoimmunity to Myeloid Lysosomal Enzymes in the Pathogenesis of Vasculitis. In *Immune Functions of the Vessel Wall*. Edited by Hansson GK and Libby P. Amsterdam: Harwood Academic Publishers, 1996:99–120.
2. Westlin WF, Gimbrone MA: Neutrophil-mediated damage to human vascular endothelium. Role of cytokine activation. *Am J Pathol* 1993, 142:117–128
3. Savage COS, Pottinger BE, Gaskin G, Pusey CD, Pearson JD: Autoantibodies developing to myeloperoxidase and proteinase 3 in systemic vasculitis stimulate neutrophil cytotoxicity towards cultured endothelial cells. *Am J Pathol* 1992, 141:335–342.
4. Muller Kobold AC, Van der Geld Y, Limburg PC, Cohen Tervaert JW, Kallenberg CGM: Molecular basis of renal disease. Pathophysiology of ANCA-associated glomerulonephritis. *Nephrol Dial Transplant* 1999, 14:1366–1375.
5. Cotran RS, Pober JS: Recent insights into mechanisms of vascular injury. Implications for the pathogenesis of vasculitis. In *Endothelial Cell Dysfunctions*. Edited by Simionescu N and Simionescu M. New York: Plenum Press, 1992:183–189.
6. Van Vollenhoven RF: Adhesion molecules, sex steroids, and the pathogenesis of vasculitis syndromes. *Curr Opin Rheum* 1995, 7:4–10.
7. Cohen Tervaert JW, Kallenberg CGM: Cell adhesion molecules in vasculitis. *Curr Opin Rheum* 1997, 9:16–25.
8. Springer TA: Traffic signals for lymphocyte recirculation and leukocyte emigration: the multistep paradigm. *Cell* 1994, 76:301–314.
9. Springer TA: Traffic signals on endothelium for lymphocyte recirculation and leukocyte emigration. *Annu Rev Physiol* 1995, 57:827–872.
10. Sundy JS, Haynes BF: Pathogenic mechanisms of vessel damage in vasculitis syndromes. *Rheum Dis Clin* 1995, 21:861–881.
11. Frenette PS, Wagner DD: Adhesion molecules — part II: blood vessels and blood cells. *N Engl J Med* 1996, 335:43–45.
12. Takeuchi T, Amano K, Sekine H, Koide J, Abe T: Upregulated expression and function of integrin adhesive receptors in Systemic Lupus Erythematosus patients with vasculitis. *J Clin Invest* 1993, 92:3008–3016.
13. Gutfleisch J, Baumert E, Wolff-Vorbeck G, Schlesier M, Strutz HJ, Peter HH: Increased expression of CD 25 and adhesion molecules on peripheral blood lymphocytes of patients with Wegener's granulomatosis and ANCA positive vasculitides. *Adv Exp Med Biol* 1993, 336:397–404.
14. Haller H, Eichhorn J, Pieper K, Göbel U, Luft FC: Circulating leukocyte integrin expression in Wegener's granulomatosis. *J Am Soc Nephrol* 1996, 7:40–48.
15. Muller Kobold AC, Mesander G, Stegeman CA, Kallenberg CGM, Cohen Tervaert JW: Are circulating neutrophils intravascularly activated in patients with anti-neutrophil cytoplasmic antibody (ANCA)-associated vasculitides? *Clin Exp Immunol* 1998, 114:491–499.
16. Muller Kobold AC, Kallenberg CGM, Cohen Tervaert JW: Monocyte activation in Wegener's granulomatosis. *Ann Rheum Dis* 1999, 58:237–245.
17. Riecken B, Gutfleisch J, Schlesier M, Peter HH: Impaired granulocyte oxidative burst and decreased expression of leucocyte adhesion molecule-1 (LAM-1) in patients with Wegener's granulomatosis. *Clin Exp Immunol* 1994, 96:43–47.
18. Brady HR: Leukocyte adhesion molecules and kidney diseases. *Kidney Int* 1994, 45:1285–1300.
19. Foreman KE, Vaporciyan AA, Bonish BK, Jones ML, Johnson KJ, Glovsky MM, Eddy SM, Ward PA: C5a-induced expression of P-selectin in endothelial cells. *J Clin Invest* 1994, 94:1147–1155.
20. Li H, Cybulsky MI, Gimbrone MA Jr, Libby P: Inducible expression of vascular cell adhesion molecule-1 by vascular smooth muscle cells *in vitro* and within rabbit atheroma. *Am J Pathol* 1993, 143:1551–1559.

21. Leung DYM, Cotran RS, Kurt-Jones E, Burns JC, Newburger JW, Pober JS: Endothelial cell activation and high interleukin-1 secretion in the pathogenesis of acute Kawasaki disease. *Lancet* 1989, ii:1298–1302.
22. Burrows NP, Molina FA, Terenghi G, Clark PK, Haskard DO, Polak JM, Jones RR: Comparison of cell adhesion molecule expression in cutaneous leucocytoclastic and lymphocytic vasculitis. *J Clin Pathol* 1994, 47:939–944.
23. Bradley JR, Lockwood CM, Thiru S: Endothelial cell activation in patients with systemic vasculitis. *Q J Med* 1994, 87:741–745.
24. Sais G, Vidaller A, Jucgla A, Condom E, Peyri J: Adhesion molecule expression and endothelial cell activation in cutaneous leukocytoclastic vasculitis. An immunohistologic and clinical study in 42 patients. *Arch Dermatol* 1997, 133: 443–50.
25. Lhotta K, Neumayer HP, Joannidis Geissler D, König P: Renal expression of intercellular adhesion molecule-1 in different forms of glomerulonephritis. *Clin Sci* 1991, 81:477–481.
26. Seron D, Cameron JS, Haskard DO: Expression of VCAM-1 in the normal and diseased kidney. *Nephrol Dial Transplant* 1991, 6:917–922.
27. Fuiano G, Sepe V, Stanziale P, Balletta M, Comi N, Magri P, Dal Canton A: Expression of intercellular adhesion molecule in idiopathic crescentic glomerulonephritis. *Contrib Nephrol* 1991, 94:81–88.
28. Chow J, Hartley RB, Jagger C, Dilly SA: ICAM-1 expression in renal disease. *J Clin Pathol* 1992, 45:880–884.
29. Bruyn JA, Dinklo NJCM: Distinct patterns of expression of intercellular adhesion molecule-1, vascular cell adhesion molecule-1, and endothelial-leukocyte adhesion molecule-1 in renal disease. *Lab Invest* 1993, 69:329–335.
30. Briscoe DM, Cotran RS: Role of leukocyte-endothelial cell adhesion molecules in renal inflammation: *in vitro* and *in vivo* studies. *Kidney Int* 1993, 44(suppl 42):S27–34.
31. Brouwer E, Huitema MG, Heeringa P, Cohen Tervaert JW, Weening JJ, Kallenberg CGM: Upregulation of adhesion molecules in renal biopsies from patients with Wegener's granulomatosis. *Clin Exp Immunol* 1993, 93, (suppl.1), 22.
32. Pall AA, Howie AJ, Adu D, Richards GM, Inward CD, Milford DV, Richards NT, Michael J, Taylor CM: Glomerular vascular cell adhesion molecule-1 expression in renal vasculitis. *J Clin Pathol* 1996, 49:238–242.
33. Patey N, Lesavre P, Halbwachs-Mecarelli L, Noël LH: Adhesion molecules in human crescentic glomerulonephritis. *J Pathol* 1996, 179:414–420.
34. Rastaldi MP, Ferrario F, Tunesi S, Yang L, D'Amico G: Intraglomerular and interstitial leukocyte infiltration, adhesion molecules, and interleukin-1a expression in 15 cases of antineutrophil cytoplasmic autoantibody-associated renal vasculitis. *Am J Kidney Dis* 1996, 27:48–57.
35. Panegyres PK, Faull RJ, Russ G, Appleton SL, Wangel AG, Bluberg PC: Endothelial cell activation in vasculitis of peripheral nerve and skeletal muscle. *J Neurol Neurosurg Psychiatry* 1991, 55:4–7.
36. Coll-Vinent B, Cebrian M, Cid MC, Font C, Esparza J, Juan M, Yague J, Urbano-Marquez A, Grau JM: Dynamic pattern of endothelial cell adhesion molecule expression in muscle and perineural vessels from patients with classic polyarteritis nodosa. *Arth Rheum* 1998, 41:435–444.
37. Wawryk SO, Ayberk H, Boyd AW, Rode J: Analysis of adhesion molecules in the immunopathogenesis of giant cell arteritis. *J Clin Pathol* 1991, 44:497–501.
38. Flipo RM, Cardon T, Copin MC, Vandecandelaere M, Duquesnoy B, Janin A: ICAM-1, E-selectin, and TNF a expression in labial salivary glands of patients with rheumatoid arthritis. *Ann Rheum Dis* 1997, 56:41–44.
39. Collins T: Endothelial nuclear factor-kappa B and the initiation of the atherosclerotic lesion. *Lab Invest* 1993, 68:499–508.
40. Takano T, Brady HR: The endothelium in glomerular inflammation. *Curr Opin Nephrol Hypert* 1995, 4:277–286.
41. Bradley JR, Johnson DR, Pober JS: Endothelial activation by hydrogen peroxide. Selective increases of intercellular adhesion molecule-1 and major histocompatibility complex class I. *Am J Pathol* 1993, 142:1598–1609.
42. Marui N, Offerman MK, Swerlick R, Kunsch C, Rosen CA, Ahmad M, Alexander RW, Medford RM: Vascular cell adhesion molecule-1 (VCAM-1) gene transcription and expression are regulated through an antioxidant sensitive mechanism in human vascular endothelial cells. *J Clin Invest* 1993, 92:1866–1874.

43. Melder RJ, Koenig GC, Witwer BP, Safabakhsh N, Munn LL, Jain RK: During angiogenesis, vascular endothelial growth factor regulate natural killer cell adhesion to tumor endothelium. *Nature Med* 1996, 2:992–997.

44. Nagel T, Resnick N, Atkinson WJ, Dewey CF, Gimbrone MA Jr: Shear stress differentially upregulates ICAM-1 expression in cultured vascular endothelial cells. *J Clin Invest* 1994, 94:885–891.

45. Mayet WJ, Meyer Zum Büschenfelde KH: Antibodies to proteinase 3 increase adhesion of neutrophils to human endothelial cells. *Clin Exp Immunol* 1993, 94:440–446.

46. Mayet WJ, Schwarting A, Orth T, Duchmann R, Meyer Zum Büschenfelde KH: Antibodies to proteinase 3 mediate expression of vascular cell adhesion molecule-1 (VCAM-1). *Clin Exp Immunol* 1996, 106:259–267.

47. Sibelius U, Hattar K, Schenkel A, Noll T, Csernok E, Gross WL, Mayet WJ, Piper HM, Seeger W, Grimminger F: Wegener's granulomatosis: anti-proteinase 3 antibodies are potent inductors of human endothelial cell signaling and leakage response. *J Exp Med* 1998, 187:497–503.

48. Belizna C, Cohen Tervaert JW. Specificity, pathogenecity, and clinical value of antiendothelial cell antibodies. *Sem Arth Rheum* 1997, 27:98–109.

49. Muller Kobold AC, van Wijk RT, Franssen CFM, Molema G, Kallenberg CGM, Cohen Tervaert JW. *In vitro* upregulation of E-selectin and induction of interleukin-6 in endothelial cells by autoantibodies in Wegener's granulomatosis and microscopic polyangiitis. *Clin Exp Rheumatol* 1999, 17:433–440.

50. Carvalho D, Savage COS, Isenberg D, Pearson JD: IgG anti-endothelial cell autoantibodies from patients with systemic lupus erythematosus or systemic vasculitis stimulate the release of two endothelial cell-derived mediators, which enhance adhesion molecule expression and leukocyte adhesion in an autocrine manner. *Arth Rheum* 1999, 42:631–640.

51. Mayet WJ, Csernok E, Szymkowiak C, Gross WL, Meyer zum Büschenfelde KH: Human endothelial cells express proteinase 3, the target antigen of anti-cytoplasmic antibodies in Wegener's granulomatosis. *Blood* 1993, 82:1221–1229.

52. King WJ, Adu D, Daha MR, Brooks CJ, Radford DJ, Pall AA, Savage COS: Endothelial cells and renal epithelial cells do not express the Wegener's autoantigen, proteinase 3. *Clin Exp Immunol* 1995, 102:98–105.

53. Gearing AJH, Newman W: Circulating adhesion molecules in disease. *Immunology Today* 1993, 14:506–512.

54. Goldberger A, Middleton KA, Oliver JA, Paddock C, Yan HC, DeLisser HM, Albelda SM, Newman PJ: Biosynthesis and processing of the cell adhesion molecule PECAM-1 includes production of a soluble form. *J Biol Chem* 1994, 269:17183–17191.

55. Martin S, Rieckmann P, Melchers I, Wagner R, Bertrams J, Voskuyl AE, Roep B, Zielasek J, Heidenthal E, Weichselbraun I, Gallatin WM, Kolb H: Circulating forms of ICAM-3 (cICAM-3). Elevated levels in autoimmune diseases and lack of association with cICAM-1. *J Immunol* 1995, 154:1951–1955.

56. Ferrara N: Missing link in angiogenesis. *Nature* 1995, 376:467.

57. Koch AE, Halloran MM, Haskell CK, Shah MR, Polverini PJ: Angiogenesis mediated by soluble forms of E-selectin and vascular cell adhesion molecule-1. *Nature* 1995, 376:517–519.

58. Spertini O, Callegari P, Cordey AS, Hauert J, Joggi J, von Fliedner V, Schapira M: High levels of the shed form of L-selectin are present in patients with acute leukemia and inhibit blast cell adhesion to activated endothelium. *Blood* 1994, 84:1249–1256.

59. Hoffman GS, Ahmed AE: Surrogate markers of disease activity in patients with Takayasu's arteritis. A preliminary report from The International Network for the Study of the Systemic Vasculitides (INSSYS). *Int J Cardiol* 1998, 66 (suppl. 1):S191–194.

60. Boehme MWJ, Schmitt WH, Youinou P, Stremmel WR, Gross WL: Clinical relevance of elevated serum thrombomodulin and soluble E-selectin in patients with Wegener's granulomatosis and other systemic vasculitides. *Am J Med* 1996, 101:387–394.

61. Noguchi S, Numano F, Gravanis MB, Wilcox JN: Increased levels of soluble forms of adhesion molecules in Takayasu's arteritis. *Int J Cardiol* 1998, 66 (suppl. 1):S23–33.

62. Carson CW, Beall LD, Hunder GG, Johnson CM, Mewman W: Serum ELAM-1 is increased in vasculitis, scleroderma, and systemic lupus erythematosus. *J Rheumatol* 1993, 20:809–814.

63. Maccioni P, Boiardi L, Meliconi R, Salvarani C, Uguccioni MG, Rossi F, Pulsatelli L, Facchini A: Elevated soluble intercellular adhesion molecule 1 in the serum of patients with polymyalgia rheumatica: influence of steroid treatment. *J Rheumatol* 1994, 21:1860–1864.

64. Jennette JC, Falk RJ, Andrassy K, Bacon PA, Churg J, Gross WL, Hagen EC, Hoffman GS, Hunder GG, Kallenberg CGM et al.: Nomenclature of systemic vasculitides. Proposal of an international consensus conference. *Arth Rheum* 1994, 37:187–192.

65. Watts RA, Jolliffe VA, Carruthers DM, Lockwood CM, Scott DG: Effect of classification on the incidence of polyarteritis nodosa and microscopic polyangiitis. *Arth Rheum* 1996, 39:1208–1212.

66. Coll-Vinent B, Grau JM, Lopez-Soto A, Oristrell J, Font C, Bosch X, Mirapeix E, Urbano-Marquez A, Cid MC: Circulating soluble adhesion molecules in patients with classical polyarteritis nodosa. *Br J Rheumatol* 1997, 36:1178–1183.

67. Furukawa S, Imai K, Matsubara T, Yone K, Yachi A, Okumura K, Yabuta K: Increased levels of circulating intercellular adhesion molecule 1 in Kawasaki disease. *Arth Rheum* 1992, 35:672–677.

68. Kim DS, Lee KY. Serum soluble E-selectin levels in Kawasaki disease. *Scand J Rheumatol* 1994, 23:283–286.

69. Nash MC, Shah V, Dillon MJ: Soluble cell adhesion molecules and von Willebrand factor in children with Kawasaki disease. *Clin Exp Immunol* 1995, 101:13–17.

70. Spertini O, Schleiffenbaum B, White-Owen C, Ruiz P Jr, Tedder TF: ELISA for quantitation of L-selectin shed from leukocytes *in vivo*. *J Immunol Methods* 1992, 156:115–123.

71. Kanekura S, Kitajima I, Nishi J, Yoshinaga M, Miyata K, Maruyama I: Low shed L-selectin levels in Kawasaki disease with coronary artery lesions: comment on the article by Furukawa et al. *Arth Rheum* 1996, 39:534–535.

72. Hauschild S, Schmitt WH, Kekow J, Szymkowiak C, Gross WL: Hohe serumspiegel von ICAM-1 bei der aktiven generalisierten Wegenerschen Granulomatose. *Immun Infekt* 1992, 20:84–85.

73. Stegeman CA, Cohen Tervaert JW, Huitema MG, de Jong PE, Kallenberg CGM: Serum levels of soluble adhesion molecules intercellular adhesion molecule 1, vascular cell adhesion molecule 1, and E-selectin in patients with Wegener's granulomatosis. Relationship to disease activity and relevance during followup. *Arth Rheum* 1994, 37:1228–1235.

74. Mrowka C, Sieberth HG: Detection of circulating adhesion molecules ICAM-1, VCAM-1 and E-selectin in Wegener's granulomatosis, systemic lupus erythematosus and chronic renal failure. *Clin Nephrol* 1995, 43:288–296.

75. Pall AA, Adu D, Drayson M, Taylor CM, Richards NT, Michael J: Circulating soluble adhesion molecules in systemic vasculitis. *Nephrol Dial Transplant* 1994, 9:770–774.

76. Yaqoob M, West DC, McDicken I, Bell GM: Monitoring of endothelial leukocyte adhesion molecule-1 in anti-neutrophil-cytoplasmic-antibody–positive vasculitis. *Am J Nephrol* 1996, 16:106–113.

77. Becvar R, Paleckova A, Tesar V, Rychlik I, Masek Z: Von Willebrand factor antigen and adhesive molecules in Wegener's granulomatosis and microscopic polyangiitis. *Clin Rheum* 1997, 16:324–325.

78. Tesar V, Jelinkova E, Masek Z, Jirsa M, Zabka J, Bartunkova J, Stejskalova A, Janatkova I, Zima T: Influence of plasma exchange on serum levels of cytokines and adhesion molecules in ANCA-positive renal vasculitis. *Blood Purification* 1998, 16:72–80.

79. Söylemezoglu O, Sultan N, Gursel T, Buyan N, Hasanoglu E: Circulating adhesion molecules ICAM-1, E-selectin, and von Willebrand factor in Henoch-Schönlein purpura. *Arch Dis Child* 1996, 75:507–511.

80. Willis FR, Smith GC, Beattie TJ: Plasma E-selectin and ICAM-1 in acute Henoch-Schönlein purpura. *Arch Dis Child* 1997, 77:94.

81. Wang CR, Liu MF, Tsai RT, Chuang CY, Chen CY: Circulating intercellular adhesion molecules-1 and autoantibodies including anti-endothelial cell, anti-cardiolipin, and anti-neutrophil cytoplasma antibodies in patients with vasculitis. *Clin Rheum* 1993, 12:375–380.

82. Voskuyl AE, Martin S, Melchers I, Zwinderman AH, Weichselbraun I, Breedveld FC: Levels of circulating intercellular adhesion molecule-1 and -3 but not circulating endothelial leucocyte adhesion molecule are increased in patients with rheumatoid vasculitis. *Br J Rheumatol* 1995, 34:311–315.

83. Lai CKW, Wong KC, Chan CHS, Ho SS, Chung SY, Haskard DO, Lai KN: Circulating adhesion molecules in tuberculosis. *Clin Exp Immunol* 1993, 94:522–526.

84. Blann AD, McCollum CN: Circulating endothelial cell/leukocyte adhesion molecules in atherosclerosis. *Thromb Haemostasis* 1994, 72:151–154.

85. DeSouza CA, Dengel DR, Macko RF, Cox K, Seals DR: Elevated levels of circulating cell adhesion molecules in uncomplicated essential hypertension. *Am J Hypertens* 1997, 10:1335–1341.

86. Hackman A, Abe Y, Insull W, Pownall H, Smith L, Dunn K, Gotto AM, Ballantyne CM: Levels of soluble cell adhesion molecules in patients with dyslipidemia. *Circulation* 1996, 93:1334–1338.

87. Blann AD, Sanders PA, Herrick A, Jayson MIV: Soluble L-selectin in the connective tissue diseases. *Br J Haematol* 1996, 95:192–194.

88. Scheinman RI, Cogswell PC, Lofquist AK, Baldwin AS: Role of transcriptional activation of IkappaBa in mediation of immunosuppression by glucocorticoids. *Science* 1995, 270:286–290.

89. Auphan N, DiDonato JA, Rosette C, Helmberg A, Karin M: Immunosuppression by glucocorticoids: inhibition of NF-kappaB activity through induction of IkappaBa synthesis. *Science* 1995, 270:286–290.

90. Baldwin AS Jr: The NF-kappa B and I kappa B proteins: new discoveries and insights. *Annu Rev Immunol* 1996, 14:649–683.

91. Neurath MF, Petterson S, Meyer Zum Büschenfelde KH, Strober W: Local administration of antisense phosphorothioate oligonucleotides to the p65 subunit of NF-kappaB abrogates established experimental colitis in mice. *Nature Med* 1996, 2:998–1004.

92. Ferran C, Millan MT, Csizmadia V, Cooper JT, Brostjan C, Bach FH, Winkler H: Inhibition of NF-kappaB by pyrrolidine dithiocarbamate blocks endothelial cell activation. *Biochem Biophys Res Commun* 1995, 214:212–223.

93. Read MA, Neish AS, Luschinskas FW, Palombella VJ, Maniatis T, Collins T: The proteasome pathway is required for cytokine-induced endothelial-leukocyte adhesion molecule expression. *Immunity* 1995, 2:493–506.

94. Grisham MB, Palombella VJ, Elliot PJ, Conner EM, Brand S, Wong HL, Pien C, Mazzola LM, Destree A, Parent L, Adams J: Inhibition of NF-kappaB activation *in vitro* and *in vivo*: role of 26S proteasome. *Methods Enzym* 1999, 300:345–363.

95. Rothlein R, Jaeger JR: Clinical Applications of Antileukocyte Adhesion Molecule Monoclonal Antibodies. In *Therapeutic Immunology*. Edited by Austen KF, Burakoff SJ, Rosen FS, Strom TS. Cambridge: Blackwell Science, 1996, 347–353.

96. Tuomanen E: A spoonful of sugar to control inflammation. *J Clin Invest* 1994, 93:917.

97. Bennett CF, Condon TP, Grimm S, Chan H, Chiang MY: Inhibition of endothelial cell adhesion molecule expression with anti-sense oligonucleotides. *J Immunol* 1994, 152:3530–3540.

98. Gerritsen ME, Carley WW, Ranges GE, Shen CP, Phan SA, Ligon GF, Perry CA: Flavonoids inhibit cytokine-induced endothelial cell adhesion protein gene expression. *Am J Pathol* 1995, 147:278–292.

99. Wahl SM, Allen JB, Hines KL, Imamichi T, Wahl AM, Furcht LT, McCarthy JB: Synthetic fibronectin peptides suppress arthritis in rats by interrupting leukocyte adhesion and recruitment. *J Clin Invest* 1994, 94:655–662.

100. Brouwer E, Huitema MG, Klok PA, Cohen Tervaert JW, Weening JJ, Kallenberg CGM: Antimyeloperoxidase-associated proliferative glomerulonephritis: an animal model. *J Exp Med* 1993, 177:905–914.

101. Coers W, Brouwer E, Vos JTWM, Chand A, Huitema S, Heeringa P, Kallenberg CGM, Weening JJ: Podocyte expression of MHC class I and II and intercellular adhesion molecule-1 (ICAM-1) in experimental pauci-immune crescentic glomerulonephritis. *Clin Exp Immunol* 1994, 98:279–286.

102. Muller Kobold AC, Cohen Tervaert JW, Klok PA, Kallenberg CGM: Intervention in experimental anti-MPO associated crescentic glomerulonephritis by monoclonal antibodies against adhesion molecules. *Clin Exp Immunol* 1995, 101 (suppl 1):53.

103. Cohen Tervaert JW, Cybulsky MI, Gimbrone MA Jr: Differential expression of VCAM-1 in a rabbit model of pulmonary granulomatous vasculitis. *Faseb J* 1993, 7:A344.

104. Barton PA, Imlay MM, Flory CM, Warren JS: Role of intercellular adhesion molecule-1 in glucaninduced pulmonary granulomatosis in the rat. *J Lab Clin Med* 1996, 128:181–193.

105. Kilgore KS, Powers KL, Imlay MM, Malani A, Allen DI, Beyer JT, Anderson MB, Warren JS: The carbohydrate sialyl Lewis^x (sLe^x) sulfated glycomimetic GM2941 attenuates glucan-induced pulmonary granulomatous vasculitis in the rat. *J Pharmacol Exp Ther* 1998, 286:439–446.

106. Devall L, Davis J, Cornicelli J, Newton R, Saxena U: Modulation of leukocyte adhesion in the glucan rat lung vasculitis model. *Faseb J* 1995, 9:A270.

107. Li H, Iiyama M, Iiyama K, DiChiara M, Gurtner GC, Milstone DS, Cybulsky MI: A hypomorphic VCAM-1 mutation rescues the embryonic lethal null phenotype and reveals a requirement for VCAM-1 in inflammation. *Faseb J* 1996, 10:A1281.

108. Elliott JD, Lockwood CM, Brettman L, Waldmann H: Antiadhesion molecule (anti CD 18) therapy for autoimmune inflammation. *J Autoimmunity* 1999 (supplement): 23.

14 Experimental Induction of Vascular Disease

Ilan Krause, Miri Blank, and Yehuda Shoenfeld

CONTENTS

I. INTRODUCTION

Animal models are of great value in evaluating pathogenic mechanisms and experimental treatments that cannot be tested directly on humans. In recent years several *in vivo* experimental models of human vascular diseases have been developed which contributed to our understanding the etio-pathogenesis of various vascular diseases. The spectrum of animal models entails spontaneous occurring vasculitis, viral or bacterial infections-mediated vascular disease, drug and chemical-induced vasculitis, and various immune manipulations leading to vascular inflammation and injury.[1-3] This chapter will focus on the induction of experimental vascular diseases mediated by pathogenic autoantibodies, among them anti-neutrophil cytoplasmic antibodies, anti-glomerular basement membrane, anti-endothelial cells, and anti-phospholipid antibodies.

II. ANIMAL MODELS OF ANCA-ASSOCIATED VASCULITIS

Anti-neutrophil cytoplasmic antibodies (ANCA) have been an increasingly prominent part of the literature of autoimmune diseases for more than 15 years. Since the first description of ANCA in patients with segmental necrotizing glomerulonephritis,[4] ANCA has been demonstrated in a number of primary vasculitic syndromes.[2,5] In most cases of systemic vasculitis, the primary target antigens for ANCA are proteinase-3 (PR-3) and myeloperoxidase (MPO).[6] Both enzymes are present in secretory granules of neutrophils and monocytes. It is now well established that anti-PR-3 is a sensitive marker of Wegener's granulomatosis (WG), whereas anti-MPO is predominantly found in microscopic polyangiitis and Churg-Strauss syndrome.[5] As well as being useful diagnostic tools, their strong association with primary vasculitic syndromes suggests an important role for ANCA in the pathophysiology of the associated disease. Indeed, in recent years several animal studies have been reported on ANCA and vasculitis using various experimental approaches.[2,3]

A. SPONTANEOUS VASCULITIS IN MRL AND SCG MICE

The MRL/lpr mouse strain was first proposed as a model for an accelerated membranoproliferative glomerulonephritis associated with anti-DNA production,[7] and has been used as an experimental model for the study of systemic lupus erythematosus (SLE) and rheumatoid arthritis. These mice spontaneously develop lymphoproliferation, proliferative glomerulonephritis, and systemic necrotizing vasculitis of small and medium-sized arteries that particularly affect the kidneys and gallbladder.[8] In addition, significant vasculopathy in the central nervous system, including vascular occlusions and perivascular infiltrates in the choroid plexus, was reported.[9] The spontaneous development of tissue injury is associated with T-cell accumulation with polyclonal B-cell stimulation, resulting in the appearance of rheumatoid factor and various autoantibodies including anti-DNA, Sm, and histones.[10] It was also reported that 20% of female MRL/lpr mice are positive for ANCA;[11] however, monoclonal IgG antibodies derived from these mice were found to be polyreactive, recognizing MPO, lactoferrin, and DNA.[11] The occurrence of vasculitis in many organs in MRL/lpr mice has been attributed to a deficiency in apoptosis.[12] It is assumed that lpr mice have a genomic deletion in parts of the *Fas* gene that results in deficient apoptosis. As a result, T-cells which are normally deleted by apoptosis are accumulating, leading to induction of vasculitis. A recombinant inbred strain of mice, derived from BxSB and MRL/lpr strains, has been termed SCG/Kj.[13] These mice develop spontaneous crescentic glomerulonephritis (58% in females and 34% in males) associated with necrotizing vasculitis of small and medium-sized arteries and arterioles in many organs, including the spleen, ovary, uterus, heart, and stomach. However, in contrast to MRL/lpr mice, necrotizing vasculitis is not found in the kidneys. Serum from SCG/Kj mice produce a perinuclear ANCA staining pattern (pANCA) and react with MPO by ELISA. Transfer of MPO-specific hybridomas derived from SCG/Kj mice into the peritoneum of nude mice induced proteinuria, although histologically no evidence of glomerulonephritis or peritonitis was found.[3]

B. ANTI-MPO IN HgCl$_2$-INDUCED VASCULITIS

Exposure to mercuric chlorid (HgCl$_2$) of susceptible rat strains, usually of the Th2-responder type such as the Brown Norway rat, induces an autoimmune syndrome mediated by T-cell-dependent polyclonal B-cell activation.[14] The HgCl$_2$-induced autoimmune syndrome is characterized by lymphoproliferation, high IL-4 production, and hypergammaglobulinemia particularly affecting the IgE class.[15] In addition, a multitude of IgG autoantibodies appear in this model including antibodies to DNA, thyroglobulin, and components of the glomerular basement membrane (GBM).[16] The model of HgCl$_2$-induced vasculitis has several characteristics that resemble aspects of human systemic necrotizing vasculitis involving small to medium-sized vessels accompanied by fibrinoid necrosis of the vessel wall and inflammatory cell infiltration. Tissue injury in multiple organs has been observed — including the lungs, liver, skin, gut, and pancreas — that increases in severity over time.[17] An important role of autoreactive CD4+ T-cells has been demonstrated. It was shown that CD4+ T-cell transfer into healthy animals can induce the disease,[18] but CD4+ OX22 high T-cells are protective against HgCl$_2$-induced vasculitis since their depletion aggravates the severity of tissue injury.[19] Treatment with cyclosporine during the early phase of the disease diminished tissue injury and attenuated the levels of autoantibodies, while late administration of the drug caused marked exacerbation of tissue injury, though development of anti-GBM and anti-MPO autoantibodies was completely suppressed.[20] These observations suggest that HgCl$_2$-induced vasculitis is primarily T-cell dependent, however, the rapid onset of tissue injury, which can be observed as early as 24 hours after the first injection of HgCl$_2$, implicates that other cells (e.g., mast cells[20,21]) are involved, especially during the induction phase of the disease.[22] It was also shown that neutrophils are necessary for the induction of the vasculitis and that the degree of vasculitis correlates with neutrophil number.[23] Anti-MPO is detectable from Day 10 after HgCl$_2$ administration, reaching a peak on Day 12 and later resolve.[24] The role of anti-MPO in HgCl$_2$-induced vasculitis is unclear.

It was shown that transfer of serum from $HgCl_2$-treated rats into normal animals fails to induce vasculitis,[1] implying that it might not be primarily involved in the pathogenesis of tissue injury.

C. Anti-MPO Associated Glomerulonephritis

In 1993 Brouwer et al. reported a model for pauci-immune necrotizing crescentic glomerulonephritis in Brown Norway rats which closely resembles the human anti-MPO-associated pauci-immune glomerulonephritis.[25] The disease was induced in MPO-immunized rats by unilateral kidney perfusion with a neutrophil lysosomal enzyme extract primarily consisting of MPO plus H_2O_2, the substrate of MPO, 5 weeks after immunization. MPO, IgG, and C3 were present along the glomerular basement membrane at 24 hours after perfusion, but were absent at 4 and 10 days. The immunized rats developed a proliferative glomerulonephritis characterized by intra- and extracapillary cell proliferation periglomerular granulomatous inflammation and formation of giant cells.[25] Granulomatous vasculitis of small vessels was found at 10 days after perfusion. Yang et al.,[26] who repeated the study in spontaneously hypertensive and Brown Norway rats, reported that pathological lesions and deposits of IgG, C3, and MPO were continuously found in immunized rats perfused with MPO + H_2O_2 or MPO alone. The degree of histologic injury was proportional in intensity to the amount of IgG immune deposits. Their results imply that this rat model might be an example of immune complex-mediated rather than pauci-immune glomerulonephritis. Differences in the immunization procedure or the composition of neutrophil lysosomal extracts might have accounted for the differences in the results. In a recent study it was shown that upon systemic injection of neutrophil lysosomal extract to MPO-immunized rats, a necrotizing vasculitis in the lungs and gut is developed.[27] The results indicate that release of products from activated neutrophils in the presence of anti-MPO autoantibodies may be relevant to the pathogenesis of anti-MPO-associated vasculitides.

D. Induction of Experimental WG by Idiotypic Immunization

According to Jerne's theory,[28,29] the idiotypic determinant of each autoantibody is complemented by those of another, creating an idiotypic network through which immunoglobulin expression might be controlled. This is manifested by the generation of anti-idiotypic antibodies of two functional subsets: those that recognize determinants in the V region and do not involve the combining site for the elicit antigen, and those that represent an internal image of the elicit antigen. We and others[30-40] have shown that immunization of naive mice with an autoantibody (Ab1) results in generation of anti-idiotypic antibody (i.e., Ab2), and 2 to 3 months later the mice develop anti-anti-idiotypic antibodies (i.e., Ab3). Ab3 may simulate Ab1 in its binding properties. The generation of Ab3 is followed by the emergence of the full-blown serological, immunohistochemical, and clinical manifestations of the respective autoimmune disease (Figure 14.1). Employing the above methods, several models for Id-associated vasculitides were developed. Wegener's granulomatosis (WG) is a granulomatous vasculitis that involves the upper respiratory tract, lungs, and kidneys, as well as skin abnormalities, peripheral neuropathy, and joint disease. WG is closely associated with the presence of anti-neutrophil cytoplasmic antibodies (ANCA), which are predominantly directed against proteinase-3 (PR-3).[6,41] Immunization of naive BALB/c mice with purified ANCA from two patients with active WG led to the development of anti-human ANCA and anti-anti-human ANCA (mouse ANCA) with specificity both to PR3 and to MPO, as well as anti-endothelial autoantibodies. Mouse ANCA were capable of inducing adhesion of neutrophils to fibronectin and activating the respiratory burst in neutrophils. Moreover, the mice that were immunized with human ANCA also developed either sterile microabscesses in the lungs after 8 months, or developed proteinuria (but not hematuria) associated with mononuclear perivascular infiltration in the lungs and diffuse granular deposition of immunoglobulins in the kidneys.[42,43] It was also shown that the IgG-ANCA-immunized mice develop high levels of IL-4, IL-6, and TNFα, but not IL-1β, IL-2, or interferon-γ.[44] This suggests that a Th2-type immune response is responsible for the initiation of

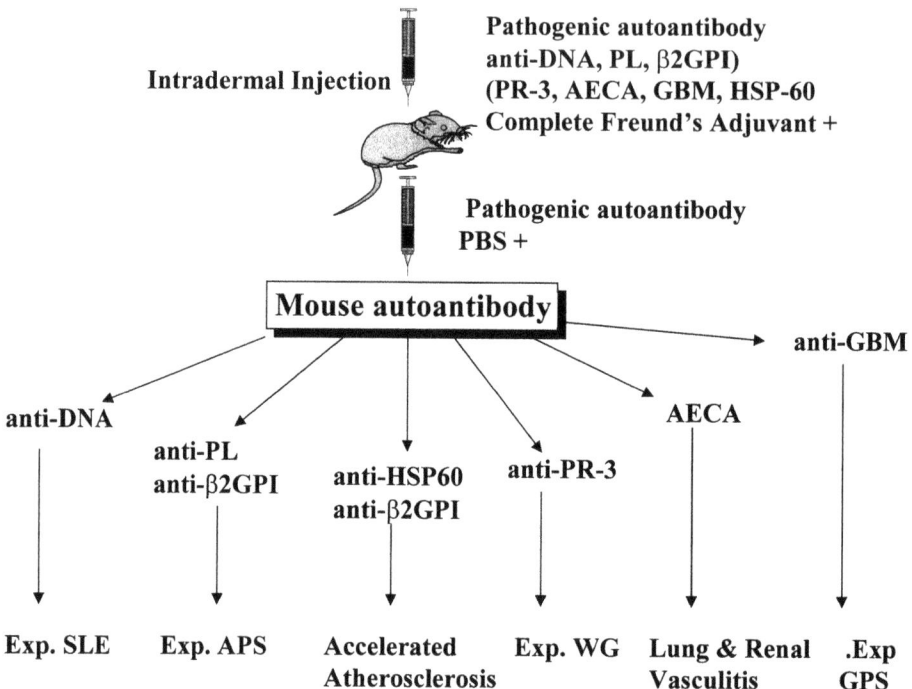

FIGURE 14.1 Induction of autoimmune disease by idiotypic immunization. Mice are immunized by an intradermal injection of a pathogenic autoantibody, in complete Freund's adjuvant (Ab1), followed by a boost injection after 3 weeks. The mice develop anti-idiotypic antibody (Ab2) and later on anti-anti-idiotypic antibody (Ab3) which may simulate Ab1 in its binding properties, and is followed by the emergence of the full-blown serological, immunohistochemical and clinical manifestations of the respective autoimmune disease (AECA — antiendothelial cell antibodies, APS — antiphospholipid syndrome, GBM — glomerular basement membrane, GPS — Goodpasture's syndrome, HSP — heat-shock proteins, PL — phospholipid, PR-3 — Proteinase 3, SLE — systemic lupus erythematosus, WG — Wegener's granulomatosis).

experimental autoimmune lung vasculitis similar to WG in humans. Those findings provide evidence for a direct role of ANCA in the pathogenesis of Wegener's-associated vasculitides.

III. EXPERIMENTAL GOODPASTURE'S SYNDROME (GPS)

GPS is a severe autoimmune disease characterized by a triad of glomerulonephritis, pulmonary hemorrhage, and anti-glomerular basement membrane (GBM) autoantibodies directed against the noncollagenous domains (NC1) on Type IV collagen.[45] Anti-GBM autoantibodies were demonstrated in the HgCl$_2$-induced vasculitis in Brown Norway rats.[16] The anti-GBM components were deposited in the kidneys and were associated with the development of proteinuria and minor inflammatory changes. Anti-basement membrane antibodies have also been demonstrated in tissues other than the kidneys, but were not associated with tissue injury.[46] Abbate et al.[47] studied the renal and pulmonary effects of immunization with alpha3(IV) NC1 collagen in Wistar-Kyoto (WKY) rats. The immunized rats developed proteinuria, linear IgG deposition in GBM, and crescentic glomerulonephritis, and the effects were dose-dependent. Pulmonary hemorrhage was detectable in 35% of immunized rats. These findings documented that glomerulonephritis and lung hemorrhage can be elicited in WKY rats by immunization with alpha3(IV) NC1. Employing our method of idiotypic immunization, we immunized naive BALB/c mice with either mouse IgG anti-NC1 monoclonal antibody, or with IgG serum fraction derived from patients with GPS. The mice developed mouse anti-NC1 antibodies of IgG isotype.[48,49] The presence of circulating anti-NC1 antibodies coincided in some of the mice with hematuria and proteinuria, as well as pathological changes in the kidneys. The results show that specific idiotypic manipulation can induce mouse anti-NC1 autoantibodies and pathological changes resembling human GPS.

IV. ANTI-ENDOTHELIAL CELL ANTIBODIES-INDUCED VASCULITIS

Anti-endothelial cell autoantibodies (AECA) have been a subject for an extensive research in the last decade.[50-52] AECA were detected in sera from patients with connective-tissue and autoimmune diseases such as SLE,[53] rheumatoid arthritis,[54] mixed connective tissue disease,[54] systemic sclerosis,[53] and systemic vasculitide.[55,56] The analysis of the antigens recognized by AECA showed that the antibodies are directed against a heterogeneous family of both constitutive and nonconstitutive surface endothelial proteins.[50] Although there are no definite conclusions concerning the clinical significance of AECA, they might well be among the driving mechanisms for vascular injury, and among the factors that may initiate the pathogenesis of vascular abnormalities. Recently we[57-59] and others,[60-63] were able to demonstrate that AECA from different sources (e.g., antiphospholipid syndrome, WG, systemic sclerosis, or Takayasu's arteritis) have a potential to activate endothelial cells (EC). Pretreatment of human umbilical vein EC with AECA led to an increased secretion of IL-6 and von-Willerband factor — which are markers of EC activation — as well as to increased ability of EC to bind human U937 monocytic cells, and increased expression of adhesion molecules. It can be hypothesized that those *in vitro* studies provide evidence for a pathogenic role of AECA in inducing vascular inflammation. In line with this assumption, we actively immunized naive mice with purified human AECA derived from a WG patient's plasma in an attempt to induce the production of mouse-AECA and autoimmune vasculitis in a murine model.[64] IgG was purified by absorption on a PR-3 affinity column, resulting in the depletion of anti-neutrophil cytoplasmic Ab activity. The absorbed IgG fraction displayed a high titer of AECA as evidenced by a cyto-ELISA against unfixed human umbilical vein endothelial cells. Three months after a boost injection with the human AECA, the mice developed endogenous AECA, but not Abs to PR-3, cardiolipin, or DNA. Histologic examination of lungs and kidneys revealed both lymphoid cell infiltration surrounding arterioles and venules, and deposition of immunoglobulins at the outer part of blood vessel walls. This experimental animal model of vasculitis, a product of our method of idiotypic manipulation, provides the first direct proof of the pathogenicity of AECA.

V. AUTOIMMUNE-MEDIATED ATHEROSCLEROSIS

Atherosclerosis is a multifactorial condition that results in the formation of lipid-laden lesions in the arterial system.[65] The implications of the complications of atherosclerosis cannot be overemphasized, being the major cause of mortality in the Western world. The basic cellular elements that play a part, at least initially, are endothelial cells, macrophages, T-lymphocytes, and smooth-muscle cells.[65] Subsequently, the monocytes differentiate into macrophages expressing the scavenger receptor(s). This allows the unregulated influx of oxidized lipoproteins in the cells, leading to foam cell formation.[66] Oxidized LDL (oxLDL) has attracted major interest in view of its various effects on different cellular components, attesting to its immunogenicity and probable causal effect on atherosclerosis progression.[66] This chain of events resembles the development of chronic inflammatory conditions and even some immune-mediated diseases. This concept has brought attention to the involvement of the immune system in atherogenesis.[67-69] Indeed, recent literature is rich in reports documenting the importance of immune mediators in the progression of the atherosclerotic process.[70]

An autoimmune reaction against heat shock protein 60 (Hsp60) expressed by endothelial cells in areas that are subject to increased hemodynamic stress was proposed as an initiating event in atherogenesis.[67] Humoral and T-cell-mediated immune responses against Hsp60 have both been demonstrated early in the disease. In addition, several clinical studies pointed to an association of SLE with premature atherogenesis.[71] The high occurrence of antiphospholipid syndrome (APS) (arterial and venous thrombosis, recurrent fetal loss, and thrombocytopenia) in patients with SLE had prompted the question of whether APS might be a risk factor for early atherosclerosis. Although no prospective controlled studies have yet documented an association between antiphospholipid antibodies (aPL) and long-term atherosclerotic complications, indirect data have pointed to a possible linkage between the two conditions. Patients with APS secondary to SLE have recently been shown to posses markers of lipid peroxidation, indicating a proatherogenic potential.[72] Furthermore, it has been shown that aPL from APS patients induces monocyte adherence to human EC, an effect being mediated by the adhesion molecules ICAM-1, VCAM-1, and E-selectin.[57,61,63] Bearing in mind that the initiation of human atherosclerotic lesions results from monocyte adhesion to EC, it is tempting to speculate that aPL may promote atherosclerosis *in vivo* by this mechanism.[73] In order to prove the proatherogenic effect of aPL *in vivo*, George et al. immunized LDL receptor-deficient (LDL-RD) mice with either β2GPI or ovalbumin.[74] All β2GPI-immunized mice developed high titers of anti-β2GPI antibodies, as well as specific lymph node proliferations to β2GPI. Atherosclerosis was enhanced in β2GPI-immunized in comparison with ovalbumin-immunized mice. The average lesion size in the β2GPI-immunized mice fed an atherogenic diet was larger than the ovalbumin-immunized mice. The atherosclerotic plaques in the β2GPI-immunized mice appeared to be more mature, and denser infiltration of CD4 lymphocytes was present in the subendothelium of the aortic sinuses from this group of mice. The results of the study provided the first direct evidence of the proatherogenic effect of β2GPI immunization and established a new model for immune-mediated atherosclerosis. Similar results were obtained using apolipoprotein E-(ApoE) deficient mice.[75]

In another study, applying the idiotypic manipulation method, George et al. assessed the effect of immunization with anti-cardiolipin (aCL) antibodies (i.e., Ab1, leading to the production of mouse aCL-Ab3) on the progression of atherosclerosis. Two groups of LDL-receptor knockout mice (LDL-RKO) were immunized with IgG purified from the serum of an APS patient or with normal human IgG, respectively. The aCL-immunized mice developed high titers of self aCL as compared with the normal human IgG-immunized mice. The extent of fatty streak formation was significantly higher in the aCL-immunized mice in comparison with the human IgG-injected mice. The results of the study show that mouse aCL induced by immunization with human aCL from an APS patient enhance atherogenesis in LDL-RKO mice, and further support the role of aPL in atherosclerosis development in patients with APS.

In another study, C57BL/6J mice were immunized with recombinant heat shock protein-65 (HSP-65) and HSP-65-rich mycobacterium tuberculosis (MT). A rapid cellular immune response to HSP-65 was evident in the immunized mice, accompanied by enhanced early atherosclerosis. Immunohistochemical analysis of atherosclerotic lesions from the immunized mice revealed infiltration of CD4 lymphocytes compared with the relatively lymphocyte-poor lesions in controls. This model, which supports the involvement of HSP-65 in atherogenesis, furnishes a valuable tool to study the role of the immune system in atherogenesis.

REFERENCES

1. Mathieson, P. W., Qasim, F. J., Esnault, V. L., Oliveira, D. B., Animal models of systemic vasculitis, *J Autoimmun*, 6, 251, 1993.
2. Heeringa, P., Brouwer, E., Cohen Tervaert, J. W., Weening, J. J., Kallenberg, C. G., Animal models of anti-neutrophil cytoplasmic antibody associated vasculitis, *Kidney Int*, 53, 253, 1998.
3. Kettritz, R., Yang, J. J., Kinjoh, K., Jennette, J. C., Falk, R. J., Animal models in ANCA-vasculitis, *Clin Exp Immunol*, 101 Suppl. 1, 12, 1995.

4. Davies, D. J., Moran, J. E., Niall, J. F., Ryan, G. B., Segmental necrotising glomerulonephritis with antineutrophil antibody: possible arbovirus aetiology?, *Br Med J Clin Res Ed*, 285, 606, 1982.

5. Kallenberg, C. G., Brouwer, E., Weening, J. J., Tervaert, J. W., Anti-neutrophil cytoplasmic antibodies: current diagnostic and pathophysiological potential, *Kidney Int*, 46, 1, 1994.

6. Jennette, J. C., Falk, R. J., Small-vessel vasculitis, *N Engl J Med*, 337, 1512, 1997.

7. Gutierrez Ramos, J. C., Andreu, J. L., Moreno de Alboran, I., Rodriguez, J., Leonardo, E., Kroemer, G., Marcos, M. A., Martinez, C., Insights into autoimmunity: from classical models to current perspectives, *Immunol Rev*, 118, 73, 1990.

8. Moyer, C. F., Strandberg, J. D., Reinisch, C. L., Systemic mononuclear-cell vasculitis in MRL/Mp-lpr/lpr mice. A histologic and immunocytochemical analysis, *Am J Pathol*, 127, 229, 1987.

9. Smith, H. R., Hansen, C. L., Rose, R., Canoso, R. T., Autoimmune MRL-1 pr/1pr mice are an animal model for the secondary antiphospholipid syndrome, *J Rheumatol*, 17, 911, 1990.

10. Cohen, P. L., Eisenberg, R. A., Lpr and gld: single gene models of systemic autoimmunity and lymphoproliferative disease, *Annu Rev Immunol*, 9, 243, 1991.

11. Harper, J. M., Lockwood, C. M., Cooke, A., Antineutrophil cytoplasmic antibody in MEL/lpr/lpr mice, *Cli Exp Immunol*, 93 (Suppl 1), 22, 1993.

12. Watanabe Fukunaga, R., Brannan, C. I., Copeland, N. G., Jenkins, N. A., Nagata, S., Lymphoprolif-eration disorder in mice explained by defects in Fas antigen that mediates apoptosis, *Nature*, 356, 314, 1992.

13. Kinjoh, K., Kyogoku, M., Good, R. A., Genetic selection for crescent formation yields mouse strain with rapidly progressive glomerulonephritis and small vessel vasculitis, *Proc Natl Acad Sci U S A*, 90, 3413, 1993.

14. Druet, P., Pelletier, L., Hirsch, F., Rossert, J., Pasquier, R., Druet, E., Sapin, C., Mercury-induced autoimmune glomerulonephritis in animals, *Contrib Nephrol*, 61, 120, 1988.

15. Prouvost Danon, A., Abadie, A., Sapin, C., Bazin, H., Druet, P., Induction of IgE synthesis and potentiation of anti-ovalbumin IgE antibody response by HgCl2 in the rat, *J Immunol*, 126, 699, 1981.

16. Pusey, C. D., Bowman, C., Morgan, A., Weetman, A. P., Hartley, B., Lockwood, C. M., Kinetics and pathogenicity of autoantibodies induced by mercuric chloride in the brown Norway rat, *Clin Exp Immunol*, 81, 76, 1990.

17. Mathieson, P. W., Thiru, S., Oliveira, D. B., Mercuric chloride-treated brown Norway rats develop widespread tissue injury including necrotizing vasculitis, *Lab Invest*, 67, 121, 1992.

18. Pelletier, L., Pasquier, R., Rossert, J., Vial, M. C., Mandet, C., Druet, P., Autoreactive T cells in mercury-induced autoimmunity. Ability to induce the autoimmune disease, *J Immunol*, 140, 750, 1988.

19. Mathieson, P. W., Thiru, S., Oliveira, D. B., Regulatory role of OX22high T cells in mercury-induced autoimmunity in the brown Norway rat, *J Exp Med*, 177, 1309, 1993.

20. Qasim, F. J., Mathieson, P. W., Thiru, S., Oliveira, D. B., Cyclosporin A exacerbates mercuric chloride-induced vasculitis in the brown Norway rat, *Lab Invest*, 72, 183, 1995.

21. Oliveira, D. B., Gillespie, K., Wolfreys, K., Mathieson, P. W., Qasim, F., Coleman, J. W., Compounds that induce autoimmunity in the brown Norway rat sensitize mast cells for mediator release and interleukin-4 expression, *Eur J Immunol*, 25, 2259, 1995.

22. Qasim, F. J., Thiru, S., Mathieson, P. W., Oliveira, D. B., The time course and characterization of mercuric chloride-induced immunopathology in the brown Norway rat, *J Autoimmun*, 8, 193, 1995.

23. Qasim, F. J., Mathieson, P. W., Sendo, F., Thiru, S., Oliveira, D. B., Role of neutrophils in the pathogenesis of experimental vasculitis, *Am J Pathol*, 149, 81, 1996.

24. Esnault, V. L., Mathieson, P. W., Thiru, S., Oliveira, D. B., Martin Lockwood, C., Autoantibodies to myeloperoxidase in brown Norway rats treated with mercuric chloride, *Lab Invest*, 67, 114, 1992.

25. Brouwer, E., Huitema, M. G., Klok, P. A., de Weerd, H., Tervaert, J. W., Weening, J. J., Kallenberg, C. G., Antimyeloperoxidase-associated proliferative glomerulonephritis: an animal model, *J Exp Med*, 177, 905, 1993.

26. Yang, J. J., Jennette, J. C., Falk, R. J., Immune complex glomerulonephritis is induced in rats immunized with heterologous myeloperoxidase, *Clin Exp Immunol*, 97, 466, 1994.

27. Heeringa, P., Foucher, P., Klok, P. A., Huitema, M. G., Cohen Tervaert, J. W., Weening, J. J., Kallenberg, C. G., Systemic injection of products of activated neutrophils and H2O2 in myeloperox-idase-immunized rats leads to necrotizing vasculitis in the lungs and gut, *Am J Pathol*, 151, 131, 1997.

28. Jerne, N. K., Towards a network theory of the immune system, *Ann Immunol Paris*, 125c, 373, 1974.

29. Jerne, N. K., Roland, J., Cazenave, P. A., Recurrent idiotopes and internal images, *Embo J*, 1, 243, 1982.
30. Mendlovic, S., Brocke, S., Shoenfeld, Y., Ben Bassat, M., Meshorer, A., Bakimer, R., Mozes, E., Induction of a systemic lupus erythematosus-like disease in mice by a common human anti-DNA idiotype, *Proc Natl Acad Sci U S A*, 85, 2260, 1988.
31. Mendlovic, S., Fricke, H., Shoenfeld, Y., Mozes, E., The role of anti-idiotypic antibodies in the induction of experimental systemic lupus erythematosus in mice, *Eur J Immunol*, 19, 729, 1989.
32. Shoenfeld, Y., Mozes, E., Pathogenic idiotypes of autoantibodies in autoimmunity: lessons from new experimental models of SLE, *Faseb J*, 4, 2646, 1990.
33. Shoenfeld, Y., Idiotypic induction of autoimmunity: a new aspect of the idiotypic network, *Faseb J*, 8, 1296, 1994.
34. Tincani, A., Balestrieri, G., Allegri, F., Cattaneo, R., Fornasieri, A., Li, M., Sinico, A., G, D. A., Induction of experimental SLE in naive mice by immunization with human polyclonal anti-DNA antibody carrying the 16/6 idiotype, *Clin Exp Rheumatol*, 11, 129, 1993.
35. Rombach, E., Stetler, D. A., Brown, J. C., Rabbits produce SLE-like anti-RNA polymerase I and anti-DNA autoantibodies in responses to immunization with either human or murine SLE anti-DNA antibodies, *Autoimmunity*, 13, 291, 1992.
36. Bakimer, R., Fishman, P., Blank, M., Sredni, B., Djaldetti, M., Shoenfeld, Y., Induction of primary antiphospholipid syndrome in mice by immunization with a human monoclonal anticardiolipin antibody (H-3), *J Clin Invest*, 89, 1558, 1992.
37. Yodfat, O., Blank, M., Krause, I., Shoenfeld, Y., The pathogenic role of anti-phosphatidylserine antibodies: active immunization with the antibodies leads to the induction of antiphospholipid syndrome, *Clin Immunol Immunopathol*, 78, 14, 1996.
38. Blank, M., Krause, I., Ben Bassat, M., Shoenfeld, Y., Induction of experimental anti-phospholipid syndrome associated with SLE following immunization with human monoclonal pathogenic anti-DNA idiotype, *J Autoimmun*, 5, 495, 1992.
39. Blank, M., Faden, D., Tincani, A., Kopolovic, J., Goldberg, I., Gilburd, B., Allegri, F., Balestrieri, G., Valesini, G., Shoenfeld, Y., Immunization with anticardiolipin cofactor (beta-2-glycoprotein I) induces experimental antiphospholipid syndrome in naive mice, *J Autoimmun*, 7, 441, 1994.
40. Blank, M., Cines, D. B., Arepally, G., Eldor, A., Afek, A., Shoenfeld, Y., Pathogenicity of human anti-platelet factor 4 (PF4)/heparin *in vivo*: generation of mouse anti-PF4/heparin and induction of thrombocytopenia by heparin, *Clin Exp Immunol*, 108, 333, 1997.
41. Falk, R. J., Jennette, J. C., ANCA small-vessel vasculitis, *J Am Soc Nephrol*, 8, 314, 1997.
42. Blank, M., Tomer, Y., Stein, M., Kopolovic, J., Wiik, A., Meroni, P. L., Conforti, G., Shoenfeld, Y., Immunization with anti-neutrophil cytoplasmic antibody (ANCA) induces the production of mouse ANCA and perivascular lymphocyte infiltration, *Clin Exp Immunol*, 102, 120, 1995.
43. Tomer, Y., Gilburd, B., Blank, M., Lider, O., Hershkoviz, R., Fishman, P., Zigelman, R., Meroni, P. L., Wiik, A., Shoenfeld, Y., Characterization of biologically active antineutrophil cytoplasmic antibodies induced in mice. Pathogenetic role in experimental vasculitis, *Arthritis Rheum*, 38, 1375, 1995.
44. Tomer, Y., Barak, V., Gilburd, B., Shoenfeld, Y., Cytokines in experimental autoimmune vasculitis: evidence for a Th2 type response, *Cli Exp Rheumatol*, (in press), 1999.
45. Bolton, W. K., Goodpasture's syndrome, *Kidney Int*, 50, 1753, 1996.
46. Bernaudin, J. F., Druet, E., Belair, M. F., Pinchon, M. C., Sapin, C., Druet, P., Extrarenal immune complex type deposits induced by mercuric chloride in the Brown Norway rat, *Clin Exp Immunol*, 38, 265, 1979.
47. Abbate, M., Kalluri, R., Corna, D., Yamaguchi, N., McCluskey, R. T., Hudson, B. G., Andres, G., Zoja, C., Remuzzi, G., Experimental Goodpasture's syndrome in Wistar-Kyoto rats immunized with alpha3 chain of type IV collagen, *Kidney Int*, 54, 1550, 1998.
48. Shoenfeld, Y., Gilburd, B., Hojnik, M., Damianovich, M., Hacham, S., Kopolovic, Y., Polak-Charcon, P., Goldberg, I., Afek, A., Hun-Chi, L., Induction of Goodpasture antibodies to noncollagenous domain (NC1) of type IV collagen in mice by idiotypic manipulation, *Hum Antibodies Hybridomas*, 6, 122, 1995.
49. Shoenfeld, Y., Pathogenicity of anti-basement membrane (NC1) antibodies: an experimental Goodpasture's syndrome, *Isr J Med Sci*, 32, 29, 1996.
50. Meroni, P. L., Khamashta, M. A., Youinou, P., Shoenfeld, Y., Mosaic of anti-endothelial antibodies. Review of the first international workshop on anti-endothelial antibodies: clinical and pathological significance Milan, 9 November 1994, *Lupus*, 4, 95, 1995.

51. Adler, Y., Salozhin, K., Le Tonqueze, M., Shoenfeld, Y., Youinou, P., Anti-endothelial cell antibodies: a need for standardization, *Lupus*, 3, 77, 1994.

52. Youinou, P., Meroni, P. L., Khamashta, M. A., Shoenfeld, Y., A need for standardization of the anti-endothelial-cell antibody test, *Immunol Today*, 16, 363, 1995.

53. Rosenbaum, J., Pottinger, B. E., Woo, P., Black, C. M., Loizou, S., Byron, M. A., Pearson, J. D., Measurement and characterisation of circulating anti-endothelial cell IgG in connective tissue diseases, *Clin Exp Immunol*, 72, 450, 1988.

54. Bodolay, E., Bojan, F., Szegedi, G., Stenszky, V., Farid, N. R., Cytotoxic endothelial cell antibodies in mixed connective tissue disease, *Immunol Lett*, 20, 163, 1989.

55. del Papa, N., Meroni, P. L., Barcellini, W., Sinico, A., Radice, A., Tincani, A., D, D. C., Nicoletti, F., Borghi, M. O., Khamashta, M. A. et al., Antibodies to endothelial cells in primary vasculitides mediate *in vitro* endothelial cytotoxicity in the presence of normal peripheral blood mononuclear cells, *Clin Immunol Immunopathol*, 63, 267, 1992.

56. Ferraro, G., Meroni, P. L., Tincani, A., Sinico, A., Barcellini, W., Radice, A., Gregorini, G., Froldi, M., Borghi, M. O., Balestrieri, G., Anti-endothelial cell antibodies in patients with Wegener's granulomatosis and micropolyarteritis, *Clin Exp Immunol*, 79, 47, 1990.

57. George, J., Blank, M., Levy, Y., Meroni, P., Damianovich, M., Tincani, A., Shoenfeld, Y., Differential effects of anti-beta2-glycoprotein I antibodies on endothelial cells and on the manifestations of experimental antiphospholipid syndrome, *Circulation*, 97, 900, 1998.

58. Levy, Y., Gilburd, B., George, J., Del Papa, N., Mallone, R., Damianovich, M., Blank, M., Radice, A., Renaudineau, Y., Youinou, P., Wiik, A., Malavasi, F., Meroni, P. L., Shoenfeld, Y., Characterization of murine monoclonal anti-endothelial cell antibodies (AECA) produced by idiotypic manipulation with human AECA, *Int Immunol*, 10, 861, 1998.

59. Blank, M., Krause, I., Goldkorn, T., Praprotnik, S., Livne, A., Langevich, P., Kaganovsky, E., Morgenstern, S., Cohen, S., Barak, V., Eldor, A., Weksler, B., Shoenfeld, Y., Monoclonal anti-endothelial cell antibodies from Takayasu's arteritis activate endothelial cells from large vessels, *Arthritis Rheum*, (in press), 1999.

60. Carvalho, D., Savage, C. O., Black, C. M., Pearson, J. D., IgG antiendothelial cell autoantibodies from scleroderma patients induce leukocyte adhesion to human vascular endothelial cells *in vitro*. Induction of adhesion molecule expression and involvement of endothelium-derived cytokines, *J Clin Invest*, 97, 111, 1996.

61. Simantov, R., LaSala, J. M., Lo, S. K., Gharavi, A. E., Sammaritano, L. R., Salmon, J. E., Silverstein, R. L., Activation of cultured vascular endothelial cells by antiphospholipid antibodies, *J Clin Invest*, 96, 2211, 1995.

62. Del Papa, N., Guidali, L., Sironi, M., Shoenfeld, Y., Mantovani, A., Tincani, A., Balestrieri, G., Radice, A., Sinico, R. A., Meroni, P. L., Anti-endothelial cell IgG antibodies from patients with Wegener's granulomatosis bind to human endothelial cells *in vitro* and induce adhesion molecule expression and cytokine secretion, *Arthritis Rheum*, 39, 758, 1996.

63. Del Papa, N., Guidali, L., Sala, A., Buccellati, C., Khamashta, M. A., Ichikawa, K., Koike, T., Balestrieri, G., Tincani, A., Hughes, G. R., Meroni, P. L., Endothelial cells as target for antiphospholipid antibodies. Human polyclonal and monoclonal anti-beta 2-glycoprotein I antibodies react *in vitro* with endothelial cells through adherent beta 2-glycoprotein I and induce endothelial activation, *Arthritis Rheum*, 40, 551, 1997.

64. Damianovich, M., Gilburd, B., George, J., Del Papa, N., Afek, A., Goldberg, I., Kopolovic, Y., Roth, D., Barkai, G., Meroni, P. L., Shoenfeld, Y., Pathogenic role of anti-endothelial cell antibodies in vasculitis. An idiotypic experimental model, *J Immunol*, 156, 4946, 1996.

65. Ross, R., The pathogenesis of atherosclerosis: a perspective for the 1990s, *Nature*, 362, 801, 1993.

66. Witztum, J. L., The oxidation hypothesis of atherosclerosis, *Lancet.*, 344, 793, 1994.

67. Wick, G., Schett, G., Amberger, A., Kleindienst, R., Xu, Q., Is atherosclerosis an immunologically mediated disease?, *Immunol Today*, 16, 27, 1995.

68. Libby, P., Hansson, G. K., Involvement of the immune system in human atherogenesis: current knowledge and unanswered questions, *Lab Invest*, 64, 5, 1991.

69. George, J., Harats, D., Gilburd, B., Shoenfeld, Y., Emerging cross-regulatory roles of immunity and autoimmunity in atherosclerosis, *Immunol Res*, 15, 315, 1996.

70. Cook, P. J., Lip, G. Y., Infectious agents and atherosclerotic vascular disease, *Qjm*, 89, 727, 1996.

71. Jonsson, H., Nived, O., Sturfelt, G., Outcome in systemic lupus erythematosus: a prospective study of patients from a defined population, *Medicine (Baltimore)*, 68, 141, 1989.

72. Iuliano, L., Pratico, D., Ferro, D., Pittoni, V., Valesini, G., Lawson, J., FitzGerald, G. A., Violi, F., Enhanced lipid peroxidation in patients positive for antiphospholipid antibodies, *Blood*, 90, 3931, 1997.

73. Shoenfeld, Y., Harats, D., George, J., Atherosclerosis and the antiphospholipid syndrome: a link unravelled?, *Lupus*, 7 Suppl 2, S140, 1998.

74. George, J., Afek, A., Gilburd, B., Blank, M., Levy, Y., Aron-Maor, A., Levkovitz, H., Shaish, A., Goldberg, I., Kopolovic, J., Harats, D., Shoenfeld, Y., Induction of early atherosclerosis in LDL-receptor-deficient mice immunized with beta2-glycoprotein I, *Circulation*, 98, 1108, 1998.

75. Afek, A., George, J., Shoenfeld, Y., Gilburd, B., Levy, Y., Shaish, A., Keren, P., Janackovic, Z., Goldberg, I., Kopolovic, J., Harats, D., Enhancement of atherosclerosis in beta-2-glycoprotein I-immunized apolipoprotein E-deficient mice, *Pathobiology*, 67, 19, 1999.

15 Hormones and Vascular Disease

Joan T. Merrill and Robert G. Lahita

CONTENTS

I. INTRODUCTION

The complexity of hormone effects on the vasculature illustrates the dynamic nature of this transportation organ. Like the international highway system, the bloodstream seems to require continuous repair, reorganization, and remodeling. Much is left to learn about signaling mechanisms which maintain the equilibrium of the vascular network, and there is only rudimentary evidence in support of a logical chain of command. It remains unclear how competing instructions that seem to bombard arteries and veins from a myriad of hormones are prioritized, or how net decisions on vascular tone or smooth muscle proliferation are made. The law of parsimony would suggest a simple summation and subtraction of positive and negative signals acting at a final common pathway. Certainly, at individual decision points, such as activation of gene transcription or a cell surface receptor, signal summation must be operative. However, in the overall regulation of blood vessels it is apparent that this simplest form of hierarchy cannot exist. A multiplicity of nonoverlapping signals can activate different but sometimes overlapping panels of cell surface receptors, or induce the transcription of alternative proteins performing the same or opposing functions.[1-7]

On the other hand, two observations support the hypothesis that there is an underlying homeostatic buffering system that can sort and accommodate conflicting instructions to the vasculature from wide-ranging hormonal and/or pro-inflammatory inputs. First, despite the redundancy of cell signaling pathways, there are well-established cross-modulating interfaces between major networks within the cell.[2,7-10] Secondly, although hormonal imbalances produced by menopause or chronic inflammation seem to inevitably lead to vascular disease, the ability of the vasculature to maintain relative homeostasis for many years following the loss of critical mediators suggests that there is a sophisticated infrastructure connecting the signaling pathways, which, when stressed, has the ability to compensate.

This chapter will suggest examples of the complexity in signaling mechanisms triggered by a wide range of hormones in regulating the vasculature and each other. We will then focus more on the central role of sex hormones in vascular health and disease, and review some ways in which the effects of inflammatory diseases on vascular health may in fact be related to hormone function.

II. HORMONES EXERT SIGNIFICANT INFLUENCE

Vascular integrity is maintained by the combined input of many hormones arising from different regions of the body as a result of various stimuli. Some examples (but by no means a complete list) include:

A. HORMONES FROM THE BRAIN

Human vascular endothelial cells have recently been found to directly express oxytocin receptors. These vascular receptors for a pituitary hormone mediate a vasodilatory effect which involves mobilization of intracellular calcium and release of nitric oxide.[11] In addition, oxytocin induces a calcium and protein kinase C-dependent cell proliferation response in endothelial cells.[11] Vasopressin also acts on human vascular smooth muscle cells[12] and may influence the permeability and growth of vascular endothelium.[12] Corticotropin-releasing hormone and urocortin, a related hormone, stimulate the same receptors, causing increased vascular permeability, possibly through histamine-mediated effects.[13] In addition, brain natriuretic peptide may influence arterial tone in a manner similar to nitroglycerin.[14] Vasodilation induced by this hormone may be partially mediated by either nitric oxide or prostaglandin release.[14]

B. HORMONES FROM THE GONADS

Sex steroids exert a myriad of effects at the genomic level, regulating circulating levels of coagulation proteins and plasma lipids and other vascular regulatory molecules.[15,16] Estrogens induce favorable changes in lipids and lipoproteins, increasing HDL-cholesterol and decreasing both LDL-cholesterol and lipoprotein (a).[16] Estrogens may have an antioxidant effect, inhibiting peroxidation of vascular smooth muscle membrane phospholipids, thereby inhibiting peroxidation-induced cell growth and migration.[16,17] Estrogen enhances blood vessel dilation,[15,16] which may involve multiple mechanisms of action. Human chorinonic gonadotrophin opposes this action of estrogen, decreasing both contractile and endothelium-dependent relaxation responses by a mechanism that involves inhibition of extracellular calcium ion influx.[18] In addition, estrogens mediate the expression of endothelial cell adhesion molecules, plasminogen activator inhibitor type 1[15] serum fibrinogen, factor VII, and plasminogen activator inhibitor-1 (PAI-1).[15,16,19] Moreover, estrogens maintain endothelial cell integrity, decrease insulin resistance, have calcium antagonist activities, inhibit adrenergic responses, and downregulate platelet and monocyte reactivity.[16] Estrogen may also modulate the renin-angiotensin system, relaxin, serotonin, and homocysteine.[16]

C. HORMONES SECRETED BY VASCULAR CELLS

Basic fibroblast growth factor (bFGF), epidermal growth factor (EGF), and vascular endothelial growth factor (VEGF) may play important roles in the maintenance of blood vessel functions, not only by controlling cell growth and differentiation, but also by mediating production of local vasodilators such as nitric oxide.[12,20] Actions of these hormones may be carried out through the MAP Kinase signaling cascade,[20] at least in a bovine model. Vascular endothelial growth factor may be a secondary mediator of both vasopressin[12] and human chorionic gonadotropin[21] effects on the vascular system. PTH-related protein is produced in vascular smooth muscle, where it is thought to have vasorelaxant properties[22,23] and may play a role in the normal development of the cardiovascular system.[22]

III. HOMEOSTATIC MECHANISMS

As suggested earlier, signal summation would be the simplest form of signal-sorting hierarchy, but the existence of cross-talk between major, multifunctional signaling pathways introduces a higher level of complexity to homeostasis. Activation of two opposing pathways at once in a cell can result in dampening or even abrogation of one or both, depending on their relative intensities. This is illustrated by the interface of protein kinase C and protein kinase A pathways which are often used by conflicting external stimuli and have been found to exhibit this sort of cross-modulating effect.[2,8,9] Just as signaling cascades may interact in an intricate intracellular network in the laying down of memory in the brain,[24] a similar complexity may regulate the net contribution of each kinase to information processing in regulation of the vasculature. Indeed, this is a widespread phenomenon in biologic systems, where positive signals may induce thier own negative feedback regulation.[8] It has been demonstrated in the regulation of nitric oxide-related pathways[10] which mediate estrogen-induced vasodilatory responses, and is likely to operate, by inference, in various vascular-control systems that use the same signaling cascades.[3-6]

IV. HORMONES AND OTHER VASCULAR MEDIATORS CAN COUNTERREGULATE EACH OTHER

Estrogen reduces angiotensin-converting enzyme and angiotensin II.[25] Cross-modulation of vascular cell growth may also be organized within hormone families. Angiotensin 1 is implicated in the pathogenesis of hypertension and atherosclerosis by its effects on blood pressure, fluid homeostasis, and vascular cell growth.[26] However, a metabolite of Angiotensin I, Ang-(l-7), has contradictory effects. This hormone has been found to stimulate the synthesis and release of vasodilator prostaglandins, augment the hypotensive actions of bradykinin, and increase the release of nitric oxide.[27] A similar dichotomy of effects has been described for the tissue factor pathway inhibitors (TFPI). TFPI-1 exhibits antiproliferative actions after vascular smooth muscle injury, whereas TFPI-2 is mitogenic for smooth muscle cells.[28] Single hormones may also have dual effects exerted concomitantly. Estrogen raises HDL cholesterol and lowers lipoprotein(a), which may in turn affect endothelium-dependent vasomotor responsiveness.[15] A single hormone may also have contradictory actions depending on the dose. Estradiol has a biphasic effect on vascular permeability.[29] In *in vitro* studies of cultured human umbilical vein endothelial cells, nanomolar concentrations of estradiol decreased permeability and micromolar concentrations increased permeability.[29] These effects appear to be mediated by dual signaling mechanisms related to endothelial nitric oxide syntheses.[29] In addition, differences in local vasculature responses may influence the effects of a hormone. For example, vasopressin has been found to induce opposite changes in blood flow in the skin and in the muscular circulation.[30]

The homeostasis of vascular growth, tone, and permeability is influenced by differential input mediated by many hormones arising from different regions of the body, possibly in response to different problems. There is evidence for a homeostatic buffering system by alternative signals generated within families of hormones, some metabolites of the others, acting at alternative cellular receptors. Finally, a single hormone may have biphasic, dose-related effects that lead to alternative outcomes in signaling to the cells. Within the cells, the activation of alternative signaling pathways by different hormones may not be entirely parallel events: cross-modulation between conflicting signals to cells may induce equal signals to dampen each other, or a stronger signal to eliminate a weaker one. This concept has been well demonstrated at the level of intracellular signaling cascades.[2,7-10,31]

The interrelationship among inflammatory mediators, hormones, and the vasculature cannot be overstressed. Although it is beyond the scope of this chapter to review all three-way interactions involved, some examples of the entangled vascular-hormonal-inflammatory axis are in order. For instance, several hormones enhance production of nitric oxide, which, along with being a vasodilator, is a potent proinflammatory mediator. In addition, nitric oxide signals back to modulate further endocrine secretion.[32] Corticotropin-releasing hormone and urocortin from the brain, which affect vascular permeability, have additional proinflammatory actions such as activation of mast cells.[13] The signaling pathways activated by vasculature-modulating hormones are not distinct from those induced by inflammatory mediators.[6,7] Clearly, then, the established connections between hormones and autoimmunity, between hormones and vascular regulation, and between inflammation and vascular diseases are no coincidence.

V. SEX STEROIDS AND THE VASCULATURE

Endothelial cells of both arteries and veins express estrogen receptors.[33-35] The evolutionary conservation of these receptors in different species suggests a common (and therefore critical) mechanism for estrogen regulation of endothelial function.[33,35] Steroid effects on blood vessels had been thought to depend on delayed, genomic mechanisms, but it is now apparent that there are both genomic and immediate effects of steroids acting directly on the vascular wall.[36]

The relationship between female hormones and the vasculature derives logically from the nature of the reproductive cycle. Endometrial proliferation, secretion, angiogenesis, and shedding is modulated by steroid hormones.[37] Global effects of estrogen and progesterone on vascular tone throughout the body may have arisen from the requirements of reproduction. For example, uterine artery blood flow on the side of a developing ovarian follicle has been found to increase during the menstrual cycle with no significant change in the contralateral vessel, correlating with changes in local serum estradiol and progesterone concentrations. Maximum blood flow during the midluteal phase is consistent with a preparation for optimal vascularity during implantation of the blastocyst.[38]

A. INFLAMMATORY MEDIATORS OF SEX STEROID VASCULAR EFFECTS

As the menstrual cycle progresses, sequential modification of the endometrial architecture is brought about by signaling changes that regulate its growth and differentiation, and requires coordination between the steroid hormones and vascular-based elements that are central to immune defense and inflammation, such as HLA-DR and adhesion molecules.[37] Menstruation is a process that involves an orchestrated destruction of epithelium, endothelium, and vascular matrix, leading to controlled bleeding, tissue extrusion, and subsequent repair.[37] Endometrial proteinases and coagulation proteins such as tissue factor (TF) are known to contribute to this process.[37] Vascular and cellular differentiation of the endometrial stroma may have evolved by adaptation of the inflammatory (granulation tissue) reaction.[39]

The cyclic inflammation required for induction of menstruation and/or invasion and implantation of the uterine wall by an embryo requires counteraction in order to protect a pregnancy from immune attack. This sets a precedent and requirement for regulation and counterregulation of a vascular-based inflammatory response by hormones. As an example of counterregulation, progesterone is thought to be important in suppressing the inflammatory reaction that would be expected in response to the presence of a foreign body, such as an embryo. Populations of macrophages and neutrophils in the uterus are under the control of estrogen and progesterone, and progesterone can antagonize the ability of estrogen to recruit macrophages and neutrophils into the mouse uterus.[40] Progesterone may also suppress IL-8 and COX-2 expression,[41] suggesting a model in which progesterone withdrawal at the time of menstruation promotes these inflammatory mediators in preparation for the increased tissue inflammation that accompanies the extrusion process. An intrinsic connection between hormone and inflammatory regulatory pathways is also suggested by the increased concentrations of activated pelvic macrophages and lymphocytes, and the elevated levels of specific cytokines and growth factors which accompany pathologic states such as endometriosis.[42] Progesterone and Danazol have been reported to inhibit spontaneous or cytokine-induced IL-6 secretion by endometriotic cells.[43]

B. COMPLEX EFFECTS OF SEX HORMONES ON INFLAMMATION

Estrogen replacement in postmenopausal women has been associated with higher C-reactive protein levels[44,45] and decreases of endothelin-1, plasminogen activator inhibitor-1, soluble thrombomodulin, von Willebrand factor, alpha-1 acid glycoprotein, and clottable fibrinogen, as well as a minor decrease in soluble E-selectin levels.[15,45,46] In addition, estrogen lowers inflammatory adhesion molecules including ICAMs, and VCAMs.[47,48] In one experimental rodent model, down-modulation of E-selectin and IL-6 gene expressions in endothelial cells by estrogen reduced cellular infiltration in acute anterior uveitis.[49] 17β-estradiol and a receptor-selective analogue LY117018 inhibit endothelial vascular cell adhesion molecule (VCAM)-1 expression at the mRNA level, and may inhibit endothelial adhesiveness towards monocytoid cells induced by LPS stimulation.[19]

On the basis of this growing literature, it has been suggested that a complex network of endometrial cytokines is normally regulated by hormones produced during the ovulatory cycle.[42] However, communication is a two-way street and, in return, inflammatory mediators also have impact on hormones. For example, LPS induces a lengthening of the follicular phase in monkeys that is associated with decreased estradiol concentrations and increased LH and FSH.[50]

Intrinsic to reproduction and the preservation of the species, then, are relationships between hormones and vasculature, inflammatory mediators and vasculature, and hormones and inflammatory mediators which set the stage for a significant hormonal impact on the vascular diseases of autoimmunity.

C. ESTROGEN AND ATHEROSCLEROSIS

Epidemiological observations, clinical studies, and basic laboratory research suggest that estrogen replacement therapy is associated with beneficial cardiovascular effects in postmenopausal women.[51-54] Estrogen has a multitude of biological effects *in vitro* that may account for this apparent benefit, most of which remain to be proven in randomized clinical trials. These include favorable effects on the lipid profile, direct effects on vascular endothelium, and improved fibrinolysis.[51-53] Estrogens have been shown to have both indirect and direct effects on the vasculature, which may improve arterial function and reduce or reverse atheroma formation. Indirect metabolic effects include changes in lipids, lipoproteins, glucose and insulin metabolism, coagulation, and fibrinolysis. Direct arterial effects include regulation of endothelium-dependent processes, ion channels, the renin-angiotensin system, and vascular remodeling processes.

Review of the literature on effects of menopause provides clinical evidence in support of the following changes which can be attributed to the lack of estrogen: increased total cholesterol and triglycerides; decreased high density lipoprotein (HDL) and HDL subfraction 2; increased low density lipoprotein, particularly in the small, dense subfraction; increased lipoprotein (a); increased insulin resistance; decreased insulin secretion; decreased insulin elimination; increased android fat distribution; impaired vascular function; increased factor VII and fibrinogen; and reduced sex-hormone-binding globulin.[55] Many of these changes are ameliorated by estrogen replacement.

Most clinical evidence, however, is derived from observational studies which suffer from important limitations of bias. The only published controlled, prospective trial of hormone replacement effects on cardiovascular outcomes, the Heart Estrogen-Progestin Replacement Study (HERS), had a negative result, showing no net benefit of estrogen plus progestin treatment over a four-year period in women who already had established coronary disease.[56] In addition, there appeared to be increased risk for cornonary thrombotic events limited to the first year of treatment in this higher risk group of women.[56] This does not suggest lack of cardioprotective benefits overall for estrogen or ineffectiveness of estrogen replacement therapy in general so much as it illustrates the complexities in acute and chronic effects of estrogen, and strongly suggests that current hormone replacement strategies may involve both patient selection and timing issues. In fact, there are two timing issues: (1) The increased risk of estrogen-induced thrombotic risk may outweigh its protective effects on atherosclerosis in women with established plaque, at least for the first years before longer-term cardioprotective effects can begin to kick in and have major impact on vascular equilibrium, (2) given the biphasic nature of many of estrogen's effects there may also be pharmacokinetic issues with the dosing and timing of estrogen therapy which are as yet poorly understood.

Pre-menopausal protection from cardiovascular disease occurs in the context of cycling the sex steroid hormones. The impact of cycling on the net protective mechanisms along with the optimal cardioprotective dosing of estrogen replacement remain to be determined. Unfortunately, it will not be possible for clinical trials to address these issues without established, clinically validated surrogate laboratory markers for both thrombotic and cardiovascular risk. A number of candidate markers for estrogen effects on the vasculature have been identified, but their clinical validity is not proven. That there is not one regimen of hormones that would suit all women should be intuitively obvious from the fact that dosage adjustments are frequently needed to ameliorate side effects such as breast enlargement and tenderness, or to increase therapeutic effects such as hot flashes. The same issues are likely to apply in optimization of cardioprotective factors and minimization of thrombotic risk, but such considerations are rarely discussed in the literature.

Fundamental mechanistic studies which compare the cellular and molecular events by which hormones affect diseased as opposed to healthy blood vessels will also be needed to define the role of postmenopausal hormone replacement therapy in primary vs. secondary cardiovascular disease prevention, and to better interpret the outcome of the HERS trial. For example, most studies suggest that estrogen inhibits the neointimal response to acute injury in normal blood vessels, but this vasoprotective effect was not seen in vessels with preexisting atherosclerosis.[54] On the other hand, one placebo-controlled study has suggested that short-term administration of 17beta-estradiol is effective in improving effort-induced myocardial ischemia in female patients with coronary artery disease.[57] Finally, acute administration of conjugated equine estrogens prior to induction of ischemia in dogs attenuated ventricular arrhythmias of ischemia as well as those of reperfusion.[58]

D. SPECIFIC EFFECTS OF ESTROGEN ON THE VASCULATURE

1. Estrogen Effects on Vascular Construction and Maintenance

Studies in the rat carotid injury model have shown that estrogen inhibits neointima formation with effects on all three layers of the vascular wall, including inhibition of medial smooth muscle cell growth and migration, stimulation of regrowth of endothelium, and inhibition of adventitial cell migration into neointima.[54,59-62] Vascular smooth muscle cells are present in early atherosclerosis and become the dominant cell type in progressive plaque. In sexually mature female pigs, significant inhibition of coronary vascular smooth muscle cell proliferation was found with physiologic concentrations of beta-estradiol.[63] Myointimal hyperplasia in allografts from E2-treated-rat aortic transplant recipients was 3- to 4-fold less than that from the placebo-treated recipients.[64] The effects of estradiol on vascular smooth muscle cells depends on their phenotype. Estradiol delays the cell cycle reentry of the contractile smooth muscle cells, but once cells have differentiated to the synthetic phenotype it promotes their replication.[65]

The pathways by which estrogen exerts its effects on vascular reconstruction may be complex. Estrogen may have an indirect, antioxidant effect, inhibiting peroxidation of vascular smooth muscle membrane phospholipids, thereby inhibiting peroxidation-induced cell growth and migration.[17] There is also some suggestion that estrogen may inhibit the influence of TGF-beta1 on vascular smooth muscle cell growth.[62] However, vascular smooth muscle cells also have estrogen receptors and may have direct responses to estrogen. On the other hand, estradiol did not alter proliferation in porcine coronary vascular smooth muscle cells obtained from sexually mature male or oophorectomized female animals.[63] This animal model demonstrates the possibility that there may be specific gender-related differences in cell proliferation in response to estrogen.

Vascular endothelial growth factor is an endothelial-specific mitogen with potent angiogenic activity. 17β-estradiol and tamoxifen may modulate vascular endothelial growth factor transcription.[66] Levels of this mitogen vary throughout the menstrual cycle and are elevated in women with endometriosis.[66] Another mitogen for vascular smooth muscle cells is endothelin-1. There is some evidence that reduced endothelin-1 production by endothelial cells may be involved in the vasoprotective effect of estrogen.[67,68] Some experiments suggest that 17β-estradiol enhances release of basic fibroblast growth factor by human coronary artery endothelial cells.[69] However, 17β-estradiol, its metabolites, and progesterone have been found to inhibit cardiac fibroblast growth *in vitro*.[59]

2. Estrogen and Lipoproteins

Estrogen replacement therapy is known to raise HDL cholesterol, lower lipoprotein (a), and reduce LDL.[15]

3. Estrogen and Vasoconstriction/Vasodilation

It has been understood for many years that sex hormones modulate vasodilator responses of arteries supplying the uterus with blood. Recently it has been shown that sex hormones such as estrogen modulate vasomotor responses of other arteries, including coronary arteries.[70] Estrogen causes favorable changes in vascular tone, decreasing mean arterial pressure and systemic vascular resistance, while increasing heart rate and cardiac output.[71-78] Administration of HRT prospectively in 68 women was associated with an increase in blood flow in the peripheral arteries, which was related directly to serum E2 levels.[79] There appears to be an ongoing maintenance effect by estrogen on subduing vascular reactivity, indicated by the finding that resistance to blood flow in cerebral vessels of postmenopausal women rapidly changes after the suspension of hormone replacement therapy.[80] Effects of estrogen on vasoconstriction may be ubiquitous. One study has suggested that uterine artery blood velocity increases on the side of a developing ovarian follicle during the progression of a menstrual cycle with no significant change in the contralateral vessel.[38] These changes correlated with changes in serum estradiol and progesterone concentrations. 17β-estradiol also has direct and indirect coronary vascular smooth muscle relaxing properties.[57]

Low-dose estradiol may protect against vasospasm by stimulating endothelium-derived nitric oxide release and inhibiting coronary artery contractility through activation of calcium channels in arterial smooth muscle cells.[81-85] At higher, pharmacologic concentrations, estradiol causes vasodilation principally by endothelium-independent mechanisms in a gender-independent fashion,[82] which may involve a number of pathways such as ATP-dependent K+ channels.[82,83,86] *In vitro* studies using human arteries have deomonstrated that 17β-estradiol significantly reduces contractile effects induced by histamine, serotonin, and angiotensin II.[87,88] Estrogen has been found to downregulate angiotensin I receptor expression.[26] Estrogen replacement therapy reduces angiotensin-converting enzyme mRNA and activity, with an associated reduction in plasma angiotensin II, a decrease in the metabolism of the vasodilator bradykinin, and an increase in the production of vasorelaxant angiotensin.[25]

Endothelin-1 is a potent vasoconstrictor as well as a mitogen for vascular smooth muscle cells. Low doses of estrogen have been found to inhibit thrombin-induced endothelin-1 release.[89] Estrogen replacement therapy results in an increased ratio of nitric oxide to endothelin-1,[67] and a growing literature now attributes a significant proportion of the vasodilatory effects of estrogen in both humans and animal models to nitric oxide-dependent mechanisms.[32,90-102]

Gender differences in the incidence of stroke and migraine may be related to circulating levels of estrogen. Myogenic tone of rat cerebral arteries differs between males and females. This difference appears to result from estrogen enhancement of endothelial nitric oxide (NO) production.[97] Experimental evidence in ewes suggests that during the follicular phase of a normal menstrual cycle, an increased local estrogen-to-progesterone ratio during the follicular phase locally elevates nitric oxide production in uterine but not systemic vasculature[99] which could increase uterine blood flow. These responses can be partly reproduced with estrogen administration. Coronary flow rates of ovariectomized female rabbits were 40 to 50% greater in animals treated with estradiol than in control animals,[98] and these changes were reversed by an inhibitor of nitric oxide synthase.[98] The estrogen-stimulated nitric oxide pathway is subject to complex regulation by several major signaling pathways, which illustrates the effects of multiple inputs on hormonal regulation of the vasculature.[10]

E. ESTRADIOL MAY HAVE A BIPHASIC EFFECT ON VASCULAR STATES

Estrogens increase the cation selectivity across endothelial cell cultures.[103] These effects may be important for protection of blood vessels when there are sudden changes in ion levels across the wall, such as during ischemia or reperfusion. *In vitro* studies of cultured human umbilical vein endothelial cells suggest that at nanomolar concentrations estradiol decreases permeability, but at micromolar concentrations it increases permeability.[29] These effects appear to be mediated by dual signaling mechanisms related to a constitutive endothelial nitric oxide synthase (decrease in permeability) and an inducible nitric oxide synthase (increase in permeability).[29]

Vascular remodeling occurs during all stages of atherosclerotic progression. Antiatherosclerotic drugs may function by restoring regulation of the processes involved in remodeling of the extracellular matrix. An important group of enzymes involved in these processes are the matrix metalloproteinases (MMPs). Estrogens have been demonstrated to possess antiatherosclerotic properties at low concentrations while being associated with plaque formation at high concentrations. 17β-estradiol appears to be a specific stimulator of MMP-2 release from human vascular cells.[104] The concentration dependence of this effect has been suggested as a basis for the differential effects of low and high estrogen levels on vascular integrity.

It has been suggested that reendothelialization of damaged blood vessels protects against the vascular injury response. Estrogen protects against neointimal injury in the balloon-injured rat, in part by facilitating the reendothelialization of the damaged vessel,[105] but this, too, may involve a biphasic effect. Endothelin-1 may play a role in reendothelialization as a mitogen for vascular smooth muscle cells. Low doses of estrogen can inhibit thrombin-induced endothelin-1 release while higher estrogen levels do not.[89]

As mentioned previously, estrogen replacement causes a net decrease in vascular adhesion molecule expression, whereas *in vitro* studies have suggested that 17β-estradiol can augment expression of adhesion molecules.[106] If a biphasic response to estradiol exists, this might explain the promotion of granulocyte adhesion to endothelium that characterizes autoimmune states with a predominance in women, such as leukocytoclastic vasculitis.[106]

The potential for dose- and kinetic-induced differences in the effects of estrogen on the vasculature derive logically from the cyclic roles of estrogen in the circulation, and the cyclic nature of estrogen concentrations in healthy premenopausal women. This may help to explain the confusing results of the HERS trial, and strongly suggests the need for pharmacokinetic analysis to optimize estrogen replacement strategies. An additional consideration will be to more fully evaluate the vascular effects of different delivery systems for estrogen replacement. It is clear that non-oral estrogen therapies fail to invoke the hepatic response associated with oral therapy.[107] Since changes in hepatic protein synthesis are minimized, plasma levels of binding globulins and other proteins tend to be normal.[107] Many of the perturbations of the hemostatic system seen with oral therapy are avoided, but without the stimulation of hepatic synthesis of apolipoproteins, plasma lipoprotein levels are found to be unchanged or reduced. Decreased fasting levels of triglycerides might be considered desirable, but the cardioprotective increase in levels of high-density lipoproteins is absent.[107] Direct effects of estrogens on the vascular receptors are preserved, leading to improved vascular function. Given these combined, theoretical advantages and disadvantages, the net effect of non-oral estrogen therapies on the risk of cardiovascular disease remains difficult to predict and introduces more variables into the question of post-menopausal hormone replacement.

F. PROGESTERONE AND THE VASCULATURE

1. Progesterone Effects on Vascular Construction and Maintenance

Functional nuclear progesterone receptors have been identified in endothelial cells and demonstrated to inhibit endothelial proliferation.[108] This involved reduction in cyclin-dependent kinase activity. In addition, treatment of endothelial cells with progestins altered the expression of cyclin E and A in accordance with G1 arrest.[108] In addition, progesterone may inhibit arterial smooth muscle proliferation.[109]

2. Progesterone and Lipoproteins

Combining estrogen and progesterone treatment does not appear to reverse the beneficial effects of estrogen replacement on plasma lipoproteins,[110,111] including increases in HDL-cholesterol and increases in apo A-1 levels and LCAT activity.[111] On the other hand, one study suggested that hormone replacement therapy with lower (2.5-mg) doses of progesterone had a better effect on lipid profiles than a higher (5 mg) dose after 12 months of treatment.[110] It has further been suggested that progesterones do not counteract the beneficial effect of 17β-estradiol on LDL oxidation when used in hormone replacement therapy.[112] Progesterone has two possible cardioprotective effects on macrophages: it acutely inhibits cholesterol ester formation, and it prevents glucocorticoid-induced increases in acyl-CoA-cholesterol-acyl transferase gene expression.[113]

3. Progesterone and Vasoconstriction/Vasodilation

In addition to 17β-E2, progesterone and other progestins can reduce vascular tone,[114,115] probably due to blockade of voltage-dependent and/or receptor-operated calcium channels.[114] Estrogen and progesterone replacement have been found to decrease coronary artery reactivity in rheusus monkeys through direct interactions with estrogen and progesterone receptors in coronary artery vascular smooth muscle cells.[116] On the other hand, long-term combined oral hormone replacement therapy with both estrogen and progesterone was found to be without beneficial effects on endothelial vasomotor function in healthy postmenopausal women[117] and in an ovariectomized rabbit model,[98] supporting the view that progesterone at pharmacologic doses may attenuate some of the beneficial effects of unopposed estrogen replacement.

In fact, progesterone may antagonize a number of benefical effects of estrogen on the vasculature, including the inhibition by estrogen of monocytoid cell adhesion,[118] estradiol mediated decreases in endothelial cell barrier properties, and adhesion molecules.[119,120]

G. ANDROGENS AND THE VASCULATURE

Male gender is an independent risk factor for coronary artery disease, and androgen administration has been associated with increased atherosclerosis in experimental animals.[121]

1. Androgen Effects on Vascular Construction and Maintenance

Dihydrotestosterone has been found to up-regulate vascular endothelial growth factor (VEGF) mRNA at a level comparable to that observed with growth factors,[122] and increases VEGF biological activity.[122] Conversely, *in vitro* and animal models suggest that androgen reduces vascular endothelial growth factor levels in normal and malignant prostatic tissue, and may therefore differentially regulate prostatic angiogenesis by this mechanism.[123,124]

Thromboxane A2 (TXA2) has been implicated as an important mediator of cardiovascular diseases. Aortas obtained from male rats or dogs are more sensitive to TXA2 mimetics compared with those obtained from testosterone, with significantly ($p < 0.05$) increased TXA2 receptor density in cultured rat aortic smooth muscle cells and guinea pig coronary artery smooth muscle cells, more so in males than in females.[125] Further studies in the rat indicate that smooth muscle cells possess an androgen receptor and that gender-related differences exist in the regulation of expression of thromboxane A2 receptors by androgens.[125]

The weak androgen dehydroepiandrosterone (DHEA) is known to have antiatherosclerotic properties.[126] DHEA has been found to inhibit endothelial cell proliferation *in vitro,* and may protect endothelial cells against LDL-induced cytotoxic effects.[126] DHEA and its sulfate metabolite DHEA-S are the most abundant steroids in humans, and their serum concentrations progressively decrease with age. DHEA-S may have protective or antiatherogenic effects of its own on vasculature, inhibiting smooth muscle cell proliferation and migration.[127] Although DHEA is an androgen in its own right, it is a natural precursor for both male and female hormones and, therefore, its net effect in men or women may be metabolism-dependent.

2. Androgens and Lipoproteins

Lipoprotein levels are adversely affected by androgens, increasing the risk of atherosclerotic disease. The increasing abuse of anabolic steroids and reports of cases of sudden death and myocardial infarction among bodybuilders are consistent with an increase in cardiovascular risk for this population. In one study, twelve competitive bodybuilders were recruited for a comprehensive study on the cardiovascular risks associated with the use of anabolic steroids.[128] The use of these androgens was associated with decreases in HDL cholesterol and apolipoprotein A-I levels. However, androgens were also associated with reduced LDL cholesterol and apolipoprotein B levels. Despite the significantly higher total and HDL cholesterol ratio, the low serum total cholesterol levels (within the fifth percentile) and low plasma triglyceride levels in members of the steroid group raise questions concerning the exact role of androgens in increasing the risk of cardiovascular disease. On the other hand, whether low serum cholesterol reflects appropriate elimination of cholesterol from the body or whether the cholesterol, in the absence of its transporter, HDL, is in actuality accumulating in the arterial walls also remains to be determined.

3. Androgens and Vasoconstriction/Vasodilation

Since endothelial dysfunction is an important event in the atherogenic process, it is of interest that androgen deprivation is associated with enhanced vascular reactivity in adult men.[121,129] In fact, short-term administration of testosterone induces a sex-independent vasodilation in coronary conductance and resistance arteries in canines *in vivo*.[130] Acute testosterone-induced coronary vasodilation of epicardial and resistance vessels is mediated in part by endothelium-derived NO. ATP-sensitive K+ channels appear to play a role in the vasodilatory effect of testosterone in resistance arteries.[130] Estradiol supplementation improves endothelium-dependent vasodilation in women, probably because of augmented NO production/release, but not in men.[131] Thus, there may be gender-specific differences in the effects of estrogen therapy on endothelial functions and NO production/release, with men more reliant on androgen mediation for these functions. At higher concentrations, however, both estradiol and testosterone can cause vasodilation, by endothelium-independent mechanisms, in a gender independent fashion,[82] suggesting that each could be considered a therapy in select clinical circumstances. In addition, the weaker androgen, DHEA, has been found to reverse induced-hypoxic pulmonary vasoconstriction in isolated ferret lungs, suggesting that it, too, might serve as a potential therapeutic modality.[132]

H. Sex Hormones, Immune Activation, and the Vascular System

Estrogen receptors have been identified in human monocytes, B-cells and T-cells, suggesting a direct role for estrogens in the regulation of immune cell activation.[133] It has been found that B-cell activities are augmented by estrogen whereas T-cell reactivity is suppressed,[134] an argument favoring the hypothesis that although estrogen has some potential to adversely affect autoimmunity, the net effects might be complex. In rats, endotoxin-induced expression of adhesion molecules associated with an influx of inflammatory cells varies with reproductive condition, increasing in pregnant but not in cyclic animals.[135] Similarly, in cultures of human umbilical cell endothelial cells, 17beta-estradiol augments TNF-alpha-induced expression of endothelial leukocyte adhesion molecule-1, intercellular adhesion molecule-1, and vascular cell adhesion molecule-1.[106] Estrogen stimulates transcription of basic fibroblast growth factor which acts at its receptor to activate signaling cascades that are regulators of inflammation.[136] Both estrogen and progesterone may have significant regulatory impact on one such critical inflammatory juncture, involving MAP Kinases.[136-138] Nitric oxide release in the vasculature is enhanced by estrogens, suggesting several pro-inflammatory actions of this hormone. 17β-estradiol enhances pokeweed mitogen-induced differentiation of mononuclear cells whereas testosterone inhibits this.[139]

Estrogen has been found to decrease inducible MHC class II antigen expression in the media of vascular allografts, accompanied by decreased macrophage infiltration.[64] In addition, 17β-estradiol, a major estrogen metabolite, may inhibit apoptosis in cultured endothelial cells,[140] and low doses of 17β-estradiol have been found to significantly inhibit basal IL-6 secretion by human umbilical vein endothelial cells.[141]

Inflammation, and inflammation-induced coagulation mechanisms are known to be predictors of cardiovascular events.[142-148] Because of this, there may be indirect effects of sex steroids on the overall metabolic equilibrium of the vasculature through immune-modulating effects. Such hormone-immune interactions have been thought to be partially accountable for the increased cardiovascular risk in patients with autoimmune diseases, however, the relationships may be unpredictable. For example, it has been found that estrogen can improve markers of fibrinolysis and vascular inflammation in arteries of postmenopausal women.[15] In addition, estrogen seems to have other antiinflammatory properties that may have beneficial impact on cardiovascular risk. Focal attachment of monocytes to endothelial cells is observed in early atherosclerotic lesions. Minimally oxidized low-density lipoprotein significantly increases the adhesion of monocytoid cells to endothelial layers, and estrogen may inhibit this interaction in a dose-dependent manner.[118] Atherosclerotic plaque demonstrates features similar to inflammation. Endothelial cell activation by inflammatory cytokines induces expression of cellular adhesion molecules, augmenting leukocyte adhesion and recruitment and the subsequent development of atherosclerosis. One study has observed a statistically significant increase in all cell adhesion molecules in men with coronary artery disease and postmenopausal women with heart disease not receiving estrogen replacement, as compared with postmenopausal women with heart disease receiving estrogen.[149] Although this contradicts other findings which suggest that estrogen can augment adhesion molecule activity,[106,135] these issues may resolve around the multiple signaling pathways and dose-responsiveness of estrogen therapies. Estrogen then, may either augment or help to limit the inflammatory response to injury by modulating the expression of endothelial adhesion molecules. Taken together, these findings suggest the possibility of at least some beneficial effects of hormone replacement therapy on atherosclerosis in the context of its beneficial effects on chronic, low-grade vascular inflammation. How this might translate into a dosing and timing schedule remains to be determined.

I. EFFECTS OF SEX-STEROID THERAPIES ON VASCULAR INFLAMMATION

Hormonal factors linked to age, gender, reproductive status, and sex hormone metabolism are undoubtedly involved in regulating the onset of autoimmune diseases.[150-153] For example, systemic lupus erythematosus, a disease characterized by immune complex-mediated pathology linked to excess Th2 cytokine production such as IL-10, primarily affects women in the reproductive years. Rheumatoid arthritis, a disease characterized by cell-mediated inflammation linked to enhanced Th1 and deficient Th2 cytokine production, is also more common in women, with a peak incidence at menopause. Changes in the production of estrogen and progesterone may play a major role in modulating Th1/Th2 cytokine balance.[153] Studies in murine autoimmune models suggest an increase in interleukin-1 (IL-1) and tumour necrosis factor-alpha (TNF-alpha) secretion in mice with experimental SLE and a reduction in IL-2, IL-4, and interferon-gamma (INF-gamma) levels as compared with the levels detected in healthy controls.[154] Treatment with physiological doses of estradiol can exert dichotomous effects on different manifestations of the lupus disease in these mice. In one study of MRL/l mice, immune complex-mediated glomerulonephritis was significantly accelerated by estrogen, accompanied by polyclonal B cell activation with increased production of circulating immune complexes and antibodies to double-stranded DNA.[134] In contrast, T-cell-mediated lesions such as focal sialadenitis, renal vasculitis, and periarticular inflammation were all significantly ameliorated in mice exposed to estrogen.[134] Thus, administration of estrogen can lead to differential outcomes of SLE morbidity.

Some justification for an estrogen-mediated model of autoimmunity in human disease is suggested by the finding that estrogen may cause a polychlonal increase in production of IgG, including IgG anti-dsDNA, in SLE patients' by enhancing B-cell activity, and by promoting IL-10 production in monocytes.[155] In the inflammatory processes associated with lupus nephritis, mesangial cells and invading immune cells cause the release of large amounts of nitric oxide in the glomerulus.[156] Vascular endothelial growth factor and its receptor tyrosine kinase may be regulated by nitric oxide, suggesting one mechanism by which estrogen might be additive to renal pathology in autoimmune renal disease.[156]

Calcineurin is a critical protein phosphatase involved in the regulation of interleukin 2 gene activation. One study[157] has found increased calcineurin mRNA expression and phosphatase activity in response to estradiol in cultured T-cells from lupus patients as compared to healthy and other autoimmune controls. These results suggest that estrogen-induced changes in lupus T-cell calcineurin signaling could alter proinflammatory cytokine gene regulation and T-B-cell interactions in a disease-specific manner. Interestingly, one report suggests that an estrogen receptor in nonreproductive organs may have antigenic similiarity to calcineurin.[158] As an integrated model, it has been speculated that calcineurin might be an estrogen receptor variant, preferentially upregulated in lupus T-cells, with some relationship to other signaling defects which have been identified in the T-cells of this population.[159]

The literature on Raynaud's phenomenon, which may occur as a primary disorder or as a manifestation of lupus, scleroderma, or other connective tissue diseases, describes a complex and confusing picture of abnormalities suggesting a multifactorial etiology. Current research suggests that the underlying disorder is related to a local fault at the level of the digital microcirculation.

Digital cutaneous neurones show a deficient release of the vasodilatory calcitonin gene-related peptide. Vasoconstricting substances such as catecholamines, endothelin-1, and 5-hydroxytrypt-amine, which may all be released in response to cold exposure, could cause digital artery closure and the associated symptoms of Raynaud's phenomenon. In some cases, this could trigger a cascade of neutrophil and platelet activation, which through the release of inflammatory mediators might contribute to the endothelial damage seen with more severe Raynaud's.[160] Both endothelium-dependent vasodilatation and endothelium-independent vasodilatation are impaired in patients with Raynaud's phenomenon secondary to systemic sclerosis, whereas intima-media thickness is increased. Short-term estrogen administration has been found to improve endothelial dysfunction in a small series of these patients.[161,162]

Effects of the menstrual cycle on heat loss, heat production, and core and skin temperature responses to cold are suggested by the finding that there is extensive peripheral vasoconstriction in the follicular phase of the cycle which elevates internal body temperature.[163] Furthermore, the temperature in the fingers can have a significant effect on the total control of body temperature during cold transients.[163] Other hormones which have been at least circumstantially implicated in the pathogenesis of Raynaud's include prolactin and DHEA-S, which have been found to correlate with disease severity in patients with systemic sclerosis.[164] These findings support the involvement of estrogen in the pathogenesis of SLE, however, the conclusion that estrogen replacement therapy is therefore ill-advised in patients with SLE may be premature given the well-established increased risk for atherosclerosis in these women.

The most definitive (in terms of size) prospective evaluation of estrogen-induced autoimmune risk suggested a statistically significant but clinically insignificant increase in risk for the development of lupus in a cohort of 69,435 postmenopausal women, followed for 14 years, with varying exposure to hormone replacement therapy.[165] Several retrospective studies suggest that HRT appears to be well tolerated and safe in postmenopausal patients with established SLE, at least those without renal disease. Therefore, the potential cardioprotective effects of estrogen may well outweigh any minor deleterious effect on disease activity in the general postmenopausal lupus patient.[166-169] On the other hand, lupus patients may have abnormal levels and/or metabolism of several sex steroids, suggesting a different reason for adverse hormone-mediated event. In a study of 23 SLE patients and 44 normal controls, increased 16 alpha-hydroxylation of estrogens was found in both males and females with SLE as compared to normal subjects.[152] Furthermore, decreased levels of androgens were observed in women with SLE, with the lowest levels in patients who had active disease.[151]

The immune system is directly affected by the relative metabolism of sex steroids. More estrogen metabolites of the C-16 variety can bind to lymphocytes.[150] Differential effects of sex steroids on immune responses may contribute significantly to a permissive environment that sets the stage for autoimmunity in women. These studies suggested that sex hormones may have a role in the treatment of some autoimmune disorders. Ongoing prospective clinical trials of dehydroepiandrosterone (Genelabs, Inc.) as therapy for systemic lupus and the NIH-funded SELENA trial evaluating the safety of estrogen replacement or oral contraceptive use in lupus arose from these considerations.

VI. CONCLUSIONS

Male gender is an independent risk factor for coronary artery disease, suggesting either a protective effect of estrogens and/or a deleterious effect of androgens on hemodynamics and vascular maintenance. Conversely, female hormones are thought to confer increased risk for the vascular inflammatory states which characterize many autoimmune diseases and may thereby contribute to the premature atherosclerosis seen in these susceptible women. Furthermore, there are many examples of differential, gender-specific effects of sex hormones on the vasculature, suggesting that gender-primed vascular receptors contribute an additional level of complexity to the effects of sex steroids.[63,170] Clearly, the net clinical effects of sex steroids and their gender-influenced vascular reception are complicated and not completely predictable at this time. This suggests that hormone-derived treatments aimed at reducing atherosclerotic risk and/or treating autoimmune diseases are possible, but will require more extensive pharmacokinetic analysis in order to be optimized for safety and efficacy.

REFERENCES

1. Green KM; Kim JH; Wang WH; Day BN; and Prather RS; Effect of myosin light chain kinase, protein kinase A, and protein kinase C inhibition on porcine oocyte activation. *Biol Reprod* 1999; 61(1):111–119.

2. Edgar VA; Sterin-Borda L; Cremaschi GA; and Genaro AM; Role of protein kinase C and cAMP in fluoxetine effects on human T-cell proliferation. *Eur J Pharmacol* 1999; 372(1):65–73.

3. Shih SC; Mullen A; Abrams K; Mukhopadhyay D; and Claffey KP; Role of protein kinase C isoforms in phorbol ester-induced vascular endothelial growth factor expression in human glioblastoma cells. *J Biol Chem* 1999; 274(22):15407–14.

4. Hata Y; Rook SL; and Aiello LP; Basic fibroblast growth factor induces expression of VEGF receptor KDR through a protein kinase C and p44/p42 mitogen-activated protein kinase- dependent pathway. *Diabetes* 1999; 48(5):1145–55.

5. Pfister MF; Forgo J; Ziegler U; and Biber J; Murer, cAMP-dependent and -independent downregulation of type II Na-Pi cotransporters by PTH. *Am J Physiol* 1999; 720–5.

6. Kelly MJ; Lagrange AH; and Wagner EJ; Ronnekleiv Rapid effects of estrogen to modulate G protein-coupled receptors via activation of protein kinase A and protein kinase C pathways. *Steroids* 1999; 64(1–2):64–75.

7. Atta-ur-Rahman; Harvey K; and Siddiqui RA; Interleukin-8: An autocrine inflammatory mediator. *Curr Pharm Des* 1999; 5(4):241–53.

8. Nishizuka Y; Studies and perspectives of protein kinase C. *Science* 1986; 233(4761):305–12.

9. Schopf S and Bringmann A; Reichenbach A; Protein kinases A and C are opponents in modulating glial Ca2+ — activated K+ channels. *Neuroreport* 1999; 10(6):1323–7.

10. Jun CD; Pae HO; Kwak HJ; Yoo JC; Choi BM; Oh CD; Chun JS; Paik SG; Park YH; and Chung HT; Modulation of nitric oxide-induced apoptotic death of HL-60 cells by protein kinase C and protein kinase A through mitogen-activated protein kinases and CPP32-like protease pathways. *Cell Immunol* 1999; 194(1):36–46.

11. Thibonnier M; Conarty DM; Preston JA; Plesnicher CL; Dweik RA; and Erzurum SC; Human vascular endothelial cells express oxytocin receptors. *Endocrinology* 1999; 140(3):1301–9.

12. Tahara A; Saito M; Tsukada J; Ishii N; Tomura Y; Wada K; Kusayama T; Yatsu T; Uchida W; and Tanaka A; Vasopressin increases vascular endothelial growth factor secretion from human vascular smooth muscle cells. *Eur J Pharmacol* 1999; 368(1):89–94.

13. Singh LK; Boucher W; Pang X; Letourneau R; Seretakis D; Green M; and Theoharides TC; Potent mast cell degranulation and vascular permeability triggered by urocortin through activation of corti-cotropin-releasing hormone receptors. *J Pharmacol Exp Ther* 1999; 288(3):1349–56.

14. Zellner C; Protter AA; Ko E; Pothireddy MR; DeMarco T; Hutchison SJ; Chou TM; Chatterjee K; and Sudhir K; Coronary vasodilator effects of BNP: mechanisms of action in coronary conductance and resistance arteries. *Am J Physiol* 1999; 276(3 Pt 2):H1049–57.

15. Koh KK; Cardillo C; Bui MN; Hathaway L; Csako G; Waclawiw MA; Panza JA; and Cannon RO; 3rd Vascular effects of estrogen and cholesterol-lowering therapies in hypercholesterolemic postmeno-pausal women. Circulation 1999; Jan 26;99(3):354–60.

16. Nasr A and Breckwoldt M; Estrogen replacement therapy and cardiovascular protection: lipid mech-anisms are the tip of an iceberg. *Gynecol Endocrinol* 1998; Feb;12(1):43–59.

17. Dubey RK; Tyurina YY; Tyurin VA; Gillespie DG; Branch RA; Jackson EK; and Kagan VE; Estrogen and tamoxifen metabolites protect smooth muscle cell membrane phospholipids against peroxidation and inhibit cell growth. *Circ Res* 1999; 84:229–39.

18. Ezimokhai M; The alterations of vascular smooth muscle reactivity *in vitro* by human chorionic gonadotrophin. *Res Exp Med (Berl)* 1998; Dec;198(4):187–98.

19. Simoncini T; De Caterina R; and Genazzani AR; Selective estrogen receptor modulators: different actions on vascular cell adhesion molecule-1 (VCAM-1) expression in human endothelial cells. Department of Reproductive Medicine and Child Development, University of Pisa, Italy. *J Clin Endocrinol Metab* 1999; Feb;84(2):815–8.

20. Zheng J; Bird IM; Melsaether AN; and Magness RR; Activation of the mitogen-activated protein kinase cascade is necessary but not sufficient for basic fibroblast growth factor- and epidermal growth factor-stimulated expression of endothelial nitric oxide synthase in ovine fetoplacental artery endothelial cells. *Endocrinology* 1999; Mar;140(3):1399–407.

21. Chiocchio SR; Suburo AM; Vladucic E; Zhu BC; Charreau E; Decima EE; and Tramezzani JH; Differential effects of superior and inferior spermatic nerves on testosterone secretion and spermatic blood flow in cats. *Endocrinology* 1999; Mar;140(3):1036–43.

22. Qian J; Lorenz JN; Maeda S; Sutliff RL; Weber C; Nakayama T; Colbert MC; Paul RJ; Fagin JA; and Clemens TL; Reduced blood pressure and increased sensitivity of the vasculature to parathyroid hormone-related protein (PTHrP) in transgenic mice overexpressing the PTH/PTHrP receptor in vascular smooth muscle. *Endocrinology* 1999; Apr;140(4):1826–33.

23. Maeda S; Sutliff RL; Qian J; Lorenz JN; Wang J; Tang H; Nakayama T; Weber C; Witte D; Strauch AR; Paul RJ; Fagin JA; and Clemens TL; Targeted overexpression of parathyroid hormone-related protein (PTHrP) to vascular smooth muscle in transgenic mice lowers blood pressure and alters vascular contractility. *Endocrinology* 1999; Apr;140(4):1815–25.

24. Micheau J and Riedel G; Protein kinases: which one is the memory molecule? *Cell Mol Life Sci* 1999; Apr;55(4):534–48.

25. Gallagher PE; Li P; Lenhart JR; Chappell MC; and Brosnihan KB; Estrogen regulation of angiotensin-converting enzyme mRNA. *Hypertension* 1999; Jan;33(1 Pt 2):323–8.

26. Nickenig G; Baumer AT; Grohe C; Kahlert S; Strehlow K; Rosenkranz S; Stablein A; Beckers F; Smits JF; Daemen MJ; Vetter H; and Bohm M; Estrogen modulates AT1 receptor gene expression *in vitro* and *in vivo. Circulation* 1998; Jun 9;97(22):2197–201.

27. Ferrario CM; Angiotension-(1-7) and antihypertensive mechanisms. *J Nephrol* 1998; Nov–Dec;11(6):278–83.

28. Shinoda E; Yui Y; Hattori R; Tanaka M; Inoue R; Aoyama T; Takimoto Y; Mitsui Y; Miyahara K; Shizuta Y; and Sasayama S; Tissue factor pathway inhibitor-2 is a novel mitogen for vascular smooth muscle cells. *J Biol Chem* 1999; Feb 26;274(9):5379–84.

29. Cho MM; Ziats NP; Pal D; Utian WH; and Gorodeski GI; Estrogen modulates paracellular permeability of human endothelial cells by eNOS- and iNOS-related mechanisms. *Am J Physiol* 1999; Feb;276(2 Pt 1):C337–49.

30. Hayoz D; Hengstler J; Noel B; and Brunner HR; Vasopressin induces opposite changes in blood flow in the skin and the muscular circulation. *Adv Exp Med Biol* 1998; 449:447–9.

31. May LG; Johnson S; Krebs S; Newman A; and Aronstam RS; Involvement of protein kinase C and protein kinase A in the muscarinic receptor signalling pathways mediating phospholipase C activation, arachidonic acid release and calcium mobilisation. *Cell Signal* 1999; Mar;11(3):179–87.

32. Prevot V; Croix D; Rialas CM; Poulain P; Fricchione GL; Stefano GB; and Beauvillain JC; Estradiol coupling to endothelial nitric oxide stimulates gonadotropin-releasing hormone release from rat median eminence via a membrane receptor. *Endocrinology* 1999; Feb;140(2):652–9.

33. Venkov CD; Rankin AB; and Vaughan DE; Identification of authentic estrogen receptor in cultured endothelial cells. A potential mechanism for steroid hormone regulation of endothelial function. *Circulation* 1996; Aug 15;94(4):727–33.

34. Kim-Schulze S; McGowan KA; Hubchak SC; Cid MC; Martin MB; Kleinman HK; Greene GL; and Schnaper HW; Expression of an estrogen receptor by human coronary artery and umbilical vein endothelial cells. *Circulation* 1996; Sep 15;94(6):1402–7.

35. Register TC and Adams MR; Coronary artery and cultured aortic smooth muscle cells express mRNA for both the classical estrogen receptor and the newly described estrogen receptor beta. *J Steroid Biochem Mol Biol* 1998; Feb;64(3–4):187–91.

36. Christ M and Wehling M; Cardiovascular steroid actions: swift swallows or sluggish snails? *Cardiovasc Res* 1998; Oct;40(1):34–44.

37. Bulletti C; De Ziegler D; Albonetti A; and Flamigni C; Paracrine regulation of menstruation. *J Reprod Immunol* 1998; Aug;39(1–2):89–104.

38. Tan SL; Zaidi J; Campbell S; Doyle P; and Collins W; Blood flow changes in the ovarian and uterine arteries during the normal menstrual cycle. *Am J Obstet Gynecol* 1996; Sep;175(3 Pt 1):625–31.

39. Finn CA; Menstruation: a nonadaptive consequence of uterine evolution. *Q Rev Biol* 1998; Jun;73(2):163–73.

40. Tibbetts TA; Connelly OM; and O'Malley BW; Progesterone via its receptor antagonizes the pro-inflammatory activity of estrogen in the mouse uterus. *Biol Reprod* 1999; May;60(5):1158–65.

41. Critchley HO; Jones RL; Lea RG; Drudy TA; Kelly RW; Williams AR; and Baird DT; Role of inflammatory mediators in human endometrium during progesterone withdrawal and early pregnancy. *J Clin Endocrinol Metab* 1999; Jan;84(1):240–8.

42. Taylor RN; Ryan IP; Moore ES; Hornung D; Shifren JL; and Tseng JF; Angiogenesis and macrophage activation in endometriosis. *Ann N Y Acad Sci* 1997; Sep 26;828:194–207.

43. Akoum A; Lemay A; Paradis I; Rheault N; and Maheux R; Secretion of interleukin-6 by human endometriotic cells and regulation by proinflammatory cytokines and sex steroids. *Hum Reprod* 1996; Oct;11(10):2269–75.

44. Cushman M; Meilahn EN; Psaty BM; Kuller LH; Dobs AS; and Tracy RP; Hormone replacement therapy, inflammation, and hemostasis in elderly women. *Arterioscler Thromb Vasc Biol* 1999; Apr;19(4):893–9 I.

45. Cushman M; Meilahn EN; Psaty BM; Kuller LH; Dobs AS; and Tracy RP; Hormone replacement therapy, inflammation, and hemostasis in elderly women. *Arterioscler Thromb Vasc Biol* 1999; Apr;19(4):893–9.

46. van Baal WM; Kenemans P; Emeis JJ; Schalkwijk CG; Mijatovic V; van der Mooren MJ; Vischer UM; and Stehouwer CD; Long-term effects of combined hormone replacement therapy on markers of endothelial function and inflammatory activity in healthy postmenopausal women. *Fertil Steril* 1999; Apr;71(4):663–70.

47. Koh KK; Bui MN; Mincemoyer R; and Cannon RO; Effects of hormone therapy on inflammatory cell adhesion molecules in postmenopausal healthy women. *Am J Cardiol* 1997; Dec 1;80(11):1505–7.

48. Caulin-Glaser T; Farrell WJ; Pfau SE; Zaret B; Bunger K; Setaro JF; Brennan JJ; Bender JR; Cleman MW; Cabin HS; and Remetz MS; Modulation of circulating cellular adhesion molecules in postmenopausal women with coronary artery disease. *J Am Coll Cardiol* 1998; Jun;31(7):1555–60.

49. Miyamoto N; Mandai M; Suzuma I; Suzuma K; Kobayashi K; and Honda Y; Estrogen protects against cellular infiltration by reducing the expressions of E-selectin and IL-6 in endotoxin-induced uveitis. *J Immunol* 1999; Jul 1;163(1):374–9.

50. Xiao E; Xia-Zhang L; Barth A; Zhu J; and Ferin M; Stress and the menstrual cycle: relevance of cycle quality in the short- and long-term response to a 5-day endotoxin challenge during the follicular phase in the rhesus monkey. *J Clin Endocrinol Metab* 1998; Jul;83(7):2454–60.

51. Stevenson JC; Various actions of oestrogens on the vascular system. *Maturitas* 1998; Sep 20;30(1):5–9.

52. Maxwell SR; Women and heart disease. *Basic Res Cardiol* 1998; 93 Suppl 2:79–84.

53. Blum A and Cannon RO; Effects of oestrogens and selective oestrogen receptor modulators on serum lipoproteins and vascular function. *Curr Opin Lipidol* 1998; Dec;9(6):575–86.

54. Oparil S and Arthur C; Corcoran Memorial Lecture. Hormones and vasoprotection. *Hypertension* 1999; Jan;33(1 Pt 2):170–6.

55. Spencer CP; Godsland IF; and Stevenson JC; Is there a menopausal metabolic syndrome? *Gynecol Endocrinol* 1997; Oct;11(5):341–55.

56. Hulley S; Grady D; Bush T; Furberg C; Herrington D; Riggs B; and Vittinghoff E; Randomized trial of estrogen plus progestin for secondary prevention of coronary heart disease in postmenopausal women. Heart and Estrogen/progestin Replacement Study (HERS) Research. *JAMA* 1998; Aug 19;280(7):605–13.

57. Rosano GM; Caixeta AM; Chierchia S; Arie S; Lopez-Hidalgo M; Pereira WI; Leonardo F; Webb CM; Pileggi F; and Collins P; Short-term anti-ischemic effect of 17beta-estradiol in postmenopausal women with coronary artery disease. *Circulation* 1997; Nov 4;96(9):2837–41.

58. McHugh NA; Solowiej A; Klabunde RE; and Merrill GF; Acute coronary vascular and myocardial perfusion effects of conjugated equine estrogen in the anesthetized dog. *Basic Res Cardiol* 1998 Dec;93(6):470–6.

59. Dubey RK; Gillespie DG; Jackson EK; and Keller PJ; 17Beta-estradiol, its metabolites, and progesterone inhibit cardiac fibroblast growth. *Hypertension* 1998; Jan;31(1 Pt 2):522–8.

60. Akkad A and Al-Azzawi F; The effect of oestrogen on intimal hyperplasia in cultured human ovarian veins. *Hum Reprod* 1998; Jun;13(6):1449–54.

61. Selzman CH; Gaynor JS; Turner AS; Johnson SM; Horwitz LD; Whitehill TA; and Harken AH; Ovarian ablation alone promotes aortic intimal hyperplasia and accumulation of fibroblast growth factor. *Circulation* 1998; Nov 10;98(19):2049–54.

62. Selzman CH; Gaynor JS; Turner AS; Whitehill TA; Horwitz LD; and Harken AH; Estrogen replacement inhibits intimal hyperplasia and the accumulation and effects of transforming growth factor beta1. *J Surg Res* 1998; Dec;80(2):380–5.

63. Moraghan T; Antoniucci DM; Grenert JP; Sieck GC; Johnson C; Miller VM; and Fitzpatrick LA; Differential response in cell proliferation to beta estradiol in coronary arterial vascular smooth muscle cells obtained from mature female versus male animals. *Endocrinology* 1996; Nov;137(11):5174–7.

64. Saito S; Foegh ML; Motomura N; Lou H; Kent K; and Ramwell PW; Estradiol inhibits allograft-inducible major histocompatibility complex class II antigen expression and transplant arteriosclerosis in the absence of immunosuppression. *Transplantation* 1998; Dec 15;66 (11):1424–31.

65. Song J; Wan Y; Rolfe BE; Campbell JH; and Campbell GR; Effect of estrogen on vascular smooth muscle cells is dependent upon cellular phenotype. *Atherosclerosis* 1998; Sep;140(1):97–104.

66. Shifren JL; Tseng JF; Zaloudek CJ; Ryan IP; Meng YG; Ferrara N; Jaffe RB; and Taylor RN; Ovarian steroid regulation of vascular endothelial growth factor in the human endometrium: implications for angiogenesis during the menstrual cycle and in the pathogenesis of endometriosis. *J Clin Endocrinol Metab.* 1996; Aug;81(8):3112–8.

67. Best PJ; Berger PB; Miller VM; and Lerman A; The effect of estrogen replacement therapy on plasma nitric oxide and endothelin-1 levels in postmenopausal women. *Ann Intern Med* 1998; Feb 15;128(4):285–8.

68. Akishita M; Kozaki K; Eto M; Yoshizumi M; Ishikawa M; Toba K; Orimo H; and Ouchi Y; Estrogen attenuates endothelin-1 production by bovine endothelial cells via estrogen receptor. *Biochem Biophys Res Commun* 1998; Oct 9;251(1):17–21.

69. Albuquerque ML; Akiyama SK; and Schnaper HW; Basic fibroblast growth factor release by human coronary artery endothelial cells is enhanced by matrix proteins, 17beta-estradiol, and a PKC signaling pathway. *Exp Cell Res* 1998; Nov 25;245(1):163–9.

70. Williams JK; Delansorne R; and Paris J; Estrogens, progestins, and coronary artery reactivity in atherosclerotic monkeys. *J Steroid Biochem Mol Biol* 1998; 65(1–6):219–24.

71. McCrohon JA; Adams MR; McCredie RJ; Robinson J; Pike A; Abbey M; Keech AC; and Celermajer DS; Hormone replacement therapy is associated with improved arterial physiology in healthy post-menopausal women. *Clin Endocrinol (Oxf)* 1996; Oct;45(4):435–41.

72. Leonardo F; Medeirus C; Rosano GM; Pereira WI; Sheiban I; Gebara O; Bellotti G; Pileggi F; Chierchia SL Leonardo F; Medeirus C; Rosano GM; Pereira WI; Sheiban I; Gebara O; Bellotti G; Pileggi F; and Chierchia SL; Effect of acute administration of estradiol 17 beta on aortic blood flow in menopausal women. *Am J Cardiol* 1997; Sep 15;80(6):791–3.

73. De Meersman RE; Zion AS; Giardina EG; Weir JP; Lieberman JS; and Downey JA; Estrogen replacement, vascular distensibility, and blood pressures in postmenopausal women. *Am J Physiol* 1998; May;274(5 Pt 2):H1539–44.

74. Arora S; Veves A; Caballaro AE; Smakowski P; and LoGerfo FW; Estrogen improves endothelial function. *J Vasc Surg* 1998; Jun;27(6):1141–6; discussion 1147.

75. Bush DE; Jones CE; Bass KM; Walters GK; Bruza JM; and Ouyang P; Estrogen replacement reverses endothelial dysfunction in postmenopausal women. *Am J Med* 1998 Jun;104(6):552–8.

76. Al-Khalili F; Eriksson M; Landgren BM; and Schenck-Gustafsson K; Effect of conjugated estrogen on peripheral flow-mediated vasodilation in postmenopausal women. *Am J Cardiol* 1998; Jul 15;82(2):215–8.

77. Magness RR; Phernetton TM; and Zheng J; Systemic and uterine blood flow distribution during prolonged infusion of 17beta-estradiol. *Am J Physiol* 1998; Sep;275(3 Pt 2):H731–43.

78. Cacciatore B; Paakkari I; Toivonen J; Tikkanen MJ; and Ylikorkala O; Randomized comparison of oral and transdermal hormone replacement on carotid and uterine artery resistance to blood flow. *Obstet Gynecol* 1998; Oct;92(4 Pt 1):563–8.

79. Lau TK; Wan D; Yim SF; Sanderson JE; and Haines CJ; Prospective, randomized, controlled study of the effect of hormone replacement therapy on peripheral blood flow velocity in postmenopausal women. *Fertil Steril* 1998; Aug;70(2):284–8.

80. Penotti M; Farina M; Castiglioni E; Gaffuri B; Barletta L; Gabrielli L; and Vignali M; Alteration in the pulsatility index values of the internal carotid and middle cerebral arteries after suspension of postmenopausal hormone replacement therapy: a randomized crossover study. *Am J Obstet Gynecol* 1996; Sep;175(3 Pt 1):606–11.

81. Wellman GC; Bonev AD; Nelson MT; and Brayden JE; Gender differences in coronary artery diameter involve estrogen, nitric oxide, and Ca(2+)-dependent K+ channels. *Circ Res* 1996; Nov;79(5):1024–30.

82. Hutchison SJ; Sudhir K; Chou TM; and Chatterjee K; Sex hormones and vascular reactivity. *Herz* 1997 Jun;22(3):141–50.

83. Darkow DJ; Lu L; and White RE; Estrogen relaxation of coronary artery smooth muscle is mediated by nitric oxide and cGMP. *Am J Physiol* 1997; Jun;272(6 Pt 2):H2765–73.

84. Collins P; Beale CM; and Rosano GM; Oestrogen as a calcium channel blocker. *Eur Heart J* 1996 Aug;17 Suppl D:27–31.

85. Binko J and Majewski H; 17 beta-Estradiol reduces vasoconstriction in endothelium-denuded rat aortas through inducible NOS. *Am J Physiol* 1998; Mar;274(3 Pt 2):H853–9.

86. Kitazawa T; Hamada E; Kitazawa K; and Gaznabi AK; Non-genomic mechanism of 17 beta-oestradiol-induced inhibition of contraction in mammalian vascular smooth muscle. *J Physiol* (Lond) 1997; Mar 1;499 (Pt 2):497–511.

87. Brosnihan KB; Li P; Ganten D; and Ferrario CM; Estrogen protects transgenic hypertensive rats by shifting the vasoconstrictor-vasodilator balance of RAS. *Am J Physiol* 1997; Dec;273(6 Pt 2):R1908–15.

88. Mugge A; Barton M; Fieguth HG; and Riedel M; Contractile responses to histamine, serotonin, and angiotensin II are impaired by 17 beta-estradiol in human internal mammary arteries *in vitro*. *Pharmacology* 1997; Mar;54(3):162–8.

89. Wingrove CS and Stevenson JC; 17 beta-Oestradiol inhibits stimulated endothelin release in human vascular endothelial cells. *Eur J Endocrinol* 1997; Aug;137(2):205–8.

90. Holm P; Korsgaard N; Shalmi M; Andersen HL; Hougaard P; Skouby SO; and Stender S; Significant reduction of the antiatherogenic effect of estrogen by long-term inhibition of nitric oxide synthesis in cholesterol-clamped rabbits. *J Clin Invest* 1997; Aug 15;100(4):821–8.

91. Caulin-Glaser T; Garcia-Cardena G; Sarrel P; Sessa WC; and Bender JR; 17 beta-estradiol regulation of human endothelial cell basal nitric oxide release, independent of cytosolic Ca2+ mobilization. *Circ Res* 1997; Nov;81(5):885–92.

92. Guetta V; Quyyumi AA; Prasad A; Panza JA; Waclawiw M; and Cannon RO; The role of nitric oxide in coronary vascular effects of estrogen in postmenopausal women. *Circulation* 1997; Nov 4;96(9):2795–801.

93. Kleinert H; Wallerath T; Euchenhofer C; Ihrig-Biedert I; Li H; and Forstermann U; Estrogens increase transcription of the human endothelial NO synthase gene: analysis of the transcription factors involved. *Hypertension* 1998; Feb;31(2):582–8.

94. Kauser K; Sonnenberg D; Diel P; Rubanyi GM; Effect of 17beta-oestradiol on cytokine-induced nitric oxide production in rat isolated aorta. *Br J Pharmacol* 1998; Mar;123(6):1089–96.

95. Hernandez I; Delgado JL; Carbonell LF; Perez MC; and Quesada T; Hemodynamic effect of 17 beta-estradiol in absence of NO in ovariectomized rats: role of angiotensin II. *Am J Physiol* 1998; Apr;274(4 Pt 2):R970–8.

96. Otter D and Austin C; Effects of 17beta-oestradiol on rat isolated coronary and mesenteric artery tone: involvement of nitric oxide. *J Pharm Pharmacol* 1998; May;50(5):531–8.

97. Geary GG; Krause DN; and Duckles SP; Estrogen reduces myogenic tone through a nitric oxide-dependent mechanism in rat cerebral arteries. *Am J Physiol* 1998; Jul;275(1 Pt 2):H292–300.

98. Gorodeski GI; Yang T; Levy MN; Goldfarb J; and Utian WH; Modulation of coronary vascular resistance in female rabbits by estrogen and progesterone. *J Soc Gynecol Investig* 1998; Jul–Aug;5(4):197–202.

99. Vagnoni KE; Shaw CE; Phernetton TM; Meglin BM; Bird IM; and Magness RR; Endothelial vasodilator production by uterine and systemic arteries. III. Ovarian and estrogen effects on NO synthase. *Am J Physiol* 1998; Nov;275(5 Pt 2):H1845–56.

100. Vacca G; Battaglia A; Grossini E; Mary DA; Molinari C; and Surico N; The effect of 17beta-oestradiol on regional blood flow in anaesthetized pigs. *J Physiol (Lond)* 1999; Feb 1;514 (Pt 3):875–84.

101. Chen Z; Yuhanna IS; Galcheva-Gargova Z; Karas RH; Mendelsohn ME; and Shaul PW; Estrogen receptor alpha mediates the nongenomic activation of endothelial nitric oxide synthase by estrogen. *J Clin Invest* 1999; Feb;103(3):401–6.

102. Bolego C; Cignarella A; Zancan V; Pinna C; Zanardo R; and Puglisi L; Diabetes abolishes the vascular protective effects of estrogen in female rats. *Life Sci* 1999; 64(9):741–9.

103. Cho MM; Ziats NP; Abdul-Karim FW; Pal D; Goldfarb J; Utian WH; and Gorodeski GI; Effects of estrogen on tight junctional resistance in cultured human umbilical vein endothelial cells. *J Soc Gynecol Investig* 1998; Sep–Oct;5(5):260–70.

104. Wingrove CS; Garr E; Godsland IF; and Stevenson JC; 17beta-oestradiol enhances release of matrix metalloproteinase-2 from human vascular smooth muscle cells. *Biochim Biophys Acta* 1998; Mar 5;1406(2):169–74.

105. White CR; Shelton J; Chen SJ; Darley-Usmar V; Allen L; Nabors C; Sanders PW; Chen YF; and Oparil S; Estrogen restores endothelial cell function in an experimental model of vascular injury. *Circulation* 1997; Sep 2;96(5):1624–30.

106. Winkler M; Kemp B; Hauptmann S; and Rath W; Parturition: steroids, prostaglandin E2, and expression of adhesion molecules by endothelial cells. *Obstet Gynecol* 1997; Mar;89(3):398–402.

107. Crook D; The metabolic consequences of treating postmenopausal women with non-oral hormone replacement therapy. *Br J Obstet Gynaecol* 1997; Nov;104 Suppl 16:4–13.

108. Vazquez F; Rodriguez-Manzaneque JC; Lydon JP; Edwards DP; O'Malley BW; and Iruela-Arispe ML; Progesterone regulates proliferation of endothelial cells. *J Biol Chem* 1999; Jan 22;274(4):2185–92.

109. Lee WS; Harder JA; Yoshizumi M; Lee ME; and Haber E; Progesterone inhibits arterial smooth muscle cell proliferation. *Nat Med* 1997; Sep;3(9):1005–8.

110. Aygen EM; Basbug M; Tayyar M; and Kaya ; The effects of different doses of medroxyprogesterone acetate on serum lipids, lipoprotein levels and atherogenic index in the menopausal period. *Gynecol Endocrinol* 1998; Aug;12(4):267–72.

111. Vadlamudi S; MacLean P; Israel RG; Marks RH; Hickey M; Otvos J; and Barakat H; Effects of oral combined hormone replacement therapy on plasma lipids and lipoproteins. *Metabolism* 1998; Oct;47(10):1222–6.

112. Mueck AO; Seeger H; and Lippert TH; Estradiol inhibits LDL oxidation: do the progestins medroxyprogesterone acetate and norethisterone acetate influence this effect? *Clin Exp Obstet Gynecol* 1998; 25(1–2):26–8.

113. Cheng W; Lau OD; and Abumrad NA; Two antiatherogenic effects of progesterone on human macrophages; inhibition of cholesteryl ester synthesis and block of its enhancement by glucocorticoids. *J Clin Endocrinol Metab* 1999; Jan;84(1):265–71.

114. Glusa E; Graser T; Wagner S; and Oettel M; Mechanisms of relaxation of rat aorta in response to progesterone and synthetic progestins. *Maturitas* 1997; Dec 15;28(2):181–91.

115. Gerhard M; Walsh BW; Tawakol A; Haley EA; Creager SJ; Seely EW; Ganz P; and Creager MA; Estradiol therapy combined with progesterone and endothelium-dependent vasodilation in postmenopausal women. *Circulation* 1998; Sep 22;98(12):1158–63.

116. Minshall RD; Stanczyk FZ; Miyagawa K; Uchida B; Axthelm M; Novy M; and Hermsmeyer K; Ovarian steroid protection against coronary artery hyperreactivity in rhesus monkeys. *J Clin Endocrinol Metab* 1998; Feb;83(2):649–59.

117. Sorensen KE; Dorup I; Hermann AP; and Mosekilde L; Combined hormone replacement therapy does not protect women against the age-related decline in endothelium-dependent vasomotor function. *Circulation* 1998; Apr 7;97(13):1234–8.

118. Suzuki A; Mizuno K; Asada Y; Ino Y; Kuwayama T; Okada M; Mizutani S; and Tomoda Y; Effects of 17beta-estradiol and progesterone on the adhesion of human monocytic THP-1 cells to human female endothelial cells exposed to minimally oxidized LDL. *Gynecol Obstet Invest* 1997; 44(1):47–52.

119. Fujimoto J; Sakaguchi H; Hirose R; and Tamaya T; Significance of sex steroids in roles of cadherin subfamily and its related proteins in the uterine endometrium and placenta. *Horm Res* 1998; 50.

120. Fujimoto J; Sakaguchi H; Hirose R; and Tamaya T; Sex steroidal regulation of vessel permeability associated with vessel endothelial cadherin (V-cadherin). *J Steroid Biochem Mol Biol* 1998; Oct;67(1):25–32.

121. Herman SM; Robinson JT; McCredie RJ; Adams MR; Boyer MJ; and Celermajer DS; Androgen deprivation is associated with enhanced endothelium-dependent dilatation in adult men. *Arterioscler Thromb Vasc Biol* 1997; Oct;17(10):2004–9.

122. Sordello S; Bertrand N; and Plouet J; Vascular endothelial growth factor is up-regulated *in vitro* and *in vivo* by androgens. *Biochem Biophys Res Commun* 1998; Oct 9;251(1):287–90.

123. Levine AC; Liu XH; Greenberg PD; Eliashvili M; Schiff JD; Aaronson SA; Holland JF; and Kirschenbaum A; Androgens induce the expression of vascular endothelial growth factor in human fetal prostatic fibroblasts. *Endocrinology* 1998; Nov;139(11):4672–8.

124. Joseph IB; Nelson JB; Denmeade SR; and Isaacs JT; Androgens regulate vascular endothelial growth factor content in normal and malignant prostatic tissue. *Clin Cancer Res* 1997; Dec;3(12 Pt 1):2507–11.

125. Higashiura K; Mathur RS; and Halushka PV; Gender-related differences in androgen regulation of thromboxane A2 receptors in rat aortic smooth-muscle cells. *J Cardiovasc Pharmacol* 1997; Mar;29(3):311–5.

126. Mohan PF and Benghuzzi H; Effect of dehydroepiandrosterone on endothelial cell proliferation. *Biomed Sci Instrum* 1997; 33:550–5.

127. Furutama D; Fukui R; Amakawa M; and Ohsawa N; Inhibition of migration and proliferation of vascular smooth muscle cells by dehydroepiandrosterone sulfate. *Biochim Biophys Acta* 1998; Feb 27;1406(1):107–14.

128. Dickerman RD; McConathy WJ; and Zachariah NY; Testosterone, sex hormone-binding globulin, lipoproteins, and vascular disease risk. *J Cardiovasc Risk* 1997; Oct–Dec;4(5–6):363–6.

129. McCredie RJ; McCrohon JA; Turner L; Griffiths KA; Handelsman DJ; and Celermajer DS; Vascular reactivity is impaired in genetic females taking high-dose androgens. *J Am Coll Cardiol* 1998; Nov;32(5):1331–5.

130. Chou TM; Sudhir K; Hutchison SJ; Ko E; Amidon TM; Collins P; and Chatterjee K; Testosterone induces dilation of canine coronary conductance and resistance arteries *in vivo*. *Circulation* 1996; Nov 15;94(10):2614–9.

131. Kawano H; Motoyama T; Kugiyama K; Hirashima O; Ohgushi M; Fujii H; Ogawa H; and Yasue H; Gender difference in improvement of endothelium-dependent vasodilation after estrogen supplementation. *J Am Coll Cardiol* 1997; Oct;30(4):914–9.

132. Farrukh IS; Peng W; Orlinska U; and Hoidal JR; Effect of dehydroepiandrosterone on hypoxic pulmonary vasoconstriction: a Ca(2+)-activated K(+)-channel opener. *Am J Physiol* 1998; Feb;274(2 Pt 1):L186–95.

133. Suenaga R; Evans, MJ; Mtiamura K; Rider V; and Abdou NI; Peripheral Blood T cells and monocytes and B cell lines derived from patients with lupus express estrogen receptor transcripts similar to those of normal cells. *J Rheumtol* 1998; 25: 1305–12.

134. Carlsten H; Nilsson N; Jonsson R; Backman K; Holmdahl R; and Tarkowski A; Estrogen accelerates immune complex glomerulonephritis but ameliorates T cell-mediated vasculitis and sialadenitis in autoimmune MRL lpr/lpr mice. *Cell Immunol* 1992; Oct 1;144(1):190–202.

135. Faas MM; Bakker WW; Valkhof N; van der Horst MC; and Schuiling GA; Reproductive condition and the low-dose endotoxin-induced inflammatory response in rats. Glomerular influx of inflammatory cells and expression of adhesion molecules. *Biol Reprod* 1997; Jun;56(6):1400–6.

136. Kim-Schulze S; Lowe WL Jr; and Schnaper HW; Estrogen stimulates delayed mitogen-activated protein kinase activity in human endothelial cells via an autocrine loop that involves basic fibroblast growth factor. *Circulation* 1998; Aug 4;98(5):413–21.

137. Yue TL; Wang X; Louden CS; Gupta S; Pillarisetti K; Gu JL; Hart TK; Lysko PG; and Feuerstein GZ; 2-Methoxyestradiol, an endogenous estrogen metabolite, induces apoptosis in endothelial cells and inhibits angiogenesis: possible role for stress-activated protein kinase signaling pathway and Fas expression. *Mol Pharmacol* 1997; Jun;51(6):951–62.

138. Morey AK; Pedram A; Razandi M; Prins BA; Hu RM; Biesiada E; and Levin ER; Estrogen and progesterone inhibit vascular smooth muscle proliferation. *Endocrinology* 1997; Aug;138(8):3330–9.

139. Sthoeger ZM; Chiorazzi N; and Lahita RG; Regulation of the immune response by sex hormones. I. *In vitro* effects of estradiol and testosterone on pokeweed mitogen-induced human B cell differentiation. *J Immunol* 1988; Jul 1;141:91–8.

140. Alvarez RJ; Gips SJ; Moldovan N; Wilhide CC; Milliken EE; Hoang AT; Hruban RH; Silverman HS; Dang CV; and Goldschmidt-Clermont PJ; 17Beta-estradiol inhibits apoptosis of endothelial cells. *Biochem Biophys Res Commun* 1997; Aug 18;237(2):372–81.

141. Keck C; Herchenbach D; Pfisterer J; and Breckwoldt M; Effects of 17beta-estradiol and progesterone on interleukin-6 production and proliferation of human umbilical vein endothelial cells. *Exp Clin Endocrinol Diabetes* 1998; 106(4):334–9.

142. Pahor M; Elam MB; Garrison RJ; Kritchevsky SB; and Applegate WB; Emerging noninvasive biochemical measures to predict cardiovascular risk. *Arch Intern Med* 1999; Feb 8;159(3):237–45.

143. Zimmermann J; Herrlinger S; Pruy A; Metzger T; and Wanner C; Inflammation enhances cardiovascular risk and mortality in hemodialysis patients. *Kidney Int* 1999; Feb;55(2):648–58.

144. Bhakdi S; Complement and atherogenesis: the unknown connection. *Ann Med* 1998; Dec;30(6):503–7.

145. Libby P; The interface of atherosclerosis and thrombosis: basic mechanisms. *Vasc Med* 1998; 3(3):225–9.

146. Ross R; Atherosclerosis — an inflammatory disease. *N Engl J Med* 1999; Jan 14;340(2):115–26.

147. Kinlay S; Selwyn AP; Libby P; and Ganz P; Inflammation, the endothelium, and the acute coronary syndromes. *J Cardiovasc Pharmacol* 1998; 32 Suppl 3:S62–6.

148. Jean WC; Spellman SR; Nussbaum ES; and Low WC; Reperfusion injury after focal cerebral ischemia: the role of inflammation and the therapeutic horizon. *Neurosurgery* 1998; Dec;43(6):1382–96; discussion 1396–7.

149. Caulin-Glaser T; Farrell WJ; Pfau SE; Zaret B; Bunger K; Setaro JF; Brennan JJ; Bender JR; Cleman MW; Cabin HS; and Remetz MS; Modulation of circulating cellular adhesion molecules in postmenopausal women with coronary artery disease. *J Am Coll Cardiol* 1998; Jun;31(7):1555–60.

150. Lahita RG; The effects of sex hormones on the immune system in pregnancy. *Am J Reprod Immunol* 1992; Oct–Dec;28(3–4):136–7.

151. Lahita RG; Bradlow HL; Ginzler E; Pang S; and New M; Low plasma androgens in women with systemic lupus erythematosus. *Arthritis Rheum* 1987; Mar;30:241–8.

152. Lahita RG; Bradlow HL; Kunkel HG; and Fishman J; Increased 16 alpha-hydroxylation of estradiol in systemic lupus erythematosus. *J Clin Endocrinol Metab* 1981; 53:174–8.

153. Wilder RL; Hormones, pregnancy, and autoimmune diseases. *Ann N Y Acad Sci* 1998; May 1;840:45–50.

154. Dayan M; Zinger H; Kalush F; Mor G; Amir-Zaltzman Y; Kohen F; Sthoeger Z; and Mozes E; The beneficial effects of treatment with tamoxifen and anti-oestradiol antibody on experimental systemic lupus erythematosus are associated with cytokine modulations. *Immunology* 1997; Jan;90(1):101–8.

155. Kanda N; Tsuchida T; and Tamaki K; Estrogen enhancement of anti-double-stranded DNA antibody and immunoglobulin G production in peripheral blood mononuclear cells from patients with systemic lupus erythematosus. *Arthritis Rheum* 1999; Feb;42(2):328–37.

156. Frank S; Stallmeyer B; Kompfer H; Schaffner C; and Pfeilschifter J; Differential regulation of vascular endothelial growth factor and its receptor fms-like-tyrosine kinase is mediated by nitric oxide in rat renal mesangial cells. *Biochem J* 1999; Mar 1;338(Pt 2):367–374.

157. Rider V; Foster RT; Evans M; Suenaga R; and Abdou NI; Gender differences in autoimmune diseases: estrogen increases calcineurin expression in systemic lupus erythematosus. *Clin Immunol Immunopathol* 1998; Nov;89(2):171–80.

158. Rao BR; Isolation and characterization of an estrogen binding protein which may integrate the plethora of estrogenic actions in non-reproductive organs. *J Steroid Biochem Mol Biol* 1998; Apr;65 (1–6):3–41.

159. Kammer GM and Tsokos GC; Emerging concepts of the molecular basis for estrogen effects on T lymphocytes in systemic lupus erythematosus. *Clin Immunol Immunopathol* 1998; Dec;89(3):192–5.

160. Turton EP; Kent PJ; and Kester RC; The aetiology of Raynaud's phenomenon. *Cardiovasc Surg* 1998; Oct;6(5):431–40.

161. Lekakis J; Mavrikakis M; Papamichael C; Papazoglou S; Economou O; Scotiniotis I; Stamatelopoulos K; Vemmos C; Stamatelopoulos S; and Moulopoulos S; Short-term estrogen administration improves abnormal endothelial function in women with systemic sclerosis and Raynaud's phenomenon. *Am Heart J* 1998; Nov;136(5):905–12.

162. Lekakis J; Papamichael C; Mavrikakis M; Voutsas A; and Stamatelopoulos S; Effect of long-term estrogen therapy on brachial arterial endothelium-dependent vasodilation in women with Raynaud's phenomenon secondary to systemic sclerosis. *Am J Cardiol* 1998; Dec 15;82(12):1555–7, A8.

163. Gonzalez RR and Blanchard LA; Thermoregulatory responses to cold transients: effects of menstrual cycle in resting women. *J Appl Physiol* 1998; Aug;85(2):543–53.

164. Straub RH; Zeuner M; Lock G; Scholmerich J; and Lang B; High prolactin and low dehydroepiandrosterone sulphate serum levels in patients with severe systemic sclerosis. *Br J Rheumatol* 1997; Apr;36(4):426–32.

165. Sanchez-Guerrero J; Liang MH; Karlson EW; Hunter DJ; and Colditz GA; Postmenopausal estrogen therapy and the risk for developing systemic lupus erythematosus. *Ann Intern Med* 1995; Mar 15;122(6):430–3.

166. Mok CC; Lau CS; Ho CT; Lee KW; Mok MY; and Wong RW; Safety of hormonal replacement therapy in postmenopausal patients with systemic lupus erythematosus. *Scand J Rheumatol* 1998; 27(5):342–6.

167. Kreidstein S; Urowitz MB; Gladman DD; and Gough J; Hormone replacement therapy in systemic lupus erythematosus. *J Rheumatol* 1997; Nov;24(11):2149–52.

168. Arden NK; Lloyd ME; Spector TD; and Hughes GR; Safety of hormone replacement therapy (HRT) in systemic lupus erythematosus (SLE). *Lupus* 1994; Feb;3(1):11–3.

169. Buyon JP; Oral contraceptives in women with systemic lupus erythematosus. *Ann Med Interne* (Paris) 1996; 147(4):259–64.

170. McNeill AM; Duckles SP; and Krause DN; Relaxant effects of 17 beta-estradiol in the rat tail artery are greater in females than males. *Eur J Pharmacol* 1996; Jul 25;308(3):305–9

Section II

Clinical Manifestations

16 Vascular Manifestations in Necrotizing and Granulomatous Vasculitides

Karim Raza, David M. Carruthers, and Paul A. Bacon

CONTENTS

I. INTRODUCTION

This chapter is an overview of the primary necrotizing and granulomatous vasculitides. It is not intended as an exhaustive review of the clinical and laboratory features of the individual vasculitides; we hope to provide an understanding of the general approach to the patient with suspected vasculitis with particular reference to our assessment of such patients. We will deal selectively with primary systemic vasculitis, with giant cell arteritis (GCA), Takayasu's arteritis (TA), and Kawasaki's disease being covered in chapters by Cid (Chapter 17), Numano (Chapter 18), and Lehman (Chapter 27). In addition to the primary systemic vasculitides with which this chapter deals, essentially identical vasculitis may occur secondary to the connective tissue diseases or rheumatoid arthritis (RA). These

TABLE 16.1
The Spectrum of Vasculitis

Type of Vasculitis	Example
Primary systemic	Polyarteritis nodosa
	Wegener's granulomatosis
	Churg-Strauss syndrome
	Microscopic polyangiitis
	Henoch-Schönlein purpura
Secondary	Vasculitis with:
	Rheumatoid arthritis
	Systemic lupus erythematosus
	Antiphospholipid antibody syndrome
	Sjögren's syndrome
	Dermatomyositis
	Systemic sclerosis
Localized	Cutaneous polyarteritis nodosa
	Primary angiitis of the central nervous system
Pseudo	Cholesterol emboli
	Atrial myxoma
	Subacute bacterial endocarditis
	Amyloidosis

must be distinguished from the pseudo-vasculitic syndromes, the notorious mimics of vasculitis such as cholesterol emboli, atrial myxoma, and subacute bacterial endocarditis (SBE) (Table 16.1).

The vasculitides is a heterogeneous group of diseases characterized by inflammation and necrosis of blood vessel walls. Vessel wall inflammation leads to luminal occlusion, or aneurysm formation and possible rupture, with resultant end organ ischemia or infarction. The manifestations of a "vasculitic syndrome" depend in part on the size, site, and number of blood vessels involved. It is important to appreciate, however, that the clinical features of a vasculitic syndrome are not confined to those directly consequent upon vasculitis. Asthma in Churg-Strauss syndrome (CSS) and synovitis in Wegener's granulomatosis (WG), for example, do not have vasculitis — as defined histologically — as their basis; nevertheless, these are important features of each vasculitic syndrome. Just as the clinical spectrum of the vasculitides varies, the spectrum of disease seen within individual vasculitic syndromes is also diverse. This is schematically illustrated for WG and rheumatoid disease (Figure 16.1).

Necrotizing vasculitis, granulomatous lesions, and serositis can all be seen in WG. The disease may begin with granulomatous airways disease and later progress to a necrotizing vasculitic phase, as Wegener initially proposed.[1] Conversely, necrotizing vasculitis may be the first manifestation of disease. However, all features may be present simultaneously or some patients may actually present with synovitis, only later progressing to a "typical" picture of WG. Indeed, a patient may present anywhere through this spectrum and the disease may alter with time with different components of the illness assuming predominance. Similarly, in rheumatoid disease, synovitis, granulomata and necrotizing vasculitis may be seen though the synovitis is dominant in this syndrome.

The majority of studies relating to the systemic vasculitides have been in the setting of tertiary referral centers. Although a U.K. study of patients with WG has shown that the spectrum of disease is similar in a district hospital and in a tertiary referral center,[2] it must be appreciated that the experience of referral centers often demonstrates bias. This needs to be taken into account when interpreting published data, much of which is presented in this chapter.

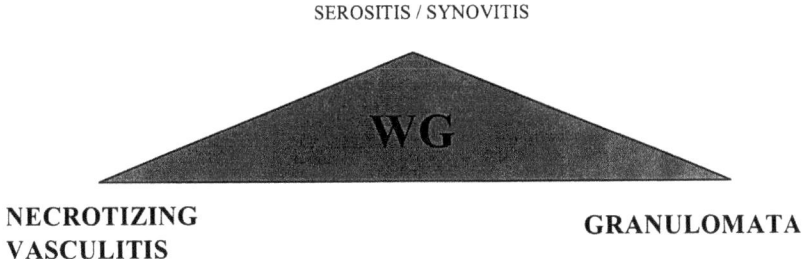

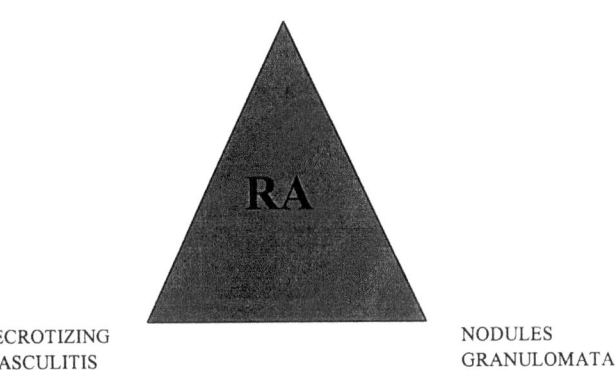

FIGURE 16.1 The spectrum of disease in Wegener's granulomatosis (WG) and rheumatoid arthritis (RA). In WG necrotizing vasculitis and granulomata are common, whereas serositis and synovitis are less so. Conversely, in RA, although necrotizing vasculitis and granulomata are seen, synovitis is a more common feature of the disease.

II. CLASSIFICATION AND EPIDEMIOLOGY

A. HISTORICAL ASPECTS

The systemic vasculitides were probably first recognized as early as 1755 by Michaelis and Martin (referred to by Lamb[3]). The first description of the syndrome now known as Henoch-Schönlein purpura (HSP) was by Heberden in 1801.[4] In 1837, Schönlein noted the association of joint pain and purpura and termed the condition purpura rheumatica.[5] Henoch subsequently noted the importance of gastrointestinal and renal involvement.[6] Kussmaul and Maier in 1866 described an apparently new disease entity characterized by a severe systemic illness involving fever, anorexia, myalgia, muscle weakness, abdominal pain, and oliguria. Numerous nodules were found along the course of small muscular arteries at autopsy, and the disorder was termed periarteritis nodosa.[7] After these early observations, it was not until the first half of the 20th century that many of the vasculitic syndromes we now recognize were described. In 1936 Wegener described his eponymous form of granulomatous vasculitis,[1] and in 1951 Churg and Strauss identified a form of vasculitis associated with asthma and eosinophilia.[8] These were all thought to be variants rather than separate entities, however, and until recently the term "polyarteritis nodosa" (PAN), first introduced by Ferrari in 1903,[9] continued to be used to describe any type of systemic vasculitis.

As the number of syndromes increased, the need grew for a classification system to distinguish between them and enable the study of etiology, natural history, therapy, and prognosis of the

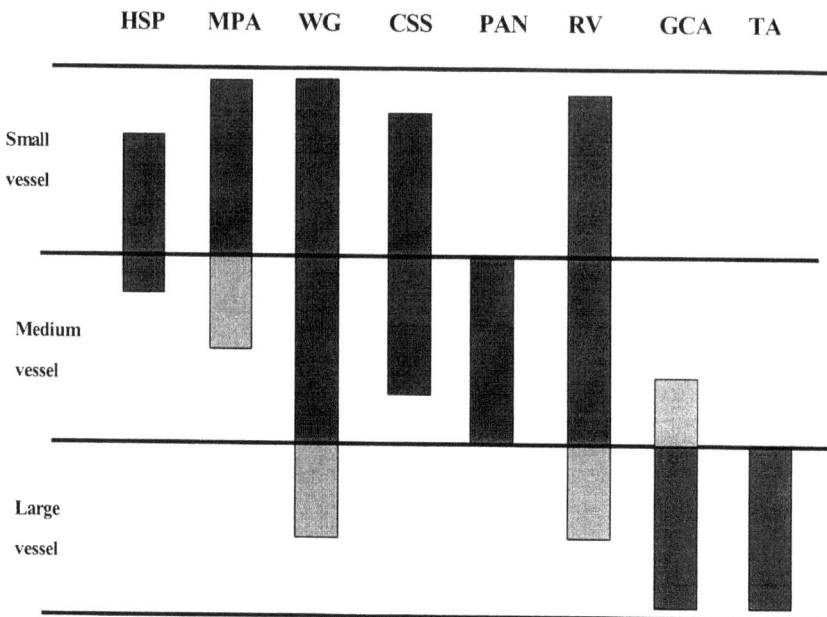

FIGURE 16.2 The spectrum of vasculitis by vessel size — common (dark shading) and uncommon (pale shading). Henoch-Schönlein purpura (HSP), microscopic polyangiitis (MPA), Wegener's granulomatosis (WG), Churg-Strauss syndrome (CSS), polyarteritis nodosa (PAN), rheumatoid vasculitis (RV), giant-cell arteritis (GCA), Takayasu's arteritis (TA).

vasculitides. In the absence of an understanding of pathogenic mechanisms, early classification systems, including the first by Zeek in 1952,[10] were based principally on the size of vessel involved. However, as shown (Figure 16.2), such classifications are frustrated by the fact that the vasculitic syndromes, and in particular WG, do not respect vessel size boundaries.

B. Classification in the 1990s

Significant advances in classification were made in the 1990s. The American College of Rheumatology (ACR) published a series of papers in 1990 addressing the issue of classification, and proposed criteria for seven types of systemic vasculitis: PAN, CSS, WG, hypersensitivity vasculitis, HSP, GCA, and TA.[11] A study was made of 807 patients with primary vasculitis, excluding Kawasaki disease, and clinical and laboratory features that would distinguish the seven groups, were identified. These criteria provided an important standard by which patients diagnosed with a systemic vasculitis could be classified into disease groups, facilitating epidemiological and therapeutic studies. There are, however, a number of concerns regarding these criteria. They were not tested against the general population or patients with other connective tissue or rheumatic diseases, so their utility is in distinguishing one type of primary vasculitis from another rather than enabling diagnosis. Because the criteria selected for classification were those that distinguished between vasculitides, the full spectrum of manifestations is not included in each instance, and important but less distinctive clinical features are not recognized. Thus, they do not help the clinician make an early diagnosis in individual patients. A third reservation about these criteria is the lack of inclusion of microscopic polyangiitis (MPA) as a disease entity as distinct from hypersensitivity vasculitis and PAN where most of the ACR cases probably hide. The characteristics of MPA were clearly established by Davson et al.[12] who suggested that the segmental necrotizing glomerulonephritis (GN) observed in PAN was linked to a microscopic form of the disease that was distinct from the PAN described by Kussmaul and Maier.[7] Further work by Savage et al.[13] defined the syndrome of MPA as a clinically

TABLE 16.2
Chapel Hill Consensus Conference on the Nomenclature of Systemic Vasculitis: Definitions for Polyarteritis Nodosa, Wegener's Granulomatosis, Churg-Strauss Syndrome, Microscopic Polyangiitis, and Henoch-Schönlein Purpura

Vasculitis	Definition
Polyarteritis nodosa	Necrotizing inflammation of medium sized or small arteries without glomerulonephritis or vasculitis in arterioles, capillaries or venules.
Wegener's granulomatosis	Granulomatous inflammation involving the respiratory tract, and necrotizing vasculitis affecting small to medium sized vessels (e.g., capillaries, venules, arterioles, and arteries). *Necrotizing glomerulonephritis is common.*
Churg-Strauss syndrome	Esinophil-rich and granulomatous inflammation involving the respiratory tract, and necrotizing vasculitis affecting small to medium sized vessels, and associated with asthma and esinophilia.
Microscopic polyangiitis	Necrotizing vasculitis, with few or no immune deposits, affecting small vessels (i.e., capillaries, venules, or arterioles). *Necrotizing arteritis involving small and medium sized arteries may be present. Necrotizing glomerulonephritis is very common. Pulmonary capillaritis often occurs.*
Henoch-Schönlein purpura	Vasculitis, with IgA-dominant immune deposits, affecting small vessels (i.e., capillaries, venules, or arterioles). *Typically involves skin, gut and glomeruli, and is associated with arthralgia or arthritis.*

Source: From Jennette, J.C. et al., Nomenclature of systemic vasculitides — proposal of an international consensus conference, *Arthritis Rheum,* 37, 187, 1994. With permission.

separate entity. Lack of inclusion of MPA in the ACR criteria is in part a reflection of the fact that the importance of the distinction between MPA and PAN has been fully appreciated only relatively recently outside the field of nephrology.

These issues were clarified in 1993 when an international group met in Chapel Hill, North Carolina, to develop a consensus for clear definitions of the nomenclature of the systemic vasculitides. The Chapel Hill Consensus Conference (CHCC) definitions were based on clinical and histological features, as well as the size of the vessel involved (Table 16.2).[14] The CHCC criteria represent an important advance in the definition of vasculitic syndromes, incorporating the separate definition of MPA. The inclusion of the category of MPA, and restriction of PAN from a relatively broad group as classified by the ACR[15] to a much narrower one, represents a significant change. The most important distinguishing feature is the presence of vasculitis in small vessels (arterioles, venules, and capillaries) in MPA. In contrast, PAN excludes patients with GN or small vessel vasculitis while including patients with necrotizing inflammation of medium-sized or small arteries only.[14] The definition of MPA also requires few or no immune deposits in the blood vessels, allowing distinction from HSP and cryoglobulinemic vasculitis. The distinction between these disease entities is important from both therapeutic and prognostic perspectives.

The vasculitides, initially described as the rare condition periarteritis nodosa, and subsequently termed polyarteritis nodosa, became increasingly recognized but for some time continued to be grouped under the term polyarteritis nodosa (Figure 16.3). With the description of distinct vasculitic syndromes, the diseases recognized as polyarteritis nodosa became more confined until the present and very restricted CHCC definition of this entity which now appears a rare syndrome again.[16]

Newer diagnostic tools, such as immunological tests for anti-neutrophil cytoplasmic antibodies (ANCA), have advanced understanding of these disorders with the realization that the ANCA-associated diseases (WG, CSS, MPA) have many features in common. However, at a recent revision meeting, the Chapel Hill group did not feel that ANCA could be used in the current definitions despite their utility in diagnosis because ANCA-negative cases would then be excluded.

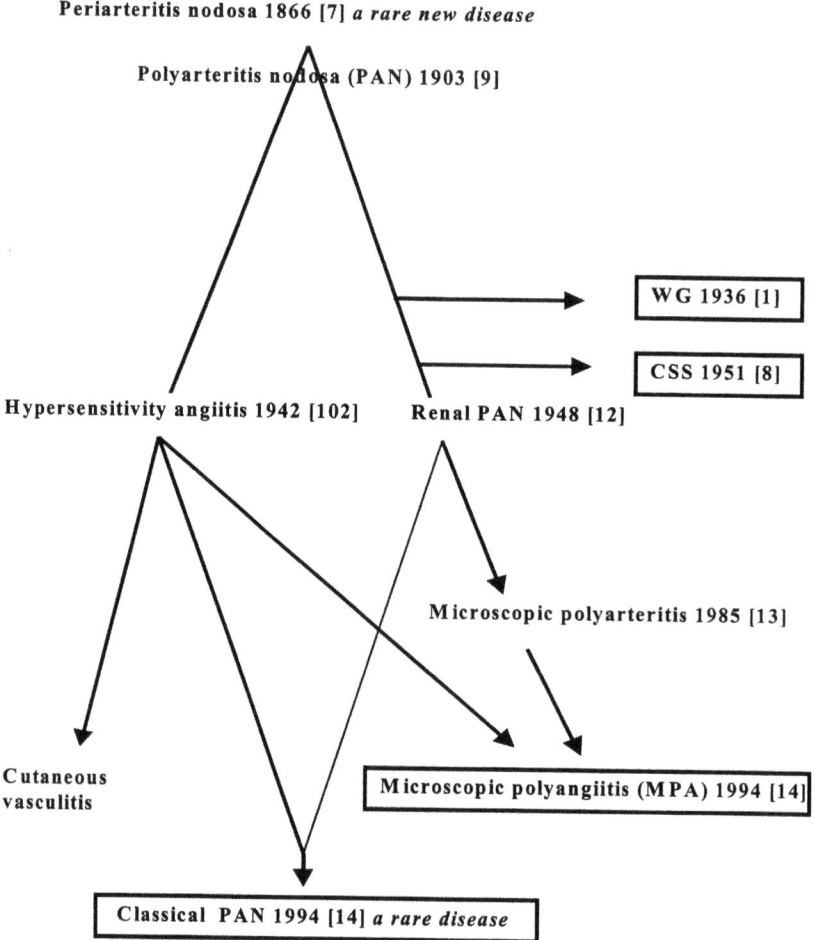

FIGURE 16.3 A historical perspective on the classification of vasculitis. Wegener's granulomatosis (WG), Churg-Strauss syndrome (CSS). Modified from Bacon, P. A., Savage, C., Adu, D., Microscopic polyarteritis (MPA), in *TheVasculitides,* Ansell, B. M., Bacon, P.A., Lie, J. T., Yazici, H., Eds., Chapman & Hall, London, 1996, Chap. 10. With permission.

In spite of these advances, there remains significant overlap among different disease entities, both within and between classification systems. The classification of the vasculitic syndromes has undergone considerable change since the first system in 1952, and will continue to evolve as understanding of disease pathogenesis develops.

C. Epidemiology

Epidemiological study of the systemic vasculitides is hampered by the rarity of these disorders, as well as changing classification criteria and disease definitions. Nevertheless, there are a number of studies providing estimates of their annual incidence. Studies from Olmstead County, U.S.A., suggest an annual incidence of 9.0/million for PAN,[18] and 4.0/million for WG.[19] There are areas, particularly those with a high rate of hepatitis B virus (HBV) infection, where the incidence of PAN may be much higher. In the Alaskan Eskimo population, for example, PAN incidence has been estimated at 77/million.[19] In the U.K., data from the Bath/Bristol area in the 1970s estimated an incidence of PAN of 4.6/million, WG of 0.5/million, and an overall incidence of systemic vasculitis of 10/million.[20] During 1988 to 94, the incidence of systemic vasculitis, excluding giant cell arteritis (GCA), in a single homogenous U.K. health authority area was determined to be greater at 42/million.[21] Specific disease annual incidences were WG (ACR criteria) 8.5/million, PAN (ACR criteria) 2.4/million, MPA (CHCC definition) 3.6/million, CSS (ACR criteria) 1.8/million, and adult HSP (ACR criteria) 13.0/million.[17] Other studies have estimated the incidence of GCA in the U.K. as 13/million adults.[22] Thus, in the U.K., the total incidence of primary systemic vasculitis may be at least 50/million, with an apparent increase in incidence between the 1970s and 1990s. In part, this may relate to increased disease recognition, but there may also be an increasing disease incidence, particularly in the elderly.

Classification criteria can have a profound impact on the estimated incidence and prevalence of disease, as illustrated in the cases of PAN and MPA. In Norfolk, U.K., for the period 1988 to 94, there were eight patients who met the ACR (1990) criteria for a diagnosis of PAN; these patients also met the CHCC definition for MPA, but not for PAN.[16] A further five patients met the CHCC definition for MPA but not the ACR (1990) criteria for PAN. Adopting the CHCC definitions, PAN appears to be becoming an increasingly rare disease, with no patients in the Norfolk study meeting the definition.[16] This may be a real phenomenon related to the diminution in cases of HBV infection in England, but is likely, in large part, to reflect changes in classification and definition. Other factors in addition to classification criteria may have a profound impact on estimates of disease incidence and prevalence. After the introduction of ANCA testing in 1987, the incidence of MPA in Leicester, U.K. increased from 0.5/million (1980 to 86) to 3.3/million (1987 to 89).[23]

Data on geographical and ethnic differences in the epidemiology of the systemic vasculitides are scarce. GCA is the most common primary vasculitis in North America and Europe, with a lower incidence in Southern Europe and Asia. In Olmstead County, U.S.A., the age- and sex-adjusted incidence of GCA in adults over 50 years of age was 178/million.[24] This population contains a high proportion of people of Scandinavian origin, which may explain the high incidence of GCA. In northwestern Spain, the incidence of GCA was 66/million adults aged over 50 years.[25] Takayasu's arteritis is said to be more common in Japan, India, and the Far East than in Europe and North America, though recent data challenge this view.[26] By contrast, WG and GCA are said to be rare in India.

III. A GENERAL APPROACH TO THE PATIENT WITH SUSPECTED VASCULITIS

In our opinion, the most important issue is to make an early diagnosis of the presence of some sort of vasculitis, confirm it by biopsy wherever possible, and assess the extent and severity of disease. This allows therapy to be commenced early, before irreversible tissue damage has developed. The precise details of classification, which are important for long-term prognosis, can then be determined at leisure. An algorithm for our approach to the patient with suspected vasculitis is shown in Figure 16.4.

A. CLINICAL

The systemic vasculitides are multisystem diseases and, as a consequence, have protean manifestations and a wide differential diagnosis, including infectious and neoplastic disorders.

1. Disease Activity and Damage

The clinical features seen with active disease reflect the inflammatory process in the organ involved. The consequence of persistent inflammation, if not treated with appropriate immunosuppressive therapy, is the development of organ damage including the formation of fibrotic scars. The clinical manifestations of disease activity span a spectrum that overlaps with those of damage. This is

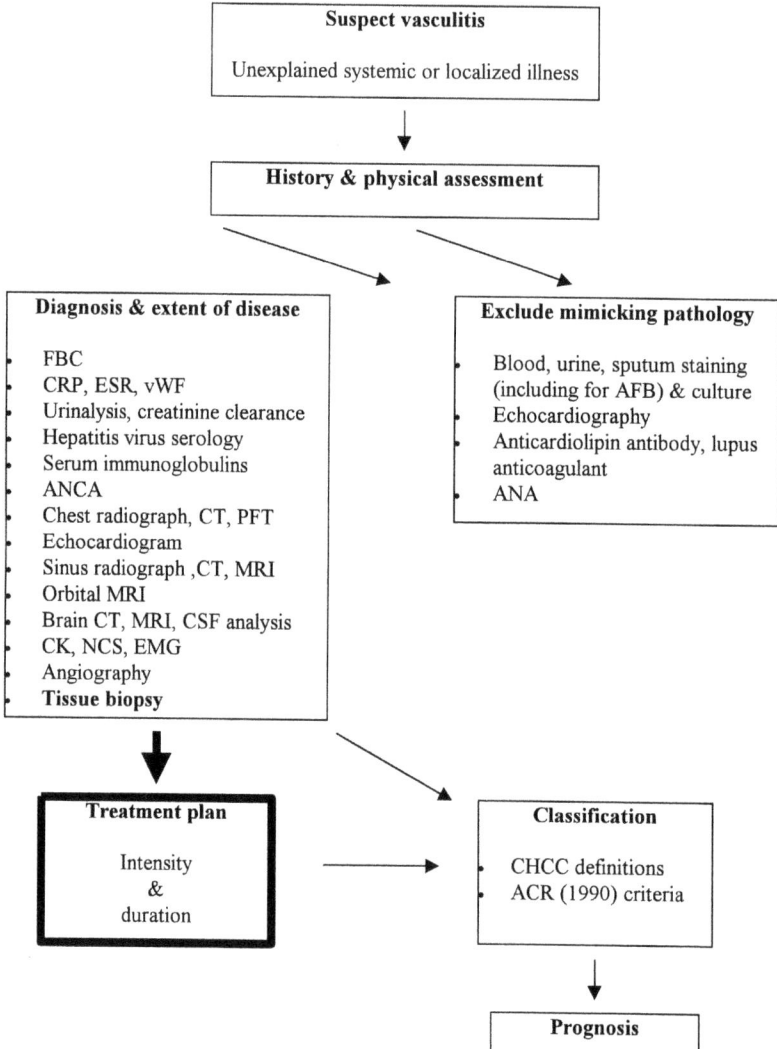

FIGURE 16.4 An approach to a patient with suspected vasculitis. Full blood count (FBC), C reactive protein (CRP), anti-neutrophil cytoplasmic antibody (ANCA), computerized tomography (CT), pulmonary function tests (PFT), magnetic resonance imaging (MRI), cerebrospinal fluid (CSF), creatine kinase (CK), nerve conduction studies (NCS), electromyography (EMG), acid fast bacilli (AFB), American College of Rheumatology (ACR), Chapel Hill Consensus Conference (CHCC).

illustrated in MPA, where disease activity in the form of vasculitic GN and damage in the form of fibrotic glomeruli may both manifest as hypertension. On the other hand, there are features which are more specific for either activity or damage. A urinary sediment with casts, for example, would be suggestive of an active vasculitic GN, and active nasal disease in WG is associated with crusting and epistaxis. The consequence of untreated active disease in the latter case is destruction of nasal cartilage with the development of the typical saddle nose appearance, representing irreversible damage. The differentiation between activity and damage has important implications for therapy (as discussed by Carruthers et al. in Chapter 34) as the former, by definition, is reversible and so merits the use of immunosuppressive therapy, whereas the irreversible nature of damage means that aggressive immunosuppression is inappropriate. The goal for successful management therefore lies in the early recognition of active inflammation, thus allowing the institution of treatment to prevent the development of organ damage.

A number of clinical tools have been developed which allow the differentiation between activity and damage and provide quantitative measures of these parameters, useful in the management of patients. The most widely used measure of disease activity, and the standard in the large multicenter European collaborative trials in progress, is the Birmingham Vasculitis Activity Score (BVAS).[27] BVAS consists of a set of clinical items divided into nine organ-based systems. Each item has a weighted score attached to it, and each system is ascribed a maximum score. An item (e.g., dyspnoea) is scored in BVAS if it is present, and considered by the physician to be secondary to *active* vasculitis as opposed to other pathology such as intercurrent infection, drug toxicity, or damage related to the vasculitis. The advantage of routine application of a disease index such as BVAS is that it can lead the clinician unfamiliar with these complex multisystem diseases to a clearer picture of disease extent and severity than is apparent at first glance. A number of other measures of activity have been developed specifically for use in WG (the Groningen Index[28] and the Disease Extent Index[29]) but their utility in other vasculitides is less clear.

Damage measured using the Systemic Necrotizing Vasculitis Damage Index (SNVDI)[30] includes no items covering upper airways damage, a significant feature of WG. This is included in the Vasculitis Damage Index (VDI),[31] which divides items into ten organ-based systems with an additional category for drug-induced damage. The VDI is largely based on clinical assessment, though there is some requirement for investigations including imaging (e.g., orbital wall destruction requiring the use of either plain radiography, computerized tomography (CT), or magnetic resonance imaging (MRI)). Though there is significant overlap with the SNVDI, the VDI has been shown to be more sensitive to change.[31] The development of internal organ system damage has important prognostic implications with high damage scores associated with more severe disease.[32] In addition, most disease-related damage tends to occur early after presentation,[32] highlighting the need for early diagnosis and institution of treatment.

Features of both activity and damage are incorporated in the Five Factor Score (FFS) developed by Guillevin et al.[33] which includes the following five items: serum creatinine > 140µmol/l, proteinuria >1g/day, severe gastrointestinal tract involvement, cardiomyopathy, and central nervous system involvement. The FFS has been found to correlate with mortality in PAN, CSS, and MPA.[33,34] Recognition of involvement of these systems at the stage of early active inflammation allows for the institution of appropriate therapy while there is still reversibility.

2. General Clinical Features

The presentation of systemic vasculitis may be nonspecific, with symptoms such as malaise, fever, and weight loss. This, together with the fact that these disorders may mimic other conditions, often leads to diagnostic delay. The large National Institutes of Health (NIH) study of 158 patients with WG showed that while the diagnosis was made within 3 months of onset of disease in 42% of patients, it was delayed for 5 to 16 years in 8%.[35] A recent survey of a patient group in the U.K. suggests that there is still a significant delay in time to diagnosis.

In addition to nonspecific symptoms, features of specific organ involvement must be sought. These become more overt with increasing duration of inflammation at that site, and more specific once irreversible damage has occurred as a consequence of active inflammation. However, waiting for characteristic signs such as nasal bridge collapse to develop is leaving the diagnosis too late. The pattern of organ involvement often changes with disease duration. This is illustrated in WG where involvement of the kidney and eye is less frequent at disease onset (18% and 15% of patients, respectively) but common later in the course of the disease (77% and 52% of patients, respectively).[35]

There is considerable variation in disease course between the vasculitic syndromes. While PAN is usually an acute disease that develops within days or weeks, MPA and WG often have an initial grumbling course.[13,35] In addition to a difference in onset, the long-term course of the vasculitides vary, with WG and MPA characterized by episodes of relapse and remission, but PAN often being a monophasic illness. Savage et al.[13] reported that 12 of 33 (36.4%) patients with MPA relapsed. Others have shown less frequent relapses in this disease (25.3%), with the median time to relapse being 24 months.[36] In WG the relapse rate appears higher at 44%, with a median time to relapse of 42 months.[36] PAN, on the other hand, has a lower relapse rate of the order of 10 to 20%. There is also a difference between the relapse rates in the different phases of a vasculitic syndrome. With advances in therapy, in the ANCA-associated group, vasculitis of the kidney is often seen as monophasic, while the more granulomatous aspects of disease such as airway involvement relapse more frequently. The pattern of organ involvement at relapse does not necessarily mimic the original presentation, and new organs may be involved.[36] In addition, the clinical features at relapse are usually less severe than at initial presentation, with less damage accumulated after relapse than at presentation.[32] A possible explanation for this observation is earlier recognition of a relapse due to heightened clinical awareness.

The prognosis of many vasculitides has improved significantly following the introduction of cyclophosphamide (CP),[37] changing them from diseases with high early mortalities to those with a chronic grumbling courses characterized by relapse and remission. However, the issue of early and late drug toxicity has become increasingly recognized and must be taken into account in clinical assessment. A full discussion of clinical features which may have an iatrogenic basis is beyond the scope of this chapter, though the following serve to illustrate the spectrum. Bone marrow suppression, with an associated risk of infection, is a potential complication of many immunosuppressive agents. The features of ensuing infection can often be difficult to distinguish from, and indeed may precipitate a flare of, active vasculitis. Of the late manifestations, bladder carcinoma is an increasingly recognized complication of CP,[38] and the resultant hematuria needs to be distinguished from the glomerular hematuria seen with GN.

3. Specific Vasculitides

a. Polyarteritis Nodosa (PAN)

PAN affects men and women equally, with an average age at onset of between 40 and 60 years. The majority of patients present with constitutional symptoms and, although the clinical presentation may be with limited disease, most have severe manifestations with multiorgan involvement and appear acutely ill. Myalgia is frequent and muscle tenderness is usual. Arthralgia is often present and is often associated with myalgia. Arthritis is generally asymmetrical, involving the lower limbs.[39] The skin is involved in 25 to 60% of patients with systemic PAN[40] and may take one of several forms, including livedo reticularis, which is common, and purpura, which is typically petechial or papular but may be bullous or vesicular. Subcutaneous nodules are seen but are uncommon and transient.

Mononeuritis multiplex, the most frequent feature (70%) in a series of 182 PAN patients,[41] may also present at disease onset.[42] Motor and sensory signs are usually asymmetric and affect predominantly the lower limbs, especially the sciatic nerve and its peroneal and tibial branches.[40] Motor deficit often occurs abruptly. Symmetrical peripheral sensory neuropathy may occur but is less common, as are cranial nerve palsies which occur in less than 2% of patients. Central nervous system involvement is rare, but ischemic stroke and cerebral hemorrhage have been described and may be due to either vasculitis or malignant hypertension.

Renal involvement occurs in between 30 to 80% of patients.[40] Nephropathy is secondary to small or medium vessel arteritis, with stenosis and aneurysm formation and consequent renal infarcts. In contrast to MPA, GN is not a feature. Hypertension develops as a result of renal artery involvement and affects 33% of patients.[41] Involvement of the ureter, due to periureteral vasculitis and secondary fibrosis, is rare but can lead to renal insufficiency.[43] Renal or perirenal hematomas may result from the rupture of microaneurysms.[44] Orchitis is a classic symptom, and indeed is one of the ACR criteria for the classification of PAN, though is more common in PAN related to HBV.[45]

Gastrointestinal vasculitis is one of the most severe manifestations of PAN, with marked abdominal pain secondary to bowel ischemia being an early feature. Diarrhea, hemorrhage, and perforation, which occurs in about 5% of patients, may be seen.[46,47] Involvement of the small bowel is more common than of the colon or stomach. Infarction and hematoma of the liver can occur.[48] Acalculous cholecystitis is found in 17% of patients,[49] and pancreatitis has been reported.[50] Clinically significant cardiac disease is uncommon in PAN but when present usually manifests as congestive cardiac failure. Pulmonary involvement is rare in PAN.

b. Churg-Strauss Syndrome (CSS)

The mean age of onset of CSS is 35 to 40 years,[40] with a reported male:female ratio ranging from 1.1 to 3.[51] CSS is characterized by the presence of asthma, which commonly predates the development of vasculitis. Based on a series of 16 patients and a review of a further 138 from the literature, Lanham et al.[51] identified three phases of CSS, though not all patients progress sequentially through them. The initial phase, which may last for many years, consists of allergic rhinitis and nasal polyposis, frequently followed by asthma. In contrast with other forms of asthma, it usually begins relatively late in life, around the age of 35 years.[51] The severity and frequency of asthma attacks often increase until the onset of the vasculitis. The second phase of the disease is characterized by constitutional symptoms, a peripheral blood eosinophilia, and a tissue eosinophilia which may manifest as an eosinophilic pneumonia with pulmonary infiltrates on chest radiography (Figure 16.5). Indeed, the development of constitutional symptoms in a patient with asthma should raise suspicion of CSS. The eosinophilic infiltrative disease may relapse and remit for years before systemic vasculitis develops. The vasculitic phase usually develops within three years of the onset of the asthma, but may be delayed. A shorter duration of asthma prior to the onset of vasculitis is associated with a poorer prognosis. Interestingly, dramatic remission of the asthma has been reported when vasculitis emerges.

As with all the diseases discussed, vasculitis commonly affects several organ systems in any individual. Of 23 patients with CSS seen over a 14-year period, systemic vasculitis involving two or more extra-pulmonary organs occurred in 22 patients.[52] Arthralgia, arthritis, myalgia, and myositis are all relatively common.[52] Cutaneous disease is also frequently seen. In the original report by Churg and Strauss, 54% of patients had nodules, and 62% had purpura,[8] though other studies have reported lower rates of cutaneous disease, with nodules and purpura being seen in only 9% and 26% of patients, respectively.[52]

The nervous system is the most common extra-pulmonary site of disease, involved in 18 of 23 patients in one report.[52] The clinical features of peripheral neuropathy in CSS have been studied; the initial symptom was an acute onset of tingling or painful paraesthesia in the legs in 23 of 28 patients and in the arms in the other 5.[53] In the initial phase, a mononeuritis multiplex is usually seen which often evolves into an asymmetrical or symmetrical peripheral neuropathy.[53]

Gastrointestinal tract and cardiac involvement represent the most severe end of the spectrum and account for much of the mortality seen in CSS. The gastrointestinal tract is involved in about 50% of patients,[8] with symptoms including abdominal pain, diarrhea, and bleeding occurring commonly, while perforation and infarction are seen less often.[46] Cardiac involvement has been found in up to 64% of autopsy cases,[8] with pathological findings including eosinophilic pericarditis, interstitial myocarditis, endomyocardial fibrosis, or epicardial coronary vasculitis. Clinically evident cardiac disease is much less common, but it is important to look specifically for this (e.g., with echocardiography) before there is severe myocardial dysfunction and irreversible damage. This is particularly so in patients with high or persistent eosinophilia, since this cell is probably directly involved in cardiac pathology.

Estimates of the proportion of patients with CSS who have renal involvement varies widely from 16% to 84%.[54,55] Although renal disease in CSS is generally considered to be less severe than

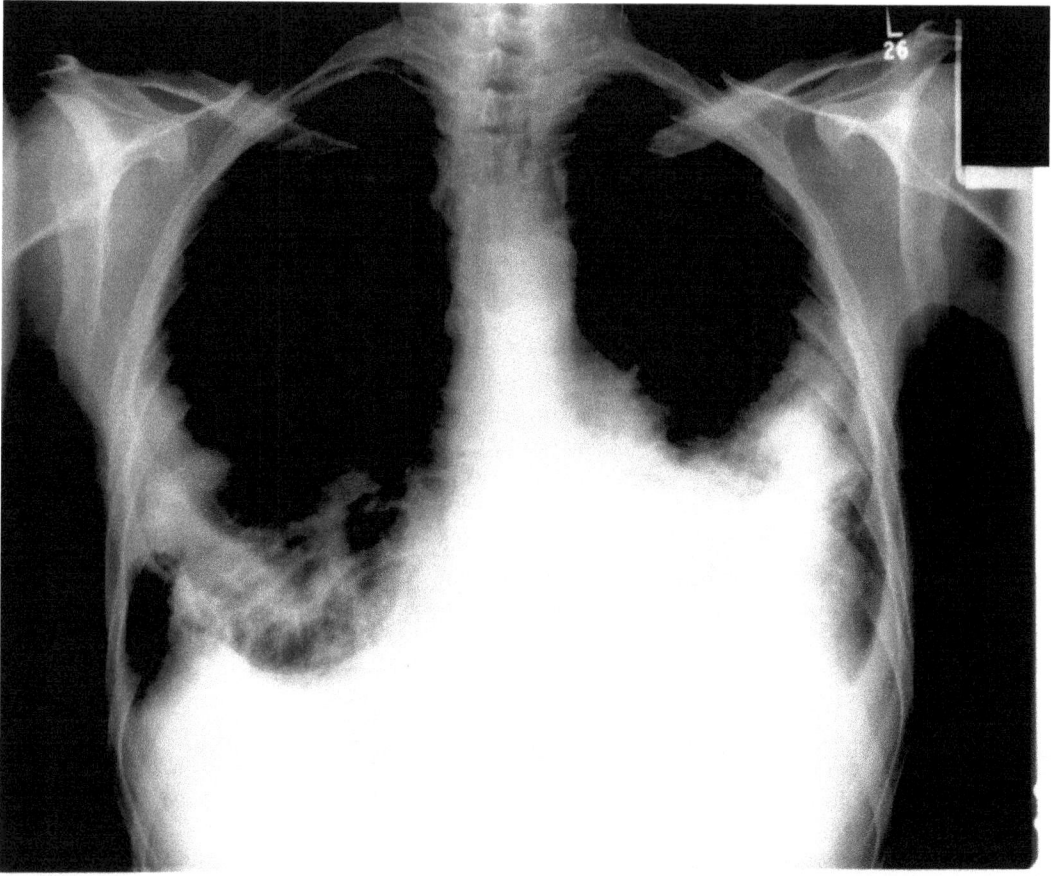

FIGURE 16.5 Pulmonary infiltrates in a patient with Churg-Strauss syndrome.

in MPA or WG, the histological picture is identical and the progression can be the same. In a series of 19 patients with CSS treated at the Hammersmith Hospital, U.K., four had a serum creatinine > 500μmol/l and two required dialysis, highlighting the potential severity of renal disease in this condition.[55]

c. Wegener's Granulomatosis (WG)

Data from the NIH suggests that WG affects both sexes equally, and occurs with a mean age of 41 years.[35] There is some evidence for a higher rate of onset in the winter,[2,56] though this has not been confirmed in other studies.[57]

In WG there is a predilection for involvement of the upper and lower respiratory tracts and kidneys, forming the classical triad described in this condition. Disease confined to the respiratory tract is well recognized. This may progress to generalized disease with renal involvement.[58] Nasal involvement is characterized by inflammatory rhinitis, with mucosal ulceration, epistaxis, and crusting. Destruction of the nasal cartilage by inflammatory tissue causes nasal septal perforation and the characteristic saddle nose deformity (Figure 16.6). Sinusitis is common and the damaged mucosal membranes may be a focus of recurrent bacterial infection. In addition to the direct morbidity, such infection may drive flares of systemic vasculitis. Otitis media may lead to a conductive deafness. Sensori-neural deafness with vasculitic involvement of the eighth cranial nerve may also be seen, though it is a less common cause of hearing loss. Salivary gland involvement has been described.[59] The subglottic region of the trachea is often affected by granulomatous

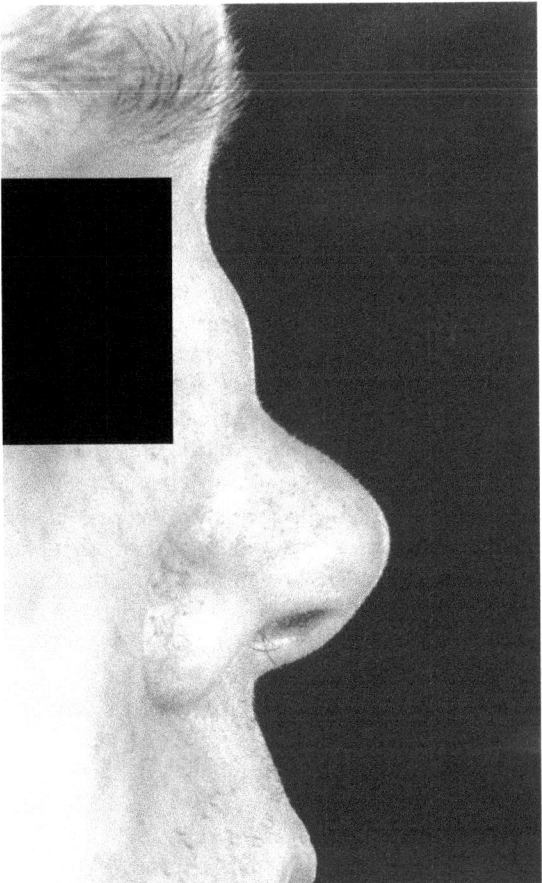

FIGURE 16.6 Saddle nose deformity in a patient with Wegener's granulomatosis.

tissue which can cause significant tracheal stenosis with hoarseness, stridor, and respiratory compromise. Such tracheal involvement is more common in children where it is seen in almost 50% of cases compared to 15% of adults.[60] A failure to respond to immunosuppression may necessitate a tracheostomy.

Pulmonary symptoms are found in 60 to 80% of patients and include cough, dyspnea, hemoptysis, and chest pain. Granulomatous pulmonary inflammation produces nodular radiographic densities which may cavitate. Alveolar capillaritis, on the other hand, may cause fleeting inflitrates through to massive pulmonary hemorrhage. The severity may be initially underestimated since large falls in hemoglobin may be seen with clinically very limited hemoptysis. This symptom must therefore be taken seriously in all cases, particularly as it is often associated with rapidly progressive renal involvement — the "pulmonary-renal syndrome."

In a series of patients from the NIH, 18% had renal disease at onset but 77% subsequently developed GN.[35] The GN is characterized by focal necrosis, crescent formation, and the absence or paucity of immune deposits.[61] The most common early abnormality is microscopic hematuria. Macroscopic hematuria and the nephrotic syndrome are uncommon. In many cases the GN is rapidly progressive and may lead to irreversible renal failure.

Ocular involvement may manifest as conjunctivitis, scleritis, uveitis, retinal vasculitis, or optic neuritis. Proptosis due to retro-orbital granulomatous tissue is occasionally seen and is particularly important because of the risk of optic nerve ischemia and visual loss.

Skin involvement manifests as nail-fold infarcts, purpuric rashes, and ulcers. Arthralgia and arthritis are often seen. Both peripheral and central nervous system involvement may occur, with mononeuritis multiplex being the most usual manifestation. Gastrointestinal manifestations are uncommon in WG, though cholecystitis, inflammatory ileocolitis, hemorrhage, and bowel infarction have all been described.[62,63]

d. Microscopic Polyangiitis (MPA)

Men are affected more frequently than women with the male:female ratio ranging from 1 to 1.8.[13,64] The average age of onset is approximately 50 years. MPA shares many features with the vasculitis of WG, though with little granulomatous disease.[13] An indolent initial course with symptoms such as arthralgia may be seen several months or years before the more severe systemic phase of disease.[13] Constitutional features are seen at diagnosis in 56 to 76% of patients.[13,65] Cutaneous involvement is common and was present in 62% of patients in one study, manifesting as purpura (41%), livedo (13%), nodules (13%), and urticaria (4%).[34] Arthralgia and myalgia were also seen.

The kidneys are usually affected with GN and, indeed, this is one of the major characteristics of MPA. Impaired renal function is common (a serum creatinine value of >120μmol/l was seen in 70% in one study[34]) and patients not infrequently present with renal failure, particularly the elderly. Microscopic hematuria and proteinuria are often found. Hypertension affects fewer patients and is less severe than in classical PAN. In a recent French study, renal manifestations were seen in 79% of 85 patients with MPA and, of these, 81% had proteinuria with 15% having the nephrotic syndrome, 67% had hematuria, and 34% had hypertension.[34] As in WG, the renal disease may deteriorate rapidly and is associated with increased mortality.[34]

Pulmonary involvement, seen in a quarter of patients in the study by Guillevin et al.,[34] may manifest as pulmonary hemorrhage, which can be massive and fatal; pneumonitis; or pleuritis. The concurrence of kidney and lung involvement constitutes a pulmonary-renal syndrome similar to that observed in Goodpasture's syndrome or WG.[66]

Peripheral nerve and gastrointestinal involvement are seen but are less frequent than in PAN. As in all the vasculitic illnesses, gastrointestinal involvement in MPA has protean manifestations including abdominal pain, weight loss, hematemesis, melena, perforation, cholecystitis, appendicitis, and pancreatitis.[34] In contrast to WG, ocular and nasopharyngeal symptoms are less common in MPA.

e. Henoch-Schönlein Purpura (HSP)

HSP is a small-vessel vasculitis that is more frequent in children than adults. The median age of onset is 4 years, and in school-aged children its incidence is as high as 13.5/100,000.[67] It is often preceded by an upper respiratory tract infection and is more common in the winter.[68]

The most common feature is a vasculitic rash (Figure 16.7), which usually occurs in dependent or pressure-bearing areas such as the legs or buttocks. It is usually apparent at presentation, and almost invariably develops during the course of the disease. Bleeding into the lesions may occur, especially in the elderly. In young children, facial involvement and subcutaneous edema are also features. Arthralgia or arthritis is the second most common symptom, frequently affecting the ankles and knees. It precedes the rash in 25% of children. Renal involvement in the form of GN is seen in 50% of patients and is serious in 10%.[69] Usually, renal disease occurs within three months of the onset of rash. The spectrum of renal disease varies from isolated microscopic hematuria to a nephritic/nephrotic syndrome with renal failure. Abdominal pain with gastrointestinal bleeding also occurs; the duodenum is the most commonly involved area, though gastric, jejunal, colonic, and rectal erosions may be seen.[67] Intussusception, either ileoileal or ileocolic, occurs in 1 to 5% of patients and is usually a consequence of the development of a submucosal hematoma.[70] Other gastrointestinal complications of HSP include major hemorrhage, intestinal perforation,[71] pancreatitis,[72] and protein-losing enteropathy.[73] Renal and gastrointestinal diseases are less common in children aged under 2 years.[74]

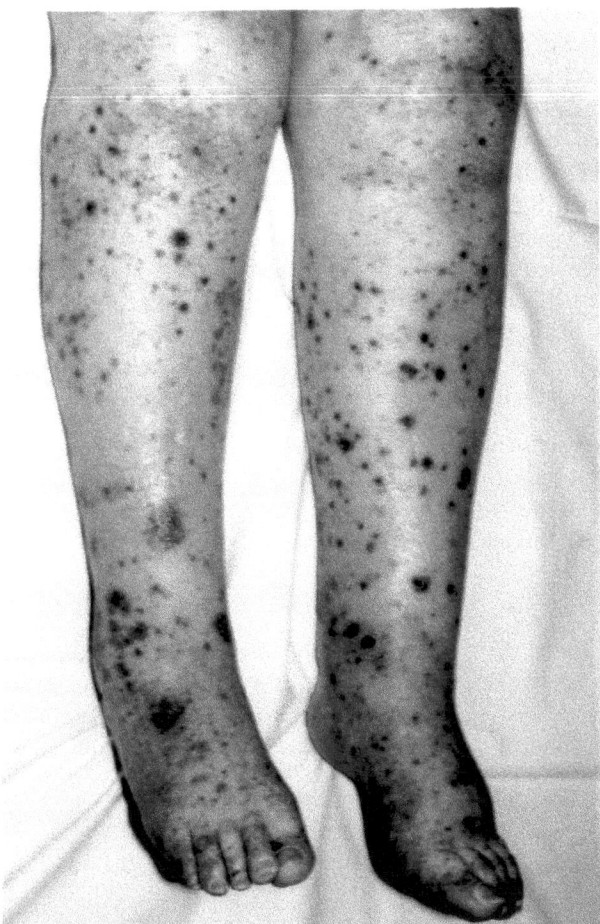

FIGURE 16.7 Vasculitic rash in a patient with Henoch-Schönlein purpura.

The disease course of HSP is variable, and though uniphasic in the majority, is polyphasic in 10 to 20% and has a chronic, continuous course in less than 5%. The prognosis of HSP is usually very good, although there is some morbidity and even mortality associated with gastrointestinal and renal diseases.[74]

f. Localized Vasculitis

The vasculitic syndromes discussed so far are multisystem diseases. There are, however, rare instances when only a single organ is involved. In some cases, localized vasculitis is the first manifestation of systemic disease, with multiple organs involved at a later stage.[75] In other instances it may represent a truly localized disease. These cases are more than just a clinical curiosity. They help shed light on factors determining tissue tropism in vasculitis. A long-term remission that has been reported in cases of localized vasculitis following surgical resection of involved tissue[76,77] is consistent with the hypothesis that the local microenvironment attracts and maintains inflammatory cells, with its surgical excision being sufficient to remove the factors that initiate and maintain relapse.

Cerebral.   Primary angiitis of the central nervous system (PACNS) is rare. It primarily affects the leptomeninges and cerebral cortex with involvement of small- and medium-sized arteries as well as veins and venules. A spectrum of histological appearances may be seen ranging from a granulomatous to a necrotizing angiitis.[78] From the early descriptions of the disease in 1959, and up to 1986, only 46 cases were reported in the literature.[79] However, with the greater availability of cerebral angiography, the disease has become increasingly described. The clinical features of pathologically documented cases have been reviewed.[78] The disease is more common in men (69% vs. 31%), with a mean age of onset of 46 years. Symptoms include decreased cognition (83%), diffuse neurologic dysfunction (68%), headache (56%), seizure (30%), stroke (14%), and cerebral hemorrhage (12%).[78] Although cerebrospinal fluid (CSF) analysis, MRI, and cerebral angiography are useful in the assessment of patients with suspected PACNS, histologic confirmation with biopsy of the leptomeninges and underlying cortex remains the gold standard and is important to exclude mimicking conditions, including lymphoproliferative diseases and sarcoidosis.[80] Early experience with PACNS led to the conclusion that it was a progressive disease that was almost always fatal,[78] an impression clearly influenced by the fact that most cases were identified postmortem. A recent analysis, however, suggested a considerably more favorable prognosis, at least for a subgroup of patients.[81]

Limited PAN. Although usually a systemic disease, localized forms of PAN are recognized at sites such as skin,[82] appendix,[83] gallbladder,[84] and testis.[75] There is little data available to help predict which patients will progress to systemic disease, though one report has suggested that seropositivity for rheumatoid factor or antinuclear antibody may be associated with such progression.[85]

B. INVESTIGATIONS

Early recognition so that prompt treatment can be instituted to reverse disease activity and prevent organ damage is the key to managing patients with vasculitis (as discussed by Carruthers et al. in Chapter 34). This requires a high index of clinical suspicion for these syndromes. Investigation of patients *suspected* on clinical grounds to have vasculitis must be directed towards:

1. Defining the presence of active vasculitis.
2. Defining the extent of organ injury.
3. Classifying the vasculitis.

In patients with *known* vasculitis, investigations are important in determining disease activity. In this context, investigations are often necessary to distinguish between active vasculitis and concurrent infection which may be indistinguishable on the basis of clinical assessment alone.

Organ involvement with active vasculitis may be suggested by clinical features. However, despite a lack of symptoms and signs in a particular organ, abnormalities may be found on laboratory investigation. Patients with WG and no clinical respiratory features may have pulmonary nodules on chest radiography. Patients with PAN and no abdominal symptoms or signs may have abnormalities on mesenteric angiography. Even renal involvement can antedate clinical evidence of disease. There is no consensus as to how far patients should be investigated for occult disease, but the following serve as useful principles. First, the greater the clinical index of suspicion of an abnormality and the importance of documenting its presence from the viewpoint of therapy or prognosis, the greater the justification for extensive and invasive investigation. Thus, for example, in a patient presenting with apparently isolated gallbladder PAN diagnosed histologically following cholecystectomy, extensive investigation including mesenteric and renal angiography, and nerve conduction studies (NCS), would be appropriate to determine whether the disease was truly limited to the gallbladder as this information would have important prognostic and therapeutic implications. Second, the utility of investigation at presentation is that it provides a baseline from which subsequent investigations can be compared.

1. Blood Tests

A number of laboratory abnormalities are common to most of the vasculitides. High values of inflammatory markers such as the erythrocyte sedimentation rate (ESR) or better, the C-reactive protein (CRP), are generally seen during active systemic vasculitis. Such markers clearly lack specificity and may be raised in other conditions, including infection. It should be noted, however, that with more localized disease, inflammatory markers may be normal.[76]

The full blood count is often abnormal in patients with vasculitis. Anemia is common and may be multifactorial, related, for example, to chronic disease and blood loss. A thrombocytosis may reflect the ongoing inflammatory process. Esinophilia is common in CSS and may be seen in PAN and WG. It serves as a useful marker for disease activity in these conditions.

A number of blood tests reflect involvement of particular organs. Serum creatinine may be raised in patients with renal involvement, though a rise above the upper limit of normal is not seen until 50% of renal function is lost and more sensitive assessments of renal function, such as creatinine clearance, should also be used. Liver function tests are often abnormal, reflecting hepatic disease which is often subclinical. Creatine kinase (CK) may be elevated in patients with involvement of skeletal muscle or myocardium.

The difficulty often encountered in distinguishing between active vasculitis and infection has led to interest in a number of blood tests including procalcitonin (PCT). PCT has recently been proposed as a useful discriminator between infection (where the PCT concentration is high) and active vasculitis (where the PCT concentration is normal).[86] Others have had difficulty confirming this and further work is required.

High levels of von-Willebrand factor (vWF), stored in endothelial granules and released on endothelial cell stimulation or injury, reflect the extent of vascular damage. In our experience vWF estimation has a rather limited utility in monitoring disease activity, taking much longer (often months) to normalize after the induction of remission than the CRP or even the ESR. However, it can be useful in initial disease assessment, and in distinguishing late flares from infection.

ANCA are assuming an increasing role in the diagnosis of patients with suspected vasculitis. The first description of antibodies to neutrophil cytoplasmic antigens was in patients with segmental necrotizing GN.[87] Since then, considerable effort has focused on their study, both as a tool to aid the diagnosis and classification of vasculitic syndromes and in terms of their role in disease pathogenesis. ANCA comprise a heterogeneous group of autoantibodies routinely detected by indirect immunofluorescence, which distinguishes three types assigned the acromyms c (cytoplasmic pattern) ANCA, p (perinuclear pattern) ANCA, and a (atypical) ANCA. van der Woude et al.[88] showed that one such antibody, directed against proteinase 3 (PR3) in neutrophil azurophilic granules and giving a cANCA staining pattern, was apparently specific and relatively sensitive for active WG. Wider experience has shown it can be present in other vasculitides as well as non-vasculitic diseases, including infection. The sensitivity of cANCA, which depends on the extent and activity of disease, is about 50% in patients with limited disease, and approaches 95% for those with active WG with renal involvement. The pANCA staining pattern is often mediated by autoantibodies to myeloperoxidase (MPO), but may involve antibodies to lactoferrin and other components of the neutrophil granule. Approximately 80% of patients with MPA and CSS have pANCA, and in these diseases the dominant specificity is for MPO. However, as pANCA can occur in other more common disorders such as RA and inflammatory bowel disease, its positive predictive value is limited when compared to that of cANCA unless the detailed antibody specificity is further defined. ANCA by immunofluorescence has several potential clinical applications. It is seen to have utility as a screening tool, though the result must be interpreted in light of the clinical condition of the patient. In addition, a positive ANCA in a patient with known vasculitis is helpful in indicating a high risk of renal disease. Furthermore, there is some evidence that in patients with ANCA positive vasculitis, a rising titer may predict disease relapse,[89] though this on its own should not lead to a change in immunosuppressive therapy.

Serum immunoglobulins should be measured; high levels of IgA are seen in HSP. Hepatitis B and C virus serology should always be checked and, if indicative of current infection, it raises the possibility of PAN or cryoglobulinemic vasculitis. Other viruses, including CMV, parvovirus,[90] and HIV[91] have been associated with vasculitis and investigation for these may be appropriate.

2. Radiology and Other Organ System Investigations

Pulmonary. Pulmonary involvement may be evidenced by abnormalities on a plain chest radiograph. These may take the form of diffuse infiltrates (e.g., in CSS) or pulmonary nodules which may cavitate (e.g., in WG). Occasionally, abnormalities may not be seen on the plain radiograph, and if clinically suspected should be investigated by CT; we have seen several patients with WG in whom plain chest radiographs were normal but CT demonstrated nodules, a finding that influenced patient management. Pulmonary function tests (PFT) may show reduced lung volumes with a restrictive pattern and reduced transfer factor for carbon monoxide (CO) in patients with pulmonary infiltrates or fibrosis. Pulmonary hemorrhage produces the characteristic "bat's wing" picture on plain radiograph and is associated with an increased CO transfer factor. Biopsy of focal pulmonary lesions, either transthoracic CT-guided or open, is often necessary. Unfortunately, the simpler transbronchial biopsy is not usually helpful. Involvement of the subglottic region in WG can be demonstrated by an abnormality in the flow volume loop.

Renal. In addition to measurement of the serum creatinine and creatinine clearance, urine microscopy should be performed for red blood cells and casts. Red blood cell morphology can give an indication of whether the hematuria is glomerular or nonglomerular. In cases of suspected PAN, angiography is useful for demonstrating the presence of narrowed tapered arteries and small aneurysms, often at the branching point of vessels. Renal biopsy is often required in cases of suspected vasculitis.

Gastrointestinal. Gastrointestinal vasculitis is notoriously difficult to confirm. Mesenteric angiography, CT scanning of the abdomen,[92] and radiolabeled white cell scans have been used in some instances, but laparoscopy or laparotomy with resection of ischemic looking bowel for histological assessment may be necessary. Abdominal ultrasound is useful for intussusception in HSP.

Cardiovascular. Cardiovascular disease should be investigated with an estimate of CK which may be elevated secondary to myocarditis. A 12-lead electrocardiogram may reveal an arrhythmia, pericarditis, or left ventricular hypertrophy. A plain chest radiograph may show an increase in the cardio-thoracic ratio. Echocardiography can demonstrate left ventricular hypertrophy or regional or global wall movement abnormality and is also useful in excluding vasculitic mimics such as SBE and atrial myxoma. Involvement of large arteries with TA or GCA can be investigated with conventional or MR angiography, which may show areas of stenosis, occlusion, dilatation, or wall thickening. The differentiation from atherosclerotic disease, particularly in the elderly population, may be difficult. Occasionally, cardiac catheterization, coronary angiography, and myocardial biopsy may be necessary.

Neuromuscular. Peripheral nerve involvement can be assessed with motor and sensory NCS. Sensory nerve action potentials are usually reduced in amplitude, while the conduction velocity is often maintained, consistent with the predominantly axonal degeneration usually seen.[53] Biopsy of the sural nerve is often carried out, with the yield highest if prior electrical testing has suggested involvement of this nerve. Electromyography (EMG) can provide evidence of myositis and, if performed unilaterally, allows for open muscle biopsy from the contralateral limb for histological diagnosis. The use of MRI also allows assessment of muscle involvement and determination of the most appropriate site for biopsy. Central nervous system involvement should be investigated with MRI, which may reveal evidence of infarction or, less commonly, hemorrhage, and is more sensitive than CT.[78] Cerebral angiography is useful, but may be normal in up to 40% of pathologically documented cases of PACNS.[93,94] CSF analysis is abnormal in 80 to 90% of patients with pathologically defined PACNS, with a modest pleocytosis and elevated protein level.[78] Increased IgG and the presence of oligoclonal bands are occasionally detected.

Other. The detailed assessment of patients with systemic vasculitis often requires a combined approach from several specialties. Assessment of the nose, throat, eyes, and retro-orbital region may require specialist endoscopy, CT or MRI, and slit lamp examination or ultrasound to assess the posterior chamber of the eye.

Future Directions.   Advances in understanding the pathology of vasculitis will allow alternative, and more specific, means of imaging sites of active vasculitis. The process of vascular endothelial cell activation, with the expression of adhesion molecules for leucocytes, is important for the localization of inflammatory responses and vascular injury. The use of radiolabeled monoclonal antibodies with specificities for these molecules may allow imaging of such endothelial cell activation.[95] We are currently assessing methods of measuring vascular endothelial function in patients with vasculitis. Using the noninvasive technique of high resolution ultrasound to measure the increase in brachial artery diameter in response to increased blood flow,[96] a process mediated by the flow-dependent release of nitric oxide from the vascular endothelium,[97] we have shown impaired vascular endothelial function in primary systemic vasculitis.[98] Preliminary data suggests that such changes may be reversible with suppression of the vasculitic process and we are exploring this further.

3. Histology

The gold standard for a positive diagnosis of vasculitis remains the histological finding of fibrinoid necrosis or the presence of granulomata and vessel wall inflammation.[99] Clearly the highest yield is from biopsy of affected tissue, as defined either clinically or on the basis of investigations. Biopsy is usually of skin, nasal mucosa, lung, peripheral nerve, kidney, or temporal artery. In rare instances it is necessary to biopsy other tissues such as brain and leptomeninges in suspected cerebral vasculitis.[78] In the rare instance where vasculitis is suspected because of an unexplained nonspecific systemic illness with no pointers towards a particular organ to biopsy, blind biopsy has been carried out of tissue such as rectum,[100] the superficial branch of the peroneal nerve combined with the peroneus brevis muscle,[101] and the minor salivary glands.

In addition to its utility in the diagnosis of vasculitis, histology is often useful in determining whether relapse has occurred. It can sometimes be difficult, with clinical assessment and the use of investigations including imaging, to determine whether an abnormality represents activity or damage. An ill-defined nodule in the lung of a patient with WG and previous pulmonary involvement may represent a fibrotic scar or an area of active vasculitis. In some cases the only way to confirm or refute the presence of active vasculitis is through biopsy and histological assessment.

IV. CONCLUSION

Manifestations of the primary systemic vasculitides span a wide spectrum, and the clinical and laboratory features of individual vasculitides often overlap. Common to all vasculitides, and an important concept in their management, is the observation that active inflammation can progress to the development of irreversible damage. This underlies the need for vigilance on the part of the clinician to consider the diagnosis of vasculitis in a patient with an unexplained systemic illness, to investigate and make the diagnosis early, and to institute early treatment to prevent damage.

REFERENCES

1. Wegener, F., Uber generalisierte, septische Gefasserkrankungen, *Verhandlungers der Deutschen Gesellschaft fur Pathologie,* 29, 202, 1936.
2. Carruthers, D.M., Watts, R.A., Symmons, D.P.M., Scott, D.G.I., Wegener's granulomatosis- increased incidence or increased awareness? *Br. J. Rheumatol.,* 35, 142, 1996.
3. Lamb, A., Periarteritis nodosa — a clinical and patholoigical review of the diseases, *Arch. Intern. Med.,* 14, 481, 1914.

4. Heberden, W., Anonymous Commertarii de Marlbaun. *Historia et Curatione*, Payne, London, 1801.
5. Schönlein, J., *Allgemeine und specielle Pathologie und Therapie*, Herisau, Wurzburg, 1837.
6. Henoch, E., Uber eine eigenthumliche form von Purpura, *Klin. Wochenschr.,* 11, 641, 1874.
7. Kussmaul, A., Maier, R., Uber eine bisher nicht beschriebene eigenthumliche Arterienerkrankung (Periarteritis nodosa), die mit Morbus Brightu und rapid fortschreitender allgemeiner Muskellahmung einhergeht, *Deutsche Archive Klinical Medizin,* 1, 484, 1866.
8. Churg, J., Strauss, L., Allergic granulomatosis, allergic angiitis and periarteritis nodosa, *Am. J. Pathol.,* 27, 277, 1951.
9. Ferrari, E., Uber Polyarteritis acuta nodosa (sogenannte Periarteritis nodosa) und ihre Beziehungen zur Polymyositis un Polyneuritis acuta, *Beitreib pat Anatomie,* 34, 350, 1903.
10. Zeek, P., Periarteritis nodosa — a critical review, *Am. J. Clin. Pathol.,* 22, 777, 1952.
11. Fries, J.F., Hunder, G.G., Bloch, D.A., Michel, B.A., Arend, W.P., Calabrese, L.H., Fauci, A.S., Leavitt, R.Y., Lie, J.T., Lightfoot, R.W., Masi, A.T., McShane, D.J., Mills, J.A., Stevens, M.B., Wallace, S.L., Zvaifler, N.J., The American College of Rheumatology 1990 criteria for the classification of vasculitis-summary, *Arthritis Rheum.,* 33, 1135, 1990.
12. Davson, J., Ball, J., Platt, R., The kidney in periarteritis nodosa, *QJM,* 17, 175, 1948.
13. Savage, C., Winearls, C., Evans, D., Rees, A., Lockwood, C., Microscopic polyarteritis: presentation, pathology and prognosis, *QJM,* 56, 467, 1985.
14. Jennette, J.C., Falk, R.J., Andrassy, K., Bacon, P.A., Churg, J., Gross, W.L., Hagen, E.C., Hoffman, G.S., Hunder, G.G., Kallenberg, C.G.M., McCluskey, R.T., Sinico, R.A., Rees, A.J., Vanes, L.A., Waldherr, R., Wiik, A., Nomenclature of systemic vasculitides — proposal of an international consensus conference, *Arthritis Rheum.,* 37, 187, 1994.
15. Lightfoot, R.W., Michel, B.A., Bloch, D.A., Hunder, G.G., Zvaifler, N.J., Mcshane, D.J., Arend, W.P., Calabrese, L.H., Leavitt, R.Y., Lie, J.T., Masi, A.T., Mills, J.A., Stevens, M.B., Wallace, S.L., The American College of Rheumatology 1990 criteria for the classification of polyarteritis nodosa, *Arthritis Rheum.,* 33, 1088, 1990.
16. Watts, R.A., Jolliffe, V.A., Carruthers, D.M., Lockwood, M., Scott, D.G.I., Effect of classification on the incidence of polyarteritis nodosa and microscopic polyangiitis, *Arthritis Rheum.,* 39, 1208, 1996.
17. Watts, R., Scott, D., Classification and epidemiology of the vasculitides, *Ballieres Clin. Rheumatol.,* 191, 1997.
18. Kurland, L., Chuang, T., Hunder, G., The Epidemiology of Systemic Arteritis, in *The Epidemiology of the Rheumatic Diseases*, Lawrence, R., Shulman, L., Eds., Gower Publishing, New York, 1984.
19. Michet, C., Epidemiology of vasculitis, *Rheum. Dis. Clin. North Am.,* 261, 1990.
20. Scott, D., Bacon, P., Elliott, P., Tribe, C., Wallington, T., Systemic vasculitis in a district general hospital 1972-1980 — clinical and laboratory features, classification and prognosis of 80 cases, *QJM,* 51, 292, 1982.
21. Scott, D.G.I., Watts, R.A., Classification and epidemiology of systemic vasculitis, *Br. J. Rheumatol.,* 33, 897, 1994.
22. Jonasson, F., Cullen, J., Elton, R., Temporal arteritis: a 14-year epidemiological, clinical and prognostic study, *Scott. Med. J.,* 24, 111, 1979.
23. Andrews, M., Edmunds, M., Campbell, A., Walls, J., Feehally, J., Systemic vasculitis in the 1980s — is there an increasing incidence of Wegeners granulomatosis and microscopic polyarteritis, *J. R. Coll. Physicians Lond.,* 24, 284, 1990.
24. Salvarani, C., Gabriel, S.E., Ofallon, W.M., Hunder, G.G., The incidence of giant-cell arteritis in Olmsted county, Minnesota — apparent fluctuations in a cyclic pattern, *Ann. Intern. Med.,* 123, 192, 1995.
25. Gonzales-Gay, M., Alonso, M., Aguero, J., Bal, M., Fernandez-Camblor, B., Sanchez-Andare, A., Temporal arteritis in a north-western area of Spain: study of 57 biopsy proven patients, *J. Rheumatol.,* 19, 277, 1992.
26. Weyand, C., Goronzy, J., Molecular approaches towards pathologic mechanisms in giant cell arteritis and Takayasu's arteritis, *Curr. Opin. Rheumatol.,* 7, 30, 1995.
27. Luqmani, R., Bacon, P., Moots, R., Janssen, B., Pall, A., Emery, P., Birmingham Vasculitis Activity Score (BVAS) in systemic necrotizing vasculitis, *QJM,* 87, 671, 1994.
28. Kallenberg, C., Cohen Tervaert, J., Stegeman, C., Criteria for disease activity in Wegener's granulomatosis: a requirement for longitudinal clinical studies, *APMIS,* Suppl. 19, 37, 1990.

29. Reinhold-Keller, E., Kekow, J., Schnabel, A., Schmitt, W., Heller, M., Beigel, A., Duncker, G., Gross, W., Influence of disease manifestation and antineutrophil cytoplasmic titer on the response to pulse cyclophosphamide therapy in patients with Wegener's granulomatosis, *Arthritis Rheum.*, 37, 919, 1994.

30. Abu-Shakra, M., Smythe, H., Lewtas, J., Badley, E., Weber, D., Keystone, E., Outcome of polyarteritis nodosa and Churg-Strauss syndrome — an analysis of 25 patients, *Arthritis Rheum.*, 37, 1798, 1994.

31. Exley, A., Bacon, P., Luqmani, R., Kitas, G., Gordon, C., Savage, C., Adu, D, Development and initial validation of the vasculitis damage index (VDI) for the standardised clinical assessment of damage in the systemic vasculitides, *Arthritis Rheum.*, 40, 371, 1997.

32. Exley, A., Carruthers, D., Luqmani, R., Kitas, G., Gordon, C., Janssen, B., Savage, C., Bacon, P., Damage occurs early in systemic vasculitis and is an index of outcome, *QJM*, 90, 391, 1997.

33. Guillevin, L., Lhote, F., Gayraud, M., Cohen, P., Jarousse, B., Lortholary, O., Thibult, N., Casassus, P., Prognostic factors in polyarteritis nodosa and Churg-Strauss syndrome: a prospective study in 342 patients, *Medicine (Baltimore)*, 75, 17, 1996.

34. Guillevin, L., Durand-Gasselin, B., Cevallos, R., Gayraud, M., Lhote, F., Callard, P., Amouroux, J., Casassus, P., Jarousse, B., Microscopic polyangiitis. Clinical and laboratory findings in eighty-five patients, *Arthritis Rheum.*, 42, 421, 1999.

35. Hoffman, G.S., Kerr, G.S., Leavitt, R.Y., Hallahan, C.W., Lebovics, R.S., Travis, W.D., Rottem, M., Fauci, A.S., Wegener granulomatosis — an analysis of 158 patients, *Ann. Intern. Med.*, 116, 488, 1992.

36. Gordon, M., Luqmani, R.A., Adu, D., Greaves, I., Richards, N., Michael, J., Emery, P., Howie, A.J., Bacon, P.A., Relapses in patients with a systemic vasculitis, *QJM*, 86, 779, 1993.

37. Fauci, A.S., Katz, P., Haynes, B.F., Wolff, S.M., Cyclophosphamide therapy of severe systemic necrotising vasculitis, *N. Engl. J. Med.*, 301, 235, 1979.

38. Talar-Williams, C., Hijazi, Y.M., Walther, M.M., Lineham, W.M., Hallahan, C.W., Lubensky, I., Kerr, G.S., Hoffman, G.S., Fauci, A.S., Sneller, M.C., Cyclophosphamide-induced cystitis and bladder cancer in patients with Wegener granulomatosis. *Ann. Intern. Med.*, 124, 477, 1996.

39. Cohen, R., Con, D., Ilstrup, D., Clinical features, prognosis and response to treatment in polyarteritis, *Mayo Clin. Proc.*, 55, 146, 1980.

40. Lhote, F., Guillevin, L., Polyarteritis nodosa, microscopic polyangiitis, and Churg-Strauss syndrome. Clinical aspects and treatment, *Rheum. Dis. Clin. North Am.*, 21, 911, 1995.

41. Guillevin, L., Lhote, F., Jarrousse, B., Fain, O., Treatment of polyarteritis nodosa and Churg-Strauss syndrome — a metaanalysis of 3 prospective controlled trials including 182 patients over 12 years, *Ann. Med. Interne* (Paris), 143, 405, 1992.

42. Cohen Tervaert, J., Kallenberg, C., Neurologic manifestations of systemic vasculitides, *Rheum Dis. Clin. North Am.*, 19, 913, 1993.

43. Azar, N., Guillevin, L., Du, L.T.H., Herreman, G., Meyrier, A., Godeau, P., Symptomatic urogenital manifestations of polyarteritis nodosa and Churg-Strauss angiitis — analysis of 8 of 165 patients, *J. Urol.*, 142, 136, 1989.

44. Smith, D.L., Wernick, R., Spontaneous rupture of a renal artery aneurysm in polyarteritis nodosa-critical review of the literature and report of a case, *Am. J. Med.*, 87, 464, 1989.

45. Guillevin, L., Le Thi Huong, D., Gayraud, M., Systemic vasculitis of the polyarteritis nodosa group and infections with hepatitis B virus: A study in 98 patients, *Eur. J. Intern. Med.*, 1, 97, 1990.

46. Bailey, M., Chapin, W., Licht, H., Reynolds, J.C., The effects of vasculitis on the gastrointestinal tract and liver, *Gastroenterol. Clin. North Am.*, 27, 747, 1998.

47. Camilleri, M., Pusey, C., Chadwick, V., Rees, A., Gastrointestinal manifestations of systemic vasculitis, *QJM*, 206, 141, 1983.

48. Bookman, A.A.M., Goode, E., Mcloughlin, M.J., Cohen, Z., Polyarteritis nodosa complicated by a ruptured intrahepatic aneurysm, *Arthritis Rheum.*, 26, 106, 1983.

49. Fauci, A., Vasculitis, *J. Allergy Clin. Immunol.*, 72, 211, 1983.

50. Bocanegra, T., Vasey, F., Espinoza, L., Germain, B., Pancreatic pseudocyst: a complication of necrotizing vasculitis (polyarteritis nodosa), *Br. J. Rheumatol.*, 37, 1363, 1980.

51. Lanham, J.G., Elkon, K.B., Pusey, C.D., Hughes, G.R., Systemic vasculitis with asthma and eosinophilia — a clinical approach to the Churg-Strauss syndrome, *Medicine*, 63, 65, 1984.

52. Reid, A., Harrison, B., Watts, R., Watkin, S., McCann, B., Scott, D., Churg-Strauss syndrome in a district hospital, *QJM*, 91, 219, 1998.

53. Hattori, N., Ichimura, M., Nagamatsu, M., Li, M., Yamamoto, K., Kumazawa, K., Mitsuma, T., Sobue, G., Clinicopathological features of Churg-Strauss syndrome associated neuropathy, *Brain,* 122, 427, 1999.

54. Guillevin, L., Guittard, T., Bletry, O., Godeau, P., Rosenthal, P., Systemic necrotizing angiitis with asthma — causes and precipitating factors in 43 cases, *Lung,* 165, 165, 1987.

55. Clutterbuck, E., Evans, D., Pusey, C., Renal involvement in Churg-Strauss syndrome, *Nephrol. Dial. Transplant.,* 5, 161, 1990.

56. Raynauld, J., Bloch, D., Fries, J., Seasonal variation in the onset of Wegener's granulomatosis, polyarteritis nodosa and giant cell arteritis, *J. Rheumatol.,* 20, 1524, 1993.

57. Cotch, M., Hoffman, G., Yerg, D., The epidemiology of Wegener's granulomatosis, *Arthritis Rheum.,* 39, 87, 1996.

58. Fauci, A.S., Haynes, B.F., Katz, P., Wolff, S.M., Wegener's granulomatosis — prospective clinical and therapeutic experience with 85 patients for 21 years, *Ann. Intern. Med.,* 98, 76, 1983.

59. Specks, U., Colby, T.V., Olsen, K.D., Deremee, R.A., Salivary-gland involvement in Wegener's granulomatosis, *Arch. Otolaryngol. Head Neck Surg.,* 117, 218, 1991.

60. Duna, G., Galperin, C., Hoffman, G., Wegener's granulomatosis, *Rheum. Dis. Clin. North Am.,* 21, 949, 1995.

61. Jennette, J., Antineutrophil cytoplasmic antibody-associated diseases: a pathologist's perspective, *Am. J. Kidney Dis.,* 18, 164, 1991.

62. Haworth, S.J., Pusey, C.D., Severe intestinal involvement in Wegener granulomatosis, *Gut,* 25, 1296, 1984.

63. McNabb, W.R., Lennox, M.S., Wedzicha, J.A., Small intestinal perforation in Wegener's granulomatosis, *Postgrad. Med. J.,* 58, 123, 1982.

64. D'Agati, V., Chander, P., Nash, M., Mancilla-Jimnez, R., Idiopathic microscopic polyarteritis nodosa: Ultrastructural observations on the renal vascular and glomerular lesions, *Am. J. Kidney Dis.,* 7, 95, 1986.

65. Adu, D., Howie, A., Scott, D., Bacon, P., McGonigle, R., Micheal, J., Polyarteritis and the kidney, *QJM,* 62, 221, 1987.

66. Niles, J.L., Bottinger, E.P., Saurina, G.R., Kelly, K.J., Pan, G.L., Collins, A.B., McCluskey, R.T., The syndrome of lung hemorrhage and nephritis is usually an ANCA-associated condition, *Arch. Intern. Med.,* 156, 440, 1996.

67. Kato, S., Shibuya, H., Neganuma, H., Nekagawa, H., Gastrointestinal endoscopy in Henoch-Schönlein purpura, *Eur. J. Pediatr.,* 151, 482, 1992.

68. Meadow, S., Glasgow, E., White, R., Moncreiff, M., Cameron, J., Ogg, C., Schönlein-Henoch nephritis, *QJM,* 41, 241, 1972.

69. Koskimies, O., Rapola, J., Savilahti, E., Vilska, J., Renal involvement in Schönlein-Henoch purpura, *Acta Paediatr.,* 63, 357, 1974.

70. Robson, W., Leung, A., Henoch-Schönlein purpura, *Adv. Pediatr.,* 41, 163, 1994.

71. Smith, H., Krupski, W., Spontaneous intestinal perforation in Schönlein-Henoch purpura, *South Med. J.,* 73, 603, 1980.

72. Puppala, A., Cheng, J., Steinheber, F., Pancreatitis — a rare complication of Schönlein-Henoch purpura, *Am. J. Gastroenterol.,* 69, 101, 1978.

73. Reif, S., Jain, A., Santiago, J., Rossi, T., Protein losing enteropathy as a manifestation of Henoch-Schönlein purpura, *Acta Paediatr.,* 80, 482, 1991.

74. Allen, D., Diamond, L., Howell, D., Anaphylactoid purpura in children (Schönlein-Henoch syndrome): Review with follow-up of the renal complications, *Am. J. Dis. Child.,* 99, 833, 1960.

75. Shurbaji, M., Epstein, J., Testicular vasculitis: implications for systemic disease, *Hum. Pathol.,* 19, 186, 1988.

76. Raza, K., Exley, A.R., Carruthers, D.M., Buckley, C., Hammond, L.A., Bacon, P.A., Localized bowel vasculitis — post-operative cyclophosphamide or not? *Arthritis Rheum.,* 42, 182, 1999.

77. Berger, J., Romano, J., Menkin, M., Norenberg, M., Benign focal cerebral vasculitis: case report, *Neurology,* 45, 1731, 1995.

78. Calabrese, L., Duna, G., Lie, J., Vasculitis in the central nervous system, *Arthritis Rheum.,* 40, 1189, 1997.

79. Calabrese, L., Mallek, J., Primary angiitis of the central nervous system: report of eight new cases, review of the literature and proposal for diagnostic criteria, *Medicine* (Baltimore), 67, 20, 1988.

80. Parisi, J., Moore, P., The role of biopsy in vasculitis of the central nervous system, *Semin. Neurol.,* 14, 341, 1994.

81. George, T., Duna, G., Rybicki, L., Calabrese, L., A reappraisal of primary angiitis of the central nervous system: pathologically verusus angiographically defined cases, *Arthritis Rheum.,* 38, S340, 1995.

82. Minkowitz, G., Smoller, B., McNutt, S., Benign cutaneous polyarteritis nodosa. Relationship to systemic polyarteritis nodosa and to hepatitis B infection, *Arch. Dermatol.,* 127, 1520, 1991.

83. Plaut, A., Asymptomatic focal arteritis of the appendix. Eighty-eight cases. *Am. J. Pathol.,* 27, 247, 1950.

84. Ito, M., Sano, K., Inaba, H., Hotchi, M., Localized necrotizing arteritis. A report of two cases involving the gallbladder and pancreas, *Arch. Pathol. Lab. Med.,* 115, 780, 1991.

85. Burke, A., Sobin, L., Virmani, R., Localized vasculitis of the gastrointestinal tract, *Am. J. Surg. Pathol.,* 19, 338, 1995.

86. Schwenger, W., Sis, J., Nowak, R., van der Woude, F., Andrassy, K., CRP levels in ANCA positive vasculitis can be specified by measurement of procalcitonin (PCT), *Clin. Exp. Immunol.,* 112, 23, 1998.

87. Davies, D.J., Moran, J.E., Niall, J.F., Ryan, G.B., Segmental necrotizing glomerulonephritis with anti-neutrophil antibody — possible arbovirus etiology, *BMJ,* 285, 606, 1982.

88. van der Woude, F.J., Lobatto, S., Permin, H., Vandergiessen, M., Rasmussen, N., Wiik, A., Vanes, L.A., Vanderhem, G.K., The, T.H., Autoantibodies against neutrophils and monocytes — tool for diagnosis and marker of disease activity in Wegener's granulomatosis, *Lancet,* 1, 425, 1985.

89. Petterson, E., Heigl, Z., Antineutrophil cytoplasmic antibody (cANCA and pANCA) titers in relation to disease activity in patients with necrotizing vasculitis: A longutidinal study, *Clin. Nephrol.,* 37, 219, 1992.

90. Finkel, T.H., Torok, T.J., Ferguson, P.J., Durigon, E.L., Zaki, S.R., Leung, D.Y.M., Harbeck, R.J., Gelfand, E.W., Saulsbury, F.T., Hollister, J.R., Anderson, L.J., Chronic parvovirus B19 infection and systemic necrotizing vasculitis — opportunistic infection or etiologic agent, *Lancet,* 343, 1255, 1994.

91. Gisselbrecht, M., Cohen, P., Lortholary, O., Jarrousse, B., Gayraud, M., Lecompte, I., Ruel, M., Gherardi, R., Guillevin, L., Human immunodeficiency virus-related vasculitis — clinical presentation of and therapeutic approach to eight cases, *Ann Med Interne* (Paris), 149, 398, 1998.

92. Qasim, F., Peat, D., Hughes, M., Lockwood, C., Four cases of perforated bowel in patients with systemic vasculitis, *Clin. Exp. Immunol.,* 112, 28, 1998.

93. Calabrese, L.H., Furlan, A.J., Gragg, L.A., Ropos, T.J., Primary angiitis of the central nervous system-diagnostic criteria and clinical approach, *Cleve. Clin. J. Med.,* 59, 293, 1992.

94. Vollmer, T.L., Guarnaccia, J., Harrington, W., Pacia, S.V., Petroff, O.A.C., Idiopathic granulomatous angiitis of the central nervous system — diagnostic challenges, *Arch. Neurol.,* 50, 925, 1993.

95. Haskard, D., McHale, J., Harari, O., Marshall, D., Imaging vascular activation, *Clin. Exp. Immunol.,* 112, 5, 1998.

96. Celermajer, D., Sorensen, K., Gooch, V., Spiegelhalter, D., Miller, O., Sullivan, I., Lloyd, J., Deanfield, J., Non-invasive detection of endothelial dysfunction in children and adults at risk of atherosclerosis, *Lancet,* 340, 1111, 1992.

97. Joannides, R., Haefeli, W., Linder, L., Richard, V., Bakkali, E., Thuillez, C., Luscher, T., Nitric oxide is responsible for flow-dependent dilatation of human peripheral conduit arteries *in vivo, Circulation,* 91, 1314, 1995.

98. Raza, K., Thambyrajah, J., Townend, J.N., Exley, A.R., Hortas, C., Filer, A., Carruthers, D.M., Bacon, P.A., Suppression of inflammation in primary systemic vasculitis restores vascular endothelial function: lessons for atherosclerotic disease?, *Circulation,* 102, 1470, 2000.

99. Lie, J., Biopsy diagnosis of systemic vasculitis, *Baillieres Clinin. Rheumatol.,* 11, 219, 1997.

100. Tribe, C., Scott, D., Bacon, P., Rectal biopsy in the diagnosis of systemic vasculitis, *J. Clin. Pathol.,* 34, 843, 1981.

101. Puechal, X., Said, G., Hilliquin, P., Coste, J., Jobdeslandre, C., Lacroix, C., Menkes, C., Peripheral neuropathy with necrotizing vasculitis in rheumatoid arthritis, *Arthritis Rheum.,* 38, 1618, 1995.

17 Vascular Manifestations in Giant-Cell Arteritis

Maria C. Cid, José Hernández-Rodríguez, and Josep M. Grau

CONTENTS

I. INTRODUCTION

Giant-cell (temporal) arteritis (GCA) is a chronic granulomatous vasculitis involving large and medium-sized vessels. The characteristic involvement of the carotid artery branches determines some of the typical manifestations of the disease and facilitates its histopathologic diagnosis, usually obtained from a temporal artery biopsy.[1,2]

Closely related to GCA is polymyalgia rheumatica (PMR), a clinically defined syndrome consisting of aching and stiffness in the neck, shoulders, or pelvic girdle occurring in about 50% of patients with GCA. PMR can also exist as a separate entity with no evidence of vascular involvement.[1,2]

II. EPIDEMIOLOGY

GCA typically occurs in people older than 50 years, and its frequency increases with age. In most series it is two times more frequent in women than in men. It clearly predominates in Caucasians, and the highest prevalence is found in northern Europe and in populations with similar ethnic background. GCA is not an uncommon disease. Recent epidemiological studies conducted in northern Europe and North America disclose an annual incidence rate of 19.1 to 27 cases per 100,000 population older than 50 years,[3-6] reaching 49 per 100,000 in individuals in their eighties.[6] In Mediterranean countries the annual incidence is lower, about 6 to 10 cases per 100,000.[7,8] PMR seems to be even more frequent with an average annual incidence rate of 52.2 per 100,000 persons aged 50 and older.[1]

Cyclic fluctuations in the incidence of GCA, occurring every 6 to 7 years, have been reported and suggest the influence of an environmental agent as a triggering factor.[6] It appears that the reported incidence of GCA is increasing in different countries.[6] Although the occurrence of GCA may be, in fact, higher, other factors, such as a longer life expectancy and a better awareness of the atypical or less frequent disease presentation patterns by attending physicians, may contribute to the increase in reported incidences.

III. PATHOLOGY

GCA involves large and medium-sized arteries. The arterial wall is invaded by an inflammatory infiltrate composed by T-lymphocytes and macrophages, frequently organized into a granulomatous reaction with the presence of multinucleated giant cells[9] (Figure 17.1). Sparse polymorphonuclear leukocytes can be occasionally observed, and B-lymphocytes as well as NK cells are virtually absent. The inflammatory infiltrates may extend across the entire vessel wall, but usually predominate at the adventitia and at the junction between the intima and media where the granulomatous reaction is more prominent. The internal elastic lamina appears disrupted by inflammatory infiltrates, and giant cells usually accumulate in its vicinity (Figure 17.2). In well-developed lesions, the lumen is occluded by intimal hyperplasia.

The inflammatory lesions are typically segmentary and are preferentially distributed along the carotid artery and vertebral branches.[9] The more severely involved arteries are the superficial temporal arteries, vertebral arteries, and ophthalmic and posterior ciliary arteries. Intracranial vessels are usually spared. While this distribution generates most of the classical clinical manifestations of the disease, necropsy studies have shown that inflammatory infiltrates can be almost

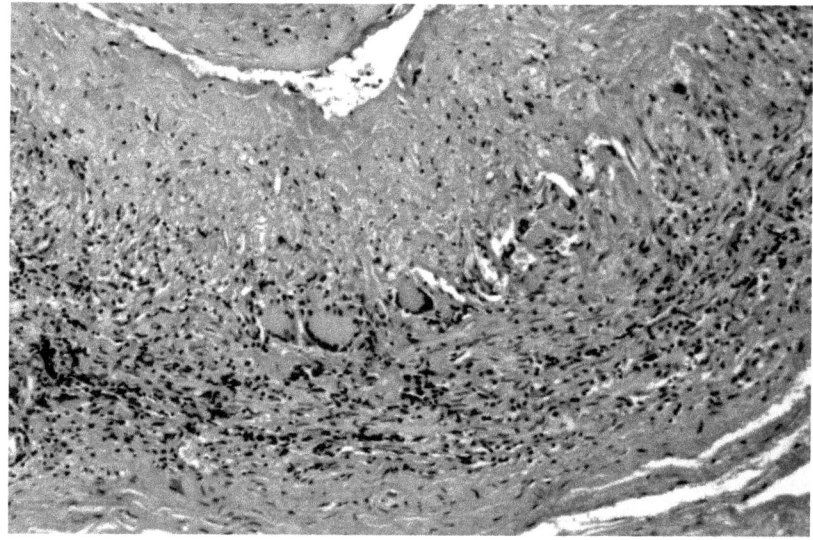

FIGURE 17.1 The arterial wall is invaded by an inflammatory infiltrate with predominance of mononuclear cells. A granulomatous reaction with plenty of multinucleated giant cells can be observed. Hematoxylin-eosin. 100 ×.

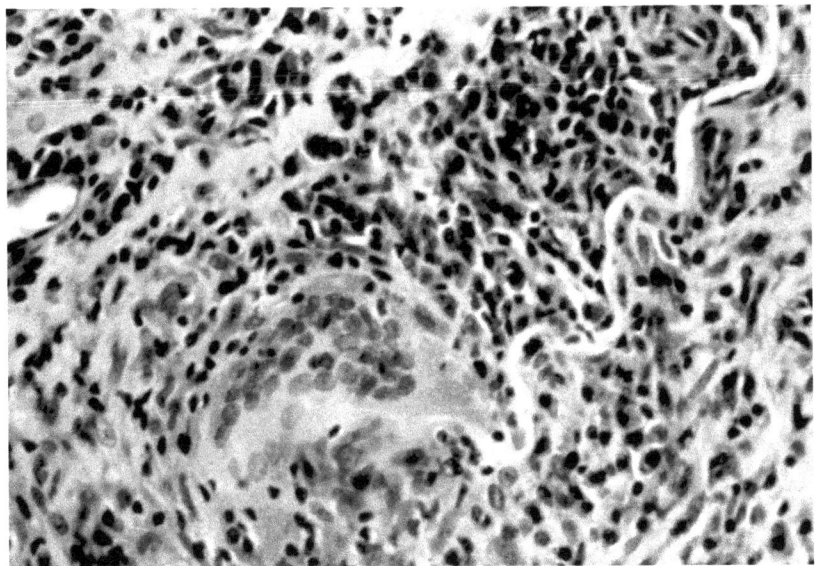

FIGURE 17.2 Multinucleated giant cells distribute in close vicinity with the internal elastic lamina which appear fragmented. Hematoxylin-eosin. 250 ×.

invariably detected in the aorta and its major tributaries.[10] However, large vessel involvement is clinically apparent in fewer than 10% of cases.[11,12]

The histopathologic substrate of PMR is a chronic synovitis and bursitis of proximal joints.[13,14] Synovitis is usually mild and the inflammatory infiltrates are composed by CD4 T-lymphocytes and macrophages with scarce neutrophils. As in GCA, B-lymphocytes are absent and there is no significant participation of the synovial lining cells. Muscle biopsies do not disclose specific abnormalities.

IV. PATHOGENESIS

A. GENETIC PREDISPOSITION

Epidemiological data reveal a predominance of GCA and PMR in Caucasians, a higher prevalence in certain geographic areas such as northern Europe, and sporadic occurrence of familial cases suggesting the existence of a genetic component in the pathogenesis of GCA.[1,2]

Over the years, several investigators have reported a higher prevalence of the HLA class II antigen DR4 in patients with GCA than in the general population, and also in patients with isolated PMR.[15,16] This association has been observed in North America, in northern Europe, and in Mediterranean countries. Interestingly, patients with PMR, alone or in combination with GCA, have a stronger association with the HLA-DR4 antigen.[16] The allelic variant DRB1*0401 is the most frequent in GCA patients, and a four-amino-acid motif located at the second hypervariable region of the polymorphic DRβ chain has been proposed as a disease-related sequence which can be mapped at the antigen-binding pocket of the DR molecule.[17]

B. IMMUNOPATHOGENIC MECHANISMS

Immunopathologic studies have demonstrated that activated macrophages and CD4 T-lymphocytes are the major constituents of GCA inflammatory infiltrates.[18] Analysis of cytokines produced by infiltrating cells indicates a T-helper1-type functional differentiation of CD4 lymphocytes.[19] Activated lymphocytes actively produce interferon γ, a cytokine which has been demonstrated to be crucial for macrophage activation and granuloma formation.[20] Therefore, both morphologically and functionally, GCA lesions exhibit a delayed-type hypersensitivity reaction pattern. A number of additional cytokines such as IL-1, TNFα, GM-CSF, and IL-6 have been domonstrated to be produced in GCA lesions.[19]

Expansion of CD4 T-lymphocyte clones derived from temporal artery biopsy specimens has shown that a minority of infiltrating lymphocytes obtained from different temporal artery segments share identical sequences at the third complementary determining region of the T-cell receptor, whereas these sequences are undetectable in lymphocytes isolated from peripheral blood.[21] This observation suggests that a minority of infiltrating T-lymphocytes undergo clonal expansion, presumably as a consequence of specific immune recognition of a disease-relevant antigen. In addition, identification of dendritic cells with a putative antigen-presenting function in temporal artery lesions further suggests that GCA lesions may develop as a consequence of a T-cell-mediated immune response directed against antigens residing in the arterial wall.[18] Preliminary attempts to identify putative causing agents by molecular techniques have been performed but the results are not conclusive.[22]

C. Mechanisms of Vascular Injury

Activated macrophages produce oxygen radicals, nitric oxide, and proteolytic enzymes that partic-ipate in the disruption of the vessel wall and in tissue destruction.[23] Lipid peroxidation products resulting from tissue oxidative damage can be detected in infiltrating mononuclear cells and smooth muscle cells of the media in temporal arteries from patients with GCA, indicating the potential role of reactive oxygen species in generating vessel wall injury.[23] The expression of inducible nitric oxide synthase by infiltrating macrophages has been detected in GCA, and the presence of perox-ynitrite-modified proteins in the vessel wall may indicate a possible role of nitric oxide in tissue damage.[23] Matrix metalloproteases and neutrophil elastase have been demonstrated to be produced in GCA and may contribute to the rupture of the internal elastic lamina, a characteristic histopatho-logic finding in GCA.[23,24]

D. Vascular Response to Inflammation

Vessel wall components actively react to cytokines and growth factors released by infiltrating leukocytes amplifying the inflammatory response through several mechanisms. Endothelial cell adhesion molecule expression induced by proinflammatory cytokines contributes to the recruitment of additional leukocytes.[2,25] Endothelial cell response to angiogenic growth factors results in exten-sive neovascularization of the vessel wall in GCA[25] (Figure 17.3). Neovessels are more prominent at the adventitial layer and within the inflammatory infiltrates, especially at the intima/media junction.[25] Inflammation-induced angiogenesis may have a protective role at distal sites where providing new blood supply may prevent organ ischemia.[2] However, newly formed microvessels intensively express endothelial adhesion molecules and contribute to the recruitment of additional leukocytes, amplifying and perpetuating the inflammatory reaction.[25]

Vascular response to inflammation leads eventually to vessel occlusion with subsequent ischemia of the tissues supplied by involved vessels. In GCA, vessel occlusion results mostly from intimal hyperplasia. A correlation between the expression of TGFβ and PDGF and the degree of intimal hyperplasia and clinical manifestations derived from vessel occlusion have been demon-strated.[22,26,27]

V. CLINICAL MANIFESTATIONS

Patients with GCA may present with a wide variety of clinical features which are summarized in Table 17.1. Disease-related manifestations may appear rapidly or may develop insidiously. A delay of weeks or even months between the beginning of clinical symptoms and diagnosis is common.

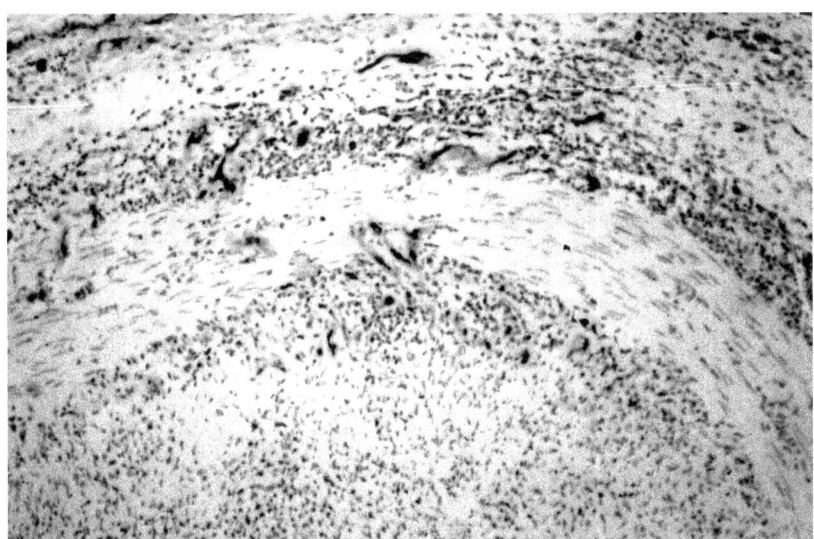

FIGURE 17.3 Inflammation-induced angiogenesis is prominent in giant cell arteritis lesions. Neovessels, identified with the lectin *Ulex europaeus*, are mainly located at the adventitial layer and within the inflammatory infiltrates at the intima/media junction. Avidin-biotin-peroxidase technique. 100 ×.

A. CLINICAL FINDINGS DERIVED FROM THE INVOLVEMENT OF CRANIAL ARTERIES

Headache is one of the most common and characteristic symptoms and occurs in about 60 to 98% of cases. The intensity of headache is highly variable. It may be diffuse but frequently predominates at the temporal areas. Scalp tenderness is also common. Patients may also present with a variety of bizarre aches in the craniofacial area, including ocular pain, earache, toothache, odynofagia, odontalgia, and carotidynia. When these symptoms predominate, a substantial delay in diagnosis is common. About 40% of patients experience jaw claudication when eating, a symptom considered characteristic of GCA, but it may be seen occasionally in other vascular diseases such as polyarteritis nodosa and amyloidosis. Other manifestations such as facial swelling, tongue pain, or edema are less frequently seen (Table 17.1).[1,28,29]

Temporal arteries may appear swollen, hard, or pulseless at physical examination (Figure 17.4). Sometimes just a slight asymmetry, decrease, or irregularity in pulse can be noticed in temporal or other cranial arteries. Inflammatory signs are very specific but are less frequently found.

Visual loss is the most frequent ischemic complication in GCA and occurs in about 15% of cases.[30,31] It develops in most cases as a consequence of anterior ischemic optic neuropathy due to the inflammatory involvement of posterior ciliary arteries supplying the optic nerve. Less frequently, central retinal artery thrombosis may also occur. Retrobulbar neuritis and cortical blindness have been occasionally reported. Visual loss can be bilateral or unilateral, complete or partial. It usually appears suddenly and it is frequently preceded by transient visual loss (*amaurosis fugax*) or diplopia.[31] Less common ischemic complications include cerebrovascular accidents due to the involvement of carotid or vertebral tributaries, and scalp or tongue necrosis. Ischemic complications tend to accumulate in particular patients and, frequently, are early events during the course of the disease.[30] A strong systemic inflammatory response is associated with a lower risk of developing ischemic complications.[31]

B. SYMPTOMATIC INVOLVEMENT OF OTHER VASCULAR TERRITORIES

Nearly 10% of patients present symptomatic involvement of other vascular territories. This includes bruits, asymmetry in blood pressure detection, and, in more severe cases, limb claudication[11] (Figure

TABLE 17.1
Clinical Findings in a Series of 250 Patients
with Giant Cell (Temporal) Arteritis

General Features

Age (mean, range)	75 (50–94)
Sex (male/female)	178/72
Cranial symptoms (%)	86
Headache	77
Jaw claudication	44
Scalp tenderness	39
Facial pain	18
Abnormal temporal arteries	74
Ocular pain	8
Tongue pain	5
Earache	18
Trismus	1
Carotidynia	5
Toothache	5
Odynofagia	12
Ischemic events (%)	23
Blindness	14
Amaurosis fugax	10
Transient diplopia	4
Cerebrovascular accident	2
Symptomatic large vessel involvement (%)	5
Polymyalgia rheumatica (%)	48
Systemic manifestations (%)	74
Fever	47
Weight loss	61

Note: According to the authors' experience.

17.5). When clinical manifestations derived from large vessel involvement predominate and appear in women in their fifties, distinction from Takayasu arteritis may be difficult.[2]

Patients with GCA present a higher incidence of aortic aneurysms, which may appear as late complications in patients apparently in sustained remission.[12] About 17% of patients with GCA may develop aortic aneurysms, and half of them may die as a consequence of its rupture.[12] Myocardial or mesenteric infarction due to GCA can be infrequently seen. Occasionally, GCA lesions in arteries supplying the female genital tract have been casually discovered in surgical resections. These patients may or may not disclose concomitantly classical GCA-related disease manifestations.

C. Polymyalgia Rheumatica

Approximately 50% of patients with GCA present symptoms of PMR, a syndrome clinically defined by the presence of aching and stiffnes in the neck, shoulders, or pelvic girdle. Pain is exacerbated with movement, and morning stiffness is a prominent finding. Proximal muscles are usually tender. PMR can develop simultaneously with cranial symptoms or may emerge months or even years earlier. Sometimes PMR may be the only clinical manifestation of GCA. Temporal artery biopsies disclosing GCA can be demonstrated in about 10% of patients with apparently isolated PMR, and the majority of them have some abnormalities at physical examination of the temporal arteries.

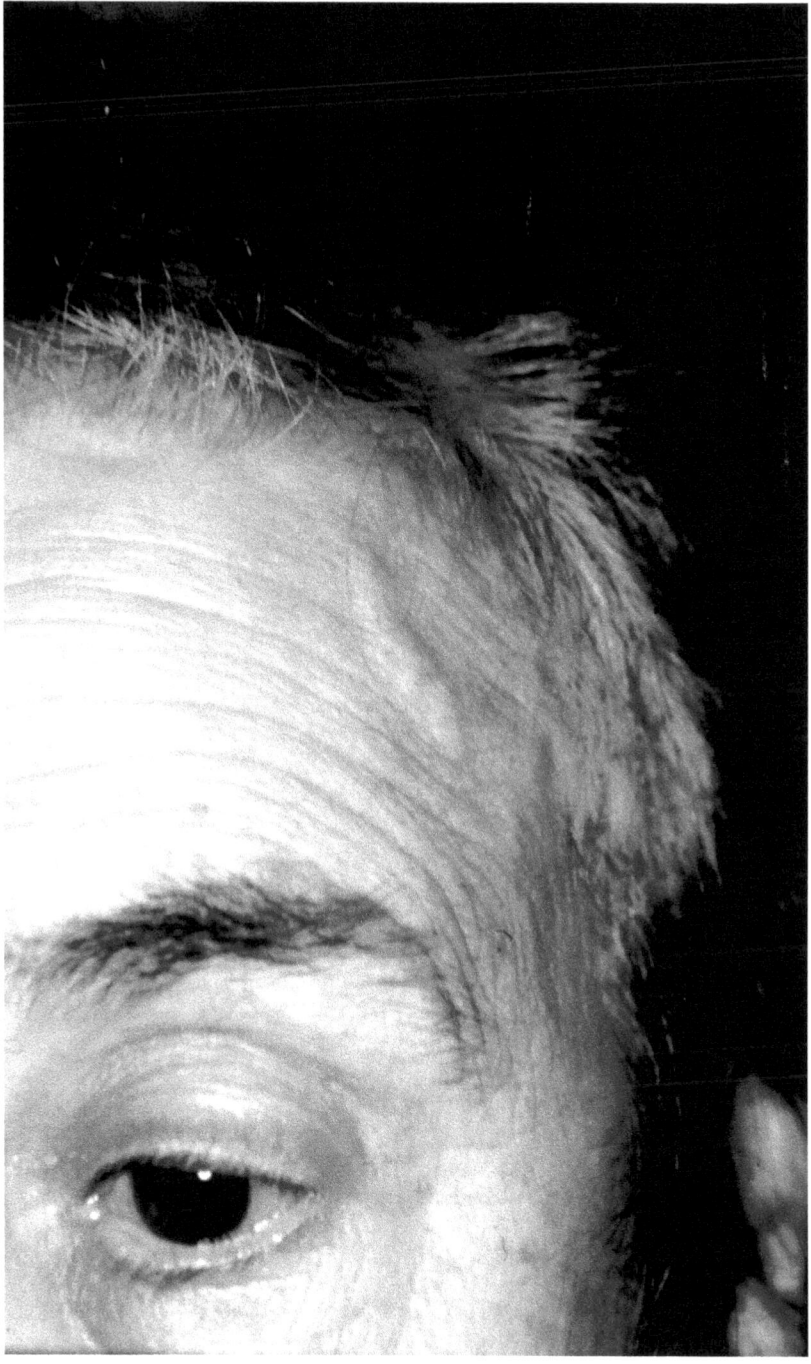

FIGURE 17.4 A swollen, hard, and pulseless superficial temporal artery highly suggests the diagnosis of giant cell arteritis.

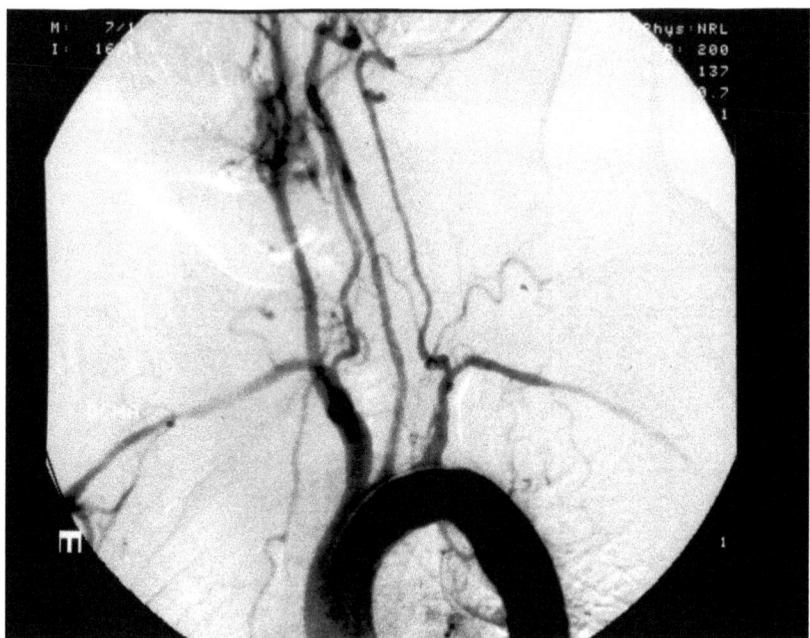

FIGURE 17.5 Large-vessel involvement in giant-cell arteritis. The angiogram shows a stenotic left subclavian artery in a patient with biopsy-proven temporal arteritis who presented with subclavian bruit and limb claudication.

Peripheral synovitis is developed by 23% of patients with GCA. Knees, wrists, and metacarpophalangeal joints are the most frequently involved. Peripheral manifestations usually occur in patients with PMR, but may also appear in patients without proximal symptoms. Other associated manifestations include tenosynovitis, carpal tunnel syndrome, and distal swelling with pitting edema.[32-34] Some patients develop a clinical picture indistinguishable from seronegative rheumatoid arthritis.[34]

PMR can exist as an isolated entity without any evidence of vascular inflammation. Patients with isolated PMR have a similar epidemiologic distribution, a similar immunogenetic background, and disclose the same biological abnormalities as patients with GCA.

D. Systemic Manifestations

Patients with GCA or PMR frequently experience malaise, anorexia, and weight loss.[1,2,33] Nearly 50% of patients with GCA have fever. In some patients fever or constitutional symptoms are the most prominent finding. About 10% of patients present with fever of unknown origin with very mild or no cranial manifestations.[1]

VI. LABORATORY FINDINGS

With a few exceptions, both GCA and PMR are characterized by a strong acute phase reaction. ESR is usually accelerated, frequently over 100 mm/h. Protein electrophoresis shows an increase in $\alpha 2$ globulins. Plasma concentrations of acute phase proteins such as C-reactive protein, haptoglobin, and fibrinogen are also elevated. Thrombocytosis and anemia of chronic disease type are common, and some patients have abnormal liver function tests, particularly increased levels of alkaline phosphatase.[1,33] Nonspecific immunological abnormalities such as decreased numbers of circulating CD8 lymphocytes and elevated levels of soluble interleukin-2 receptors are common in both diseases.[33]

TABLE 17.2
Criteria for the Diagnosis of GCA

1. Age greater than 55
2. Positive response within 48 hours to corticosteroid therapy
3. Length of history greater than 2 weeks
4. Positive temporal artery biopsy
5. Proximal symmetrical girdle or upper arm muscle pain, stiffness, or tenderness
6. Jaw claudication
7. Clinical abnormality of a temporal artery (tenderness, thickening, redness)
8. Systemic symptoms or signs (malaise, anorexia, weight loss, anemia, pyrexia)
9. Recent onset headache
10. Visual disturbance (loss, diplopia, blurring)

Note: Criteria 1 to 3 plus any three criteria from 5 to 10 are required for clinical diagnosis. Criterion 4 refers to histolopathologic diagnosis.

Several monocyte and/or endothelial cell activation products can be detected at raised concentrations in plasma from patients with GCA and PMR. These include cytokines such as IL-6 and TNFα, soluble adhesion molecules such as ICAM-1, and vWF antigen.[1,2,36-38]

VII. DIAGNOSIS

Histopathologic examination of a temporal artery biopsy provides the definitive diagnosis of GCA.[9] When the area to be excised is carefully selected, a 2–3 cm fragment is removed, and multiple histologic sections are examined, temporal artery biopsy has an elevated sensitivity for the diagnosis of GCA.[39,40] When negative, excision of the contralateral artery may increase diagnostic sensitivity. Occasionally, temporal artery biopsy reveals temporal artery involvement by other vasculitides such as necrotizing vasculitis or by other disorders such as amyloidosis.[9] A normal temporal artery biopsy does not completely exclude GCA given the segmental distribution of inflammatory infiltrates. For that reason, criteria for the clinical diagnosis of GCA have been established (Table 17.2).[41] However, according to follow-up studies, only in a minority of patients with a negative temporal artery biopsy is the diagnostic suspicion sustained, and they receive long-term corticosteroid therapy.[39] Given the frequent existence of overlapping features among vasculitides, criteria sets have been established in order to classify vasculitis patients in specific categories. Criteria for the classification of GCA are depicted in Table 17.3.[42]

TABLE 17.3
American College of Rheumatology Criteria for the Classification of Giant Cell (Temporal) Arteritis

1. Age at disease onset, 50 years.
2. New onset of headache or new type of localized pain in the head.
3. Temporal artery tenderness or decreased pulsation.
4. ESR, 50 mm/hour (Westergren).
5. Temporal artery biopsy showing vasculitis with a predominance of mononuclear cells or granulomatous inflammation, usually with multinucleated giant cells.

Note: A patient is considered to have GCA if at least 3 of the above criteria are present. The presence of any 3 or more criteria yields a sensitivity of 93.5% and a specificity of 91.2%.

TABLE 17.4
Criteria for the Diagnosis of Polymyalgia Rheumatica

1. Persistent pain (for at least 1 month) involving two of the following: neck, shoulders, pelvic girdle.
2. Morning stiffness for > 1 hour.
3. Rapid response to prednisone at ≤20 mg/day.
4. Absence of other diseases capable of causing the musculoskeletal symptoms.
5. Age over 50 years.
6. ESR > 40 mm/hour.

Note: Diagnosis of polymyalgia rheumatica is made if all the above criteria are satisfied.

The diagnosis of PMR relies, at present, on clinical criteria.[33] One of the most widely used criteria sets is exposed in Table 17.4.[43] The diagnosis of PMR requires a careful evaluation to exclude other disorders which may occasionally present with similar symptoms. These include rheumatoid arthritis, inflammatory myopathies, polyarteritis nodosa, and chronic infection.

Magnetic resonance imaging studies are able to detect subdeltoid and subacromial bursitis in PMR patients. These findings are even more frequent than joint synovitis. MRI could then be a useful tool in the evaluation of patients with suspected PMR, but its sensitivity and specificity needs to be evaluated in larger studies.[33]

VIII. TREATMENT AND COURSE

Corticosteroid therapy is the treatment of choice for GCA, and it induces a dramatic amelioration of disease manifestations within a few days. The most widely recommended initial dose is 40 to 60 mg/day. The presence of transient ocular manifestations such as *amaurosis fugax* or diplopia must be considered a medical emergency and treatment must be started immediately, even before the histological confirmation of GCA is obtained. It has been demonstrated that previous corticosteroid treatment for several days, even weeks, does not clear the inflammatory infiltrates and, therefore, does not hinder the histopathologic diagnosis.[44] When visual loss is established, corticosteroid pulses of 1 gm/day for 3 days are recommended by some authors, although it has not been clearly demonstrated that this dose is really more effective than the standard treatment.[45] Early treatment, within the first 12 to 24 hours, appears to be the major determinant of visual recovery, which can be expected in 12% of cases.[45]

The starting dose is maintained for 2 to 4 weeks and then progressively tapered to 5 mg/week, approximately. Although most patients do well with a daily maintenance dose of 10 mg, some patients may require higher doses. Tapering is guided mainly by clinical evaluation. ESR is a useful parameter in the follow-up of GCA, but therapeutic decisions must not rely solely on ESR values. Yet, it must be taken into account that ESR values of 30 to 40 can be considered normal in aged people.[1,2] The endorsed initial dose for patients with isolated PMR is 15 mg/day. Guidelines for reduction are the same as those recommended for GCA.[1,33] Some PMR patients with mild symptoms may respond to nonsteroidal antiinflammatory drugs.[32]

The total duration of therapy may vary, but most patients require 1 to 2 years. Reduction below the maintenance doses must be very slow in order to avoid the relapses which are common during the first two years of treatment. Approximately 30% of patients require low-dose corticosteroid therapy for several years, some perhaps indefinitely.[1,2]

In a majority of patients, ESR quickly normalizes after the beginning of corticosteroid therapy. However, other inflammatory markers such as IL-6, C-reactive protein, haptoglobin, and vWFAg persist elevated in most patients in clinically apparent remission, probably indicating a persistent low-level inflammatory activity.[1,2,38] The long-term clinical consequences of this remaining activity is unknown. It is not clear, at present, whether persistent low-level inflammatory activity should influence therapeutic decisions.

Iatrogenic complications derived from corticosteroid therapy are not infrequent in both GCA and PMR.[1,28,33,46] For that reason the usefulness of other immunesuppressive drugs as corticosteroid sparing agents is currently being tested in clinical trials, but their efficacy has not yet been proven. In patients with severe corticosteroid side-effects, other immunesuppressive drugs such as azathioprine, cyclosporin, or methotrexate can be tried.

Several studies suggest that, overall, GCA does not influence the long-term survival of patients. However, deathly complications such as cerebrovascular accidents, aneurysm rupture, or myocardial infarction directly related to GCA may occur in some patients.[12,47]

ACKNOWLEDGMENTS

The data generated by the authors have been supported by grants from Fondo de Investigación Sanitaria (FIS 98/0443 and FIS 00/0689).

REFERENCES

1. Hunder, GG, Giant-cell arteritis and polymyalgia rheumatica, *Med. Clin. North. Am.,* 1997; 81: 195–219
2. Cid, MC, Large vessel vasculitides, *Curr. Opin. Rheumatol.,* 1998; 10: 18–28.
3. Baldursson, O, Steinsson, K, Bjornsson, J, Giant-cell arteritis in Iceland: an epidemiologic and histologic analysis, *Arthritis Rheum.,* 1994; 37: 1007–1012.
4. Noltorp, S, Svensson, B, High incidence of polymyalgia rheumatica and giant-cell arteritis in a Swedish community, *Clin. Exp. Rheumatol.,* 1991; 9: 351–354.
5. Nordborg, E, Bengtsson, BA, Epidemiology of biopsy-proven giant-cell arteritis, *J. Intern. Med.,* 1990; 227: 233–236.
6. Salvarani, C, Gabriel, SE, O'Fallon, WM, Hunder, GG, The incidence of giant-cell arteritis in Olmsted County, Minnesota: apparent fluctuations in a cyclic pattern, *Ann. Intern. Med.,* 1995; 123: 192–194.
7. González-Gay, MA, Alonso, MD, Agüero, JJ, Bal, M, Fernámdez-Camblor, B, Sánchez–Andrade, A, Temporal arteritis in a Northwestern area of Spain: study of 57 biopsy-proven patients, *J. Rheumatol.,* 1992; 19: 277–280.
8. Sonnenblick, M, Nesher, G, Friedlander, Y, Rubinow, A, Giant-cell arteritis in Jerusalem: a 12-year epidemiological study, *Br. J. Rheumatol.,* 1994; 33: 938–941.
9. Lie, JT, Histopathologic specificity of systemic vasculitis, *Rheum. Dis. Clin. North Am.,* 1995; 21: 883–909.
10. Ostberg, G, Morphological changes in the large arteries in polymyalgia arteritica, *Acta Med. Scand.,* 1972; 533: 135–164.
11. Klein, RG, Hunder, GG, Stanson, AW, Sheps SG, Large artery involvement in giant-cell (temporal) arteritis, *Ann. Intern. Med.,* 1975; 83: 806–812.
12. Evans, JM, O'Fallon, WM, Hunder, GG, Increased incidence of aortic aneurysm and dissection in giant cell (temporal) arteritis, *Ann. Intern. Med.,* 1995; 122: 502–507.
13. Meliconi, R, Pulsatelli, L, Uguccioni, M, Salvarani, C, Macchioni, P, Melchiorri, C, Focherini, C, Frizziero, L, Facchini, A, Leukocyte infiltration in synovial tissue from the shoulder of patients with polymyalgia rheumatica: quantitative analysis and influence of corticosteroid treatment, *Arthritis Rheum.,* 1996; 39: 1199–1207.
14. Meliconi, R, Pulsatelli, L, Melchiorri, C, Frizziero, L, Salvarani, C, Macchioni, P, Uguccioni, M, Focherini, MC, Facchini, A, Synovial expression of cell adhesion molecules in polymyalgia rheumatica, *Clin. Exp. Immunol.,* 1997; 107: 494–500.
15. Bignon, JD, Barrier, J, Soulillou, JP, Martin, PH, Grolleau, JY, HLA-DR4 and giant-cell arteritis, *Tissue Antigens,* 1984; 24: 60–62.

16. Cid, MC, Ercilla, MG, Vilaseca, J, Sanmartí, J, Villalta, J, Ingelmo, M, Urbano-Márquez, A, Poly-myalgia rheumatica: a syndrome associated with the HLA-DR4 antigen, *Arthritis Rheum.*, 1988; 31: 678–682.

17. Weyand, CM, Hicok, KC, Hunder, GG, Goronzy, JJ, The HLA-DRB1 locus as a genetic component in giant cell arteritis: mapping of a disease-linked sequence motif to the antigen binding site of the HLA-DR molecule, *J. Clin. Invest.*, 1992; 90: 2355–2361.

18. Cid, MC, Campo, E, Ercilla, G, Palacín, A, Vilaseca, J, Villalta, J, Ingelmo, M, Immunohistochemical analysis of lymphoid and macrophage cell subsets and their immunologic activation markers in temporal arteritis, *Arthritis Rheum.*, 1989; 32: 884–893.

19. Weyand, CM, Hicok, KC, Hunder, GG, Goronzy, JJ, Tissue cytokine patterns in patients with poly-myalgia rheumatica and giant-cell arteritis, *Ann. Intern. Med.*, 1994; 121: 484–491.

20. Weyand, CM, Tetzlaff, N, Björnsson, J, Brack, A, Younge, B, Goronzy, JJ, Disease patterns and tissue cytokine profiles in giant cell arteritis, *Arthritis Rheum.*, 1997; 40: 19–26.

21. Weyand, CM, Shonberger, J, Oppitz, U, Hunder, NNH, Hicok, KC, Goronzy, JJ, Distinct vascular lesions in giant cell arteritis share identical T cell clonotypes, *J. Exp. Med.*, 1994; 179: 951–960.

22. Gabriel, S, Espy, M, Erdman, D, Björnsson, J, Smith, TF, Hunder, GG, The role of parvovirus B19 in the pathogenesis of giant-cell arteritis. A preliminary evaluation, *Arthritis Rheum.*, 1999; 42: 1255–1258.

23. Weyand, CM, Goronzy, JJ, Arterial wall injury in giant cell arteritis, *Arthritis Rheum.*, 1999; 42: 844–853.

24. Font, C, Cebrián, M, Cid, MC, Coll-Vinent, B, Sánchez, E, López–Soto, A, Grau, JM, Polymorpho-nuclear leukocytes and E-selectin expression in inflammatory lesions of giant cell arteritis, *Arthritis Rheum.*, 1996; 39 (suppl): S67.

25. Cid, MC, Cebrián, M, Font, C, Coll-Vinent, B, Hernández-Rodríguez, J, Esparza, J, Urbano-Márquez, A, Grau, JM, Cell adhesion molecules in the development of inflammatory infiltrates in giant-cell arteritis. Inflammation-induced angiogenesis as the preferential site of leukocyte/endothelial cell interactions, *Arthritis Rheum.*, 2000; 43: 184–194.

26. Cid, MC, New developments in the pathogenesis of systemic vasculitis, *Curr. Opin. Rheumatol.*, 1996; 8:1–11.

27. Kaiser, M, Weyand, CM, Björnsson, J, Goronzy, JJ, Platelet-derived growth factor, intimal hyperplasia, and ischemic complications in giant cell arteritis, *Arthritis Rheum.*, 1998; 41: 623–633.

28. Huston, KA, Hunder, GG, Lie, JT, Kennedy, RH, Elveback, LR, Temporal arteritis. A 25-year epidemiological, clinical and pathologic study, *Ann. Intern. Med.*, 1978; 88: 162–167.

29. Calamia, KT, Hunder, GG, Clinical manifestations of giant cell arteritis, *Clin. Rheum. Dis.*, 1980; 6: 389–403.

30. Hayreh, SS, Podhajsky, PA, Zimmerman, B, Ocular manifestations of giant cell arteritis, *Am. J. Ophthalmol.*, 1988; 125: 509–520.

31. Cid, MC, Font, C, Oristrell, J, de la Sierra, A, Coll-Vinent, B, López-Soto, A, Vilaseca, J, Urbano-Márquez, A, Grau, JM, Association between strong inflammatory response and low risk of developing visual loss and other cranial ischemic complications in giant cell (temporal) arteritis, *Arhritis Rheum.*, 1998; 41: 26–32.

32. Chuang, TY, Hunder, GG, Ilstrup, DM, Kurland, LT, Polymyalgia rheumatica: a 10-year epidemiologic and clinical study, *Ann. Intern. Med.*, 1982; 97: 672–680.

33. Salvarani, C, Macchioni, P, Boiardi, L, Polymyalgia rheumatica, *Lancet*, 1997; 350: 43–47.

34. Salvarani, C, Hunder, GG, Musculoskeletal manifestations in a population-based cohort of patients with giant-cell arteritis, *Arthritis Rheum.*, 1999; 42: 1259–1266.

35. Salvarani, C, Cantini, F, Macchioni, P, Olivieri, I, Niccoli, L, Padula, A, Boiardi, L, Distal muscu-loskeletal manifestations in polymyalgia rheumatica, *Arthritis Rheum.*, 1998; 41: 1221–1226.

36. Roche, EN, Fullbright, JW, Wagner, A, Hunder, GG, Goronzy, JJ, Weyand, CM, Correlation between interleukin-6 production and disease activity in polymyalgia rheumatica and giant cell arteritis, *Arthritis Rheum.*, 1993; 36: 1286–1294.

37. Coll-Vinent, B, Vilardell, C, Font, C, Oristrell, J, Hernández-Rodríguez, J, Yagüe, J, Urbano-Márquez, A, Grau, JM, Cid, MC, Circulating soluble adhesion molecules in patients with giant cell arteritis. Correlation between soluble intercellular adhesion molecule-1 (ICAM-1) concentrations and disease activity, *Ann Rheum. Dis.*, 1999; 58: 189–192.

38. Cid, MC, Monteagudo, J, Oristrell, J, Vilaseca, J, Pallarés, L, Cervera, R, Font, C, Font, J, Ingelmo, M, Urbano-Márquez, A, Von Willebrand factor in the outcome of temporal arteritis, *Ann. Rheum. Dis.,* 1996; 55: 927–930.

39. Vilaseca, J, González, A, Cid, MC, López-Vivancos, J, Ortega, A, Clinical usefulness of temporal artery biopsy, *Ann. Rheum. Dis.,* 1987; 46: 282–285.

40. Cid, MC, Campo, E, Diagnostic value of the temporal artery biopsy, *Med. Clin.* (Barc.), 1989; 92: 95–97.

41. Ellis, ME, Ralston, WS, The ESR in the diagnosis and management of the polymyalgia rheumatica/giant cell arteritis syndrome, *Ann. Rheum. Dis.,* 1983; 42: 168–170.

42. Hunder, GG, Bloch, DA, Michel, BA, Stevens, MB, Arend, WP, Calabrese, LH, Edworthy, SM, Fauci, AS, Leavitt, RY, Lie, JT, Lightfoot, RW, Masi, AT, McShane, DJ, Mills, JA, Wallace, SL, Zvaifler, NJ, The American College of Rheumatology 1990 criteria for the classification of giant cell arteritis, *Arthritis Rheum.,* 1990; 33: 1122–1128.

43. Healey, LA, Long-term follow-up of polymyalgia rheumatica: evidence for synovitis, *Semin. Arthritis Rheum.,* 1984; 13: 322–328.

44. Achkar, AA, Lie, JT, Hunder, GG, O'Fallon, WM, Gabriel, SE, How does previous corticosteroid treatment affect the biopsy findings of giant cell (temporal) arteritis? *Ann. Intern. Med.,* 1994; 120: 987–992.

45. González-Gay, MA, Blanco, R, Rodríguez-Valverde, V, Martínez-Taboada, VM, Delgado-Rodríguez, M, Figueroa, M, Uriarte, E, Permanent visual loss and cerebrovascular accidents in giant cell arteritis, *Arthritis Rheum.,* 1998; 41: 1497–1504.

46. Delecoeuillerie, G, Joly, P, Cohen de Lara, A, Paolaggi, JB, Polymyalgia rheumatica and temporal arteritis: a retrospective analysis of prognostic features and different corticosteroid regimens (11 year survey of 210 patients), *Ann. Rheum. Dis.,* 1988; 47: 733–739.

47. Save-Söderbergh, J, Malmvall, BE, Andersson, R, Bengtsson, BA, Giant cell arteritis as a cause of death, *JAMA,* 1986; 255: 493–496.

18 Vascular Manifestations in Takayasu's Arteritis

Fujio Numano, M.D., Ph.D.

CONTENTS

0-8493-1335-X/01/$0.00+$.50
© 2001 by CRC Press LLC

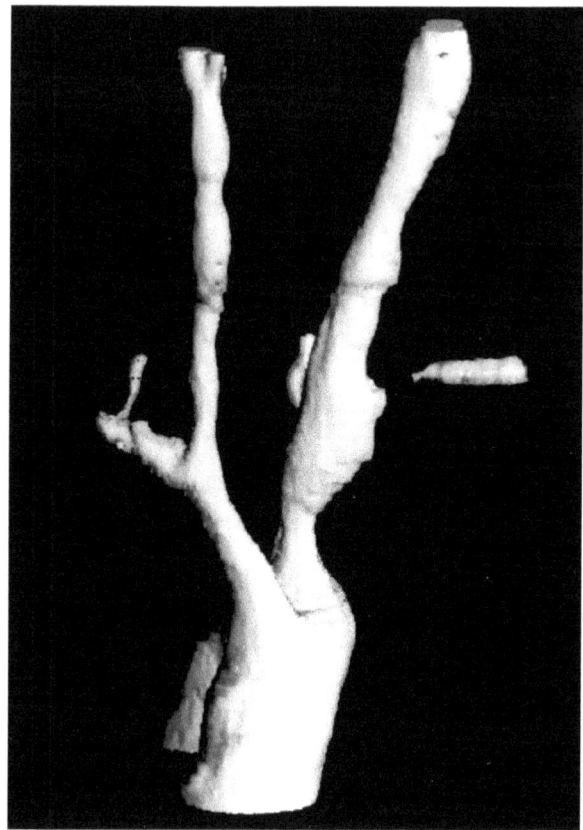

FIGURE 18.1 3D-CT picture of 24-year-old male patient with Takayasu's arteritis.

I. PREFACE

A. DEFINITION

Takayasu's arteritis is a systemic chronic vasculitis which frequently involves the aorta and/or its major branches and as well as the coronary and pulmonary arteries. These chronic inflammatory conditions cause arterial stenosis and/or occlusion of the arteries, resulting from thrombus formation presenting the characteristic clinical picture of weakness or absence of pulses (Figure 18.1).[1-6]

On the other hand, rapid inflammation causes dilatation and/or aneurysmal formation of vessel wall, developing into serious morbid conditions such as dissecting aneurysms and aortic regurgitation due to the dilatation of ascending aorta. Other clinical manifestations documented are coarctation of aorta, renovascular hypertension, cerebral bleeding, ischemic cerebral and heart disease, congestive heart failure, pulmonary infarction, cataracts, blindness, and nephrotic syndrome.[1,6-8]

The disease has a chronic progressive course generally, and often presents nonspecific inflammatory conditions such as intermittent fever, fatigue, and malaise existing months to years prior to the onset of full-blown vascular disease.[9,10] The etiology of this morbid condition is still unknown. Today it is generally accepted that it is a multifactorial disease, and autoimmune mechanism may play an important role in the initiation and the progression of the morbid condition.[8,10] Recent studies demonstrated a close association of HLA with this disease, which may solve the puzzle of racial differences of this condition.[1,11-13]

Sex differences in prevalence have also been noted as the other characteristics of this disease, in addition to the findings that female subjects of reproductive age are most often affected.

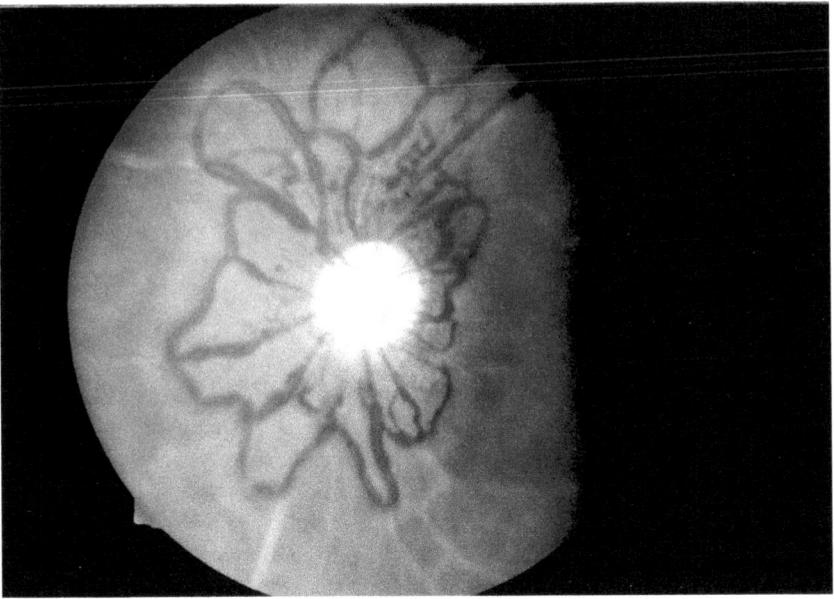

FIGURE 18.2 Typical coronary anastomosis of retinal vessels observed in a patient with Takayasu's arteritis. (Courtesy of Dr. K. Sano.)

In fact, Takayasu's arteritis is frequently found in certain Asian countries including Japan,[9] Korea,[14] China,[15] India,[16] Thailand,[17] Turkey,[18] and Israel.[19] It is also found in South and Central American countries, including Mexico,[20] Columbia,[21] Brazil,[22] and Peru,[23] but rarely among Caucasian peoples.

B. History

The first case of this morbid condition was reported by Mikito Takayasu in 1905 at the Japan Ophthalmology Society Meeting,[8,24,25] describing an interesting eyeground view of a 21-year-old female characterized by coronary anastomosis of retinal central vessels (Figure 18.2). This report was independently corroborated at the same meeting by K. Onishi and T. Kagoshima with their own cases presenting the same characteristic eyeground. In these cases it was also pointed out that the pulse could not be palpated in both radial arteries (K. Onishi) or in the left radial artery (T. Kagoshima). Today, this condition has been elucidated as vasculitis and the characteristic ophthalmic condition resulted from the ischemia of retinal vessels. Reviewing old Japanese medical literature, this very same condition was documented as early as 1830 in the book called *Kitsuo-Idan* by Dr. Rokushu Yamamoto.[25]

The systemic pathological study was first reported by K. Ohta for a 25-year-old female patient with Takayasu arteritis. It was made clear that this disease was caused by vasculitis involving mainly the aorta and its main branches, and also included pulmonary arteritis.[25,26] The inflammatory changes were confirmed not only in the medial layer but also in both the intima and adventitia of the arteries, and thus characterized as "pan aortitis." The clinical features of 31 cases with Takayasu arteritis were summarized by Shimizu and Sano in 1951 and reported as "pulseless disease,"[2] emphasizing pulselessness, coronary anastomosis in the retinal vasculature, and accentuated carotid sinus reflex as the triad of clinical features. Caccamize and Whiteman, thereafter, introduced this disease in the *American Heart Journal*,[3] contributing much to establish the descriptive apellation of "pulseless disease" in Western countries.

Ross and Mckussich and Ask-Upmark classified the pulseless conditions into three types: "young female arteritis," "syphilitic aortitis," and "various other pathological conditions such as severe arteriosclerosis."[4,27] "Young female arteritis" can be equivalent to Takayasu's arteritis and can be identified with four similar cases reported by Frovig where concomitant cerebral and ocular manifestations were observed.[28] Ueda stressed an involvement of autoimmune mechanism as one of the main causes of this condition, which has become a trigger for HLA analysis in search of the relationship to genetic failure.[29]

II. PATHOGENESIS

A. PATHOLOGICAL FEATURES

Though more than 50% of patients demonstrated angiographically confirmed involvement of the entire aorta,[1,11,30] pathological study revealed that there were usually intact areas between the affected area of arteries (skipped lesions), and active productive inflammatory areas were sometimes encountered in neighboring old fibrous areas. However, recent autopsy cases have made clear that skipped lesions were disappearing and, in turn, atherosclerotic lesions were more often evident.[31]

Nasu histologically classified Takayasu's arteritis into the three types: granulomatous inflammation, diffuse productive inflammation, and fibrotic type, which are characterized according to the progression of Takaysu's arteritis[32] (Figure 18.3a). Hotchi, examining autopsy cases, classified its inflammatory lesions into acute exudative (including suppurative), chronic nonspecific productive, and granulomatous inflammation. He stressed elastico phagia (Figure 18.3B) as the important characteristic features of Takayasu's arteritis.[31] These inflammatory lesions originate as shown in (Figure 18.3C); significant accumulation of T-cells first, and later macrophages are commonly seen in the outer side of the media and/or its neighboring adventitia around vaso vasorum. Recent studies have demonstrated positive production of inflammatory cytokines and/or adhesion molecules around these areas, which may give rise to chemotactic activity of monocytes and T-cells.[33,34] This may suggest an autoimmune process or a reaction to viral infection.[35,36] Destruction of medial smooth muscle cells and elastic fiber, fibrotic changes, and fibrocellular thickening of the intima are followed (Figure 18.3C). With fibrous thickening in all three layers, the fibrotic type is completed (Figure 18.3D). The fibrocellular changes in intima also accelerate atherosclerotic changes. The invasion into intima by monocytes, lipids, and/or various inflammatory substances from blood streams result in stenotic changes and thrombogenic surfaces.

These complications with atherosclerosis have made it difficult to diagnose Takayasu arteritis, particularly in elderly patients. Confirmation of thickened adventitia is the best clue for differential diagnosis. Acute progress of inflammation destroys the medial structure rapidly causing formation of aneurysms, and sometimes dissected aneurysms.

B. HLA AND THE AUTOIMMUNE MECHANISM

The racial and geographically different distributions observed in Takayasu's arteritis suggest ethnic difference in the susceptibility to and/or clinical manifestation of this disease. Moreover, familial occurrence of Takayasu's arteritis has been reported, including three monozygotic twin sisters in Japan, India, and Brazil,[1,12,23] strongly suggesting some genetic factor(s) being involved in its pathogenesis.

Worldwide investigation has been conducted in search of an association of HLA class antigen with Takayasu's arteritis, because HLA genes are the best candidates in determing the susceptibility to the disease. HLA genes are highly polymorphic and show remarkable ethnic or geographic differences in allele and haplotype frequencies.[37,38] Moreover, HLA allelic differences determine the susceptibility to autoimmune diseases. Takayasu's arteritis reveals several characteristic features

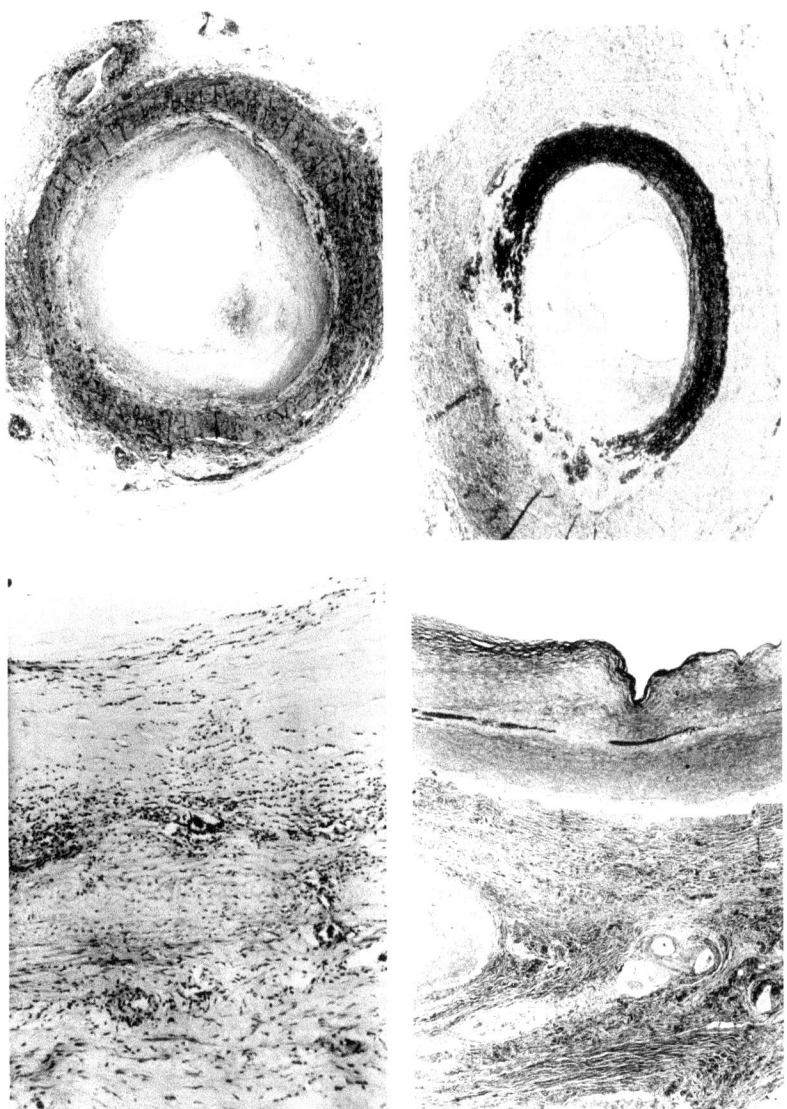

FIGURE 18.3 Histological features of Takayasu's arteritis. (A) Subclavian artery in a 48-year-old female patient with Takayasu arteritis: atherosclerotic changes in intima, totally destructed medial layer and thickened adventitia with cellular infiltration from vasa vasorum (H. E. Stain × 10). (B) Segmental destruction of the media, reactive fibrous thickening of the intima, and perivascular fibrosis. Elastica van Gieson (by Dr. Hotchi, ref. 31). (C) Cellular infiltration is remarkable from adventitia to medical layer. (D) Typical fibrous intimal thickening, destructed and fibrous media and thickened adventitia.

of autoimmune disorder and complications with other autoimmune diseases such as Behçet disease, SLE, ulcerative colitis, and autoimmune endocrine disorders.[39,40] Previous reports in serological HLA typing revealed the close association of Takayasu's arteritis with HLA-B52 and DR2 in Japanese;[41,42] B5 in Indians;[43] B52, DR7, and DQ2 in Koreans;[44] and DR4 in Caucasians.[45]

Recent progress in PCR-based HLA-DNA oligo typing techniques enables analyzation of the polymorphisms in HLA genes at the DNA level,[46] and Kimura confirmed the close association of Takayasu's arteritis with HLA-B52[01], B39[02], DPB_1* 0901, and DRB1* 1502 in Japanese[13] (Figure 18.4) (Table 18.1). DRB1* 1502 and DPB_1* 0901 show strong linkage disequilibrium with B5201

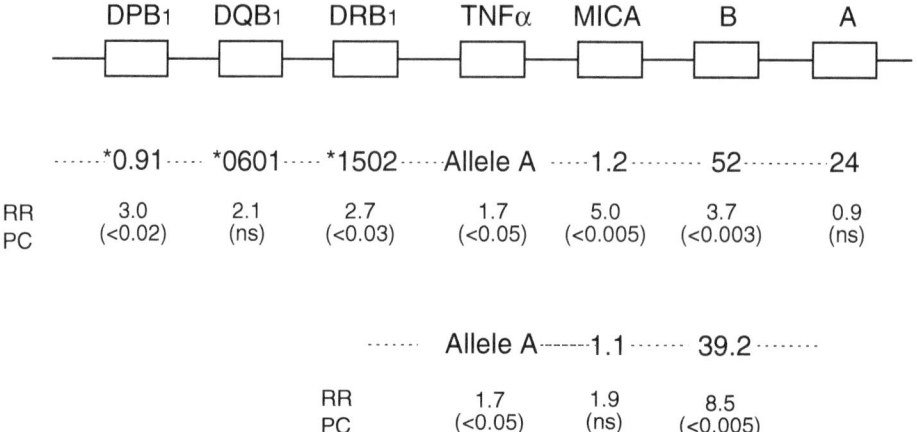

FIGURE 18.4 Association of HLA, TNFα, MICA gene with Takayasu's arteritis.

in Japanese. Furthermore, analysis of MIC genes, which are located near the HLA B locus, exhibited even stronger association with the disease, suggesting primary genetic factors could be located between MIC and the HLA B locus gene (Table 18.2).[47] Although the frequency of B3902 is very low among the general population in Japan, the statistical significance was clearly observed between the patients with Takayasu's arteritis and control subjects. This significance was even greater in patients without HLA-B52 than in those who were HLA-B52 positive. It will be interesting to study a frequency of B3902 in South Americans in whom B39 frequency in known to be high. The distribution of HLA-B52 and B39 antigens are different in different ethnic groups[13] (Table 18.3). The disease-associated B39.2 was different from the nondisease-associated B39.1 by two amino acid residues at the 63rd and 67th positions: Asn and Cys in B39.1 and Glu and Ser in B39.2, respectively. On the other hand, sequencing analysis of B52 from patients showed that B*5201, B52, and B3902 share the structure of B pocket in the peptide binding groove of the HLA-B molecule, which might be effective in presenting, for instance, molecules of retrovirus reverse

TABLE 18.1
Association of HLA and MIC-DNA Type with Japanese Patients of Takayasu's Arteritis

HLA	Patients (n = 64)	Controls (n = 492)	RR	PC
B52	65.7%	24.2%	3.7	<0.003
B39.1	7.8	4.5	1.8	ns
B39.2	6.3	0.6	10.9	<0.03
DRB_1 *1502	46.9	24.2	2.7	<0.03
DQB_1 *0601	57.8	39.4	2.1	ns
DPB_1 *0901	45.3	20.9	3.0	<0.02
MICA	**(n = 81)**	**(n = 160)**	**RR**	**PC**
1.1	28.4%	17.5%	1.9	ns
1.2	79.0	43.1	5.1	<0.005

TABLE 18.2
Odds Ratio of Risk in Japanese Patients of Takayasu's Arteritis

B52	vs.	B39.2	Patients (n = 64)	Controls (n = 492)	Odds Ratio	PC
+		+	1	1	14.2	<0.06
+		−	34	121	4.0	<0.00001
−		+	3	2	21.2	<0.00001
−		−	26	368	1.0	
B52	**vs.**	**MICA 1.2**	**(n = 81)**	**(n = 160)**		
+		+	45	31	7.8	<0.0001
+		−	0	0		<0.02
−		+	19	38	2.6	
−		−	17	91		

transcripture, thereby leading to destruction of vessels by killer cells. Interestingly, B52 and B39.2 also share the structure Glu at the 63rd position and Ser at the 67th position.

Recently, Weck reported that murine r-herpes virus causes severe large-vessel arteritis.[48] Through pathological examination of the affected vessels from patients with Takayasu's arteritis, Seko reported the accumulation of T-cells or perforin-secreting cells and heat shock protein in aortic lesions. These infiltrating T-cells are with killer activity and are identified as T-cells.[49] Tanaka also postulated the leading role of cytomegalo virus in inflammatory aortic disease.[50] These data suggest several viruses as the disease-causing agents that induce the autoimmune mechanism in vasculitis.[51,52]

TABLE 18.3
Frequencies of HLA-B52 and B39 Antigens in Various Ethnic Groups

Ethnic Group[a]	B52	B39
Japanese[b]	24.2%	5.1%
Korean	4.9	3.5
Thais	6.1	3.5
Northern Han	4.2	3.5
Indian	13.2	3.1
Mexican	7.2	12.8
Amerinds	6.0	32.8
Aborigine	0.0	29.1
African blacks	5.1	9.3
German	2.1	3.9
Italian	5.3	6.8
Spanish	4.1	1.2

[a] Frequency data were obtained from 11th IHWS,[4] except for Japanese.
[b] Frequency data were obtained from our control panel.

TABLE 18.4
Female:Male Ratio of Patients with Takayasu's Arteritis

Nation (Reporter)	Total (No.)	Female	Male	F/M Ratio
Japan (Dept. Welfare)	2148	1909(89%)	239(11%)	9.0:1
Korea (Park Y.B.)	47	40(85%)	7(15%)	5.7:1
China (Zheng D.)	500	370(74%)	130(26%)	2.8:1
Thailand (Suwanwela N.)	63	43(68%)	20(32%)	2.2:1
India (Sharma B.K.)	106	65(61%)	41(39%)	1.6:1
Israel (Rosenthal T.)	56	32(57%)	18(43%)	1.8:1
Turkey (Turkoglu C.)	14	11(78%)	3(22%)	3.7:1
Mexico (Reyes P.A.)	237	207(87%)	30(13%)	6.9:1
Brazil (Sato E.I.)	73	61(84%)	12(16%)	5.1:1
Colombia (Igresias G.)	35	26(74%)	9(26%)	2.9:1

Source: Takayasu Arteritis I, *Heart & Vessels,* 1992; Takayasu Arteritis II, *Int. J. Card.,* 54, 1996; Takayasu Arteritis III, *Int. J. Card.,* 56, 1998.

C. HYPERESTROGENISM

Another characteristic feature of Takayasu's arteritis is sex difference. More than 80% of patients are female, which has led Takayasu's arteritis to be referred to as "young female arteritis"[5,8,11] (Table 18.4). Numano, observing medial smooth muscle atrophy, necrosis, calcification, and inflammatory reaction in the aortas of rabbits treated with high doses of estrogen, proposed hyperestrogenism as being involved in the pathogenesis of the disease.[53] The author confirmed constantly high levels of urinary total estrogens in young female patients with Takayasu's arteritis. He posturated that high frequency of aortic regurgitation could be induced by destruction of the aortic wall in combined effects of hyperestrogenism and rapid blood flow from cardiac contraction (Figure 18.5).[53] Aortic regurgitation is the most serious complication in Japan. A recent national survey in Japan clearly demonstrated female predominence (female : male = 9:1), and onset ages of female patients were between the teens and the twenties. Male patients, on the other hand, did not show this characteristic age distribution (unpublished data). However, an international survey of Takayasu's arteritis presented the different sex ratios. Japan, Korea, and South American countries revealed predominantly female patients, while India, Thailand, China, Israel, and Turkey did not show a remarkable female predominance[15-23] (Table 18.4).

Sharma reported that Indian female patients were similar to Japanese female patients in suffering from involvements of the aortic arch and its branches, whereas Indian male patients showed predominantly abdominal aortic involvement, more frequent hypertension, and its complication.[54] Deutch, who first described the racial differences, also observed a high frequency of abdominal aorta in males.[25,55] These data, in turn, stress the different definitions for Takayasu's arteritis in Japan than in other countries.[30]

IV. CLINICAL MANIFESTATIONS

Takayasu's arteritis is a systemic vascular disease that causes a variety of symptoms and complaints reflecting the sites of vessels involved, which makes diagnosis of this disease more difficult. Table 18.5 summarizes the chief clinical symptoms obtained from two national surveys in Japan.[9] Japanese patients exhibit the complaints of abnormal blood flow in cerebral or opthalmological and/or upper extremities, such as dizziness, faulty vision, palpitation, pulselessness, and neck pain. In addition, many patients expressed complaints of general inflammatory conditions such as general malaise and fibrilla.[1,9] There are many reports where patients were accidentally found during their regular

TABLE 18.5
Clinical Symptoms of Takayasu's Arteritis

	1973 to 1975 (Major Complaint at the Initial Consultation) Case (%)	1982 to 1984 (Throughout the Course of Disease) Case (%)
Cerebrovascular disorder[a]	873/1,351 (64.6)	551/1,302 (42.3)
Ophthalmological symptom	310/1,297 (23.9)	301/1,276 (23.6)
Cardiac symptom	742/1,344 (55.2)	536/1,296 (41.4)
Hypertension	606/1,336 (45.4)	734/1,318 (55.7)
Vascular disorder in the extremities[b]	969/1,341 (72.3)	930/1,261 (73.8)
Acute pain[c]	492/1,292 (38.1)	288/1,255 (22.9)
Systemic symptom	885/1,324 (66.8)	769/1,280 (60.1)

[a] Cerebral ischemia in the present survey.

[b] Ischemia in the extremities in the present survey.

[c] Vascular pain in the present survey.

health examinations by elevated erythrocyte sedimentation rate (ESR), difference in blood pressure for both upper extremities, or pulselessness. A subsequent survey has confirmed a clear decline of opthalmologic complaints due mainly to early diagnosis and early initiation of treatment. As already mentioned, it is quite rare in many counties to find patients whose eyegrounds show the typical retinal characteristic changes shown in Figure 18.1. The American College of Rheumatology subcommittee has, therefore, excluded this rarely seen ophthalmic condition from the criteria.[56] Nevertheless, a sizable number of patients are still suffering from ophthalmic disorders in Japan.[57] On the contrary, headache and dizziness caused by hypertension are the most commonly noted symptoms among Takayasu's patients in other Asian countries. Intermittent claudication is another serious symptom in China,[15] India,[16] and Thailand,[17] although it is very rare in Japan (Table 18.6).[9] These clear differences received much attention. A comparative survey among Asian countries was undertaken and confirmed several distinct involvements of the aorta.[11,58,59]

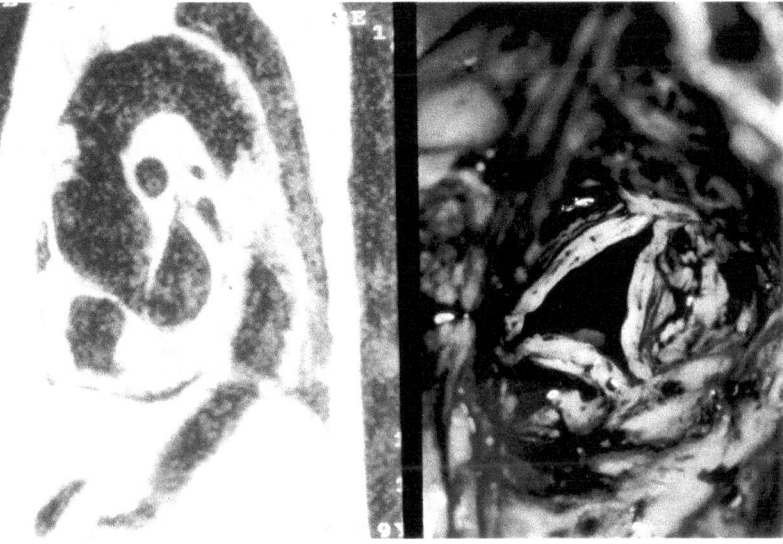

FIGURE 18.5 Aortic regurgitation due to dilation of ascending aorta in Takayasu's arteritis.

TABLE 18.6
Main Complications

	Japan	India	P Value
Hypertension	44/75 (59%)	90/101 (89%)	P < 0.01
Cerebrovascular disease	3/53 (5.6%)	11/96 (11%)	NS
Retinopathy	15/100 (30%)	74/102 (73%)	P < 0.01
Aortic regurgitation	35/66 (53%)	7/94 (7.5%)	P < 0.01
Congestive heart failure	6/60 (10%)	13/100 (13%)	NS

A. CLINICAL PRESENTATIONS

Cardiac Manifestation. Cardiac manifestation has become the most serious complication in Japan, while the classic ophthalmic condition has decreased. Chest pain, dizziness, arrythmia, and short breath due to ischemic heart disease have increased among patients with Takayasu's arteritis.[9] Accelerated coronary atherosclerosis becomes more evident as patients age and it produces these ischemic conditions.[60,61]

Congestive heart disease and arrhythmia due to aortic regurgitation is now the number-one cause of death among Takayasu's patients. Aortic regurgitation is the result of a dilated ascending aorta as shown in Figure 18.5.[9,11,62,63] It is the most important task for physicians to apply careful judgment at the inflammatory stage, and to determine the appropriate timing for a Bental operation (see Surgical Treatment).

Pulmonary Manifestations. Pulmonary disease in Takayasu's arteritis is usually due to the involvement of the pulmonary artery and includes symptoms of dyspnea, pleurisy, and hemoptysis. The right pulmonary artery in the upper lung field is most often involved. Easy thrombus formation is one of the characteristic pathological conditions that is responsible for the relatively high frequency of pulmonary infarction. As it is a slowly progressive condition, however, many patients may be unaware of pulmonary infarction. A pulmonary synchigram is very useful to confirm patients' lung conditions. This is because the infarction frequently starts in the pulmonary (functional) artery, not in the bronchial nutritional arteries.[61,64]

Nonvascular pulmonary intraparenchymal changes can also occur occasionally. These descriptions are of acute interstitial pneumonia, interstitial pulmonary fibrosis, and alveolar damage with focal hyaline membrane formation on pathological examination of lung specimens. A favorable response to steroid therapy has been reported with interstitial pneumonia and pneumonic consolidation.

Renal Manifestations. Renal involvement is usually characterized by renovascular hypertension. Sharma reported renal artery involvement involving ostia and a variable length of proximal renal artery in 48% of patients in India.[16] The various therapeutic modalities suggested for treatment of renal artery stenosis include percutaneous angioplasty, vascular bypass graft, and autotransplantation of the kidney. The prolonged clinical course of Takayasu's arteritis has brought attention to the nephrotic syndrome in Japan.[9] The presence of proteinuria, hypercholesteremia, can be characterized in renal dysfunction. It is thought that nonspecific ischemic glomerular lesions are generated from long-standing arterial narrowing and mesangial deposits of IgM, IgG, and IgA. The usual clinical manifestations of glomerular involvement are microscopic hematuria and proteinuria in the nonnephrotic range.[65]

Neurological Manifestation. The common neurologic manifestations are headache, paraesthesia, visual disturbances, syncope, hemiplegia, seizure, hypertensive encephalopathy, and paraplegia. Although cerebral vascular accident was once the number-one cause of death among patients in Japan, such a desperate condition is less frequently seen today because of well-controlled blood pressure. However, in other Asian countries, hypertension is still frequently reported, and cerebral vascular accident is the most prevalent serious complication in Takayasu arteritis.[14-19] Serious illness and death in younger patients can occur from central nervous system involvement. Cerebral vascular disease is either due to an uncontrolled hypertension or as a consequence of carotid or brachiocephalic obstruction.

Complication with Other Autoimmune Diseases. The autoimmune mechanism is now considered to play an important role in the pathogenesis of Takayasu's arteritis. There have been several papers reporting Takayasu's arteritis complicated with other autoimmune diseases, or collagen diseases such as SLE, colitis ulcerosa, and Behçet disease.[66-69]

B. REGIONAL DIFFERENCES

An international annual survey completed recently on Takayasu's arteritis revealed that the main characteristic features seen in Japan did not always coincide with those in patients of other nationalities. There are many different characteristic clinical manifestations among Asian populations.[11-23] Clinical manifestations and angiographic findings were compared among Japanese, Korean, and Indian patients.[58,59] Most Japanese patients present weak or absent radial pulse and/or ischemic symptons of cervical arteritis. Most Korean, Chinese, and Indian patients, however, present the complaints suggestive of lesions in the abdominal aorta with involvement of renal arteries, leading to renovascular hypertension. These characteristic manifestations are confirmed by comparative studies on angiograms under the new criteria[70] (Figure 18.6).

In comparison of angiograms, Japanese patients frequently show an involvement of the ascending aorta and aortic arch with their branches, and in only a very few cases some limited involvement of the abdominal aorta. In contrast, Indian and Thai patients exhibit an involvement of the abdominal aorta far more frequently than Japanese ($p < 0.01$) (Table 18.7).[58,70] In addition, a large number of cases demonstrated a suggestive progression of vasculitis from the abdominal aorta to the thoracic aorta. In a separate study the clinical manifestations were compared in Japanese and Indian patients. While dizziness, vertigo, and pulselessness were common in Japanese, headache and hypertension were common in Indians. Electrocardiographic findings showed that left ventricular hypertrophy was more frequent in Indian patients, probably due to the higher frequency of hypertension. These

TABLE 18.7
Anatomical Distribution of Vascular Lesions

	Japan	India	P Value
Ascending aorta	34	9	$P < 0.01$
Aortic arch	14	19	NS
Descending thoracic aorta	36	29	$P < 0.05$
Brachiocephalic artery	22	15	$P < 0.05$
Vertebral artery (right/left)	26 (16/10)	10 (3/7)	$P < 0.01$
Subclavian artery (right/left)	67 (25/42)	86 (26/60)	NS
Common carotid artery (right/left)	68 (29/39)	30 (11/19)	$P < 0.01$
Abdominal aorta	38	75	$P < 0.05$
Renal artery (right/left)	27 (13/14)	122 (59/63)	$P < 0.01$
Celiac artery	1	7	NS
Superior mesenteric artery	5	15	NS
Inferior mesenteric artery	2	3	NS
Iliac artery (right/left)	0	28 (16/12)	$P < 0.01$
Total	340	448	

different manifestations suggest the different involvement of vascular sites. Angiographic analysis confirmed that an involvement of the ascending aorta, the aortic arch, and the branchiocepharic, vertebral, and common carotid arteries was observed mainly in Japanese patients. On the other hand, an involvement of the abdominal aorta and renal arteries was observed mainly in Indian patients. These angiographical differences reflect the higher frequency of aortic regurgitation, pulselessness, dizziness, and vertigo among Japanese patients, and hypertension of renal vascular origin, retinopathy, and headache among Indian patients. The comparison of anatomical findings between Japanese and Indian patients coincides with these clinical characteristic manifestations.[58,65,70]

IV. DIAGNOSIS

A. DIAGNOSTIC CRITERIA

Diagnosis of Takayasu's arteritis is often delayed due to a nonspecific presentation. The prevalence of this disease has been widely variable in different geographical regions of the world. Due to the inflammatory or systemic features of this disease, undiagnosed patients are kept under investigation for rheumatoid arteritis, Behçet disease, ankylosing spondylitis, infective endocarditis, artherosclerotic disease, fever of unknown origin, essential hypertension, coarctation of the aorta, and cardiomyopathy before the final diagnosis is established. In Japan, young female patients were occasionally misdiagnosed with tuberculosis for elevated ESR and malaise. Ishikawa proposed his criteria in 1988.[71] Table 18.8 is the guideline for clinical diagnosis by the Committee of Takayasu's Arteritis of the Ministry of Health and Welfare of Japan.[7] These criteria consisted of an obligatory criterion of age being less than 40 years old, two major criteria of left and right subclavian arterial lesions, and nine minor criteria including hypertension, a high ESR, and arteriographic demonstration of lesions for different arteries. In addition to the obligatory criterion, the presence of two major or one major plus two or more minor criteria, or four or more minor criteria, suggest a high probability of Takayasu's arteritis. Ishikawa's criteria were solely based on observations of Japanese

---

TABLE 18.8
Guidelines for Making a Clinical Diagnosis of Takayasu's Arteritis

1. Symptoms
    (1) Cerebral ischemia: vertigo (especially when looking upward), fainting spells, visual disturbance (especially at direct sunshine)
    (2) Ischemia of the extremities: cold fingers, easy fatiguability of the upper extremities
    (3) Stenosis of the aorta or renal arteries: headache, vertigo, shortness of breath, which are considered due to hypertension
    (4) Generalized symptoms: slight fever may be recognized at the onset of the disease
2. Important findings for diagnosis
    (1) Abnormalities of the pulse of the upper extremities (weak or diminution and/or right/left difference of the radial pulse)
    (2) Abnormalities of the pulse of the lower extremities (accentuation or decrease of the pulse)
    (3) Vascular murmur in the arteries of the neck, back, or abdomen
    (4) Ophthalmologic abnormalities
3. Abnormalities in laboratory examinations
    (1) Increased erythrocytes sedimentation rate
    (2) Positive C-reactive protein
    (3) Increase in gamma-globulin levels in the serum
4. Important diagnostic points
    (1) Prevalent in young women
    (2) Final clinical diagnosis can be made by an aortography
5. Differential diagnosis to be made: Buerger's disease, arteriosclerosis, collagen disease, congenital vascular abnormalities

Research Committee of Takayasu's arteritis. The Japanese Ministry of Health and Welfare, 1997.

TABLE 18.9
Modified Diagnostic Criteria for Takayasu's Arteritis*

Three major criteria:

1. Left mid subclavian artery lesion	The most severe stenosis or occlusion present in the mid portion from the point 1 cm proximal to the vertebral artery orifice up to that 3 cm distal to the orifice determined by angiography
2. Right mid subclavian artery lesion	The most severe stenosis or occlusion present in the mid portion from the right vertebral artery orifice to the point 3 cm distal to orifice determined by angiography
3. Characteristic signs and symptoms of at least one month duration	These include limb claudication, pulselessness or pulse differences in limbs, an unobtainable or significant blood presence difference (>10 mmHg systolic blood presence difference in limb), fever, neck pain, transient amaurosis, blurred vision, syncope, dysponea or palpitations.

Ten minor criteria

1. High ESR	Unexplained persistent high ESR > 20 mm/h (Westergren) at diagnosis or presence of the evidence in patients history
2. Carotid artery tenderness	Unilateral or bilateral tenderness of common arteries on palpation. Neck muscle tenderness is unacceptable.
3. Hypertension	Persistent blood pressure > 140/90 mmHg brachial or > 160/90 mmHg popliteal
4. Aortic regurgitation or Annuloaortic ectasia	By auscultation or doppler echocardiology or angiography. By angiography or two-dimension echocardiography.
5. Pulmonary artery lesion	Lobar or segmental arterial occlusion or equivalent determined by angiography or perfusion scintigraphy, or presence of stenosis, aneurysm, luminal irregularity or any combination in pulmonary trunk or in unilateral or bilateral pulmonary arteries determined by angiography.
6. Left mid common carotid lesion	Presence of the most severe stenosis or occlusion in the mid portion of 5 cm in length from the point 2 cm distal to its orifice determined by angiography.
7. Distal brachiocephalic trunk lesion	Presence of the most severe stenosis or occlusion in the distal third determined by angiography
8. Descending thoracic aorta lesion	Narrowing, dilation or aneurysm, luminal irregularity or any combination deteremined by angiography; tortuosity alone is unacceptable.
9. Abdominal aorta lesion	Narrowing, dilation or aneurysm, luminal irregularity or aneurysm combination.
10. Coronary artery lesion	Documented on angiography below the age of 30 years in the absence of risk factors like hyperlipidemia or diabetes mellitus

Note: The presence of two major or one major and two minor criteria or four minor criteria suggests a high probability of Takayasu's arteritis.

* Sharma et al., 1995.

patients; therefore, it was not concerned about the geographical and racial variations which resulted in underdiagnosis in some parts of the world.[71] Other criteria suggested by the American College of Rheumatology in 1990[56] consist of six aspects: age being less than 40 years, claudication for an extremity, decreased brachial artery pulse, greater than 10 mmHg difference in systolic pressure between arms, a bruit over subclavian arteries or aorta, and angiographic evidence of narrow or occlusion of the aorta or its primary or proximal branches. The presence of three of the six criteria is required for the diagnosis. The patients in whom the abdominal aorta is predominantly involved can be underdiagnosed. In these criteria, ophthalmologic findings and/or symptoms were excluded, perhaps due to low frequency. However, it should be noted that in Japan there are still more than 20% of patients with complaints of visual disturbance such as cataracts or blindness.[57] Table 18.9 is Ishikawa's criteria modified by Sharma et al. in 1995.[72] These modifications include (a) removal of the obligatory criterion of age, (b) the characteristic signs and symptoms being made one of the major criteria, (c) removal of age from defining hypertension, (d) deletion of the absence of aorto-iliac lesion from the ninth minor criterion, and (e) an addition of the tenth minor criterion of coronary artery lesion in patients younger than age 30. The presence of two major or one major plus two minor criteria or four minor criteria, should suggest a high probability of Takayasu's arteritis. Three sets of criteria were compared for sensitivity and specificity in 106 angiographically proven patients.[72] An adoption of these criteria is likely to diagnose sooner, thereby preventing a high morbidity and mortality occurring due to severe hypertension, retinal damage, cardiac or renal failure, and devastating effects of irreversible vascular occlusion associated with the disease.

B. Angiographic Classifications

Nasu classified the autopsy findings of Japanese patients into four types.[68] Type I primarily involves the branches from the aortic arch. Type II included an involvement of the abdominal aorta, and particularly of the renal arteries. Type III involved the whole aorta and its branches.[73] However, a recent international survey demonstrated that an involvement of the descending and/or abdominal aorta and its branches is more significant in Asians and South Americans than in Japanese. Thus, a new classification for Takayasu arteritis was established in 1994[70] (Figure 18.6). Type I involves primarily the aortic arch and its branches. Type IIa involves the ascending aorta, aortic arch, and its branches. Type IIb involves the ascending aorta, aortic arch with its branches, and thoracic descending aorta. Type III involves the thoracic descending aorta, abdominal aorta, and/or renal arteries. This type can be significant when considering the spread of vascular lesions and was not defined in Nasu's classification. Type IV affects only the abdominal aorta and/or renal arteries. Type V affects the combined features of both Type IIb and II. Furthermore, an involvement of coronary or pulmonary artery should be indicated as C(+) or P(+), respectively. Table 18.10 compares the angiographic findings in five countries.[14,15,17,58,59] The frequency of Type IIa was significantly higher among Japanese patients, while the frequencies of Type IV and Type V cases were higher in Indian and Thai patients. Nearly half of all three countries are Type V, the combined type of vascular distribution. Patients in Central and South American countries, though small in number, appeared to be similar to Japanese types.[21,22]

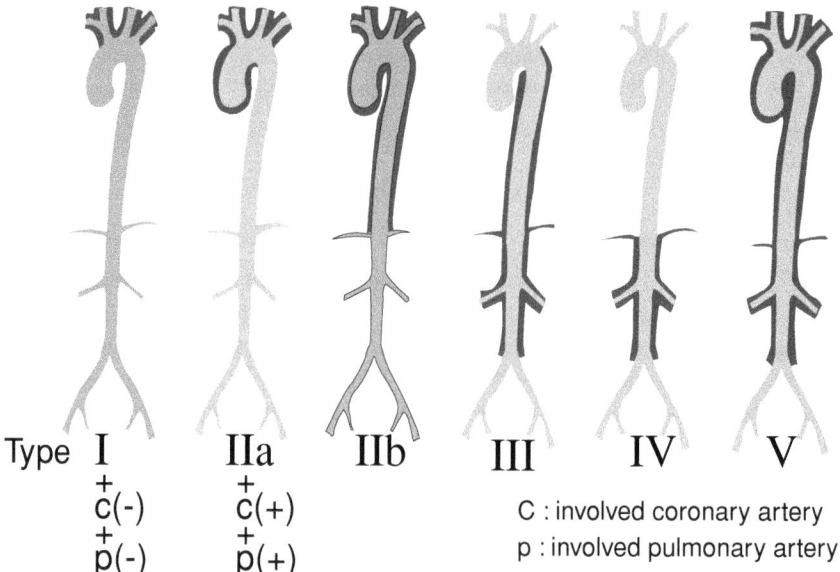

FIGURE 18.6 New classification of angiogram in Takayasu's arteritis. (International Conference on Takayasu's arteritis. Tokyo, 1994.)

TABLE 18.10
Angiographic Classification of Takayasu's Arteritis
(Int. Conf. On Takayasu Arteritis 1994)

Type	Japan	Colombia	Brazil	India	Thailand
I	19 (24%)	12 (35%)	6 (21%)	7 (7%)	0
II a	9 (11%)	4 (11%)	1 (4%)	1 (1%)	0
II b	8 (10%)	2 (6%)	0	6 (6%)	7 (11%)
III	1 (1%)	7 (20%)	4 (14%)	29 (28%)	12 (19%)
V	42 (54%)	10 (29%)	16 (54%)	56 (55%)	42 (67%)
Total	80	35	28	102	63

C. LABORATORY TESTS AND IMAGING MODALITIES

1. Laboratory Tests

Inflammatory conditions of Takayasu's arteritis are expressed in elevated ESR and positive CRP as well as subjective complaints of neck pain, malaise, fibrilla, and fatigue. Changes in these indicators are well correlated with its inflammatory condition and curative response to steroid therapy. A national survey in Japan (Table 18.11) indicates 88% of patients with the accelerated ESR (>20mm/h) and 69% with positive CRP (>20 titer).[9] Gamma-globulinemia and leucocytosis (52% and 44%, respectively) are suggestive of autoimmune disorders. Total T-cell count is significantly higher in Takayasu arteritis patients as compared to control subjects. Hematologic data of anemia are common, often multifactorial, and probably related to chronic inflammation. Leukocytosis and thrombocytosis indicate the active stage of Takayasu arteritis. Relatively large numbers of patients exhibit an increase of ASO titer and positive RA,[9] which may suggest the common mechanism with rheumatic diseases. Thrombogenic tendency is also remarkable at acute inflammatory stage.[9] Accelerated platelet aggregation, hyperfibrinemia, expression of adhesion molecules (VCAM-1, ECAM-1), and accelerated coagulability are valuable information in assessing the clinical condition of these patients.[74]

TABLE 18.11
Findings of Laboratory Examinations in Patients with Takayasu's Arteritis

	1973 to 1975 (at the Initial Consultation) Case (%)	1982 to 1984 (at Deterioration) Case (%)
Elevated erythrocyte sedimentation	868/1,193 (72.8)	997/1,130 (88.2)
Increased WBC	437/1,249 (35.0)	506/1,160 (43.6)
Anemia	563/1,175 (47.9)	629/1,149 (54.7)
Increase in γ globulin	483/1,008 (47.9)	502/972 (51.6)
Increase in ASLO	155/1,067 (14.5)	142/920 (15.4)
CRP Positive	666/1,287 (51.7)	800/1,153 (69.4)
RA Positive	108/1,185 (9.1)	119/1,010 (11.8)
Positive Wassermann reaction	23/1,105 (2.1)	25/863 (2.9)
Positive tuberculin reaction	366/532 (68.8)	241/342 (70.5)
Increase in cardiothoracic ratio	413/1,028 (40.2)	
Aortic calcification	239/1,160 (20.6)	251/1,142 (22.0)
Abnormal ECG	538/1,221 (44.1)	578/1,169 (49.4)

2. Imaging Modalities

When CT Scan shows calcification in the vessel walls in young patients, this finding is helpful in the diagnosis of this disease. Carefully taken CT reveals not only wall thickness, appearance of the vessel, intraluminal thrombus, and the lumen, but also the thickness of adventitia, which helps in making the differential diagnosis of Takayasu's arteritis from atherosclerotic change. This can also be a convenient follow-up method for patients undergoing medical treatment.[75-77] Stenosis, dilatation, aneurysms, and hematoma caused by vascular rupture can also be well demonstrated by this imaging. Spiral CT angiography can demonstrate even more clearly the visualization of the blood vessels by three-dimensional reconstruction in multiple planes[78] (Figure 18.1).

Magnetic resonance imaging is a noninvasive procedure requiring no contrast. It produces more detailed information concerning dilatation, stenosis, occlusion, irregularity of vessel wall, and aneurysmal formation in multiple planes. It can demonstrate vascular flow as well. When compared to angiography, a high detection rate (95%) of the lesions can be expected for the aorta, which contributes to diagnose Takayasu's arteritis even in the early stage;[76] however, it is less sensitive for smaller vessels. Magnetic resonance angiography has its main advantages of being noninvasive and requiring no intravascular contrast.[79] It shows better correlation with angiography of the findings of brachiocephalic arteries. In addition, it has been successful in the evaluation of circulation in the head and neck. It has been very useful in Japan in follow-up of dilatation of the aortic wall, especially the ascending aorta, which is causative of aortic regurgitation. Digital Subtraction Angiography (DSA) can also clearly demonstrate its vascularization; however, one has to be aware of the size of vessels examined for correct diagnosis. It is necessary to check vascularization of the affected lesion very carefully when surgical treatment is under consideration. CT Scan, MR imaging, and MR angiography have limited applications and less sensitive modes for detection of the lesions. Nevertheless, these techniques are noninvasive procedures that can provide reasonable details of intraluminal thrombus, vascular wall, and surrounding tissue. Therefore, these techniques can be considered for the screening of suspected patients.

D. DIFFERENTIAL DIAGNOSIS

1. Atherosclerosis

It can sometimes be a problem, particularly among older patients, to differentiate Takayasu's arteritis from atherosclerotic disorders. An angiogram cannot differentiate noted stenosis or obstruction from atherosclerosis. The presence of inflammatory markers, abnormalities in lung scintigrams, and thickened adventitia in CT are helpful clues to differentiate one from another. It should be emphasized that patients with Takayasu's arteritis tend to accelerate atherosclerotic changes because the inflammation itself is considered a serious risk factor of atherosclerosis.

2. Congenital Vascular Abnormalities

The information from angiographical imaging and the presence of inflammatory markers are valuable for differentiation.

3. Arteritis Syphilitica

Although this is a rarely seen condition nowadays, it is recommended that one be aware of it. A positive Wassermann reaction should rule it in or out.

4. Renal Arterial Stenosis

Renovascular hypertension is not common in Japan, but is frequently encountered in Asian countries among Takayasu's arteritis patients. A renal angiogram provides the most helpful information in establishing a definitive diagnosis. Fibromuscular stenosis should be carefully differentiated by MRI angiography.

5. Tuberculosis

Diagnosis of Takayasu's arteritis in young patients was sometimes delayed or patients were misdiagnosed with tuberculosis based on elevated ESR or chest X-ray findings. A positive PPD should be confirmatory.

6. Collagen Diseases

It is reasonable to evaluate possible complications with lupus erythematosus or Sjogren syndromes, particularly in patients presenting remarkably elevated inflammatory markers. It makes it rather difficult to differentiate Takayasu's arteritis from vascular Behçet when other characteristic symptoms are not evident. However, it should be noted that Takayasu's arteritis is sometimes complicated with collagen diseases.[66-69]

7. Buerger Disease

Although it is sometimes considered to be somewhat related with or similar to Takayasu's arteritis, Buerger disease is a chronic vasculitis and is seen far more frequently among young males rather than females.[80,81] Buerger disease is characterized with more peripheral vascular disorders, particularly lesions on the lower limbs. Raynaud's phenomenon, cyanosis, and ulcers in peripheral lesions are frequently encountered. Recent studies indicated the presence of a close association between Buerger disease and HLA B54 and/or MIC genes.[47]

V. TREATMENT AND PROGNOSIS

A. TREATMENT

Since the etiology of Takayasu's arteritis is still unknown, its treatment is primarily a medical and symptomatic one.[82] However, if diagnosed as Takayasu's arteritis, the indication of surgical treatment should always be kept in mind. Renovascular hypertension, coarctation of the aorta, severe ischemic condition of retinal arteries, aortic regurgitation, a dissected aneurysm require prompt surgical treatment because they are totally out of medical treatment.[82,83] Surgical treatment, however, should be applied when the inflammatory condition is under reasonable control.

1. Medical Treatment

Steroid Therapy. Significant improvement can be achieved by steroids treatment, particularly at the acute stage or active stage. Starting with prednisolone, 20 to 30 mg/day, then reduction of 5 mg/day over 2 to 3 weeks should be attempted when feasible, judging from ESR and CRP values as well as symptoms. The target maintenance dose is 5 to 10 mg/day.[82] Once this maintenance dose is achieved, taper it for a time, and then discontinue totally. It has been generally possible in our experience to maintain half of the patients free from steroids. However, some Japanese patients presenting difficulty in tapering steroids were found to have an HLA haplotype of A24-B52-DR2. It seems necessary to use a larger dose (30 to 40 mg/day) for a longer period with these patients.[83]

Immunosuppressive Therapy. Although immunosuppressive treatment was tried in Japan for a long time, its effect was less than remarkable, and several serious adverse effects were reported. Nowadays an immunosuppressive drug is used, mostly in combination therapy with steroids, for patients presenting resistance to steroid treatment. Conventionally, 100mg of cyclosporin is administered daily or every other day together with 10 to 20 mg/day of steroids.

Antithrombotic Therapy.   This is the essential treatment together with steroid therapy. Thrombus formation is easily induced on the rough surface of the vessel wall, and active inflammation accelerates thrombus formation even more. When thrombus formation is under progress or already being completed, anticoagulant therapy with or without fibrinolytic treatment is necessary. A daily dose of 20 to 30 mg of Waffarin, 10 units of Defibrase/day, and 10 to 20 mg of Argatroban are given intravenously.

Antiplatelet therapy should also be considered for all patients for protection from subsequent thrombus formation. The small dose (81 mg/day) of acetyl salicylic acid (Children's Bufferin) is the most popular medication.[84] Other antiplatelet drugs such as dipyridamole, ticlopidin, and cilostazol are also used in Japan.

Others.   As treatment is mainly symptomatic, it is often necessary to use medications such as Digitalis, antiangina, anti-hypertensive, and also to improve cerebral metabolism in addition to steroids and antithrombotic therapies. However, introduction here is only with respect to the treatment of arteritis. This disease requires the long-term observation of patients, even after they are completely free from symptoms and steroid therapy has long been discontinued, because it can flare up due to the common cold or other infectious pathogens.

Vascular changes can progress silently and asymptomatically for some time. Therefore, careful evaluation of all patients on a regular basis is vitally important. If there are signs that patients are complicated with aortic regurgitation, ischemic heart disease, and hypertension, vigorous treatment plans need to be set to protect patients from developing more desperate conditions.

2. Noninvasive Intervention

Recent progress in catheterization has made angioplasty therapy possible, and it has become recognized as the effective noninvasive procedure for vascular disease. Pericutaneous transluminal (coronary) angioplasty (PTA) is widely applied today in numerous patients suffering from coronary, atherosclerotic, or other vascular disorders. There have also been a few reports dealing with PTA performed successfully in Takayasu's patients complicated with renovascular hypertension.[85,86] However, this procedure seems most effective for atherosclerotic disorders, and less for Takayasu arteritis, because the thickened adventitia and fibrous intima in vessel walls seem to reduce the therapeutic effect. Stenting has recently been applied successfully.[87]

3. Surgical Treatment

Surgical procedures are essential for treatment in the following situations: coarctation of the aorta, severe hypertension in the upper half of the body, severe aortic regurgitation, congestive heart failure, renovascular hypertension, severe visual disturbance due to an ischemic condition, developing aneurysmal formation, and dissecting aneurysms.[88,89] The Bental operation is a very effective procedure, but the timing of the operation must be carefully evaluated in order to protect patients from subsequent severe aortic regurgitation.[90] Grafting is also available to improve their prognosis. When such a surgical procedure is considered, the outcome should indicate a better prognosis.[90]

B. PROGNOSIS

By early diagnosis and early initiation of treatment, the prognosis of this disease has improved remarkably. It is, however, very important to follow the patients carefully at regular intervals to check for complications. The most frequent concerns are heart failure due to aortic regurgitation, thrombus formation leading to cerebral thrombosis, myocardial infarction, severe visual disturbance, and hypertension leading to cerebral bleeding. Congestive heart failure with or without arrhythmia is the number-one cause of death in Japan, whereas cerebral vascular complication is the most serious in other Asian countries. It is noteworthy that improved life expectancy for patients has lighted on a new complication, such as renal dysfunction characterized by nephrotic syndrome.

REFERENCES

1. Numano, F., Takayasu's arteritis, clinical characteristics and the role of genetic factors in its pathogenesis, *Vascular Med.,* 1, 227, 1996.
2. Shimizu, K. and Sano, K., Pulseless disease, *J. Neuropathol. Clin. Neurol.,* 1, 37, 1951.
3. Cacamise, W. C. and Whiteman, J. F., Pulseless disease. Preliminary case report, *Am. Heart J.,* 44, 629, 1952.
4. Ross, R. S. and Mckusick V. A., Aortic arch syndromes: diminished or absent pulses in arteries arising from the arch of the aorta, *Arch. Int. Med.,* 92, 701, 1953.
5. Judge, R. D., Currier, R. D., Gracie, W. A., and Figley, M. R., Takayasu's arteritis and the aortic arch syndrome, *Am. J. Med.,* 32, 379–392, 1962.
6. Virmani, R., Lande, A., and McAllister, H. A. Jr., Pathological aspects of Takayasu's arteritis. In: Lande, A., Berkman, Y. M., and McAllister, H. A. Jr., eds., *Aortitis: Clinical, Pathologic, and Radiographic Aspects, Raven,* 55–79, 1986.
7. Sekiguchi, M., Suzuki, An overview on Takayasu arteritis, *Heart & Vessels,* Suppl. 7, 6, 1992.
8. Numano, F., Introductory remarks for this special issue on Takayasu arteritis, *Heart & Vessels,* Suppl. 7, 3, 1992.
9. Koide, K., Takayasu arteritis in Japan, *Heart & Vessels,* Suppl. 7, 48, 1992.
10. Nagasawa, T., Current status of large and small vessel vasculitis in Japan, *Int. J. Card.,* 54, S91, 1996.
11. Numano, F., Differences in clinical presentation and out come in different countries for Takayasu's arteritis, *Current Opinion in Rhematology,* 9, 12, 1997.
12. Numano, F., Hereditary factors of Takayasu arteritis, *Heart & Vessels,* Suppl. 7, 68, 1992.
13. Kimura, A., Kitamura, H., Date, Y., and Numano, F., Comprehensive analysis of HLA genes in Takayasu arteritis in Japan, *Int. J. Card.,* 54, S65, 1996.
14. Park, Y. B., Hong, K. J., Choi, D. W., Sohn, D. W., Oh, B. H., Lee, M. M., Choi, Y. S., Seo, J. D., Lee, Y. W., and Park, J. H., Takayasu arteritis in Korea. Clinical and angiographic features, *Heart & Vessels,* Suppl. 7, 55, 1992.
15. Zheng, D., Fan, D., and Lieu, L., Takayasu arteritis in China, *Heart & Vessels,* Suppl. 7, 32, 1992.
16. Sharma, B. K., Sagar, S., Singh, A. P. et al., Takayasu arteritis in India, *Heart & Vessels,* Suppl. 7, 37, 1992.
17. Piyachon, C. and Suwanwela, N., Takayasu arteritis in Thailand: Clinical and Imaging Features, *Int. J. Card.,* 54, S117, 1996.
18. Turkoglu, C., Memis, A., and Payzing et al., Takayasu arteritis in Turkey, *Int. J. Card.,* 54, S135, 1996.
19. Rosenthal, T., Morag, B., and Itzchak Y., Takayasu arteritis in Israel, *Heart & Vessels,* Suppl. 7, 44, 1992.
20. Dabague, J. and Reyes P. A., Takayasu arteritis in Mexico, *Int. J. Card.,* 54, S103, 1996.
21. Canas, C. A. D., Jimenez, C. A. P., Ramirez, L. A., Uribe, O., Tobon, I., and Torrenegra, A., Takayasu arteritis in Columbia, *Int. J. Card.,* 66, S73, 1998.
22. Sato, E. I., Hatta, F. S., Levy-Neto, M., and Fernandes, S., Demographic, clinical and angiographic data of patients with Takayasu arteritis in Brazil, *Int. J. Card.,* 66, S67, 1998.
23. Lupi-Herrea, E., Sanchez-torres, G., Marcushamer, J., Horwitz, S., and Vela, J. E., Takayasu's arteritis-clinical study of 107 cases, *Am. Heart J.,* 93, 94, 1977.
24. Takayasu, M., A case with peculiar changes of retinal central vessels (in Japanese), *Acta Soc. Ophthal. Jpn.,* 12, 554, 1908.
25. Numano F., Takayasu arteritis — five doctors in history of Takayasu arteritis, *Int. J. Card.,* 54, S1, 1996.
26. Ohta, K., Ein Seltener Fall on becder seitigen carotis-subclavianverschluss Ein Beitrag Zur Pathologie der anastomosis peripapillaris des auges mitfehlendem radial plus, *Trans. Soc. Pathol. Jap.,* 30, 680, 1940.
27. Ark-Upmark, E. and Fajers, C. M., Further observation on Takayasu's syndrome, *Acta Med. Scand.,* 155, 275, 1956.

28. Froving, A. G., Bilateral obliteration of the common carotid artery, *Acta Psychiat. Neural.,* 39, 19746.

29. Ueda, H., Clinical and pathological studies of aortic syndrome, *Jap. Heart J.,* 9, 76, 1968.

30. Numano, F., Takayasu arteritis — beyond pulselessness, *Jap. J. Int. Med.,* 38, 226, 1999.

31. Hotchi, M., Pathological studies on Takayasu arteritis, *Heart & Vessels,* Suppl. 7, 11, 1992.

32. Nasu, T., Pathology of pulseless disease, a systematic study and critical review of 21 autopsy cases reported in Japan, *Angiology,* 14, 225, 1963.

33. Noguchi, S., Numano, F., Gravanis, M. B. et al., Increased levels of soluble forms of adhesion molecules in Takayasu arteritis, *Int. J. Card.,* 66, S23, 1998.

34. Wilcox, J., Local expression of inflammatory cytokines in human atherosclerotic plaques, *J. Atheroscl. Throm.,* 1, Suppl. 10–13, 1992.

35. Wilcox, J. N. and Scott, N. A., Potential role of the adventitia in arteritis and atherosclerosis, *Int. J. Card.,* 54, S21, 1996.

36. Wissler, R. W., PDAY Group, Athero arteritis: a combined immunological and lipid imbalance, *Int. J. Card.,* 54, S37, 1996.

37. Bodmer, J. G., Marsh, S. G. E., Albert, E. D., Bodmev, W. F., Bontrop, R. E., and Charron, D., Nomenclature for factors of the HLA system, *Tissue Antigen,* 46, 1, 1995.

38. Imanishi, T., Akaza, T., Kimura, A.,Tokunaga, K., and Gojohori, T., Reference tables: Allele frequencies and haplotype frequencies for HLA and compliment foci in various ethnic groups, *HLA 1991,* Vol. 1, Oxford University Press, 1065, 1992.

39. Numano, F., Okawara, M., Inomata, H., Kobayashi, Y., Takayasu's arteritis, *Lancet,* 356, 1023, 2000.

40. Sharma, B. K., Jain, S., and Sagar, S., Systemic manifestation of Takayasu arteritis: The expand spectrum, *Int. J. Card.,* 54, S149, 1996.

41. Isohisa, I., Numano, F., Maezawa, H., and Sasazuki, T., HLA-B52 in Takayasu disease, *Tissue Antigen,* 12, 246, 1978.

42. Numano, F., Isohisa, I., Maezawa, H., and Sasazuki, T., HLA antigen in Takayasu disease, *Am. Heart J.,* 98, 153, 1979.

43. Mehra, M. K., Rajalingam, R., Sagar, S., Jain, S., and Sharma, B. K., Direct role of HLA-B5 in influencing susceptibility to Takayasu aortoarteritis, *Int. J. Card.,* 54, S55, 1996.

44. Park, M. H., and Park Y. B., HLA typing of Takayasu arteritis in Korea, *Heart & Vessels,* Suppl. 7, 81, 1992.

45. Volkman, D. J., Mann, D. L., and Fanci, A. S., Association between Takayasu's arteritis and B-cell alloantigen in North American, *N. Eng. J. Med.,* 306, 464, 1982.

46. Yoshida, M., Kimura, A., Numano, F., and Sasazuki, T., Polymerase-chain reaction-based analysis of polymorphism in the HLA-B gene, *Human Immunol.,* 34, 257, 1992.

47. Kimura, A., Kobayashi, Y., Takahashi, M., Ohbuchi, N., Kitamura, H., Nakamura, T., Yasukochi, Y., and Numano, F., MIC A gene polymorphism in Takayasu arteritis and Buerger Disease, *Int. J. Card.,* 66, S107, 1998.

48. Weck, K. E., Dal Canto, A. J., Gould, J. D., O'Guin, A. K., Roth, K. A., Saffitz, J. E., Speck, S. H., and Virgin, H. W., Murine r-herpes virus 68 causes severe interferon-r responsiveness: A new model for virus-induced vascular disease, *Nature Med.,* 3, 1346, 1997.

49. Seko, Y., Minota, S., Kowasaki, A., Shinkai, Y., Maeda, K., and Tagita, H., Perforin-secreting killer cell infiltration and expression of a 65-KD heat-shock protein in aortic tissues of patients with Takayasu arteritis, *J. Clin. Invest.,* 93, 750, 1994.

50. Tanaka, S., Komori, K., Okadome, K., Sugimachi, K., and Mon, R., Detection of active cytomegalo virus megalo virus infection in inflammatory aortic aneurysms with RNA polymerase chain reaction, *J. Vasc. Surg.,* 20, 235, 1994.

51. Numano, F., Takayasu arteritis, Buerger disease and inflammatory abdominal aortic aneurysms — Is there a common pathway in their pathogenesis, *Int. J. Card.,* 66, S5, 1998.

52. Wekerle, H., The viral triggering of auto immune disease, *Nat. Med.,* 4, 770, 1998.

53. Numano, F. and Shimamoto, T., Hyper secretion of estrogen in Takayasu disease, *Am. Heart J.,* 81, 591, 1971.

54. Sharma, B. K. and Jain, S., A possible role of sex in determining distribution of lesions in Takayasu arteritis, *Int. J. Card.,* 66, S81, 1998.

55. Deutsch, V., Wexler, L., and Deutsch, H., Takayasu arteritis — an angio graphic study with remarks on ethnic distribution of 102 cases, *Am. Roentgenol. Rad. Ther.,* 122, 18, 1974.

56. Arend, W. P., Michael B. A., and Bloch, D. A., The American College of Rhematology 1990 criteria for the classification of Takayasu's arteritis, *Arthritis Rheum.,* 33, 1129, 1990.

57. Kiyosawa, M. and Baba, T., Ophthalmological findings in patients with Takayasu disease, *Int. J. Card.,* 66, S141, 1998.

58. Moriwaki, R., Noda, M., Yojima, M., Sharma, B. K., and Numano, F., Clinical manifestation of Takayasu arteritis in India and Japan — New classification of Angiographic findings, *Angiology,* 48, 369, 1997.

59. Yajima, M. and Numano, F., Comparative studies of the patients with Takayasu arteritis in Japan, Korea and India, *Jap. Circ. J.,* 88, 1994.

60. Matsubara, O., Kuwat, Nemoto, T., Kasuga, T., and Numano F., Coronary artery lesions in Takayasu arteritis: Pathological consideration, *Heart & Vessels,* Suppl. 7, 26, 1992.

61. Lie, J. T., Pathology of isolated non classical and catastrophic manifestation of Takayasu arteritis, *Int. J. Card.,* 66, S11, 1998.

62. Hashimoto, Y., Oniki, T., Aerbajinai, W., and Numano, F., Aortic regurgitation in patients with Takayasu arteritis: assessment by color doppler echocardiography, *Heart & Vessels,* Suppl. 7, 111, 1992.

63. Hashimoto, Y., Tanaka, M., Hata, A., Kakuta, T., Maruyama, Y., and Numano, F., Four years follow-up study in patients with Takayasu arteritis and severe aortic regurgitation: assessment by echocardiography, *Int. J. Card.,* 54, 173, 1996.

64. Matsubara, O., Yoshimura, M., Tamura, A., Kasuga, T., Yamada, I., Numano, F., and Mark, E. J., Pathological features of the pulmonary artery in Takayasu arteritis, *Heart & Vessels,* Suppl. 7, 18, 1992.

65. Sharma, B. K., Jain, S., and Radotora, B. D., An autopsy study of Takayasu arteritis in India, *Int. J. Card.,* 66, S85, 1998.

66. O'Duffy, J. D., Behcet's disease, *Current Opinion in Rhematology,* 6, 39, 1994.

67. Hayasaka, S., Kurome, H., and Noda, S., HLA antigens in a Japanese family with Behcet's disease, *Arch. Clin. Exp. Ophthal.,* 232, 589, 1994.

68. Ishikawa, H., Kondo, Y., Yusa, Y., Ejiri, Y., and Sato, Y., An autopsy case of ulcerative colitis associated with Takayasu's arteritis with a review of 13 Japanese cases, *Gastroenter. Jap.,* 28, 100, 1993.

69. Numano, F., Miyata, T., and Nakajima, T., Ulcerative Colitis, Takayasu Arteritis and HLA, *Int. Med.,* 35, 521, 1996.

70. Hata, A., Noda, M., Moriwaki, R., and Numano, F., Angiographic findings of Takayasu arteritis: New classification, *Int. J. Card.,* 4, S155, 1996.

71. Ishikawa, K., Diagnostic approach and proposed criteria for the clinical features of arteritis syndrome in Japanese women older than 40 year, *J. Am. Coll Card.,* 12, 964, 1988.

72. Sharma, B. K., Jain, S., Suri, S., and Numano, F., Diagnostic criteria for Takayasu Arteritis, *Int. J. Cardiology,* 54, S141, 1996.

73. Nasu, T., Takayasu tranco-arteritis: Pulseless disease or aortitis syndrome, *Acta Path. Jpn.,* 32, 117, 1982.

74. Noguchi, S., Numano, F., Gravanis, M. B., and Wilcox, J. N., Increased levels of soluble form of adhesion molecules in Takayasu arteritis, *Int. J. Card.,* 66, S23, 1998.

75. Park, J. H., Conventional and CT, Angiographic diagnosis of Takayasu arteritis, *Int. J. Card.,* 54, S165, 1996.

76. Hata, A. and Numano, F., Magnetic resonance imaging of vascular changes in Takayasu arteritis, *Int. J. Card.,* 52, 45–52, 1995.

77. Hayashi, K., Fukushima, T., and Matsunaga, N., Takayasu arteritis, decrease in aortic wall thickening following steroid therapy, *Br. Radol.,* 59, 281, 1986.

78. Rubin, C. D. and Jeffrey, R. B. Jr., 35 Spiral CT Angiography of the Abdomen and Thorax, in: *Spiral CT: Principles, Techniques and Clinical Application,* Fishman, E. K., Jeffrey, R. B. Jr., Eds, Raven Press Ltd, NY, 1995, pp 183.

79. Flamm, S. D., White, R. D., and Hoffman, G. S., The clinical application of edema weighted magnetic resonance imaging in the assessment of Takayasu's arteritis, *Int. J. Card.,* 66, S151, 1998.

80. Mishima, Y., Thrombo angiitis obliterans (Buerger's disease), *Int. J. Card.,* 54, S185, 1996.

81. Suzuki, S., Yamada, I., and Himeno, Y., Angiographic findings in Buerger disease, *Int. J. Card.,* 54, S189, 1996.

82. Ito, S., Medical treatment of Takayasu arteritis, *Heart & Vessels,* Suppl. 7, 133, 1992.

83. Moriwaki, R. and Numano, F., Takayasu arteritis, follow up studies for 20 years, *Heart & Vessels,* Suppl. 7, 138, 1992.

84. Numano, F., Maruyama, Y., Koyama, T., and Numano, F., Antiaggregative aspirin dosage at the affected vessel wall, *Angiology,* 37, 695, 1986.

85. Khalilullah, M. and Tyagi, S., Percutaneous transluminal angio plasty in Takayasu arteritis, *Heart & Vessels,* 7, 146, 1992.

86. Zheng, D., Liu, L., Dai, R., Wu, H., and Liu, G., Percutaneous transluminal renal angioplasty in aorta arteritis, *Int. J. Card.,* 66, S205, 1998.

87. Bali, H. K., Jain, S., Jain, A., and Sharma, B. K., Stent supported angioplasty in Takayasu arteritis, *Int. J. Card.,* 66, S243, 1998.

88. Weaver, F. A. and Yellin, A. E., Surgical treatment of Takayasu arteritis, *Heart & Vessels,* Suppl. 7, 154, 1992.

89. Tada, Y., Sato, O., Ohshima, A., Miyata, T., and Shindo, S., Surgical treatment of Takayasu arteritis, *Heart & Vessels,* Suppl. 7, 159, 1992.

90. Amano, J., Suzuki, A., Tanaka, H., and Sunamori, M., Surgical treatment for annulo aortic ectasia in Takayasu arteritis, *Int. J. Card.,* 66, S197, 1998.

19 Vascular Manifestations in Systemic Lupus Erythematosus

Josep Font, Ricard Cervera, and Miguel Ingelmo

CONTENTS

I. INTRODUCTION

Systemic lupus erythematosus (SLE) is the most diverse of the systemic autoimmune diseases because it may affect any organ of the body and display a broad spectrum of clinical and immunological manifestations.[1,2] A pathologic hallmark of SLE is the appearance of diverse vascular lesions. Although the etiology of the processes which initiate SLE remains uncertain, there is a growing understanding of the cellular and molecular events that are responsible for vascular injury. In this chapter we will review the main SLE clinical manifestations due to vascular involvement, as well as the most accepted pathogenic mechanisms of vascular disease in this condition.

II. CLINICAL MANIFESTATIONS

Any type of vessel in any tissue may be affected in SLE. Thus, the clinical manifestations due to vascular involvement are protean and can affect many different organs.[3-5] Some vascular manifestations are due to thrombosis mediated by antiphospholipid antibodies (aPL). Other manifestations

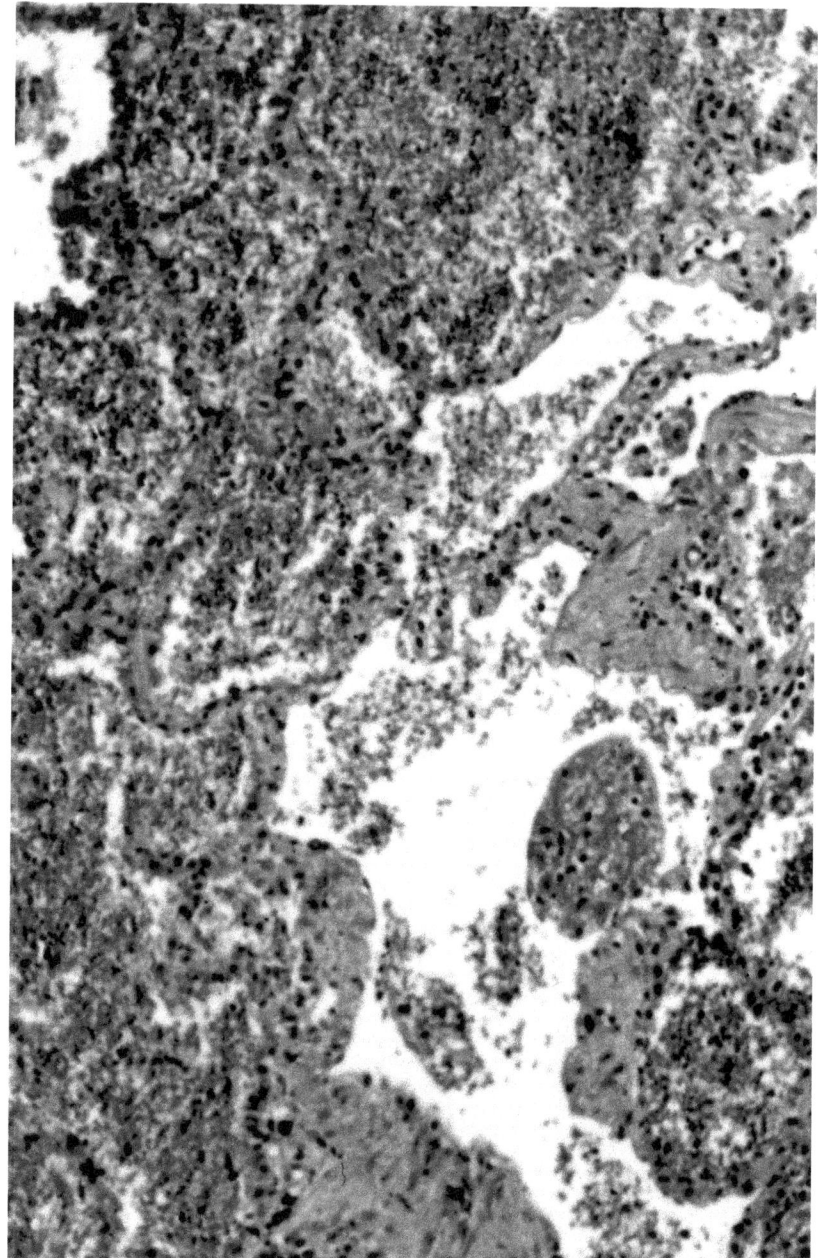

FIGURE 19.1 Pulmonary capillaritis.

are produced by inflammation of the vessel walls (vasculitis) and can be classified according to the vessel size:

1. Vasculitis affecting small vessels such as venules, capillaries, and arterioles causes purpura in skin, mononeuritis multiplex in peripheral nerves, myalgias in skeletal muscles, mucosal hemorrhage in the gut, glomerulonephritis in the kidneys, and alveolar hemorrhage in the lungs, among other manifestations (Figure 19.1).
2. Vasculitis affecting visceral arteries, e.g., in the liver, kidney, heart, gut, pancreas, and spleen, causes infarction and hemorrhage with resultant pain, dysfunction, and release

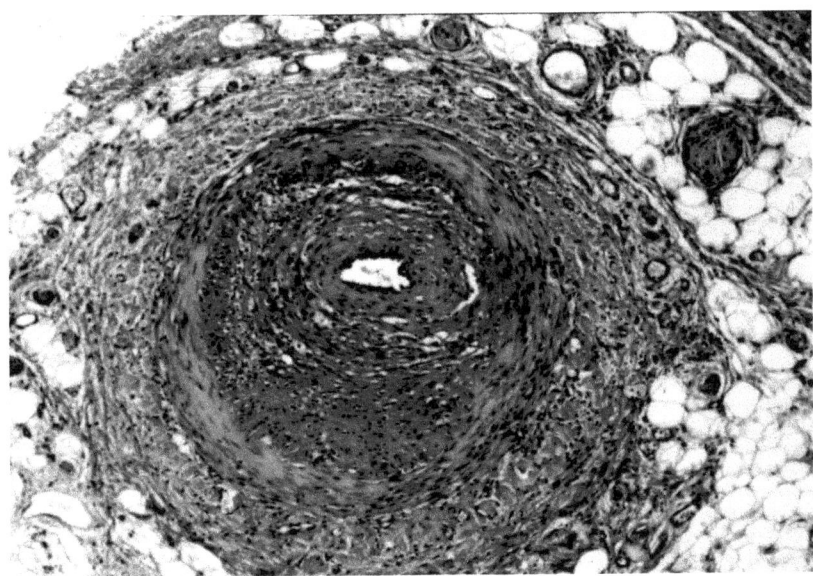

FIGURE 19.2 "Polyarteritis nodosa-like" necrotizing vasculitic lesion affecting the colon.

of intracellular enzymes into the blood. This is a "polyarteritis nodosa-like" necrotizing vasculitis (Figure 19.2).

3. Vasculitis affecting the aorta and its major branches causes ischemic effects in whole organs and body regions. Takayasu's arteritis has been reported to coexist with SLE in a few cases, probably being a coincidental occurrence of overlapping autoimmune diseases.

Most of these clinical manifestations are similar to those described in other vasculitic syndromes and are reviewed in depth in other chapters. In this chapter, we will focus on the most representative vasculitic manifestations in SLE, e.g., cutaneous, peripheral nervous system, muscular, and systemic manifestations.

A. CUTANEOUS MANIFESTATIONS

The skin is the most frequent target organ for the expression of peripheral inflammatory vascular disease in SLE. The most common cutaneous vasculitic manifestations of SLE are due to a leukocytoclastic vasculitis that produces palpable purpura and petechial lesions, generally involving the lower extremities.[6,7] These lesions are frequently asymptomatic. The development of lesions is episodic; and they may leave residual hyperpigmentation secondary to hemosiderin deposition.

Another common type of vasculitic skin lesions in SLE are urticaria-like lesions which may or may not contain petechiae. Generally, these erythematous and edematous lesions persist for more than 24 hours, in contrast to transient common urticaria, the duration of which is less than 4 to 6 hours. These urticaria-like vasculitic lesions usually are nonpruritic, but may be associated with a burning sensation.[8]

A less common group of SLE vasculitic skin lesions includes erythematosus macular and papular lesions. In this category also are classical erythema multiforme lesions (persistent erythematous macules and papules, with target or iris lesions), which have been seen in a small subset of patients. Another uncommon cutaneous manifestation of vasculitis is subcutaneous nodules. Necrotizing panniculitis, secondary to vasculitic lesions involving the subcutaneous adipose tissue, also has been noted occasionally.[9]

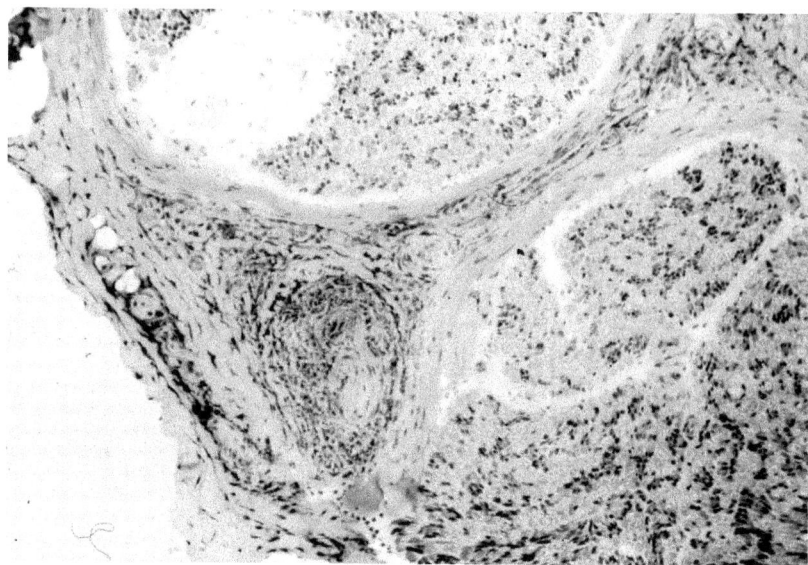

FIGURE 19.3 "Polyarteritis nodosa-like" necrotizing vasculitic lesion affecting a peripheral nerve.

These manifestations of cutaneous vasculitis are not specific or unique to SLE, but represent the spectrum of lesions that can be produced by vasculitic involvement of the skin. Recognition of their significance as lesions of vasculitis are, however, important.

B. Peripheral Nervous System Manifestations

Peripheral nervous system involvement in SLE is well recognized, although uncommon, and several forms of neuropathy have been described. Limited evidence suggests that the etiology of at least some forms of neuropathies is related to inflammatory vascular disease of the *vasa nervorum*[10] (Figure 19.3).

C. Muscular Manifestations

Patients with SLE often have muscle involvement. However, classical myositis, with proximal muscle weakness, striking elevation of muscle enzymes, and characteristic electromyographic changes, is relatively uncommon. In contrast, a smoldering myopathy with focal lymphocytic infiltrates and minimal or no myonecrosis is more common. The presence of inflammatory vascular disease within muscle blood vessels, either alone or in association with myositis, has been described.

D. Systemic Manifestations

In addition to peripheral inflammatory vascular disease (i.e., involving skin, nerve, or muscle), patients can develop vascular inflammation of other organs (i.e., systemic vasculitis). Single or multiple organ systems may be involved. Since the inflammatory vascular disease of SLE appears to affect predominantly small vessels, the manifestations tend to be subacute, insidious, and slowly progressive over time. A subset of patients, however, particularly those with larger vessel involvement (indistinguishable from polyarteritis nodosa) or severe diffuse small vessel involvement, have a more precipitous onset of the clinical manifestations of their vasculitis and a more aggressive course.

Inflammatory vascular disease syndrome ("lupus vasculitis") has been observed to more frequently affect the kidneys, lungs, gastrointestinal tract (stomach, small bowel, colon), and pancreas, among other organs. This process consists of deposits, in the vascular lumina and walls of an eosinophilic, strongly periodic, acid-Schiff-positive, homogeneous proteinaceous material, which

TABLE 19.1
Pathologic and Clinical Spectrum of Vascular Injury in Systemic Lupus Erythematosus*

Pathology	Pathogenesis	Clinical phenomenon
Capillaritis+	Immune complex deposition	+Glomerulonephritis, pulmonary alveolar hemorrhage
Vasculitis++	Activation of complement, neutrophils, and endothelium Modeled by Arthus lesion	++Cutaneous purpura, polyarteritis nodosa-like systemic and cerebral vasculitis
Leukothrombosis	Intravascular activation of complement, neutrophils, and vascular endothelium Absence of local immune complex deposition Modeled by Shwartzman lesion	Widespread vascular injury, hypoxia, cerebral dysfunction, systemic inflammatory response syndrome
Atheromatosis	Glucocorticoids OX-LDL-Ab Nephrotic syndrome	Transient ischemic attacks, acute myocardial infarction
Thrombosis	Antibodies to anionic phospholipid-protein complexes interact with endothelial cells, platelets, or coagulation factors Modeled by antiphospholipid syndrome Disseminated intravascular platelet aggregation	Arterial and venous thrombosis, fetal wastage, thrombocytopenia, pulmonary hypertension Thrombotic thrombocytopenic purpura

* Capillaritis, or microvascular angiitis, and lupus vasculitis share a similar pathogenesis but are associated with different clinical phenomena, designated here as + and ++ (adapted from Reference 3).

is to be distinguised from microvascular thrombosis. Immunofluorescence miscroscopy shows the deposit to be a mixture of IgG, IgA, and IgM immunoglobulins and complement components, a finding that was not observed in a group of non-SLE patients with various vascular lesions.[11]

III. PATHOPHYSIOLOGY OF VASCULAR MANIFESTATIONS

The pathophysiology of vascular disease in SLE can be classified into two broad categories: inflammatory and thrombotic.[3] The former may or may not be associated with local deposition of immune complexes, and the latter is generally associated with circulating aPL. Although they are not mutually exclusive, inflammatory and thrombotic vasculopathy coexist infrequently in the same patient. Additionally, vascular lesions due to atheromatosis are becoming more and more common nowadays, mainly due to steroid therapy (Table 19.1).

A. INFLAMMATORY VASCULAR DISEASE

Advances in cellular and molecular biology have increased understanding of how cytokines and adhesion molecules mediate the complex interactions between leukocytes and endothelial cells that characterize the inflammatory response.[12] These advances have also provided important insights into the pathogenesis of vasculitis.

1. Cytokines

Both quantitative and qualitative abnormalities in cytokine production have been described in vasculitic syndromes associated with SLE. Elevated serum levels of interleukin (IL)-1, IL-2, IL-6, and tumor necrosis factor (TNF)-α, and increased production of TNF-α by circulating mononuclear cells has been reported in patients with SLE and vasculitis. More recent studies have focused on the *in situ* production of proinflammatory cytokines in active vasculitic lesions.[13]

2. Adhesion Molecules

The importance of adhesion molecules as mediators of leukocyte-endothelial interactions and inflammatory vascular injury is illustrated by the results of studies of the Shwartzman reaction. In 1928, Shwartzman observed that animals given an intravenous injection of bacterial culture filtrate developed hemorrhagic vasculitis in skin sites where the same culture filtrate had been injected intradermally 24 hours previously. It has since been shown that endotoxin, or a combination of IL-1 and TNF-α, can be substituted for culture filtrates.[14] No immune complexes are detected in the skin lesion, suggesting that the Shwartzman reaction may be a model for vasculitic processes in which immune complex deposition is limited or absent.

Increased expression of adhesion molecules by circulating leukocytes has been observed in a number of autoimmune diseases associated with vasculitis.[15] In patients with active SLE, increased expression of CD11b/CD18 can be detected on circulating neutrophils, and this correlates with disease activity.[16] Other studies have found upregulated expression of CD11a/CD18 (LFA-1) and VLA-4 on peripheral blood lymphocytes from a subgroup of SLE patients with active vasculitis, suggesting that these molecules may be involved in the pathogenesis of vasculitis in SLE.[17] Increased expression of ICAM-1 and VCAM-1 by microvasculature endothelium has been detected in tissues from a number of inflammatory states, including synovium from patients with rheumatoid arthritis, skin from patients with SLE, and vasculitis.[18]

3. Immune Complexes

SLE is the most important immune complex-mediated autoimmune human disease. Localization of immune complexes in tissues, either by deposition from the circulation or *in situ* formation, is the major pathogenic event in much of the tissue.

The formation of antigen-antibody immune complexes is part of the normal humoral immune response. Immune complex formation normally does not lead to pathogenic inflammatory responses because complexes are rapidly cleared by complement-dependent mechanisms. Immune complexes containing immunoglobulin G (IgG) and IgM activate complement via the classic pathway resulting in their incorporation of C3b. C3b-containing immune complexes bind to complement receptor-1 (CR1) on erythrocytes, and are rapidly cleared from the circulation by Kupffer cells and macrophages in the liver and spleen.[19]

The consequences of pathogenic intravascular immune complex formation became apparent with the use of horse-derived antisera to treat infectious diseases such as diphtheria and scarlet fever. Patients treated with horse antiserum developed a serum sickness characterized by fever, arthralgias, lymphadenopathy, urticarial rash, and, occasionally, nephritis.

A second type of animal model for immune complex-mediated vasculitis is the Arthus reaction. In this model, a focal cutaneous vasculitis develops at the site where an animal has been injected with an antigen to which it was previously immunized. Immune complexes form in the vessel wall when performed circulating antibodies react with the injected antigen. A cascade of inflammatory responses ensues which result in vessel damage. The Arthus reaction has been extensively used to investigate the role of neutrophils and complement in the pathogenesis of immune complex-mediated tissue damage.[11]

The study of animal models of immune complex disease has allowed the delineation of mechanisms by which the deposition of immune complexes can result in vasculitis.[4] The ability of immune complexes to activate complement is believed to be of primary importance in the initiation of vascular damage. Antibodies of the IgM and IgG1, IgG2, and IgG3 isotypes can activate complement through the classic pathway, whereas IgE, IgA, and IgG4 antibodies activate complement through the alternate pathway. Immune complexes containing activated complement components are ultimately deposited in blood vessel walls at sites of increased vascular permeability. The increased vascular permeability is thought to result from the release of vasoactive amines by platelets and IgE-triggered mast cells. Once the immune complexes are deposited, vessel damage can occur by a number of interacting mechanisms. The activation of complement by immune deposits can lead to endothelial damage through formation of the C5b-9 membrane attack complex. Complement activation also results in the production of chemotactic factors (e.g., C5a) that recruit neutrophils and monocytes into the area and stimulate the clotting and kinin pathways leading to vessel thrombosis and further inflammation. Immune complexes deposited in vessel walls can directly interact with inflammatory cells through Fcγ receptors present on neutrophils and monocytes. This interaction leads to cellular activation and the release of cytokines, oxygen radicals, and proteolytic enzymes, which further escalate the inflammatory vascular damage.[3,4]

Vasculitis in SLE most commonly results from the local deposition of immune complexes, particularly those containing antibodies to DNA, in blood vessel walls.[20] The pathologic consequences of immune complex deposition in SLE include both a microvascular angiitis (either glomerulonephritis or pulmonary capillaritis with or without pulmonary hemorrhage) and necrotizing vasculitis (e.g., cutaneous purpura, polyarteritis nodosa-like, cerebral).

4. Direct Autoantibody Attack

Autoantibodies directed against constituents of vessel walls (e.g., endothelial cells and basement membrane) mediate vascular injury. The interaction of an autoantibody with vascular autoantigens may require synergistic events, such as endothelial alterations to expose basement membrane antigens, or induction of expression of surface membrane antigens on endothelial cells. Once autoantibodies bind to antigens in vessel walls, the effect is *in situ* immune complex formation. Therefore, the resultant pathogenic events share a common final pathway with injury induced by immune complexes that arrive in vessels walls by deposition from the circulation, namely, activation of humoral and cellular mediators leading to acute vascular inflammation.

a. Antiendothelial Cell Autoantibodies

Antiendothelial cell autoantibodies (AECA) have been incriminated as pathogenic factors in vascular injury in patients with autoimmune vasculitis and glomerulonephritis, including Kawasaki disease, rheumatoid vasculitis, IgA nephropathy, hemolytic uremic syndrome, Wegener's granulomatosis, and microscopic polyarteritis. The titers of AECA correlated with disease activity. Patients with Wegener's granulomatosis and microscopic polyangiitis also have circulating antineutrophil cytoplasmic antibodies (ANCA), and there is controversy over whether the AECA or ANCA, both or neither, are involved in the pathogenesis of the vasculitis.[21,22] Del Papa et al.[23] observed that AECA from patients with Wegener's granulomatosis are not toxic to endothelial cells, but caused endothelial cells to upregulate adhesion molecules and to release proinflammatory cytokines. These events could synergize with ANCA by the mechanisms discussed in the next section.

b. Antineutrophil Cytoplasmic Antibodies

Inflammatory vasculopathy independent of immune complex deposition also may occur as a result of ANCA or lymphocyte responses. A pathogenic role for ANCA in vasculitis has been suggested by demonstration of the activation of polymorphonuclear leukocytes and enhanced adhesion to endothelial cells by antibodies to proteinase-3 or myeloperoxidase.[24] Lymphocytes directly reacting to antigen may release cytokines that result in tissue damage and a mononuclear inflammatory disease. These mechanisms of vascular injury, however, are more typical of Wegener's granulomatosis and Sjögren's syndrome, respectively, than of SLE.

B. THROMBOTIC NONINFLAMMATORY VASCULAR DISEASE

The majority of thrombotic noninflammatory vascular manifestations in SLE are associated with the presence of aPL (antiphospholipid syndrome), but thrombotic thrombocytopenic purpura (TTP) has also been occasionally described in some patients.[25]

1. Antiphospholipid Syndrome

The pathophysiology of this syndrome is extensively reviewed in another chapter.

2. Thrombotic Thrombocytopenic Purpura

SLE exacerbations are infrequently accompanied by TTP with complete or incomplete features of the clinical pentad: fever, microangiopathic hemolytic anemia, thrombocytopenia, renal disease, and neurologic dysfunction. In the absence of aPL, the characteristic pathology of TTP (eosinophilic hyaline microthrombi) has been identified in patients with SLE.[25,26] Large multimers of von Willebrand factor (vWF) that are capable of mediating disseminated intravascular platelet aggregation have been demonstrated in patients with chronic, relapsing TTP as well as SLE. A consequence of the endothelial cell activation or injury observed in SLE may be the release of vWF multimers or other mediators of platelet aggregation that are capable of initiating a TTP-like illness.[27]

C. ATHEROMATOSIS

Pathophysiology of atheromatosis in SLE and other autoimmune diseases is reviewed in depth in Chapter 5.

IV. CONCLUDING REMARKS

Recently, Belmont et al.[3] suggested a unifying hypothesis to account for the diverse, episodic, and variably distributed nature of SLE vascular lesions. Inflammatory lesions would require either circulating immune complexes or significant complement activation of neutrophils, while thrombotic lesions would require aPL. An additional biologic factor, however, is required to explain the waxing and waning nature of disease exacerbations and the limitation of lesions to one, or a few, vascular beds. Immune complexes, activated neutrophils, or aPL may be necessary, but likely are not sufficient to explain vascular pathology in SLE. Because they may be present in the absence of disease activity and can travel throughout the general circulation, they are incapable of explaining the relapsing and focal nature of vascular injury.

The specificity of vascular injury in SLE may depend on the endogenous capacity of vascular endothelium to respond to stimuli. When activated, endothelial cells can express E-selectin, increased ICAM-1, and an inducible form of nitric oxide synthase (iNOS). There is a restriction to this endothelial cell capacity, however, such as the upregulation of endothelial cells' adhesion molecules being limited to postcapillary venules. Therefore, it is possible that the episodic and focal nature of vascular pathology in SLE is dependent on the presence or absence, as well as the nature, of endothelial cell activation. Endothelial cell permissiveness for immune complex deposition or *in situ* formation can result in vasculitis. Activation of endothelial cell adhesion molecules by cytokines, immune complexes, complement components, AECA, or aPL can result in leuko-thrombosis if there is simultaneous activation of neutrophils and complement. Abnormal iNOS synthesis may also have a role in permitting neutrophil-endothelial cell interaction and the Shwartzman-like lesion. Additionally, endothelial cell activation may lead to the expression of membrane-associated coagulation proteins that are the target of aPL.

Vascular injury in SLE may require immune complex formation, complement activation, or aPL production. Additionally, the endothelial cell response would be responsible for the clinical character of a disease exacerbation by determining the timing and organ distribution of vascular pathology.

REFERENCES

1. Cervera, R, Khamashta, MA, Font, J, et al., Systemic lupus erythematosus: Clinical and immunological patterns of disease expression in a cohort of 1000 patients. *Medicine* (Baltimore), 1993; 72: 113–124.
2. Cervera, R, Khamashta, MA, Font, J, et al., Morbidity and mortality in systemic lupus erythematosus. A multicenter prospective study of 1,000 patients. *Medicine* (Baltimore), 1999; 78: 167–175.
3. Belmont, HM, Abramson, SB, Lie, JT, Pathology and pathogenesis of vascular injury in systemic lupus erythematosus. Interactions of inflammatory cells and activated endothelium, *Arthritis Rheum.*, 1996; 39: 9–22.
4. Sneller, MC, Fauci, AS, Pathogenesis of vasculitis syndromes, *Med. Clin. North Am.*, 1997; 81: 221–241.
5. Calabrese, LH, Duna, GF, Lie, JT, Vasculitis in the central nervous system, *Arthritis Rheum.*, 1997; 40: 1189–1201.
6. Drenkard, C, Villa, AR, Reyes, E, Abelló, M, Alarcón-Segovia, D, Vasculitis in systemic lupus erythematosus, *Lupus*, 1997; 6: 235.
7. Watson, R, Cutaneous lesions in systemic lupus erythematosus, *Med. Clin. North Am.*, 1989; 73: 1091–1111.
8. Sontheimer, RD, Systemic lupus erythematosus and the skin. In: *Systemic Lupus Erythematosus*, Lahita, RG, (Editor), 3rd Edition, Academic Press, 1999; 631–656.
9. Marteus, PB, Moder, RG, Ahmed, I, Lupus panniculitis: clinical perspectives from case series, *J. Rheumatol.*, 1999; 26: 68–72.
10. Boumpas, DT, Austin, IH, Fessler, BJ, et al., Systemic lupus erythematosus: emerging concepts. *Ann. Intern. Med.*, 1995; 122: 940–950.
11. Breedveld, FC, Vasculitis associated with connective tissue disease, *Bailliere's Clin. Rheum.*, 1997; 11: 315–334.
12. Croustein, B, Weissman, G, The adhesion molecules of inflammation, *Arthritis Rheum.*, 1993; 36: 147–153.
13. Tsokos, GG, Kovacs, B, Liossis, SNC, Lymphocytes, cytokines, inflammation and immune trafficking, *Curr. Op. Rheumatol.*, 1997; 9: 380–386.
14. Movat, HZ, Burrowes, CE, Cybulsky, MI, et al., Acute inflammation and a Shwartzman-like reaction induced by interleukin-1 and tumor necrosis factor: Synergistic action of the cytokines in the induction of inflammation and microvascular injury, *Am. J. Pathol.*, 1987; 129: 463.
15. McMurray, RW, Adhesion molecules in autoimmune diseases, *Semin. Arthritis Rheum.*, 1996; 25: 215–235.
16. Buyon, JP, Shadick, N, Berkman, R, et al., Surface expression of Gp 165/95, the complement receptor CR3, as a marker of disease activity in systemic lupus erythematosus, *Clin. Immunol. Immunopathol.*, 1988; 46: 141.
17. Takeuchi, T, Amano, K, Sekine, H, et al., Upregulated expression and function of integrin adhesive receptors in systemic lupus erythematosus patients with vasculitis, *J. Clin. Invest.*, 1993; 92: 3008.
18. Belmont, HM, Buyon, J, Giorno, R, et al., Up-regulation of endothelial cell adhesion molecules characterizes disease activity in systemic lupus erythematosus: the Shwartzman phenomenon revisited, *Arthritis Rheum.*, 1994; 37: 376.
19. Hebert, LA, Cosio, FG, Birmingham, DJ, et al., Biologic significance of the erythrocyte complement receptor: a primate prerequisite, *J. Lab. Clin. Med.*, 1991; 118: 301.
20. Hahn, BH, Antibodies to DNA, *N. Engl. J. Med.*, 1998; 338: 1359–1368.
21. Navarro, M, Cervera, R, Font, J, et al., Anti-endothelial cell antibodies in systemic autoimmune diseases: prevalence and clinical significance, *Lupus*, 1997; 6: 521–526.
22. Cervera, R, Navarro, M, López-Soto, A, et al., Antibodies to endothelial cells in Behçet's disease: cell-binding heterogeneity and association with clinical activity, *Ann. Rheum. Dis.*, 1994; 53: 265–267.
23. Del Papa, N, Guidali, L, Sironi, M, et al., Anti-endothelial cell IgG antibodies from patients with Wegener's granulomatosis bind to human endothelial cells *in vitro* and induce adhesion molecule expression and cytokine secretion, *Arthritis Rheum.*, 1996; 39: 758–766.
24. Hoffman, GS, Specks, U, Antineutrophil cytoplasm antibodies, *Arthritis Rheum.*, 1998; 41: 1521–1537.

25. Musio, F, Bohen, E, Review of thrombotic thrombocytopenic purpura in the setting of systemic lupus erythematosus, *Semin. Arthritis Rheum.,* 1998; 28: 1–19.
26. Brunner, HI, Freedman, M, Silverman, Close relationship between systemic lupus erythematosus and thrombotic thrombocytopenic purpura in childhood, *Arthritis Rheum.,* 1999; 42: 2346–2355.
27. Jorfén, M, Callejas, JL, Formiga, F, Cervera, R, Font, J, Ingelmo, M, Fulminant thrombotic thrombocytopenic purpura in systemic lupus erythematosus, *Scand. J. Rheumatol.,* 1998; 27: 76–77.

20 Vascular Manifestations in the Antiphospholipid Syndrome

Ronald A. Asherson and Ricard Cervera

CONTENTS

I. INTRODUCTION

Antiphospholipid syndrome (APS) is defined as the occurrence of venous and arterial thromboses, often multiple, and recurrent fetal losses frequently accompanied by a moderate thrombocytopenia in the presence of antiphospholipid antibodies (aPL), namely lupus anticoagulant (LA), anticardiolipin antibodies (aCL), or both. Diagnosis of this syndrome is based on the presence of any of these clinical manifestations together with the detection of aPL. However, it is recommended that an aPL test be positive on at least two occasions more than three months apart. Chronic biological false-positive serological tests for syphilis (BFP-STS) may be present in some of these patients, because these tests also detect the presence of aPL. Other autoantibodies have also been detected in many patients with an APS, such as anti-β2 glycoprotein I (GPI), antimitochondrial (M5 type), antiendothelial cell, antiplatelet, antierythrocyte, and antinuclear antibodies.

The APS may be seen in patients having neither clinical nor laboratory evidence of any other definable condition (primary APS), or it may be associated with other diseases (secondary APS). Systemic lupus erythematosus (SLE) is the disorder with which the secondary APS is most commonly associated. Less frequently it may also be encountered in other groups of patients.[1]

The clinical picture of APS is characterized by venous and arterial thromboses, fetal losses, and thrombocytopenia. Single vessel involvement or multiple vascular occlusions may give rise to a wide variety of presentations. Any combination of vascular occlusive events may occur in the same individual, and the time interval between them varies considerably from weeks to months or even years. Rapid chronological occlusive events, occuring over days to weeks, have been termed the "catastrophic" APS.[2,3]

II. LARGE-VESSEL MANIFESTATIONS

A. VENOUS OCCLUSIONS

Venous occlusions, particularly affecting the deep veins of the lower limbs (deep vein thrombosis, DVT), are the most common clinical manifestation of APS.[4] Less commonly, a superficial thrombophlebitis may be seen, and the mottled appearance of *livedo reticularis* frequently appears in this group of patients, usually in the upper thighs. It is due to dilatation of superficial dermal vessels consequent on deeper arterial vascular occlusions. Chronic venous stasis and malleolar ulceration may result after episodes of deep vein thrombosis. On occasion, other large veins may be thrombosed, e.g., subclavian, external jugular, ileo-femoral, or even the vena cava itself (both inferior and superior).[5-7] Unusual vessels may be involved in catastrophic APS.

Venous occlusions occurring at sites of venous access, e.g., indwelling venous catheters or underlying compressive lesions, are not uncommon in patients with the aPL procoagulopathy. Particular care should be taken by these patients to exercise frequently in situations requiring prolonged immobilization, e.g., prolonged bed rest, particularly following surgical procedures, long air journeys, the wearing of plaster casts on limbs because of fractures, etc. Certain times predispose to excessive hypercoagulability, e.g., pregnancy and the puerperium (up to six weeks post delivery). The administration of certain drugs (particularly sulphur-containing compounds or oral contraceptives) may also be added risk factors, and care should be taken with their administration to these susceptible patients. In some there may be other risk factors present, e.g., protein s/c deficiencies, factor V Leiden mutation, or hyperhomocysteinemia.

B. ARTERIAL OCCLUSIONS

These were first described in 1965,[4] and other authors followed with single-case reports of this association.[5,6] Asherson et al.,[7] in reviewing six patients with large vessel occlusive disease with gangrene, found four who were aPL positive. The thoracic branches of the aorta may be affected, and an "aortic arch syndrome" with absent brachial pulse has been documented. The patient was shown to have developed occluded axillary and subclavian arteries.[8] Unilateral Raynaud's phenomenon was also found to be due to an occluded subclavian artery in another reported case,[9] while an earlier case had a BFP-STS.[10] Occlusion of the abdominal aorta itself has been reported on several occasions, and renal artery involvement results in hypertension.[11,12] Narrowing of the ileo-femoral arteries with resultant claudication and eventual gangrene of the extremities has also been documented on many occasions.[13,14] Of course, other splanchnic vessels may be affected by the coagulopathy with resultant end organ infarction should the blood supply to the organ be affected and severely compromised (e.g., hepatic, renal, splenic, mesenteric, etc). The aPL could be an added risk factor in patients with atherosclerotic vascular disease.

Aortitis, with thickening between the renal arteries and the iliac bifurcation, has been documented in one case in association with aPL.[15]

III. NEUROLOGIC MANIFESTATIONS

A. THROMBOTIC INFARCTIONS

Thrombotic infarctions in APS are second only to DVT in frequency. They are often multiple, recurrent, and, most commonly, affect the territory of the middle cerebral artery, with lesions occurring predominantly in the frontal and parietal lobes. The vertebro-basilar system may be affected less frequently. After a first ischemic stroke, the presence of aCL has been shown to be associated with an increased risk of recurrence of stroke over two years and of other thromboembolic events and death.[16] Patients with the highest IgG aCL titers have been shown to have the shortest times to subsequent thrombo-occlusive events.[17] Recurrent stroke and thrombo-occlusive events frequently occur in the first year in patients with aPL and an index cerebral ischemic event.[18,19] aPL-associated stroke occurs more often in younger people, and is more frequent in females.[17]

B. SNEDDON'S SYNDROME

The association of livedo and ischemic stroke, accompanied on occasion by hypertension, has been known as Sneddon's syndrome since 1965.[20] It is, however, an infrequent cause of cerebral ischemia, accounting for only 0.26% of all cases of cerebrovascular ischemia.[21] The syndrome is more frequent in women, it is usually diagnosed in the fourth or fifth decade, and there is a familial clustering in some patients. It clearly may be a manifestation of primary APS,[22] although confusion in nomenclature has occurred.[23,24] Focal and segmental intimal hyperplasia and recanalization of thrombi has been seen histologically.[21] Some investigators have stressed that early inflammatory reactions (endothelitis) of small arteries occur, and these are followed by subendothelial cell proliferation leading to partial or complete occlusion.[25]

C. TRANSIENT ISCHEMIC ATTACKS

Transient cerebro-ocular ischemia resulting in amaurosis fugax or transient paresthesias, and motor weakness, or vertigo, have all been described in patients with aPL.

D. MULTIINFARCT DEMENTIA

Many patients with multiinfarct dementia and aPL have been documented.[26] The clinical manifestations of dementia associated with APS is no different than those encountered in patients with vascular dementia of any other cause, including Binswanger's subcortical arteriosclerotic encephalopathy, cerebral amyloid angiopathy, and Alzheimer's disease.

E. ACUTE ISCHEMIC ENCEPHALOPATHY

Acute ischemic encephalopathy has been observed and reported.[27] Patients are acutely ill, confused, and obtunded with an asymmetrical quadriparesis, hyperreflexia, and bilateral extensor plantar responses. Seizures may also occur. These patients have been recorded as having the highest aCL levels among a large series of patients. Plasmapheresis and immunosuppression were effective therapies in some of the patients. Small cortical hypodensities were discernible on magnetic resonance imaging (MRI) scanning in several patients. Differential diagnosis lies between acute lupus cerebritis and even steroid psychosis in those with predominantly frontal lobe symptomatology. With the unraveling of catastrophic APS, it seems likely that cerebral thrombotic microangiopathy, predominant in that condition, is the basis of acute ischemic encephalopathy, a common accompaniment of catastrophic APS itself.

F. Embolic Stroke

Embolic stroke may arise with underlying nonbacterial thrombotic endocarditis (NBTE), but may also arise from dislodging atherogenic plaques in the aorta or carotid system. Heart valves may previously have been damaged by lupus vasculitis or aPL valvulitis due to deposition of cardiolipin, aCL, and complement on the subendothelial surface of the valves, or on a congenitally abnormal valve. Cerebral embolic events in patients with aPL have been reported by many investigators.[28,29]

G. Cerebral Venous and Dural Sinus Thrombosis

Cerebral venous sinus thrombosis (CVST) or dural sinus thrombosis (DST) have a diverse spectrum of clinical manifestations, the commonest being headache, accompanied by papilledema, nausea, vomiting, and visual field loss. CVST is one of the causes of the syndrome referred to as "pseudotumor cerebri" (benign intracranial hypertension), many cases of which are idiopathic and related to disturbed cerebrospinal fluid (CSF) dynamics. Several cases of the association between CVST and aPL have been reported.[30]

H. Psychosis (Occasional)

Several cases have been recorded where APS is preceded many years prior to the occurrence of thrombotic symptoms by psychosis.[31] Increased aPL have been documented in some schizophrenic patients[32] and in those with major depression.[33] Their role in this group of conditions is undetermined at this time.

I. Cognitive Defects

It is well known that cognitive defects, including behaviorial and affective disturbances, are not uncommon in SLE patients, and are usually ascribed to a "lupus cerebritis." Recently, work in animal models has related neurologic and behavioral deficits in experimental animal models of APS to effects of aPL. On immunofluorescence staining, immunoglobulin deposits have been observed in vessel walls of brain derived from these animals.[34] Four patients with APS who presented with rapidly progressive change in mental status, confusion, memory disturbance, and emotional lability have also been reported.[35] Psychometric testing revealed severe impairment. Transient global amnesia, a syndrome of sudden unexplained short-term memory loss, associated often with stereotyped behavior, has been linked to aPL in one patient,[36] the authors suggesting that aPL-linked ischemia may underlie the process.

J. Pseudomultiple Sclerosis

Several young patients who had fluctuating and recurrent neurologic events with focal and visual neurologic symptoms have been published. High signal lesions in the periventricular white matter on T2-weighted images resembled multiple sclerosis.[37]

K. Migraine and Migranous Stroke

Headaches, often nonmigrainous in type, may precede or accompany TIA or strokes in aPL-positive patients. Migraine is, however, common in SLE. Although many investigators have commented on an association between true migraine and aPL,[38] some even suggesting that patients with aPL may be a subset of migraineurs in whom the migraine might have an immunologic basis, several other studies have not borne out any association.[39] The prevalence of aPL in 16 patients with migranous stroke was recently studied and found to be approximately 40%.[40] No other immunologic disorder was present in these patients. Migraines in these patients are usually very frequent, long-lasting, and severe, with a poor response to specific therapy.

L. Epilepsy

Epileptiform seizures are common in SLE and may precede the appearance of other serological or clinical evidence of the disease by many years. Pathogenesis may be related to hypertension, uremia, or electrolyte disturbances when the epilepsy is deemed secondary. However, it is most frequently seen concomitant with SLE activity itself and might be immunologically mediated or, as a result of ischemic vascular disease, often secondary to the hypercoagulable state associated with aPL.[41] In 1994, 221 unselected patients with SLE were studied, of whom 21 suffered from epileptic seizures not attributable to any cause other than SLE. LA was detected in 43.8% of the epileptic patients and in 20.8% of controls (p = 0.057). A statistically significant association was found between moderate-to-high titers of IgG aCL and the presence of seizures (p = 0.02).[42]

M. Movement Disorders

1. Chorea

This is an infrequent clinical manifestation of SLE (occurring in less than 4% of cases) that has been strongly linked to the presence of aPL, and its occurrence in APS has recently been reviewed and discussed.[43] It does not differ from chorea encountered with rheumatic fever (Sydenhan's) or the inherited form (Huntington's). It may antedate other manifestations or be seen during the course of APS. Chorea may appear without any obvious precipitating factors, or may be induced by oral contraceptives. In a review of 50 cases,[43] we have found that 96% were females and that the mean age was 23 years. One episode of chorea was seen in 66% of the patients, while in 34% it was recurrent. Oral contraceptive-induced chorea, chorea gravidarium, and postpartum chorea occurred in 2 to 6% of patients. It was seen bilaterally or unilaterally, and occasionally commenced on one side, to reappear on the other side within weeks to months. Computed tomography (CT) scanning is usually normal, but infarcts outside the basal ganglia themselves might be seen. MRI findings were only reported in 13 of the 50 cases, and infarcts in the caudate nuclei were seen only in three. Steroids, haloperidol, aspirin, and anticoagulation were used in several patients and all patients recovered, but the time taken in recovery varied from days to as long as a few months.

2. Hemiballismus

This rare movement disorder in an aCL-positive patient has been recorded.[44]

3. Cerebellar Ataxia

This may unusually be related to the presence of aPL.[45]

N. Spinal Syndromes

1. Transverse Myelopathy

This is uncommon in SLE (occurs in less than 1% of patients) and is generally associated with a poor prognosis. Presentation is usually acute, with paresthesia in the legs, ascending to the thorax within 24 to 48 hours. Paraplegia, back pain, and loss of sphincter control may follow. Several papers have stressed the occurrence of transverse myelitis with the presence of aPL.[46] Optic neuritis may occur simultaneously with transverse myelitis, presenting with rapid visual loss accompanied by orbital pain.[47]

2. Guillain-Barré Syndrome

A number of patients with this complication have been documented.[48] It has been suggested that aCL of the IgA isotype are associated with peak disease activity.

3. Anterior Spinal Artery Syndrome

Sparing of the posterior columns occurs in this condition, with the patient presenting with a flaccid paraplegia, sphincter disturbances, and dissociated sensory impairment. One case with positive aCL has been documented.[49]

O. OPHTHALMIC COMPLICATIONS

Small vessel occlusions affecting the choroid, retina, and optic nerve result in ischemia and even infarctions. Neovascularization leads to secondary vitreous hemorrhage, traction retinal detachments, or glaucoma. Several reports have estimated retinal vascular occlusions in 8 to 12% of patients with aPL. Optic neuropathy (acute retrobulbar optic neuritis, ischemic optic atrophy, and progressive optic atrophy) has also been linked to the presence of aPL.[50]

IV. CARDIAC MANIFESTATIONS

A. MYOCARDIAL INFARCTIONS

Myocardial infarction (MI) in SLE is usually due to accelerated atherosclerosis or vasculitis but, in recent years, since the discovery of aPL, it has become evident that MI is not an uncommon accompaniment of APS.[51] Conversely, reports of aPL in patients with MI have yielded conflicting results. While it has been reported that aCL are common in young postinfarction patients and should be regarded as markers for recurrent cardiovascular events,[52] other investigators could not confirm this finding.[53] In an analysis of 43 patients with coronary artery disease presenting under 50 years of age, it was found that 67% had primary coagulation defects.[54] Other authors[55] subsequently summarized all cases of MI with aPL reported until 1993 (60 patients) and concluded that aPL were significant risk factors in acute MI, but in selected patients only. Finnish investigators,[56] more recently have found that the presence of high aCL is an independent risk factor in MI and cardiac death.

B. UNSTABLE ANGINA

This subject has been studied, but no association between aPL positivity and either the severity of angiographic changes or an adverse clinical outcome could be found.[57]

C. CORONARY BYPASS GRAFT AND ANGIOPLASTY OCCLUSIONS

Elevated aCL levels in patients who developed late bypass vein graft occlusions have been detected.[58] Another study[59] reported increased IgA aCL levels in men with coronary artery disease treated with percutaneous transluminal coronary angioplasty who restenosed.

D. CARDIOMYOPATHY

Multiple small vascular occlusions ("thrombotic microvasculopathy") are responsible for both the acute and chronic cardiomyopathy seen in patients with aPL, the clinical picture being dependent on the rapidity of the process. Acute cardiac collapse (often together with respiratory decompensation) is frequent in patients with catastrophic APS, and is one of the most common causes of death in this group. Circulatory failure, as an isolated event, has also been reported,[60] analagous to that seen with renal thrombotic microangiopathy. Chronic cardiomyopathy may be global or localized. Segmental ventricular dysfunction can supervene. Impaired left ventricular diastolic filling has also been documented in primary APS patients.[61] This has been known to be associated with cardiomyopathy, and is an early manifestation of myocardial ischemia caused by coronary arteriolar occlusions. These may lead to myocardial fibrosis and decrease of left ventricular compliance.

E. Valvular Disease

1. Valve Thickening

Valve thickening, resulting in valve dysfunction and incompetence, is common in APS and the mitral valve is most frequently affected. Several series of studies have been published demonstrating valvulopathy in patients with primary APS[62] as well as SLE.[63]

2. Vegetations

Nonbacterial vegetations may be combined with valve thickening and are thought to reflect the same pathological process. Libman-Sacks endocarditis, as these lesions are named, may eventually heal with a fibrous plaque, sometimes with focal calcification and marked scarring, thickening, and deformity, leading to valve dysfunction. Regurgitation is common while stenosis is rare, and the mitral valve is mainly affected followed by the aortic valve. The tricuspid and pulmonary valves are less frequently affected. Usually, in APS patients, these valve lesions are not of clinical or hemodynamic significance, but with extensive deformity surgical replacement may be necessary. Thromboembolic events constitute the major danger to the patient with Libman-Sacks endocarditis and can damage the brain, kidneys, and other organs. Recently, a study on valves derived from patients with secondary APS as well as primary APS showed that subendothelial immunoglobulin deposits contained aPL.[64]

3. Pseudo-Infective Endocarditis

SLE patients in the presteroid era often had large verrucae due to Libman-Sacks endocarditis, and it was not uncommon in these to become infected. Large vegetations, however, are now rare. aPL-associated valvular lesions may, however, still serve as substrates for microbial colonization. Diagnostic and therapeutic problems may arise in patients with the so-called "pseudo-infective" endocarditis. These patients may present with fever, splinter hemorrhages, cardiac murmurs with echocardiographic evidence of valve vegetations, moderate to high levels of aPL, and repeatedly negative blood cultures.[65]

F. Intracardiac Thrombus

Several patients with aPL have been reported who developed thrombi in the ventricular cavities.[66] Clinically, patients may present with systemic or pulmonary embolic symptoms (e.g., TIA, stroke, pulmonary infarction) depending on the location of the thrombus (right or left ventricle). Thrombus tends to form on akinetic segments of the ventricle. Atrial thrombus might mimic atrial myxoma. Occasionally, a clot may form on a normal mitral valve.

G. Cyanotic Congenital Heart Disease

Three patients with cyanotic congenital heart disease and elevated aCL have been published. Two had thrombotic episodes and a BFP-STS. The three were also thrombocytopenic.[67]

H. Complications of Cardiovascular Surgery

A 10% prevalence of a hypercoagulable condition has been detected on screening 158 patients with cardiovascular surgical procedures, and these patients had a significantly higher incidence of early graft thrombosis 27% vs 1.6% (P < 0.01).[68] Other authors[69] identified 19 patients with aPL among 1,078 treated for vascular surgical problems over a 5-year period. They noted that these patients tended to be female, younger, nonsmokers, and more likely to have involvement of the upper extremity than patients who were aPL negative. In a survey over a 2-year period, another group[70] found that 26% of its patients were aPL-positive and that they were 1.8 times more likely to have undergone previous lower-extremity vascular surgical procedures, and 5.6 times more likely to have suffered occlusion of previous reconstructions. In 1995, in a 5-year study, the authors identified 71 aPL-positive patients, of whom 19 had cardiovascular surgical procedures (including lower-extremity reconstructions and fistulas, cardiac valve replacements, coronary artery bypass procedures, major amputations, carotid endarterectomies, and infrarenal aortic reconstruction). Also, 84.2% suffered major postoperative complications including thrombosis of graft, strokes, MI, pulmonary emboli, and major bleeding events.[71] The aPL positivity, therefore, identifies a subset of the population who appear to be at increased risk for thrombotic complications following cardiovascular surgery.

V. PULMONARY MANIFESTATIONS

A. Pulmonary Embolism and Infarction

DVT is the most common manifestation of the occlusive vascular complications of aPL,[72] and it is therefore not surprising that pulmonary embolism and complicating infarctions are frequently seen in this group of patients, occurring in approximately one-third of patients presenting with DVT. Rarely, thromboembolic pulmonary hypertension (PHT) supervenes.[73] As these patients manifest pleuritic pain, dyspnoea, and may also demonstrate pyrexia. The differential diagnosis between PE and lupus/infective pneumonitis with complicating pleurisy is clearly important as the therapy differs between steroids and antiinfectives versus anticoagulation. Rarely, pulmonary embolism may be complicated by adrenal collapse and acute hypoadrenalism. It is important for this complication to be recognized in PE patients demonstrating aPL, as they require intensive steroid therapy and not increases in anticoagulation.[74] Pulmonary hemorrhage may also be seen coincident with pulmonary infarction, as in the one patient reported.[75] Thromboembolic disease has also been documented in patients with right ventricular thrombus.[76]

B. Major Pulmonary Arterial Thrombosis

Although cerebral and peripheral vessels are most commonly involved in aPL-induced thrombosis, major pulmonary arterial occlusion is distinctly uncommon. One such case was reported by Luchi et al.[77] This complication has also been reported postpartum.

C. Pulmonary Microthrombosis

Although originally thought to be the cause of PHT in aPL-positive patients, this complication is uncommon and has only been documented over the past five years. Several patients who demonstrated small vessel occlusive disease of the pulmonary vasculature have been documented, all with histopathological evidence provided.[78] A mixed histological picture may be seen with evidence of pulmonary alveolar hemorrhage and "capillaritis" co-existing in the same patients.[78,79] Adult respiratory distress syndrome (ARDS) may complicate the clinical course of these patients.[80] Pulmonary microthrombosis may be part of the "antiphospholipid lung syndrome" as recently described,[81] and patients present with recurrent episodes of dyspnoea, minimal hemoptyses, and rapidly changing infiltrates on chest radiographs.[82]

D. Pulmonary "Capillaritis"

Gertner and Lie[78] coined this term to describe aPL patients who, on histopathological examination, often demonstrated alveolar hemorrhage and microvascular thromboses. Rarely, bronchiolitis obliterans may also be seen. Pulmonary capillaries are the major component in the alveolar septa, supplied only by delicate individual fibers of collagen and elastic. Polymorphonuclear neutrophil leucocytes may fill the vessel lumen and traverse the vessel wall. Immune complex deposition may be demonstrated by immunofluorescent staining, as in the one patient documented.[82] An identical picture may be seen in patients with hypersensitivity pneumonitis, Wegener's granulomatosis, and with collagen vascular disease such as SLE itself.

E. Pulmonary Hypertension

PHT is one of the most serious complications of all connective tissue disorders (CTDs), occurring with SLE, scleroderma (in particular with its CREST variety), and MCTD, and it has also been reported in the "primary" antiphospholipid syndrome. A relationship exists between thromboembolic PHT and aPL for obvious reasons. However, many patients with SLE-associated PHT have high levels of aPL. Often, however, other thromboembolic complications of APS are absent in this group of patients, as discussed by Asherson et al.,[73] making one suspect that the high levels of aPL seen in these patients may be secondary and due to extensive endothelial cell damage of the pulmonary microvasculature. It is also of interest that a percentage of patients with plexogenic PHT of the "primary" variety may also demonstrate aPL in low to moderate titers, leading investigators suspect that either the aPL may be just another immunological accompaniment of the PHT (as with positive ANA), or perhaps an indication of diffuse pulmonary endothelial cell damage.[83]

VI. RENAL MANIFESTATIONS

The kidney, like many other organs, may be affected by aPL-induced coagulopathy. Large, (veins, arteries) vessels as well as small vessels may be affected. When glomerular vessels are occluded, the condition is referred to as renal "thrombotic microangiopathy." The lesions may be encountered during the course of SLE itself, or in the absence of any defined connective tissue disorder, i.e., in primary APS.

A. Renal Vein Thrombosis

Despite the frequency of venous involvement in APS, renal vein thrombosis is distinctly uncommon. The first two such cases were reported by Asherson et al. in 1984,[84] and in the same year Mintz et al.[85] pointed out that renal vein thrombosis (RVT) was more frequently encountered in patients with nephrotic syndrome (when a leak of antithrombin III occurs, predisposing to thrombosis), as well as in patients who had suffered a previous DVT of the limbs.

Gluek et al., in 1985,[86] found three patients with RVT in 18 LA-positive patients with SLE. Inferior vena cava occlusions, occlusions of other mesenteric veins, and even adrenal failure secondary to adrenal venous thrombosis may be encountered, as in the case reported by Le Thi Huong et al.[87] That renal vein thrombosis might be bilateral and may occur in the postpartum period predominantly is evident from a recent case report in 1993.[88]

B. Major Renal Artery Occlusions

Renal artery trunk lesions have also been documented in both SLE and primary APS patients (Figure 20.1). Hypertension is a not infrequent accompaniment of this condition, may be severe,

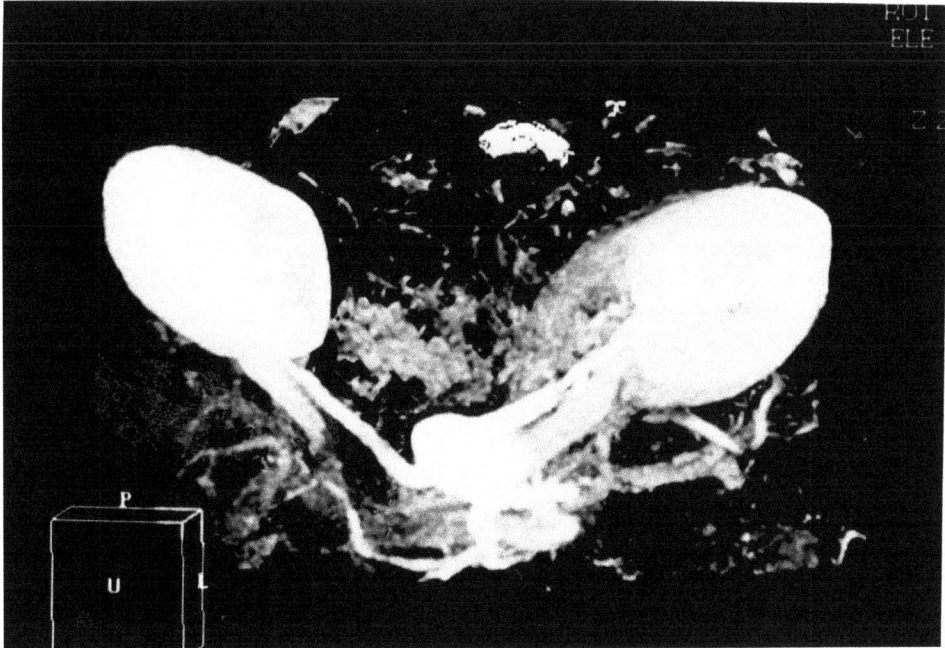

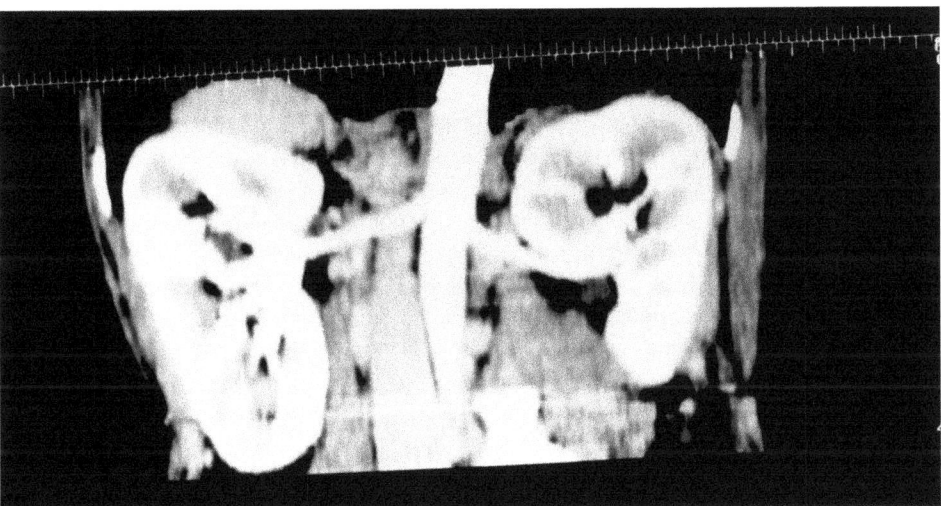

FIGURE 20.1 A. Double helicoidal renal angiotomography showing stenosis of both renal arteries. The left one shows marked stenosis along the medial and distal third. The right artery is mildly stenosed at the medial third. B. Control double helicoidal renal angiotomography showing the recanalization of both renal arteries.

and on occasion may result in oliguric renal failure. The renal artery occlusions may be unilateral[89-91] or bilateral.[92,93]

The renal artery may be occluded in patients with thrombosis of the abdominal aorta itself, as in the case described by Drew et al.[94] Some authors have used the term "fibromuscular dysplasia" to denote renal artery stenosis, and this has also been reported with aPL.[95]

C. RENAL INFARCTION

Consequent on vascular occlusive renal disease, the vessels have been documented by several investigators.[96-98] Although widely resulting from *in situ* thrombosis of the renal artery or one of its branches, as a complication of renal artery "stenosis," or fibromuscular dysplasia, it may rarely result from a possible embolus originating from a cardiac valve lesion.[99]

D. Thrombotic Microangiopathy

In SLE patients, it has been clearly demonstrated that the presence of aPL associates strongly with glomerular capillary thrombosis,[100] and that this occurs more frequently in patients suffering from proliferative glomerular nephritis. Progression to glomerular sclerosis also seems to be more frequent in patients who present initially with capillary thrombosis.

When severe or accelerated hypertension supervenes in SLE patients, even in the absence of overt nephritis,[101-103] these reno-vascular lesions have been responsible for the event. Several reports of this association have now been documented.[104-106] Ischemic glomeruli, intrarenal or arteriolar thrombosis, or simple intimal fibrosis were seen histopathologically in these patients.

Progressive loss of renal function in the absence of hypertension or overt proliferative nephritis has also been reported in several patients in whom frank-tubular interstitial lesions were described.[107] Other patients who presented with massive proteinuria only have also been documented.[108,109] Overt nephritis in these patients was not seen. Similar lesions have been demonstrated in patients with primary APS[110] and lupus-like syndrome.[111-116] Fibrin has been demonstrated in these thrombi, but no glomerular or arteriolar immune deposits have been demonstrated. Early descriptions of essentially the same lesions were documented by Kincaid-Smith et al. in the 1980s[117] in nephropathies associated with pregnancy. Similar lesions have also always been present in patients with catastrophic APS.

VII. ADRENAL MANIFESTATIONS

The first reports of an association between aPL and the adrenal gland, manifesting as hypoadrenalism (usually acute), appeared in 1988/1989 from several different centers.[118-120] An editorial was then published in 1991[121] and, at a special meeting commemorating the 200th anniversary of the birth of Thomas Addison which was published in 1994,[122] a comprehensive review of 41 reported cases was given by Asherson. In 1995 a further review appeared.[123] Histopathologically, the adrenal failure is caused by adrenal hemorrhage and infarction consequent on the hypocoagulable state. Thrombosis of adrenal veins as the primary event occurs, and the hemorrhagic infarction ensues as a secondary phenomenon. The adrenal glands may be enlarged on abdominal computed tomography, and, over the course of time, adrenal atrophy ensues. It appears that the condition is more common in patients with PAPS rather than defined SLE, and is not an uncommon accompaniment of CAPS, occurring in no less than 25% of patients reported by Asherson et al. in their recent series of 50 patients.[124] It has also been seen in isolated patients with discoid SLE, as well as with drug-induced LE. Although Addison's disease might be evident from adrenal infarction occurring years previously, the onset may often be insidious rather than acute with abdominal pain and severe hypotension.

The condition may develop following surgical procedures, even minor interventions such as cervical dilatation and curettage or tendon repair, and its effects may not only occur immediately postoperatively, but may be delayed for as long as six weeks following the procedure. In four patients reported it followed PE. The diagnosis in this latter situation is critically important as sudden collapse following PE requires immediate IV steroids rather than an increase in anticoagulation therapy. It is also not uncommon in the postpartum period along with other thromboembolic complications in aPL-positive patients. Warfarin withdrawal may be an important precipitating factor in these patients. In patients with catastrophic APS, there is often an association with ARDS, which is cytokine mediated, and it is possible that cytokine-induced thrombosis may be the basis of the condition. This has, however, not been fully investigated because of its rarity. Adrenal infarction is an important cause of abdominal pain in aPL-positive patients, along with mesenteric/renal/hepatic ischemia and infarction and thrombotic pancreatitis.

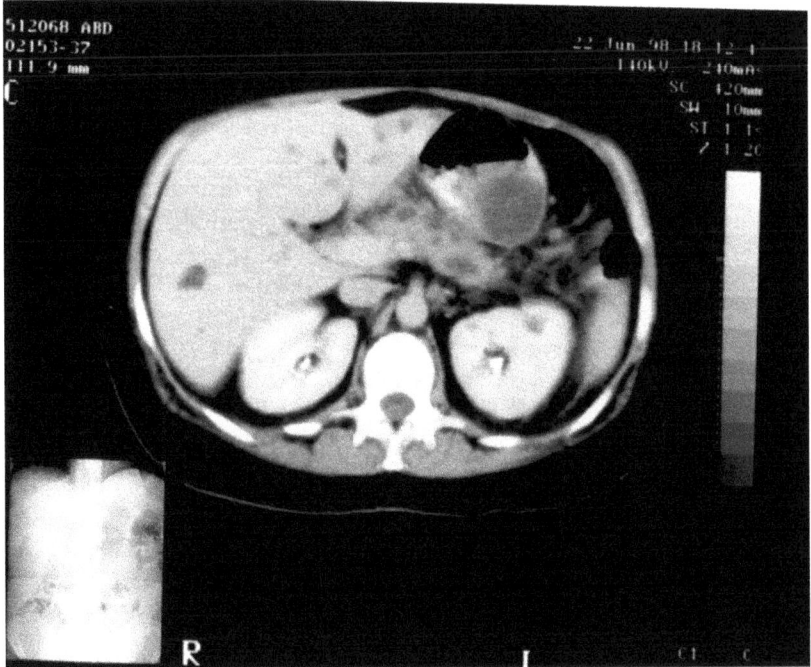

FIGURE 20.2 Abdominal CT scan showing edematous pancreas with several cysts and multiple hepatic defects shown to be infarctions.

VIII. HEPATIC AND DIGESTIVE MANIFESTATIONS

A. HEPATIC MANIFESTATIONS

Several hepatic manifestations have been described in patients with aPL. These include the Budd-Chiari syndrome, portal hypertension, obstruction of small hepatic veins (hepatic veno-occlusive disease), nodular regenerative hyperplasia, hepatic infarctions (Figure 20.2), hepatitis, alcoholic liver disease, and cirrhosis. Most of these lesions are due to vascular lesions of liver microcirculation.[125]

B. ESOPHAGEAL NECROSIS

A patient with a primary APS who thrombosed vessels at the lower end of the esophagus resulting in necrosis, septic mediastinitis, and death has been documented.[126] Bleeding esophageal varices from portal vein thromboses have also been reported.

C. GASTRIC ULCERATION

Progressive gastric ulceration with necrosis in a patient presenting with severe abdominal pain was found to be due to widespread occlusive vascular disease involving veins, small arteries, and arterioles.[127]

D. SMALL- AND LARGE-BOWEL VASCULAR OCCLUSIONS

Several cases of large bowel and intestinal infarctions in patients with aPL have been reported.[128] Peritonitis is not an uncommon accompaniment. Severe gastrointestinal hemorrhage may also result from bowel ischemia, or from an atypical duodenal ulcer.

E. Mesenteric Inflammatory Vaso-Occlusive Disease

One patient with an unusual form of vasculitis involving the mesenteric vessels — mesenteric inflammatory vaso-occlusive disease (MIVOD) — has been reported who also developed an APS with DVT, thrombocytopenia, and high titers of aCL. Small bowel infarction had occurred due to MIVOD.[129] This condition primarily affects veins and venules of the bowel and mesentery resulting in ischemic injury; almost 50% of the cases described thus far are primary or idiopathic. There is often a family history of thromboembolism in these primary cases, suggesting that an inherited hypercoagulable disorder may be present. The association of idiopathic mesenteric thrombosis and peripheral thrombosis has, in fact, been known for a long time.

F. Inflammatory Bowel Disease

Thromboembolic disease is a well recognized, although uncommon, complication of inflammatory bowel disease. It has recently been reported that the presence of aPL may be associated with thrombosis in patients with ulcerative colitis and Crohn's disease.[130]

G. Pancreatitis

Abdominal pain in patients with APS may be due to pancreatic involvement by the microangiopathy characteristic of aPL. The presentation may be acute, with abdominal pain and vomiting. Pancreatic involvement was noted in 6 of the 50 patients recently reviewed with catastrophic APS.[3] However, in only one was the diagnosis made clinically. In three, microvascular thromboses of pancreatic vessels was noted at *post mortem,* and in two, pancreatic enzymes were found to be elevated.

H. Cholecystitis

Two patients presenting with acute cholecystitis in the absence of gallstones have been reported in the course of catastrophic APS[3] (Figure 20.3).

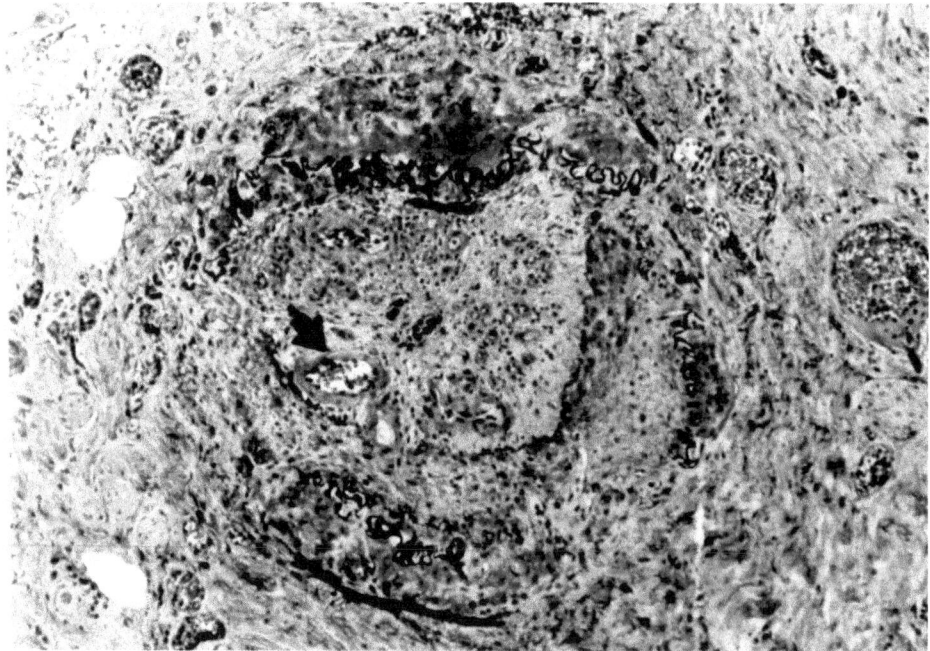

FIGURE 20.3 Gallbladder showing thrombosed artery with areas of neovascularization within the thrombus.

I. OCCLUSION OF SPLENIC VESSELS

Occlusion of splenic vessels has been reported in combination with other vascular occlusions.[128] Splenic infarction may supervene. Splenic atrophy is a rare event, even in SLE, but one such patient with long-standing SLE and aCL who developed this complication has been documented.[131]

IX. OBSTETRIC MANIFESTATIONS

A. MATERNAL COMPLICATIONS

Several reports have suggested that women with aPL are more likely to develop toxemia of pregnancy and pre-eclampsia, as well as HELLP syndrome. The postpartum cardio-pulmonary syndrome, chorea gravidarum, postpartum cerebral infarct following aspirin withdrawal, and maternal death have also been reported in patients with aPL. Clinical thrombosis, both arterial and venous, is associated with pregnancy and the post-partum period in these women, and therefore pregnancy is a challenge to both mother and baby.[132]

B. FETAL COMPLICATIONS

In 1989 a review of all previous clinical reports was published.[133] A total of 183 patients diagnosed with aPL had 652 pregnancies. Pregnancy failure occurred in 305 at unspecified gestational age (47%), 129 ended as spontaneous abortion (20%), and 129 ended as fetal death (20%). Only 89 (13.7%) of the pregnancies resulted in the delivery of a viable infant. Viable infants, however, are not necessarily untouched by the effects of aPL. Intrauterine growth retardation is significantly more frequent in mothers with aPL. Increased incidence of severe early onset preeclampsia and abruptio placenta may precipitate premature birth. Abnormal uterine artery flow velocity may predict poor outcome in cases of aPL, and elevated maternal serum alpha fetoprotein levels may be harbingers of fetal death. The potential for transplacental passage of the procoagulant tendency (by transplacental transfer of immunoglobulin G) has been reinforced by reports of neonatal stroke, multiple placental vascular thromboses (Figure 20.4), and disseminated neonatal thrombosis in infants delivered of mothers with aPL.[132]

X. DERMATOLOGIC MANIFESTATIONS

Several cutaneous manifestations have been described in patients with aPL. These include *livedo reticularis*, skin ulcerations, small painful leg ulcers of livedoid vasculitis, cutaneous necrosis, macules and nodules, multiple subungual hemorrhages, gangrene and digital necrosis, anetoderma, discoid LE, intravascular coagulation necrosis of the skin associated with cryofibrinogenemia and diabetes mellitus, and pyoderma gangrenosum. Most of these lesions are due to vascular lesions of skin microcirculation.[134]

XI. CATASTROPHIC ANTIPHOSPHOLIPID SYNDROME

Although single cases of this unusually widespread subset of APS demonstrating extensive microvasculopathy had previously been published,[135,136] it was in 1992 that it was first attempted to define its clinical and serological features as well as its course, and when the term "catastrophic" was introduced to describe its presentation.[2] Since the original description, several reviews analyzing the major features of this condition have been published, and at the present time a total of 50 patients conforming to this diagnosis have been reported.[3,137,138] Most patients are either suffering from primary APS or SLE. A minority of cases with Sjögren's syndrome, rheumatoid arthritis, or systemic sclerosis have also occurred. Patients with catastrophic APS are generally admitted to

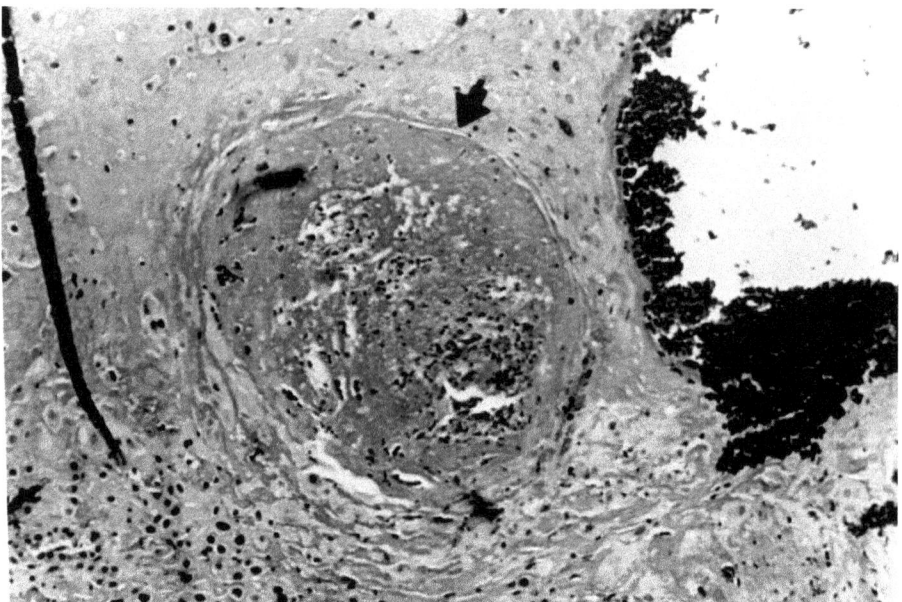

FIGURE 20.4 Placenta showing decidual vessel occluded by thrombus.

intensive care units and are critically ill, with multiorgan failure affecting all major organs. They may have been previously suffering from SLE or primary APS, well controlled on a variety of regimens, or the condition may arise *de novo* in a previously healthy individual — perhaps examples of primary APS with no previous history of thrombotic events. The pathogenesis of catastrophic APS is multifactorial and has been discussed in a recent editorial.[139] Multiorgan thrombosis may be "triggered" by an infection[140] (usually gram negative) or drug administration (e.g., thiazide diuretics, captropril, oral contraceptives). Surgical procedures (major or minor) or anticoagulation withdrawal may also be triggering events. Often two or three of these triggering factors are evident e.g., infection followed by a surgical procedure coincident with anticoagulation withdrawal, the so called "double" or "treble" hit hypothesis.

Kitchens,[141] in a recent paper, suggested that ongoing thrombosis was dependent on the widespread coagulopathy itself. He proposed the term "thrombotic storm," which seemed to occur in these patients. The proteins governing coagulation are consumed during the process of haemostasis and these include mainly Protein C and S and Antithrombin III, and the newly formed clots themselves produce activated coagulation factors including prothrombin activation products F1 and 2, thrombin antithrombin complex, and protein C activation peptide.

The fibrinolytic system is also under stress during times of trauma, surgery, or during pregnancy, and vascular clearance of fibrin is impaired. This is a process referred to as "fibrinolytic shutdown," mediated by an increase in plasminogen activator inhibitors (PAI). Multiorgan failure is the mode of presentation, and the frequency of organ involvement is summarized in Table 20.1.

A. RENAL

Renal failure is evident in 70% of patients and may be accompanied by hypertension (on occasion of the accelerated or malignant variety). However, oliguric renal failure leading to demise is unusual.

B. PULMONARY

A picture of adult respiratory distress syndrome (ARDS) dominates the clinical presentation, although multiple pulmonary emboli, pulmonary infiltrations, or alveolar hemorrhage may also be encountered, as may be pulmonary arterial microthrombotic lesions, in a minority of patients.

TABLE 20.1
**Frequency of Organ Involvement
in the Catastrophic APS**

Renal	70%
Pulmonary	66%
Central Nervous System	56%
Skin	50%
Cardiac	50%
Gastrointestinal	38%
Adrenal	26%

C. CENTRAL NERVOUS SYSTEM

The vast majority of patients end up in a coma, having been confused and disorientated prior to this. Seizures may be seen in a minority of patients. The majority of patients demonstrate cerebral microthrombi, with a minority only manifesting major cerebral infarctions resulting from large vessel occlusive disease.

D. SKIN

Dermatological complications include livedo reticularis, digital ischemia or frank gangrene, superficial skin necrosis, and ischemic ulceration of limbs, all dependent upon small vessel occlusive disease affecting the dermis, which may be frequently encountered. Several dermatological presentations may be present in one patient e.g., livedo reticularis and gangrene.

E. CARDIAC

The outstanding feature is cardiac microangiopathy leading to hypotension and a reduced ejection fraction because of myocardial ischemia and hypofunction. It should also be stressed that the excessive cytokines produced in this condition may lead to diminished cardiac function. Frank myocardial infarction (MI) is unusual but might accompany the thrombotic microangiopathy itself. Valve lesions (mitral/aortic) or intracardiac thrombosis (atrium, ventricle), such as seen in patients with a "simple" APS, may also be encountered in this group of patients.

F. GASTROINTESTINAL

Abdominal pain as a presenting feature occurs in approximately one-third of patients and is usually due to mesenteric ischemia. Hepatic involvement with a transaminitis is very common, but actual hepatic infarction is rare. Thrombotic pancreatitis has also been reported. Ischemic ulceration of the esophagus, stomach and duodenum, bowel, or colon may lead to perforation/ulceration and death from mediastinitis or peritonitis.

G. ADRENAL

A high frequency of adrenal involvement is encountered in CAPS patients which is due to hemorrhagic infarction of the adrenal glands. Adrenal hyperfunction is not always evident clinically, and a high index of suspicion is required in order to effect a correct diagnosis and institute appropriate replacement therapy with corticosteroids. Adrenal venous occlusion is the basic pathophysiological etiology, with secondary compromise of the arterial circulation due to edema resulting from the venous occlusive situation. One of the interesting predisposing causes of this condition is PE, and sudden collapse with hypotension in an aPL-positive patient is *not* due to recurrent thromboembolism and does not require increased anticoagulation, but steroid supplements.

The clinical manifestations of catastrophic APS are due to the thrombotic occlusions themselves affecting organ function (e.g., kidney, brain, heart, etc.) as well as the "cytokine storm" which ensues as a result of extensive tissue damage. It is the excess production of cytokines such as TNF Alpha, IL-I, and IL-6 which is responsible for some of the major clinical manifestations.[142] These include ARDS, cerebral edema causing the initial confusion, and myocardial dysfunction in addition to the microangiopathy present. CAPS is different from simple APS because of unusual sites of vessels involved, e.g., testicular/scrotal vessels, splanchnic vessels, great veins of the arm and neck, etc.

Disseminated intravascular coagulation (DIC) may be a feature of catastrophic APS and was seen in approximately 30% of the original series. At times, distinction between thrombotic thrombocytopenic purpura (TTP) and DIC may be difficult as these conditions may also present with multiorgan microvascular occlusive disease,[143] and excessive cytokine production may also be evident in these patients.

Serologically, more than 50% of patients demonstrate high levels of aCL and/or lupus anticoagulants. This isotype is almost always IgG, although a patient with IgM aCL and catastrophic APS has been reported. The antinuclear antibodies (ANA) may be low positive in primary APS patients (21:160) or higher in those suffering from SLE, who will also demonstrate antibodies to dsDNA. Anti Ro, anti La, or RNP may also be positive in a minority of patients with SLE.

XII. VASCULITIS

The association of aPL and vasculitis is unusual (Table 20.2). There is a difference between a "true" vasculitis, histopathologically, with its typical inflammatory cell infiltration of vessel walls, and a "reactive" cellular infiltrate which may accompany primary vascular occlusions (noninflammatory thrombosis). This has been stressed in several publications.[144-146]

Vasculitis is commonly encountered in SLE patients, as is the presence of aPL. It is not surprising, therefore, that these two conditions may coexist in some SLE patients. Vasculitic events may occur in up to 20% of SLE patients and typically involve the microvasculature of the skin and kidneys (less frequently, vessels of the heart and lungs). Medium and large-size vasculature involvement is unusual. Necrotizing vasculitis of the polyarteritis nodosa-type might be very rarely encountered, and may affect particularly the cerebral vasculature and, even more infrequently,

---

TABLE 20.2
Vasculitis and Antiphospholipid Antibodies

1. Vasculitis (large/medium size vessel) with aPL in SLE. Rarely, PAN-type of necrotizing vasculitis may be seen (cerebral vasculature mainly).
2. "Pseudo" vasculitis (secondary to organizing thrombus) in PAPS or SLE; coexisting atherosclerosis may be present in older patients.
3. "Capillaritis" (quasivasculitis) indicative of necrotizing glomerulonephritis or lung (pulmonary capillaritis ± alveolar hemorrhage)
4. Aortitis
5. Leucocytoclastic vasculitis of skin vessels reported in PAPS.
6. Systemic vasculitides and aPL/APS; coexistence of two conditions
    — PAN; Microscopic polyarteritis
    — Giant Cell arteritis
    — Takayasu's arteritis
    — Relapsing polychondritis

systemic vessels, e.g., renal. Fibrinoid necrosis will be demonstrated in these patients histologically.[147] Among three patients reported was one with SLE.[147] The remaining two had no evidence of SLE but conformed to primary APS.[148] Both also demonstrated leucocytoclastic vasculitis affecting the small skin vessels. Clinically, recurrent cutaneous nodules appeared in one. It thus appears from these and other reports[149,150] that a *cutaneous leucocytoclastic vasculitis* may be seen in patients with a primary APS, both being manifestations of the underlying immunological disorder.

In another patient described,[151] aPL, vasculitis and atherosclerosis coexisted. A BFP-STS had been found in this 63-year-old female at the age of 28 years. aPL had therefore been present for many years. Atherosclerotic lesions of the abdominal aorta with stenosis, iliac arteries, and the inferior mesenteric arteries were affected by the atherosclerotic process. It is likely that the inflammatory infiltrate in this case was consequent on the healing process and organization of thrombus in this patient. "True" vasculitis was not present thrombosis atherosclerosis, and a mild perivascular infiltrate was demonstrated.

"Aortitis" in a male with PAPS was recently documented.[152] This patient manifested abdominal and back pain accompanied by fever, and demonstrated abdominal aortic parietal thickening between the renal arteries and the iliac bifurcation. Histologically, the pain and fever responded to corticosteroid therapy. CT scans returned to normal after six weeks of therapy. This patient did not conform to a diagnosis of Takayasu's arteritis.

The association of aPL with classical polyarteritis nodosa is rare. Several well-documented cases have been published.[153,154] The topic was recently reviewed by Norden et al.[155] A patient who developed microscopic polyarteritis in the puerperium has also been reported.[156] Another, also with microscopic polyarteritis and a DVT as well as lupus anticoagulant, was also documented.[157]

Elevated aCL was demonstrated in a patient with giant cell arteritis.[158] McHugh et al.[159] found that 50% of their patients with temporal arteritis had elevated IgG aCL, and suggested that the presence of aCL in polymyalgia rheumatica patients might predict which patients were at increased risk for developing temporal arteritis. In their series of patients, they also described a 32-year-old female with typical Takayasu's arteritis and elevated aCL. Two further such patients were documented from Japan.[160] The first had complete occlusion of the subclavian arteries, narrowing of the common carotid, and occlusion of the infrarenal abdominal aorta. Their second case showed changes in the ascending aorta and common carotid arteries, and also had an aortic valve involvement with histological changes typical of Takayasu's arteritis.

Sera of 34 patients with Takayasu's arteritis were screened for aCL.[161] A total of 41% were found to have raised IgG aCL, and 5 of the 14 patients had values of more than 40 GPL. None, however, had clinical features of primary APS.

Relapsing polychondritis, another of the systemic vasculitides, has also been associated with lupus anticoagulant positivity.[162,163]

In summary, it seems that the presence of aCL and lupus anticoagulant in patients with vasculitis represents a coexistence of the two conditions.

REFERENCES

1. Asherson, RA, Cervera, R, Piette, JC, Shoenfel, Y, The antiphospholipid syndrome: history, definition, classification, and differential diagnosis. In: Asherson, RA, Cervera, R, Piette, JC, Shoenfeld, Y, eds., *The Antiphospholipid Syndrome,* CRC Press, Boca Raton, 1996.
2. Asherson, RA, The catastrophic antiphospholipid syndrome, *J. Rheumatol.,* 1992; 19: 508–512.
3. Asherson, RA, Cervera, R, Piette, JC, et al., Catastrophic antiphospholipid syndrome: clinical and laboratory features of 50 patients. *Medicine* (Baltimore), 1998: 77: 195–207.
4. Alarcon-Segovia, D, Osmindson, PJ, Peripheral vascular syndromes associated with systemic lupus erythematosus, *Ann. Intern. Med.,* 1965: 62: 907–919.

5. Jindal, BK, Martin, MFR, Gayner, A, Gangrene developing after minor surgery in a patient with undiagnosed systemic lupus erythematosus and lupus anticoagulant, *Ann. Rheum. Dis.*, 1983: 42: 347–349.

6. Hall, S, Buettner, H, Luthra, HA, Occlusive retinal vascular disease in systemic lupus erythematosus, *J. Rheumatol.*, 1984: 11: 846–850.

7. Asherson, RA, Derksen, RHWM, Harris, EN, et al., Large vessel occlusion in gangrene and systemic lupus erythematosus and lupus-like disease. A report of six cases, *J. Rheumatol.*, 1986: 13: 740–747.

8. Asherson, RA, Harris, EN, Gharavi, AE, Aortic arch syndrome associated with anticardiolipin antibodies and the lupus anticoagulant — comment on Ferrantè paper, *Arthritis Rheum.*, 1985: 28: 594–595.

9. Asherson, RA, Ridley, MG, Khamashta, MA, Hughes, GRV, Gangrene en il lupus eritematosa sistemico, *Piel.*, 1988: 2: 409–412.

10. Lessof, MH, Glynn, LE, The pulseless syndrome, *Lancet*, 1959: 1: 799–801.

11. Drew, P, Asherson, RA, Zuk, RJ, et al., Aortic occlusion in systemic lupus erythematosus associated with antiphospholipid antibodies, *Ann. Rheum. Dis.*, 1987: 46: 612–616.

12. McGee, GS, Pearce, WH, Sharma, L, Green, D, Yas, JJT, Antiphospholipid antibodies and arterial thrombosis, *Arch. Surg.*, 1992: 127: 342–346.

13. Setoguchi, M, Fujishima, Y, Abe, I, Kobayashi, K, Fujishima, M, Aorto-iliac occlusion associated with the lupus anticoagulant. 1997: 4: 357–364.

14. Hohlfeld, J, Schneider, M, Hein R, et al., Thrombosis of the terminal aorta, deep vein thrombosis, recurrent fetal loss, and antiphospholipid antibodies, *VASA*, 1996: 25: 194–197.

15. Fain, O, Mathieu, E, Seror, O, et al., Aortitis: A new manifestation of primary antiphospholipid syndrome, *Br. J. Rheumatol.*, 1995: 34: 686–696.

16. Stern, BJ, Brey, RL, Anticardiolipin antibodies are associated with an increased risk of stroke occurrence, *Neurol.*, 1994; 44 (Suppl 2): A327.

17. Levine, SR, Brey, RL, Sawaya, KL, et al., Recurrent stroke and thrombo-occlusive events in the antiphospholipid syndrome, *Ann. Neurol.*, 1995; 38: 119–124.

18. Coull, BM, Goodnight, SH, Antiphospholipid antibodies, prethrombotic state and stroke, *Stroke*, 1990; 21: 1370–1374.

19. Brey, RL, Hait, RG, Sherman, DG, Tegeler, CH, Antiphospholipid antibodies and cerebral ischemia in young people, *Neurol.*, 1990; 40: 1190–1196.

20. Sneddon, IB, Cerebrovascular lesions and livedo reticularis, *Br. J. Dermatol.*, 1965; 77: 180–185.

21. Rebollo, M, Val, FJ, Garijo, F, et al., Livedo reticularis and cerebro-vascular lesions (Sneddon's syndrome). Clinical, radiological and pathological features in eight cases, *Brain*, 1983; 106: 965–979.

22. Brey, RL, Escalante, A, Futrell, N, Asherson, RA, Cerebral Thrombosis and Other Neurologic Manifestations in the Antiphospholipid Syndrome. In: *The Antiphospholipid Syndrome,* Asherson, RA, Cervera, R, Piette, J-C, Shoenfeld, Y., Eds., 1996; pp 133–150.

23. Asherson, RA, Mayou, S, Black, M, et al., Livedo reticularis, connective tissue disease, anticardiolipin antibodies and CNS complications, *Arthritis Rheum.*, 1987; 30(Suppl 4): S69.

24. Asherson, RA, Cervera, R, Sneddon's and the "Primary" Antiphospholipid Syndrome: confusion clarified, *J. Stroke Cerebrovasc. Dis.*, 1993; 3: 121–122.

25. Stockhammer, G, Felber, SR, Zelger, B, et al., Sneddon's Syndrome: Diagnosis by skin biopsy and MRI in 17 patients, *Stroke*, 1993; 24: 685–690.

26. Asherson, RA, Mercey, D, Phillips, G, et al., Recurrent stroke and multiinfarct dementia in systemic lupus erythematosus: association with antiphospholipid antibodies, *Ann. Rheum. Dis.*, 1987; 46: 605–611.

27. Briley, DP, Coull, BM, Goodnight, SH, Neurological disease associated with antiphospholipid antibodies, *Ann. Neurol.*, 1989; 25: 221–227.

28. D'Alton, JG, Preston, DN, Bormanis, J, et al., Multiple transient ischemic attacks, lupus anticoagulant and verrucous endocarditis, *Stroke*, 1985; 16: 512–514.

29. Anderson, D, Bell, D, Lodge, R, Grant, E, Recurrent cerebral ischemia and mitral valve vegetation in a patient with antiphospholipid antibodies, *J. Rheumatol.*, 1987; 14: 839–841.

30. Levine, SR, Kieran, S, Puzio, K, Feit, H, Patel, SC, Welch, KYA, Cerebral venous thrombosis with lupus anticoagulant. Report of two cases, *Stroke*, 1987; 18: 801–804.

31. Jurtz, G, Muller, N, The antiphospholipid syndrome and psychosis, *Am. J. Psychiat.,* 1994; 151: 1841–1842.

32. Sirota, P, Schild, K, Firer, M, et al., The diversity of autoantibodies in schizophrenic patients and their first degree relatives: analysis of multiple case families. In: Abstracts of the First International Congress of the International Society of Neuro-Immune Modulation. Florence, *ISNIM,* 1991 p. 389.

33. Maes, M, Meltzer, H, Jacobs, J, et al., Autoimmunity in depression: increased antiphospholipid autoantibodies, *Acta Psychiatr. Scand.,* 1993; 87: 160–166.

34. Ziporen, L, Eilam, D, Shoenfeld, Y, Korczyn, AD, Neurologic dysfunction associated with antiphospholipid antibodies: animal models, *Neurology,* 1996; 46: A459.

35. Mikdashi, JA, Chase, C, Kay, GG, Neurocognitive deficits in antiphospholipid syndrome, *Neurology,* 1996; 46: A359.

36. Montalban, J, Arboix, A, Staub, H, et al., Transient global amnesia and antiphospholipid antibodies, *Clin. Exp. Rheumatol.,* 1989: 7: 85–87.

37. Scott, TF, Hess, D, Brillman, J, Antiphospholipid antibody syndrome mimicking multiple sclerosis clinically and by magnetic resonance imaging, *Arch. Intern. Med.,* 1994; 154: 917–920.

38. Hogan, MJ, Brunet, DG, Ford, PM, Lillicrap, D, Lupus anticoagulant, antiphospholipid antibodies and migraine, *Can. J. Neurol. Sci.,* 1988; 15; 420–425.

39. Montalbán, J, Cervera, R, Font, J, et al., Lack of association between anticardiolipin antibodies and migraine in systemic lupus erythematosus, *Neurology,* 1992; 42: 681–682.

40. Silvestrini, M, Matteis, M, Troisi, E, Cupini, LM, Zaccari, G, Bernardi, G, Migrainous stroke and the antiphospholipid antibodies, *Eur. Neurol.,* 1994; 34: 316–319.

41. Montalbán, J, López, M, Jordana, R, Ordi, J, Gallart, R, Codina, A, Anticuerpos antifosfolípido en la epilepsia tardía, *Rev. Neurol.* (Barc.), 1991; 19: 119–121.

42. Herranz, MT, Rivier, G, Khamashta, MA, Blaser, KV, Hughes, GRV, Association between antiphospholipid antibodies and epilepsy in patients with systemic lupus erythematosus, *Arthritis Rheum.,* 1994; 37: 568–571.

43. Cervera, R, Asherson, RA, Font, J, et al., Chorea in the antiphospholipid syndrome. Clinical, neurologic and immunologic characteristics of 50 patients from our clinics and the recent literature, *Medicine* (Baltimore), 1997; 76: 203–212.

44. Tam, L-S, Cohen, MG, Li, EK, Hemiballismus in systemic lupus erythematosus: possible association with antiphospholipid antibodies, Lupus, 1995; 4: 67–69.

45. Singh, PR, Piasaa, K, Qumar, A, et al., Cerebellar ataxia in systemic lupus erythematosus: three case reports, *Ann. Rheum. Dis.,* 1988; 97: 954–956.

46. Lavalle, C, Pizarro, S, Drenkard, C, Sánchez-Guerrero, J, Alarcón-Segovia, D, Transverse myelitis: manifestation of systemic lupus erythematosus strongly associated with antiphospholipid antibodies, *J. Rheumatol.,* 1990; 17: 34–37.

47. Oppenheimer, S, Hofbrand, BI, Optic neuritis and myelopathy in systemic lupus erythematosus, *Can. J. Neurol. Sci.,* 1986; 13: 129–132.

48. Harris, EN, Englert, H, Derue, G, Hughes, GRV, Gharavi, AE, Antiphospholipid antibodies in acute Guillain-Barré syndrome, *Lancet,* 1983; ii: 1361–1362.

49. Marcusse, HN, Hahn, J, Tan, WD, Breedveld, FC, Anterior spinal artery syndrome in systemic lupus erythematosus, *Br. J. Rheumatol.,* 1989; 28: 344–346.

50. Montehermoso, A, Cervera, R, Font, J, Ramos-Casals, M, García-Carrasco, M, Formiga, F, Callejas, JL, Jorfán, M, Griñó, MC, Ingelmo, M, Association of antiphospholipid antibodies with retinal vascular diseases in systemic lupus erythematosus, *Semin. Arthritis Rheum.,* 1999; 28: 326–332.

51. Asherson, RA, Cervera, R, Antiphospholipid antibodies and the heart: lessons and pitfalls for the cardiologist, *Circulation,* 1991; 84: 920–923.

52. Hamsten, A, Norberg, R, Bjorkholm, M, et al., Antibodies to cardiolipin in young survivors of myocardial infarction: an association with recurrent cardiovascular events, *Lancet,* 1986; ii: 113–116.

53. Sletnes, KE, Smith, P, Abdelnoor, M, et al., Antiphospholipid antibodies after myocardial infarction and their relation to mortality, reinfarction, and non-haemorrhagic stroke, *Lancet,* 1992; 339: 451–453.

54. Bick, RL, Ishmail, Y, Baker, WF, Coagulation abnormalities in precocious coronary artery thrombosis and in patients failing coronary artery bypass grafting and percutaneous transcoronary angioplasty, *Semin. Thromb. Hemost.,* 1993; 10: 412–417.

55. Baker, WF, Bick, RL, Antiphospholipid antibodies in coronary artery disease: a review, *Semin. Thromb. Hemost.,* 1994; 20: 27–45.

56. Vaarala, O, Mänttäri, M, Manninen, V, et al., Anticardiolipin antibodies and risk of myocardial infarction in a prospective cohort of middle-aged men, *Circulation,* 1995; 91: 23–27.

57. Díaz, MN, Becker, RC, Anticardiolipin antibodies in patients with unstable angina, *Cardiology,* 1994; 84: 380–384.

58. Morton, KE, Gavaghan, TP, Krilis, SA, et al., Coronary artery bypass graft failure: an autoimmune phenomenon?, *Lancet,* 1986; ii: 1353–1356.

59. Eber, B, Schumacher, M, Auer-Grumbach, P, Toplak, H, Klein, W, Increased IgM anticardiolipin antibodies in patients with restenosis after percutaneous transluminal coronary angioplasty, *Am. J. Cardiol.,* 1992; 69: 1255–1258.

60. Brown, JH, Doherty, CC, Allen, DC, Morton, P, Fatal cardiac failure due to myocardial microthrombi in systemic lupus erythematosus, *Br. Med. J.,* 1988; 296: 1505.

61. Hasnie, AMA, Stoddard, MF, Gleason, CB, et al., Diastolic dysfunction is a feature of the antiphospholipid syndrome, *Am. Heart J.,* 1995; 129: 1009–1113.

62. Cervera, R, Khamashta, MA, Font, J, et al., High prevalence of significant heart valve lesions in patients with the 'primary' antiphospholipid syndrome, *Lupus,* 1992; 1: 43–47.

63. Khamashta, MA, Cervera, R, Asherson, RA, et al., Association of antibodies against phospholipids with heart valve disease in systemic lupus erythematosus, *Lancet,* 1990; 335: 1541–1544.

64. Ziporen, L, Goldberg, I, Arad, M, et al., Libman-Sacks endocarditis in the antiphospholipid syndrome: immunopathologic findings in deformed heart valves, *Lupus,* 1995; 5: 196–205.

65. Font, J, Cervera, R, Pare, C, et al., Non-infective verrucous endocarditis in a patient with "primary" antiphospholipid syndrome, *Br. J. Rheumatol.,* 1991; 30: 305–307.

66. O'Neill, D, Magaldi, J, Dobkins, D, Greco, T, Dissolution of intracardiac mass lesions in the primary antiphospholipid antibody syndrome, *Arch. Intern. Med.,* 1995; 155: 325–327.

67. Martínez-Levín, M, Fonseca, C, Arugo, MC, Maya, A, Reyes, PA, Ruiz-Argüelles, A, Antiphospholipid syndrome in patients with cyanotic congenital heart disease, *Clin. Exp. Rheumatol.,* 1995; 13: 489–491.

68. Donaldson, MC, Weinberg, D, Belkin, M, et al., Screening for hypercoagulable states in vascular surgical practice: a preliminary study, *J. Vasc. Surg.,* 1990; 11: 825–831.

69. Shortell, CK, Ouriel, K, Green, RM, et al., Vascular disease in the antiphospholipid syndrome: a comparison with the patient population with atherosclerosis, *J. Vasc. Surg.,* 1992; 15: 158–166.

70. Taylor, IM, Chitwood, RW, Dalman, RL, et al., Antiphospholipid antibodies in vascular surgery patients: a cross-sectional study, *Ann. Surg.,* 1994; 226: 545–551.

71. Ciocca, RG, Choi, J, Graham, AM, Antiphospholipid antibodies lead to increased risk in cardiovascular surgery, *Ann. J. Surg.,* 1995; 170: 198–200.

72. Ordi-Ros, JM, O'Callaghan, A, Vilardell-Tarres, M, Thrombotic manifestations in the antiphospholipid syndrome, In: *The Antiphospholipid Syndrome,* Asherson, RA, Cervera, R, Piette, J-C, Shoenfeld, Y., Eds., CRC Press, Boca Raton, pp. 107–118.

73. Asherson, RA, Higgenbottam, TW, Dinh Xuan AT, et al., Pulmonary hypertension in a lupus clinic. Experience with twenty-four patients, *J. Rheumatol.,* 1990; 17: 1292–1296.

74. Asherson, RA, The catastrophic antiphospholipid syndrome, 1998. A review of the clinical features, possible pathogenesis and treatment, *Lupus,* 1998; 7: 1–8.

75. Howe, HS, Boey, ML, Fong, KY, Feng, PH, Pulmonary haemorrhage, pulmonary infraction and the lupus anticoagulant, *Ann. Rheum. Dis.,* 1988; 47: 869–872.

76. Ryan, J, Lasarda, D, Spero, J, et al., Thrombolysis of right atrial thrombus with pulmonary embolism in anticardiolipin syndrome, *Am. Heart. J.,* 1995; 130: 905–907.

77. Luchi, ME, Asherson, RA, Lahita, RG, Primary idiopathic pulmonary hypertension complicated by pulmonary arterial thrombosis: association with antiphospholipid antibodies, *Arthritis Rheum.,* 1992; 35: 700–705.

78. Gertner, E, Lie, JT, Pulmonary capillaritis, alveolar haemorrhage and recurrent microvascular thrombosis in primary antiphospholipid syndrome, *J. Rheumatol.,* 1993; 20: 1224–1228.

79. Brucato, A, Baudo, F, Barberis, M, et al., Pulmonary hypertension secondary to thrombosis of the pulmonary vessels in a patient with primary antiphospholipid syndrome, *J. Rheumatol.,* 1994; 21: 942–944.

80. Ghosh, E, Walters, HD, Joist, JH, et al., Adult Respiratory Distress Syndrome associated with antiphospholipid antibody syndrome, *J. Rheumatol.,* 1993; 20: 1406–1408.

81. Asherson, RA, Cervera, R, The antiphospholipid antibody lung syndrome, submitted.

82. Crausman, RS, Achenbach, GA, Pluss, WT, et al., Pulmonary capillaritis and alveolar haemorrhage associated with the antiphospholipid syndrome, *J. Rheumatol.,* 1995; 22: 554–556.

83. Asherson, RA, Cervera, R, Antiphospholipid antibodies and the lung, *J. Rheumatol.,* 1995; 22: 62–66.

84. Asherson, RA, Lanham, JG, Hull, RG, Boey, ML, Gharavi, AE, Hughes, GRV, Renal vein thrombosis in systemic lupus erythematosus: association with the "lupus anticoagulant," *Clin. Exp. Rheumatol.,* 1984; 2: 75–79.

85. Mintz, G, Accvedo-Vazquez, E, Guttierres-Espinosa, G, Avclar-Garnica, F, Renal vein thrombosis and inferior vena cava thrombosis in systemic lupus erythematosus, *Arthritis Rheum.,* 1984; 27: 539–544.

86. Glueck, HJ, Kant, KS, Weiss, MA, Pollak, VH, Miller, MA, Coots, M, Thrombosis in systemic lupus erythematosus. Relation to the presence of circulating anticoagulants, *Arch. Intern. Med.,* 1985; 145: 1389–1395.

87. Le, Thi Huong Du, Wechsler, B, Piette, J-C, et al., Le syndrome des antiphospholipides: une nouvelle cause d'hèmorragic bilatèrale des surrènales. Revue de la littèrature à propos de 4 cas, *Presse. Med.,* 1993; 22: 249–254.

88. Asherson, RA, Buchanan, B, Baguley, E, Hughes, GRV, Postpartum bilateral renal vein thrombosis in the primary antiphospholipid syndrome, *J. Rheumatol.,* 1993; 20: 874–876.

89. Ostuni, PA, Lazzarin, P, Pengo, V, Ruffati, A, Schiavon, F, Gambari, P, Renal artery thrombosis and hypertension in a 13-year-old girl with antiphospholipid syndrome, *Ann. Rheum. Dis.,* 1990; 49: 184–187.

90. Asherson, RA, Noble, GE, Hughes, GRV, Hypertension, renal artery stenosis and the "primary" antiphospholipid syndrome, *J. Rheumatol.,* 1991; 18: 1413–1415.

91. Kupferminc, MJ, Lee, MJ, Green, D, Peaceman, AM, Severe postpartum, cardiac and renal syndrome associated with antiphospholipid antibodies, *Obstet. Gynecol.,* 1994; 83: 806–807.

92. Ames, PRJ, Cianciaruso, B, Bellizzi, V, et al., Bilateral renal occlusion in a patient with primary antiphospholipid syndrome: thrombosis, vasculitis or both?, *J. Rheumatol.,* 1992; 19: 1802–1806.

93. Remondino, GI, Hysler, E, Pissano, MN, et al., A reversible bilateral renal artery occurrence in association with antiphospholipid syndrome, *Lupus,* 9: 65–67.

94. Drew, P, Asherson, RA, Zuk, RJ, Goodwin, EJ, Hughes, GRV, Aortic occlusion in systemic lupus erythematosus associated with antiphospholipid antibodies, *Ann. Rheum. Dis.,* 1987; 46: 612–616.

95. Mandreoli, M, Zuccala, A, Zucchelli, P, Fibromuscular dysplasia of the renal arteries associated with antiphospholipid auto-antibodies: two case reports, *Am. J. Kidney. Dis.,* 1992; 20: 500–503.

96. Asherson, RA, Hughes, GRV, Derksen, RHWM, Renal infarction associated with antiphospholipid antibodies in systemic lupus erythematosus and "lupus-like" disease, *J. Urol.,* 1988; 140: 1028.

97. Sonpal, GM, Sharma, A, Miller, A, Primary antiphospholipid antibody syndrome, renal infarction and hypertension, *J. Rheumatol.,* 1993; 20: 1221–1223.

98. Arnold, MH, Schreiber, L, Splenic and renal infarction in systemic lupus erythematosus: association with anticardiolipin antibodies, *Clin. Rheumatol.,* 1988; 7: 406–410.

99. Mandreoli, M, Zucchelli, P, Renal vascular disease in patients with primary antiphospholipid antibodies, *Nephrol. Diab. Transplant.,* 1993; 8: 1277–1280.

100. Kant, KS, Pollak, VH, Weiss, MA, Blueck, HJ, Miller, MA, Hess, HV, Glomerular thrombosis in systemic lupus erythematosus: prevalence and significance, *Medicine,* 1981; 60: 71–86.

101. Herreman, G, Bonnet, F, Helman, A, Glaser, P, Puech, H, Godeau, P, Hypertension artèrielle maligne et lupus èrythèmateux dissèminè. A propos d'un cas d'èvolution favorable, *Rev. Med. Interne.,* 1980; 1: 231–235.

102. Jouquan, J, Pennec, Y, Mottier, D, et al., Accelerated hypertension associated with lupus anticoagulant and false-positive VDRL in systemic lupus erythematosus, *Arthritis Rheum.,* 1986; 29: 147.

103. Julkunen, H, Kaaja, R, Jouhikainen, T, Teppo, A, Friman, C, Malignant hypertension and antiphospholipid antibodies as presenting features of SLE in a young woman using oral contraceptives, *Br. J. Rheumatol.,* 1991; 30: 471–472.

104. Kleinknecht, D, Bobrie, G, Meyer, O, Noel, LH, Callard, P, Ramdane, M, Recurrent thrombosis and renal vascular disease in patient with a lupus anticoagulant, *Nephrol. Diab. Transplant.,* 1989; 4: 854–858.

105. Ramdane, M, Gryman, R, Bacques, O, Callard, P, Kleinknecht, D, Ischèmic rènale corticale, thrombose auriculaire droite et occlusion coronaire au cours d'un syndrome des anticorps antiphospholipides, *Nèphrologie*, 1989; 10: 189–193.

106. Cacoub, P, Wechsler, B, Piette, J-C, et al., Malignant hypertension in antiphospholipid syndrome with overt lupus nephritis, *Clin. Exp. Rheum.*, 1993; 11: 479–485.

107. Leaker, B, McGregor, A, Griffiths, M, Smith, M, Neild, GH, Isenberg, D, Insidious loss of renal function in patients with anticardiolipin antibodies and absence of overt nephritis, *Br. J. Rheumatol.*, 1991; 30: 422–425.

108. Spronk, PE, Bootsma, H, Nikkels, PG, Kallenberg, CGM, A new class of lupus nephropathy associated with antiphospholipid antibodies, *Br. J. Rheumatol.*, 1994; 33: 686–687.

109. Scolari, P, Savoldi, S, Constantino, E, et al., Antiphospholipid syndrome and glomerular thrombosis in the absence of overt lupus nephritis, *Nephrol. Diab. Transplant.*, 1993; 8: 1274–1276.

110. Amigo, MC, Garcia-Torrès, R, Robles, M, Bochicchio, T, Reyes, PA, Renal involvement in primary antiphospholipid syndrome, *J. Rheumatol.*, 1992; 19: 1181–1185.

111. Becquemont, L, Thervet, E, Rondeau, E, Lacave, R, Mougenot, B, Sraer, JD, Systemic and renal fibrinolytic activity in a patient with anticardiolipin syndrome and renal thrombotic microangiopathy, *Am. J. Nephrol.*, 1990; 10: 254–258.

112. D'Agati, V, Kunis, C, Williams, G, Appel, GB, Anticardiolipin antibody and renal disease: a report of three cases, *J. Am. Soc. Nephrol.*, 1990; 1: 777–784.

113. Hughson, MD, Nadasdy, T, McCarty, GA, Sholer, C, Min, KW, Silva, F, Renal thrombotic microangiopathy in patients with systemic lupus erythematosus and the antiphospholipid syndrome, *Am. J. Kidney. Dis.*, 1992; 20: 150–158.

114. Lacueva, J, Enriquez, R, Cabezuelo, JB, Arenas, MD, Teruel, A, Gonzalcz, C, Acute renal failure as first clinical manifestation of the primary antiphospholipid syndrome, *Nephron*, 1993; 64: 479–480.

115. Domrongkitchaiporn, S, Cameron, EC, Jetha, N, Kassen, BO, Sutton, RAL, Renal microangiopathy in the primary antiphospholipid syndrome: a case report with literature review, *Nephron*, 1994; 68: 128–132.

116. Isenberg, DA, Griffiths, M, Neild, GH, Woman with livedo reticularis, renal failure and benign urinary sediment, *Nephrol. Diab. Transplant.*, 1995; 10: 295–297.

117. Kincaid-Smith, P, Fairley, KF, Kloss, M, Lupus anticoagulant associated with renal thrombotic microangiopathy and pregnancy-related renal failure, *Q. J. Med.*, 1988; 69: 795–815.

118. Grottolo, A, Ferrari, V, Mariarosa, M, et al., Primary adrenal insufficiency, circulating lupus anticoagulant and anticardiolipin antibodies in a patient with multiple abortions and recurrent thrombotic episodes, *Hematologia*, 1988; 73: 517–519.

119. Asherson, RA, Hughes, GRV, Recurrent deep vein thrombosis and Addison's disease in "primary" antiphospholipid syndrome, *J. Rheumatol.*, 1989; 16: 378–380.

120. Carette, S, Jobin, F, Acute adrenal insufficiency as a manifestation of the anticardiolipin syndrome, *Ann. Rheum. Dis.*, 1989; 48: 430–431.

121. Asherson, RA, Hughes, GRV, Addison's disease and antiphospholipid antibodies, *J. Rheumatol.*, 1991; 18: 1–3.

122. Asherson, RA, Hypoadrenalism and the antiphospholipid antibodies. A new cause of "idiopathic" Addison's disease in advanced: Advances in Thomas Addison's diseases, Bhatt, HR, James, VHT, Besser, GM, Bottazzo, GF, Keen, HJ, Eds., *Endocrinol. Ltd.*, Bristol, 1994; 1: 87–101.

123. Arnason, JA, Graziano, FM, Adrenal insufficiency in the antiphospholipid antibody syndrome, *Semin. Arthritis Rheum.*, 1995; 26: 109–116.

124. Asherson, RA, Cervera, R, Piette, J-C, et al., Catastrophic antiphospholipid syndrome. Clinical and laboratory features of 50 patients, *Medicine* (Baltimore), 1998; 77: 195–207.

125. Asherson, RA, Adrenal, hepatic, and other intraabdominal manifestations in the antiphospholipid syndrome. In: Asherson, RA, Cervera, R, Piette, JC, Shoenfeld, Y, Eds., *The Antiphospholipid Syndrome,* CRC Press, Boca Raton, 1996; pp. 183–193.

126. Cappell, M, Oesophageal necrosis and perforation associated with the anticardiolipin antibody syndrome, *Am. J. Gastroenterol.*, 1994; 89: 1241–1245.

127. Kalman, DR, Khan, A, Romain, PL, Nompleggi, DJ, Giant gastric ulceration associated with antiphospholipid antibody syndrome, *Am. J. Gastroenterol.*, 1996; 91: 1244–1247.

128. Asherson, RA, Morgan, S, Harris, EN, et al., Arterial occlusion causing large bowel infarction: a reflection of clotting diathesis in SLE, *Clin. Rheumatol.,* 1986; 5:102–106.

129. Gül, A, Inanc, M, Öcal, L, Konice, M, Aral, O, Lie, JT, Primary antiphospholipid syndrome associated with mesenteric inflammatory veno-occlusive disease, *Clin. Rheumatol.,* 1996; 15: 207–210.

130. Vianna, JL, D'Cruz, D, Khamashta, MA, Asherson, RA, Hughes, GRV, Anticardiolipin antibodies in a patient with Crohn's disease and thrombosis, *Clin. Exp. Rheumatol.,* 1992; 10: 165–168.

131. Pettersson, T, Julkunen, H, Asplenia in a patient with systemic lupus erythematosus and antiphospholipid antibodies, *J. Rheumatol.,* 1992; 19: 115.

132. Salafia, CM, Starzyk, KA, López-Zeno, J, Parke, A, Fetal losses and other obstetric manifestations in the antiphospholipid syndrome. In: Asherson, RA, Cervera, R, Piette, J-C, Shoenfeld, Y, Eds., *The Antiphospholipid Syndrome,* CRC Press, Boca Raton, 1996; pp 117–131.

133. Triplett, DA, Antiphospholipid antibodies and recurrent pregnancy loss, *Am. J. Reprod. Immunol.,* 1989; 20: 52–67.

134. Francès, C, Blétry, O, Piette, J-C, Dermatologic manifestations in the antiphospholipid syndrome. In: Asherson, RA, Cervera, R, Piette, JC, Shoenfeld, Y, Eds., *The Antiphospholipid Syndrome,* CRC Press, Boca Raton, 1996; pp 201–211.

135. Ingram, SB, Goodnight, SH, Bennet, RM, An unusual syndrome of a devastating non-inflammatory vasculopathy associated with anticardiolipin antibodies. Report of two cases, *Arthritis Rheum.,* 1987; 30: 1167–1171.

136. Greisman, SG, Thayaparan, R-S, Godwin, TA, Lockshin, MD, Occlusive vasculopathy in systemic lupus erythematosus associated with anticardiolipin antibodies, *Arch. Intern. Med.,* 1991; 151: 389–392.

137. Asherson, RA, Piette, J-C, The catastrophic antiphospholipid syndrome 1996: acute multi-organ failure associated with antiphospholipid antibodies. A review of 31 patients, *Lupus,* 1996; 5: 414–417.

138. Asherson, RA, The catastrophic antiphospholipid syndrome 1998. A review of the clinical features, possible pathogenesis and treatment, *Lupus,* 1998; 1–8.

139. Asherson, RA, Triplett, D, Pathogenesis of the catastrophic antiphospholipid syndrome, *Am. J. Haem.,* 2000; 63: 154.

140. Asherson, RA, Shoenfeld, Y, The role of infections in the catastrophic antiphospholipid syndrome — molecular mimicry?, Editorial, *J. Rheumatol.,* 2000; 27: 12–15.

141. Kitchens, CS, Thrombotic storm: when thrombosis begets thrombosis, *Am. J. Med.,* 1998; 104: 381–385.

142. Belmont, HM, Abramson, SB, Lie, JT, Pathology and pathogenesis of vascular injury in systemic lupus erythematosus. Interactions of inflammatory cells and activated endothelium, *Arthritis Rheum.,* 1998; 39: 9–22.

143. Asherson, RA, Cervera, R, Font, J, Multi-organ thrombotic disorders in systemic lupus erythematosus. A common link?, *Lupus,* 1992; 1: 199–203.

144. Lie, JT, Vasculopathy in the Antiphospholipid Syndrome: thrombosis or vasculitis, or both, *J. Rheumatol.,* 1989; 16: 713–715.

145. Lie, JT, Vasculitis in the phospholipid syndrome: culprit or consort?, *J. Rheumatol.,* 1994; 21: 397–399.

146. Lie, JT, Vasculopathy in the antiphospholipid syndrome revisited. Thrombosis is the culprit and vasculitis the consort, *Lupus,* 1996; 5: 368–271.

147. Alarcon-Segovia, D, Cardiel, MH, Reyes, E, Antiphospholipid arterial vasculopathy, *J. Rheumatol.,* 1989; 16: 762–767.

148. Asherson, RA, Khamashta, MA, Ordi-Ros, et al., The "primary" antiphospholipid syndrome: major clinical and serological features, *Medicine,* 1989; 68: 366–374.

149. Alarcon-Segovia, D, Sanchez-Guerrero, J, Correction of thrombocytopenia with small dose aspirin in the primary antiphospholipid syndrome, *J. Rheumatol.,* 1989; 9: 169–172.

150. Jeffrey, P, Asherson, RA, Rees, J, Recurrent deep vein thrombosis, thromboembolic pulmonary hypertension and the "primary" antiphospholipid syndrome, *Clin. Exp. Rheumatol.,* 1989; 7: 567–573.

151. Goldberger, E, Elder, RC, Swartz, RA, et al., Vasculitis in the antiphospholipid syndrome. A cause of ischemia responding to corticosteroids, *Arthritis Rheum.,* 1992; 35: 569–572.

152. Fain, O, Mathieu, E, Seror, O, et al., Aortitis: a new manifestation of primary antiphospholipid syndrome, *Br. J. Rheumatol.,* 1995; 34: 686–696.

153. Praderio, L, de Angelo, A, Taccagni, G, et al., Association of lupus anticoagulant with polyarteritis nodosa: report of a case, *Haematalogica*, 1990; 75: 387–390.

154. Dasgupta, B, Almond, MK, Tanqueray, A, Polyarteritis and the antiphospholipid syndrome, *J. Rheumatol.*, 1997; 36: 1210–1211.

155. Norden, DK, Ostrov, BE, Shafritz, AB, Von Feldt, JM, Vasculitis associated with antiphospholipid syndrome, *Semin. Arthritis. Rheum.*, 1995; 24: 273–281.

156. Weidensaul, D, Vassa, N, Luger, A, Walker, SE, McMurray, RW, Primary antiphospholipid syndrome and microscopic polyarteritis in the puerperium: a case report, *Int. Arch. Allergy. Immunol.*, 1994; 103: 311–316.

157. Cohney, S, Savige, J, Stewart, MR, Lupus anticoagulant in anti-neutrophil cytoplasmic — antibody associated polyarteritis, *Am. J. Nephrol.*, 1995; 15: 157–160.

158. Cid, MC, Cervera, R, Font, J, et al., Recurrent arterial thrombosis in a patient with giant cell arteritis and raised anticardiolipin antibody levels, *Br. J. Rheumatol.*, 1988; 27: 164–166.

159. Cid, MC, Cervera, R, Font, J, Campo, E, Lopez-Soto, A, Recurrent arterial thrombosis in a patient with giant cell arteritis and raised anticardiolipin antibody levels, *Br. J. Rheumatol.*, 1988; 27: 164–166.

160. Yokoi, K, Hosoi, E, Akaike, M, Shigekiyo, T, Saito, S, Takayasu's arteritis associated with antiphospholipid antibodies. Report of two cases, *Angiology*, 1996; 47: 315–319.

161. Misra, R, Aggarwal, A, Chag, M, Sinha, N, Shrivastava, S, Raised anticardiolipin antibodies in Takayasu's arteritis, *Lancet*, 1994; 343: 1644–1645.

162. Balsa-Criado, A, Gonzalez-Hernandez, T, Cuesta, MV, Aguado, P, Garcia, S, Gijon, J, Lupus anticoagulant in relapsing polychondritis, *J. Rheumatol.*, 1990; 17: 1426–1427.

163. Empson, M, Adelstein, S, Garsia, R, Britton, W, Relapsing polychondritis presenting with recurrent venous thrombosis in association with anticardiolipin antibody, *Lupus*, 1998; 7: 132–134.

21 Vascular Manifestations in Sjögren's Syndrome

Ann L. Parke

CONTENTS

I. INTRODUCTION

In 1888 W.B. Hadden presented an elderly woman with a "crocodile skin tongue" to the London Medical Society. This patient demonstrated the severe consequences of xerostomia (dry mouth), which improved when she was treated with a few drops of tincture of Jaforandi (pilocarpine).[1] This was probably the earliest description of what is now known as Sjögren's syndrome. It was to be another 50 years before Hans Sjögren, a Swedish ophthalmologist, presented his paper describing sicca complaints in several post menopausal women,[2] but the credit is appropriate as it was Sjögren who first recognized the systemic nature of this disease.

Sjögren's syndrome is a systemic disease that may accompany other systemic connective tissue diseases when it is known as secondary Sjögren's syndrome. It may also occur alone, without other well-defined connective tissue diseases, when it is known as primary Sjögren's syndrome. Even though this is a systemic disease, it is the sicca complaints that have been used to define it. Each of the sets of criteria that have been developed for Sjögren's syndrome include subjective complaints and objective tests of dry mouth (xerostomia) and dry eyes (xerophthalmia).[3-5] This rather limited approach to defining a systemic disease has been one of the factors that has contributed to the confusion surrounding Sjögren's syndrome. As there are many causes of xerostomia and xerophthalmia, this approach has also resulted in a nonspecific heterogeneous group of patients who have been grouped together under the Sjögren's umbrella. Recently, some progress towards specificity has been made as the European criteria now require either a positive lip biopsy or antibodies to Ro and/or La antigens for a definite diagnosis of Sjögren's syndrome.[6]

Even though Sjögren's syndrome is a systemic disease, the exocrine gland is the main site of pathology. Typical pathological changes that occur in the exocrine glands of patients include a focal infiltrate of cells, which are predominantly T-helper cells.[7] These cellular infiltrates usually aggregate around ducts.[8] Other studies have determined that glandular epithelial cells are abnormally activated, expressing DR antigen[9] as well as secreting chemokines and cytokines.[10,11] The epithelial cell is now considered to be the site of primary pathology,[12] and the cellular infiltrate a secondary phenomenon. In animal models it has been demonstrated that androgens can reduce glandular inflammation and increase glandular function.[13,14] It has been shown that the epithelial cell is the cellular target for the androgen effect.[15] Many aspects of the etiopathogenesis of Sjögren's syndrome remain unanswered, including the pronounced sicca complaints even in patients with residual glandular tissue, which suggest a defect in the neuro-endocrine control.[16,17]

As this is a truly systemic disease affecting many organs and presenting with a multitude of clinical complaints, the clinical picture can sometimes be confusing and the diagnosis missed completely, especially if the patient has another connective tissue disease. This chapter will not discuss the vascular manifestation that may occur as a consequence of an accompanying connective tissue disease, i.e., systemic lupus erythematosus (SLE), rheumatoid arthritis (RA), and systemic sclerosis (SS), but will concentrate primarily on the vascular manifestations that have been described in primary Sjögren's syndrome. These vascular manifestations can be divided into inflammatory and noninflammatory disease.[18] Inflammatory vascular disease includes vasculitis, which can occur as a consequence of circulating immune complexes and may be part of a mixed cryoglobulinemia. In the noninflammatory category, Sjögren's patients may develop a phospholipid antibody syndrome resulting in a noninflammatory, bland, thrombotic disease found in both the arterial and venous systems, and/or Raynaud's phenomenon.

II. RAYNAUD'S PHENOMENON

Raynaud's phenomenon occurs in up to 30% of patients with Sjögren's syndrome.[19] This vasospastic condition presents clinically with color changes and ischemia of extremities on exposure to cold and emotion. It is a recurrent phenomenon which, when associated with an underlying connective tissue disease, may result in endothelial damage, loss of capillary vasculature, and thickening of the soft tissues of the affected extremities.[20] The precise pathogenesis of this syndrome is still unclear, but recent studies have demonstrated an increase in vasocontrictive peptides including endothelin-1, and a deficiency of vasodilating calcitonin gene-related peptide.[21,22] There is also some evidence that patients with Raynaud's phenomenon have dysfunction of the autonomic nervous system, with some degree of sympathetic hyperactivity being found even in those who do not have an associated connective tissue disease and who are considered to have primary Raynaud's disease.[23] Recent studies have suggested an association between helicobacter pylori infection and Raynaud's phenomomen with the demonstration of fewer vasospastic attacks after the eradication of the infection.[24]

It is important to not confuse true Raynaud's phenomenon with the ischemic that occurs in patients with cryoglobulinemia and/or Waldenstrom's macroglobulinemia. In these patients vasospasm is not the primary pathology, and ischemia occurs as a consequence of vasculitis or sludging due to a hyperviscosity syndrome from the macroglobulinemia.

III. ANTIPHOSPHOLIPID SYNDROME

Antiphospholipid syndrome is defined as the association of antibodies to phospholipid/protein complexes and a constellation of clinical complaints, including recurrent arterial and venous thrombosis, recurrent late fetal loss, and thrombocytopenia.[25-27] The basic pathology contributing to these clinical complaints is a bland noninflammatory thrombosis,[28] and animal models that develop clinical features identical to human antiphospholipid syndrome suggest that the antiphospholipid antibodies are directly involved in the pathological changes that are characteristic of this syndrome.[29,30] Antiphospholipid antibodies do occur in SS patients but the thrombotic syndrome is more frequently found in patients with secondary disease, especially patients fulfilling revised ARA criteria for SLE. An early report documented a devastating noninflammatory vasculopathy in two patients with the clinical features of Sjögren's syndrome. The first patient was also considered to have a lupus-like disease, whereas the clinical features of the second patient were more suggestive of primary Sjögren's syndrome with a catastrophic antiphospholipid syndrome.[31]

IV. VASCULITIS

Although the basic pathology of Sjögren's syndrome is an infiltrate of T-cells in glandular tissues, there are also B-cell abnormalities characterized by B-cell hyperactivity and autoantibody production.[32,33] It is, therefore, not surprising that vasculitis is also a pathological feature of Sjögren's syndrome. Alexander states that up to 30% of Sjögren's patients have vasculitis which may often be subtle and therefore missed.[34] Previous studies have determined that primary Sjögren's patients producing antibody to Ro (part of the extractable nuclear antigen) are more likely to experience extraglandular manifestations including vasculitis.[35] Alexander and colleagues have identified two basic pathologies that contribute to the vasculitis of Sjögren's syndrome.[36,37] As would be expected, a small vessel leucocytoclastic vasculitis has been well described, but these authors have also demonstrated a mononuclear inflammatory disease they considered to be an early pathology, and which may transform into neutrophilic vasculitis.[34,36,37] Uniform deposition of immunoglobulin and/or complement in affected vessel walls is not routinely found in Sjögren's vasculitis, but work by Alexander et al. suggests that immunoglobulin containing plasma cells with adjacent immunoglobulin has been identified.[34]

Sjögren's vasculitis is usually a small-vessel vasculitis that may present in a variety of ways, but most typically with palpable purpura in the lower extremities. Some Sjögren's patients without vasculitis may develop dependent purpura, but these patients have macroglobulinemic purpura that occurs because of elevated levels of gammaglobulin, leading to capillary fragility and vessel leakage with resulting hemosiderin deposition.[38] Those patients with a true vasculitis may develop other cutaneous manifestations of their inflammatory pathology, such as urticarial-like lesions and erythematous lesions including erythema multiform and erythema nodosum-like lesions.[39] Although the renal manifestations of Sjögren's syndrome are many, glomerulonephritis is comparatively uncommon but may occur in the setting of a vasculitis.[40]

Other features of a systemic vasculitis occur in these patients, including neurological disease. Peripheral neuropathies, including the more typical mononeuritis multiplex, are almost certainly a consequence of vasculitis, and it has been suggested that the responsible pathology is usually a mononuclear cell vasculitis.[41] Central nervous system (CNS) involvement in patients with primary Sjögren's syndrome has been the subject of much debate. Alexander has suggested that CNS involvement is comparatively common,[42] but subsequent reports have determined that CNS involvement in primary Sjögren's syndrome patients is extremely rare.[43,44] We have had two patients with primary Sjögren's syndrome and systemic vasculitis that have demonstrated CNS involvement as a consequence of their vasculitis.

Case 1

Mrs. PP was a 56-year-old woman who had had sicca complaints for ten years. She had been diagnosed with primary Sjögren's syndrome on the basis of a positive lip biopsy, antibodies to Ro and La, and objective tests that demonstrated dry eyes and dry mouth. She also had a purpuric rash which was predominately found on the lower limbs, and on biopsy had been proven to be a leucocytoclastic vasculitis. Cryoglobulins were not present, but she had an elevation of all immunoglobulins and an IgM kappa chain monoclonal spike. Bone marrow biopsy was normal. The vasculitis and Sjögren's syndrome were well controlled for many years with modest doses of prednisone and plaquenil. In 1997 she suddenly complained of weakness and numbness in one leg. This was followed by numbness of one hand. An EMG confirmed the presence of a mononuritis multiplex. She then experienced a devastating cerebral bleed, which was responsible for her demise.

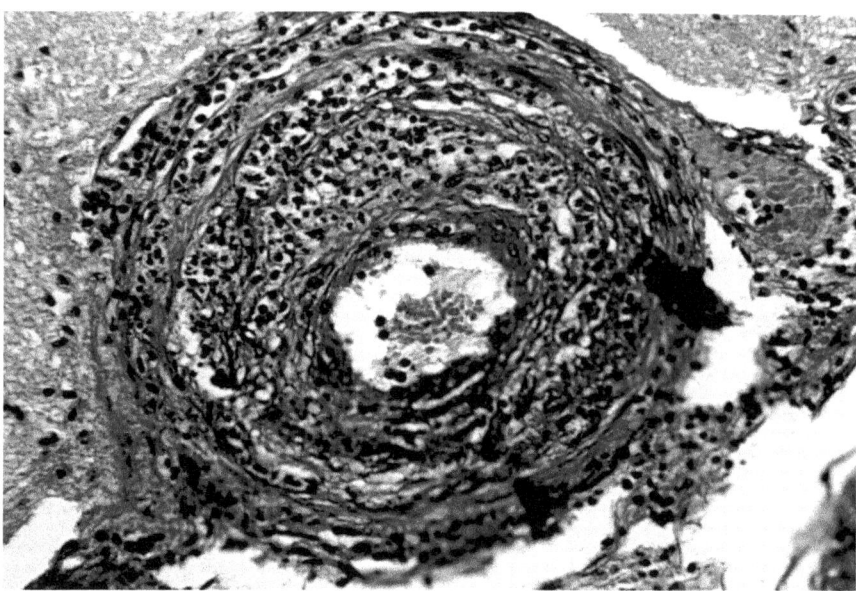

FIGURE 21.1 Cerebral vasculitis in a patient with Primary Sjögren's syndrome.

An autopsy study was performed that demonstrated that she had a systemic vasculitis, which was also found in the cerebral vessels (Figure 21.1). This patient with primary Sjögren's syndrome had not only developed a peripheral neuropathy, but had also had involvement of the central nervous system as a consequence of her underlying vasculitis.

CASE 2

Mrs. DK was a 76-year-old woman diagnosed with Sjögren's syndrome on the basis of a positive lip biopsy, sicca complaints, and recurrent parotid glandular swelling for many years. She did not have antibodies to Ro and La, but had cryoglobulinemia and an IgM kappa monoclonal spike. She had vasculitis which initially presented as palpable purpura, and which responded well to modest doses of prednisone. She then developed an episode of dizziness which was accompanied by some confusion. An MRI of the head showed multiple defects in the brain (Figure 21.2A), including a large defect in the cerebellum (Figure 21.2B). The patient was given three large boluses of corticosteroids and seemed to stabilize. She then developed new central nervous system manifestations and eventually became very confused. An MRI at this time showed multiple new lesions. The patient eventually succumbed to her illness and an autopsy was not performed.

V. HEPATITIS C

In some Sjögren's syndrome patients, vasculitis may be a consequence of a mixed cryoglobuline- mia, and it is important to evaluate patients with cryoglobulins for the presence of chronic infection, in particular hepatitis C.[45,46] It has now been determined that hepatitis C infection is very wide- spread, and that 85% of hepatitis C-infected patients will persist with chronic infection resulting in the development of chronic liver disease.[47] Chronic hepatitis C may be associated with patho- logical glandular changes similar to those found in Sjögren's syndrome,[48] posing the question of whether this chronic infection is a cause of a falsely positive glandular biopsy or whether chronic hepatitis C infection may result in Sjögren's syndrome. Evaluating patients for the presence of antibody to hepatitis C has therefore become an important part of the initial work-up of patients with Sjögren's syndrome.[45,49,50]

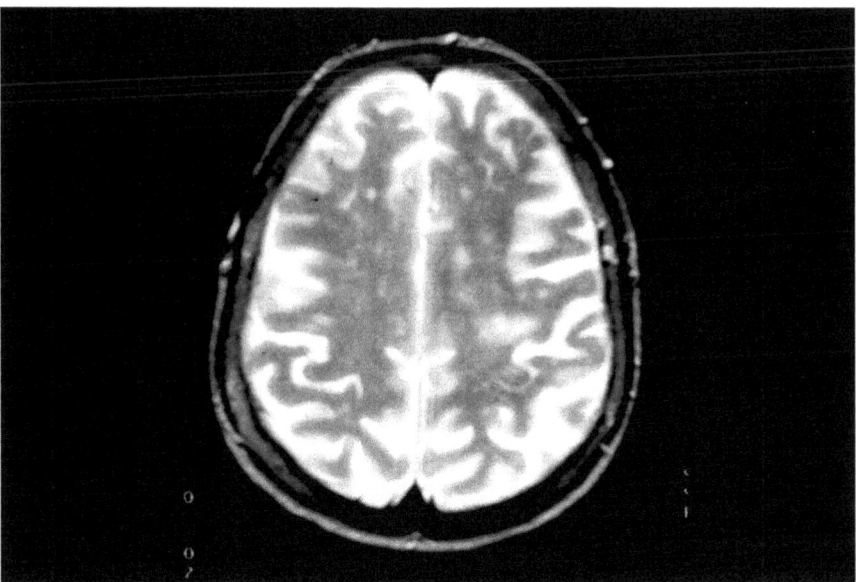

FIGURE 21.2A Multiple cerebral defects consistent with a diagnosis of vasculitis.

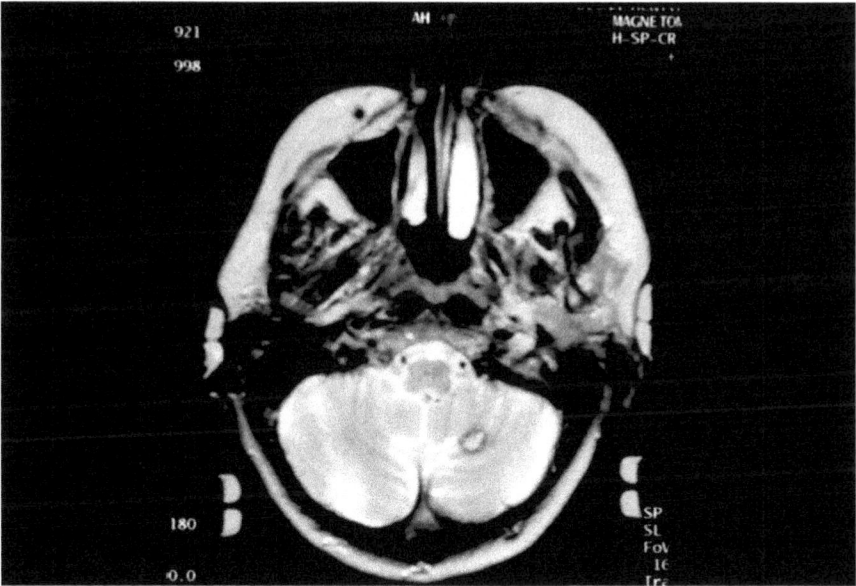

FIGURE 21.2B Large defect in the cerebellum in a patient with vasculitis.

Previous studies have determined that approximately 19% of primary Sjögren's syndrome patients have evidence of liver disease,[51] and other studies have determined that 19% of patients with sicca syndrome complaints have evidence of hepatitis C infection.[52] In the study by Jorgensen et al., it was determined that hepatitis C-positive patients were less likely to produce antibodies to Ro and La antigens, but were more likely to have rheumatoid factor and cryoglobulins.[52] Also, 83% of these hepatitis C-positive sicca patients had evidence of viral RNA found in their saliva. Not surprisingly, hepatitis C-positive Sjögren's patients had evidence of chronic active hepatitis on liver biopsy, but Jorgensen et al. also demonstrated that the hepatitis C-positive patients were more likely to have neurological complaints.[52]

A consequence of long-standing Sjögren's syndrome is an increased relative risk for developing malignant lymphoma,[53,54] which are almost always B-cell tumors. Recent studies have suggested that persistent hepatitis C infection may be directly implicated in the development of B-cell lymphoid malignancies and Waldenstrom's macroglobulinemia.[55-59] In a recent study of 50 patients with B-cell malignancies, Izumi et al. demonstrated that eight patients (16%) were positive for hepatitis C viral-RNA.[55] This figure is much higher than the 1% reported in healthy blood donors in Japan, leading these authors to conclude that there is an association between the persistence of hepatitis C viral infection and the development of B-cell malignancies.[55]

VI. CASTLEMAN'S DISEASE

Another type of lymphoproliferative disorder, originally described in 1956, is Castleman's disease.[60] Pathological studies have defined two subtypes of Castleman's disease: hyaline-vascular type and plasma cell type.[61] In the hyaline vascular type, vascular changes include the presence of thick-walled vessels with prominent endothelial cells, and interfollicular proliferation of capillaries and small venules.[62] Although the association of this rather rare lymphoproliferative syndrome with Sjögren's syndrome is unusual, there have been reports documenting Sjögren's syndrome associated with Castleman's disease.[63]

VII. SUMMARY

Vascular disease is not a major feature of Sjögren's syndrome as the predominant site of pathology is the exocrine gland and, in particular, the glandular epithelial cell. Inflammatory vascular disease does occur in primary Sjögren's syndrome and may cause the usual devastating consequences that are more commonly associated with other autoimmune diseases. Mixed cryoglobulinemia can result in vasculitis, and in patients with Sjögren's syndrome mixed cryoglobulinemia occurs more frequently in those who are infected with hepatitis C. The recent realization that chronic hepatitis C infection can produce glandular pathology that is similar to that found in Sjögren's syndrome has broadened our concept of this syndrome, and it is one more example of an association between a viral infection and Sjögren's syndrome.[56,64,65] As the etiology of this common syndrome remains obscure, such clues are extremely important.

REFERENCES

1. Hadden, W.B., On "dry mouth," or suppression of the salivary and buccal secretions, *Trans. Clin. Soc. London*, 21, 176, 1888.
2. Sjögren, H., Zur kenntnis der kerato conjunctivitis sicca keratitis filiformis bei hypofunction der tränendrüsen, *Acta Ophthalmol.* (Suppl. II) 1, 1933.
3. Vitali, C., Bombardieri, S., Moutsopoulos, H.M. et al., Preliminary criteria for the classification of Sjögren's syndrome: Results of a prospective concerted action supported by the European Community. *Arthritis Rheum.*, 36, 340, 1993.
4. Fox, R.I., Robinson, C.A., Curd, J.G., Kozin, F., Howell, F.V., Sjögren's syndrome: proposed criteria for classification. *Arth. Rheum.*, 29, 577, 1986.
5. Manthrope, R., Andersen, V., Jensen, O.A. et al., Editorial comments to the four sets of criteria for Sjögren's syndrome. *Scand. J. Rheumatol.*, (Suppl.) 61, 31, 1986.
6. Vitali, C., Bombardieri, S., The European classification criteria for Sjögren's syndrome (SS): proposal for modification of the rules for classification suggested by the analysis of the receiver operating characteristics (ROCS) curve of the criteria performance. *J. Rheum.*, 24 (Suppl.):S18, 1997.
7. Skopouli, F.N., Fox, P.C., Galanopoulou, V. et al., T-cell subpopulations in the labial minor salivary gland histopathologic lesion of Sjögren's syndrome. *J. Rheumatol.*, 18, 210, 1991.
8. Chisholm, D.M., Mason, D.K., Labial salivary gland biopsy in Sjögren's syndrome. *J. Clin. Pathol.*, 21, 656, 1968.

9. Fox, R.I., Bumol, T., Fantozzi, R. et al., Expression of histocompatibility antigen HLA-DR by salivary gland epithelial cells in Sjögren's syndrome. *Arthritis Rheum.*, 29, 1105, 1986.

10. Mustafa, W., Ziiu, J., Deng, G., Diab, A., Link, H., Frithiof, L., Klinge, B., Augmented levels of macrophage and Th1 cell-related cytokine mRNA in submandibular glands of MRL/lpr mice with autoimmune sialoadenitis, *Clin. Exp. Immunol.*, 112, 389, 1998.

11. Cuello, C., Palladinetti, Tedia, N., Di Girolamo, N., Lloyd, A.R., McCluskey, P.J., Wakefield, D., Chemokine expression and leucocyte infiltration in Sjogren's syndrome, *B. J. Rheum.*, 37, 779, 1998.

12. Moutsopoulos, H.M., Sjögren's syndrome: autoimmune epithelitis. *Clin. Immunol. Immunopathol.*, 72, 162, 1994.

13. Ariga, H., Edwards, J., Sullivan, D.A., Androgen control of autoimmune expression in lacrimal glands of MRL/Mp-lpr/lpr mice. *Clin. Immunol. Immunopathol.*, 53, 499, 1989.

14. Sato, E.H., Ariga, H., Sullivan, D.A., Impact of androgen therapy in Sjögren's syndrome: Hormonal influence on lymphocyte populations and Ia expression in lacrimal glands of MRL/Mp-lpr/lpr mice. *Invest. Ophthamol. Vis. Sci.*, 33, 2537, 1992.

15. Ono, M., Rocha F.J., Sullivan, D.A., Immunocytochemical location and hormonal control of androgen receptors in lacrimal tissues of the female MRL/Mp-lpr/lpr mouse model of Sjögren's syndrome. *Exp. Eye Res.*, 61, 659, 1995.

16. Walcott, B., Claros, N., Patel, A., Peterson, E., Brink, P.R., Changes in innervation and membrane properties of lacrimal acinar cells in the NZB/NZW F1 mouse occur before lymphocytic infiltration. *J Rheumatol,* (Abstract #34) vol 24., (Suppl. 50) 1997.

17. Meneray, M.A., Bennett, D.J., Nguyen, D.H., Beuerman R.W., Effect of sensory denervation on the structure and physiologic responsiveness of rabbit lacrimal gland. *Cornea,* 17, 99, 1998.

18. Manthorpe, R., Asmussen, K., Oxholm, P., Primary Sjögren's Syndrome: Diagnostic criteria, clinical features, and disease activity. *J. Rheumatol.*, (Suppl.) 24, 8, 1997.

19. Grassi, W., De Angelis, R., Lapadula, G., Leardini, G., Scarpa, R., Clinical diagnosis found in patients with Raynaud's phenomenon; a mulicentre study, *Rheumatol. Int.*, 18 (1), 17, 1998.

20. Mourad, J.J., Priollet, P., Physiopathology of Raynaud's phenomenon: current data, *Rev. Med. Interne,* 18, (8), 611, 1997

21. Turton, E.P., Kent, P.J., Kester, R.C., The aetiology of Raynaud's phenomenon. *Cardiovasc. Surg.,* Oct 6 (5), 431, 1998.

22. Guilmot, J.L., Diot, E., Lasfargues, G., Boissier, C., *Rev. Prat.,* 48, 1647, 1998.

23. Pancera, P., Sansone, S., Presciuttini, B., Montagna, L., Ceru, S., Lunardi, C., Lechi, A., Autonomic nervous system dysfunction in sclerodermic and primary Raynaud's phenomenon. *Clin. Sci.,* (Colch) Jan., 96 (1), 49, 1999.

24. Gasbarrini, A., Massari, I., Serricchio, M., Tondi, P., De Luca, A., Franceschi, F., Ojetti, V., Dal Lago, A., Flore, R., Santoliquido, A., Gasbarrini, G., Pola, P., Helicobacter pylori eradication amerliorates primary Raynaud's phenomenon, *Dig. Dis. Sci.*, 43 (8) 1641, 1998.

25. Bowie, E.J., Thompson, J.H. Jr., Pascuzzi, C.A., et al., Thrombosis in systemic lupus erythematosus despite circulating anticoagulants. *J. Lab. Clin. Med.,* 62, 416, 1963.

26. Asherson, R.A., Khamashta, M.A., Ordi-Ros, J., et al., The "primary" antiphospholipid antibody syndrome: major, clinical and serologic features. *Medicine* (Baltimore), 68, 366, 1989.

27. Alarcon-Segovia, D., Sanches-Guerrero, J., Primary antiphospholipid syndrome, *J. Rheumatol.*, 16, 482, 1989.

28. Lie, J.T., Pathology of the antiphospholipid syndrome. *The Antiphospholipid Syndrome*, 8, 89, 1996.

29. Blank M., Cohen, J., Toder, V. et al., Induction of antiphospholipid syndrome by passive transfer of anticariolipin antibodies. *Proc. Nat. Acad. Sci. U.S.A.,* 88, 3069, 1991.

30. Gharavi, A.E., Sammaritano, L.R., Wen, J. et al., Induction of antiphospholipid autoantibodies by immunizations with B2 glycoprotein I (apolipoprotein H). *J. Clin. Invest.*, 90, 1105, 1992.

31. Ingram, S.B., Goodnight, S.H. Jr., Bennett, R.M., An unusual syndrome of a devastating noninflammatory vasculopathy associated with anticardiolipin antibodies: Report of two cases, *Arthritis Rheum.*, 30 (10), 1167, 1987.

32. Harley, J.B., Alexander, E.L., Bias, W.B., Fox, O.F., Provost, T.T., Reichlin, M., Yamagata, H., Arnett, F.C., Anti-Ro (SS-A) and anti-La (SS-B) in patients with Sjögren's syndrome. *Arthritis Rheum.*, 29, 196, 1986.

33. Bloch, K.J., Buchanan, W.W., Wohl, M.J., Bunim, J.J., Sjögren's syndrome. A clinical, pathological and serological study of sixty-two cases. *Medicine (Baltimore)*, 44, 187, 1965.
34. Alexander, E.L., Inflammatory vascular disease in Sjögren's syndrome. *Sjögren's Syndrome Clinical and Immunological Aspects,* Springer-Verlag, 6, 129, 1987.
35. Alexander, E.L., Arnett, F.C., Provost, T.T., Stevens, M.B., (1983a) Sjögren's syndrome: Association of anti-Ro (SS-A) antibodies with vasculitis, hematologic abnormalities, and serologic hyperreactivity. *Ann. Intern. Med.,* 98, 155, 1983.
36. Molina, R., Provost, T.T., Alexander, E.L., Two histopathologic prototypes of inflammatory vascular disease in Sjögren's syndrome; differential association with seroactivity to rheumatoid factor and antibodies to Ro (SS-A) and with hypocomplementemia. *Arthritis Rheum.,* 28, 1251, 1985.
37. Alexander, E.L., Moyer, C., Travlos, G.S., Roths, J.B., Murphy, E.D., Two histopathologic types of inflammatory vascular disease in MRL/Mp autoimmune mice. *Arthritis Rheum.,* 28, 1146, 1985.
38. Strauss, W.G., Purpura hyperglobulinemia of Waldenstrom. *NEJM,* 260, 857, 1959.
39. Alexander, E.L., Provost, T.T., Cutaneous manifestations of primary Sjögren's syndrome: a reflection of vasculitis and association with anti-Ro (SS-A) antibodies. *J. Invest. Dermatol.,* 80, 386, 1983.
40. Moutopoulos, H.M., Balow, J.E., Cawley, T.J., Stahl, N.I., Autonovych, T.T., Chused, T.M., Immune complex glomerulonephritis in sicca syndrome. *Am. J. Med.,* 64, 955 1978.
41. Alexander, E.L., Lijewski, J.E., Jerdan, M.S., Alexander, G.E., Evidence of an immunopathogenic basis for central nervous system disease in primary Sjögren's syndrome, *Arthritis Rheum.,* 29, 1223, 1986.
42. Alexander, G.E., Provost, T.T., Stevens, M.B., Alexander, E.L., Sjögren's syndrome: Central nervous system manifestations. *Neurology,* 31, 1391, 1981.
43. Binder, A., Snaith, M.L., Isenberg, D., Sjögren's syndrome: a study of its neurological complication. *Br. J. Rheumatol.,* 27, 275, 1988.
44. Moutsopoulos, H.M., Sarmas, J.H., Talal, N., Is central nervous system involvement a systemic manifestation of primary Sjögren's syndrome? *Rheum. Dis. Clin. North Am.,* 19, 909, 1993.
45. King, P.D., McMurray, R.W., Becherer, P.R., Sjögren's syndrome without mixed cryoglobulinemia is not associated with hepatitis C virus infection, *Am. J. Gastroenterol.,* 89, 1047, 1994.
46. Ramos-Casals, M., Cervera, R., Yague, J., Garcia-Carrasco, M., Trego, O., Jimenez, S., Morla, R.M., Font, J., Ingelmo, M., Cryoglobulinemia in primary Sjogren's syndrome: prevalence and clinical characteristics in a series of 115 patients. *Semin. Arthritis Rheum.,* Dec., 28 (3), 200, 1998.
47. Bizollon, T., Ducerf, C., Trepo, C., Mutimer, D., Hepatitis C virus recurrence after liver tranplantation. *Gut,* Apr. 44 (4), 575, 1999.
48. Haddad, J., Deny, P., Munz-Gotheil, E. et al., Lymphocytic sialadenitis of Sjögren's syndrome associated with chronic hepatitis C virus liver disease. *Lancet,* 339, 321, 1992.
49. Durand, J.M., Lefevre, P., Kaplanski, G. et al., Sjögren's syndrome and hepatitis C virus infection. *Clin. Rheumatol.,* 14, 570, 1995.
50. Verbaan, H., Carlson, J., Eriksson, S., Larsson, A., Liedholm, R., Manthrope, R., Tabery, H., Widell, A., Lindgren, S., Extrahepatic manifestation of chronic hepatitis C infection and interrelationship between primary Sjögren's syndrome and hepatitis C in Swedish patients. *Ann. Intern. Med.,* 245, 127, 1999.
51. Ramos, M., Cervera, R., Garcia-Carrasco, M., Miret, C., Munoz, F.J., Primary Sjögren's syndrome: clinical and immunologic study of 80 patients. *Med. Clin.* (Barc), May 3, 108 (17), 652, 1997.
52. Jorgensen, C., Legouffe, M.C., Perney, P., Coste, J., Tissot, B., Segarra, C., Bologna, C., Bourrat, L., Combe, B., Blanc, F., Sany, J., Sicca syndrome associated with hepatitis C virus infection. *Arthritis Rheum.,* 39, 1166, 1996.
53. Talal, N., Bunim, J.J., The development of malignant lymphoma in the course of Sjögren's syndrome. *Am. J. Med.,* 36, 529, 1964.
54. Kassan, S.S., Thomas, T.L., Moutsopoulos, H. M., Measured risk of lymphoma in sicca syndrome. *Ann. Int. Med.,* 89, 888, 1978.
55. Izumi, T., Sasaki, R., Tsunoda, S., Akutsu, M., Okamoto, H., Miura, Y., B cell malignancy and hepatitis C virus infection, *Leukemia,* 11 (Suppl. 3) 516, 1997.
56. Gonzalez-Amaro, R., Garcia-Monzon, C., Garcia-Buey, L., Moreno-Otero, R., Alonso, J.L., Yague, E., Pivel, J.P., Lopez-Cabrera, M., Fernandes-Ruiz, E., Sanchez-Madrid, F., Induction of tumor necrosis factor production by human hepatocytes in chronic viral hepatitis. *J. Exp. Med.,* 179, 841, 1994.

57. Ferri, C. et al., Hepatitis C virus infection in patients with non-Hodgkin's lymphoma. *Br. J. Haematol.*, 88, 392, 1994.

58. Santini, G. et al., Waldenström macroglobulinemia: a role of HCV infection? *Blood*, 82, 2932, 1993.

59. Pozzato, G. et al., Low-grade malignant lymphoma, hepatitis C virus infection, and mixed cryoglobulinemia, *Blood*, 84, 3047, 1994.

60. Castleman, B., Towne, V.W., Localized mediastinal lymph node hyperplasia resembling thymoma. *Cancer*, 9, 822, 1956.

61. Keller, A.R., Hochholzer, L., Castleman hyaline-vascular and plasma cell types of giant lymph node hyperplasia of the mediastinum and other locations. *Cancer*, 29, 670, 1972.

62. Tavoni, A., Vitali, C., Baglioni, P., Gerli, Rl, Marchetti, G., Di Munno, O. et al., Multicentric Castleman's disease in a patient with primary Sjögren's syndrome. *Rheumatol. Int.*, 12, 251, 1993.

63. Higashi, K., Matsuki, Y., Hidaka, T.B., Aida, S., Suzuki, K., Nakamura, H., Primary Sjogren's syndrome associated with hyaline-vascular type of Castleman's disease and autoimmune idiopathic thrombocytopenia. *Scand. J. Rheumatol.*, 26 (6), 482, 1997.

64. Itescu, S., Winchester, R., Diffuse infiltrative lymphocytosis syndrome: a disorder occurring in human immunodeficiency virus infection that may present a sicca syndrome. *Rheum. Dis. Clin. North Am.*, 18, 683, 1992.

65. Venables, P.J.W., Rigby S.P., Viruses in the Etiopathogenesis of Sjögren's syndrome. *J. Rheum.*, Vol 24 (Suppl.) 50, 3, 1997.

22 Vascular Manifestations of Progressive Systemic Sclerosis

Christopher P. Denton and Carol M. Black

CONTENTS

I. SCLERODERMA

A. INTRODUCTION

The designation "collagen-vascular disease," although rather misleading when applied to most autoimmune rheumatic diseases, is perhaps most applicable to the scleroderma spectrum of disorders. It links two hallmark pathological features: deposition of excessive collagen-rich extracellular matrix, and vascular dysfunction. Scleroderma describes a group of human diseases characterized by the development of thickened sclerotic skin. The term scleroderma is often used as a synonym for systemic sclerosis (SSc), but it is probably more appropriate to consider a scleroderma spectrum of disorders which includes a number of diseases with similar clinical and pathological features. These similarities lend support to the view that there are likely to be common etiological factors and pathogenic processes operating in these conditions despite their clinical diversity.

Systemic sclerosis should be considered uncommon rather than rare. In the U.K. there are approximately 300 new cases per year, and the population prevalence has been estimated to be 100 per million. Both of these figures are significantly lower than estimates of disease frequency in the U.S. The epidemiology of scleroderma is reviewed in several publications.[1,2] Recent epidemiological analyses of survival in systemic sclerosis suggest a reduction in mortality compared with earlier studies, although greater awareness of the milder forms of the disease may partly account for this. Limited cutaneous systemic sclerosis is approximately twice as common as the diffuse subtype.[3]

B. CLASSIFICATION

Disorders which comprise the scleroderma spectrum are shown in Table 22.1. Two groups are recognized that comprise localized scleroderma and systemic forms of the disease. For the latter group, the term systemic sclerosis is probably more appropriate than systemic scleroderma since it emphasizes that internal organ pathology often occurs and is generally the most important aspect

---

TABLE 22.1
Classification of the Scleroderma-Spectrum Disorders

Localized

Morphea
  localized
  generalized
Linear scleroderma

Systemic

Limited cutaneous systemic sclerosis
Diffuse cutaneous systemic sclerosis
Overlap syndromes*
Systemic sclerosis *sine scleroderma*

Raynaud's phenomenon

Autoimmune Raynaud's phenomenon**
Primary Raynaud's phenomenon

* Features of systemic sclerosis together with those of at least one other autoimmune rheumatic disease, e.g., SLE, RA, or polymyositis.
** Raynaud's phenomenon associated with antinuclear antibodies (or other SSc-associated autoimmune serology), usually also abnormal nail-fold caillaroscopy.

---

of these systemic forms. Localized scleroderma disorders can be further divided: linear scleroderma, most commonly occurring in childhood, causes abnormalities of the skin and subcutaneous tissues which often follow a dermatomal distribution and are found predominantly on one side of the body.[4] Sometimes linear scleroderma affecting the scalp is accompanied by marked abnormalities of underlying mesenchymally derived tissues including the skull; this subtype is often referred to descriptively as *en coup de sabre*. Morphoea describes patches of sclerotic skin which develop on the trunk and limbs at sites of previously normal texture.[5] Single plaques can occur, and are usually termed localized morphoea. In other cases skin changes are much more widespread, often symmetrically involving the trunk and limbs and leading to widespread skin sclerosis. It is particularly important to distinguish between severe generalized morphoea and diffuse systemic sclerosis. In generalized morphoea there is typically relative sparing of the hands and face, and the absence of major vascular symptoms and visceral manifestations. Nevertheless, widespread morphoea is certainly not a benign condition, and powerful immunosuppressive and antifibrotic therapies may be necessary, along the lines of those employed to treat diffuse cutaneous systemic sclerosis.

Systemic sclerosis is generally subdivided into diffuse cutaneous and limited cutaneous subsets — usually abbreviated dcSSc and lcSSc, respectively.[3] A third important but much rarer group are those patients who develop the vascular features and visceral fibrosis typical of systemic sclerosis, but who do not exhibit significant skin involvement. This group is sometimes described as *systemic sclerosis sine scleroderma*.[6] Diffuse cutaneous scleroderma comprises approximately one-third of individuals with systemic sclerosis and is generally the more severe form of the disease. It is therefore the most important subset in which to establish an early definitive diagnosis.[1] The central criterion for diagnosis of this subset is the extension of skin sclerosis proximal to the wrists, particularly over the proximal limbs and trunk, although usually sparing the upper back. In the more common limited cutaneous subset, skin sclerosis is confined to the hands and, to a lesser extent, the face and neck. Skin sclerosis score[7] is a cornerstone for scleroderma classification, particularly among patients with diffuse cutaneous scleroderma. Maximum skin score and rate of increase in skin score correlates with outcome, including mortality.[8]

Other groups of patients must also be considered when classifying scleroderma disorders. First, there is a group of patients with overlap syndromes who demonstrate some of the clinical features of systemic sclerosis, or more unusually localized scleroderma, but who also have manifestations of other autoimmune rheumatic diseases such as systemic lupus erythematosus (SLE), dermatomyositis, or rheumatoid arthritis. This heterogeneous group poses an important management problem and also provides indirect evidence that similar etiological factors and pathogenetic processes may be involved in these different conditions. It has been suggested that immunogenetic associations can be used to predict the ultimate clinical phenotype in patients in the early stages of an overlap syndrome that has features of more than one autoimmune rheumatic disease.[9] In classifying the scleroderma spectrum, patients with Raynaud's phenomenon (RP) must also be considered. Some cases can readily be determined to be primary RP and will not develop features of any other connective tissue disorder. Some Raynaud's patients, however, will develop one of the autoimmune rheumatic disorders, especially systemic sclerosis. This group is sometimes designated *autoimmune Raynaud's* and is characterized by abnormal nailfold capillaroscopic findings and the presence of positive antinuclear antibodies. Individuals with definite RP who also demonstrate one of the hallmark autoantibodies of scleroderma, such as anti-centromere, anti-topoisomerase I, anti-RNA polymerase I or III antibodies, are sometimes designated prescleroderma patients.[10]

C. CLINICAL FEATURES OF SCLERODERMA SPECTRUM DISORDERS

The major clinical features of scleroderma arise through the effects of the pathological processes of vascular perturbation, inflammation, and fibrosis occurring within lesional tissues. The extent and distribution of these changes varies between different conditions within the scleroderma spectrum. These different disorders have widely differing prognoses and clinical features, and their grouping together may be somewhat inappropriate. The most important distinction is between the localized (skin-restricted) forms of scleroderma and the systemic forms of the condition. Within the systemic forms it is imperative for effective management that the differences between the two main subsets of diffuse and limited disease are appreciated.

1. Generalized Scleroderma Disorders

These conditions are those to which the term "systemic sclerosis" can be most appropriately applied. Typically, a patient with diffuse cutaneous systemic sclerosis presents with pain, stiffness, and swelling of the extremities. This is followed by subjective tightness of the skin over the hands, often extending proximally and associated with pruritis. The vascular symptoms of Raynaud's phenomenon typically begin around the time of the skin sclerosis.

The clinical presentation of limited cutaneous systemic sclerosis is usually less dramatic than that of diffuse disease. Typically, Raynaud's phenomenon precedes any other manifestation by several years. Sclerodactyly, sclerosis of skin around the face and neck and esophageal problems are clues of progression to established scleroderma. The severity of the Raynaud's and the presence of features such as pitting scars and ulcers also occur in limited scleroderma. Telangiectasia and calcinosis are less useful in early diagnosis since they point towards well-established disease.

2. Localized Scleroderma Disorders

Localized scleroderma may develop at any age, although it comprises a greater proportion of childhood onset scleroderma cases than in adult disease. In adulthood, morphoea is generally benign with one or a few patches of texturally abnormal skin. These lesions progress in a characteristic sequence of skin inflammation accompanied by an inflammatory infiltrate, and later skin fibrosis with accompanying hyper- or hypo-pigmentation. Lesions tend to progress circumferentially and all stages of the pathology are present in an active established lesion. Following a period of thickened fibrosis of the affected skin, this usually evolves into atrophic scar tissue. Generalized morphoea is more significant with similar histological appearances, but there is a more widespread distribution, often involving the trunk and limbs. Lesions often appear to follow vascular or neural territories although the significance of this is unclear. Linear scleroderma is primarily a childhood-onset disease and typically develops to involve one limb or one side of the body. A variant which involves deeper structures and may have a developmental basis is the *en coup de sabre* lesion of the skull. In childhood these regional forms of localized scleroderma are far more significant than in adults due to their impact on the growth of the affected tissues.[11]

II. VASCULAR MECHANISMS IN SSc PATHOGENESIS

A. Vascular Abnormalities in Early SSc

The pathological features of vascular damage, immune cell activation, and fibrosis are believed to be closely linked in scleroderma.[12] Many histological features are often shared in both localized and generalized disease, but the remainder of this discussion will focus on systemic sclerosis. Detailed studies suggest that in both the skin and internal organs one of the earliest features is endothelial cell injury, initially at the ultrastructural level,[13] and that this is temporally and spatially associated with activation of perivascular fibroblasts and the subsequent deposition of increased amounts of structurally normal extracellular matrix components.[14] Inflammation is associated with early lesions leading to tissue edema and leucocytic infiltration. Mononuclear cells predominate, with monocytes/macrophages among the earliest cells within lesional tissue,[15] followed later by lymphocytes, mainly carrying phenotypic markers of activated T-lymphocytes and including a significant proportion of Ro+ "memory" cells.[16,17]

TABLE 22.2
Endothelial Cell Products which May Play a Role in Scleroderma

Growth Factors and Cytokines

Platelet-derived growth factor
Transforming growth factor-β*
Connective tissue growth factor
Insulin like growth factor (s)
Basic fibroblast growth factor
Interleukin-1α and β*
Interleukin-6
Colony stimulating factor(s)
Platelet activating factor

Extracellular Matrix Proteins, Adhesion Molecules, and Matricellular Proteins

Collagens: types III, IV and V
Sulphated proteoglycans
Fibronectin
Thrombospondin
E-selectin
P-selectin
Intercellular adhesion molecule-1 (ICAM-1)
Vascular cell adhesion molecule-1 (VCAM-1)

Coagulation Pathway Factors and Cofactors

von Willebrand factor
Antithrombin III
Thrombomodulin
Protein S

Vasoactive Mediators

Nitric oxide (endothelial-dependent relaxation factor)
Endothelin (endothelial-dependent vasoconstriction factor)
Prostanoids (prostacyclin (PGI_2) and prostaglandin species)

* Precursor molecule produced by endothelial cells my require activation by other
cell types to generate the active cytokine.

B. ENDOTHELIAL CELL DYSFUNCTION IN SCLERODERMA

Vascular abnormalities form one of the three central features of the pathology of systemic sclerosis, along with immunological activation and extracellular matrix deposition. Endothelial cell perturbation is a consequence of the vascular injury occurring in scleroderma. Other endothelial cell changes may influence disease manifestations through their effects on inflammation, vascular tone, and hemostasis via the mechanisms outlined above.

There is considerable evidence of endothelial cell dysfunction in scleroderma.[13,18,19] Markers of endothelial cell damage and activation are present at altered levels in the blood of patients with scleroderma spectrum disorders, including von Willebrand factor,[20] thrombomodulin,[21] endothelin-1 (ET-1),[22-24] and the soluble forms of endothelial cell surface adhesion molecules ICAM-1, VCAM-1, and E-selectin.[25-27] Although initially thought to be derived mainly from endothelial cells, soluble levels of these markers are now recognized as also reflecting activation of other cell types depending on the potential sources of these markers.[28] Thus, VCAM-1 is expressed on lymphoid cells, especially antigen-presenting dendritic cells,[29] and on epithelial cells including renal tubular epithelium.[30] ICAM-1 is expressed and released by a wide range of cells including fibroblasts. Indeed, ICAM-1 expression and shedding is increased by scleroderma fibroblasts *in vitro*.[31] Endothelin-1 has been shown to be released by scleroderma fibroblasts *in vitro*,[32] although levels secreted are very low and it is likely that endothelial cell-derived ET-1 accounts for the majority of that in circulation. Not all markers of endothelial cell function are increased in scleroderma; several authors report reduced levels of angiotensin-converting enzyme (ACE)[33] and possibly also thrombomodulin. The ACE results might be confounded by the fact that functional assays may be disturbed by the ACE inhibiting drugs, which are in common clinical use in systemic sclerosis.[34] Some studies have suggested that levels of these markers of endothelial cell damage or activation are a reflection of clinical status, perhaps correlating with either disease activity or severity. Thus E-selectin and VCAM-1 levels have been correlated in individual patients with changes in the severity of lung, renal, and skin disease, and it has also been suggested that E-selectin levels may be elevated prior to the development of renal scleroderma crisis.[27] Some investigators have suggested that ET-1 levels may reflect both the extent of skin sclerosis and the presence of vascular disease in scleroderma, although other series have not found such associations.[23]

Another indirect indicator that endothelial cell damage occurs in scleroderma is the high prevalence of antiendothelial cell autoantibodies in this disease.[35] This is a common feature of a number of connective tissue disorders, particularly those with a prominent vascular component such an systemic lupus erythematosus and vasculitis. The significance of these antibodies remains uncertain, and the antigens to which they bind are heterogeneous, both within and between sera. Functional effects *in vitro* have been demonstrated for these antibodies present in systemic sclerosis sera, and also in samples from patients with Wegener's granulomatosis.[36] These effects include upregulation of adhesion molecule expression, increased leucocyte adherence, and induction of cytokine release by endothelial cells.[37] Preliminary studies suggest that AECA activity varies longitudinally in individual cases with scleroderma, and that these autoantibodies may be undetectable at some stages of disease.[38] Other studies have suggested that they are clinically associated with vascular manifestations of scleroderma.[38,39] Other antibodies such as anti-U1-RNP, which are not specific for endothelial cell-expressed antigens, may also modulate EC properties.[40]

Support for early endothelial cell changes in scleroderma is provided by the studies of early lesional tissue from biopsy specimens. In both the skin[17] and internal organs[41] there is histological evidence of endothelial injury as an early event. Damage has also been shown at an ultrastructural level in early lesional tissue from the skin, kidney, lung, and gut in systemic sclerosis.[43,44] In the skin and other tissues studied, endothelial cell surface adhesion molecules are expressed in biopsies from clinically uninvolved tissue, adding further weight to the view that endothelial activation is central to the initial pathogenic events.[45,46] The early demonstration of microvascular injury and endothelial cell damage in scleroderma led to the proposition of a vascular hypothesis to explain disease, suggesting that vascular, and particularly endothelial cell events, may underlie the development of these disorders.[47] Recent studies have suggested that there is defective endothelium-dependent vasodilatation of the pulmonary circulation in SSc, even in those without evidence of pulmonary hypertension, providing further support for a generalized abnormality of EC function in this disease that might precede other disease manifestations.[48]

C. LINKS BETWEEN ENDOTHELIAL CELL AND FIBROBLAST DYSFUNCTION

The *in vitro* properties of fibroblasts and endothelial cells strongly suggest that functional interactions, or cross-talk, between these cells *in vivo* might be important. Such interactions could be mediated directly by soluble products of each cell type acting on the other, or indirectly through their effect on the extracellular matrix or cell shape, or through recruitment of other cellular elements such as platelets or leucocytes. The feasibility of such an interplay is supported by the close juxtaposition of endothelial cells and fibroblasts in most tissues, and by the range of soluble products of each cell type which might influence the other.[49]

Endothelial cells have been reported to produce a large number of cytokines and growth factors. These include IL-1,[50] IL-6,[51] bFGF,[52] ET-1,[53] IL-8, MCP-1, IGF-1, GM-CSF,[54] TGF-β,[55] and CTGF.[56] All of these factors have been shown to modulate fibroblast properties, and would be candidate mediators for endothelial cell — induced modulation of fibroblast properties. The potent mitogenic effect of endothelial cell-conditioned medium is believed to arise through a combination of endothelial cell-derived mitogenic factors.[57,58] It is possible that feedback inhibitory signals from connective tissue cells, such as fibroblasts or smooth muscle cells, act on endothelial cells to reduce the secretion of activating factors. It has been shown that ET-1 secretion is inhibited in co-culture with mesenchymal cells.[59]

Fibroblast products are also diverse, and their production and release are modulated by extrinsic influences. However, studies of mRNA levels by northern hybridization, *in situ* hybridization, and RT-PCR suggest that several relevant factors may be synthesized, including IL-1, IL-6, and IGF-1.[60-62] It is less clear to what extent these mRNA transcripts are translated, or whether any proteins synthesized are released in an active form so that they can modulate endothelial cell properties. Theoretically, however, the case is strong since these factors are known to modulate endothelial cell properties. Other studies have obtained direct evidence of functional interactions between endothelial cells and fibroblasts. [52,63]

D. OXIDANT STRESS IN SCLERODERMA PATHOGENESIS

Oxidative stress has received considerable attention as a potentially important mechanism involved in triggering or sustaining the abnormal properties of cells involved in SSc pathogenesis. Mechanisms by which reactive oxygen species might contribute to vascular damage, immune activation/autoantibody generation, and fibroblast activation have all been proposed. There is additional *in vivo* evidence of increased oxidative stress in SSc patients. One attractive link between the vascular and immune manifestations of SSc, and perhaps the environment, follows from the demonstration that SSc-associated autoantigens are selectively fragmented by oxidant stress in heavy metal-catalyzed oxidation reactions. Since the tissue hypoxia associated with RP might provide the necessary oxidant stress, and the immunogenetic determination of the ability of an individual to respond to particular antigenic determinants has been clearly shown,[64] perhaps environmental heavy metals could provide an additional component to the pathogenetic pathway. Such a link between vascular aspects, the immune system, and the environment at least provides a plausible model. It seems likely that the combined research strategies currently being employed in many laboratories worldwide will allow more complete models to be developed and ultimately tested. Some of the observations that support a role for reactive oxygen species in the development of SSc are listed in Table 22.3.

A mechanistic link between vascular dysfunction and autoimmunity may be provided by oxidant stress-induced fragmentation of protein antigens; this has been proposed for scleroderma hallmark antigens in the presence of heavy metal ions.[69] It has also been suggested that antioxidant agents may be beneficial for the treatment of Raynaud's phenomenon and SSc, and there are preliminary data supporting this for both dietary supplementation and using synthetic antioxidant drugs. It is noteworthy that antioxidant strategies appear to be especially helpful to the vascular manifestations of systemic sclerosis.

E. PLATELET DYSFUCTION IN SCLERODERMA

Platelet dysfunction may be important in the pathogenesis of systemic sclerosis, and ultrastructural abnormalities have recently been reported.[71] There is evidence for altered platelet function in Raynaud's phenomenon and scleroderma;[72] however, it is unclear whether the changes in platelet function which are observed in systemic sclerosis are a primary characteristic of this disease or whether they are secondary to vascular changes.[73] Platelet degranulation releases mediators which

TABLE 22.3
Oxidant Stress in the Pathogenesis of Systemic Sclerosis

Evidence	Reference
Elevated Isoprostanes in Urine	
Increased urinary levels of oxidative metabolites of prostaglandins in patients with SSc suggests *in vivo* oxidative stress.	Stein et al.[65]
Reduced Micronutrient Antioxidants in SSc	
Levels of vitamin C, vitamin E, and other dietary antioxidants lower in SSc patients — suggests increased susceptibility to reactive oxygen species.	Herrick et al.[66]
Reduced *in vitro* LDL Oxidation Lag-Time in SSc	
Oxidation lag time *in vitro* is reduced for LDL isolated from SSc patients' serum. Suggests greater susceptibility to oxidation *in vivo*. Oxidized LDL are potentially injurious to endothelial cells.	Bruckdorfer et al.[67]
Oxidant Stress Effects on Fibroblasts	
Increased fibroblast proliferation and matrix synthesis induced by oxidative stress *in vitro*.	Farber et al.[68]
Fragmentation of SSc-Associated Autoantigens	
Oxidative fragmentation of SSc-associated autoantigens in the presence of heavy metal ions.	Casciola-Rosen et al.[69]
Beneficial Effects of Antioxidant Administration	
Many patients report subjective benefit from diet rich in antioxidant nutrients. The synthetic antioxidant probucol has apparent benefit in treatment of Raynaud's phenomenon.	Denton et al.[70]

are implicated in scleroderma pathogenesis, including TGFβ and PDGF,[74] and this could provide an important mechanistic link between vascular and other features of the disorder. Altered rheological properties of platelets have been reported in Raynaud's phenomenon, and several agents with apparent efficacy have effects on platelet properties.[75]

F. Immune Dysfunction in Scleroderma

Some of the clearest evidence of immune perturbation comes from the frequent occurrence of autoantibodies of defined specificity in the sera of scleroderma patients. These include a range of antibodies, directed against nuclear antigens and some of these are apparently restricted to scleroderma such as anti-topoisomerase-1 antibody, or at least highly associated, e.g., anti-RNA polymerase I, or III; anticentromere; antifibrillarin (U3-RNP); and anti-PM-Scl antibody.[77] There are important clinical associations for these different antibodies. Some of the differences in the autoantibody profile may be explained in terms of Class II MHC haplotype.[78] This lends support to the view that they might be a reflection of host susceptibility to scleroderma or specific complications of the disease. There is considerable current interest in other potential genetic susceptibility or severity markers. Hopefully, studies will identify new clinically useful associations which may be helpful both in understanding scleroderma pathogenesis and in identifying subgroups of patients at increased risk of certain disease complications who can be closely followed prospectively. Further clarification of the molecular mechanisms underlying the Class II MHC associations seen in scleroderma has come from detailed studies of the epitopes recognized in association with particular MHC haplotypes. Several groups have associated the ability of lymphocytes to recognize particular antigenic epitopes on topoisomerase and CENT (kinetochore) antigens with particular Class II haplotypes.[78] Similar studies have demonstrated, however, that normal individuals with equivalent haplotypes are also able to respond to these antigens *in vitro,* albeit after a longer period of antigen exposure. This suggests that ability to respond to these antigens is not restricted to those who develop scleroderma. Elegant studies of T-cell receptor heterogeneity in scleroderma peripheral blood, and in lymphocytes isolated from bronchoalveolar lavage fluid, have also produced interesting data, although, again, without a definite conclusion. There is evidence of restricted clonality, especially among the γδ T-cells, which is suggestive of an antigen-driven process.[79] Overall, it may be concluded that although there is a considerable body of indirect evidence for immunological involvement in scleroderma pathogenesis, direct evidence is less persuasive.[80,81]

III. CLINICAL CONSEQUENCES OF VASCULAR PATHOLOGY IN SSc

A. RAYNAUD'S PHENOMENON

Episodic acral vasospasm precipitated by cold or emotional stress (Raynaud's phenomenon) is a common occurrence in otherwise healthy individuals. Some series estimate its prevalence to be up to 15% of the female population, with a much lower frequency in males. It represents a disorder of vasomotor regulation, and probably has a complex pathogenesis. The relevance of Raynaud's phenomenon to scleroderma is that it is almost universal in patients with established scleroderma. It may precede onset of SSc, especially the lcSSc subset, by many years, whereas in dcSSc it generally first manifests around the time of the onset of other features of the disorder, or sometimes a period of time after the onset of other disease features. One particularly interesting group of patients are those individuals who have Raynaud's phenomenon in association with one of the hallmark autoantibodies of SSc, such as anticentromere or antitopoisomerase-1. A substantial number of such individuals will subsequently (typically within three to five years) develop other features of SSc, so these individuals may represent a prescleroderma state. It must be noted, however, that they may also develop features of other autoimmune rheumatic disorders. Autoimmune Raynaud's may represent a prescleroderma condition. It has been suggested that Raynaud's phenomenon leads to the development of other disease features; although this may be true, it cannot be a universal occurrence given that the large majority of Raynaud's sufferers do not develop any serious subsequent disease, and also that Raynaud's may develop after the onset of other features of SSc.

B. LUNG DISEASE

1. Pulmonary Hypertension

Pulmonary vascular disease is now recognized as a frequent complication of scleroderma. The overall prevalence is still unclear, but it is undoubtedly observed much more frequently now that noninvasive methods of detection are available such as echocardiography, especially in combination with Doppler estimation of the peak pulmonary arterial systolic pressure (from the velocity of retrograde flow into the right atrium in the presence of tricuspid regurgitation). In a recent cross-sectional study this technique was shown to give estimated pressures which correlate reasonably well with measurements obtained at right heart catheterization.[83] Recent studies have suggested that there are significant diurnal variations in PA pressure and single time-point assessment may be misleading.[84] Overall prevalence of pulmonary hypertension is difficult to assess, with frequencies of between 5 and 30% being reported in different series.[85]

Conventionally, pulmonary hypertension (PHT) in scleroderma is divided into isolated PHT, in which there is no additional pulmonary pathology. This pattern of disease is most characteristic of limited cutaneous SSc, especially in the classical CREST form of this subset with florid cutaneous telangiectasis, and often characterized serologically by the presence of anticentromere antibodies. It has recently been reported that antiendothelial cell antibodies may be more prevalent in these cases.[86] Some cases of isolated PHT diffuse cutaneous SSc, and these have been associated with antibodies to U3-RNP.[87] The remaining cases occur in the context of established pulmonary fibrosis. This is termed secondary PHT. Survival analyses suggest that these two patterns of disease progress at different rates. Other mechanisms for the development of PHT may also operate, such as thromboembolic disease, perhaps associated with antiphospholipid antibodies, and an inflammatory vasculopathy. The latter is implicated in cases in which immunosuppressive therapy has been associated with improvement in apparent isolated PHT in scleroderma.

There are considerable similarities between the histological features of isolated PHT in scleroderma and primary pulmonary hypertension. There is evidence of subintimal cell proliferation, endothelial hyperplasia, and obliteration of small intrapulmonary vessels. It has been suggested that initial proliferative changes lead to the characteristic plexiform pathology of rapidly progressive pulmonary hypertension, with remodeling leading to the concentric obliterative lesions which predominate at necropsy in patients succumbing to severe SSc-associated PHT.[88] The role of circulating vasoconstrictors is unclear; circulating endothelin-1 appears to be elevated in SSc,[23] but a specific association with pulmonary vascular disease is disputed.[24] Intravascular thrombosis may also contribute to the development or progression of PHT in SSc, although studies have failed to demonstrate the reduced levels of thrombomodulin which are found in primary pulmonary hypertension.[89] In fact, thrombomodulin levels have been reported to be increased in SSc, perhaps due to EC damage.[90] Survival analysis suggests that patients with SSc-associated PHT may have a better prognosis that those with primary pulmonary hypertension, especially with mild to moderate elevation in PA pressure.[91]

2. Lung Fibrosis

In addition to abnormalities in the pulmonary circulation which occur in association with pulmonary hypertension, studies of biopsy material from lungs of patients with SSc suggest that there may be an early endothelial lesion preceding the development of fibrotic changes in the lung interstitium.[43] This is sometimes apparent by electron microscopy, even before the development of any histological abnormality. This is similar to the lesions observed at the earliest stages of the disease or in prelesional territories of the skin, and provide evidence that some of the earliest pathogenic events in SSc may involve endothelial cell structure or function. Moreover, the recently reported impairment of endothelium-dependent pulmonary vasodilatation in SSc patients at risk of interstitial lung disease suggests that vascular dysfunction may be premonitory to fibrotic lung disease.

C. SCLERODERMA RENAL DISEASE

Several patterns of renal pathology are recognized in scleroderma, and all involve vascular abnormalities. Even patients without evidence of renal impairment may have altered renal blood flow.[92] The most clearly defined is the scleroderma renal crisis (SRC) which describes the occurrence of acute renal failure in a scleroderma patient in whom no other cause for the nephropathy is present. Accelerated hypertension usually occurs, further compounding the renal pathology. However, many SSc patients demonstrate less severe renal complications, probably associated with reduced renal blood flow and the consequent reduction in glomerular filtration rate.[93] The mechanism for this slowly-progressive form of chronic renal disease in SSc is unclear. Co-morbidity may account for renovascular disease in SSc, and for the renal manifestations of overlap syndromes such as vasculitis or glomerulonephritis, especially in SLE/SSc overlap cases, and for treatment-related complications (e.g., cyclosporin A, D-penicillamine, and antithymocyte globulin).

1. Acute Renal Crisis

This generally occurs in patients with diffuse SSc within five years of disease onset. Patients generally present clinical features of severe hypertension including headaches, visual disturbances, hypertensive encephalopathy (especially seizures), and pulmonary edema. The overall incidence of SRC varies between different SSc subsets and disease stages. In high risk patients the incidence may be as great as 20%, but, overall, it is probably less than 10%.[93] Traub[94] proposed the following criteria to diagnose scleroderma renal crisis: abrupt onset of arterial hypertension greater than 160/90 mmHg, hypertensive retinopathy of at least grade III severity, rapid deterioration of renal function and elevated plasma renin activity. Other typical features include the presence of a microangiopathic hemolytic blood film (MAHA) and hypertensive encephalopathy, often complicated by generalized convulsions. It is often useful to perform a renal biopsy once hypertension has been adequately controlled. This provides prognostic information, and allows histological confirmation of the diagnosis and exclusion of other causes for abrupt onset renal failure, such as glomerulonephritis. Histologically, SSc renal crisis usually shows fibrinoid necrosis and mucoid or fibromucoid proliferative intimal lesions (when extensive, termed "onion-skinning") in renal arteries, particularly the arcuate and interlobular vessels; glomerular thrombi occur and, ultimately, glomerulosclerosis. The extent of the glomerular lesion can be useful in predicting the degree of functional recovery that can ultimately occur. Occasionally, a similar pattern of renal dysfunction occurs without hypertension (normotensive renal crisis), suggesting that the pathological features are not simply the end-organ consequences of raised arterial pressure.[95]

Symptoms of the crisis usually present abruptly and it should be regarded as a life-threatening medical emergency requiring prompt intervention. The pulse rate is increased and patients develop headaches, visual phenomena, and convulsions due to accelerated hypertension. Symptoms and signs of left ventricular failure may follow rapidly. The glomerular filtration rate and renal blood flow are decreased, and serum creatinine increases. Oliguria and anuria may follow, and death from renal failure can occur within a short time in untreated patients. Proteinuria is almost universal; although it may present long before the renal crisis develops, it often increases with the crisis, though not to nephrotic levels. Microscopic hematuria and granular casts may be present and, as in other forms of accelerated hypertension, SRC may be complicated by microangiopathic hemolytic anemia.

Although renal crisis usually occurs in patients with established SSc, it can occasionally be the presenting feature of the disease. For this reason the hands and face of any patient presenting with unexplained severe or accelerated hypertension should be examined for clues which might suggest an underlying connective tissue disorder such as SSc. Clinical suspicions should be followed up with appropriate investigations, particularly autoimmune serology and nailfold capillaroscopy.

Once diagnosed, an acute renal SSc crisis must be treated as a medical emergency. The patient should be admitted immediately, and reasonable blood pressure control is a priority. However, extreme caution must be taken to avoid precipitous or excessive drops in arterial pressure, and also to prevent relative or actual hypovolemia associated with the vasodilatation of constricted vascular beds, both of which can further diminish renal perfusion and compound the SSc lesion with acute tubular necrosis. For this reason, powerful parenteral antihypertensives (e.g., intravenous nitroprusside or labetolol) should be avoided; an internal jugular or subclavian venous cannula should be inserted to monitor central venous filling pressure, and an indwelling arterial cannula for pressure monitoring should be considered, especially if sclerodermatous involvement of the upper limb causes difficulties in using a sphygmomanometer. It is also imperative to avoid administration of potentially nephrotoxic agents such as nonsteroidal antiinflammatory drugs and/or X-ray contrast dyes. Hypertension should be treated using ACE inhibitors; it has been suggested that quinapril may be preferable to other agents, although historically most patients have received either captopril or enalapril.[96] Calcium channel blockers should be used to reduce both diastolic and systolic pressure by 10 to 15 mmHg per day until baseline levels of diastolic pressure at 80 to 90 mmHg are achieved. Sublingual nifedipine, or hydralazine subcutaneously can be used if the patient is vomiting. Intravenous prostacyclin, which may directly benefit the microvascular lesion, is often administered from diagnosis. Renal function should be closely monitored by twice weekly creatinine clearance and daily serum creatinine until the condition either stabilizes or requires renal replacement therapy.

Regular full blood count, clotting screen and, fibrin degradation product estimations are important to detect and monitor microangiopathic hemolytic anemia (MAHA), which often reflects activity of the disease process. Short-term hemodialysis should be given if necessary, and peritoneal dialysis often works well if long-term renal replacement therapy is needed. Interestingly, it has been observed that after a renal crisis, skin sclerosis and other features of SSc improve,[97] particularly if a patient is undergoing maintenance dialysis. The basis for this is uncertain; it may result from the removal or inactivation of circulating mediators, or may simply reflect the natural history of the disease. Considerable recovery in renal function often occurs after an acute crisis, sometimes allowing dialysis to be discontinued, and improvement can continue for up to two years. Therefore, any decisions regarding renal transplantation should not be made before this time.

Plasma renin activity (PRA) increases markedly with the onset of renal injury and may rise acutely to extreme levels, but there is no convincing evidence that a rise precedes the onset of scleroderma renal crisis. One series reported 13 cases in which plasma renin activity was measured prior to the development of the renal crisis; none of the patients had significantly increased levels.[94] Similar results have been reported by others.[98,99] A functional Raynaud's-like renal vasoconstriction may be superimposed on more chronic structural changes; this hypothesis is consistent with the data provided by Kovalchik et al.,[42] who performed renal biopsies on nine patients with scleroderma and normal renal function. Plasma renin activity was slightly elevated in three of four patients with microscopic vascular damage, was normal in the other, but rose significantly in all four after cold pressor testing. The resting and cold pressor levels remained normal in patients without microscopic changes. Xenon clearance studies provide additional support for the importance of functional vascular narrowing.[99,100] In these studies, renal cortical perfusion was found to be decreased in systemic sclerosis patients, and much more so at times of renal crisis. Decreased perfusion is likely to cause ischemia of the juxtaglomerular apparatus, increased renin secretion, and the formation of large amounts of angiotensin II which, in turn, causes both renal and generalized vasoconstriction. Thus, although increased renin secretion is probably a secondary phenomenon, it certainly adds to the vicious circle of vascular constriction and damage.

Endothelin-1 levels, when measured, have also been found to be elevated in SRC, but whether this represents a primary or secondary phenomenon is unclear. Elevated levels of endothelin might simply reflect endothelial damage associated with SRC. Some support for this comes from reports of correlation between circulating soluble forms of the endothelial adhesion molecule VCAM-1 and renal dysfunction in SSc, with particularly high levels occurring in SRC.[27,102]

2. Chronic Nephropathy

Patients who survive scleroderma renal crisis may develop similar but less florid proliferative changes in the interlobular and arcuate arteries. Even those who have never had a renal crisis may show reduplication of elastic fibres, sclerosed glomeruli tubular atrophy, and interstitial fibrosis, presumably reflecting the chronic changes of scleroderma.

The renin-angiotensin axis has also been investigated in scleroderma-associated chronic renal disease. A study by Clements et al.[103] investigated some of the milder forms of renal disease associated with SSc. Renal plasma flow, assessed by PAH clearance, was diminished in many SSc patients, and plasma renin activity increased. Stress tests to determine the responsiveness of the renin-angiotensin system were performed and confirmed elevated levels in many patients. Although no factors were identified which were associated with an increased frequency of SRC, stimulated PRA levels correlated with survival. Thus, the absence of an exaggerated PRA response to sodium depletion (single dose frusemide) was associated with reduced survival. It is suggested that this might reflect the failure of a homeostatic mechanism for maintenance of intravascular volume; for example, reflecting a nonreactive vascular bed. Overall, however, elevated levels of PRA or reduced PAH did not correlate with either increased incidence of renal crises or worse survival. The widespread elevation of PRA in scleroderma is further evidence that the renin-angiotensin system is active in the disease, and perhaps explains why ACE-inhibitors are helpful in this condition.

3. Glomerulonephritis

In addition to the classical scleroderma renal crisis and chronic nephropathy, there are a small number of case reports of glomerulonephritis occurring in SSc. Interestingly, several cases have been reported in which a progressive cresentic glomerulonephritis was associated with positive antimyeloperoxidase autoantibodies.[104] A distinct glomerulonephritic process has been postulated to explain these cases. More commonly, coincident pathologies such as drug-induced glomerular injury[105] or serum sickness (such as that which has been reported following treatment with anti-thymocyte globulin), or overlap syndromes with features of other connective tissue disorders, such as systemic lupus erythematosus, are likely to underlie such features.

D. Gastrointestinal Disease

Involvement of the gastrointestinal tract is extremely frequent in scleroderma. Abnormalities have been demonstrated throughout its length, although esophageal involvement is the most frequently involved site, occurring in up to 80% of patients. Esophageal dysmotility is associated with reflux esophagitis, stricture formation, and, in some cases, epithelial metaplasia, which may predispose to adenocarcinoma. The pathological mechanism for gut involvement is incompletely understood but there is considerable histological evidence that reduced blood flow and an obliterative microangiopathy may be important components in its development of gut disease.[106] Several studies have demonstrated reduced mucosal blood flow by laser-Doppler methods.[107] Local ischemia may lead to secondary autonomic dysfunction and to fibrosis in addition to compromising neuromuscular control of motility. Severe small intestinal involvement is increasingly being recognized as an important contributor to mortality from scleroderma, especially when associated with malabsorption.[108]

Antral venous ectasia has a characteristic appearance at endoscopy, hence the synonym "watermelon stomach." It manifests as iron deficiency anemia due to recurrent or chronic hemorrhage, or as more substantial episodic hematemesis or melena. It is an important diagnosis because it is potentially life-threatening, and also because it is amenable to treatment using laser photocoagulation.[109] Chronic hemorrhage from telangiectatic lesions is now recognized as a significant cause of chronic iron deficiency in SSc.[110-112]

E. Cardiac Involvement from Scleroderma

It is likely that cardiac involvement from scleroderma, although important and potentially life-threatening, is underdiagnosed. This partly reflects uncertainty about its frequency, and also the intrinsic difficulties of detection of some specific manifestations such as paroxysmal arrhythmia or cardiac fibrosis. By analogy with advances which have occurred in the management of other important complication it is likely that cardiac scleroderma management will be greatly facilitated when clinicians are better able to identify the stage, subset, and perhaps ethnic groups which are particularly susceptible. Accurate risk-stratification will then allow screening resources to be applied in a more focused way. There have been several recent studies that have attempted to better define the pattern and frequency of cardiac involvement from scleroderma.

1. Prevalence

Although it has been recognized for many years that cardiac involvement was likely to be an important complication from SSc, the precise prevalence has not been determined. Early studies used a simple weighted scoring system for gross ECG or abnormalities and demonstrated a substantial frequency and association between the presence of these abnormalities and mortality.[113] More recently, abnormal long axis function has been suggested to be an indicator of myocardial fibrosis.[114] More comprehensive assessment using multiple modalities and examining patients who did not have cardiac symptoms suggested that almost 50% of patients attending hospital clinics with established SSc may have abnormalities in at least one cardiac investigation.[115] Abnormalities were much more frequent in patients with dcSSc than with lcSSc.[116] This is consistent with previous observations that cardiac muscle disease was associated with skeletal muscle involvement in SSc, the latter being more often seen in diffuse than limited SSc. Better methods to detect myocardial fibrosis noninvasively have been sought, including MRI, ultrasonic videodensitometry,[117] and spiral CT scan.

2. Pericardial Disease

Pericarditis is well recognized as a complication of SSc. It is particularly seen in the context of severe diffuse cutaneous SSc, and is probably most frequently encountered in patients with established or imminent scleroderma renal crisis. Echocardiographic studies often reveal small hemodynamically insignificant effusions in scleroderma patients. Therapeutic pericardiocentesis is only occasionally required.

Recently, a number of studies have attempted to define the frequency of pericardial disease in scleroderma, and to delineate more clearly the stage and subset associations. A study by Thompson and Pope[118] reported that pericardial effusions were present in 17% of patients with dcSSc and 4% with lcSSc. As suggested by earlier investigators, pericardial effusion was particularly associated with active progressive dcSSc, and most frequently seen in the context of scleroderma renal crisis.[119]

3. Cardiac Fibrosis

Autopsy studies have identified at least three patterns of myocardial involvement from systemic sclerosis. Up to 50% of patients at autopsy show features of myocardial fibrosis. Other reported histological patterns of cardiac disease include contraction band necrosis and, less frequently, inflammatory cardiomyopathy. The latter probably occurs most often in the context of an inflammatory myopathy associated with systemic sclerosis.

Fibrotic changes in the myocardium in scleroderma have been demonstrated in biopsy specimens and at necropsy. However, the precise prevalence of this complication is unclear. Noninvasive imaging techniques such as MRI or spiral CT scanning may allow this to be determined more precisely. Indirect clues of cardiac involvement may be deduced from ECG or echocardiographic studies.

4. Myocarditis

Inflammatory disease of the cardiac muscle is almost certainly underdiagnosed in patients with systemic sclerosis. It is likely that an inflammatory phase occurs in the majority of cases in which fibrosis ultimately develops, drawing analogy with the better understood sequence of pathogenic events in skin or lung fibrosis in this disease. This inflammatory process should probably be viewed as distinct from more significant myocarditis occurring in some cases with severe progressive dcSSc.

5. Electrophysiological Abnormalities

Electrophysiological cardiac abnormalities are well recognized in scleroderma. Fixed or persistent conduction defects may be easily detected, but intermittent problems, especially arrhythmias, are much more difficult to diagnose. This means that this potentially important group of complications is likely to be underreported. Interestingly, most survival studies for scleroderma demonstrate an increase in mortality above that explicable by the frequency of life-threatening renal, pulmonary, or small intestinal disease, and occult cardiac pathology is likely to be an important contributor to this increased mortality.

An early study of conduction abnormalities[120] based upon autopsy analysis suggested that the specialized conduction tissues were relatively spared from the fibrotic process in SSc. However, a well-conducted prospective study using 24-hour ambulatory ECG recordings demonstrated a prevalence of 14% for conduction disturbances and 32% for supraventricular tachycardia likely to arise from proximal AV node involvement. Another, larger study identified the presence of ventricular ectopy as strongly correlating with total mortality and sudden death.[121]

A recent study examining SSc patients without clinical features of cardiac disease by invasive electrophysiological assessment is confirmatory, providing strong support for atrial conduction defects which would be predicted to give rise to supraventricular tachycardia. Moreover, three cases of reentrant monomorphic ventricular tachycardia occurring in SSc and responding to local ablative therapy have recently been reported.

Another possible mechanism contributing to cardiac rate and rhythm disturbances is part of a cardiac autonomic neuropathy, and there is some evidence to support this[122] based upon analysis of circadian heart rate variability.[123] These may arise from either of the preceding pathological processes. Conduction defects are the most frequently observed disturbances. Typical features include QTc prolongation on a 12-lead ECG.[124] Later conduction tissue fibrosis may lead to varying degrees of heart block, including first- or second-degree block, or complete heart block necessitating pacemaker implantation. Bundle branch blocks may reflect abnormalities in the conducting tissues or may be complications of ventricular strain. Thus RBBB may be seen in association with PHT, and LBBB may occur when there is left ventricular strain from hypertension or cardiac muscle disease.

Paroxysmal dysrhythmias are much more difficult to detect than conduction abnormalities. Prolonged ambulatory ECG monitoring may be necessary for diagnosis and, once diagnosed, treatment options are limited. It seems likely, however, that serious arrhythmias from occult cardiac disease are an important cause of sudden unexplained death, which occurs with increased frequency in patients with systemic sclerosis.

6. Coronary Arterial Vasospasm — Cardiac Raynaud's

As for other vascular beds, notably the renal and pulmonary circulation, it has been suggested that episodic vasospasm may occur in the cardiac circulation, and perhaps this may have significant clinical consequences in scleroderma. One of the earliest studies to examine cold-induced vasospasm on myocardial function was negative,[125] although the end-point of echocardiographically-determined LVEF was relatively insensitive. In a markedly different study, using thallium scintigraphy to detect reversible reduction in myocardial perfusion patients who had no clinical evidence for coexistent cardiac disease demonstrated cold-induced ischemia.[126] These observations were confirmed and extended in a more recent study[127] which found that 50% of patients with longstanding Raynaud's had evidence of cold-induced coronary artery vasospasm. Interestingly, this was not observed in patients with recent onset (<5y) of Raynaud's symptoms. Some support for this mechanism has been provided by studies showing that systemically active vasoconstrictor mediators such as endothelin-1 are elevated in the arterial circulation in SSc.[128] Recent reports suggesting reduced nitric oxide synthase levels in SSc provide additional pathogenetic mechanisms.

F. Macrovascular Disease

There have been several reports that macrovascular disease may be increased in patients with SSc. This is largely based upon case reports and small series. Large cross-sectional case-control studies or longitudinal prospective cohort studies will be necessary to confirm the association. At present, even if this occurs, it is possible that it may only be found in certain populations or ethnic groups. However, it is plausible given the number of common etiopathogenetic mechanisms between the processes of atherosclerosis and systemic sclerosis, including endothelial cell perturbation, activation and damage, and subsequent fibroproliferation. One possibility is that common etiological agents predispose to both conditions.

Large vessel disease has important implications for organ-based complications of SSc such as renal disease, peripheral ischemia, and bowel involvement. Some noninvasive studies have suggested large vessel flow abnormalities in cerebral and renal circulation in SSc and, by analogy with the results of studies investigating cardiac and pulmonary blood flow variations attributable to vasomotor instability in these vascular beds, it is certainly plausible that episodic vasospasm is not restricted to the extremities.

One of the first reports suggesting an association between scleroderma and macrovascular disease was that of Youseff et al.[129] A small number of patients with severe macrovascular disease but few risk factors were reported. The same group[130] extended its observations with a retrospective cohort study of patients with limited SSc. A relative risk of 6.0 was observed compared with controls who had been matched with respect to vascular disease risk factors. Independently performed studies within the U.K. have confirmed and extended these studies. Thus, Veale et al.[131] reported a prevalence of symptomatic macrovascular disease of more than four times that observed in a population control group. A recent study from Australia has attempted to define more precisely the pattern of macrovascular disease in SSc and, interestingly, a particular predilection for the ulnar artery was observed.[132] Clearly, this particular pattern of involvement is likely to be directly relevant to the development of severe digital ischemia. It may also suggest that factors related to the vasospastic or skin sclerosis components of the disease might be involved in the development of co-existing macrovascular disesae. Recently, necropsy-based studies have reported that cerebrovascular disease, especially with vascular calcification, may be disproportionately severe in patients with limited cutaneous SSc[133] compared with macrovascular disease at other sites.

G. CUTANEOUS TELANGIECTASIS

Another common vascular manifestation of scleroderma is the development of local cutaneous dilated loops of small blood vessels termed telangiectsiae. These are often distressing for patients, and may also cause problems from hemorrhage if they are at sites prone to trauma. Hemorrhage from mucosal telangiectasiae is also becoming increasingly recognized as a clinical problem and may require local therapy if it is a recurrent problem. Gastrointestinal hemorrhage and epistaxis have both been reported. Male patients with facial telangienctasiae may experience difficulties with shaving.

Cosmetic camouflage techniques can be very effective for masking facial telangiectasiae, and appropriate advice should be offered to all patients who might benefit. Recently, the pulsed dye laser has been used with some success.[134]

It has been noted that telangiectasiae occur especially in lcSSc — sometimes termed CREST syndrome — although they are usually also present in patients with late stage dcSSc. Indeed, they may often become more florid, even in the plateau phase of dcSSc or when the skin is softening.

H. VASCULITIS IN SCLERODERMA

Vasculitis is not a feature of either of the classical forms of systemic sclerosis, although vasculopathy is almost universal. The presence of vasculitic lesions should therefore be taken as a strong indicator of an overlap syndrome, and features of other autoimmune rheumatic diseases should be sought clinically and serologically. Clinical manifestations vary according to the size of vessel involved and, as with other vasculitides, treatment is dictated by clinical activity and evidence of end-organ damage.

IV. CLINICAL ASSESSMENT OF VASCULAR MANIFESTATIONS OF SCLERODERMA

Reliable assessment of Raynaud's phenomenon is important for diagnosis and management of scleroderma. In particular, it is useful to have reproducible methods of assessment for monitoring therapeutic responses, assessing disease severity over time, and assessing patients who have Raynaud's phenomenon in the absence of a definite connective tissue disease. That is because there are a number of features that may help to predict those cases which will develop into SSc. The methods used in assessing the clinically important vascular manifestations of SSc are summarized in Table 22.4.

TABLE 22.4
Clinical Assessment of Vascular Manifestations of SSc

Raynaud's Phenomenon

Infrared thermography
Laser-Doppler flowmetry
Nailfold capillaroscopy — including quantitation
Occlusion plethymography
Iontopheresis

Large-Vessel Disease

Doppler angiology
Direct vascular imaging — MRI angiography, digital subtraction arteriography

Cardiac Disease

Electrocardiography
Echocardiography
MRI
Thallium perfusion scintigraphy
Other imaging modalities

Pulmonary Vascular Disease

CO diffusing capacity
Doppler-echocardiography
Pulmonary vascular resistance

Renal Blood Flow

GFR estimation
Doppler ultrasonography

Gut Blood Flow

Laser Doppler flowmetry
Endoscopy for mucosal vascular lesions

V. CONCLUSION

Although some have suggested that scleroderma may be primarily a vascular disease, the growing understanding of the complex processes involved in SSc pathogenesis make this unlikely.[134] There is, however, a broad range of evidence that vascular dysfunction is an important process in the pathogenesis of this condition, and many of the most important organ-based clinical features have a clearly demonstrable vascular basis. It is likely, therefore, that substantial clinical benefit will be gained if therapies directed towards the vascular dysfunction in SSc are extended and refined. It seems likely that, as with many of the systemic rheumatic diseases, there are important genetic factors influencing the natural history of the disease in individual patients, and this is likely to be the case for the vascular manifestations of the disease and to vascular processes in pathogenesis. Ultimately, better risk stratification and a clearer understanding of the initiating events may allow a more proactive management approach to vascular scleroderma.

REFERENCES

1. Silman, A. J., Scleroderma-demographics and survival. *J. Rheumatol.*, 48, 58, 1997.
2. Medsger, T. A., Epidemiology of systemic sclerosis. *Clin. Dermatol.*, 12, 207, 1994.

3. LeRoy, E. C., Black, C., Fleischmajer, R., Jablonska, S., Krieg, T., Medsger, T. A., Rowell, N., and Wollheim, F., Scleroderma (systemic sclerosis): classification, subsets and pathogenesis. *Journal of Rheumatology,* 15, 202, 1988.

4. Black, C. M., Scleroderma and fasciitis in children. *Current Opinion in Rheumatology,* 7, 442, 1995.

5. Falanga, V., Localized scleroderma. *Medical Clinics of North America,* 73, 1143, 1989.

6. Molina, J. F., Anaya, J. M., Cabera, G. E., Hoffman, E., and Espinoza, L. R., Systemic sclerosis sine scleroderma: an unusual presentation of scleroderma renal crisis. *Journal of Rheumatology,* 22, 557, 1995.

7. Black, C. M., Measurement of skin involvement in scleroderma. *Journal of Rheumatology,* 22, 1217, 1995.

8. Steen, V. D. and Medsger, T. A., Epidemiology and natural history of systemic sclerosis. *Rheumatic Diseases Clinics of North America,* 16, 6, 1995.

9. Gendi, N. S. T., Welsh, K. I., Van Venrooji, W. J., Vancheeswaran, R., Gilroy, J., and Black, C. M., HLA as a predictor of mixed connective tissue disease differentiation. Ten year clinical and immunogenetic follow-up of 46 patients. *Arthritis & Rheumatism,* 30, 259, 1995

10. Kallenberg, C. G., Early detection of connective tissue disease in patients with Raynaud's phenomenon. *Rheumatic Diseases Clinics of North America,* 16, 11, 1990

11. Black, C. M., Scleroderma and fasciitis in children, *Current Opinion in Rheumatology,* 7, 442, 1995.

12. Black, C. M., The aetiopathogenesis of systemic sclerosis: thick skin-thin hypotheses. The Parkes Weber Lecture 1994. *Journal of the Royal College of Physicians of London,* 29, 119, 1995.

13. Pearson, J. D., The endothelium: its role in scleroderma. *Annals of the Rheumatic Diseases,* 50, Suppl. 4, 866, 1991

14. Kahaleh, M. B. and Yin, T. G., Enhanced expression of high-affinity interleukin-2 receptors in scleroderma: possible role for IL-6. *Clinical Immunology & Immunopathology,* 62, 97, 1992.

15. Kraling, B. M., Maul, G. G., and Jimenez, S. A., Mononuclear cellular infiltrates in clinically involved skin from patients with systemic sclerosis of recent onset predominantly consist of monocytes/macrophages. *Pathobiology,* 63, 48, 1995

16. Fleischmajer, R., Perlish, J. S., and Reeves, J. R. T., Cellular infiltrates in scleroderma skin. *Arthritis & Rheumatism,* 20, 975, 1977.

17. Prescott, R. J., Freemont, A. J., Jones, C. J., Hoyland, J., and Fielding, P., Sequential dermal microvascular and perivascular changes in the development of scleroderma. *Journal of Pathology,* 166, 255, 1992.

18. Blann, A. D., Illingworth, K., and Jayson, M. I., Mechanisms of endothelial cell damage in systemic sclerosis and Raynaud's phenomenon. *Journal of Rheumatology,* 20, 1325–1330, 1993.

19. Herrick, A. L., Illingworth, K., Blann, A., Hay, C. R., Hollis, S., and Jayson, M. I., Von Willebrand factor, thrombomodulin, thromboxane, beta-thromboglobulin and markers of fibrinolysis in primary Raynaud's phenomenon and systemic sclerosis. *Annals of the Rheumatic Diseases,* 55, 122, 1996.

20. Marasini, B., Cugno, M., and Agostoni, A., Plasma levels of tissue-type plasminogen activator and von Willibrand factor in patients with Raynaud's phenomenon. *Arthritis & Rheumatism,* 255-256, 1991.

21. Soma, Y., Takehara, K., Sato, S., and Ishibashi, Y., Increase in plasma thrombomodulin in patients with systemic sclerosis. *Journal of Rheumatology,* 20, 1444, 1993.

22. Kahaleh, M. B., Endothelin, an endothelial-dependent vasoconstrictor in scleroderma. Enhanced production and profibrotic action. *Arthritis & Rheumatism,* 34, 978, 1991.

23. Vancheeswaran, R., Magoulas, T., Efrat, G., Wheeler-Jones, C., Olsen, I., Penny, R., and Black, C. M., Circulating endothelin-1 levels in systemic sclerosis subsets-a marker of fibrosis or vascular dysfunction? *Journal of Rheumatology,* 21, 1838, 1994.

24. Morelli, S., Ferri, C., Polettini, E., Bellini, C., Gualdi, G. F., Pittoni, V., Valesini, G., and Santucci, A., Plasma endothelin-1 levels, pulmonary hypertension, and lung fibrosis in patients with systemic sclerosis. *American Journal of Medicine,* 99, 255, 1995.

25. Sfikakis, P. P., Tesar, J., Baraf, H., Lipnick, R., Klipple, G., and Tsokos, G. C., Circulating intercellular adhesion molecule-1 in patients with systemic sclerosis. *Clinical Immunology & Immunopathology,* 68, 88, 1993.

26. Blann, A. D., Herrick, A., and Jayson, M. I., Altered levels of soluble adhesion molecules in rheumatoid arthritis, vasculitis and systemic sclerosis. *British Journal of Rheumatology,* 34, 814, 1995.

27. Denton, C. P., Bickerstaff, M. C., Shiwen, X., Carulli, M. T., Haskard, D. O., Dubois, R. M., and Black, C. M., Serial circulating adhesion molecule levels reflect disease severity in systemic sclerosis. *British Journal of Rheumatology*, 34, 1048, 1995.

28. Gearing, A. J. H. and Newman, W., Circulating adhesion molecules in disease. *Immunology Today*, 14, 506, 1993.

29. Clark, E. A., Grabstein, K. H., and Shu, G. L., Cultured human follicular dendritic cells. Growth characteristics and interactions with B lymphocytes. *Journal of Immunology*, 148, 3327, 1992.

30. Seron, P., Cameron, J. S., and Haskard, D. O., Expression of VCAM-1 in normal and diseased tissue. *Nephrology, Dialysis and Transplantation*, 6, 917, 1991.

31. Shi-Wen, X., Panesar, M., Vancheeswaran, R., Mason, J., Haskard, D., Black, C. M, Olsen, I., and Abraham, D., Expression and shedding of intercellular adhesion molecule 1 and lymphocyte function-associated antigen 3 by normal and scleroderma fibroblasts. Effects of interferon-gamma, tumor necrosis factor alpha, and estrogen. *Arthritis & Rheumatism*, 37, 1689, 1994.

32. Kawaguchi, Y., Suzuki, K., Hara, M., Hidaka, T., Ishizuka, T., Kawagoe, M., and Nakamura, H., Increased endothelin-1 production in fibroblasts derived from patients with systemic sclerosis. *Annals of the Rheumatic Diseases*, 53, 506, 1994.

33. Matucci-Cerinic, M., Pignone, A., Lotti, T., Spillantini, G., Curradi, C., Leoncini, G., Iannone, F., Falcini, F., and Cagnoni, M., Reduced angiotensin converting enzyme plasma activity in scleroderma. A marker of endothelial injury? *Journal of Rheumatology*, 17, 328, 1990.

34. Medsger, T. A., Treatment of systemic sclerosis. *Annals of the Rheumatic Diseases*, 50, Suppl. 4, 877, 1991.

35. Rosenbaum, J., Pottinger, B. E., Woo, P., Black, C. M., Loizou, S., Byron, M. A., and Pearson, J. D., Measurement and characterisation of circulating anti-endothelial cell IgG in connective tissue diseases. *Clinical & Experimental Immunology*, 72, 450, 1988.

36. Del Papa, N., Guidali, L., Sironi, M., Shoenfeld, Y., Mantovani, A., Tincani, A., Balestrieri, G., Antonella, R., Sinico, R. A., and Meroni, P. L., Anti-endothelial cell IgG antibodies from patients with Wegener's granulomatosis bind to human endothelial cells *in vitro* and induce adhesion molecule expression and cytokine secretion. *Arthritis & Rheumatism*, 39, 758, 1996.

37. Carvalho, D., Savage, C. O., Black, C. M., and Pearson, J. D., IgG antiendothelial cell autoantibodies from scleroderma patients induce leukocyte adhesion to human vascular endothelial cells *in vitro*. Induction of adhesion molecule expression and involvement of endothelium-derived cytokines. *Journal of Clinical Investigation*, 97, 111, 1996.

38. Denton, C. P., Carvalho, D., Stratton, R., Black, C. M., and Pearson, J. D., A longitudinal study of anti-endothelial cell antibody activity in systemic sclerosis. *British Journal of Rheumatology*, 35, S41, 1996.

39. Salojin, K. V., Le Tonqueze, M., Saraux, A., Nassonov, E. L., Dueymes, M., Piette, J. C., and Youinou, P. Y., Antiendothelial cell antibodies: useful markers of systemic sclerosis. *Am. J. Med.*, 102, 178, 1997.

40. Negi, V. S., Tripathy, N. K., Misra, R., and Nityanand, S., Antiendothelial cell antibodies in scleroderma correlate with severe digital ischemia and pulmonary arterial hypertension. *J. Rheumatol.*, 25, 462, 1998.

41. Okawa-Takatsuji, M., Aotsuka, S., Fujinami, M., Uwatoko, S., Kinoshita, M., and Sumiya, M., Up-regulation of intercellular adhesion molecule-1 (ICAM-1), endothelial leucocyte adhesion molecule-1 (ELAM-1) and class II MHC molecules on pulmonary artery endothelial cells by antibodies against U1-ribonucleoprotein. *Clin. Exp. Immunol.*, 116:174, 1999.

42. Kovalchik, M. T., Guggenham, S. J., Silverman, M. H., Robertson, J. S., and Steigerwald, J. C., The kidney in progressive systemic sclerosis. *Annals of Internal Medicine*, 89, 881, 1978.

43. Harrison, N. K., Myers, A. R., Corrin, B., Soosay, G., Dewar, A., Black, C. M., and du Bois, R. M., Structural features of interstitial lung disease in systemic sclerosis. *American Review of Respiratory Disease*, 144, 707, 1991.

44. Kaye, S. A., Seifalian, A. M., Lim, S. G., Hamilton, G., and Black, C. M., Ishaemia of the small intestine in patients with systemic sclerosis: Raynaud's phenomenon or chronic vasculopathy? *Quarterly Journal of Medicine*, 87, 495, 1994.

45. Claman, H. N., Giorno, R. C., and Seibold, J. R., Endothelial and fibroblastic activation in scleroderma. The myth of the "uninvolved skin." *Arthritis & Rheumatism*, 34, 1495, 1991.

46. Freemont, A. J., Hoyland, J., Fielding, P., Hodson, N., and Jayson, M. I., Studies of the microvascular endothelium in uninvolved skin of patients with systemic sclerosis: direct evidence for a generalized microangiopathy. *British Journal of Dermatology*, 126, 561, 1992.

47. Kahaleh, M. B., The role of vascular endothelium in fibroblast activation and tissue fibrosis, particularly in scleroderma (systemic sclerosis) and pachydermoperiostosis (primary hypertrophic osteoarthropathy). *Clinical & Experimental Rheumatology,* 10, Suppl. 7, 51, 1992.

48. Cailes, J., Winter, S., du Bois R. M., and Evans, T. W., Defective endothelially mediated pulmonary vasodilation in systemic sclerosis. *Chest,* 114, 178, 1998.

49. Kahaleh, M. B. and Yin, T. G., Enhanced expression of high-affinity interleukin-2 receptors in scleroderma: possible role for IL-6. *Clinical Immunology & Immunopathology,* 62, 97, 1992.

50. Cozzolini, F., Torcia, M., Aldinucci, D., Ziche, M., Almerigogna, F., Bani, D., and Stern, D. M., Interleukin-1 is an autocrine regulator of human endothelial cell growth. *Proceedings of the National Academy of Sciences of the United States of America,* 87 6487, 1990.

51. Brooks, R. A., Burrin, J. M., and Kohner, E. M., Characterisation of release of bFGF from bovine retinal endothelial cell monolayer cultures. *Biochemical Journal,* 276, 113, 1991.

52. Wagner, O. F. and Christ, G., Polar secretion of ET-1 by cultured endothelial cells. *Journal of Biological Chemistry,* 267, 16066, 1992.

53. Swerlick, R. A. and Lawley, T. J., Role of microvascular endothelial cells in inflammation. *Journal of Investigative Dermatology,* 100, 111S, 1993

54. Antonelli-Orlidge, A., Saunders, K. B., Smith, S. R., and D'Amore, P. A., An activated form of transforming growth factor β is produced by cocultures of endothelial cells and pericytes. *Proceedings of the National Academy of Sciences of the United States of America,* 86, 4544, 1989.

55. Bradham, D. M., Igarashi, A., Potter, R. L., and Grotendorst, G. R., Connective tissue growth factor: a cysteine-rich mitogen secreted by human vascular endothelial cells is related to the SRC-induced immediate early gene product CEF-10. *Journal of Cell Biology,* 114, 1285, 1991.

56. McNeil, P. L., Muthukrishna, L., Warder, E., and D'Amore, P. A., Growth factors are released by mechanically wounded endothelial cells. *Journal of Cell Biology,* 109, 811, 1989.

57. Eguchi, K., Migita, K., Nakashima, M., Ida, H., Terada, K., Sakai, M., Kawakami, A., Aoyagi, T., Ishimaru, T., and Nagataki, S., Fibroblast growth factors released by wounded endothelial cells stimulate proliferation of synovial cells. *Journal of Rheumatology,* 19, 1925, 1992.

58. Villanueva, A. G., Farber, H. W., Rounds, S., and Goldstein, R. H., Stimulation of fibroblast collagen and total protein formation by an endothelial cell-derived factor. *Circulation Research,* 69, 134, 1991.

59. Stewart, D. J., Langleburn, D., Cernacek, P., and Ciaflone, K., Endothelin release is inhibited by co-culture of endothelial cells with cells of the vascular media. *American Journal of Physiology,* 259, H1928, 1990.

60. Eckes, B., Hunzelmann, N., Ziegler-Heitbrock, H. W., Urbanski, A., Luger, T., Krieg, T., and Mauch, C., IL-6 expression by fibroblasts grown in three-dimensional gel cultures. *FEBS Letters,* 298, 229, 1992.

61. Kupper, T. S. and Groves, R. W., The interleukin-1 axis and cutaneous inflammation. *Journal of Investigative Dermatology,* 105, 62S, 1995

62. Weber, C., Alon, R., Moser, B., and Springer, T. A., Sequential regulation of $\alpha4\beta1$ and $\alpha5\beta1$ integrin avidity by CC chemokines in monocytes: implications for transendothelial chemotaxis. *Journal of Cell Biology,* 134 1063, 1996.

63. Guarda, E., Myers, P. R., Brilla, C. G., Tyagi, S. C., and Webber, K. T., Endothelial cell induced modulation of cardiac fibroblast collagen metabolism. *Cardiovascular Research,* 27, 1004, 1993.

64. Kuwana, M., Kaburaki, J., and Okano, Y., The HLA-DR and DQ genes control the autoimmune response to DNA topoisomerase I in systemic sclerosis (scleroderma). *Journal of Clinical Investigation,* 92, 1296, 1993

65. Stein, C. M., Tanner, S. B., and Awad, J. A., Evidence of free radical-mediated injury (isoprostane overproduction) in scleroderma. *Arthritis and Rheumatism,* 39, 1146-50, 1996.

66. Herrick, A. L., Rieley, F., and Schofield, D., Micronutrient antioxidant status in patients with primary Raynaud's phenomenon and systemic sclerosis. *Journal of Rheumatology,* 21, 1477, 1994.

67. Bruckdorfer, K. R., Hillary, J. B., Bunce, T. et al., Increased susceptibility to oxidation of low-density lipoproteins isolated from patients with systemic sclerosis. *Arthritis and Rheumatism,* 38, 1060, 1995

68. Farber, J. L., Kyle, M. E., and Coleman, J. B., Mechanisms of cell injury by activated oxygen species. *Laboratory Investigation,* 62, 67, 1990.

69. Casciola-Rosen, L., Wigley, F., and Rosen, A., Scleroderma autoantigens are uniquely fragmented by metal-catalyzed oxidation reactions: implications for pathogenesis. *Journal of Experimental Medicine,* 185, 71, 1997.

70. Denton, C. P., Bunce, T. D., Dorado, M. B., Roberts, Z., Wilson, H., Howell, K., Bruckdorfer, K. R., and Black, C. M., Probucol treatment improves symptoms and reduced lipoprotein oxidation susceptibility in Raynaud's phenomenon. *Rheumatology*, 38, 309, 1999.

71. Maeda, M., Kachi, H., and Mori, S., Ultrastructural observation of platelets from patients with progressive systemic sclerosis. *Journal of Dermatology*, 25, 222, 1998.

72. Lau, C. S., McLaren, M., Saniabadi, A., and Belch, J. J., Increased whole blood platelet aggregation in patients with Raynaud's phenomenon with or without systemic sclerosis. *Scandanavian Journal of Rheumatology*, 22, 97, 1993.

73. Goodfield, M. J., Orchard, M. A., and Rowell, N. R., Whole blood platelet aggregation and coagulation factors in patients with systemic sclerosis. *British Journal of Haematology*, 84, 675, 1993.

74. Gay, S., Jones, R. E., and Huang, G., Immunohistologic demonstration of platelet-derived growth factor and *sis*-oncogene expression in scleroderma. *Journal of Investigative Dermatology*, 92, 301, 1989.

75. Rademaker, M., Meyrick Thomas, R. H., Kirby, J. D., and Kovacs, I. B., The anti-platelet effect of nifedipine in patients with systemic sclerosis. *Clinical and Experimental Rheumatology*, 10, 57, 1992.

76. Bona, C. and Rothfield, N., Autoantibodies in scleroderma and tight skin mice. *Current Opinion in Immunology*, 6, 931, 1994.

77. Lee, B. and Craft, J. E., Molecular structure and function of autoantigens in systemic sclerosis. *International Reviews of Immunology*, 12, 129, 1995.

78. Reveille, J. D., Owerbach, D., Goldstein, R., Moreda, R., Isern, R. A., and Arnett, F. C., Association of polar amino-acids at position 26 of the HLA-DQB1 first domain with the anticentromere antibody response in systemic sclerosis. *Journal of Clinical Investigation*, 89, 1208, 1992.

79. White, B. and Yurovsky, V. V., Oligoclonal expansion of V delta 1+ gamma/delta T-cells in systemic sclerosis patients. *Annals of the New York Academy of Sciences*, 756, 382, 1995.

80. Piela-Smith, T. H. and Korn, J. H., Lymphocyte modulation of fibroblast function in systemic sclerosis. *Clinics in Dermatology*, 12, 369, 1994

81. Denton, C. P., Korn, J. H., Black, C. M., and de Crombrugghe, B., Systemic sclerosis: current pathogenetic concepts and future prospects for targeted therapy. *Lancet*, 347, 1453, 1996.

83. Denton, C. P., Cailes, J. B., Phillips, G. D., Wells, A. U., Black, C. M., and du Bois, R. M., Comparison of Doppler-echocardiography and right heart catheterisation to assess pulmonary hypertension in systemic sclerosis. *British Journal of Rheumatology*, 36, 239, 1997.

84. Raeside, D. A., Chalmers, G., Clelland, J., Madhok, R., and Peacock, A. J., Pulmonary artery pressure variation in patients with connective tissue disease: 24 hour ambulatory pulmonary artery pressure monitoring. *Thorax*, 53, 857, 1998.

85. Koh, E. T., Lee, P., Gladman, D. D., and Abu-Shakra, M., Pulmonary hypertension in systemic sclerosis: an analysis of 17 patients. *British Journal of Rheumatology*, 35, 989, 1996.

86. Sacks, D. G., Okano, Y., Steen, V. D., Curtiss, E., Shapiro, L. S., and Medsger, T. A., Isolated pulmonary hypertension in systemic sclerosis with diffuse cutaneous involvement: association with serum anti-U3RNP antibody. *Journal of Rheumatology*, 23, 639, 1996

87. Cool, C. D., Kennedy, D., Voelkel, N. F., and Tuder, R. M., Pathogenesis and evolution of plexiform lesions in pulmonary hypertension associated with scleroderma and human immunodeficiency virus infection. *Human Pathology*, 28, 434, 1997.

88. Welsh, C. H., Hassell, K. L., Badesch, D. B., Kressin, D. C., and Marlar, R. A., Coagulation and fibrinolytic profiles in patients with severe pulmonary hypertension. *Chest*, 110, 710, 1996.

89. Cacoub, P., Carmochkine, M., Dorent, R., Nataf, P., Piette, J. C., Godeau, P., Gandjbakhch, I., and Boffa, M. C., Plasma levels of thrombomodulin in pulmonary hypertension. *American Journal of Medicine*, 101, 160, 1996

90. Mercie, P., Seigneur, M., and Conri, C., Plasma thrombomodulin as a marker of vascular damage in systemic sclerosis. *Journal of Rheumatology*, 22, 1440, 1995.

91. MacGregor, A. J., Davrashvili, J., Knight, C., Denton, C. P., Lipkin, D. P., and Black, C. M., Early pulmonary hypertension in systemic sclerosis: risk of progression and consequences for survival. *Arthritis and Rheumatism*, 39, S151, 1996.

92. Rivolta, R., Mascagni, B., Berruti, V., Quarto Di Palo, F., Elli, A., Scorza, R., and Castagnone, D., Renal vascular damage in systemic sclerosis patients without clinical evidence of nephropathy. *Arthritis and Rheumatism*, 39, 1030, 1996.

93. Steen, V. D. and Medsger, T. A., Case-control study of corticosteroids and other drugs that either precipitate or protect from the development of scleroderma renal crisis. *Arthritis and Rheumatism*, 41, 1613, 1998.

94. Traub, X., Hypertension and renal failure (scleroderma renal crisis) in progressive systemic sclerosis. Review of a 25 year experience with 68 cases. *Medicine*, 62, 335, 1983.

95. Helfrich, D. J., Banner, B., Steen, V. D., and Medsger, T. A., Renal failure in normotensive patients with systemic sclerosis. *Arthritis and Rheumatism*, 32, 1128, 1989.

96. Lopez-Ovejero, J. A., Lopez-Ovejero, J. A., Saal, S. D., D'Angelo, W. A., Cheigh, J. S., Stenzel, K. H., and Laragh, J. H., Reversal of vascular and renal crises of sderoderma by oral angiotensin-converting enzyme blockade. *New England Journal of Medicine*, 300, 1417, 1979.

97. Denton, C. P., Abdullah, A., Sweny, P., and Black, C. M., Acute renal failure occurring in scleroderma treated with cyclosporin A — a report of three cases. *British Journal of Rheumatology*, 33, 90–2, 1994.

98. Fleischmajer, R. and Gould, A. P., Serum renin and renin substrate levels in scleroderma. *Proc. Soc. Exp. Biol. Med.*, 150, 374, 1975.

99. Fiocco, U., Montanaro, D., Filippi, R., Peserico, A., Borsatti, A., and Todesco, S., Plasma renin activity in progressive systemic sclerosis. *Bollettino della Societa Italiana di Biologia Sperimentale*, 54, 2507, 1978.

100. Urai, L., Nagy, Z., Szinay, G., and Waltner, W., Renal function in scleroderma. *British Medical Journal*, 2, 1264, 1958

101. Cannon, P. J., Hassar, M., Case, D. B., Casarella, W. J., Sommers, S. C., and LeRoy, E. C., The relationship of hypertension and renal failure in scleroderma (progressive systemic sclerosis) to structural and functional abnormalities of the renal cortical circulation. *Medicine*, 53, 1, 1974.

102. Stratton, R. J., Coghlan, J. G., Pearson, J. D., Burns, A., Sweny, P., Abraham D. J., and Black, C. M., Different patterns of endothelial cell activation in renal and pulmonary vascular disease in scleroderma. *Quarterly Journal of Medicine*, 91, 561, 1998.

103. Clements, P. J., Lachenbruch, P. A., Furst, D. E., Maxwell, M., Danovitch, G., and Paulus, H. E., Abnormalities of renal physiology in systemic sclerosis. A prospective study with 10-year followup. *Arthritis and Rheumatism*, 37, 67, 1994.

104. Anders, H. J., Wiebecke, B., Haedecke, C., Sanden, S., Combe, C., and Schlondorff, D., MPO-ANCA-Positive crescentic glomerulonephritis: a distinct entity of scleroderma renal disease? *American Journal of Kidney Disease*, 33, 3, 1999.

105. Karpinski, J., Jothy, S., Radoux, V., Levy, M., and Baran, D., D-penicillamine-induced crescentic glomerulonephritis and antimyeloperoxidase antibodies in a patient with scleroderma. Case report and review of the literature. *American Journal of Nephrology*, 17, 528, 1997.

106. Belch, J. J., Land, D., Park, R. H., McKillop, J. H., and MacKenzie, J. F., Decreased oesophageal blood flow in patients with Raynaud's phenomenon. *British Journal of Rheumatology*, 27, 426, 1988.

107. Kaye, S. A., Seifalian, A. M., Lim, S. G., Hamilton, G., and Black, C. M., Ischaemia of the small intestine in patients with systemic sclerosis: Raynaud's phenomenon or chronic vasculopathy? *Quarterly Journal of Medicine*, 1994, 87, 495.

108. Kaye, S. A., Lim, S. G., Taylor, M., Patel, S., Gillespie, S., and Black, C. M., Small bowel bacterial overgrowth in systemic sclerosis: detection using direct and indirect methods and treatment outcome. *British Journal of Rheumatology*, 34, 265, 1995.

109. Liberski, S. M., McGarrity, T. J., Hartle, R. J., Varano, V., and Reynolds, D., The watermelon stomach: long-term outcome in patients treated with Nd:YAG laser therapy. *Gastrointestinal Endoscopy*, 40, 584, 1994

110. Murphy, F. T., Enzenauer, R. J., and Cheney, C. P., Watermelon stomach. *Arthritis and Rheumatism*, 42, 573, 1999.

111. Khanlou, H., Malhotra, A., Friedenberg, F., and Rothstein, K., Jejunal telangiectasias as a cause of massive bleeding in a patient with scleroderma. *Reviews in Rheumatology*, 66, 119, 1999.

112. Duchini, A. and Sessoms, S. L., Gastrointestinal hemorrhage in patients with systemic sclerosis and CREST syndrome. *American Journal of Gastroenterology*, 1998, 93, 1453.

113. Clements, P. J., Lachenbruch, P. A., Furst, D. E., Paulus, H. E., and Sterz, M. G., Cardiac score. A semiquantitative measure of cardiac involvement that improves prediction of prognosis in systemic sclerosis. *Arthritis and Rheumatism*, 34, 1371, 1991.

114. Henein, M. Y., Cailes, J., O'Sullivan, C., du Bois, R. M., and Gibson, D. G., Abnormal ventricular long-axis function in systemic sclerosis. *Chest,* 108, 1533, 1995.

115. Morelli, S., Ferri, C., Polettini, E., Bellini, C., Gualdi, G. F., Pittoni, V., Valesini, G., and Santucci, A., Plasma endothelin-1 levels, pulmonary hypertension, and lung fibrosis in patients with systemic sclerosis. *American Journal of Medicine,* 99, 255, 1995.

116. Candell-Riera, J., Armadans-Gil, L., Simeon, C. P., Castell-Conesa, J., Fonollosa-Pla, V., Garcia-del-Castillo, H., Vaque-Rafart, J., Vilardell, M., and Soler-Soler, J., Comprehensive noninvasive assessment of cardiac involvement in limited systemic sclerosis. *Arthritis and Rheumatism,* 39, 1138, 1996.

117. Ferri, C., Di Bello, V., Martini, A., Giorgi, D., Storino, F. A., Bianchi, M., Bertini, A., Paterni, M., Giusti, C., and Pasero, G., Heart involvement in systemic sclerosis: an ultrasonic tissue characterisation study. *Annals of the Rheumatic Diseases,* 57, 296, 1998.

118. Thompson, A. E. and Pope, J. E., A study of the frequency of pericardial and pleural effusions in scleroderma. *British Journal of Rheumatology,* 37, 1320, 1998.

119. Satoh, M., Tokuhira, M., Hama, N., Hirakata, M., Kuwana, M., Akizuki, M., Ichikawa, Y., Ogawa, S., and Homma, M., Massive pericardial effusion in scleroderma: a review of five cases *British Journal of Rheumatology,* 34, 564, 1995.

120. Ridolfi, R. L., Bulkley, B. H., and Hutchins, G. M., The cardiac conduction system in progressive systemic sclerosis. Clinical and pathologic features of 35 patients. *American Journal of Medicine,* 61, 361, 1976.

121. Kostis, J. B., Seibold, J. R., Turkevich, D., Masi, A. T., Grau, R. G., Medsger, T. A., Steen, V. D., Clements, P. J., Szydlo, L., and D'Angelo, W. A., Prognostic importance of cardiac arrhythmias in systemic sclerosis. *American Journal of Medicine,* 84, 1007, 1988.

122. Autonomic dysfunction in systemic sclerosis: time and frequency domain 24 hour heart rate variability analysis. Ferri, C., Emdin, M., Giuggioli, D., Carpeggiani, C., Maielli, M., Varga, A., Michelassi, C., Pasero, G., L'Abbate, A., *British Journal of Rheumatology,* 36, 669, 1997.

123. Morelli, S., Sgreccia, A., Ferrante, L., Barbieri, C., Bernardo, M. L., Perrone, C., and De Marzio, P., Relationships between electrocardiographic and echocardiographic findings in systemic sclerosis (scleroderma). *International Journal of Cardiology,* 57:151, 1996.

124. Sgreccia, A., Morelli, S., Ferrante, L., Perrone, C., De Marzio, P., De Vincentiis, G., and Scopinaro, F., QT interval and QT dispersion in systemic sclerosis (scleroderma). *Journal of Internal Medicine,* 243, 127, 1998.

125. Siegel, R. J., O'Connor, B., Mena, I., and Criley, J. M., Left ventricular function at rest and during Raynaud's phenomenon in patients with scleroderma. *American Heart Journal,* 108, 1469, 1984.

126. Long, A., Duffy, G., and Bresnihan, B., Reversible myocardial perfusion defects during cold challenge in scleroderma. *British Journal of Rheumatology,* 25, 158, 1986.

127. Lekakis, J., Mavrikakis, M., Emmanuel, M., Prassopoulos, V., Papazoglou, S., Papamichael, C., Moulopoulou, D., Kostamis, P., Stamatelopoulos, S., and Moulopoulos, S., Cold-induced coronary Raynaud's phenomenon in patients with systemic sclerosis. *Clinical and Experimental Rheumatology,* 1998, 16, 135.

128. Kazzam, E., Waldenstrom, A., Hedner, T., Hedner, J., and Caidahl, K., Endothelin may be pathogenic in systemic sclerosis of the heart. *International Journal of Cardiology,* 60, 31, 1997.

129. Youssef, P., Englert, H., and Bertouch, J., Large vessel occlusive disease associated with CREST syndrome and scleroderma. *Annals of the Rheumatic Diseases,* 52, 564–569. 1993.

130. Youssef, P., Brama, T., Englert, H., and Bertouch, J., Limited scleroderma is associated with increased prevalence of macrovascular disease. *Journal of Rheumatology,* 1995, 22, 469–72.

131. Veale, D. J., Collidge, T. A., and Belch, J. J., Increased prevalence of symptomatic macrovascular disease in systemic sclerosis. *Annals of the Rheumatic Diseases,* 54, 853, 1995

132. Stafford, L., Englert, H., Gover, J., and Bertouch, J., Distribution of macrovascular disease in scleroderma. *Annals of the Rheumatic Diseases,* 57, 476, 1998.

133. Campbell, P. M. and LeRoy, E. C., Pathogenesis of systemic sclerosis: a vascular hypothesis. *Seminars in Arthritis and Rheumatism,* 4, 351, 1975.

134. Ciatti, S., Varga, J., and Greenbaum, S. S., The 585 nm flashlamp-pumped pulsed dye laser for the treatment of telangiectases in patients with scleroderma. *Journal of the American Academy of Dermatology,* 35, 487, 1996.

23 Vascular Manifestations in Rheumatoid Arthritis, Dermato/Polymyositis, and Mixed Connective Tissue Disease

Jean-Charles Piette and Camille Francès

CONTENTS

I. RHEUMATOID ARTHRITIS

Rheumatoid vasculitis is frequently found postmortem in rheumatoid arthritis (RA), but its heterogeneous clinical manifestations are observed in no more than 1 to 3% of unselected cases, and 6–10% of in-patients.[1-4] However, given the high prevalence of RA, rheumatoid vasculitis might be the most frequent systemic vasculitis.[5]

Rheumatoid vasculitis is usually diagnosed by pathological examination of skin, muscle or nerve, or, as recently proposed, by labial salivary gland biopsy.[6] It mainly affects small- and medium-sized arteries with various aspects: (a) acute fibrinoid necrosis of the vessel wall invaded by polymorphonuclear leucocytes, very similar to that of polyarteritis nodosa; (b) mononuclear vessel wall infiltrate and; (c) intimal proliferation leading to occlusion and sometimes recanalization, as observed in systemic sclerosis.[3] These lesions occur either singly or in combinations. The latter aspect is usually considered as sequelae of a former inflammation. The pathophysiology of rheumatoid vasculitis is thought to result from vessel wall deposition of immune complexes, as attested by the presence of immunoglobulins and complement within necrotic lesions. Antibodies to the collagen-like region of C1q, antiendothelial cell antibodies, and antilactoferrin ANCA might be of peculiar relevance.[7-10]

Patients who develop clinical manifestations are more frequently men with long-standing RA, destructive joint disease, rheumatoid nodules, ANA, hypocomplementemia, and high titers of serum rheumatoid factor and immune complexes.[11,12] The presence of DRB1*0401 might also be a risk factor.[13,14] It has been suggested that abrupt withdrawal or quick tapering of steroids may precipitate the emergence of rheumatoid vasculitis, but when systemic manifestations occur, synovitis is frequently inactive. Patients with Felty's syndrome are more likely to develop rheumatoid vasculitis.

Clinically, rheumatoid vasculitis mainly involves the skin and the peripheral nervous system.[3,4] The most frequently observed dermatological manifestations are distal microinfarcts, located close to the nails. These infarcts usually result from digital obliterative endarteritis, thought to be a benign variant of rheumatoid vasculitis, and in the absence of associated vascular manifestations they do not require aggressive management.[15] Skin involvement by severe, i.e., active, vasculitis features skin with necrosis or ulcers of abrupt onset located on lower limbs, large gangrenes affecting digits or toes, and palpable purpura or livedo.[3,4] Within peripheral neuropathies the presence of a symmetrical distal, painful, sensitive neuropathy affecting lower and sometimes upper limbs was not usually regarded as ominous. However, this statement has been recently disputed.[16] On the opposite, asymmetrical sensory-motor mononeuritis multiplex of abrupt onset, thought to result from a vasculitis-induced vasa nervorum injury and leading to muscle atrophy, carry a poor prognosis. Interestingly, a very similar distinction between these two types of neuropathies has been recently proposed by our group in the setting of hepatitis C virus (HCV) -related disorders. The former is a usual feature of HCV-related cryo and the latter is a manifestation of the rare HCV-related "true" polyarteritis nodosa. Other organs or tissues may rarely be involved by rheumatoid vasculitis:[3,4]

- Central nervous system, featuring as seizures or strokes[17]
- Gut, leading to gut infarction and/or perforation[18]
- Heart, resulting in myocardial infarction; a granulomatous aortitis may accompany coronary arteritis[19]
- Eye, with necrotizing scleritis as the most severe manifestation[20]
- Muscle, responsible for proximal pain and weakness associated with elevated serum muscle enzymes, in fact rarely observed compared to the frequent histological involvement[21]

Though all organs or tissues may be affected by rheumatoid vasculitis, it should be noted that renal involvement is extremely rare,[22] contrary to the usual form of polyarteritis nodosa. Fever and weight loss are frequently present during vasculitis flares.

There is no consensus about treatment strategies in rheumatoid vasculitis;[23] this reflects both the rarity of this condition and its heterogeneity. The more severe forms require high-dose steroids, initiated as methylpredisolone infusion and usually associated with immunosuppressive agents such as cyclophosphamide — either oral or intravenous — azathioprine, or chlorambucil.[3,4,20,23] In limited "mild" vasculitis, management includes control of RA, local wound care, and reducing trauma to involved areas. Despite intensive regimens, 20 to 40% of patients with true rheumatoid vasculitis die within five years.[16] However, other studies have reported a limited impact of rheumatoid vasculitis on the survival of patients with rheumatoid arthritis.[4,24] Whether the use of methotrexate or of the recently introduced etanercept reduces the incidence of rheumatoid vasculitis has not been yet determined.

II. DERMATO/POLYMYOSITIS

Dermatomyositis and polymyositis are the main subsets of a large group of acquired disorders characterized by inflammatory infiltrates within the skeletal muscles, frequently leading to muscle weakness.

Though usually considered as a whole, this group in fact encompasses major heterogeneity, especially with regards to the pathogenic role of vascular lesions. Several attempts have therefore been made to classify the diverse forms of inflammatory myopathies. Bohan and Peter initially proposed to identify five subsets: polymyositis (PM), dermatomyositis (DM), polymyositis or dermatomyositis associated with malignancy, childhood DM (or PM) associated with vasculitis, and myositis with associated collagen-vascular disease.[25] Due to the identification of inclusion-body myositis (IBM), new diagnostic criteria have been proposed by Dalakas.[26] Japanese authors recently proposed a set of criteria to improve classification of patients between PM and DM.[27]

The distinction between PM and DM is much more than of academic importance, given that the increased risk of malignancy is mainly observed in adult DM.[28] Furthermore, there is now strong evidence that DM and PM are separate disorders resulting from distinct immune processes, i.e., mainly humoral in DM, and cellular in PM.[26] In DM, muscle histopathologic examination mainly shows perifascicular myofibril atrophy, endothelial hyperplasia of intramuscular blood vessels, early capillary depletion, and deposition of immune complexes in the walls of muscle arteries and capillaries. The muscle inflammatory infiltrates observed in DM are predominantly located to perivascular areas or interfascicular septa, and are mainly made of B and T-CD4 lymphocytes.[26,29,30] On the opposite, in PM and IBM, muscle histopathologic examination shows no endothelial abnormalities and the cellular infiltrates are mainly located in the fascicles, surrounding or invading individual muscle fibers. Contrary to DM, the PM infiltrate is made of T-CD8, macrophages, and natural killer cells.[26,29,30] In summary, the elementary muscular lesion of DM, not PM, is microvasculitis leading to muscle microinfarcts.

On a clinical ground, small vessel involvement plays a role in the development of some extramuscular manifestations observed in DM. This applies to dermatological lesions,[31] and especially to the periungueal abnormalities of great value in a patient presenting with suspected myositis.[32] Often visible to the naked eye, they are precisely depicted by nailfold microscopy as enlarged capillary loops and hemorrhages, and have been correlated to disease outcome.[33] On the opposite, the discovery of multiple splinter subungueal hemorrhages in a patient presenting with acute muscle pain should alert for possible trichinosis. Skin ulcerations may occur in the course of DM.[34] Raynaud's phenomenon is more prevalent when myositis overlaps with another connective tissue disorder, mainly scleroderma. Associated vascular manifestations may be present in such circumstances according to the overlapping disease, including antiphospholipid-related thrombotic events when it features with a clinical or biological lupus component. Coming back to "pure" DM, visceral involvement rarely results from a vascular mechanism in adult cases.[35] On the other hand, childhood DM may be complicated by a true vasculitis affecting the gastrointestinal tract and leading to life-threatening ulceration or hemorrhage, or sometimes the heart, eye, and skin.[36,37] It should be noted that the importance of vasculitis in childhood DM was pointed more than 20 years ago by Bohan and Peter.[25]

The last point to be discussed is the significance of the occurrence of venous thrombosis or pulmonary embolism in patients with myositis. It may be facilitated by decubitus, myositis-related heart failure, or profound hypoalbuminemia observed in some patients with acute edematous myositis. The main risk is to overlook an occult malignancy, which may manifest as recurrent deep or superficial thrombophlebitis.[38] The possible demonstration of antiphospholipid antibodies should be considered cautiously, especially in the elderly, given their frequent occurrence in cancer patients.[39,40] Within myositis, age is indeed the major factor suggestive of a possible underlying malignancy, while cancer is very rare in patients with either childhood DM; clearcut overlapping connective tissue disorder; antisynthetase antibodies, namely anti-Jo1; and/or interstitial lung involvement.[41,42]

III. MIXED CONNECTIVE TISSUE DISEASE

Since its initial individualization 30 years ago by Sharp et al., the field of mixed connective tissue disease (MCTD) remains a matter of debate, especially with regard to the use of the term MCTD versus undifferentiated connective tissue disease.[43-45] Today it is generally agreed that distinct patients initially feature with Raynaud's phenomenon, sausage-shaped fingers, polyarthralgias or arthritis, myalgias, and high titers of antibodies directed to U1 RNP. Over years, some have a protracted unchanged benign course, while others develop additional clinical and biological manifestations suggestive of a "true" MCTD or a definite disorder, mainly SLE, RA, or scleroderma.[46] Therefore, the initial presentation of UCTD cannot be regarded as indicative of a benign prognosis.

Due to nomenclature problems and potential overlap with definite connective tissue disorders, it is difficult to summarize "specific" vascular manifestations associated with MCTD. All patients with UCTD have Raynaud's phenomenon. Nailfold capillary microscopy frequently shows a scleroderma pattern, but it has been said that the presence of dystrophic, branched, "bushy" capillaries was very suggestive of the disorder.[47] When performed, hand angiography frequently shows obstruction of ulnar arteries, superficial arches, or digital arteries,[48] but this examination is of little clinical usefulness. Severe visceral involvement by a vasculitic process has been reported, but it cannot be regarded as specific.[49] Conversely, compared to other CTD, patients with MCTD have increased prevalence of primary pulmonary hypertension (PPH),[50] formerly called "plexogenic,"[51] i.e., PH unrelated to chronic causes of hypoxia, left ventricular failure, or repeated pulmonary embolism. Many reported cases originated from Japan.[50,52] PH complicating MCTD usually occurs in the absence of interstitial lung involvement, contrary to what is observed in systemic sclerosis, with the exception of the CREST variant.[53] Patients progressively develop exertional dyspnea, and increased second pulmonary sound can be heard on examination. PH is easily detected by echocardiogram and Doppler examination, but cardiac catheterization remains mandatory, at least in severe forms. Catheterization not only allows a precise measurement of pulmonary artery pressure/resistance and response to acute drug testing,[54] but it also has a role to exclude confounding causes of PH, mainly occult pulmonary embolism detected by pulmonary angiogram. It should be kept in mind that patients with MCTD have an increased prevalence of aPL[55] and are therefore prone to develop thromboembolic events. The problem is far from easy, given that it has been recently shown that IgG aCL are specifically associated with PH-related deaths in a long-term study of patients with MCTD.[56] None of these aCL-positive patients had thromboembolic manifestations. However, in this study pulmonary involvement was statistically associated with PH, though the four autopsied patients had little or no interstitial fibrosis.[56] Whatever the context, MCTD, SLE, or Primary APS, the pathogenic role of aPL in the occurrence of PPH remains unclear.[51] On the opposite, the recent demonstration of an increased production of proinflammatory cytokine by pulmonary artery endothelial cells induced by supernatants from monocytes stimulated with U1-RNP autoantibodies, and the up-regulation of ICAM-1, ELAM-1, and class II MHC molecule expression directly provoked by U1-RNP autoantibodies on these endothelial cells might offer more relevant clues to the pathophysiology of MCTD-associated PPH.[52,57] Beside chronic anticoagulation and oxygen administration, empirical management of patients with MCTD and PPH ranges from oral calcium channel blocker administration to continuous intravenous prostacyclin infusion[58,59] and monthly cyclophosphamide pulses.[60,61] Diverse surgical procedures are discussed in advanced forms refractory to medical regimens. Atrial septectomy is used by several teams.[62] Transplantation, either lung or heart-lung, may cure the disease,[62,63] but mortality remains high and donors scarce. Such risky procedures should be discussed on an individual basis, keeping in mind that the prognosis of patients with MCTD and PPH is poor. PPH should be regarded as a very specific vascular cause of death in MCTD.

REFERENCES

1. Panush, RS, Katz, P, Longley, S, Carter, R, Love, J, Stanley, H, Rheumatoid vasculitis: diagnostic and therapeutic decisions. *Clin. Rheumatol.*, 1983, 2:321–30.
2. Danning, CL, Illei, GG, Boumpas, DT, Vasculitis associated with primary rheumatologic diseases. *Curr. Opin. Rheumatol.*, 1998, 10:58–65.
3. Scott, DG, Bacon, PA, Tribe, CR, Systemic rheumatoid vasculitis: a clinical and laboratory study of 50 cases. *Medicine* (Baltimore), 1981, 60:288–97.
4. Vollertsen, RS, Conn, DL, Ballard, DJ, Ilstrup, DM, Kazmar, RE, Silverfield, JC, Rheumatoid vasculitis: survival and associated risk factors. *Medicine* (Baltimore), 1986, 65:365–75.

5. Watts, RA, Carruthers, DM, Symmons, DP, Scott, DG, The incidence of rheumatoid vasculitis in the Norwich Health Authority. *Br. J. Rheumatol.*, 1994, 33:832–3.

6. Flipo, RM, Janin, A, Hachulla, E, Houvenagel, E, Foulet, A, Cardon, T, Desbonnet, A, Grardel, B, Duquesnoy, B, Delcambre, B, Labial salivary gland biopsy assessment in rheumatoid vasculitis. *Ann. Rheum. Dis.*, 1994, 53:648–52.

7. Siegert, CE, Daha, MR, van der Voort, EA, Breedveld, FC, IgG and IgA antibodies to the collagen-like region of C1q in rheumatoid vasculitis. *Arthritis Rheum.*, 1990, 33:1646–54.

8. Heurkens, AH, Daha, MR, Breedveld, FC, Anti-endothelial cell antibodies in patients with rheumatoid vasculitis. *Arthritis Rheum.*, 1989, 32:1191–2.

9. van der Zee, JM, Heurkens, AH, van der Voort, EA, Daha, MR, Breedveld, FC, Characterization of anti-endothelial antibodies in patients with rheumatoid arthritis complicated by vasculitis. *Clin. Exp. Rheumatol.*, 1991, 9:589–94.

10. Coremans, IE, Hagen, EC, Daha, MR, van der Woude, FJ, van der Voort, EA, Kleijburg-van der Keur, C, Breedveld, FC, Antilactoferrin antibodies in patients with rheumatoid arthritis are associated with vasculitis. *Arthritis Rheum.*, 1992, 35:1466–75.

11. Scott, DG, Bacon, PA, Allen, C, Elson, CJ, Wallington, T, IgG rheumatoid factor, complement and immune complexes in rheumatoid synovitis and vasculitis: comparative and serial studies during cytotoxic therapy. *Clin. Exp. Immunol.*, 1981, 43:54–63.

12. Voskuyl, AE, Zwinderman, AH, Westedt, ML, Vandenbroucke, JP, Breedveld, FC, Hazcs, JM, Factors associated with the development of vasculitis in rheumatoid arthritis: results of a case-control study. *Ann. Rheum. Dis.*, 1996, 55:190–2.

13. Weyand, CM, Hicok, KC, Conn, DL, Goronzy, JJ, The influence of HLA-DRB1 genes on disease severity in rheumatoid arthritis. *Ann. Intern. Med.*, 1992, 117:801–6.

14. Voskuyl, AE, Hazes, JM, Schreuder, GM, Schipper, RF, de Vries, RR, Breedveld, FC, HLA- DRB1, DQA1, and DQB1 genotypes and risk of vasculitis in patients with rheumatoid arthritis. *J. Rheumatol.*, 1997, 24:852–5.

15. Watts, RA, Carruthers, DM, Scott, DG, Isolated nail fold vasculitis in rheumatoid arthritis. *Ann. Rheum. Dis.*, 1995, 54:927–9.

16. Puechal, X, Said, G, Hilliquin, P, Coste, J, Job-Deslandre, C, Lacroix, C, Menkes, CJ, Peripheral neuropathy with necrotizing vasculitis in rheumatoid arthritis. A clinicopathologic and prognostic study of 32 patients. *Arthritis Rheum.*, 1995, 38:1618–29.

17. Bathon, JM, Moreland, LW, DiBartolomeo, AG, Inflammatory central nervous system involvement in rheumatoid arthritis. *Semin. Arthritis Rheum.*, 1989, 18:258–66.

18. Babian, M, Nasef, S, Soloway, G, Gastrointestinal infarction as a manifestation of rheumatoid vasculitis. *Am. J. Gastroenterol.*, 1998, 93:119–20.

19. Gravallese, EM, Corson, JM, Coblyn, JS, Pinkus, GS, Weinblatt, ME, Rheumatoid aortitis: a rarely recognized but clinically significant entity. *Medicine* (Baltimore), 1989, 68:95–106.

20. Foster, CS, Forstot, SL, Wilson, LA, Mortality rate in rheumatoid arthritis patients developing necrotizing scleritis or peripheral ulcerative keratitis. Effects of systemic immunosuppression. *Ophthalmology*, 1984, 91:1253–63.

21. Voskuyl, AE, van Duinen, SG, Zwinderman, AH, Breedveld, FC, Hazes, JM, The diagnostic value of perivascular infiltrates in muscle biopsy specimens for the assessment of rheumatoid vasculitis. *Ann. Rheum. Dis.*, 1998, 57:114–7.

22. Helin, HJ, Korpela, MM, Mustonen, JT, Pasternack, AI, Renal biopsy findings and clinicopathologic correlations in rheumatoid arthritis. *Arthritis Rheum.*, 1995, 38:242–7.

23. Luqmani, RA, Watts, RA, Scott, DG, Bacon, PA, Treatment of vasculitis in rheumatoid arthritis. *Ann. Med. Interne* (Paris), 1994, 145:566–76.

24. Voskuyl, AE, Zwinderman, AH, Westedt, ML, Vandenbroucke, JP, Breedveld, FC, Hazes, JM, The mortality of rheumatoid vasculitis compared with rheumatoid arthritis. *Arthritis Rheum.*, 1996, 39:266–71.

25. Bohan, A, Peter, JB, Bowman, RL, Pearson, CM, A computer-assisted analysis of 153 patients with polymyositis and dermatomyositis. *Medicine* (Baltimore), 1977, 56:255–286.

26. Dalakas, MC, Polymyositis, Dermatomyositis, and Inclusion-Body Myositis. *N. Engl. J. Med.*, 1991, 325:1487–1498.

27. Tanimoto, K, Nakano, K, Kano, S, Mori, S, Ueki, H, Nishitani, H, Sato, T, Kiuchi, T, Ohashi, Y, Classification criteria for polymyositis and dermatomyositis. *J. Rheumatol.*, 1995, 22:668–74; Published erratum appears in *J. Rheumatol.*, 1995, 22:1807.

28. Sigurgeirsson, B, Lindelof, B, Edhag, O, Allander, E, Risk of cancer in patients with dermatomyositis or polymyositis. A population-based study. *N. Engl. J. Med.*, 1992, 326:363–367.

29. Dalakas, MC, Clinical benefits and immunopathological correlates of intravenous immune globulin in the treatment of inflammatory myopathies. *Clin. Exp. Immunol.*, 1996, 104 (Suppl. 1):55–60.

30. Plotz, PH, Rider, LG, Targoff, IN, Raben, N, O'Hanlon, TP, Miller, FW, Myositis: Immunologic contributions to understanding cause, pathogenesis, and therapy. *Ann. Intern. Med.*, 1995, 122:715–724.

31. Crowson, AN, Magro, CM, The role of microvascular injury in the pathogenesis of cutaneous lesions of dermatomyositis. *Hum. Pathol.*, 1996, 27:15–9.

32. Callen, JP, Dermatomyositis. *Lancet*, 2000, 355:53–7.

33. Silver, RM, Maricq, HR, Childhood dermatomyositis: serial microvascular studies. *Pediatrics*, 1989, 83:278–83.

34. Yosipovitch, G, Feinmesser, M, David, M, Adult dermatomyositis with livedo reticularis and multiple skin ulcers. *J. Eur. Acad. Dermatol. Venereol.*, 1998, 11:48–50.

35. Riemekasten, G, Opitz, C, Audring, H, Barthelmes, H, Meyer, R, Hiepe, F, Burmester, GR, Beware of the heart: the multiple picture of cardiac involvement in myositis. *Rheumatology* (Oxford), 1999, 38:1153–7.

36. Pachman, LM, Maryjowski, MC, Juvenile dermatomyositis and polymyositis. *Ann. Rheum. Dis.*, 1984, 10:95–115.

37. Takeda, T, Fujisaku, A, Jodo, S, Koike, T, Ishizu, A, Fatal vascular occlusion in juvenile dermatomyositis. *Ann. Rheum. Dis.*, 1998, 57:172–3.

38. Prandoni, P, Lensing, AWA, Büller, HR, Cogo, A, Prins, MH, Cattelan, AM, Cuppini, S, Noventa, F, Ten Cate, JW, Deep-vein thrombosis and the incidence of subsequent symptomatic cancer. *N. Engl. J. Med.*, 1992, 327:1128–1133.

39. Piette, JC, Cacoub, P, Antiphospholipid syndrome in the elderly: caution (Editorial). *Circulation*, 1998, 97:2195–6.

40. Asherson, RA, Cervera, R, Antiphospholipid antibodies and malignancies. *Cancer and Autoimmunity*, Shoenfeld, Y and Gershwin, E, Eds., Elsevier, Amsterdam, 2000:93–103.

41. Love, LA, Leff, RL, Fraser, DD, Targoff, IN, Dalakas, M, Plotz, PH, Miller, FW, A new approach to the classification of idiopathic inflammatory myopathy — myositis-specific autoantibodies define useful homogeneous patient groups. *Medicine* (Baltimore), 1991, 70:360–374.

42. Fieschi, C, Piette, JC, Myositis and neoplasia. *Cancer and Autoimmunity*, Shoenfeld, Y and Gershwin, E, Eds., Elsevier, Amsterdam, 2000:85–92.

43. Sharp, GC, Irvin, WS, LaRoque, RL, Velez, C, Daly, V, Kaiser, AD, Holman, HR, Association of autoantibodies to different nuclear antigens with clinical patterns of rheumatic disease and responsiveness to therapy. *J. Clin. Invest.*, 1971, 50:350–9.

44. Sharp, GC, Hoffman, RW, Clinical, immunologic, and immunogenetic evidence that mixed connective tissue disease is a distinct entity: comment on the article by Smolen and Steiner. *Arthritis Rheum.*, 1999, 42:190–1.

45. Kahn, MF, Mixed connective tissue disease dispute. *Lupus*, 1995, 4:258.

46. Hayem, G, Kahn, MF, Syndrome de Sharp et connectivites mixtes. *Maladies et Syndromes Systémiques*, Kahn, MF, Peltier, AP, Meyer, O, Piette, JC, Eds., Flammarion Médecine-Sciences, Paris, 2000:575–596.

47. Granier, F, Vayssairat, M, Priollet, P, Housset, E, Nailfold capillary microscopy in mixed connective tissue disease. Comparison with systemic sclerosis and systemic lupus erythematosus. *Arthritis Rheum.*, 1986, 29:189–95.

48. Peller, JS, Gabor, GT, Porter, JM, Bennett, RM, Angiographic findings in mixed connective tissue disease. Correlation with fingernail capillary photomicroscopy and digital photoplethysmography findings. *Arthritis Rheum.*, 1985, 28:768–74.

49. Marshall, JB, Kretschmar, JM, Gerhardt, DC, Winship, DH, Winn, D, Treadwell, EL, Sharp, GC, Gastrointestinal manifestations of mixed connective tissue disease. *Gastroenterology*, 1990, 98:1232–8.

50. Sawai, T, Murakami, K, Kasukawa, R, et al., Histopathological study of mixed connective tissue disease from 32 autopsy cases in Japan. *Jpn. J. Rheumatol.,* 1997, 7:179–292.
51. Piette, JC, Hunt, BJ, Pulmonary hypertension and antiphospholipid antibodies. In: *Hughes' Syndrome,* Khamaohta, MD, Ed., Springer-Verlag, London, 2000:96–104.
52. Okawa-Takatsuji, M, Aotsuka, S, Uwatoko, S, Kinoshita, M, Sumiya, M, Increase of cytokine production by pulmonary artery endothelial cells induced by supernatants from monocytes stimulated with autoantibodies against U1-ribonucleoprotein. *Clin. Exp. Rheumatol.,* 1999, 17:705–12.
53. Galie, N, Manes, A, Uguccioni, L, Serafini, F, De Rosa, M, Branzi, A, et al., Primary pulmonary hypertension: insights into pathogenesis from epidemiology. *Chest,* 1998, 114(3 Suppl):184S-194S.
54. Jolliet, P, Thorens, JB, Chevrolet, JC, Pulmonary vascular reactivity in severe pulmonary hypertension associated with mixed connective tissue disease. *Thorax,* 1995, 50:96–7.
55. Merkel, PA, Chang, YC, Pierangeli, SS, Convery, K, Harris, EN, Polisson, RP, The prevalence and clinical associations of anticardiolipin antibodies in a large inception cohort of patients with connective tissue diseases. *Am. J. Med.,* 1996, 101:576–583.
56. Burdt, MA, Hoffman, RW, Deutscher, SL, Wang, GS, Johnson, JC, Sharp, GC, Long-term outcome in mixed connective tissue disease: longitudinal clinical and serologic findings. *Arthritis Rheum.,* 1999, 42:899–909.
57. Okawa-Takatsuji, M, Aotsuka, S, Fujinami, M, Uwatoko, S, Kinoshita, M, Sumiya, M, Up-regulation of intercellular adhesion molecule-1 (ICAM-1), endothelial leucocyte adhesion molecule-1 (ELAM-1) and class II MHC molecules on pulmonary artery endothelial cells by antibodies against U1-ribonucleoprotein. *Clin. Exp. Immunol.,* 1999, 116:174–80.
58. De la Mata, J, Gomez-Sanchez, MA, Aranzana, M, Gomez-Reino, JJ, Long-term iloprost infusion therapy for severe pulmonary hypertension in patients with connective tissue diseases. *Arthritis Rheum.,* 1994, 37:1528–33.
59. Humbert, M, Sanchez, O, Fartoukh, M, Jagot, JL, Sitbon, O, Simonneau, G, Treatment of severe pulmonary hypertension secondary to connective tissue diseases with continuous IV epoprostenol (Prostacyclin). *Chest,* 1998, 114:80S–82S.
60. Dahl, M, Chalmers, A, Wade, J, Calverley, D, Munt, B, Ten year survival of a patient with advanced pulmonary hypertension and mixed connective tissue disease treated with immunosuppressive therapy. *J. Rheumatol.,* 1992, 19:1807–9.
61. Tam, LS, Li, EK, Successful treatment with immunosuppression, anticoagulation and vasodilator therapy of pulmonary hypertension in SLE associated with secondary antiphospholipid syndrome. *Lupus,* 1998, 7:495–7.
62. Haworth, SG, Primary pulmonary hypertension. *J. R. Coll. Physicians Lond.,* 1998, 32:187–90.
63. Asherson, RA, Higenbottam, TW, Dinh Xuan, AT, Khamashta, MA, Hughes, GRV, Pulmonary hypertension in a lupus clinic: experience with 24 patients. *J. Rheumatol.,* 1990, 17:1292–1298.

24 Vascular Manifestations in Relapsing Polychondritis

Jean-Charles Piette, Philippe Vinceneux, and Camille Francès

CONTENTS

I. INTRODUCTION

Relapsing polychondritis (RP) is a rare disorder characterized by recurrent inflammatory episodes affecting nonarticular cartilaginous structures, mainly the external ear(s), nose, larynx, and tracheobronchial tree, sometimes leading to cartilage destruction.[1-4] Diverse systemic manifestations are frequently associated, involving the articles, eyes, skin, inner ear, and sometimes vessels. The pathophysiology of RP remains poorly understood. A genetic predisposition has been reported in HLA-DR4 patients, but no particular DR4 subtype was involved.[5,6] Though autoimmune phenomena are highly suspected as playing a significant role in the pathogenesis of RP, the "true" antigen has been disputed. Type II collagen, the main type of collagen present within affected cartilaginous structures, was implicated 20 years ago, and antibodies directed to type II collagen were said to be both sensitive and specific markers of the disease.[7] Their clinical relevance has been discussed, but it remains that immunization with native type II collagen induces an experimental RP in both rats and mice.[8] Interestingly, a similar genetic background, i.e., HLA-DQ6 or DQ8, has been reported as important for disease susceptibility, both in experimental transgenic mice[9] and in the human RP.[10] However, recent discoveries suggest that the cartilage antigen responsible for RP might in fact be matrilin-1.[11]

Cardiac and/or vascular involvement is encountered in 29% of patients with RP according to a recent literature review of 500 patients, including 180 from our unit.[4] It should be classified into three subsets according to the vessels involved, i.e., aorta and large arteries, microvasculature, and veins.

II. AORTA AND LARGE ARTERIES[1,12-17]

Acquired aneurysms affecting the thoracic aorta are a very peculiar feature of RP, with the exception of Takayasu's arteritis. Despite a possible surgical repair, they carry a poor long-term prognosis.

They occur in about 5% of patients both in literature and in our experience.[2,4,18] In such cases, the mean age at onset of RP is about 35 years, i.e., about 8 years earlier than commonly observed in this disorder.[15] Aneurysms are usually located in the ascending aorta, originating from a dilated aortic annulus. Nowadays, they are frequently diagnosed either when a diastolic murmur is detected, when a systematic frontal and lateral chest X-ray shows a possible dilatation of the aorta, or on a systematic echocardiogram survey.[4,18] However, in rare instances, aortic regurgitation may develop in RP without dilatation of the aortic root.[18,19] Later, large thoracic aneurysms may be responsible for mediastinal symptoms, and may sometimes lead to severe aortic failure or even fatal rupture.[18] Embolic events are rarely encountered.[20] Aneurysms may be disclosed in the absence of any serum inflammatory response, when RP seems to remain under control.[15] Development of arterial aneurysms is a late event in the course of RP, occurring seven years after RP onset in a literature review.[15] Modern imaging techniques such as CT scan or MRI offer elegant tools for early diagnosis of thoracic aneurysms. Histopathological studies, obtained either after surgical repair or post-mortem, show intimal hyperplasia and adventitial fibrosis. The lesions, however, predominantly affect the media with major alterations of the elastic fibers and the presence of inflammatory cells, mainly lymphocytes sometimes accompanied by giant cells, rarely polymorphonuclears.[16,18,21-24] Calcium deposits may be observed.[16] Involvement of aortic vasa vasorum has been reported in some cases.[24] RP-related aneurysms sometimes extend from the thoracic to the abdominal aorta, but "pure" abdominal aneurysms are rare.[1,17,22,25] Very few patients have features really suggestive of Takayasu's arteritis due to the coexistence of aneurysms with stenosis affecting the aorta and/or its major branches. Case reports have described aortic dissection or cystic medial necrosis,[13,17,26,27] abdominal aortic occlusion within RP-associated antiphospholipid syndrome or not,[1,28-30] and even aortic wall ossification with hematopoiesis.[31]

Large arteries may be affected by aneurysms, stenosis, or both.[4,12,14,22] The former originate from contiguous aortic involvement or develop as independent saccular lesions involving cerebral,[13,32] coronary,[17] iliofemoral,[33] or upper limb[12,17] arteries. Rupture may be their presenting, and sometimes fatal, manifestation.[25,34] Pathological features are similar to those reported in the aortic wall.[12,33] It should be noted that such patients are prone to develop false aneurysms after arterial puncture,[35] leading to the preferential use of nontraumatic methods such as Döppler and angio-MRI for their imaging. Inflammatory stenotic or occlusive lesions may also affect carotid,[36] cerebral,[37] celiac/mesenteric,[12,13,37] coronary,[1,13] iliac, or limb[12,22,37,38] arteries. Renal artery lesions rarely lead to systemic hypertension.[39] Some patients feature with an aortic arch syndrome.[38,40] Two locations warrant a special mention. Temporal artery lesions sometimes mimic Horton's disease, including on pathological grounds, but diverse histological aspects may also be observed, including in middle-aged patients.[12,15,34,41] Several cases of lower-limb artery inflammatory involvement affecting young patients have been reported, sometimes even leading to amputation.[12,42] Conversely, arterial embolic events are extremely rare.[20] Contrary to Takayasu's arteritis and Behçet's disease, the pulmonary artery is unaffected by RP, except in one case displaying deep pits in both the main pulmonary artery and the aorta walls at autopsy.[43]

In our experience, the prevalence of Raynaud's phenomenon in RP is about 10% in the absence of associated connective tissue disorders and therefore similar to that observed in healthy subjects.

III. MICROVASCULATURE

The occurrence of microvasculitis is not a rare event in RP.[1,2,4,14] It has been said, indeed, that 5 to 14% of cases develop cutaneous leucocytoclastic vasculitis,[1,14] sometimes with typical features of polyarteritis nodosa (PAN) on biopsy. In our experience, of 127 RP patients devoid of any associated potentially confounding condition, dermatological involvement was present in 45 (35.4%) cases (unpublished data). On histological examination, leucocytoclastic vasculitis was the most frequent figure, corresponding to various clinical aspects such as, in decreasing order, purpura, urticarial papules, sterile pustules, nodules on the limbs, livedo reticularis, skin ulcerations, or erythema elevatum diutinum (mucosal aphthae and superficial phlebitis were not biopsied). Lymphocytic vasculitis was rarely encountered. It should be noted that RP-related dermatological involvement may also correspond to other histological abnormalities such as neutrophilic infiltrates, panniculitis, or skin vessels thrombosis. The prevalence of skin lesions was as high as 91% in patients with coexistent RP and myelodysplasia, a condition mainly restricted to men older than 60 years,[44] with leucocytoclastic vasculitis and Sweet's syndrome-like images as the most common histological features (unpublished data). Moreover, it has been said that up to 10% of RP cases are associated with or complicated by a severe systemic vasculitic process affecting the kidneys with "pauci-immune" crescentic focal or diffuse glomerulonephritis sometimes leading to dialysis,[13] eyes,[45] and/or the central or peripheral nervous system leading to various forms of injuries such as strokes, mononeuritis multiplex, or cranial neuropathies.[14,23,37] Contrary to aortic aneurysms, systemic vasculitis may occur early in the course of RP.

Though pathological demonstrations remain extremely scarce, microvasculitis might be responsible for some of the more classical manifestations of RP, such as audiovestibular or scleral involvement; this is supported by the frequent clustering of these very diverse visceral injuries.[12-14] Micro-aneurysms[46] or kidney infarctions[1] have been rarely reported. RP-associated visceral lesions usually belong to the scope of micropolyangiitis, and this is in agreement with the possible presence of perinuclear ANCA in patients with RP.[47] Two cases of Churg-Strauss syndrome associated with RP have been reported.[41,48] The limitations of the classifications proposed for vasculitides have been clearly emphasized, especially with regard to those based on the size of the vessels involved.[49] This especially applies to RP, which may affect all of them, from aorta to capillaries, and even veins.

IV. VEINS

Initially published as isolated case reports, the occurrence of venous thrombosis is observed in more than 10% of patients with RP.[4] Thrombophlebitis may affect either superficial or deep veins. The former manifests as a typical reddened, warm, tender cord extending along a superficial vein of the limbs, or as nodular dermatological lesions located on lower limbs assumed to result from superficial thrombophlebitis by histological examination only. Deep venous thrombosis may be complicated by pulmonary embolism or by recurrences.[1,12,50,51] Various sites may be involved, including retinal veins[45] or superior vena cava obstruction in a patient who has a large aneurysm of the ascending aorta.[22] The pathophysiology of RP-associated venous thrombosis is multifactorial. Beside nonspecific factors such as bed rest, attention has recently been paid to the presence of antiphospholipid antibodies — especially in patients with associated disorders such as systemic lupus erythematosus in young women or myelodysplasia in older men[50,52] — and to the relationship between RP and Behçet's disease and, more anecdotically, to a defect in tissue plasminogen activator.[53]

V. DIAGNOSIS

The diagnosis of RP is mainly based on the patient's history and physical examination. Among diverse sets of criteria, the most commonly used are those proposed by Michet et al.[2] (Table 24.1). Frequently, a full-blown picture is already constituted when patients are sent to reference centers, no further examinations being required to ensure diagnosis. On the other hand, confirmatory tools may be needed at the initial phase of the disease, in atypical forms, or when an alternative diagnosis is discussed. To date, serological tests remain of little value. Rheumatoid factors or ANA may sometimes be present in low titers in the absence of an associated connective tissue disorder, but significant titers suggest overlap with rheumatoid arthritis, Sjögren's syndrome, or systemic lupus erythematosus.[3,54] Antibodies to cartilage detected by indirect fluorescence staining have been scarcely studied, but have been reported as fairly specific.[55] In our hands, they were found present

---

TABLE 24.1
Empirical Diagnostic Criteria for Relapsing Polychondritis[2]

Major Criteria
Proven inflammatory episodes involving auricular cartilage
Proven inflammatory episodes involving nasal cartilage
Proven inflammatory episodes involving laryngotracheal cartilage

Minor Criteria
Ocular inflammation (conjunctivitis, keratitis, episcleritis, uveitis)
Hearing loss
Vestibular dysfunction
Seronegative inflammatory arthritis

Note: Diagnosis is made by two major criteria or one major + two minor.
Histological examination of affected cartilage is not required.

---

in only 28% of 85 patients (unpublished data). Though initially claimed both sensitive and specific,[7] the determination of circulating antibodies directed to collagen II has limited clinical significance.[8] The potential interest of testing antibodies to matrilin-1 is currently under investigation.[56] Histological examination of an affected cartilage, mainly auricular, is considered of value when it shows the association of degenerative changes with the presence of an inflammatory infiltrate penetrating the cartilage from its outer surface to its depth.[1,3,4] Given that the former changes are commonly found in normal controls aged 40 or more, it is mandatory to perform any auricular biopsy during an acute flare of chondritis to objectivate the presence of inflammatory cells within cartilage.

VI. DIFFERENTIAL DIAGNOSIS

Differential diagnosis of RP will be focused on vascular manifestations. Involvement of the aortic root may also be encountered in Marfan[57] or Ehlers-Danlos syndrome, syphilis, medial cystic necrosis, or spondylarthropathies.[18] However, the main pitfalls of RP-associated large arterial involvement remain located to three disorders, i.e., Cogan's syndrome, Takayasu's arteritis, and Behçet's disease. Cogan's syndrome may be responsible for aneurysms affecting the ascending aorta complicated by aortic valve insufficiency and for diverse other arterial manifestations.[58] Though interstitial keratitis is very suggestive of Cogan's syndrome and its fluctuating audiovestibular disorder distinct from the common aspects of RP, some cases may be difficult to classify, especially among "atypical" Cogan's syndrome.[58] Takayasu's arteritis is usually considered a very distinct entity. However, due to the possible involvement of the ascending aorta, presence of dermatological manifestations and associated conditions such as spondylarthropathies or Crohn's disease also shared with RP, some cases may be difficult to classify.[59,60] Indeed, among 200 cases of RP, we have observed three patients whose arterial lesions were very suggestive of Takayasu's arteritis (unpublished data). Similar remarks could apply to Horton's disease, a condition closely related to Takayasu's arteritis. As mentioned above, temporal artery involvement has been described in several cases of RP[12,34,41] as in various other vasculitides,[61] and thoracic aortic aneuryms may also develop late in the course of Horton's disease.[62] Behçet's disease is now regarded a true vasculitis, responsible not only for thrombophlebitis affecting very diverse sites, but also for arterial aneurysms or stenosis located to pulmonary arteries and to various segments of the aorta and its main branches.[63] Similarities between Behçet's disease and RP have been noted as early as 1975,[51] and the term "M.A.G.I.C. syndrome" (Mouth And Genital ulcers with Inflamed Cartilage) proposed to qualify this overlap.[29] Beside thrombophlebitis, such patients may develop severe arterial complications.[35,64] In our opinion, M.A.G.I.C. syndrome is more closely related to RP than to Behçet's disease.

Due to the possible association of RP with a vasculitis, either systemic or located to the skin, the differential diagnosis of RP-related microvascular involvement might cover pages. Furthermore, it has been suggested by some authors that a vasculitic process might be implicated in most cases of RP,[65] but we do not agree.[66] Given that such debates are frequently more academic than practical, discussion will be limited to Wegener's granulomatosis. RP and GW often share peculiar clinical features, such as acquired saddle nose deformity, subglottic stenosis, scleral inflammation, and sometimes audiovestibular involvement or pauci-immune glomerulopathy,[13] as well as nonspecific manifestations such as arthritis or skin vasculitis.[66] However, RP and WG are regarded as distinct entities. Granulomatous vasculitis and cytoplasmic ANCA directed to proteinase 3 are potent markers of WG, whereas ANCA found in a minority of patients with RP lack this specificity.[47] The same is true for WG parenchymal lung involvement, to be distinguished from airway stricture-induced bacterial pneumonia sometimes observed in RP. Thoracic helical CT, especially using the tracheo-bronchial perspective volume rendering technique (virtual endoscopy), offers an elegant way to visualize lesions of the respiratory tree — including diffuse tracheomalacia as a peculiar feature of RP — without the hazards of classical endoscopy.[1] The borders between RP and WG, however, may sometimes remain unprecise.[67] Auricular chondritis has been described in WG,[68] and proptosis or nasal septum perforation in RP.[12,69] We consider that a true overlap between both disorders is present in rare patients.[70] Such cases should be treated as WG, i.e., with a combination of steroids and cyclophosphamide or methotrexate. Last, the differential diagnosis of both conditions now includes the syndrome recently described in patients with a recessive genetic defect affecting expression of the transporter associated with antigen presentation (TAP) genes, who develop skin vasculitis and sometimes saddle nose deformity.[71]

VII. PROGNOSIS

RP carries a severe prognosis, due in part to the frequent requirement for high-dose steroids, and to the extreme duration of the disease which, unlike rheumatoid arthritis or systemic lupus erythematosus, rarely evolves to extinction. The five- and ten-year probabilities of survival after diagnosis were 74% and 55%, respectively in the Mayo Clinic series published in 1986.[2] Recent data[3] and our experience are more encouraging. A literature review performed in 1982 revealed that death was frequently related to RP, the leading causes being airway obstruction or collapse in women versus specific cardiovascular involvement in men.[15] A male predominance was also noted among patients with RP requiring heart valve replacement.[18] In the Mayo Clinic cohort, infection (12 of 41 deaths) was the leading cause of death, followed by systemic vasculitis (7 deaths) and large artery lesions (5 deaths). For patients less than 51 years old, saddle nose deformity and systemic vasculitis were the worst prognostic factors.[2] The five-year survival rate was as low as 45% when RP was associated with systemic vasculitis.[2] For older patients, only anemia predicted outcome. It should be recalled that myelodysplasia is frequent in men with RP who are aged 60 or more, that myelodysplasia is usually accompanied by dermatological lesions corresponding to leucocytoclastic vasculitis, and that survival remains limited to a few years after onset of requirement for repeated erythrocyte transfusions.[44] Therefore, taken together, vascular manifestations should be regarded as an indicator of a poor prognosis in patients with RP.

VIII. TREATMENT

Treatment of RP remains empirical, and due to the rarity of the condition, no randomized trials are expected to be conducted.[3] This is especially true for the diverse aspects of vascular involvement, which probably result from distinct and poorly understood processes requiring distinct approaches. Therefore, the following should be considered no more than modest proposals. Concerning aortic and large artery involvement, steroids are the mainstay of therapy. Immunosuppressive agents are frequently associated, especially when steroids alone fail to control RP. Due to the poor mid-term prognosis of large artery involvement in RP, and to the beneficial effects reported in similar conditions such as Takayasu's arteritis and Behçet's disease,[59,63] we think immunosuppressive agents should probably be included in first-line strategy. However, they were used only in 8 of the 112 patients from the Mayo Clinic.[2] Literature data mainly consist of case reports, and therefore do not help to choose a drug. Methotrexate given at an average weekly dose of 17.5 mg has been recently said to be effective in a majority of patients with RP, but without specific information on vascular involvement.[3] Cyclophosphamide or azathioprine have been frequently used with various results,[1,3,12,13,25,72] but unlike methotrexate, alkylating agents carry a theoretical risk of inducing myelodysplastic syndromes in patients who are already prone to spontaneously develop this complication. Monitoring of therapy remains a difficult question. While stenotic lesions are expected to resolve, aneurysms are not. Aortic dilatation may progress despite persistently normal ESR, and it is unclear whether this reflects smoldering activity of vasculitis — as demonstrated on histological specimens in Takayasu's arteritis[59] — or the mechanical consequence of repeated left ventricular ejection. Beta-adrenergic blockade with propanolol has been shown effective in slowing the rate of aortic dilatation in patients with Marfan's syndrome,[57] and it might also be of interest for that aim in RP. Whatever drug is used, a strict control of arterial pressure is mandatory. Failure of medical therapy leads one to consider surgical procedures. The optimal date for repair of aortic aneurysms should take into account their size, rate of progression, and magnitude of associated aortic regurgitation, but it remains difficult to determine.[18] About 30 cases of aortic valve replacement have been performed in RP, associated or not with reconstruction of the ascending aorta.[12,18,20,22,24,25] Surgery is less frequently performed in other sites for arterial aneuryms or symptomatic stenoses refractory to medical management.[13,33,34,39] A careful preoperative evaluation is mandatory, both to detect silent associated heart or vascular lesions given their frequent multiplicity,[12] and to ensure safe anesthesia, taking into account upper and lower respiratory tract abnormalities.[73] Epidural analgesia may sometimes be choosen for limb arterial surgery.[33] Alternative procedures such as percutaneous transluminal angioplasty or placement of an endovascular stent graft may also be considered in some high-risk patients.[39,74] Immediate postoperative results are usually good,[18] but further prognosis is drastically darkened by the occurrence of relapsing aneurysms, either anastomotic or developing *de novo* in a previously unaffected site; vascular occlusion; prosthetic valve desinsertion secondary to ongoing inflammation; or unexpected sudden death which might result from the rupture of an unrecognized aneurysm.[1,14,17,18,22,25,26,33-35,75] Like others,[18,19] we recommend the use of immunosuppressive agents at least during the two years following surgery, though failures have been reported with cyclophosphamide, azathioprine, or cyclosporine.[17,35] Lifelong regular clinical and radiological monitoring is needed.[18]

Treatment of microvascular involvement depends on its extent. Patients with vasculitis restricted to the skin may draw benefit from colchicine or dapsone. Conversely, those who feature as systemic vasculitis, namely of the micropolyangiitis type, should receive steroids and probably cyclophosphamide or azathioprine[4,13,14] as used in micropolyangiitis unrelated to RP.[76] In the case of RP-associated myelodysplasia, neither classical immunosuppressive agents nor dapsone may be used due to their hematological side-effects. Therefore, when disease control is not achieved by steroids alone, the choice for additional treatment is mainly limited, in this peculiar setting, to cyclosporin or high-dose immunoglobulins,[4] but results are uncertain.

In conclusion, vascular involvement in RP is frequent and heterogeneous. Survival may be jeopardized by aortic aneurysms or systemic micropolyangiitis. Pathophysiology remains unknown, and especially the mysterious link between cartilage and vascular wall inflammation needs to be elucidated.

REFERENCES

1. Mc Adam, LP, O'Hanlan, MA, Bluestone, R, Pearson, CM, Relapsing polychondritis. Prospective study of 23 patients and a review of the literature. *Medicine* (Baltimore), 1976, 55: 193–215.
2. Michet, CJ, Jr, Mc Kenna, CH, Luthra, HS, O'Fallon, WM, Relapsing polychondritis. Survival and predictive role of early disease manifestations. *Ann. Intern. Med.,* 1986, 104: 74–78.
3. Trentham, DE, Le, CH, Relapsing polychondritis. *Ann. Intern. Med.,* 1998, 129: 114–122.
4. Vinceneux, P, Pouchot, J, Piette, JC, Polychondrite atrophiante. In: *Maladies et Syndromes Systémiques,* Kahn, MF, Peltier, AP, Meyer, O, Piette, JC, Ed, Flammarion Médecine-Sciences, Paris, 2000: 623–649.
5. Lang, B, Rothenfusser, A, Lanchbury, JS, Rauh, G, Breedveld, FC, Urlacher, A, et al., Susceptibility to relapsing polychondritis is associated with HLA-DR4. *Arthritis Rheum.,* 1993, 36: 660–664.
6. Zeuner, M, Straub, RH, Rauh, G, Albert, ED, Scholmerich, J, Lang, B, Relapsing polychondritis: clinical and immunogenetic analysis of 62 patients. *J. Rheumatol.,* 1997, 24: 96–101.
7. Foidart, JM, Abe, S, Martin, GR, Zizic, TM, Barnett, EV, Lawley, TJ, et al., Antibodies to type II collagen in relapsing polychondritis. *N. Engl. J. Med.,* 1978, 299: 1203–1207.
8. Cremer, MA, Rosloniec, EF, Kang, AH, The cartilage collagens: a review of their structure, organization, and role in the pathogenesis of experimental arthritis in animals and in human rheumatic disease. *J. Mol. Med.,* 1998, 76: 275–88.
9. Bradley, DS, Das, P, Griffiths, MM, Luthra, HS, David, CS, HLA-DQ6/8 double transgenic mice develop auricular chondritis following type II collagen immunization: a model for human relapsing polychondritis. *J. Immunol.,* 1998, 16: 5046–53.
10. Hüe-Lemoine, S, Caillat-Zucman, S, Amoura, Z, Bach, JF, Piette, JC, HLA-DQA1* and DQB1* alleles are associated with susceptibility to relapsing polychondritis: from transgenic mice to humans. *Arthritis Rheum.,* 1999, 42 (Suppl): S 261.
11. Hansson, AS, Heinegard, D, Holmdahl, R, A new animal model for relapsing polychondritis, induced by cartilage matrix protein (matrilin-1). *J. Clin. Invest.,* 1999, 104: 589–98.
12. Esdaile, J, Hawkins, D, Gold, P, Freedman, SO, Duguid, WP, Vascular involvement in relapsing polychondritis. *Canad. Med. Ass. J.,* 1977, 116: 1019–1022.
13. Chang-Miller, A, Okamura, M, Torres, VE, Michet, CJ, Wagoner, RD, Donadio, JV, Jr, et al., Renal involvement in relapsing polychondritis. *Medicine* (Baltimore), 1987, 66: 202–217.
14. Michet, CJ, Jr, Vasculitis and relapsing polychondritis. *Rheum. Dis. Clin. North Am.,* 1990, 16: 441–4.
15. Piette, JC, Polychondrite chronique atrophiante. Etude d'une série de 29 cas et revue de la littérature. *Thèse de Médecine,* Paris. C.H.U. Pitié-Salpêtrière, 1982.
16. Allal, J, Rossi F, Petitalot, JP, Vouhe, P, Barraine, R, Sudre, Y, Les manifestations cardiaques de la polychondrite chronique atrophiante. *Ann. Cardiol. Angéiol.,* 1985, 34: 335–337.
17. Mainguèné, C, Bouhour, JB, De Lajartre, AY, Dupon, H, Les complications cardiovasculaires de la polychondrite chronique atrophiante. A propos d'un cas anatomo-clinique. Revue de la littérature. *Ann. Cardiol. Angeiol.,* 1991, 40: 97–102.
18. Lang-Lazdunski, L, Hvass, U, Paillole, C, Pansard, Y, Langlois, J, Cardiac valve replacement in relapsing polychondritis: a review. *J. Heart Valve Dis.,* 1995, 4: 227–235.
19. Buckley, LM, Ades, PA, Progressive aortic valve inflammation occurring despite apparent remission of relapsing polychondritis. *Arthritis Rheum.,* 1992, 35: 812–814.
20. Marshall, DAS, Jackson, R, Rae, AP, Capell, HA, Early aortic valve cusp rupture in relapsing polychondritis. *Ann. Rheum. Dis.,* 1992, 51: 413–415.
21. Arkin, CR, Masi, AF, Relapsing polychondritis: review of current status and case report. *Semin. Arthritis Rheum.,* 1975, 5: 41–61.
22. Sohi, GS, Desai, AM, Ward, WW, Flowers, NC, Aortic cusp involvement causing severe aortic regurgitation in a case of relapsing polychondritis. *Cathet. Cardiovasc. Diagn.,* 1981, 7: 79–86.
23. Stewart, SS, Ashizawa, T, Dudley, AW, Jr, Goldberg, JW, Idsky, MD, Cerebral vasculitis in relapsing polychondritis. *Neurology,* 1988, 38: 150–2.
24. Thuaire, C, Benamer, H, Brochet, E, Aubry, P, Hayem, G, Vissuzaine, C, et al., Etude anatomo-clinique de l'insuffisance aortique au cours d'une polychondrite atrophiante. A propos d'une observation. *Arch. Mal. Coeur.,* 1997, 90: 995–998.
25. Hughes, RAC, Berry, CL, Seifert, M, Lessof, MH, Relapsing polychondritis. *Quart. J. Med.,* 1972, 41: 363–380.

26. Alexander, CS, Derr, RF, Sako, Y, Abnormal aminoacid and lipid composition of aortic valve in relapsing polychondritis. *Am. J. Cardiol.,* 1971, 28: 337–341.
27. Hainer, JW, Hamilton, GW, Aortic abnormalities in relapsing polychondritis. Report of a case with dissecting aortic aneurysm. *N. Engl. J. Med.,* 1969, 280: 1166–1168.
28. Balsa-Criado, A, Gonzalez-Hernandez, T, Cuesta, MV, Aguado, P, Garcia, S, Gijon, J, Lupus antico-agulant in relapsing polychondritis. *J. Rheumatol.,* 1990, 17: 1426–7.
29. Firestein, GS, Gruber, HE, Weisman, MH, Zvaifler, NJ, Barber, J, O'Duffy, JD, Mouth and genital ulcers with inflamed cartilage: MAGIC syndrome. Five patients with features of relapsing polychon-dritis and Behcet's disease. *Am. J. Med.,* 1985, 79: 65–72.
30. Quere, I, Biron, C, Dubois, A, Lupus anticoagulant and thrombosis in relapsing polychondritis. *J. Rheumatol.,* 1996, 23: 946–947.
31. Wilson, GE, Hasleton, PS, Manns, JJ, Marks, JS, Relapsing polychondritis: bone marrow and circular fibrous nodules in the aorta. *Ann. Rheum. Dis.,* 1990, 49: 795–7.
32. Strobel, ES, Lang, B, Schumacher M, Peter HH, Cerebral aneurysm in relapsing polychondritis. *J. Rheumatol.,* 1992, 19: 1482–1483.
33. Joyeux, A, Vavdin, F, Caudine, M, Thevenet, A, L'atteinte artérielle ilio-fémorale dans la polychondrite atrophiante. *J. Mal. Vasc.,* 1984, 9: 207–10.
34. Cipriano, PR, Alonso, DR, Baltaxe, HA, Gay, WA, Jr, Smith, JP, Multiple aortic aneurysms in relapsing polychondritis. *Am. J. Cardiol.,* 1976, 37: 1097–1102.
35. Du Le Thi Huong, Wechsler, B, Piette, JC, Papo, T, Jaccard, A, Jault, F, et al., Aortic insufficiency and recurrent valve prosthesis dehiscence in MAGIC syndrome. *J. Rheumatol.,* 1993, 20: 397–398.
36. Rabuzzi, DD, Relapsing polychondritis. *Arch. Otolaryng.,* 1970, 91: 188–194.
37. Herman, JH, Dennis, MV, Immunopathologic studies in relapsing polychondritis. *J. Clin. Invest.,* 1973, 52: 549–558.
38. Rajapaske, DA, Bywaters, EGL, Relapsing polychondritis and pulseless disease. *Brit. Med. J.,* 1973, 4: 488–489.
39. Koifman, P, Lasry, JL, Kadouch, R, Lagneau, P, Valleteau, M, Sténoses artérielles multiples inaugurales d'une polychondrite atrophiante. A propos d'un cas. *J. Mal. Vasc.,* 1994, 19: 320–322.
40. Giordano, M, Valentini, G, Sodano, A, Relapsing polychondritis with aortic arch aneurysm and aortic arch syndrome. *Rheumatol. Int.,* 1984, 4: 191–3.
41. Conn, DL, Dickson, ER, Carpenter, HA, The association of Churg-Strauss vasculitis with temporal artery involvement, primary biliary cirrhosis, and polychondritis in a single patient. *J. Rheumatol.,* 1982, 9: 744–748.
42. Menkes, CJ, Siaud, JR, Delrieu, F, Chouraki, L, Bellaiche, D, Delbarre, F, Polychondrite chronique atrophiante: deux cas dont l'un avec cataracte et artérite des membres inférieurs. *Ann. Med. Interne,* 1970, 121: 895–904.
43. Pappas, G, Johnson, M, Mitral and aortic valvular insufficiency in chronic relapsing polychondritis. *Arch. Surg.,* 1972, 104: 712–714.
44. Piette, JC, Papo, T, Chavanon, P, Du Le Thi Huong, Francès, C, Godeau, P, Myelodysplasia and relapsing polychondritis. *J. Rheumatol.,* 1995, 22: 1208–1209.
45. Isaak, BL, Liesegang, TJ, Michet, CJ, Jr., Ocular and systemic findings in relapsing polychondritis. *Ophthalmology,* 1986, 93: 681–689.
46. Bourbigot, B, Barrier, J, Buzelin, F, Mussini-Montpellier, J, Grolleau, JY, Guenel, J, Polychondrite récidivante avec microanévrysmes rénaux et glomérulonéphrite segmentaire nécrosante. *Rev. Med. Interne,* 1984, 5: 107–109.
47. Papo, T, Piette, JC, Le, Thi Huong Du, Godeau, P, Meyer, O, Kahn, MF, et al., Antineutrophil cytoplasmic antibodies in polychondritis. *Ann. Rheum. Dis.,* 1993, 52: 384–385.
48. Giroux, L, Paquin, F, Guerard-Desjardins, MJ, Lefaivre, A, Relapsing polychondritis: an autoimmune disease. *Semin. Arthritis Rheum.,* 1983, 13: 182–187.
49. Lie, JT, Nomenclature and classification of vasculitis: plus ça change, plus c'est la même chose. *Arthritis Rheum.,* 1994, 37: 181–186.
50. Empson, M, Adelstein, S, Garsia, R, Britton, W, Relapsing polychondritis presenting with recurrent venous thrombosis in association with anticardiolipin antibody. *Lupus,* 1998, 7: 132–134.
51. Saurat, JH, Noury-Duperrat, G, Delanoe, J, Kernbaum, S, Frottier, J, Puissant, A, Les manifestations cutanées de la polychondrite atrophiante et leurs rapports avec l'aphtose. *Ann. Dermatol. Syphiligr.,* 1975, 102: 145–56.

52. Piette, JC, Papo, T, Amoura, Z, Blètry, O, Marie, L, Saada, V, et al., Syndrome des antiphospholipides et polychondrite atrophiante. *Rev. Med. Interne,* 1997, 18: 172–173.

53. Grant, A, Menkes, CJ, Polychondrite chronique atrophiante, vascularite et grossesse. *Sem. Hop. Paris,* 1991, 67: 376–379.

54. Piette, JC, El-Rassi, R, Amoura, Z, Antinuclear antibodies in relapsing polychondritis. *Ann. Rheum. Dis.,* 1999, 58: 656–657.

55. Ebringer, R, Rook, G, Swana, GT, Bottazzo, GF, Doniach, D, Autoantibodies to cartilage and type II collagen in relapsing polychondritis and other rheumatic diseases. *Ann. Rheum. Dis.,* 1981, 40: 473–479.

56. Buckner, JH, Wu, JJ, Reife, RA, Terato, K, Eyre, DR, Autoreactivity against matrilin-1 in a patient with relapsing polychondritis. *Arthritis Rheum.,* 2000, 43: 939–43.

57. Shores, J, Berger, KR, Murphy, EA, Pyeritz, RE, Progression of aortic dilatation and the benefit of long-term beta-adrenergic blockade in Marfan's syndrome. *N. Engl. J. Med.,* 1994, 330: 1335–41.

58. Haynes, BF, Kaiser-Kupfer, MI, Mason, P, Fauci, AS, Cogan Syndrome: studies in thirteen patients, long-term follow-up, and a review of the literature. *Medicine* (Baltimore), 1980, 59: 426–441.

59. Kerr, GS, Hallahan, CW, Giordano, J, Leavitt, RY, Fauci, AS, Rottem, M, Hoffman, GS, Takayasu arteritis. *Ann. Intern. Med.,* 1994, 120: 919–29.

60. Francès, C, Boisnic, S, Blétry, O, Dallot, A, Thomas, D, Kieffer, E, et al., Cutaneous manifestations of Takayasu arteritis. A retrospective study of 80 cases. *Dermatologica,* 1990; 181: 266–72.

61. Généreau, T, Lortholary, O, Pottier, MA, Michon-Pasturel, U, Ponge, T, de Wazieres, B, et al., Temporal artery biopsy: a diagnostic tool for systemic necrotizing vasculitis. *Arthritis Rheum.,* 1999, 42: 2674–81, erratum in *Arthritis Rheum.,* 2000, 43: 929.

62. Evans, JM, O'Fallon, WM, Hunder, GG, Increased incidence of aortic aneurysm and dissection in giant cell (temporal) arteritis. A population-based study. *Ann. Intern. Med.,* 1995, 122: 502–7.

63. Le Thi Huong, D, Wechsler, B, Papo, T, Piette, JC, Blètry, O, Vitoux, JM, et al., Arterial lesions in Behçet's disease. A study in 25 patients. *J. Rheumatol.,* 1995, 22: 2103–13.

64. Fernandez-Monras, F, Fornos, C, Argimon, J, Pujadas, R, Aortitis aneurismatica en el sindrome de MAGIC. *Med. Clin.* (Barc), 1997, 109: 42–43.

65. Handrock, K, Gross, WL, Relapsing polychondritis as a secondary phenomenon of primary systemic vasculitis. *Ann. Rheum. Dis.,* 1993, 52: 895–896.

66. Piette, JC, Papo, T, Le, Thi Huong, D, Meyer, O, Relapsing polychondritis as a secondary phenomenon of primary systemic vasculitis. Reply. *Ann. Rheum. Dis.,* 1993, 52: 896–7.

67. Case Records of the Massachusetts General Hospital (case 26-1985). *N. Engl. J. Med.,* 1985, 312: 1695–1703.

68. Diaz Jouanen, E, Alarcon-Segovia, D, Chondritis of the ear in Wegener's granulomatosis. *Arthritis Rheum.,* 1977, 20: 1286–1288.

69. Neilly, JB, Winter, JH, Stevenson, RD, Progressive tracheobronchial polychondritis: need for early diagnosis. *Thorax,* 1985, 40: 78–79.

70. Cauhape, P, Aumaitre, O, Papo, T, Courant, B, Hemeret, A, Kemeny, JL, et al., A diagnostic dilemna: Wegener's granulomatosis, relapsing polychondritis or both? *Eur. J. Med.,* 1993, 2: 497–498.

71. Moins-Teisserenc, HT, Gadola, SD, Cella, M, Dunbar, PR, Exley, A, Blake, N, et al., Association of a syndrome resembling Wegener's granulomatosis with low surface expression of HLA class-I molecules. *Lancet,* 1999, 354: 1598–603.

72. Stewart, KA, Mazanec, DJ, Pulse intravenous cyclophosphamide for kidney disease in relapsing polychondritis. *J. Rheumatol.,* 1992, 19: 498–500.

73. Biro, P, Rohling, R, Schmid, S, Matter, C, Lang, M, Anesthesia in a patient with acute respiratory insufficiency due to relapsing polychondritis. *J. Clin. Anesth.,* 1994, 6: 59–62.

74. Labarthe, MP, Bayle-Lebey, P, Bazex J, Cutaneous manifestations of relapsing polychondritis in a patient receiving goserelin for carcinoma of the prostate. *Dermatology,* 1997, 195: 391–394.

75. Van Decker, W, Panidis, IP, Relapsing polychondritis and cardiac valvular involvement. *Ann. Intern. Med.,* 1988, 109: 340–1.

76. Guillevin, L, Durand-Gasselin, B, Cevallos, R, Gayraud, M, Lhote, F, Callard, P, et al., Microscopic polyangiitis: clinical and laboratory findings in 85 patients. *Arthritis Rheum.,* 1999; 42: 421–30.

25 Vascular Manifestations in Behçet's Disease

A. Olcay Aydintuğ

CONTENTS

I. INTRODUCTION

Behçet's disease (BD) is a multisystem inflammatory disorder classified among the vasculitides. It is a chronic disease of a yet unknown etiology with relapses and remissions of unpredictable duration and frequency. It was first described as a triad of recurrent oral and genital ulcers and uveitis with hypopion. Various other opthalmic and cutaneous lesions as well as musculoskeletal, vascular, gastrointestinal, neurological, pulmonary, and cardiac involvement are other well-known features of BD.[1-9] Behçet's disease has a worldwide distribution but its prevalence varies widely, being most frequent in the Far East, Middle East, and the Mediterranean basin.[3] The male to female ratio ranges between 0.63–4.9:1 in large series with an almost equal sex distribution in some, but serious and life-threatening disease is mainly seen in young males.[2,3,9-14] Disease onset is most frequent in the third and fourth decades, but it may present at any age.[2,3,13,14] It is beyond the scope of this chapter to review BD, which is detailed elsewhere;[2,3,9] instead, a description of the clinical and histopathological findings related with vascular involvement, and a brief review of the pathogenesis and treatment with emphasis on the vascular aspects will be presented.

II. CLINICAL AND HISTOPATHOLOGICAL FEATURES

Vasculitis, which can affect all types and sizes of vessels, has been suggested as the common underlying mechanism of most manifestations of BD, but histologic evidence of vasculitis is not always present in all lesions. That may be due to treatment, the stage of the disease, host susceptibility, enviromental influences, or other undefined factors.[6,8,15,16] Venous involvement is more frequent than arterial. Small-vessel vasculitis is mostly observed in mucocutaneous, opthalmic, pulmonary, and gastrointestinal lesions.[3,15-17] Kidney and peripheral nerves are rarely affected in BD. Major histopathological features of BD are predominantly perivascular inflammatory infiltrates, and a tendency to thrombus formation in both veins and arteries of every size.[15,18-20] Infiltrating inflammatory cells consist of lymphocytes, monocytes, or neutrophils, or a mixture in varying degrees, depending on the stage of the lesion when the biopsies are taken.[15] Sequential histologic observation of some mucocutaneous lesions has shown that lymphocytes and monocytes predominate in the early stage, followed by neutrophil predominance in the later stages.[21] Jorizzo, however, has suggested that the lymphocyte predominance is a feature of older lesions and that earlier lesions show varying degrees of leukocytoclastic vasculitis or neutrophilic vascular reactions.[22] Immuno-histological analysis of oral ulcers has shown that most of the cells in the perivascular infiltration are CD4+ T-lymphocytes with numerous HLA-DR+ cells.[23] Leukocytoclastic vasculitis was seen in 42% of oral and 29% of genital ulcers in one study, whereas the frequency of lymphocytic vasculitis was 25% in oral and 57% in genital ulcers.[24] The authors of this study have considered vasculitis as a secondary phenomenon to intense inflammation.

In another study, 48% of patients with cutanous lesions, including erythema nodosum (EN)-like eruptions, palpable purpura, papulopustular lesions (PPL), infiltrated erythema, Sweet-syn-drome-like eruptions, and extragenital skin ulcers, have shown venulitis or phlebitis, with 65% lymphocytic and the rest being leukocytoclastic vasculitis.[17] Vasculitis is generally mild or absent in the early or late lesions of pathergy;[25,26] however, a leukocytoclastic type or a Sweet's-like vasculitis has also been reported in positive pathergy reactions.[27] In a multicenter international study, histopathologic examination of 17 spontaneous PPL revealed perivascular and interstitial mixed infiltrate with neutrophils in 12 patients, with only 3 showing fully developed leukocytoclastic vasculitis, and a perivascular infiltrate of mononuclear cells without neutrophils in only 2 patients.[28] Vasculitis of diverse morphology can be seen in the intestinal ulcers of BD in most precapillaries, capillaries, arterioles, and venules even remote from ulcers.[3] Pulmonary vasculitis (PV) is seen in less than 5% of patients and predominantly in males.[8,11,12,14,29] Hemoptysis, dyspnea, chest pain, and cough are symptoms related to PV. Hemoptysis is one of the most serious manifestations of BD, with a fatality of 30%, mostly within 2 years.[8] Pulmonary manifestations are generally accompanied by fever and active disease elsewhere.[11,29] Small and large pulmonary arteries, veins, venules, and septal capillaries may be involved, which can be complicated by thrombosis, infarction, hemorrhage, and aneurysm formation.[8,30] The inflammatory infiltrate is transmural in the smaller vessels and mainly subintimal in the large muscular pulmonary arteries.[8]

The terms "Vasculo-Behçet" or "Angio-Behçet" describe patients with aneurysm and/or occlu-sion of large blood vessels. Vasculo-Behçet is strikingly more common in males, and is one of the major causes of morbidity and mortality.[3,7,31-36] Prevalence of vasculo-behçet in some large series are 7.7%,[31] 16%,[37] 24.5%,[7] and 27.7%.[35] In a survey of 515 BD patients from Tunisia, 22% venous thrombosis and 4% large artery involvement were reported.[34] Among 137 Turkish patients with vascular involvement, 88% had venous lesions and 12% had arterial lesions.[35] Coexistence of arterial and venous involvement is not infrequent.[34,38] A higher prevalence of pathergy positivity,[35] EN,[7,35] and eye involvement[35] have been observed in patients with large vessel disease, with contradictory results in other studies.[3] The mean durations of time from the diagnosis of BD to the appearance of vascular involvement were 1.7 and 3.3 years in two studies, with vascular lesions appearing after 23 years in one patient, and after 16.3 years in another.[7,35] Vasculo-Behçet may occasionally be the presenting manifestation of BD, making the diagnosis difficult.[33,35,38-40]

Venous involvement may develop in 30 to 40% of patients and range from superficial throm-bophlebitis (STP) to deep venous thrombosis (DVT) of the extremities, superior and inferior vena cava (SVC and IVC, respectively), their branches, and cerebral veins.[2,3,5,7,16,34,35] The mean frequency of venous involvement was 24% in a review of 11 series.[2] STP is the most common form of venous involvement; it occurs mainly in the subcutaneous veins of the extremities, usually in the lower limbs.[35,39] Venipunctures can cause upper-limb STP.[2,7] STP of BD can sometimes be clinically indistinguishable from EN. We found subcutaneous TP in 66.7% of BD patients and in none of the controls when appearently EN-like lesions were analyzed histopathologically (Figure 25.1).[41]

Patients with STP tend to have DVT and systemic vessel involvement.[35] DVT may be bilateral in almost half of the patients, and both caval systems can be involved.[7,33] Fever may accompany episodes of venous thrombosis.[2] Pathologic analysis of occluded veins shows thrombosis and periphlebitis.[2] Thrombi of BD generally are strictly adherent to the vessel walls, which may well explain the rarity of pulmonary thromboembolism in BD.[2,12,29,34,35] Chronic relapsing DVTs of the

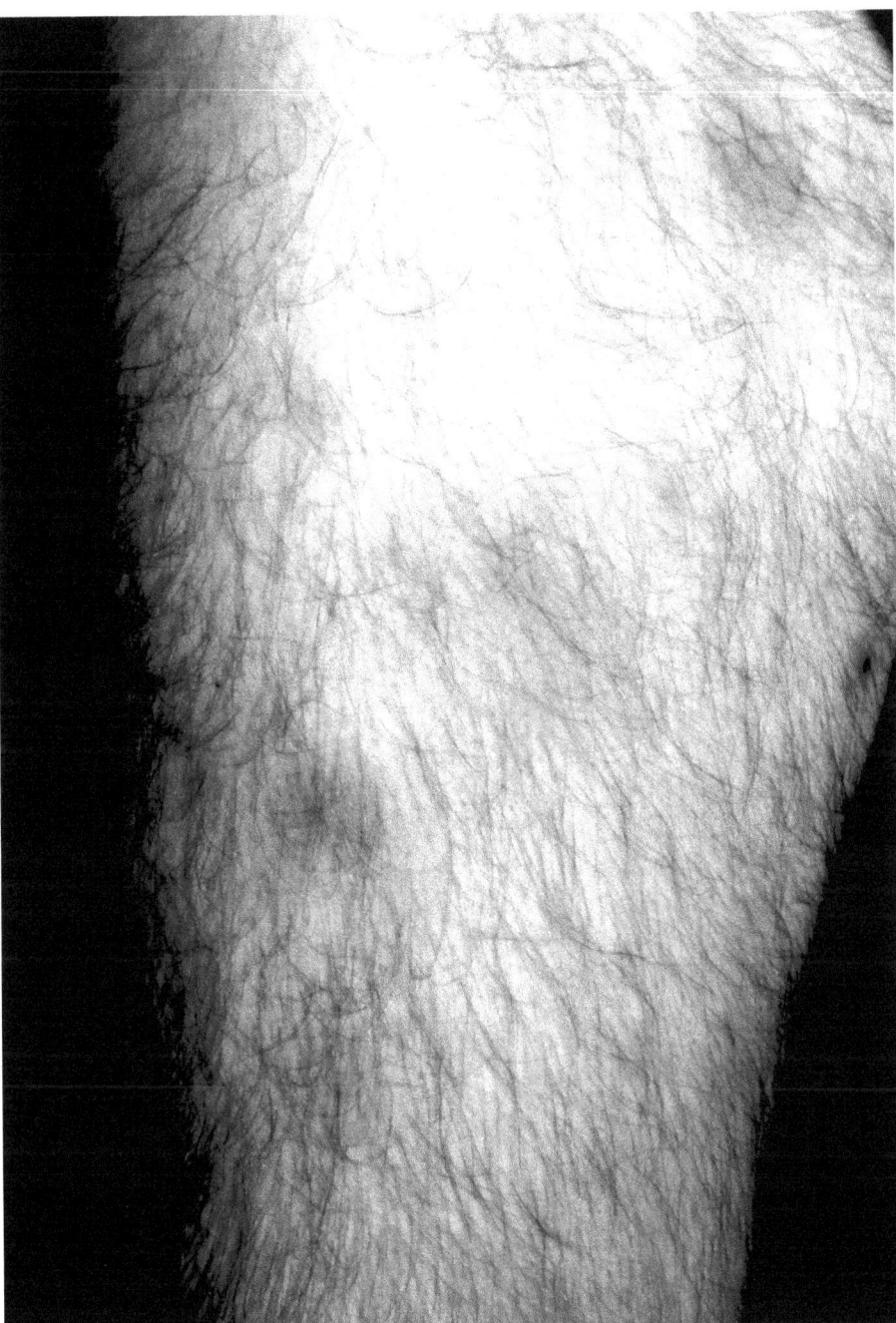

FIGURE 25.1 Subcutaneous thrombophlebitis presenting as erythema-nodosum like lesions.

lower extremities may harbor IVC thrombosis. Caval obstruction usually begins adjacent to the affected large veins, and generally presents itself with edema of the limbs and/or dilated superficial collateral veins, on the extremities or the body (Figure 25.2). Some patients with massive caval thrombosis may survive for years with few symptoms because of the development of extensive collateral veins.[2] Occluded veins can be recanalized. Postthrombotic chronic venous insufficiency and skin ulcers may develop. Noninvasive peripheral vascular examination of the lower extremities in 34 patients with BD free of vascular symptoms has revealed a more pronounced venous insuf-

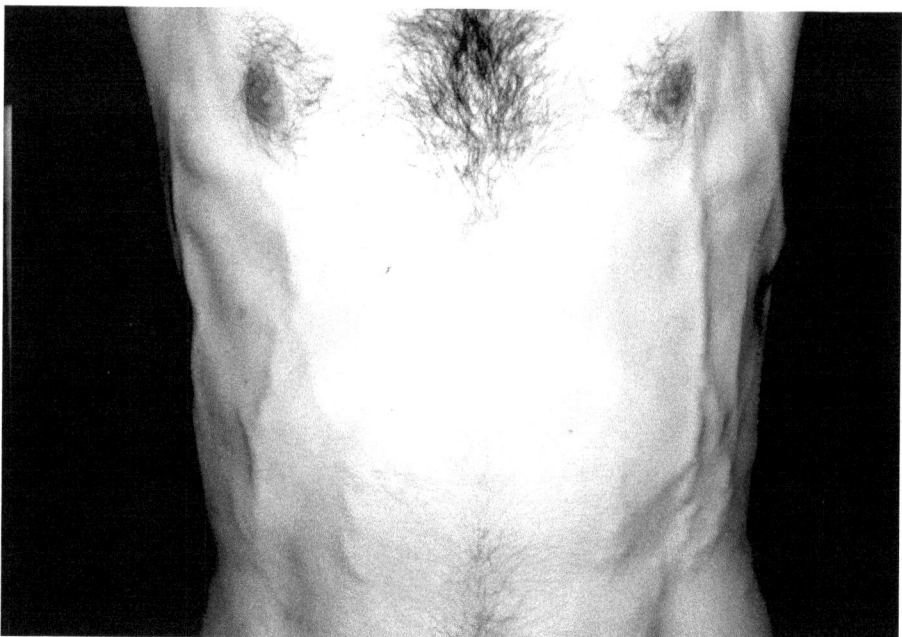

FIGURE 25.2 Collateral venous circulation on the abdominal wall caused by thrombosis of the inferior vena cava.

ficiency in BD than in the healthy controls. Asymptomatic DVT was found in three patients and in none of the controls.[42] Color Doppler USG is noninvasive and effective in diagnosing DVT, and in differentiating acute thrombosis from chronic sequela and postthrombophlebitic syndrome.

Hepatic vein thrombosis (HVT) leading to Budd-Chiari syndrome is usually related to the extension of IVC thrombosis to the ostium of the hepatic vein.[32] HVT is predominantly seen in young males, and its major features are abdominal pain, hepatomegaly, ascites, sometimes jaundice, and portal hypertension with splenomegaly. It is usually a sudden event, causing early liver failure with a 25% mortality within two weeks of onset.[32] However, spontaneous improvement with progression to liver cirrhosis may also be seen.

Cerebral vein thrombosis (CVT) can cause intracranial hypertension (pseudotumor cerebri) leading to papilledema and neurological symptoms such as persistent headache, hemi- or mono-paresis, diplopia, drowsiness, amnesia, and cranial palsies. Onset may be acute in 48 hours or progressive in weeks. The sites of CVT, in decreasing order, are superior sagittal sinus, one or both of transverse sinuses, deep cerebral veins, and caverneous sinuses. Patients with CVT are more prone to vascular involvements elsewhere. CVT has been angiographically proven in 35% of 70 patients, with BD presenting with neurological involvement and, in only one patient, it was together with meningeencephalitis.[5] Brain CT may be normal or may show smaller ventricles and focal hypodensities. An MRI is very helpful in diagnosing cerebral vasculitis or thrombosis, as well as documenting recanalization.

The prevalence of arterial occlusion in BD is 0.5%,[7] 0.25%,[37] and 1.5%[35] in some series. Arterial occlusions are generally accepted as *in situ* thrombosis associated with vasculitis. Arterial occlusions generally present acutely with serious ischemia in the distribution of the affected vessel, but chronic arterial insufficiency with insidious symptoms have also been reported.[38,43] Peripheral arterial thrombosis may cause ischemic symptoms, intermittent claudication, and sometimes frank gangrene.[38] Occlusion of the coronary, subclavian, and carotid arteries can lead to myocardial infarction, pulseless disease, and stroke, respectively. Stenosis of the femoral artery may lead to osteonecrosis of femoral head, causing hip pain.[3]

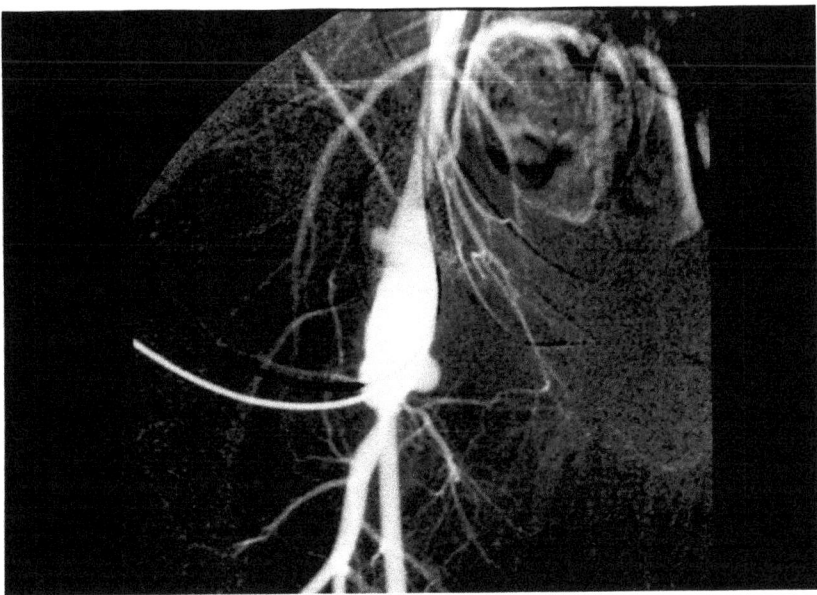

FIGURE 25.3 Right femoral arteriogram showing aneurysm of common femoral artery. (Courtesy of Prof. Dr. A. Tüzüner, Dept. of Surgery, Medical School of Ankara University.)

Large-vessel disease in the abdomen may cause mesenteric ischemia and infarction.[44,45] Hepatic arteritis may cause abdominal pain and abnormalities in liver function tests.[46] Renal artery involvement may cause hypertension. Pulmonary vascular occlusions in lobar or segmental vessels lead to pulmonary infarction and hemorrhage. Recurrent or progressive occlusions can cause irreversible pulmonary hypertension and respiratory failure. Aneurysms and arterial thromboses may coexist.[44,47] Aneurysms are more frequent than occlusions and have worse prognoses.[3,7,38,44,47] Recurrence, severity, and complications of arterial lesions generally parallel the disease activity. The most common sites for aneurysm formation are the aorta and pulmonary, femoral, popliteal, subclavian, and common carotid arteries, but every artery including, common iliac, brachial, cerebral, coronary, radial, ulnar, renal, and splenic artery, can be affected.[3,16,20,35,40,44]

Peripheral aneurysms generally appear as pulsatile and tender swellings.[18,48,49] The disappearance of an aneurysmal pulsation points to spontaneous thrombosis.[38] Aneurysms are mostly saccular, but may be dissecting as well[20] (Figure 25.3). Both true or false aneurysms can be seen.[19,34,44] Aneurysms tend to be multiple, recurrent, and prone to rupture.[34,48-51] Rupture of true aneurysms may lead to pseudoaneurysms.[50] Aneurysmal rupture is the leading cause of death.[3] Angiographically normal arteries may develop aneurysm in a week's time.[51] Cultures of aneurysms and thrombi have been negative.[18,37,53] Pulmonary aneurysms are usually bilateral, with partial thrombosis in some.[8,12,19,29] They can erode into the bronchial tree causing arterio-bronchial fistula and hemoptysis, which may require transfusion and may even lead to death. Pulmonary aneurysms may be accompanied by other aneurysms[40,53] and venous thrombosis[2,12,19,29,53] elsewhere in the body. Thrombophlebitis may precede the pulmonary manifestations by years.[8] Pulmonary aneurysms can be seen as unilateral or bilateral, mainly hilar but also peripheral, nodular, or ill-defined noncavitating opacities in chest radiographs.[12,29] Areas of hemorrhage or infarction may appear as transient micro- or macronodular infiltrates. Ventilation-perfusion scans may be misleading in such cases and may cause an erroneous diagnosis of pulmonary embolism with infarction, especially if accompanied by DVT elsewhere. Dynamic CT, high-resolution CT (HRCT), and MRI are helpful in diagnosing pulmonary lesions.[11] Pulmonary angiography not only proves arterial aneurysms and thromboses, but may show pulmonary hypertension by concomitant right-heart catheterization as well.[19] Aneurysms are probably the result of intense active inflammation in the media and adventitia along with

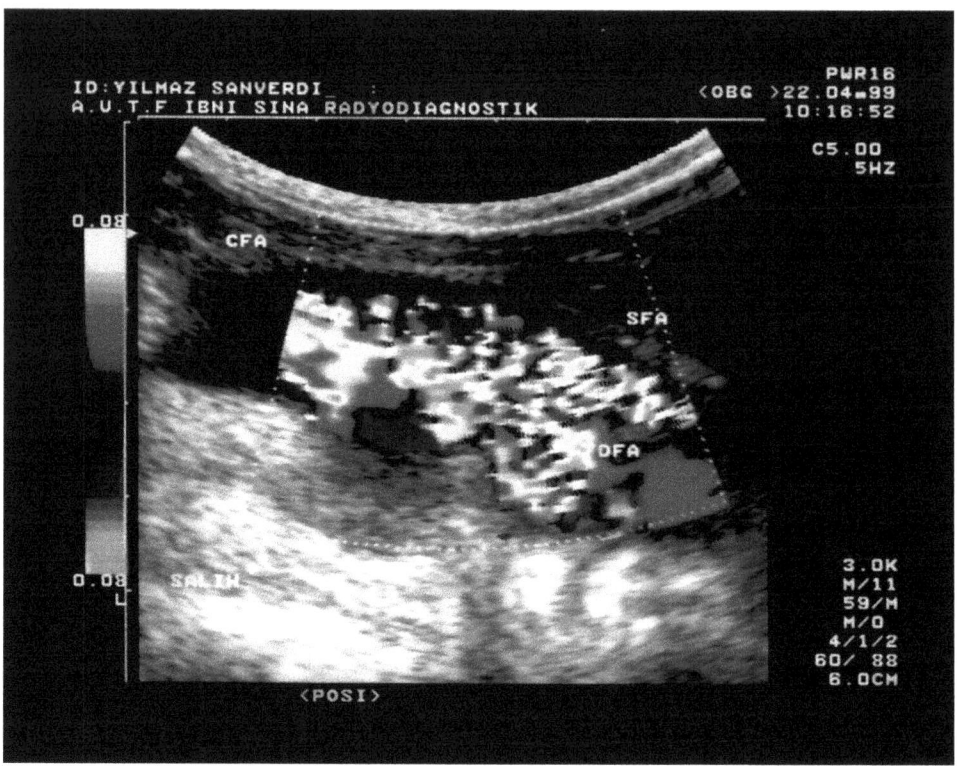

FIGURE 25.4 Doppler USG showing thrombus on the posterior wall of the aneurysmatic dilatation of the femoral artery in Figure 25.3.

deterioration of the vasa vasorum. Perivascular lymphoplasmocytic infiltration and obliterative endarteritis of the vasa vasorum, with or without fibrinoid necrosis, lead to severe destruction, fibrous thickening, and weakening of the arterial wall.[2,8,20,50,54] Electron microscopy has shown occluded capillaries by bulging degenerated or even frankly necrotic endothelial cells in the aneurysmal wall with perivascular infiltrates of lymphocytes and polymorphonuclear leukocytes.[48] Only fibrosis and thrombosis can be seen in later stages of an aneurysm.[55] Aortic wall calcification has been described in BD.[3] A pathergy-like phenomenon can affect large vessels. Arterial punctures for angiography or surgical interventions may cause further aneurysms.[56] The use of intravenous digital substraction angiography can help to prevent this unpleasant risk. MR angiography can adequately demonstrate the arterial aneurysms of BD, avoiding the risks of pseudoaneurysm formation at the puncture site for arterial angiography, and TP at the puncture site for I.V DSA.[57] Angiographic features of BD by themselves are not specific. Color Doppler USG is also helpful in demonstrating peripheral aneurysms and thromboses (Figure 25.4). These data strongly suggest that differential diagnosis of large-vessel occlusions or aneurysms unaccounted for by risk factors, especially in a young male from a certain geographic or ethnic origin, must include BD.

Although cardiac disease is randomly recognized in BD in antemortem studies, it may cause morbidity and mortality. Intracardiac thrombi,[35,58] ventricular aneurysms, and myocardial infarction due to coronary arteritis and occlusion can be seen. Silent myocardial ischemia diagnosed by abnormal Holter electrocardiography and thallium myocardial perfusion in the presence of normal coronary angiograms was observed in 25% of asymptomatic patients, most of whom had vasculo-Behçet which could be evaluated as a manifestation of probable microvascular vasculitis, although without histologic confirmation.[59] Endomyocardial fibrosis predominantly involving the right ventricle has been found to be closely linked with valvulopathy and intraventricular thrombus in patients

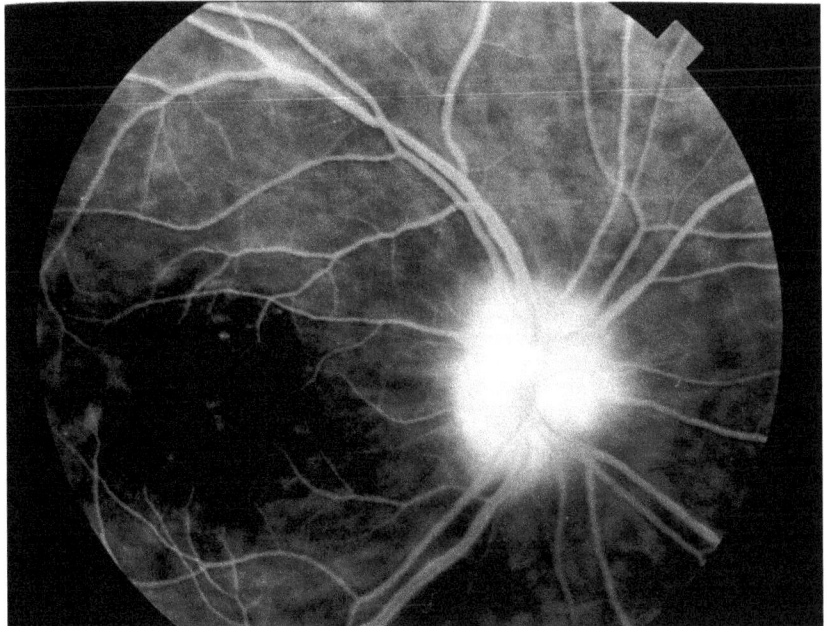

FIGURE 25.5 Fundus fluorescein angiography showing dye leakage from vasculitic vessels and hyperfluorescence at the optic disc and macula due to retinal vasculitis. (Courtesy of Prof. Dr. L. S. Atmaca, Dept. of Opthalmology, Medical School of Ankara University.)

mostly with vasculo-Behçet pattern, which implicates some sequela of vasculitis of endocardium or myocardium.[60]

Obliterative, necrotizing vasculitis of retinal veins and arteries and retinal infarcts are the main histopathological features of posterior eye involvement.[15,61] Anterior uveitis is usually accompanied by retinal vasoocclusive disease.[62] Vasculitis may present either as a periphlebitis or arteriitis obliterans, which can lead to retinal edema, exudation, and vitreus hemorrhage.[61] Repeated attacks of retinal vaso-occlusive disease can result in sight-threatening complications in almost 25% of patients.[2] Optic atrophy generally occurs at a late stage, possibly due to obliterative vasculitis occurring in the circulation-to-nerve head.[61] The risk of eye involvement, which is high in the first two years of disease, has been found higher in patients with accompanying vascular thrombosis and CNS involvement.[63] Fundus fluorescein angiography can show leakage in opthalmoscopically normal-appearing vessels, and is very helpful in early diagnosis and follow-up of retinal vasculitis[61] (Figure 25.5).

Color flow Doppler ultrasonography of penile vasculature has revealed mostly slight arterial insufficiency and venous leakage in some patients, which may implicate involvement of penile vessels.[64]

III. PATHOGENESIS

The quite frequent coexistence of thrombosis and arterial aneurysms implicates a primary vascular pathology rather than a major coagulation defect in BD. No single abnormality has been shown to account for the increased tendency to thrombus formation in BD.[65] Antiphospholipid antibodies do not seem to play a major pathogenetic role in BD.[66,67] Antineutrophil cytoplasmic antibodies (ANCA) are generally negative in BD.[66,68] Several cytokines and other soluble activation markers are increased.[69-72] An exogenous agent in a genetically predisposed patient may stimulate mononuclear cells to secrete the proinflammatory cytokines, causing further mononuclear as well as endothelial activation with a further flow of more cytokines, other inflammatory mediators, and increased expression of cellular and soluble adhesion molecules which can attract and activate lymphocytes and neutrophils.[72,73] Such an interaction may result in damage and/or functional impairment of the vascular wall and a tendency to thrombosis. Several functional and morphological abnormalities of the vascular endothelium have been described in BD. These include impairment of prostacyclin production,[74] significantly higher plasma ET-1,2[75] and von Willebrand factor levels in patients with vascular involvement,[76] elevated levels of soluble intercellular adhesion molecule-1 correlating with disease activity,[77] and higher prevalences of retinal vasculitis and acute thrombotic events in patients with antiendothelial cell antibodies (AECA) than in those without AECA.[66] These may all be secondary to endothelial cell activation and/or damage, or may be markers of inflammation rather than the cause of it.

Higher prevalances of Factor V Leiden (FVL) mutation have been reported in BD.[78,79] FVL mutation was found more frequently in BD patients with venous thrombosis when compared with patients without thrombosis,[78-80] but further investigations are necessary as no FVL mutation was found in BD in a study from France.[81]

IV. TREATMENT

Treatment is generally symptomatic and individualized. Although usually given to every patient, colchicine is effective for mucocutaneous lesions and arthralgia.[82] Colchicine may also help to prevent amyloidosis.[83] Severe and resistant vasculitic mucocutaneous lesions may benefit from steroids (20 mg/day) and azathioprine (AZA) (2.5 mg/kg/day).[9] Thalidomide, 100 to 300 mg/day, can be effective as well, but its teratogenicity is a major concern.[85] Steroids are mostly effective in the control of acute eye lesions, but their long-term effectiveness in disease control is not very clear.[9] High-dose IV pulse methylprednisolone may reverse severe vision loss in acute Behçet retinitis.[85] AZA 2.5 mg/kg/day is effective in maintaining visual acuity and preventing new eye disease.[86] Cyclosporine A, 5 mg/kg/day, is quite effective in rapid control of eye lesions, but its effectiveness may diminish over time.[87] Central nervous system involvement is generally treated with IV 1 g methylprednisolone pulses for 3 to 7 days followed by high-dose steroids (0.5–1 mg/kg/day, depending on the type and severity of the lesions) and immunosuppressives such as AZA or 2–2.5 mg/kg/day oral, or 500 to 750 mg/m^2 monthly pulses of IV cyclophosphamide.[9] High-dose steroids, along with immunosuppressives such as cyclophosphamide, are recommended for pulmonary vasculitis before irreversible damage to the arterial walls develops.[11,12,29] Some add colchicine, acetylsalicylicacid (ASA), and dipyridamole to this combination.[11] FK-506, has been effective in controlling early pulmonary small-vessel vasculitis at a dose of 0.1 mg/kg/day for eight weeks.[30] Cyclosporine A has also been suggested for pulmonary BD.[88]

The optimal treatment of major vein thrombosis is still controversial. The proposed treatments range from platelet antiaggregating drugs to anticoagulants. Low-dose ASA is recommended by Yazici in thrombophlebitis, whereas Koç et al. avoid it.[9,35] Some authors recommend anticoagulants for major vein thrombosis,[35,89] whereas others find heparin and oral anticoagulants potentially hazardous and suggest avoidance as they may cause bleeding in this vasculitic disorder.[90] Anticoagulants alone have no therapeutic effect on the vasculitic process. Furthermore, as mentioned earlier, the risk of pulmonary embolism seems to be very low in BD. Yazici recommends AZA for TP to suppress the disease activity in general.[9]

Although suggesting caution on the risk of bleeding from possible accompanying arterial aneurysms or cerebral microhematoma, Wechsler et al. have reported good results with a combined therapy of steroids and prolonged anticoagulants in patients with CVT.[5] CVT, however, may occur despite adequate chronic oral anticoagulation for limb thrombosis.[5] Multichamber cardiac thrombi have been reported to disappear without any hemorrhage, as detected by echocardiography, in a patient with pulmonary aneurysm and CVT after treatment with heparin, prednisolone, and cyclophosphamide.[58] Any BD patient presenting with hemoptysis and TP/DVT should be evaluated for PV and arterial aneurysm before considering anticoagulation as this may be harmful for PV and can cause severe hemorrhage.[8] Successful lysis of acute caval thrombosis with thrombolytic agents has been described in some cases.[91,92] Arterial lesions including pulmonary aneurysms are treated with a combination of systemic steroids (prednisolone 1 mg/kg/day) and immunosupressives such as oral or IV pulse cyclophosphamide.[9,12,55] Le Thi Huong et al. suggest avoidance of high-dose steroids for isolated arterial occlusions as their results are not good.[47] Steroids and immunosupressives usually bring symptomatic relief with an unknown effect on the development of further vascular lesions.[35] Two years of clinical remission is generally recommended before stopping immunosuppressives in serious involvements. Surgery is indicated for aneurysms whenever feasible because they can rupture. The operative therapy of arterial aneurysms, pseudoaneurysms, and thromboses is resection, or exclusion by bypass grafting. There is a tendency to disruption, thrombosis, and new aneurysm formation in the graft and operated arteries.[18,40,49,50,52,54,55] Major surgical operations are better avoided before appropriate treatment for BD is given unless a life threatening condition exists. Wound healing does not seem to be altered in BD.[93] Postoperative steroids are advised to prevent relapses of arterial lesions, with better results if steroids are combined with immunosuppressives.[47] This approach is not without risk, warranting careful follow-up. Some recommend postoperative anticoagulation in patients with bypass for lower-limb arterial lesions.[47] A judgment balancing the risk of graft thrombosis against the risk of recurrent pseudoaneurysm formation after arterial reconstruction is essential when deciding on anticoagulants.[49]

REFERENCES

1. Behçet, H., Über residivierende aphtose, durch ein virus verursachte Geschwure am Mund, am Auge und an den Genitalien, *Dermatol. Wochenschr.*, 105, 1152, 1937.
2. Chajek, T., Fainaru, M., Behçet's disease. Report of 41 cases and a review of the literature, *Medicine*, 54, 179, 1975.
3. Shimizu, T., Ehrlich, G. E., Inaba, G., Hayashi, K., Behçet Disease (Behçet Syndrome), *Semin. Arthritis Rheum.*, 8, 223, 1979.
4. Boe, J., Dalgaard, J., Scott, D., Mucocutaneous-ocular syndrome with intestinal involvement. A clinical and pathological study of four fatal cases, *Am. J. Med.*, 25, 857, 1958.
5. Wechsler, B., Vidailhet, M., Piette, J. C., Bousser, M. G., Isola, D., Bletry, O., Godeau, P., Cerebral sinus thrombosis in Behçet's disease. Clinical study and long-term follow-up of 25 cases, *Neurology*, 42, 614, 1992.
6. Hadfield, M. G., Aydin, F., Lippman, H. R., Kubal, W. S., Sanders, K. M., Neuro-Behçet's Disease, *Clin. Neuropathol.*, 15, 249, 1996.
7. Müftüoğlu, A. Ü., Yurdakul, S., Yazici, H., Tüzün, Y., Pazarli, H., Altuğ, E., Özyazgan, Y., Serdaroğlu, S., Özdoğan, H., Vascular involvement in Behçet's disease — a review of 129 cases, in *Recent Advances in Behçet's Disease*, 103, Lehner, T., Barnes, C. G., Eds., Royal Society of Medicine Services Limited, London, 1986, 256–260.
8. Raz, I., Okon, E., Chajek-Shaul, T., Pulmonary manifestations in Behçet's disease, Chest, 95, 585, 1989.
9. Yazici, H., Yurdakul, S., Hamuryudan, S., Behçet's syndrome, in *Oxford Textbook of Rheumatology*, 2nd edition, Maddison, P. J., Isenberg, D. A., Woo, P., Glass, D. N., Eds., Oxford, Hong Kong, 1998, 1394-1402.
10. Yazici, H., Tüzün, Y., Pazarli, H., Yurdakul, S., Özyazgan, N., Özdoğan, H., Serdaroğlu, S., Ersanli, M., Ülkü, B. Y., Müftüoğlu, A. Ü., Influence of age of onset and patient's sex and the prevalence and severity of manifestations of Behçet's syndrome, *Ann. Rheum. Dis.*, 43, 783, 1984.
11. Erkan, F., Çavdar, T., Pulmonary vasculitis in Behçet's disease, *Am. Rev. Respir. Dis.*, 146, 232, 1992.
12. Hamuryudan, V., Yurdakul, S., Moral, F., Numan, F., Tüzün, F., Tüzün, H., Tüzüner, N., Mat, C., Tüzün, Y., Özyazgan, Y., Yazici, H., Pulmonary arterial aneurysms in Behçet's Syndrome, *Br. J. Rheumatol.*, 33, 48, 1994.

13. Bang, D., Yoon, K. H., Chung, H. G., Choi, E. H., Lee, E. S., Lee, S., Epidemiological and clinical features of Behçet's disease in Chorea, *Yonsei Med. J.,* 38, 428, 1997.
14. Gürler, A., Boyvat, A., Türsen, Ü., Clinical manifestations of Behçet's disease. An analysis of 2147 patients, *Yonsei Med. J.,* 38, 423, 1997.
15. Lakhanpal, S., O'Duffy, J. D., Lie, J. T., Pathology, in *Behçet's Disease: A Contemporary Synopsis,* Plotkin, G. R., Calabro, J. J., O'Duffy, J. D., Eds., *Futura,* Mount Kisko, 1988, 101–142.
16. Lie, J. T., Vascular involvement in Behçet's disease: Arterial and venous and vessels of all size, *J. Rheumatol.,* 19, 341, 1992.
17. Chen, K. R., Kawahara, Y., Miyakawa, S., Nishikawa, T., Cutaneous vasculitis in Behçet's disease: a clinical and histopathologic study of 20 patients, *J. Am. Acad. Dermatol.,* 36, 689, 1997.
18. Smith, J. E., Abulafi, M., McPherson, G. A., Allison, D. J., Mansfield, A. O., False aneurysm of the abdominal aorta in Behçet's disease, *Eur. J. Vasc. Surgery,* 5, 481, 1991.
19. Durieux, P., Bletry, O., Huchon, G., Wechsler, B., Chretien, J., Godeau, P., Multiple pulmonary aneurysms in Behçet's disease and Hughes-Stovin syndrome, *Am. J. Med.,* 71, 736, 1981.
20. Matsumoto, T., Uekusa, T., Fukuda, Y., Vasculo-Behçet's disease, *Hum. Pathol.,* 22, 45, 1991.
21. Efthimiou, J., Addison, I. E., Johnson, B. V., *In vivo* leucocyte migration in Behçet's syndrome, *Ann. Rheum. Dis.,* 48, 206, 1989.
22. Jorizzo, J. L., Behçet's disease. An update based on the 1985 International conference in London, *Arch. Dermatol.,* 122, 556, 1986.
23. Çelenligil, H., Kansu, E., Ruacan, R., Eratalay, K., Characterization of peripheral blood lymphocytes and immunohistological analysis of oral ulcers in Behçet's disease, in *Behçet's Disease. Basic and Clinical Aspects,* O'Duffy, J. D., Kökmen, E., Eds., Marcel Dekker, New York, 1991.
24. Chun, S. I., Su, W. P., Lee, S., Histopathologic study of cutaneous lesions in Behçet's syndrome, *J. Dermatol.,* 17, 333, 1990.
25. Gül, A., Esin, S., Dilsen, N., Koniçe, M., Wigzell, H., Biberfeld, P., Immunohistology of skin pathergy test reaction in Behçet's disease, *Br. J. Dermatol.,* 132, 901, 1995.
26. Ergun, T., Gürbüz, O., Harvell, J., Jorizzo, J., White, W., The histopathology of pathergy: a chronologic study of skin hyperreactivity in Behçet's disease, *Int. J. Dermatol.,* 37, 929, 1998.
27. Jorizzo, J. L., Solomon, A. R., Cavalho, T., Behçet's syndrome: immunopathologic and histopathologic assessment of pathergy lesions is useful in diagnosis and follow-up, *Arch. Pathol. Lab. Med.,* 109, 747, 1985.
28. Jorizzo, J. P., Abernethy, J. L., White, W. L., Mangelsdorf, H. C., Zouboulis, C. C., Sarica, R., Gaffney, K., Mat, C., Yazici, H., Al Ialaan, A., Assad-Khalil, S. H., Kaneko, F., Jorizzo, E. A. F., Mucocutaneous criteria for the diagnosis of Behçet's disease: An analysis of clinicopathologic data from multiple international centers, *J. Am. Acad. Dermatol.,* 32, 968, 1995.
29. Eftimiou, J., Johnston, C., Spiro, S. G., Turner-Warwick, M. T., Pulmonary disease in Behçet's syndrome, *Quarter. J. Med.,* 227, 259, 1986.
30. Koga, T., Yano, T., Ichikawa, Y., Oizumi, K., Mochizuki, M., Pulmonary infiltrates recovered by FK506 in a patient with Behçet's disease. *Chest,* 104, 309, 1993.
31. Masuda, K., Inaba, G., Mizushima, Y., Yaoita, H., A nationwide survey of Behçet's disease in Japan, clinical survey, *Jpn. J. Opthalmol.,* 19, 278, 1975.
32. Bismuth, E., Hadengue, A., Hammel, P., Benhamou, J. P., Hepatic vein thrombosis in Behçet's disease, *Hepatology,* 11, 969, 1990.
33. Kansu, E., Özer, F. L., Akalin, E., Güler, Y., Zileli, T., Tanman, E., Kaplaman, E., Müftüoğlu, E., Behçet's syndrome with the obstruction of venae cavae, *Quar. J. Med.,* XLI, 151, 1972.
34. Hamza, M., Angio Behçet, in *Proceedings of the 6th International Conference on Behçet's Disease,* Godeau, P., Wechsler, B., Eds., Elsevier, Amsterdam, 1993.
35. Koç, Y., Güllü, I., Akpek, G., Akpolat, T., Kansu, E., Kiraz, S., Batman, F., Kansu, T., Balkanci, F., Akkaya, S., Telatar, H., Zileli, T., Vascular involvement in Behçet's disease, *J. Rheumatol.,* 19, 402, 1992.
36. Yazici, H., Basaran, G., Hamuryudan, V., Hizli, N., Yurdakul, S., Mat, C., Tüzün, Y., Özyazgan, Y., Dimitriyadis, I., The ten-year mortality in Behçet's syndrome, *Br. J. Rheumatol.,* 35, 139, 1996.
37. Kuzu, M. A., Özarslan, C., Köksoy, C., Gürler, A., Tüzüner, A., Vascular involvement in Behçet's disease: eight-year audit, *World J. Surg.,* 18, 948, 1994.

38. Sechas, M. N., Liapis, C. D., Gougoulakis, A. G., Mandrekas, D. P., Fotiadis, C. I., Vaiopoulos, G. A., Vascular manifestations of Behçet's disease, *Int. Angiol.,* 8, 145, 1989.

39. Haim, S., Sobel, J. D., Friedman-Birnbaum, R., Thrombophlebitis. A cardinal symptom of Behçet's syndrome, *Acta Dermato Vener.,* 54, 299, 1974.

40. Sheriff, A., Stewart, P., Mendes, D. M., The repetitive vascular catastrophes of Behçet's disease. A case report with review of the literature, *Ann. Vasc. Surg.,* 6, 85, 1992.

41. Sentürk, T., Aydintuğ, O., Kuzu, I., Düzgün, N., Tokgöz, G., Gürler, A., Tulunay, Ö., Adhesion molecule expression in erythema-nodosum-like lesions in Behçet's disease, *Rheumatol. Int.,* 18, 51, 1998.

42. Kuzu, A., Köksoy, C., Özaslan, C., Gürler, A., Tüzüner, A., Evaluation of peripheral vascular system disorders in vascular symptom-free Behçet's disease, *Cardiovasc. Surg.,* 4, 381, 1996.

43. Cooper, A. M., Naughton, M. N., Williams, B. D., Chronic arterial occlusion associated with Behçet's disease, *Br. J. Rheumatol.,* 33, 170, 1994.

44. Park, J. H., Han, M. C., Bettmann, M. A., Arterial manifestations of Behçet's disease, *Am. J. Radiol.,* 143, 821, 1984.

45. Chubachi, A., Saitoh, K., Imii, H., Miura, A. B., Kotanagi, H., Abe, T., Matsumoto, T., Case report: intestinal infarction after an aneurysmal occlusion of superior mesenteric artery in a patient with Behçet's disease, *Am. J. Med. Sci.,* 306, 376, 1993.

46. Mathur, A. K., Maslow, J., Urffer, P. A., Hepatic arteritis in Behçet's disease, *J. Rheumatol.,* 16, 11, 1989.

47. Le Thi Huong, D., Wechsler, B., Papo, T., Piette, J. C., Bletry, O., Vitoux, J. M., Kieffer, E., Godeau, P., Arterial lesions in Behçet's disease. A study in 25 patients, *J. Rheumatol.,* 22, 2103, 1995.

48. Freyrie, A., Paragona, O., Cenacchi, G., Pasquinelli, G., Guiducci, G., Faggioli, G. L., True and false aneurysms in Behçet's disease: Case report with ultrastructural observations, *J. Vasc. Surg.,* 17, 762, 1993.

49. Jenkins, A. McL., Macpherson, A. I. S., Nolan, B., Housley, E., Peripheral aneurysms in Behçet's disease, *Br. J. Surg.,* 63, 199, 1976.

50. Enoch, B. A., Castillo-Olivares, J. L., Khoo, T. C. L., Grainger, R. G., Henry, L., Major vascular complications in Behçet's syndrome, *Postgrad. Med. J.,* 44, 453, 1968.

51. Bartlett, S. T., McCarthy, W. J., Palmer, A. S., Flinn, W. R., Bergan, J. J., Yao, J. S. T., Multiple aneurysms in Behçet's disease, *Arch. Surg.,* 123, 1004, 1988.

52. Bedirhan, M. A., Onursal, E., Barlas, C., Yilmazbahan, D., Unusual complication of femoro-popliteal saphenous vein bypass-aneurysm formation, *Eur. J. Vasc. Surg.,* 5, 583, 1991.

53. Salamon, F., Weinberger, A., Nili, M., Avidor, I., Neuman, M., Zelikovsky, A., Levy, M. J., Pinkhas, J., Massive hemoptysis complicating Behçet's syndrome: The importance of early pulmonary angiography and operation, *Ann. Thorac. Surg.,* 45, 566, 1988.

54. Little, A., Zarins, C., Abdominal aortic aneurysm and Behçet's disease, *Surgery,* 91, 359, 1982.

55. Christensen, P. A., Tvedegaard, E., Strandgaard, S., Thomsen, B. S., Behçet's syndrome presenting with peripheral arterial aneurysms, *Scand. J. Rheumatol.,* 26, 386, 1997.

56. Kingston, M., Ratcliffe, J. R., Alltree, M., Merendino, K. A., Aneurysm after arterial puncture in Behçet's disease, *BMJ,* 11, 1766, 1979.

57. Berkmen, T., MR angiography of aneurysms in Behçet's disease: a report of four cases, *J. Comput. Assist. Tomogr.,* 22, 202, 1998.

58. Vanhaleweyk, G., El-Ramahi, K. M., Hazmi, M., Sieck, J. O., Zaman, L., Fawzy, M., Right atrial, right ventricular and left ventricular thrombi in Behçet's disease, *European Heart Journal,* 11, 957, 1990.

59. Güllü, I. H., Benekli, M., Müderrisoğlu, H., Oto, A., Kansu, E., Kabakçi, G., Oram, E., Bekdik, C., Silent myocardial ischemia in Behçet's disease, *J. Rheumatol.,* 23, 323, 1996.

60. Le Thi Huong, D., Wechsler, B., Papo, T., de Zettere, D., Bletry, O., Hernigou, A., Delcourt, A., Godeou, P., Piette, J. C., Endomyocardial fibrosis in Behçet's disease, *Ann. Rheum. Dis.,* 56, 205, 1997.

61. Atmaca, L., Özmert, E., Michelson, J. B., Friedlaender, M. H., Visualisation of the vasculitis of Behçet's disease, in *Behçet's Disease. Basic and Clinical Aspects,* O'Duffy, J. D., Kökmen, E., Eds., Marcel Dekker, New York, 1991.

62. Nussenblatt, R. B., Uveitis in Behçet's disease, *Int. Rev. Immunol.,* 14, 67, 1997.

63. Demiroğlu, H., Barista, I., Dündar, S., Risk factor assessment and prognosis of eye involvement in Behçet's disease in Turkey, *Opthalmology*, 104, 701, 1997.
64. Sarica, K., Süzer, O., Gürler, A., Baltaci, S., Özdiler, E., Dinçel, Ç., Urological evaluation of Behçet patients and the effect of colchicine on fertility, *Eur. Urol.*, 27, 39, 1995.
65. Hampton, K. K., Chamberlain, M. A., Menon, D. K., Davies, J. A., Coagulation and fibrinolytic activity in Behçet's disease, *Thromb. Haemostasis*, 66, 292, 1991.
66. Aydıntuğ, A. O., Tokgöz, G., D'Cruz, D. P., Gürler, A., Cervera, R., Düzgün, N., Atmaca, L. S., Khamashta, M. A., Hughes, G. R. V., Antibodies to endothelial cells in patients with Behçet's disease, *Clin. Immunol. Immunopathol.*, 67, 157, 1993.
67. Karmochkine, M., Boffa, M. C., Wechsler, B., Piette, J. C., Godeau, P., Absence of antiphospholipid antibodies in Behçet's disease, *Ann. Rheum. Dis.*, 52, 623, 1993.
68. Hamza, M., Meyer, O., Negative antineutrophil cytoplasmic antibodies in BD, *Ann. Rheum. Dis.*, 49, 817, 1990.
69. Akoğlu, T. F., Direskeneli, H., Yazici, H., Lawrence, R., TNF, soluble IL-2R and soluble CD-8 in Behçet's disease, *J. Rheumatol.*, 17, 1107, 1990.
70. Sayinalp, N., Özcebe, O. I., Özdemir, O., Haznedaroğlu, İ. C., Dündar, S., Kirazli, S., Cytokines in Behçet's disease, *J. Rheumatol.*, 23, 321, 1996.
71. Mege, J. L., Dilsen, N., Sanguedolce, V., Gül, A., Bongrand, P., Roux, H., Öcal, L., Inanç, M., Capo, C., Overproduction of monocyte derived tumor necrosis factor alpha, interleukin (IL) 6, IL-8 and increased neutrophil superoxide generation in Behçet's disease. A comparative study with Familial Mediterranean Fever and healthy subjects, *J. Rheumatol.*, 20, 1544, 1993.
72. Sahin (Özgün), S., Lawrence, C., Direskeneli, H., Hamuryudan, V., Yazici, H., Akoğlu, T., Monocyte activity in Behçet's disease, *Br. J. Rheumatol.*, 35, 424, 1996.
73. Emmi, L., Brugnolo, F., Salvati, G., Marchione, T., Immunopathological aspects of Behçet's disease (editorial), *Clin. Exp. Rheumatol.*, 13, 687, 1995.
74. Kansu, E., Sahin, G., Sahin, F., Sivri, B., Sayek, I., Batman, F., Impaired prostacyclin synthesis by vessel walls in Behçet's disease, *Lancet*, 15, 1154, 1986.
75. Koç, Y., Kansu, E., Koray, Z., Duru, S., Batman, F., Kansu, T., Akkaya, S., Eldem, B., Sahin, G., Telatar, H., Zileli, T., Endothelin-1,2 levels in Behçet's disease, in *Behçet's Disease. Proceedings of the 6th International Conference on Behçet's Disease*, Godeau, P., Wechsler, B., Eds., Elsevier, Amsterdam, 1993.
76. Yazici, H., Hekim, N., Özbakir, F., Yurdakul, S., Tüzün, Y., Pazarli, H., Müftüoğlu, A., Von Willebrand factor in Behçet's syndrome, *J. Rheumatol.*, 14, 305, 1987.
77. Aydıntuğ, A. O., Tokgöz, G., Özoran, K., Düzgün, N., Gürler, A., Tutkak, H., Elevated levels of soluble intercellular adhesion molecule-1 correlate with disease activity in patients with Behçet's Disease, *Rheumatol. Int.*, 15, 75, 1995.
78. Gül, A., Özbek, U., Öztürk, C., İnanç, M., Koniçe, M., Özçelik, T., Coagulation factor V gene mutation increases the risk of venous thrombosis in Behçet's disease, *Br. J. Rheumatol.*, 35, 1178, 1996.
79. Öner, A. F., Gürgey, A., Gürler, A., Mesci, A., Factor V Leiden mutation in patients with Behçet's disease, *J. Rheumatol.*, 25, 496, 1998.
80. Mammo, L., Al-Dalaan, A., Bahabri, S. S., Saour, J. N., Association of Factor V Leiden with Behçet's disease, *J. Rheumatol.*, 24, 2196, 1997.
81. Lesprit, P., Wechsler, B., Piette, J. C., Du-Boutin, L. T., Godeau, P., Alhenc-Gelas, M., Aiach, M., Activated protein C resistance caused by factor V Arg 506.- Gln mutation has no role in Behçet's disease, *Ann. Rheum. Dis.*, 54, 860, 1995.
82. Aktulga, E., Altaç, M., Müftüoğlu, A., Özyazgan, Y., Pazarli, H., Tüzün, Y., Yalçin, B., Yazici, H., Yurdakul, S., A double-blind study of colchicine in Behçet's disease, *Haematologica*, 65, 399, 1980.
83. Dilsen, N., Koniçe, M., Aral, O., Erbengi, T., Uysal, V., Koçak, N., Özdoğan, E., Behçet's disease associated with amyloidosis in Turkey and in the world, *Ann. Rheum. Dis.*, 47, 157, 1988.
84. Hamuryudan, V., Mat, C., Saip, S., Özyazgan, Y., Siva, A., Yurdakul, S., Zwingenberger, K., Yazici H., Thalidomide in the treatment of the mucocutaneous lesions of the Behçet's syndrome. A randomized, double-blind, placebo controlled trial, *Ann. Intern. Med.*, 128, 443, 1998.
85. Reed, J. B., Morse, L. S., Schwab, I. R., High dose intravenous pulse methylprednisolone hemisuccinate in acute Behçet retinitis, *Am. J. Opthalmol.*, 125, 409, 1998.

86. Hamuryudan, V., Özyazgan, Y., Hizli, N., Mat, C., Yurdakul, S., Tüzün, Y., Senocak, M., Yazici, H., Azathioprine in Behçet's syndrome: effects on long-term prognosis, *Arthritis Rheum.*, 40, 769, 1997.
87. Masuda, K., Nakajima, A., Urayama, A., Nakae, K., Kogure, M., Inaba, G., Double-masked trial of cyclosporin versus colchicine and long-term open study of cyclosporin in Behçet's disease, *Lancet*, i, 1093, 1989.
88. Vanstenkiste J. F., Peene, P., Verschakelen, J. A., van de Woestijne, K. P., Cyclosporin treatment in rapidly progressive pulmonary thromboembolic Behçet's disease, *Thorax*, 45, 295, 1990.
89. Wechsler, B., Piette, J. C., Behçet's disease. Retains most of its mysteries, *BMJ*, 304, 1199, 1992.
90. Bacon, P. A., Carruthers, D. M., Vasculitis associated with connective tissue disorders, *Rheumatic Dis. Clin. North Am.*, 21, 1077, 1995.
91. Kroger, K., Ansassy, M., Rudofsky, G., Postoperative thrombosis of the superior caval vein in a patient with primary asymptomatic Behçet's disease, *Angiology*, 48, 649, 1997.
92. Roguin, A., Edelstein, S., Edoute, Y., Superior vena cava syndrome as a primary manifestation of Behçet's disease. A case report, *Angiology*, 48, 365, 1997.
93. Mat, M. C., Nazarbaghi, M., Tüzün, Y., Hamuryudan, V., Hizli, N., Yurdakul, S., Özyazgan, Y., Yazici, H., Wound healing in Behçet's syndrome, *Int. J. Dermatol.*, 37, 120, 1998.

26 Vascular Manifestations in Microangiopathic Syndromes

Gale A. McCarty

CONTENTS

I. CLASSIFICATION OF MICROANGIOPATHIC SYNDROMES

A. HISTORY OF MICROANGIOPATHIES

Thrombotic microangiopathy is the hallmark of multifactorial syndromes that share variable degrees of thrombocytopenia, microangiopathic hemolytic anemia, neurologic dysfunction, renal dysfunction, and fever.[1-7] This pentad comprised the initial description of thrombotic thrombocytopenia purpura (TTP) by Moschowitz in 1925 in a young female with anemia, petechiae, fever, central nervous system paresis, and proteinuria, called "acute febrile pleiochromic anemia with hyaline thrombosis of the terminal arterioles and capillaries," and platelet aggregation in the microcirculation. In 1936 Baehr described four cases of "anemia and thrombocytopenic purpura."[1,2,8] TTP was proposed in 1947 by Singer for similar adult syndromes with thrombocytopenia, schistocytes, and neurologic dysfunction as a triad; in 1955 von Gasser described five children with thrombocytopenia, Coombs' positive hemolytic anemia, and renal failure as "hemolytic-uremic syndrome (HUS)," and Allison in 1957 described TTP in six children.[1,4,7]

B. DIFFERENTIAL DIAGNOSIS

While both TTP and HUS have been applied to pediatric and adult syndromes with microangiopathic hemolytic anemic (MAHA) characterized by schistocytes, and thrombotic microangiopathy with platelet aggregation and minimal fibrin thrombi, the designation "TTP" is more commonly applied to adult cases with neurologic symptoms, and "HUS" is used for pediatric cases with prominent renal involvement (Table 26.1). In obstetrical patients, the complex of *hemolysis, elevated liver*

TABLE 26.1
Classification Schemes for TTP/HUS

TTP

Idiopathic
Acute
Plasma-Resistant
Familial

HUS

Pregnancy-Related:
　Postpartum HUS
　HELLP Syndrome (Hemolysis, Elev. Liver Tests, Low Plts)

TABLE 26.2
Differential Diagnostic Features

Feature	TTP	HUS	HELLP
Fever	+	+	+
Skin Lesions	++	–	+
Hypertension	–	++	+
CNS Dysfunction	++	+/–	+
Renal Dysfunction	+	+++	+
Thrombocytopenia	++	+	++
Microangiopathic HA	+++	++	+
Proteinuria	+/–	+++	++
LDH Increase	++	+++	+
Bili Increase	+	+	++
Fib Increase	–	–	–
FSP Increase	–	+	–
PT/PTT Abnl.	+/–	+/–	+/–
Antiphospholipid Antibody Presence	+	+	++

enzymes, and *low platelets* comprise the "HELLP" syndrome," and a postpartum HUS similar to pregnancy-induced hypertension exists. These three "syndromes" (TTP, HUS, and HELLP) represent current parlance in the literature. A useful classification scheme that addresses the initial pentad, newer clinical features, and the growing tenet that many of these syndromes, when fully characterized and serologically investigated, likely have shared pathophysiology and possibly primary or secondary antiphospholipid antibody syndrome (APS) as their bases is presented in Table 26.2.

A variety of infectious agents have been proven to be or are strongly associated with TTP/HUS, and include primarily bacteria and viruses (Table 26.3) with an ever-increasing number of reports in individuals with HIV infections. In addition to common medications such as antibiotics and birth control pills, advances in oncologic and transplantation chemotherapeutic modalities have been associated with a myriad of TTP/HUS syndromes (Table 26.4). Due to overlapping symptomatology, occurrence in patients with multisystem disorders, and likely overlapping pathophysiology, the entity of disseminated intravascular coagulation (DIC) often requires differentiation from TTP/HUS syndromes. Many of the etiologic entities listed in Tables 26.3 and 26.4 also can produce this clinical picture. In DIC, the first-level laboratory tests as listed in Table 26.2 are done, and for further coagulation and fibrinolysis assessment, thrombiin-antithrombin, D-dimers, soluble fibrin monomers, and other studies complete the evaluation (Table 26.5).

TABLE 26.3
Infectious Agents and TTP/HUS

Bacteroides	Coxsackie
Campylobacter	Cytomegalovirus
Capnocytophagi	Epstein Barr
E. coli 0157:H7	Echovirus
Pseudomonas	HIV-1
Salmonella	Influenza
Shigella	Rubella
	Toga

TABLE 26.4
Drugs and TTP/HUS

Birth control pills	Interferon
Bone Marrow Tx Therapies	IV IgG
Cisplatin	Mitomycin C
Cyclosporin A	Monoclonals OKT3, Anti-CD3
Combination Chemotherapy	Pentostatin
FK 506	Ticlopidine
Hydroxyurea	Quinine
	Valacyclovir

TABLE 26.5
Comparative Coagulation Features

Feature	TTP/HUS	DIC
TAT	+	+
D Dimer	−	+
Sol. Fibrin Monomers	−	+
TM	+	+
PA-1	+	+
Protein C	+	+
TF	−	++

II. PATHOLOGY AND PATHOPHYSIOLOGY

TTP/HUS represents, at the microvascular cellular level, the combined results of diverse immunologic recognition, amplification, and effector mechanisms, along with thrombogenic and thrombolytic mechanisms. The time course of endothelial cell (EC) activation, destruction, necrosis, and apoptosis, along with platelet activation and aggregation — with contributions from effector mechanisms involving autoantibodies, complement, and cellular elements of the immune system — vary in intensity with the time course of the inciting disease entity, and the duration of therapies utilized to suppress tissue destruction, often instituted prior to the establishment of a true diagnosis. Clinical diagnoses are often made with concomitant administration of immunosuppression, anticoagulation, and, in some cases, antibiosis, or removal of preformed antibodies by pheresis. Tissue is not always obtained at early stages of disease. Thus, the published pathology needs to be

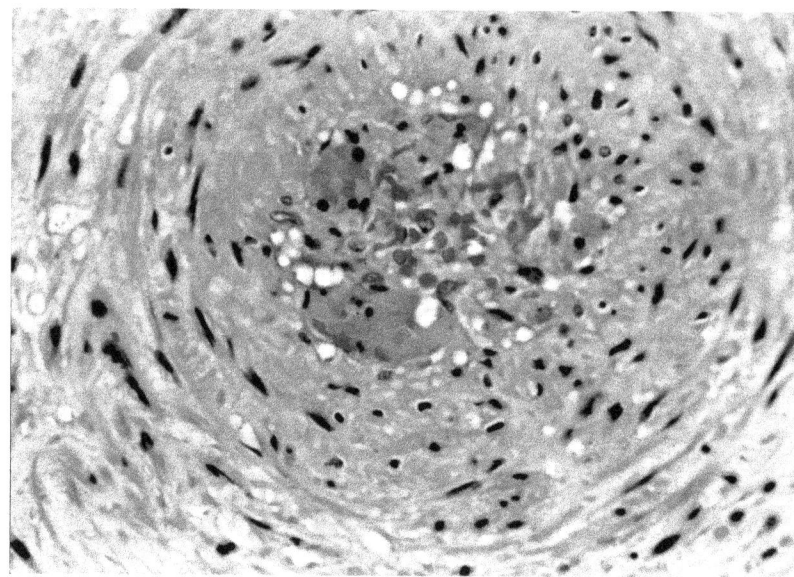

FIGURE 26.1 Thrombotic Microangiopathy in a Small Muscular Artery. The classic findings of fibrin thrombi, red cell ghosts, luminal obliteration, swollen endothelial cells, and a lack of panvascular or perivascular cellular infiltration are present.

considered with these caveats, and involved tissue may not always be accessible. Natural reparative or thrombolytic functions may already be activated in parallel with ongoing immunologic injury to ECs and platelets.

Light microscopic studies often cannot determine whether EC damage leading to exposure of subendothelial components occurred prior to platelet deposition, or if EC swelling and proliferation occurred in response to thrombosis and platelet degeneration. Figure 26.1 shows a light micrograph of a medium-sized arteriole from a patient with HELLP syndrome. Delineation of the intima from the lumen is indistinct due to vacuolar degeneration in the vessel, adherent fibrin thrombi, and a lack of panvascular or perivascular cellular infiltrate. At the electron microscopic level, microvascular ECs exhibit cytoplasmic vacuolization, lysosomal damage, and swollen mitochondria, leading to necrosis. This occurs prior to endothelial cell detachment. The sum of these processes is programmed cell death, or apoptosis. IgG, IgM, and C3 are often found by immunofluorescence when assessed, but serum complement is not often depleted in TTP and, as shown in Figure 26.1, no panvascular or perivascular inflammation is apparent. While platelet microaggregation is a fundamental pathologic lesion in classic TTP and sporadic or idiopathic HUS, fibrin thrombi rather than platelet aggregation tend to predominate in diarrhea-associated HUS and TTP/HUS syndromes reported with neoplasia.[9,10] In diarrhea-associated HUS, fibrin thrombi occur in larger vessels and can be associated with cortical necrosis in the kidneys. In adult HUS, platelet thrombi precede EC activation and proliferation, and eventuate in obliteration of the lumen and apoptosis.

1. Thrombin/Antithrombin and D-Dimers

Fibrin deposition often occurs at the periphery of the platelet plug (see Figure 26.1). Mural platelet thrombi are compressed and incorporated into vessel walls and interact with ECs leading to subendothelial hyaline degeneration, according to a recent study in vessels from eight adults with TMA.[12] Increased fibrin split products, abnormal antithrombin III but normal D-dimers, and abnormal thrombin-antithrombin (TAT) were present. Thus, acute TMA is accompanied by increased coagulation parameters and decreased fibrinolysis.

2. Thrombomodulin

In TTP/HUS and the subset of bone marrow transplantation TMA, thrombomodulin (TM) often significantly increases and can parallel worsening serum creatinine.[13] TM released in the urine occurs only with endothelial cell damage while concomitant with vWF antigen release. In TTP/HUS, the ratio of TM/creatinine parallels the vWF antigen level, whereas in bone marrow transplant TMA there is no correlation.

3. Platelet Derived Microparticles (PMP)

Microvesicular remnants from platelets are found in patients with TTP/HUS, cardiopulmonary bypass, adult respiratory distress syndrome, and idiopathic thrombocytopenia purpura (ITP).[15] In ITP there is a reciprocal relationship between the number of circulating platelets and circulating PMP. PMPs occur when platelets are activated by various agonists and then shed from the surface as lost membrane-bound particles and, due to the known phospholipid (PL) asymmetry in membranes, present phosphatidylserine (PS) on the outer leaflet of the platelet membrane. These PLs are then available for binding with existing antiphospholipid antibodies or, theoretically, could contribute with chronic damage to an antigen-driven immune response.

4. Plasminogen Activator Inhibitor-1(PAI-1)

Studies from patients with TMA and renal involvement show the induction of PAT-1 at the glomerular level, and also the expression of the corresponding membrane receptor in glomerular capillar loops and arteriolar walls.[16] By cDNA studies, local synthesis *in situ* have been confirmed. Further analyses showed that tissue PA is present in both normal and abnormal glomerular and vascular ECs, while tubular epithelial cells express a different form of PA. Thus, the local release of PAI-1 likely plays a role in the persistent deposition of fibrin.

5. Fas and CdC2 Expression

The apoptosis expressed by endothelial cells in TTP/HUS likely is a response to chronic injury, development of endothelial cell-derived membrane-bound vesicles analogous to PMPs, release of chromatin, with a noticeable lack of inflammatory cell influx.[17] Endothelial cell swelling as noted in Figure 26.1 is likely the *in vivo* counterpart of apoptosis *in vitro*. Fas transcripts are induced by platelets from plasma isolated from TTP patients, as well as those with sporadic HUS, and have exhibited microheterogeneity in certain vascular beds.[18,19] Microvascular endothelial cells from skin, kidneys, and the central nervous system are susceptible to Fas, but not pulmonary, large vessels, coronary arteriolar, or hepatic endothelial cells. Thus, there exists differential sensitivity to plasma factor induction in different endothelial cell beds, resulting in apoptotic cells achieving a procoagulant phenotype. In sporadic HUS, endothelial cell toxins and endothelial cell activation are present without necrosis or inflammation, whereas in nonsporadic HUS the obverse is true, with only necrosis and inflammation present. Apoptotic ECs shed procoagulant membrane blebs, and also have attendant decreases in prostaglandin (PGI2) levels. Anti-Fas monoclonal antibodies do not fully block the upregulation of Fas on microvascular ECs by various agonists.

6. Autoantibodies

CD36 is an 88kd platelet glycoprotein related to thrombospondin (TSP). In TTP and in a patient with a borderline elevated IgG anticardiolipin, thrombocytopenia, and two early fetal losses, who retrospectively would meet criteria for the diagnosis of APS, antibodies to CD36 were defined.[20]

7. Thrombopoietin (TPO)

TPO levels often correlated with the degree of platelet decrease in TTP, but not in ITP. In TTP and HUS, TPO is often elevated. TPO mRNA appeared to be modulated by the effective platelet count in one study, and TPO has been observed to decrease after platelet transfusion. TPO may contribute to platelet aggregation induced by shear stresses in vessels and platelet agonists, and may also bind directly to activated platelets. In ITP, platelets are consumed in the spleen, whereas in TTP and DIC they are consumed in vesicles.

8. Arginine-Nitric Oxide-Pathways

The endothelial cell can prevent platelet aggregation by the synthesis or secretion of nitric oxide (NO) and prostaglandins; this system regulates vascular tone and platelet aggregation. The endogenous inhibitor of the NO system is asymmetric dimethyl arginine (ADMA). Data from some models show that endotoxin stimulates the arginine-NO pathway, with subsequent decrease in NO and generation of NO metabolite levels.[22] In gastrointestinal infections, EC damage by endotoxin activates iNOS, increases NO, and depletes arginine, either by inhibiting enzymes by ADMA or inadequate transfer of arginine to ECs. In the HELLP syndrome, an NO donor, s-nitrosoglutamine was tried to increase platelets with some efficacy, and when arginine dietary supplementation has been used, the frequency of relapse has decreased.[22] Since bacterial and viral products cause ECs to form NO, the deoxynitrate that subsequently results can then interact with polymorphonuclear cells and modulate, via superoxide and 02- pathways, cytotoxin production, which also perpetuates vascular damage. Sera from patients with acute TMA induce the NO system in human vascular endothelial cells, whereas normal human sera does not.[14] This leads to an excess of 02-, lipid peroxidation, and thus is contributory to vasooclusive disease.

9. VWF Cleaving Proteases and vWF Multimers

In normal plasma a protease that cleaves large multimers of vWF known to aggregate platelets in the setting of high shear forces exists, and these mechanisms have been studied in TTP.[23] The protease cleaves at tyr 842-meth 843. In sera from 20 of 21 nonfamilial TTP patients, severe deficiency of this protease and inhibition by IgG fractions were noted: in five of five familial TTP patients, less severe deficiency was present, but their IgG was not inhibitory. In HUS patients there were no abnormalities noted. When EC injury occurs, an excess of large vWF multimers are released that cannot be subsequently broken down. Normal human plasma prohibits this, and is likely the basis for why plasma exchange treatment might not be as effective in HUS as it is in TTP as a first-line therapy. Requirements for larger amounts of fresh-frozen plasma (FFP), adjunctive immunoabsorption Sepaharose-protein A columns, vincristine, and splenectomy might be explained in TTP by these mechanisms. An absence of proteases was noted in one study of chronic relapsing TTP, and transient inhibition of action was noted due to an IgG fraction during a single acute episode that was not present in chronic episodes. The vWF multimers here bound to platelet gp1b/IX/V and may have activated gp IIb/IIIa. This could explain why platelet thrombi often have vWF but not fibrin, and why FFP and plasmapheresis work to eliminate the autoantibodies.

10. Antiphospholipid Antibodies

Several excellent reviews of the regulatory schemes of clotting factors have cited with exemplary case reports that various aspects of TMA actually can be attributed to the presence of various aPLs.[27] Case 1 was a patient with HELLP who, upon the development of a Budd-Chiari syndrome, was shown to have aPLs and actual serologic criteria for SLE that were not present during the initial HELLP phase. Case 3 had neither aPLs by enzyme immunoassays nor sensitive coagulation parameters determined, but the presence of cerebral sinus thrombosis postpartum and other clinical symptomatology was highly suggestive of APS. Case 5 was a classic presentation of APS with antiphosphatidylserine but not anticardiolipin antibodies. In these patients, the different specialty focus of the consultants involved in their care contributed to the terminology used to designate the etiologies for their TMA.

11. Autoantibodies to Factor H

Autoantibodies to Factor H have been recently detected in sporadic nondiarrheal-associated HUS and represent mechanisms analogous to the aforementioned vWF-cleaving protease story. This has been shown to be autosomal recessive.[28] Since Factor H modulates the alternative pathway of complement, and familial HUS and TTP are often worse in the setting of attendant severe hypo-complementemia, usually C3 reduction, it has been postulated that Factor H abnormalities might contribute to these mechanisms of injury, as a predominance of familial HUS and ITP patients exhibit hypocomplementemia (73%).[29,30] Low C3 levels are often dependent on an inherited Factor H deficiency that occurs in the majority, but not all, of the proteins. This is a point mutation in a short consensus repeat sequence with an arg-to-gly substitution in two of the domains,[1-4,6-10] These are not far from the third C3b binding site repeats at 16 to 20. This mutation causes a deletion of premature termination codons in about 50% of the Factor H proteins. Some authors think that the recurrence of HUS in allografts that have previously improved with plasma exchange and are often associated with severe hypocomplementemia are explained by these findings.

12. Activated Protein C Resistance and Factor V Leiden Mutation R506

In a study of patients with venous thrombosis and often recurrent disease during pregnancy, cleavage site abnormalities for Factor V were present in 61%.[31] Historically, a major risk factor was the provocation by exposure to oral contraceptives. These patients were not fully evaluated for the presence of aPLs, but sound historically like APS patients.

III. CLINICAL SUBSETS

A wide variety of published literature reviewed here involves case reports and small series of patients where TMA is present with clinical overlapping features. These are now more easily recognized as manifestations of HUS/TTP using the traditional definition schema as noted above, but with the additional cognizance that many of the same features and settings are associated with APS.

A. OBSTETRICAL SYNDROMES

These are often classified as preeclampsia, HUS, TTP, HUS/TTP, or pregnancy-induced hypertension. The pentad of symptoms as listed above varies in severity; commonly, preeclampsia with thrombocytopenia is termed HUS, whereas the HELLP syndrome, which is within the shared clinical spectrum, is invoked when liver chemistries are abnormal. In a recent series of 17 patients who had anticardiolipin antibodies and had one or more lupus anticoagulant tests performed, some had renal arteriolar changes, postpartum worsening (which would be atypical for preeclampsia, which improves postpartum), and were variably associated with low complement. When all clinical and laboratory features are considered, these patients likely are APS.[32] The presence of aPL affords many other levels of interactions between the coagulation scheme and the immune system as mentioned above, but additionally aPL act as PAF-like molelcules and interact with vWF multimers to shift to a procoagulant phenotype and cause recurrent thromboses. Of note is that many of the same treatments for preeclampsia, or TTP/HUS, involve the same agents: antiplatelet agents, pheresis of preformed antibodies. Figure 26.2 shows TMA in a placental vessel with nucleated RBCs denoting fetal oxidative stress, and many of the same features of endothelial cell swelling, fibrin thrombi, and obliteration of the lumen without panvascular or perivascular infiltrates that occur in Figure 26.1. The patient is an 18-year-old primipara who developed hypertension, chorea, thrombocytopenia, an intrapartum DVT, and renal insufficiency with CNS dysfunction that was initially called

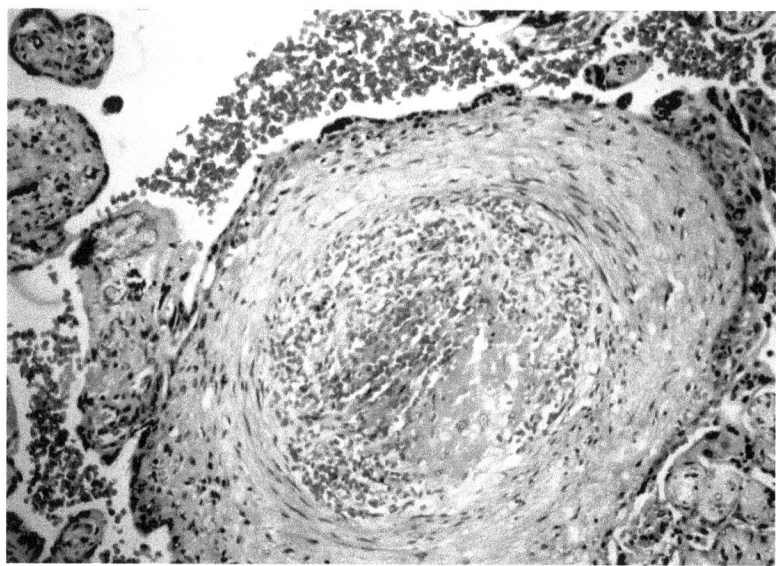

FIGURE 26.2 Thrombotic Microangiopathy in Placental Vessels. Endothelial cell swelling, fibrin thrombi, and nucleated RBCs signifying fetal distress.

preeclampsia, then "HELLP without elevated LFTs," and then eventuated into her true diagnosis of primary antiphospholipid antibody syndrome when usual therapies did not work well.

An approach to the differentiation of the TMA known as HELLP was proffered by Rose and Eldon who evolved a clinical and laboratory criteria scale[33] grading from 0 to 2 central nervous system findings from normalcy to focality, seizures, and coma; normal renal function to mild or moderate renal insufficiency; normal platelet counts to severe thrombocytopenia <20,000; and normal hemoglobin ranging to severe anemia below 9 gms. (These features are all components of both primary and secondary antiphospholipid antibody syndromes; this 1992 study did not assess aPL or lupus anticoagulant profiles.) Of the 11 patients reported in this descriptive nonrandomized study, eight were with TTP, three with HUS, and they had their disease onset 4 weeks to 15 days postpartum, all with significant microangiopathic hemolytic anemia; four had chronic renal insufficiency, seven had live births, two intrauterine fetal demises, and one a spontaneous abortion. All patients received fresh-frozen plasma, two of nine had RBC support, and five had platelet support. The main treatments included steroids in eight, pheresis in eight, aspirin in seven, vincristine in two, and splenectomy in one. Maternal mortality was 18%, and fetal loss was 3%. The general response rate ranged for these patients from 11 to 54%: for pheresis alone, 85%, for steroids alone, 25%. When pheresis was done before fresh-frozen plasma in sicker patients with CNS problems and severe thrombocytopenia, this timing was associated with a better outcome. The use of platelet transfusions was controversial, expensive, and not always effective. That was likely due to the multiple specificities of platelet-reactive or platelet-cross-reactive antibodies that could interact with platelets and result in rapid peripheral destruction.

In another study, vWF multimers and antiendothelial cell antibodies were assessed in a small series of patients with TTP, HELLP, tender hepatomegaly, but no severe CNS manifestatons.[34] When TTP vs. HELLP patients, respectively, were comparatively assessed, MAHA was present in 96 to 98%, TTP in 83 to 96%, renal disease in 76 to 88%, and CNS disease in 60–92%. The most severe thrombocytopenia was present in TTP patients, <20,000, whereas most of the HELLP patients were >100,000.

Advances in imaging have helped the diagnosis of diffuse right upper quadrant pain in patients with HELLP, and 13 of 33 were found to have intraperenchymal hematomas as well. The pain syndrome included right upper quadrant direct pain with tender hepatomegaly, and referred pain to the back and shoulder.[35] A review of 327 patients with HELLP yielded the proposal for criteria for the full vs. partial syndrome, and a designation as "partial HELLP," where 22% of patients were preeclamptic. The full syndrome is characterized by peripheral schistocytosis, LDH ≥600U/L, SGPt ≥70U/L, and platelets <100,000; the partial form has only two of these listed findings. DIC was suspected in patients with abruption, subcapsular large hematoma, and septis. By their criteria, full HELLP occurred in 67, partial HELLP in 71, and definitive alternative diagnosis could not be made in the remainder.[36] They estimated that 5% of their preeclamptic patients were HELLP.

Another report linking preeclampsia, liver infarction, and APS was noted in three patients with HELLP, positive aCL, and LAC profiles; two of three had hepatic infarction, or Budd-Chiari syndrome, this right upper quandrant pain could have been overlooked and misdiagnosed as hepatomegaly and pain not due to HELLP.[37] Two of the three mothers experienced intrauterine demise. Unfortunately, supportive or suppressive therapy for APS was not instituted in these patients. A recent review by McRae and Cines of coagulation factor normalcy and abnormalcy in pregnancy supports the theory advanced here that many of the obstetrical cases of TMA in the literature might actually represent coexistent APS.[38] When renal insufficiency progresses or presents suddenly postpartum, APS must be considered in the differential diagnosis. Often, TMA is found on renal biopsy in both primary and secondary APS.

An interesting case report documented that four years after an episode of TTP without another obvious inciting factor, a patient develped TTP/HUS, a positive LAC and aCL, and on further workup was shown to have Factor V Leiden mutation and APC resistance.[39]

A patient with HELLP diagnosed at 16 weeks of gestation was shown to have antiphosphatidylserine antibodies, and was therefore treated with conventional therapy for APS, including low-dose aspirin, steroids, and fragmin, with eventual delivery of a 3200 g male.[40] Another patient was recently described as "HELLP associated with primary APS," yet all of her symptomatology is attributable to APS. She had thrombocytopenia, an elevated aPTT, and HELLP laboratory findings. Despite anticoagulation, platelet exchange, and steroids, she progressed to severe CNS dysfunction associated with multiple small-vessel ischemic changes on MRI, which prompted further lab studies resulting in the discovery of aPLs. Traditional HELLP treatment did not save the pregnancy and she aborted; multiple fibrin thrombi were found in placental vessels. Her treatment was then changed to low-dose aspirin, heparin, and eventual warfarin to an INR of 2.5. At three months' followup she was clinically better but still had persistant aPLs.[41] An extensive discussion of HELLP syndrome was based on a patient with initially preeclamptic-HELLP symtomatology who, at biopsy, had fibrin-like hyaline deposits in hepatic sinousoids, and developed worsening thrombocytopenia with supratentorial dysfunction and clonus. She was treated with magnesium sulfate and nitroprusside, but not APS therapy. This case likely represents APS.[42]

That thrombocytopenia occurs to a variable degree in normal pregnancy as well as in HELLP pregnancies has been reemphasized in a 1998 review; platelets activate PAF, generate an increase in fibrin split products, and change fibrinopeptides and beta thromboglobulin levels. Thrombopoietin levels are known to be increased in normal and HELLP pregnancies, thus leading to megakaryogenesis. Extensive studies have shown that rather than circulating platelet mass, the premegakaryocyte mass is the major determinant of thromboglobulin levels, and these mechanisms likely determine the variability of actual platelet counts.[43]

When 13 pregnancies were studied in 11 women with TMA, 62% were shown to have these problems in the peripartum period, 23% had problems mid-pregnancy, and the remainder had postpartum events. Of nine survivors, 50% had recurrent disease, likely implying an antibody-mediated mechanism; none of these patients were assessed for APS.[44]

B. SYSTEMIC RHEUMATIC DISEASES

An extensive review of the literature regarding pathology of APS, including 59 photomicrographs from primary and secondary APS patients with clinicoserologic data, summarizes current concepts of how TMA is generated.[45] Multisystem problems in patients with rheumatic diseases should prompt determination of aPLs by both enzyme immunoassays and coagulation-based tests. The most complete review of renovascular complications of SLE is by Appel et al. and shows comparative pathology of small- and large-vessel components. When TMA due to HUS/TTP, malignancies, and hypertension are considered, preglomerular arteriolar and small interlobular arteries show vascular proliferation and glomerular capillary loop involvement. Luminal narrowing, deposition of material staining positive for fibrin, endothelial cell swelling, denudation, and fragmented or hemolyzed RBCs are most commonly noted.[46] While fibrin and variable immunofluorescence are often seen in the preglomerular spaces, these changes occur in the interlobular regions in the noninflammatory necrotizing vasculopathy that describes much of lupus renal disease with TMA components. In some patients there is luminal and vessel wall fibrin, medial myocytic smudging with fibrillar fibrin staining, and inspissated platelets. These findings are most common in proliferative glomerulopathies.[46]

Recently, five patients were reported with primary APS, four of whom presented with renal infarction; all patients had anticardiolipin and positive coagulation tests. Aspirin and ticlid were used, along with impeccable hypertension control. Most of the infarcts were cortical in location.[47]

While most vasculopathy related to APS involves TMA without panvasculitis or perivasculitis, some of the cases as published in the review above[45] and that of Lie[48] document that both primary and secondary APS can show cellular infiltration, albeit infrequently. One case of primary APS and renal vasculitis during pregnancy has been published concerning a patient with anticardiolipin antibodies.[49] Another report documents arteriolar thrombosis without vasculitis, but platelet and fibrin deposition in small arteries and arterioles; this patient responded to aspirin and steroids but not to anticoagulation.[50] A growing recognition exists that APS can be associated with diabetes, as evidenced by a patient with MAHA, TCP, APS manifested by a positive aCL and LAC, and schistocytes, and with a negative Coombs' test.[51]

Still's disease has been reported in a patient with classic HUS/TTP who failed steroids and pheresis and was treated with IV IgG. Renal biopsy showed fibrin and platelet fragments, an fusion of the podocytes, and were compared to two prior cases with TTP presentations who were treated with fresh-frozen plasma and cryoprecipitates.[53] One patient with Behçet's syndrome developed HUT/TTP manifested by schistocytes and thrombocytopenia to 40,000 in association with neurological manifestations.[54] The occurrence of hepatic venoocclusive disease accompanied the development of HUS/TTP in a patient with polymyositis; no necrosis was found in the vessel walls, but a focal lymphocytic infiltrate was present in small hepatic veins. Schistocytes were present in renal glomerular capillaries characterized by medial thickening, and an electron-dense fluffy deposit was noted that was not characterized further.[55] Similar electron-dense deposits were noted in a patient with TMA who, at the time, was negative for LAC but not tested for aPLs, and showed glomerular capillary microthrombi. Some deposition of C1q and C3 but no immunoglobulins were noted on immunofluorescence.[56]

Coagulation disorders accompanying acute renal failure with emphasis on TTP/HUS are the subject of a recent review by Schetz.[57] An upregulation of Verotoxin receptors that occurs in renal endothelial cells when compared to human vascular endothelial cells has been noted in some forms of TMA as a possible model of renovascular injury.[58] The reader is directed to an excellent review of the roles of polymorphonuclear leukocytes, platelets, and activated vascular endothelial in the critical milieu of cytokine expression, circulating immune complexes, integrins, and cell adhesion molecules that relate to other possible mechanisms of injury in these syndromes.[59] That patients with APS often are "seronegative" for aPLs and/or "plasmanegative" for LAC test abnormalities at the time of acute events, which could explain some of the above patients with clinical features suggesting APS, was recently addressed by Miret, and was discussed in the vascular manifestations of APS review cited earlier.[45,60] A consensus set of preliminary guidelines for the diagnosis of APS addressing clinical manifestations in both primary and secondary forms, and a variety of tests have recently been published, but with many caveats for exclusions, and recognition that the classical tests (IgG/M aCL, aPTT, or other LAC test) are likely to be applicable in delineation of groups of patients for study, but not diagnostic in an individual patient.[61]

C. Infectious, Postchemotherapy, and Bone Marrow Transplantation Syndromes

While a variety of infectious agents comprising Table 26.3 involve common bacterial and viral pathogens, the majority of recent reports concentrate on HIV-1 and have been elegantly reviewed by Hymes and Karpatkin.[62] In splenic endothelial cells, HIV-1 and p24 antigen transcripts were localized, but not always located where TMA was present. That certain microvascular beds are differentially susceptible to HIV is suspected. Human brain capillaries, however, are quite susceptible to infection by HIV. Proteases from HIV augment endothelial cell and mononuclear leukocytic function and upregulate integrins, increase cytokines such as TNFalpha, and thus might predispose to EC apoptosis. HIV sera causes apoptosis in microvascular EC cultures but not in large vessels, and upregulate Fas expression that is inhibitable by anti-Fas monoclonal antibodies. In 13 of 14 patient studies, treatments that were most effective were cryodepleted plasma, low-dose aspirin, and splenectomy; in one patient the HIV TMA resolved after zidouvidine therapy.[62]

Recently, 18 of 1,227 patients with HIV on a valacyclovir trial for the HIV-associated cytomegalovirus (CMV) infections developed MAHA, TCP, and later renal disease, but CNS dysfunction was not common.[63] Nine patients underwent biopsies of renal and gingival tissues, which demonstrated TMA in most patients. Normal aPTTs and PTs were present; none were assessed for aPLs. Sixteen of the 18 patients died, with 56% of deaths attributable to TTP/HUS and renal insufficiency. The CD4 counts did not correlate with either the presence or severity of TMA. Risk factors for TMA were analyzed and shown to be positively correlated with sulfimethoxasole-trimethoprim, valacyclovir, antimycobacterials, Kaposi's sarcoma, and Mycobacterium avium complex, but not with CMV. All patients experienced a gradual onset with slow progression. Their response rate to usual therapies for TTP/HUS was low, and their course was similar to another subset of patients with low response rates, those who develop the syndrome status post bone marrow transplantation (BMT). TMA in several patients was also associated with pneumococcal sepsis, in which schistocytes, aphasia, hemiparesis, and renal arteriolar disease on biopsy occurrred. These patients were treated with fresh-frozen plasma, steroids, and, unfortunately, died. Differences between HIV-ITP syndromes and HIV-TMA syndromes were that antiplatelet agents and steroids were very effective in HIV-ITP, but MAHA was more associated with HIV-TMA.

A large series of 62 patients status post allogeneic BMT who developed TTP/HUS less than 120 days after transplant was recently published.[64] MAHA alone occurred more frequently in patients who had low cyclosporin A (CSA) doses and FK506, and CNS abnormalities were also associated with positive MRI findings. CSA was thought to increase TMA by a cytotoxic effect on endothelial cells, reduction of TM generation with effective APC, and alteration of thromboxane/prostaglandin ratios, resulting in EC damage. No trials of plasmapheresis were used, mortality was high, and, in some patients, total body irradiation was used. That enterohemorrhagic E. coli O157:H7 is an emerging pathogen in these types of patients is also being recognized, with excess mortality in the young and elderly, and features compatible with TTP/HUS.[65,66]

In the syndromes with TMA due to drugs and bone marrow transplantation, Moake and Byrnes emphasize that HUS is much more frequent than TTP, and total body irradiation can also cause it.[67] Regarding specific mechanisms, CSA was thought to induce TMA by increasing vWF and platelet aggregation; other chemotherapeutic agents, especially in combination, decrease vWF multimers, and most of these syndromes are fatal. Quinine causes ITP by an antibody mechanism related to glycoprotein Ib/IX and IIb/IIIa. There have been over 90 cases of BMT HUS/TTP, primarily in the settings of leukemia, and non-Hodgkin's lymphoma. Approximately 6 to 12 months after BMT, an acute or subacute nephritis develops that resembles HUS. Plasma exchange and antiplatelet agents are often used, depending on the individual patient.

One patient undergoing hydroxyurea treatment for chronic myelogenous leukemia developed retinal, renal, and CNS TMA. Fibrin thrombi were noted in the kidneys and in brain tissue; no studies for aPLs were undertaken.[68,69] A patient being treated with IV IgG for a cancer-associated TTP-HUS syndrome developed noncardiogenic pulmonary edema thought to be precipitated by the IV IgG in another recent report.[70] TMA has also occurred post BMT when graft vs. host chemoprophylaxis was employed pretransplant.[71]

IV. TREATMENT

A. General Measures

Since the differential diagnosis of TMA includes idiopathic disease, autoimmune disorders, systemic rheumatic diseases, antiphospholipid antibody syndrome, infectious agents, drugs, and tumors, identification of the most likely inciting agent is foremost. Unfortunately, some of the aforementioned entities have overlapping symptomatology and protracted time courses. Some entities evolve quickly after an intervention, making the generation of an algorithm for treatment difficult. Utilization of full diagnostic serologies and coagulation-based testing is important and, of necessity, should be performed on initial sera and plasma samples saved and stored appropriately, as therapies started quickly for disease control such as plasma exchange or steroids will abrogate immunologic tests. Unfortunately, trainees and attending physicians alike often do not appropriately store these samples for future testing. When antibiosis is indicated, it should be undertaken. When autoimmune disorders are considered etiologic, usual therapies should be employed judiciously with appropriate monitoring to achieve immunologic control. Avoidance of other general health problems that worsen vascular disease (hypertension, smoking, hyperlipidemia, IV drug use, diabetes) is empiric.

B. Specific Measures

Aspirin is often helpful as an antiplatelet agent, as well as contributing to the reconstitution of interleukin deficits that might be present in some syndromes; one example is the interleukin 3 defect noted in APS. Except for a history of aspirin-induced anaphylaxis or aspirin allergy-nasal polyps-tartrazine dye sensitivity syndromes, there are no real contraindications to aspirin therapy, and 81 to 325 mg should be the appropriate dosing. In some situations, such as APS, low-dose aspirin can augment platelet counts relatively rapidly in a matter of days, but full efficacy may take up to three weeks. Fresh-frozen plasma, plasma exchange transfusion, or plasmapheresis are employed in many TTP/HUS situations, which may provide missing proteases and/or remove preformed autoantibodies of various specificities that may reestablish balance in an autoantiidiotypic control network for autoantibody production. For rapid suppression of autoantibody production, IV pulse methylprednisolone therapy qd or in q6h dosing is effective versus high-dose PO steroids with careful followup, H2 blockers to prevent gastritis, and calcium replacement to prevent eventual osteoporosis. Depending on the disorder involved, vincristine, azathioprine, cyclophosphamide, and other immunosuppressives may be useful. IV IgG is of help in limited cases as an adjunct, and is used when other modalities pursued hierarchically do not work. Utility depends upon the fact that IV IgG may block autoantibody binding sites, and may also be efficacious by the serendipitous provision of an immunoglobulin component that reestablishes control in the autoantiidiotypic network.

Renal transplantation has come under consideration in adults with TTP/HUS for therapy-responsive cases.[72] One recent report of iloprost IV as efficacious in 13 patients with TMA is promising but deserves confirmation.[73] Immunoabsorptive columns to remove antibodies and immune complexes in combination with immunosuppression are intriguing modalities and have recently been used successfully in BMT-associated TMA.[74] A recent review of plasma therapy from one institution over 15 years provides support for the utility of this treatment in some clinical situations, but often adjunctive therapies are needed concurrently.[75]

Earlier in this chapter the use of supplemental dietary arginine was mentioned, but further confirmatory trials are needed.[76] Recent detailed reviews of TTP/HUS management have been provided by Kaplan, and Kwaan and Soff,[77,78] and a general overview of thrombotic syndromes occurring in the setting of systemic rheumatic and autoimmune disease is provided by Fessler.[79] The fact that TTP/HUS syndromes considerably overlap with APS prompts consideration of the use of hydroxychloroquin 200 mg po bid, as it can act as a microanticoagulant at the platelet and endothelial cell levels, and has been recently shown to decrease both the symptomatology and aPL production of multiple specificities and isotypes in both primary and APS (McCarty, G.A., manuscript in submission, 2000). Future diagnosis and treatment will likely evolve as the common pathophysiology underlying immune recognition, amplification, effector, and coagulation systems are understood.

TABLE 26.6
Pathophysiology-A

Endothelial cell
  Activation, damage, necrosis
  Apoptotic cells procoagulant
Immune complex and complement deposition
Fibrin deposition
  peripheral plt. plug
Thrombomodulin
  Release with damage
Platelet-derived microvesicles
  Membrane asymmetry, PL exposure
Plasminogen Activator-1 release

TABLE 26.7
Pathophysiology-B

CD36 — Platelet Interactions
PGI2 Dysregulation
Thrombopoietin
Nitric Oxide/iNOS
VWF multimers and cleaving proteases
Autoantibodies
  Factor H
  Factor V Leiden mutation-APC
  Phospholipids

TABLE 26.8
Treatment

General:
Eliminate incitors
Reevaluate carefully-case-specific!
Parallel vs. Serial Rx

Specific:
Antiplatelet Agents
Platelet Support
Fresh/Frozen Plasma/Factors
Plasma Exchange
Plasmapheresis
IV/PO Steroids
IV IgG
Hydroxychloroquin
Immunosuppressive Therapy

Concurrent Therapy for Inciting Disease

REFERENCES

1. Moake, J.L., Thrombotic thrombocytopenic purpura. *Thromb. Haemost.,* 74(1):240–245, 1995.
2. Ruggenenti, P., Remuzzi, G., The pathophysiology and management of thrombotic thrombocytopenic purpura. *Eur. J. Haematol.,* 56(4):191–207, 1996.
3. Bell, W.R., Thrombotic thrombocytopenic purpura/hemolytic uremic syndrome relapse: frequency, pathogenesis, and meaning. *Semin. Hematol.,* 34(2):134–9, 1997.
4. Kulzer, P., Wanner, C., Thrombotic microangiopathy: a challenge with uncertain outcome. *Nephrol. Dial. Transplant.,* 13(8):2154–60, 1998.
5. Ruggenenti, P., Lutz, J., Remuzzi G., Pathogenesis and treatment of thrombotic microangiopathy. *Kidney Int. Suppl.,* 58:S97–101, 1997.
6. Zijlstra, J.G., Das, P.C., Haemolytic uraemic syndrome and thrombocytopenic thrombotic purpura [editorial]. *Int. J. Artif. Organs,* 20(4):191–4, 1997.
7. Moake, J.L., Chow, T.W., Thrombotic thrombocytopenic purpura: understanding a disease no longer rare. *Am. J. Med. Sci.,* 316(2):105–119, 1998.
8. Hollenbeck, M., Kutkuhn, B., Aul, C., Leschke, M., Willers, R., Grabensee, B., Haemolytic-uraemic syndrome and thrombotic-thrombocytopenic purpura in adults: clinical findings and prognostic factors for death and end-stage renal disease. *Nephrol. Dial. Transplant.,* 13(1):76–81, 1998.
9. Laurence, J., Dang, C., Pathologic distinctions among the thrombotic microangiopathies [letter]. *Clin. Neph.,* 50(6):393, 1998.
10. Neild, G.H., Hemolytic uremic syndrome/thrombotic thrombocytopenic purpura pathophysiology and treatment. *Kidney Int. Suppl.,* 64:S45–9, 1998.
11. George, J.N., Gilcher, R.O., Smith, J.W., Chandler, L., Duvall, D., Ellis, C., Thrombotic thrombocytopenic purpura-hemolytic uremic syndrome: diagnosis and management. *J. Clin. Apheresis,* 13(3):120–5, 1998.
12. Sagripanti, A., Carpi, A., Baicchi, U., Morganti, M., Rosaia, B., Nicolini, A., Mittermayer, C., Plasmatic parameters of coagulation activation in thrombotic microangiopathy. *Biomed. Pharmacother.,* 50(8):357–62, 1996.
13. Zeigler, Z.R., Rosenfeld, C.S., Andrews, D.F., III, Nemunaitis, J., Raymond, J.M., Shadduck, R.K., Dramer, R.E., Gryn, J.F., Rintels, P.B., Besa, E.C., George, J.N., Plasma von Willebrand Factor Antigen (vWF:AG) and thrombomodulin (TM) levels in adult thrombotic thrombocytopenic purpura/hemolytic uremic syndromes (TTP/HUS) and bone marrow transplant-associated thrombotic microangiopathy (BMT-TM). *Am. J. Hematol.,* 53(4):213–20, 1996.

14. Noris, M., Ruggenenti, P., Todeschini, M., Figliuzzi, M., Macconi, D., Zoja, C., Paris, S., Gaspari, F., Remuzzi, G., Increased nitric oxide formation in recurrent thrombotic microangiopathies: a possible mediator of microvascular injury. *Am. J. Kidney Dis.,* 27(6):790–6, 1996.

15. Galli, G., Grassi, A., Barbui, T., Platelet-derived microvesicles in thrombotic thrombocytopenic purpura and hemolytic uremic syndrome. *Thromb. Haemost.,* 75(3):427–31, 1996.

16. Xu, Y., Hagege, J., Mougenot, B., Sraer, J.D., Ronne, E., Rondeau, E., Different expression of the plasminogen activation system in renal thrombotic microangiopathy and the normal human kidney. *Kidney Int.,* 50(6):2011–9, 1996.

17. Mazzoni, M.C., Schmid-Schonbein, G.W., Mechanisms and consequences of cell activation in the microcirculation. *Cardiovasc. Res.,* 32:709–719, 1996.

18. Laurence, J., Mitra, D., Apoptosis of microvascular endothelial cells in the pathophysiology of thrombotic thrombocytopenic purpura/sporadic hemolytic uremic syndrome. *Semin. Hematol.,* 34(2):98–105, 1997.

19. Mitra, D., Jaffe, E.A., Weksler, B., Hajjar, K.A., Soderland, C., Laurence, J., Thrombotic thrombocytopenic purpura and sporadic hemolytic-uremic syndrome plasmas induce apoptosis in restricted lineages of human microvascular endothelial cells. *Blood,* 89(4):1224–34, 1997.

20. Borzini, P., Riva, M., Nembri, P., Rossi, E., Pagliaro, P., Vergani, P., Greppi, P., Tantardini, P., CD36 autoantibodies and thrombotic diathesis, thrombocytopenia and repeated early fetal losses. *Vox. Sang.,* 73(1):46–8, 1997.

21. Herlitz, H., Petersson, A., Sigstrom, L., Wennmalm, A., Westberg, G., The arginine-nitric oxide pathway in thrombotic microangiopathy. *Scand. J. Urol. Nephrol.,* 31(5):477–9, 1997.

22. Hiyoyama, K., Wada, H., Shimura, M., Nakasaki, T., Katayama, N., Nishikawa, M., Shiku, H., Tahara, T., Kato, T., Increased serum levels of thrombopoietin in patients with thrombotic thrombocytopenic purpura, idiopathic thrombocytopenic purpura, or disseminated intravascular coagulation. *Blood Coagul. Fibrinolysis,* 8(6):345–9, 1997.

23. Furlan, M., Robles, R., Galbuseara, M., Remuzzi, G., Kyrle, P.A., Brenner, B., Krause, M., Scharrer, I., Aumann, V., Mittler, U., Solenthaler, M., Lammle, B., von Willebrand factor-cleaving protease in thrombotic thrombocytopenic purpura and the hemolytic-uremic syndrome. Comment in: *N. Engl. J. Med.,* 1998 Nov 26; 339(22):1629–31; *N. Engl. J. Med.,* 339(22):1578–84, 1998.

24. Wada, H., Mori, Y.U., Shimura, M., Hiyoyama, K., Ioka, M., Nakasaki, T., Nishikawa, M., Nakano, M., Kumeda, K., Kaneko, T., Nakamura, S., Shiku, H., Poor outcome in disseminated intravascular coagulation or thrombotic thrombocytopenic purpura patients with severe vascular endothelial cell injuries. *Am. J. Hematol.,* 58(3):189–94, 1998.

25. Morita, T., Yamamoto, T., Churg, J., Mesangiolysis: an update. *Am. Kidney. Dis.,* 31(4):559–573, 1998.

26. Moake, J.L., Moschcowitz, Multimers and metalloproteinases (Editorial). *N. Engl. J. Med.,* 339:1629–33, 1998.

27. Kitchens, C.S., Thrombotic storm: when thrombosis begets thrombosis. *Am. J. Med.,* 104:381–85, 1998.

28. Sarkodee-Adoo, C., Gojo, I., Heyman, M.R., von Willebrand factor-cleaving protease in thrombotic thrombocytopenic purpura and the hemolytic-uremic syndrome [letter]. *N. Engl. J. Med.,* 340(17):1368;discussion 1369, 1999.

29. Noris, M., Ruggenenti, P., Perna, A., Orisio, S., Caprioli, J., Skerka, C., Vasile, B., Zipfel, P.F., Remuzzi, G., Hypocomplementemia discloses genetic predisposition to hemolytic uremic syndrome and thrombotic thrombocytopenic purpura: role of factor H abnormalities — Italian Registry of Familial and Recurrent Hemolytic Uremic Syndrome/Thrombotic Thrombocytopenic Purpura. *J. Am. Soc. Nephrol.,* 10(2):281–93, 1999.

30. Brenner, B., Lanin, N., Thalen, I., HELLP syndrome associated with Factor V R506Q mutation. *Br. J. Haematol.,* 92:999–1001, 1996.

31. Noris, M., Remuzzi, G., Are HUS and TTP genetically determined? *Kidney Int.,* 53(4):1085–6, 1998.

32. Kniaz, D., Eisenberg, G.M., Elrad, H., Johnson, C.A., Valaitis, J., Bregman, H., Postpartum hemolytic uremic syndrome associated with antiphospholipid antibodies. *Am. J. Nephrol.,* 12:126–133, 1992.

33. Egerman, R.S., Witlin, A.G., Friedman, S.A., Sibai, B.M., Thrombotic thrombocytopenic purpura and hemolytic uremic syndrome in pregnancy: review of 11 cases. Comment in: *Am. J. Obstet. Gynecol.,* 1997 Jun,176(6):1397–8; Comment in: *Am. J. Obstet. Gynecol.,* 1997 Aug,177(2):486; *Am. J. Obstet. Gynecol.,* 175(4 Pt 1):950–6, 1996.

34. Kaiser, C., Distler, W., TTP and HELLP syndrome; differential diagnostic problems. *Am. J. Ob. Gyn.,* 175:506–507, 1996.

35. Barton, J., Siai, B., Hepatic imaging in HELLP. *Am. J. Ob. Gyn.,* 174:1820–1825, 1996.

36. Audibert, R., Friedman, S., Frongiech, A., Sibai, B., Obstetrics: Clinical utility of strict diagnostic criteria for HELLP Syndrome. *Am. J. Ob. Gyn.,* 175:400–64, 1996.

37. Alsulyman, O.M., Castro, M.A., Zuckerman, E., McGehee, W., Goodwin, T.M., Preeclampsia and liver infarction in early pregnancy associated with the antiphospholipid syndrome. *Obstet. Gynecol.,* 88(4 Pt 2):644–6, 1996.

38. McCrae, K.R., Cines D.B., Thrombotic microangiopathy during pregnancy. *Semin. Hematol.,* 34(2):148–58, 1997.

39. Grandone, E., Margaglione, M., Pavone, G., Thrombotic thrombocytopenic purpura in pregnancy: a multifaceted disease [letter]. Comment on: *Am. J. Obstet. Gynecol.,* 1996 Oct; 175(4 Pt 1): 950–6. *Am. J. Obstet. Gynecol.,* 177(2):486, 1997.

40. McMahon, L.P., Smith, J., The HELLP Syndrome at 16 weeks' gestation: possible association with the antiphospholipid syndrome. *Aust. N. Z. J. Obstet. Gynecol.,* 37(3):13–4, 1997.

41. Nagayama, K., Izumi, N., Miyasaka, Y., Saita, K., Ono, K., Noguchi, O., Hoshinao, Y., Uchihara, M., Miyake, S., Enomoto, N., Tanaka, Y., Marumo, F., Sato, S., Hemolysis, elevated liver enzymes, and low platelets syndrome associated with primary anti-phospholipid antibody syndrome. *Intern. Med.,* 36(9):661–6, 1997.

42. Stone, J., HELLP (Grand Rounds at JHH). *JAMA,* 280:559–62, 1998.

43. Frolich, M.A., Datta, S., Corn, S.B., Thrombopoietin in normal pregnancy and pre-eclampsia. *Am. J. Ob. Gyn.,* 179:100–04, 1998.

44. Dashe, J.S., Ramin, S.M., Cunningham, F.G., The long-term consequences of thrombotic microangiopathy (thrombotic thrombocytopenic purpura and hemolytic uremic syndrome) in pregnancy. *Obstet. Gynecol.,* 91(5 Pt. 1):662–8, 1998.

45. McCarty, G.A., Vascular pathology of the antiphospholipid syndrome. In: Khamashta, M.A., Hughes GRU (Eds). *The Antiphospholipid Antibody Syndrome — Hughes Syndrome,* Springer-Verlag, London, 1999.

46. Appel, G.P., Pirani, C.L., G'Rgati, V., Renovascular complications of SLE. *J. Am. Assn. Nephro.,* 4:1499–1515, 1994.

47. Mandreoli, M., Zucchelli, P., Renal vascular disease in patients with primary antiphospholipid antibodies. *Nephrol. Dial. Transplant.,* 8:1277–1280, 1993.

48. Lie, J.T., Vasculopathy of APS revisited: thrombosis is the culprit and vasculitis is the consort. *Lupus,* 5:308–71, 1996.

49. Almeshari, K., Alfurayh, O., Akhtan, M., Primary APS and self-limited renal vasculitis during pregnancy: case report and review of the literature. *Am. J. Kid. Dis.,* 24:505–08, 1994.

50. Legerton, C., Puett, D., Sergent, J., Renal coagulopathy, thrombocytopenia, and anticardiolipin antibody: therapeutic response to cortiosteriods and aspirin but not anticoagulation. *J. Rheum.,* 21:172, 1994.

51. Morita, H., Suwa, T., Takeda, N., Ishizuka, T., Yasuda, K., Case report: diabetic microangiopathic hemolytic anemia and thrombocytopenia with antiphospholipid syndrome. *Am. J. Med. Sci.,* 311(3):148–51, 1996.

52. Trent, K., Neustrater, B.R., Lottenberg, R., Chronic relapsing thrombotic thrombocytopenic purpura and antiphospholipid antibodies a report of two cases. *Am. J. Hematol.,* 54(2):155–9, 1997.

53. Diamond, J.R., Hemolytic uremic syndrome/thrombotic thrombocytopenic purpura (HUS/TTP) complicating adult Still's disease: remission induced with intravenous immunoglobulin G. *J. Nephrol.,* 10(5):253–7, 1997.

54. Docci, D., Baldrati, L., Capponcini, C., Facchini, F., Giudicissi, A., Feletti, C., Hemolytic uremic syndrome/thrombotic thrombocytopenic purpura in a patient with Behcet's disease treated with cyclosporin. *Nephron,* 75(3):356–7, 1997.

55. Ishida, Y., Utikoshi, M., Kurosaki, M., Ohta, K., Chujo, T., Aoyama, S., Ohsawa, K., Saito, K., Yokoyama, H., Ohta, S., Hepatic veno-occlusive disease in a case of polymyositis associated with thrombotic thrombocytopenic purpura/hemolytic uremic syndrome. *Intern. Med.,* 37(8):694–9, 1998.

56. Kimura, M., Fujigaki, Y., Ohtake, T., Furuya, R., Hishida, A., Kaneko, E., A patient with thrombotic microangiopathy accompanied by glomerular subendothelial electron dense deposits. *Am. J. Nephrol.,* 18(2):155–9, 1998.

57. Schetz, M.R., Coagulation disorders in acute renal failure. *Kidney Int.,* Suppl. 66:S96–101, 1998.

58. Nangaku, M., Shankland, S.J., Couser, W.G., A new model of renal microvascular injury. *Nephrol. Hypertension,* 7:457–462, 1998.

59. Belmont, H.M., Abramson, S.B., Lie, S.L.E., Pathology and pathogenesis of vascular injury in SLE-interaction of inflammatory cells and activated endothelium. *Arthritis Rheum.,* 39(1): 9–22, 1996.

60. Miret, C., Cervena, R., Reverber, J., Garcia-Carrasco, M., Molla, M., Font, J., Inglemo, M., APS without aPL antibodies at the time of the thrombotic event: transient seronegative APS? *Clin. Exp. Rheum.,* 15:541–544, 1997.

61. Wilson, W.A., Gharavi, A.E., et al., Special Article — International Concensus Statement on Preliminary Classification of Definite APS — Report of an International Workshop. *Arthritis Rheum.,* 41:1309–11, 1999.

62. Hymes, K.B., Karpatkin, S., Human immunodeficiency virus infection and thrombotic microangiopathy. *Semin. Hematol.,* 34(2):117–25, 1997.

63. Bell, W.R., Chulay, J.D., Feinberg, J.E., Manifestations resembling thrombotic microangiopathy in patients with advanced human immunodeficiency virus (HIV) disease in a cytomegalovirus prophylaxis trial (ACTG 204). *Medicine,* 76(5):369–80, 1997.

64. Schriber, J.R., Herzig, G.P., Transplantation-associated thrombotic thrombocytopenic purpura and hemolytic uremic syndrome. *Semin. Hematol.,* 34(2):126–33, 1997.

65. Koutkia, P., Myloakis, E., Flanigan, T., Enterohemorrhagic Escherichia coli O157:H7 — an emerging pathogen. Comment in: *Am. Fam. Physician,* 1998 Apr 1;57(7):1494. *Am. Fam. Physician,* 56(3):853–6, 859–61, 1997.

66. Sutor, G.C., Schmidt, R.E., Albrecht, H., Thrombotic microangiopathies and HIV infection: report of two typical cases, features of HUS and TTP, and review of the literature. *Infection,* 27(1):12–5, 1999.

67. Moake, J.L., Byrnes, J.J., Thrombotic microangiopathies associated with drugs and bone marrow transplantation. *Hematol. Oncol. Clin. North Am.,* 10(2):485–497, 1996.

68. Shammas, F., Meyer, P., Heikkila, R., Apeland, T., Goransson, L., Berland, J., Kjellevold, K., Thrombotic microangiopathy in a patient with chronic myelogenous leukemia on hydroxyurea. *Acta Haematol.,* 97(3):184–6, 1997.

69. Gordon, L.I., Kwaan, H.C., Cancer-and drug-associated thrombotic thrombocytopenic purpura and hemolytic uremic syndrome. *Semin. Hematol.,* 34(2):140–7, 1997.

70. Suassuna, J.H., da Costa, M.A., Faria, R.A., Melichar, A.C., Noncardiogenic pulmonary edema triggered by intravenous immunoglobulin in cancer-associated thrombotic thrombocytopenic purpura-hemolytic uremic syndrome [letter]. *Nephron,* 77(3):368–70, 1997.

71. Paquette, R.L., Tran, L., Landaw, E.M., Thrombotic microangiopathy following allogeneic bone marrow transplantation is associated with intensive graft-versus-host disease prophylaxis. *Bone Marrow Transplant,* 22(4):351–7, 1998.

72. Conlon, P.J., Brennan, D.C., Pfaf, W.W., Finn, W. F., Gehr, T., Bolling, R.R., Smith, S.R., Renal transplantation in adults with thrombotic thrombocytopenic purpura/haemolytic-uraemic syndrome. *Nephrol. Dial. Transplant.,* 11(9):1810–4, 1996.

73. Saripanti, A., Carpi, A., Rosaia, B., Morelli, E., Innocenti, M., D'Acunto, G., Nicolini, A., Iloprost in the treatment of thrombotic microangiopathy: report of 13 cases. *Biomed. Pharmacother.,* 50(8):350–6, 1996.

74. Ziegler, Z.R., Shadduck, R.K., Nath, R., Andrews, D.F., III, Pilot study of combined cryosupernatant and protein A immunoadsorption exchange in the treatment of grade 3–4 bone marrow transplant-associated thrombotic microangiopathy. *Bone Marrow Transplant,* 17(1):81–6, 1996.

75. Samtleben, W., Blumenstein, M., Bosch, T., Lysaght, M.J., Schmidt, B., Plasma therapy at Kliniskum Grosshadern: a 15-year retrospective. *Artif. Organs,* 20(5):408–14, 1996.

76. Jaradat, Z.W., Marquardt, R.R., L-arginine as a therapeutic approach for the verotoxigenic Escherichia coli-induced hemolytic uremic syndrome and thrombotic thrombocytopenic purpura. *Med. Hypotheses,* 49(3):277–80, 1997.

77. Kaplan, A.A., Therapeutic apheresis for renal disorders. *Therapeutic Apheresis,* 3(1):25–30, 1999.

78. Kwaan, H.C., Soff, G.A., Management of thrombotic thrombocytopenic purpura and hemolytic uremic syndrome. *Semin. Hematol.,* 34(2):159–66, 1997.

79. Fessler, B.J., Thrombotic syndromes and autoimmune diseases. *Rheum. Dis. Clin. North Am.,* 23(2):461–479, 1997.

27 The Vasculitic Diseases of Childhood

Thomas J. A. Lehman

CONTENTS

I. INTRODUCTION

With rare exception, all of the vasculitic diseases have been reported in childhood. However, only Henoch-Schoenlein purpura (HSP) and Kawasaki disease (KD) are primarily restricted to this age group. This chapter provides a fundamental overview of these two illnesses, as well as those aspects of other vasculitic diseases that are unique to their occurrence or treatment in childhood. Polyarteritis nodosa, Wegener's granulomatosis, and Takayasu's arteritis are well described in childhood. Churg-Straus syndrome, microscopic polyangiitis, and Behçet's disease are less common but also well recognized in childhood.

Despite being well described, vasculitic illnesses are infrequent in childhood. HSP may be the most commonly observed vasculitis in childhood,[1] but others believe KD is more frequent.[2] Incidence figures for all of the vasculitides vary widely from study to study.[3-5] The absence of a rigid classification schema and the lack of definite diagnostic criteria for many of the vasculitides contribute to the difficulty in providing accurate estimates of the incidence and prevalence of many diseases.

II. KAWASAKI DISEASE

Kawasaki disease (KD) is a widespread vasculitis, primarily affecting medium-sized arteries, which has an important predilection for involvement of the coronary arteries.[2-6] Initially described as mucocutaneous lymph node syndrome by Dr. Kawasaki (in English) in 1974,[7] it is closely related to and not clearly distinct from what was previously termed infantile polyarteritis nodosa.[8,9] KD is important because it may be the most common vasculitis of childhood,[2] and because it is believed to be the most common cause of acquired childhood heart disease in countries where acute rheumatic fever has been suppressed.[10]

The diagnosis of KD is based on criteria established by the American Heart Association.[6] These include fever for more than five days, nonsuppurative conjunctivitis, significant cervical lymphadenopathy, a pleomorphic rash, oral mucosal changes, and brawny edema of the hands and feet with subsequent peeling of the skin around the fingertips and/or in the perineal region. Fever and at least four of the other criteria must be present to establish the diagnosis. Many clinicians have assumed that any febrile illness followed by peeling of the skin must be KD, but this is not correct.[11] In addition, there are other (less frequent) causes of coronary artery aneurysms in childhood. The presence of coronary artery aneurysms, while suspicious, does not establish the diagnosis of KD.[12] Presumed "atypical" cases of KD should be carefully investigated to exclude other illnesses.[13]

A. EPIDEMIOLOGY

KD has its peak incidence in the first five years of life, with a high proportion of cases occurring during the first year.[14] The disease occurs with greater frequency among Asians, and in males, but is seen in all races and both sexes.[15-18] Although there are reports of KD occurring in adolescents and adults, these cases are rare.[19] In children over ten years of age the diagnosis of KD should be regarded with relative suspicion and alternative explanations should be vigorously sought.[20-26] Very young children may be affected by KD, with reported cases as young as 20 days of age in a Japanese series of over 100,000 cases which included 1768 cases occurring before 90 days of age.[27]

The reported incidence of KD has varied both seasonally and from year to year with apparent seasonal epidemics.[14,28,29] Overall, the annual incidence in Japan is estimated to be 90/100,000 children under the age of five years. In contrast, it is estimated that only 7.6/100,000 children under five years of age were affected during an outbreak in the Chicago area.[30] However, this may be a low estimate as it is widely believed that there is significant underreporting of cases in the U.S.[31]

The increased incidence of KD among those of Asian ancestry (even when they reside in the U.S.) suggests genetic predisposition.[17] Further support for genetic factors which contribute to susceptibility comes from Japanese epidemiological studies demonstrating a higher case rate in siblings than in schoolmate controls.[32] However, there are plausible alternative explanations for this data. In Japan an HLA association was found with an increased incidence of HLA-BW22 (25.4% of patients vs. 11.8% of controls),[33] but this has not been confirmed. In the Boston area a study of Caucasian children found an increase in HLA-BW51 and not HLA-BW22, but with small numbers.[34] Shulman has proposed that KD may result from an infectious agent to which persons with a specific kappa chain Km1 allotype have an increased susceptibility.[35]

B. ETIOLOGY

The occurrence of KD in apparent epidemics,[19,28,36] and the increased incidence of contemporaneous disease in siblings[32] strongly suggest that KD has an infectious etiology. Intensive efforts to establish a retrovirus etiology in the late 1980s[37-39] were unsuccessful. At present it is believed that KD is not due to a retrovirus.[40,41] Others have proposed that KD may be the result of infection with herpes viruses,[42] paroviruses,[43-45] Epstein Barr virus,[46-49] or other viral agents.[50] Extensive testing has not confirmed any of these hypotheses.[51]

Many other possible etiologies have been proposed for KD. Mercury has been considered a possible agent.[52,53] Another frequently reported association is with house dust mites.[54-58] Again, the preponderance of the evidence is not convincing.[59]

Two curious observations continue to encourage the search for an etiologic agent: studies demonstrating that those who live near water are at greater risk of KD,[60] and studies demonstrating an association between KD and recent rug shampooing. The association with rug shampooing was first noted in an outbreak in Colorado.[61] A large number of subsequent studies have confirmed this association, although it has not been present in every outbreak.[62-66] The explanation for this association is unclear, but it suggests an etiologic agent which is facilitated by dampness.

It may be that KD is not an unusual infection, rather an unusual response to a relatively common infection. This would serve to explain the rarity of the illness after the first few years of life. Several investigations have suggested that KD may be an atypical response to streptococcus-associated enterotoxin.[10,67-69] This enterotoxin has been shown to be a "superantigen." Superantigens are by definition associated with limited Vb gene expression in the immune response.[70] Investigators have attempted to demonstrate the expected limited Vb gene expression in children with KD, but they have been unsuccessful.[71,72] Others have suggested that variant strains of psuedonomas[73] or propionobacteria may be responsible.[74]

Investigators working with animal models have demonstrated that coronary artery lesions which closely resemble those of KD can be induced in mice by injecting killed fragments of Lactobacillus casei[75-77] or Candida albicans.[78] While it is a large step from mouse to man, the onset of disease is at an age when the initial bacterial colonization of the gut is occurring, and the association of the disease with flooding and other exposures to dampness are consistent with the known natural history of Lactobacilli. Two studies of jejunal biopsies from children with KD support the concept that an unusual response to "normal" enteric flora may play a role in the pathogenesis of KD.[72,79] Despite these findings and the efforts of many investigators, the etiology of KD remains the subject of extensive speculation, but is unknown at present.

C. CLINICAL MANIFESTATIONS

Typically, KD presents as a fever greater than 38.5 C which persists despite the administration of antibiotics. Over a several-day period the fever is followed by the development of a nonsuppurative conjunctivitis (85%), marked cervical adenopathy (70%) often mimicking a cellulitis, and a pleomorphic rash (80%). Mucous membrane changes consisting of dry, cracked, red lips or a "strawberry" tongue are present in 90% of children by the third to fifth day of illness.[6] However, the mucous membrane changes are often overlooked or ascribed to other causes associated with fever. A "brawny" edema of the hands and feet, characterized by a diffuse swelling which is not limited to the joints, also becomes evident at this stage of the illness.

Laboratory evaluation during the initial phase often reveals a moderate elevation of the white blood cell count and erythrocyte sedimentation rate with a raised platelet count. The more marked elevations of these parameters that are indicative of KD typically begin around the fifth day of illness. Thrombocytopenia is extremely rare in KD and should prompt careful evaluation for alternative diagnoses — especially sepsis complicated by DIC. There are no specific laboratory tests that confirm the diagnosis of KD. Several investigators have noted that children with KD have an increased number of neutrophils with toxic granulation and degenerative vacuoles relative to normals and other febrile controls,[80,81] but this finding may not be uniformly useful. Unusual but well described clinical manifestations during the early phase of KD include aseptic meningitis,[82] facial nerve palsy,[83,84] retroperitoneal soft tissue swelling,[85] uvulitis and supraglottitis,[86] parotitis,[87] a submandibular mass,[88] uveitis,[89,90] periorbital vasculitis,[91] colitis with diarrhea,[92] and pancreatitis.[93]

A variety of illnesses may be confused with KD during this early phase. In one well-documented study, children with both group A streptococcal infection and children with measles were shown to fulfill the diagnostic criteria for KD.[60] Carbamazapine toxicity is another cause of a clinical picture resembling KD.[94] Given the breadth of the potential complications and atypical cases described in the literature, a clear resolution is not always possible.[95] The occurrence of atypical cases complicated by giant aneurysms and fatalities shifts the balance in favor of treatment once other explanations have been thoroughly explored.[13,96-98]

Between the 7th and 14th day of illness, children with KD typically experience a dramatic climb in white blood cell count, erythrocyte sedimentation rate, and platelet count. Coincident with these laboratory findings, the earliest evidence of skin peeling may be noted either around the distal fingertip or in the perineal region. These changes may persist for up to three weeks. Many children also develop a mild arthritis of the large joints two to three weeks after the onset of illness.[99] This may lead to confusion between KD and Reiter's syndrome.[100] Other manifestations that may become evident during this period include hearing loss,[101] gallbladder hydrops,[68,102-107] nephritis,[108] uveitis,[90] and urethritis. Most often these resolve without permanent sequelae. However, significant cardiac involvement often becomes clinically evident during this period.

D. CARDIAC MANIFESTATIONS

Untreated, 25% of children with KD will have significant coronary artery involvement.[22,109] Careful study of autopsy specimens has shown that inflammation of the small vessels of the heart and perivasculitis of the coronary arteries are often present, even before the tenth day of illness.[110] By two to four weeks after the onset of illness panvasculitis of the coronary arteries with aneurysm development and thrombosis may be present. Myocarditis and valvulitis are common. After the fourth week of illness granulation tissue is present in the coronary arteries. Persistent arterial stenosis and scarring may persist indefinitely.[109,111,112] Similar findings have been noted in the animal model where periadventitial inflammatory foci can be seen as early as the third day after the intraperitoneal injection of bacterial cell walls.[75,76] Evidence of severe coronary artery damage and repeated myocardial infarctions were found in mice sacrificed two years after the induction of illness.[77]

With treatment, the incidence of clinically detectable coronary artery involvement has been markedly reduced.[113] Most cardiac damage and coronary artery involvement is evident on 2-D echocardiography.[114] Appropriate adjustment must be made for the patient's size in interpreting whether or not the coronary arteries are of normal caliber.[115] Additional information may become available as our techniques for noninvasive evaluation of the coronary arteries improve. Recently, ultra-fast CT has been used for this purpose.[116] Using 2-D echocardiography, multiple studies have demonstrated that between 10 and 15% of treated children will develop coronary artery abnormalities.[111,113,117] The long-term outlook for children with documented coronary artery abnormalities is uncertain.

There are many reports of myocardial infarction occurring years after the acute illness in children with "resolved" KD.[22,109,112,118-121] Males and children afflicted during the first year of life or after five years of age appear to be at increased risk.[113,122] There is also an increased risk for cardiac involvement in those children who suffer a recurrent episode of KD.[123]

Large Japanese series suggest that children who have KD are at increased risk during the first two months after the onset of disease, but after this period the increase in mortality does not reach statistical significance.[124,125] However, numerous studies document poor coronary artery endothelial function in children who have recovered from KD.[126-129] These findings suggest increased morbidity and mortality should be expected as affected children reach the age where atherosclerosis and other factors that contribute to coronary artery disease become operative. When "recovered" children are stressed using a treadmill or drug intervention, continuing cardiovascular impairment is evident in those children who had evidence of cardiac involvement during the acute phase of their disease.[130-132] Abnormalities have also been found in some children who were not initially noted to have cardiac involvement.[126,133,134] The impaired cardiac function in these children (with normal 2-D echocardiography during the acute phase) may be due to intimal thickening that was not detected on the initial echo. This type of intimal thickening is being found in what were thought to be normal coronary arteries when the arteries are examined using intravascular ultrasound.[135]

At present, the long-term outcome of children who have KD without evidence of coronary artery involvement appears to be excellent.[109,136] The prognosis is also believed to be good for those children who have coronary artery ectasia or small aneurysms during the acute phase which resolve within a few months of recovery.[109] The prognosis for those with larger coronary artery aneurysms is less clear. Those with giant coronary artery aneurysms ($\geq$8 mm diameter) are clearly at increased risk.[109,119,137] Small series have demonstrated altered lipid profiles and decreased HDL persisting after the acute episode of KD has resolved. These findings raise additional concerns about the long-term prognosis of affected children.[138-140]

E. TREATMENT

Intravenous gammaglobulin (IVIgG) is the official recommended therapy for KD.[141-143] Although the initial rationale for its use was to provide antibodies to an unknown agent which has never been found,[144] IVIgG has been shown to truncate the acute phase of the disease and to prevent the occurrence of giant coronary artery aneurysms.[145,146] The mechanism of action of IVIgG is unknown. Many hypothetical mechanisms have been proposed. These range from a direct neutralizing effect on a toxin or infectious agent to Fc-receptor blockade, antiidiotypic antibodies, or down-regulation of cytokine synthesis.[147-149] There is little convincing experimental evidence.[150]

A variety of IVIgG dosage schedules have been used. Initially, children were given 400 mg/kg/day for four days.[151] Subsequent studies demonstrated that 1 gram/kg given on one day was more effective.[152,153] More recent studies have suggested that 2 grams/kg given on one day provides the best efficacy.[154,155] A large meta-analysis study concluded that high-dose IVIgG or low-dose IVIgG combined with aspirin were equally effective in preventing coronary artery aneurysms.[156] However, the same study found no difference in efficacy between high- or low-dose aspirin therapy when combined with IVIgG. Repeated treatment with IVIgG has been necessary in children with KD who continued to manifest active disease after the first treatment.[157] However, alternative therapy should be considered for children with persistent disease despite a second course of IVIgG. Corticosteroids have been used episodically in the treatment of KD.[158,159] However, it was initially reported that their use resulted in worsening of coronary artery aneurysms.[160,161] More recently the use of corticosteroids has been advocated for children with KD who have not responded to repeated courses of IVIgG.[162] The proper role of corticosteroids in this situation remains controversial.

At the present time high-dose IVIgG remains the treatment of choice for KD.[141] Studies of different preparations of IVIgG have shown differing frequencies of adverse reactions, but no difference in efficacy in preventing coronary artery aneurysms.[163] Since coronary artery aneurysms are an infrequent event in IVIgG-treated children, it has been difficult to accumulate sufficient numbers to be sure that a true difference between preparations has not been overlooked. Adverse reactions to IVIgG remain a significant cause of concern. Short-term allergic reactions are usually easily treated, but drastic complications have occurred in children treated with IVIgG for KD and other illnesses.[164,165]

Despite some initial reports,[166] aspirin alone, high- or low-dose, appears ineffective in blocking aneurysm formation.[167] When compared to IVIgG, aspirin alone was also ineffective in preventing damage to left ventricular cardiac contractility.[168] Much attention has been directed to the measurement of aspirin levels in children with KD.[169] During the acute phase of the illness there is decreased serum salicylate binding. This results in a decreased amount of measured serum salicylate, but it is the free form which is effective as an antiinflammatory, and this may in fact be increased in children with low levels of measured serum salicylate resulting from decreased serum protein binding.[170] Significant gastrointestinal bleeding has occurred as a complication of salicylate therapy for KD.[171] Since the study of Durongpisitkul and others[156] found no difference in efficacy between high- or low-dose aspirin therapy when combined with IVIgG, it is unlikely that high-dose aspirin therapy has any role in KD.[172,173]

F. Immunopathology

KD is a medium-sized vessel vasculitis with close pathologic similarities to infantile polyarteritis nodosa.[8,174] However, it is clinically a distinct disease. Numerous studies have attempted to elucidate the immunopathogenesis of KD. Most investigators agree immune complexes play a significant role in the initial endothelial injury.[148] The quantity of immune complexes in the circulation as demonstrated by cryoprecipitates is a predictor of disease severity.[175] Recent studies have demonstrated that these immune complexes are associated with IgG subclasses 1 and 3.[176] Simultaneous with the presence of increased immune complexes there is a marked increase in cytokine levels in the serum. TNF-alpha, IL2, IL6, and IL8 have all been shown to be increased in the early stages of KD.[177-183] Antineutrophil cytoplasmic antibodies (ANCA) have been found with increased frequency in children with KD, but antiendothelial antibodies have not.[184] The significance of these observations is uncertain.

The dramatic nature of the initial inflammatory response has led several investigators to propose that KD represents a response to a superantigen.[70,185] However, repeated studies have failed to show the expected limited Vb gene expression.[71,186] Increased atopy and increased serum IgE levels have been noted in a small proportion of KD patients,[187] but this observation does not occur with sufficient frequency to suggest it is etiologically important.

Cellular immune responses are thought to play a significant role in KD,[188] but at least one case of suspected KD has occurred in a child with acquired immune deficiency disease.[189] The well-demonstrated activation of cellular immunity at the sites of previous BCG immunization is one of the most interesting aspects of the immune response in children with KD.[190-193] This strongly suggests a generalized activation of immunomodulatory cells. In the gut, investigators have found an increased frequency of Dr-positive cells in the lamina propria of the small bowel, and a decreased number of CD8-positive cells.[194] These findings are typical of a hypersensitivity reaction in the gut. Recently, Rowley described an increased number of IgA-secreting plasma cells in the vascular endothelium of KD patients.[195] This may be further evidence that KD results from an immune response to a previously unseen antigen in the gastrointestinal tract.

III. HENOCH SCHOENLEIN PURPURA (HSP)

HSP is a second common vasculitis of childhood. It primarily affects small vessels, producing a characteristic triad of purpura (without thrombocytopenia), arthritis, and abdominal pain.[196] Frequently, the symptoms appear over a period of hours following the onset of an upper respiratory infection and the syndrome is easily diagnosed. In most cases the symptoms are self-limited and no therapy is necessary. However, a small percentage of cases are complicated by renal, intestinal, or other complications necessitating more aggressive intervention. HSP is typically an illness of younger children, affecting boys more often than girls. It may occur in clusters[3] or episodically, giving rise to widely varied estimates of its frequency.[197,198] Adults may also be affected.[199]

A. Epidemiology

The epidemiology of HSP is complex. Clustering of cases has been noted by some investigators,[3] while other investigators have concluded that such clusters are unusual.[4,200] Most feel that HSP may follow any of a wide variety of infections when they occur in a susceptible individual.[201] Studies of HLA haplotypes suggest an increased frequency of DRB1*01 and DRB1*11, but a decreased frequency of DRB1*07.[202] Although a retrospective review of renal biopsy specimens in the state of New Mexico noted a disproportionate number of specimens from American Indians,[203] no clear racial variation has been reported.

B. Etiology

HSP appears to be a large immune complex-mediated vasculitis. Multiple antigens may give rise to large immune complexes under the appropriate circumstances. Bacterial infections, especially those due to streptococci, have frequently been implicated,[201] but are clearly not the only etiologic agents. Examples of HSP which resolved with treatment of the associated infection include a tubo-ovarian abcess,[204] disseminated tuberculosis,[205] and Heliobacter pylori infections.[206] Other associated infections include coxsackie B1 virus,[207] parvovirus B19,[208] and hepatitis B and C viruses.[209,210] HSP has also been associated with cocaine abuse.[211] It is clear that no single etiology explains all the cases of HSP.[4] Indeed, in rare cases, HSP may be a paraneoplastic syndrome in both adults and children.[212-214]

C. Clinical Manifestations

HSP most often begins with a diffuse rash of palpable purpura over the buttocks and lower extremities. Because it is primarily large immune complex-mediated, the rash occurs predominantly in dependent areas and worsens with prolonged upright posture. It is not unusual for an ill child to be placed at bed rest with the foot of the bed elevated. In these circumstances the head becomes dependent and a rash may appear on the face. Although this is often interpreted as a worsening of the disease, it is merely a gravity-driven shift in the localization of the immune complexes. Diffuse edema of the effected areas leads to swelling and discomfort. Scrotal edema may be pronounced in males.[215-217] Abdominal pain usually follows the onset of rash by hours to days, but may precede it.[218-220]

Severe abdominal pain should prompt careful and thorough evaluation. Intussusception is the most common gastrointestinal complication of HSP[218] and may require surgical reduction. Perforations of both the large and small bowel can occur.[221-223] Diffuse ilieitis,[224] duodenal strictures, and even obstruction[225,226] have been reported. In one case a child with HSP developed a protein-losing enteropathy for which no other explanation was found.[227]

Severe immune complex-mediated nephritis may occur in both adults and children. In most affected individuals the renal involvement will resolve over time, but progression to renal failure may occur.[228-231] Renal compromise in children with HSP may also be the result of ureteral obstruction[232,233] or intrarenal hemorrhage.[234] Numerous schemata for predicting those at increased risk of poor renal outcome have been proposed.[235,236] Increased severity of rash, increased duration of rash, increasing age, and decreased factor XIII activity are all associated with increased risk of renal disease.[236] Nephritis has recurred following renal transplantation, even with continued immunosuppressive therapy.[237,238]

As would be expected in a large immune complex-mediated illness, mild pulmonary involvement is common. Significant pulmonary compromise including pulmonary hemorrhage has been reported[239,240] and may be fatal. Central nervous system involvement is also well documented. This may manifest as seizures secondary to vasculitis, or diffuse encephalopathy.[241] The vasculitis may be demonstrable by magnetic resonance imaging.[242,243] In rare cases HSP has been associated with intracranial hemorrhage.[244] One case of HSP-associated Guillian Barree syndrome has been reported,[245] but this may represent a rare coincidence.

A definite diagnosis of HSP is based on the American College of Rheumatology criteria.[196] Other vasculitic illnesses that may present with abdominal pain and rash must be differentiated from HSP. Autoimmune hemorrhagic edema of infancy is a leukocytoclastic vasculitis typically affecting children under the age of two years.[246] Although it often gives rise to a "typical appearing" HSP rash, there is no internal organ involvement and aggressive therapy is not indicated.[247-251] This entity may be partially responsible for reports that HSP in children less than two years of age is a less severe illness.[252,253]

Polyarteritis nodosa and poststrepotoccal glomerulonephritis may present with rash, arthritis, abdominal pain, and renal involvement.[254,255] In general, polyarteritis nodosa is a more severe disease characterized by larger vessel involvement. A definite boundary between severe HSP and mild PAN has not been well delineated. A positive test for antineutrophil cytoplasmic antibodies (ANCA) may be helpful in differentiating microscopic polyarteritis.[255,256] Michel and others have proposed a decision tree to assist in distinguishing HSP from isolated leukocytoclastic vasculitis.[257]

Most cases of HSP are short-lived and are symptomatically resolved within weeks. A small percentage of cases of HSP are associated with recurrent episodes of rash and abdominal pain over a period of years. In the absence of severe abdominal pain secondary to intussusception or vascular compromise of the gastrointestinal tract, the majority of children do well. However, chronic nephritis may ultimately result in renal failure in a small percentage of cases.

D. TREATMENT

Most of the manifestations of HSP respond to corticosteroids in small or moderate doses.[215,258] Due care should be taken in using corticosteroids in children with severe abdominal pain as their use may mask peritonitis.[259] While steroids are often adequate therapy,[236] in some cases persistent and progressive renal disease necessitates more aggressive treatment. The combination of corticosteroids with azathioprine is frequently used.[260] Others have utilized high-dose pulse methylprednisolone for children with crescenteric glomerulonephritis or nephrotic syndrome.[261] In one small uncontrolled series, pulse methylprednisolone followed by oral corticosteroids, oral cyclophosphamide, and dyprimadole was associated with a favorable outcome.[262] Efforts to avoid corticosteroid toxicity by utilizing IVIgG or cyclosporine have generally been unsatisfactory.[202,263-265] Children with chronic renal failure may under go renal transplant, but there is a risk of recurrence.[237,238]

E. IMMUNOPATHOLOGY

Abnormal clearance of polymeric IgA immune complexes and widespread IgA deposition in damaged tissues are hallmarks of HSP.[266,267] Indeed, it has been proposed that an increased percentage of IgA-secreting circulating plasma cells may assist in making the diagnosis of HSP.[268] However, increased IgA desposition in skin and other tissues is not specific for HSP.[269] There is increasing evidence of abnormal IgA1 glycosolation in children with HSP.[270-272] This abnormal glycosolation is hypothesized to interfere with the ability to clear IgA immune complexes from the serum and, hence, predispose to the development of HSP.

An increased number of large von Willebrand factor (vWF) multimers in the circulation is a second well-documented finding that is relatively unique to children with HSP.[272-277] The amount of vWF in the circulation of children with HSP seems to correlate directly with disease severity, and inversely with Factor XIII activity.[278]

Investigators have reported the presence of IgA ANCA in children with HSP,[279] and of IgA antiendothelial cell antibodies.[280] However, it has been suggested that the ANCA may be false positive results secondary to IgA rheumatoid factor-like activity in children with HSP[281] or lectin binding.[282] Anticardiolipin antibodies are not increased in children with HSP.[283]

Complement activation is not commonly associated with HSP.[284] Interestingly, there is one report of a C4-deficient family in which one member suffered from HSP and another from Wegener's granulomatosis.[285] A variety of reports have sought to distinguish factors predisposing children to renal complications of HSP. Renal disease appears to be associated with increased levels of TNF in the serum[286] and increased thrombomodulin with decreased tissue-type plaminogen activation.[287] Unlike SLE, HSP is not associated with increased circulating levels of soluble TNF receptor (sTNF-r).[288] Others have noted increased serum levels of IgD in HSP children without nephritis,[289] but increased levels of circulating VCAM in children with renal vasculitis secondary to HSP or other vasculitides.[290]

A variety of additional interesting observations regarding children with HSP has not yet been confirmed. An increase in frequency of the IL1 receptor allele IL1RN*2 was found in children with HSP compared to children with either IgA nephropathy or poststreptococcal glomerulonephritis.[291] Children with HSP have also been found to have an increased level of eosinophilic cationic protein which is not present in those with IgA nephropathy.[292]

While a full explanation of the immunopathogenesis of HSP remains to be determined, most investigators agree that HSP results from inadequate clearance of IgA immune complexes elicited by a wide variety of antigens. Abnormal IgA is likely to play a key role in this process,[293,294] perhaps as a result of abnormal glycosylation.

IV. OTHER VASCULITIDES

Virtually every form of vasculitis has been recognized in childhood with the exception that there are no convincing cases of childhood temporal arteritis. However, the remaining vasculitides have been reported only as isolated case reports or very small series in childhood. These reports add little to the prior discussions of the etiology, immunopathology, and epidemiology of these diseases in the chapters in this text that describe these diseases in adults. Therefore, the remainder of this chapter will be limited to a description of the clinical presentation and treatment of these diseases as they occur in childhood, as much as possible without repetition of information provided elsewhere.

A. POLYARTERITIS NODOSA

Polyarteritis nodosa (PAN) is well recognized in childhood.[295,296] It is a medium-sized vessel vasculitis that may affect the skin as well as muscles and visceral organs. PAN occurs at all ages, including very young children, adolescents, and adults. PAN is recognized to occur with increased frequency in association with infections, especially hepatitis B[297,298] and group A streptococcal infections.[299] It has also been reported in increased frequency in children suffering from familial Mediterranean fever, but the explanation for this association is unclear.[300]

Mild cases of PAN confined to the skin may require minimal if any therapy, while cases with significant internal organ involvement may be life-threatening and require immunosuppression. PAN tends to affect both sexes equally.[296] In reviewing the older literature, it should be remembered that many children with KD were erroneously labeled as PAN before KD became a widely recognized entity.[301] There is some concern that this situation is reversed at present.

1. Epidemiology

There are no reliable figures for the incidence or prevalence of PAN. It is not as common as either Kawasaki disease or Henoch Schoenlein purpura, but it is probable that some cases of PAN are mistaken for more common vasculitides. In reported series, males are affected as often as females, and all age groups are affected.[296] Specific criteria have been suggested for the diagnosis of PAN in childhood, but they are not widely applied.[302]

2. Etiology

PAN is thought to be a large immune complex-mediated vasculitis, much like HSP. Associations between PAN and hepatitis B virus[298] and Group A streptococcal infections[299,303-307] in childhood are well described. Despite well-documented flares of disease in association with group A streptococcal infections in some children, it has not been possible to convincingly demonstrate immune complexes containing streptococcal antigens even in these subjects. Reports of transplacental PAN, which resolves as maternal antibody levels wane, highlight the complexity of these issues.[308] PAN has also been associated with exposure to isoretinoin,[309] further suggesting that this is an immune complex-mediated vasculitis. Two cases of a PAN-like illness during an outbreak of trichinosis in which IgE immune complexes were demonstrated in the vessel wall are very suggestive in this regard.[310]

PAN has also been shown to occur with increased frequency in association with ulcerative colitis.[311-314] This may be due to increased bowel permeablility, and an increased exposure to immune complexes with gut-associated antigens. However, an increased incidence of PAN in association with familial Mediterranean fever (FMF) has also been described.[300,315-318] Whether this is a true association or an independent vasculitis associated with FMF is unclear.

3. Clinical Manifestations

Children with PAN often present initially with fever, weight loss, and arthritis. The characteristic picture includes the additional findings of abdominal pain, hypertension, and purpuric rash.[295,296,302,304] When all the characteristic findings are present the diagnosis is not difficult, though some children are misdiagnosed as "atypical" or severe HSP. However, many children present with an incomplete picture. The absence of typical daily fever spikes, the frequent occurrence of severe abdominal pain, and the different appearance of the rash all help to distinguish children with PAN from those with systemic onset JRA. Hypertension and nephritis in the presence of arthritis may suggest SLE. PAN may be associated with a positive test for ANA, but hypocomplementemia and antibodies to dsDNA should not be present.

Some children described as PAN in reports prior to 1975 are, in fact, cases of KD and should be treated as such.[301] The relationship of KD to PAN has been much discussed without clear resolution. PAN may involve the heart and has been associated with decreased left ventricular contractility on long-term follow-up.[319] Autopsy series have also demonstrated PAN to be complicated by arteritis of the epicardial coronary arteries.[320] PAN may be a cause of significant pulmonary compromise. Seven of ten fatal cases of PAN in which the lungs were carefully inspected at autopsy demonstrated bronchial artery involvement.[321] Case reports document that PAN may involve any medium-sized artery. It has been associated with widespread arterial involvement and thrombosis of multiple major vessels in childhood.[322,323]

A number of case reports describe children who have unusual clinical presentations with pathologic findings including fibrinoid necrosis of medium-sized vessels. These are often included in series of PAN, but their relationship to children who fit the classical clinical syndrome is uncertain. These range from reports of isolated central nervous system disease in an eight-month-old[324] to reports of a child with granulomatous glomerulonephritis and microscopic polyarteritis.[325] Other reports in which abdominal pain was the dominant finding include PAN presenting as abdominal perforation[326] and presenting with ureteral obstruction.[327] Kumar reported an atypical series of ten young children with apparent benign cutaneous polyarteritis, in which seven of ten had episodes of gangrene.[328]

It is not clear whether cutaneous PAN is a distinct entity or simply represents mild PAN. Children with cutaneous PAN often have fever and elevated sedimentation rate. Some have mild arthritis. Children with skin, muscle, and peripheral nerve involvement are included as cutaneous PAN in some series.[329] However, those with marked evidence of systemic illness and involvement beyond the skin are at risk of progression to "true" PAN and should probably be considered separately.[329]

4. Treatment

Corticosteroids are the mainstay of therapy for PAN. Like adults, most children respond favorably. However, some children with PAN have significant renal or other internal organ involvement necessitating more aggressive treatment. A variety of immunosuppressive agents have been used in the treatment of adults with PAN, with varying reports of success. Severe cases in childhood are often treated with intravenous cyclophosphamide.[330] Other agents including azathioprine, IVIgG,[331] and low-dose weekly methotrexate have been utilized with varying reports of success.[332]

B. Wegener's Granulomatosis in Childhood

1. Clinical Manifestations

Wegener's granulomatosis (WG) is an unusual finding in both adults and children,[333] but in large series as many as 15% of cases had their onset in childhood or adolescence.[334] Nonetheless, Wegener's is an unexpected finding in childhood. Perhaps it is for this very reason that there are so many case reports. Children most often present with recurrent episodes of sinusitis associated with fever, weight loss, and lethargy. Typically, the persistence of symptoms and the elevated sedimentation rate prompt further investigation, leading to discovery of pulmonary lesions and/or nephritis.[334-336] In one large study comparing older and younger (ages 13 to 23 years) patients with Wegener's, it was found that the younger patients had a higher frequency of unusual manifestations, including hearing loss and intracranial lesions.[335] Subglotic stenosis and nasal perforation have also been reported to occur more often in children than adults with Wegener's.[337]

A variety of unusual presentations of Wegener's have been reported in childhood. Children with pseudotumor cerebri,[338,339] orbital pseudotumor,[340] dacryoadenitis,[341] and chronic otitis complicated by exophthalmos[342] have all been described. Some children with chronic nonspecific upper airway symptoms have developed rapidly progressive subglottic stenosis resulting in death.[343]

Skin lesions are often a predominant finding in childhood. Many children have presented with unusual skin lesions found to be Wegener's on biopsy.[344-346] When they were questioned, these children had minimal complaints of malaise. Evidence of systemic involvement was detected only after the biopsy results were known. Often the diagnosis of Wegener's is not initially suspected. Children have been followed with diagnoses of HSP[347-349] or fever of unknown origin[350] for prolonged periods prior to the correct diagnosis being made. In some reports, children with typical signs of Wegener's have died without premortem diagnosis.[351]

Uveitis is a well-described complication of Wegener's and may be its first manifestation.[352] Chronic scleritis has also been a presenting ocular manifestation.[353] Other children have presented with chronic pleural effusions,[354] persistent gingivitis,[355] or fever, malaise, and weight loss without obvious localizing findings.[356] There is one case report of a child with a well-recognized systemic onset JRA of long-standing who went on to develop Wegener's,[357] but there is no known association of these illnesses. Serologic testing for the presence of antineutrophil cytoplasmic antibodies (ANCA) may be useful in raising the index of suspicion for Wegener's.[358] However, not all children with ANCAs are suffering from Wegener's.[359] Nonetheless, children with positive ANCAs should be carefully evaluated for signs or symptoms of Wegener's. Chest roentgenograms and computer-assisted tomography of the chest may be helpful in this regard.[360,361]

2. Treatment

The majority of children with Wegener's have been treated, as adults are, with prednisone and oral cyclophosphamide.[362-364] Pulse cyclophosphamide therapy has been used in childhood and found effective in inducing remission, but not in maintaining it.[365] The combination of methotrexate and prednisone has been used successfully in children.[366] Others have preferred the combination of azathioprine and prednisone.[367] A single child with Wegener's successfully treated with IVIgG has been reported.[368]

3. Prognosis

The majority of reports of Wegener's granulomatosis in childhood consist of either small series or single case reports. There are many reports of fatalities, but these often represent children whose disease was not suspected. With appropriate diagnosis and aggressive therapy the long-term prognosis for most children with Wegener's appears to be good.

C. Takayasu's Arteritis

1. Clinical Manifestations

Takayasu's arteritis (TA) is well described in childhood. It affects females far more often than males, with many cases having their onset before 20 years of age.[369-371] In many parts of the world there is a strong association between Takayasu's arteritis and tuberculosis, as manifested by a positive PPD; but in other areas this association is less clear.[369,370,372,373] Most often TA is discovered during the evaluation of a child with severe hypertension.[372,374,375] However, children may present with nonspecific symptoms including prolonged fever and malaise.[376,377] In one series that compared the manifestations of adults and children, arthritis and congestive heart failure were more frequent in those with childhood onset.[370]

The pathologic diagnosis of Takayasu's arteritis is based on the characteristic granulomatous changes in the large vessels. However, the diagnosis is made clinically on recognition of vasculitic involvement of the aortic arch and its larger branches. Although described as "pulseless" disease, early in the disease course TA is often associated only with attenuation of pulses associated with involved vessels. In some cases arterial inflammation results in stenosis, with poststenotic dilatation and seemingly bounding arterial pulses. The diagnosis is often made when widening of the aortic arch is recognized on routine radiographic examination of the chest.[378] Aortography is the most accurate method of determining the full extent of vascular involvement.[379] However, gallium scanning has also been useful in assessing areas of active vasculitis, and with a lesser morbidity than aortography.[380,381]

In the absence of significant peripheral hypertension, TA may go undetected for a prolonged period. Many children with TA spontaneously recover from the acute inflammatory phase, but are left with damaged vessels. Significant pulmonary artery involvement may be fatal.[382-384] Aortitis involving the aortic root may be associated with occlusion of the coronary ostia, resulting in myocardial infarction.[385,386] Chronic unsuspected TA has been reported presenting as unilateral finger-clubbing.[387] Central nervous system involvement in children with TA may result from either hypertensive encephalopathy secondary to renovascular hypertension, or direct intracranial vessel involvement.[375,388]

Rare cases associating TA with other rheumatic diseases are of unknown significance. Several cases of systemic lupus erythematosus and TA have been described.[389] There are also several case reports of juvenile rheumatoid arthritis and TA.[390,391] The possibility that these cases represent TA which was misdiagnosed as JRA must always be considered.[392] Similarly, it is unclear whether three reports of inflammatory bowel disease associated with TA in childhood represent coincidence, overlapping disease manifestations, or a true association.[393-395]

While hypertension is the most frequent renal manifestation of TA, children have presented with hematuria and proteinuria secondary to glomerulonephritis. Most often this is focal segmental,[396] but crescentic glomerulonephritis[397] and amyloidosis[398] have been reported.

2. Treatment

As previously described for adults, the treatment of Takayasu's arteritis in childhood consists of corticosteroids and other immunosuppressive agents to correct the inflammation, and the use of antihypertensives when necessary to correct renal vascular hypertension.[372,388] Unresponsive renovascular hypertension may require surgical treatment, and even resection and autotransplanation or cadaveric transplantation.[377,399,400] There is only a single report of the use of methotrexate as a steroid sparing agent for TA in childhood.[401]

In general, the prognosis for children with appropriately recognized and treated TA is good,[371,384] but the outcome varies from series to series.[370,373] An increased index of suspicion and prompt institution of antiinflammatory therapy are key to optimum outcome.

D. OTHER VASCULITIDES

Goodpasture's syndrome,[402] Kohlmeir Degos syndrome,[403] Mucha Haberman Disease,[404] Churg Strauss syndrome,[405,406] and Behçet's[407] all occur rarely in childhood. Since none has unique manifestations that have been appreciated in the pediatric age group, and each is described in detail elsewhere in this text, the reader is referred to the appropriate chapters for a complete description of these diseases.

V. CONCLUSIONS

With the probable exception of temporal arteritis, all of the vasculitic diseases occur in children. Two, HSP and KD, are found predominantly in children and rarely in adults. The explanation for this dichotomy is not well understood. Perhaps there is an age related vulnerability to injury caused by the responsible antigens. It may be that as the vasculature and the immune system mature, the susceptible individuals become resistant to the process which initiates these diseases. Conversely, temporal arteritis is a disease of older age groups in whom a characteristic defense mechanism may be deteriorating.

One's first thought on reviewing the vasculitic diseases in childhood is that they must represent a variety of different etiologic insults. However, certain agents such as group A streptococci have been suggestively associated with a variety of vasculitides. Perhaps in part, the variety of vasculitic syndromes we see represent not differing etiologic insults, but a genetically determined variety of host responses to a more limited number of agents. Such a finding has been demonstrated in animal models[75,408] and would explain the varying racial and geographic frequencies of these illnesses.

The major concern for physicians dealing with the vasculitides in childhood is the frequency with which they are incorrectly diagnosed or not diagnosed at all. It is important for the practicing physician to be aware that all of the vasculitic diseases may occur in childhood. Prompt recognition and prompt institution of appropriate therapy are vital to improved prognoses.

REFERENCES

1. Athreya, BH. Vasculitis in children. *Pediatric Clinics of North America.* 1995;42:1239–61.
2. Kawasaki, T. General review and problems in Kawasaki disease. *Japanese Heart Journal.* 1995;36:1–12.
3. Farley, TA, Gillespie, S, Rasoulpour, M, Tolentino, N, Hadler, JL, Hurwitz, E. Epidemiology of a cluster of Henoch-Schonlein purpura. *American Journal of Diseases of Children.* 1989;143:798–803.

4. Nielsen, HE. Epidemiology of Schonlein-Henoch purpura. *Acta Paediatrica Scandinavica.* 1988;77:125–31.

5. Watts, RA, Carruthers, DM, Scott, DG. Epidemiology of systemic vasculitis: changing incidence or definition? *Seminars in Arthritis & Rheumatism.* 1995;25:28–34.

6. Anonymous. Diagnostic guidelines for Kawasaki disease. American Heart Association Committee on Rheumatic Fever, Endocarditis, and Kawasaki Disease. *American Journal of Diseases of Children.* 1990;144:1218–19.

7. Kawasaki, T, Kosaki, F, Odawa, S, et al. A new infantile acute febrile mucocutaneous lymph node syndrome prevailing in Japan. *Pediatrics.* 54, 271, 1974.

8. Landing, BH, Larson, EJ. Are infantile periarteritis nodosa with coronary artery involvement and fatal mucocutaneous lymph node syndrome the same? Comparison of 20 patients from North America with patients from Hawaii and Japan. *Pediatrics.* 1977;59:651–62.

9. Munro-Faure, H. Necrotizing arteritis of the coronary vessels in infancy. *Pediatrics.* 23, 914, 1959.

10. Nishiyori, A, Sakaguchi, M, Kato, H, Igarashi, H, Miwa, K. Toxic shock syndrome toxin-secreting Staphylococcus aureus in Kawasaki syndrome [letter]. *Lancet.* 1994;343:299–300.

11. Kuijpers, TW, Tjia, KL, de Jager, F, Peters, M, Lam, J. A boy with chickenpox whose fingers peeled. *Lancet.* 1998;351:1782.

12. Parrillo, JE, Fauci, AS. Necrotizing vasculitis, coronary angiitis, and the cardiologist. *American Heart Journal.* 1980;99:547–54.

13. Levy, M, Koren, G. Atypical Kawasaki disease: analysis of clinical presentation and diagnostic clues. *Pediatric Infectious Disease Journal.* 1990;9:122–26.

14. Yanagawa, H, Yashiro, M, Nakamura, Y, Kawasaki, T, Kato, H. Results of 12 nationwide epidemiological incidence surveys of Kawasaki disease in Japan. *Archives of Pediatrics & Adolescent Medicine.* 1995;149:779–83.

15. Rauch, AM. Kawasaki syndrome: critical review of U.S. epidemiology. *Progress in Clinical & Biological Research.* 1987;250:33–44.

16. Salo, E. Epidemiology of Kawasaki disease in Northern Europe. *Progress in Clinical & Biological Research.* 1987;250:67–70.

17. Shulman, ST, McAuley, JB, Pachman, LM, Miller, ML, Ruschhaupt, DG. Risk of coronary abnormalities due to Kawasaki disease in urban area with small Asian population. *American Journal of Diseases of Children.* 1987;141:420–425.

18. Melish, ME. Kawasaki syndrome (the mucocutaneous lymph node syndrome). *Pediatric Annals.* 1982;11:255–68.

19. Yanagawa, H, Yashiro, M, Nakamura, Y, Kawasaki, T, Kato, H. Epidemiologic pictures of Kawasaki disease in Japan: from the nationwide incidence survey in 1991 and 1992. *Pediatrics.* 1995;95:475–79.

20. Tomiyama, J, Hasegawa, Y, Kumagai, Y, Adachi, Y, Karasawa, K. Acute febrile mucocutaneous lymph node syndrome (Kawasaki disease) in adults: case report and review of the literature. *Japanese Journal of Medicine.* 1991;30:285–89.

21. Bauer, HM, Oaks, S, Anderson, VA. Mucocutaneous lymph node syndrome in adult [letter]. *JAMA.* 1980;244:2416.

22. Burns, JC, Shike, H, Gordon, JB, Malhotra, A, Schoenwetter, M, Kawasaki, T. Sequelae of Kawasaki disease in adolescents and young adults. *Journal of the American College of Cardiology.* 1996;28:253–57.

23. Lee, TJ, Vaughan, D. Mucocutaneous lymph node syndrome in a young adult. *Archives of Internal Medicine.* 1979;139:104–5.

24. Marcella, JJ, Ursell, PC, Goldberger, M, Lovejoy, W, Fenoglio, JJJ, Weiss, et al. Kawasaki syndrome in an adult: endomyocardial histology and ventricular function during acute and recovery phases of illness. *Journal of the American College of Cardiology.* 1983;2:374–78.

25. Saxe, N, Horak, A, Goldblatt, J. Mucocutaneous lymph node syndrome in a young adult. A case report. *South African Medical Journal.* 1980;58:1011–13.

26. Todd, JK. Mucocutaneous lymph node syndrome (Kawasaki disease) in adults [letter]. *JAMA.* 1980;243:1631.

27. Tsuchida, S, Yamanaka, T, Tsuchida, R, Nakamura, Y, Yashiro, M, Yanagawa, H. Epidemiology of infant Kawasaki disease with a report of the youngest neonatal case ever reported in Japan. *Acta Paediatrica.* 1996;85:995–97.

28. Yanagawa, H, Nakamura, Y, Yashiro, M, Fujita, Y, Nagai, M, Kawasaki, T, et al. A nationwide incidence survey of Kawasaki disease in 1985–1986 in Japan. *Journal of Infectious Diseases*. 1988;158:1296–301.

29. Yanagawa, H, Nakamura, Y, Kawasaki, T, Shigematsu, I. Nationwide epidemic of Kawasaki disease in Japan during winter of 1985–86. *Lancet*. 1986;2:1138–39.

30. Anonymous. Multiple outbreaks of Kawasaki syndrome — United States. *MMWR — Morbidity & Mortality Weekly Report*. 1985;34:33–35.

31. Bronstein, DE, Besser, RE, Burns, JC. Passive surveillance for Kawasaki disease in San Diego County. *Pediatric Infectious Disease Journal*. 1997;16:1015–18.

32. Fujita, Y, Nakamura, Y, Sakata, K, Hara, N, Kobayashi, M, Nagai, M, et al. Kawasaki disease in families. *Pediatrics*. 1989;84:666–69.

33. Kato, S, Kimura, M, Tsuji, K, Kusakawa, S, Asai, T, Juji, T, et al. HLA antigens in Kawasaki disease. *Pediatrics*. 1978;61:252–55.

34. Krensky, AM, Berenberg, W, Shanley, K, Yunis, EJ. HLA antigens in mucocutaneous lymph node syndrome in New England. *Pediatrics*. 1981;67:741–43.

35. Shulman, ST, Melish, M, Inoue, O, Kato, H, Tomita, S. Immunoglobulin allotypic markers in Kawasaki disease. *Journal of Pediatrics*. 1993;122:84–86.

36. Yanagawa, H, Nakamura, Y, Yashiro, M, Ojima, T, Tanihara, S, Oki, I, et al. Results of the nationwide epidemiologic survey of Kawasaki disease in 1995 and 1996 in Japan. *Pediatrics*. 1998;102:E65.

37. Shulman, ST, Rowley, AH. Does Kawasaki disease have a retroviral aetiology? *Lancet*. 1986;2:545–46.

38. Burns, JC, Huang, AS, Newburger, JW, Reinhart, AL, Walsh, MM, Hoch, S, et al. Characterization of the polymerase activity associated with cultured peripheral blood mononuclear cells from patients with Kawasaki disease. *Pediatric Research*. 1990;27:109–12.

39. Rowley, AH, Shulman, ST, Preble, OT, Poiesz, BJ, Ehrlich, GD, Sullivan, JR. Serum interferon concentrations and retroviral serology in Kawasaki syndrome. *Pediatric Infectious Disease Journal*. 1988;7:663–66.

40. Okamoto, T, Kuwabara, H, Shimotohno, K, Sugimura, T, Yanase, Y, Kawasaki, T. Lack of evidence of retroviral involvement in Kawasaki disease [letter]. *Pediatrics*. 1988;81:599.

41. Rowley, A, Castro, B, Levy, J, Sullivan, J, Koup, R, Fresco, R, et al. Failure to confirm the presence of a retrovirus in cultured lymphocytes from patients with Kawasaki syndrome. *Pediatric Research*. 1991;29:417–19.

42. Burns, JC, Newburger, JW, Sundell, R, Wyatt, LS, Frenkel, N. Seroprevalence of human herpesvirus 7 in patients with Kawasaki disease [letter]. *Pediatric Infectious Disease Journal*. 1994;13:168–69.

43. Cohen, BJ. Human parvovirus B19 infection in Kawasaki disease [letter]. *Lancet*. 1994;344:59.

44. Nigro, G, Zerbini, M, Krzysztofiak, A, Gentilomi, G, Porcaro, MA, Mango, T, et al. Active or recent parvovirus B19 infection in children with Kawasaki disease. *Lancet*. 1994;343:1260–1261.

45. Yoto, Y, Kudoh, T, Haseyama, K, Suzuki, N, Chiba, S, Matsunaga, Y. Human parvovirus B19 infection in Kawasaki disease [letter]. *Lancet*. 1994;344:58–59.

46. Iwanaga, M, Takada, K, Osato, T, Saeki, Y, Noro, S, Sakurada, N. Kawasaki disease and Epstein-Barr virus [letter]. *Lancet*. 1981;1:938–39.

47. Kikuta, H, Sakiyama, Y, Matsumoto, S, Hamada, I, Yazaki, M, Iwaki, T, et al. Detection of Epstein-Barr virus DNA in cardiac and aortic tissues from chronic, active Epstein-Barr virus infection associated with Kawasaki disease-like coronary artery aneurysms. *Journal of Pediatrics*. 1993;123:90–92.

48. Kikuta, H, Mizuno, F, Osato, T, Konno, M, Ishikawa, N, Noro, S, et al. Kawasaki disease and an unusual primary infection with Epstein-Barr virus [letter]. *Pediatrics*. 1984;73:413–14.

49. Okano, M, Hase, N, Sakiyama, Y, Matsumoto, S. Long-term observation in patients with Kawasaki syndrome and their relation to Epstein-Barr virus infection. *Pediatric Infectious Disease Journal*. 1990;9:139–41.

50. Moynahan, EJ. Kawasaki disease: a novel feline virus transmitted by fleas? *Lancet*. 1987;1:195.

51. Rowley, AH, Wolinsky, SM, Relman, DA, Sambol, SP, Sullivan, J, Terai, M, et al. Search for highly conserved viral and bacterial nucleic acid sequences corresponding to an etiologic agent of Kawasaki disease. *Pediatric Research*. 1994;36:567–71.

52. Aschner, M, Aschner, JL. Mucocutaneous lymph node syndrome: is there a relationship to mercury exposure? [letter]. *American Journal of Diseases of Children*. 1989;143:1133–34.

53. Orlowski, JP, Mercer, RD. Urine mercury levels in Kawasaki disease. *Pediatrics*. 1980;66:633–36.

54. Freed, DL. Kawasaki disease, housedust mites, and rugs letter. *Lancet*. 1983;1:1221.

55. Fujimoto, T, Kato, H, Ichiose, E, Sasaguri, Y. Immune complex and mite antigen in Kawasaki disease [letter]. *Lancet*. 1982;2:980–981.

56. Furusho, K, Ohba, T, Soeda, T, Kimoto, K, Okabe, T, Hirota, T. Possible role for mite antigen in Kawasaki disease [letter]. *Lancet*. 1981;2:194–95.

57. Hamashima, Y, Tasaka, K, Hoshino, T, Nagata, N, Furukawa, F, Kao, T, et al. Mite-associated particles in Kawasaki disease [letter]. *Lancet*. 1982;2:266.

58. Ishii, A, Yatani, T, Kato, H, Fujimoto, T. Mite fauna, housedust, and Kawasaki disease [letter]. *Lancet*. 1983;2:102–3.

59. Jordan, SC, Platts-Mills, TA, Mason, W, Takahashi, M, Sakai, R, Rawle, F, et al. Lack of evidence for mite-antigen-mediated pathogenesis in Kawasaki disease letter. *Lancet*. 1983;1:931.

60. Burns, JC, Mason, WH, Glode, MP, Shulman, ST, Melish, ME, Meissner, C, et al. Clinical and epidemiologic characteristics of patients referred for evaluation of possible Kawasaki disease. United States Multicenter Kawasaki Disease Study Group. *Journal of Pediatrics*. 1991;118:680–686.

61. Patriarca, PA, Rogers, MF, Morens, DM, Schonberger, LB, Kaminski, RM, Burns, et al. Kawasaki syndrome: association with the application of rug shampoo. *Lancet*. 1982;2:578–80.

62. Daniels, SR, Specker, B. Association of rug shampooing and Kawasaki disease. *Journal of Pediatrics*. 1991;118:485–88.

63. Ichida, F, Fatica, NS, O'Loughlin, JE, Klein, AA, Snyder, MS, Levin, AR, et al. Epidemiologic aspects of Kawasaki disease in a Manhattan hospital. *Pediatrics*. 1989;84:235–41.

64. Ohga, K, Yamanaka, R, Kinumaki, H, Awa, S, Kobayashi, N. Kawasaki disease and rug shampoo [letter]. *Lancet*. 1983;1:930.

65. Fatica, NS, Ichida, F, Engle, MA, Lesser, ML. Rug shampoo and Kawasaki disease. *Pediatrics*. 1989;84:231–34.

66. Rauch, AM, Glode, MP, Wiggins, JWJ, Rodriguez, JG, Hopkins, RS, Hurwitz, ES, et al. Outbreak of Kawasaki syndrome in Denver, Colorado: association with rug and carpet cleaning. *Pediatrics*. 1991;87:663–69.

67. Kawai, M, Osawa, N, Yamaura, N, Ikewaki, N, Yashiro, K, Hiraishi, S, et al. Possible role of Streptococcus pyogenes in mucocutaneous lymph node syndrome. IX. Quantitation by ELISA of streptococcal pyrogenic exotoxin in the serum of MCLS patients. *Acta Paediatrica Japonica*. 1989;31:529–36.

68. Krensky, AM, Teele, R, Watkins, J, Bates, J. Streptococcal antigenicity in mucocutaneous lymph node syndrome and hydropic gallbladders [letter]. *Pediatrics*. 1979;64:979–80.

69. Leung, DY, Sullivan, KE, Brown-Whitehorn, TF, Fehringer, AP, Allen, S, Finkel, et al. Association of toxic shock syndrome toxin-secreting and exfoliative toxin-secreting Staphylococcus aureus with Kawasaki syndrome complicated by coronary artery disease. *Pediatric Research*. 1997;42:268–72.

70. Leung, DY, Giorno, RC, Kazemi, LV, Flynn, PA, Busse, JB. Evidence for superantigen involvement in cardiovascular injury due to Kawasaki syndrome. *Journal of Immunology*. 1995;155:5018–21.

71. Pietra, BA, De Inocencio, J, Giannini, EH, Hirsch, R. TCR V beta family repertoire and T-cell activation markers in Kawasaki disease. *Journal of Immunology*. 1994;153:1881–88.

72. Yamashiro, Y, Nagata, S, Oguchi, S, Shimizu, T. Selective increase of V beta 2+ T-cells in the small intestinal mucosa in Kawasaki disease. *Pediatric Research*. 1996;39:264–66.

73. Keren, G, Barzilay, Z, Alpert, G, Spirer, Z, Danon, Y. Mucocutaneous lymph node syndrome (Kawasaki disease) in Israel. A review of 13 cases: is pseudomonas infection responsible? *Acta Paediatrica Scandinavica*. 1983;72:455–58.

74. Kato, H, Fujimoto, T, Inoue, O, Kondo, M, Koga, Y, Yamamoto, S, et al. Variant strain of Propionibacterium acnes: a clue to the aetiology of Kawasaki disease. *Lancet*. 1983;2:1383–88.

75. Lehman, TJ, Walker, SM, Mahnovski, V, McCurdy, D. Coronary arteritis in mice following the systemic injection of group B Lactobacillus casei cell walls in aqueous suspension. *Arthritis & Rheumatism*. 1985;28:652–59.

76. Lehman, TJ, Mahnovski, V. Animal models of vasculitis. Lessons we can learn to improve our understanding of Kawasaki disease. *Rheumatic Diseases Clinics of North America*. 1988;14:479–87.

77. Lehman, TJ. Can we prevent long term cardiac damage in Kawasaki disease? Lessons from Lactobacillus casei cell wall-induced arteritis in mice. *Clinical & Experimental Rheumatology*. 1993;11 Suppl 9:S3–S6.

78. Murata, H. Experimental candida-induced arteritis in mice. Relation to arteritis in the mucocutaneous lymph node syndrome. *Microbiology & Immunology.* 1979;23:825–31.

79. Yamashiro, Y, Nagata, S, Ohtsuka, Y, Oguchi, S, Shimizu, T. Microbiologic studies on the small intestine in Kawasaki disease. *Pediatric Research.* 1996;39:622–24.

80. Rowe, PC, Quinlan, A, Luke, BK. Value of degenerative change in neutrophils as a diagnostic test for Kawasaki syndrome. *Journal of Pediatrics.* 1991;119:370–374.

81. Takeshita, S, Sekine, I, Fujisawa, T, Yoshioka, S. Studies of peripheral blood toxic neutrophils as a predictor of coronary risk in Kawasaki disease — the pathogenetic role of hematopoietic colony-stimulating factors (GM-CSF, G-CSF). *Acta Paediatrica Japonica.* 1990;32:508–14.

82. Dengler, LD, Capparelli, EV, Bastian, JF, Bradley, DJ, Glode, MP, Santa, S, et al. Cerebrospinal fluid profile in patients with acute Kawasaki disease. *Pediatric Infectious Disease Journal.* 1998;17:478–81.

83. Kleiman, MB, Passo, MH. Incomplete Kawasaki disease with facial nerve paralysis and coronary artery involvement. *Pediatric Infectious Disease Journal.* 1988;7:301–2.

84. Nigro, G, Midulla, M. Facial nerve paralysis associated with Kawasaki syndrome letter. *Pediatric Infectious Disease Journal.* 1988;7:889–90.

85. Hester, TO, Harris, JP, Kenny, JF, Albernaz, MS. Retropharyngeal cellulitis: a manifestation of Kawasaki disease in children. *Otolaryngology — Head & Neck Surgery.* 1993;109:1030–1033.

86. Kazi, A, Gauthier, M, Lebel, MH, Farrell, CA, Lacroix, J. Uvulitis and supraglottitis: early manifestations of Kawasaki disease. *Journal of Pediatrics.* 1992;120:564–67.

87. Seyedabadi, KS, Howes, RF, Yazdi, M. Parotitis associated with Kawasaki syndrome letter. *Pediatric Infectious Disease Journal.* 1987;6:223.

88. Ruef, C. Mucocutaneous lymph node syndrome (Kawasaki syndrome) mimicking a suppurative parapharyngeal space infection. Case report and review of the literature. *Helvetica Paediatrica Acta.* 1989;43:307–12.

89. Lapointe, N, Chad, Z, Lacroix, J, Jacob, JL, Urbanski, P, Polomeno, R, et al. Kawasaki disease: association with uveitis in seven patients. *Pediatrics.* 1982;69:376–78.

90. Smith, LB, Newburger, JW, Burns, JC. Kawasaki syndrome and the eye. *Pediatric Infectious Disease Journal.* 1989;8:116–18.

91. Felz, MW, Patni, A, Brooks, SE, Tesser, RA. Periorbital vasculitis complicating Kawasaki syndrome in an infant. *Pediatrics.* 1998;101:E9.

92. Chung, CJ, Rayder, S, Meyers, W, Long, J. Kawasaki disease presenting as focal colitis. *Pediatric Radiology.* 1996;26:455–57.

93. Lanting, WA, Muinos, WI, Kamani, NR. Pancreatitis heralding Kawasaki disease. *Journal of Pediatrics.* 1992;121:743–44.

94. Hicks, RA, Murphy, JV, Jackson, MA. Kawasaki-like syndrome caused by carbamazepine. *Pediatric Infectious Disease Journal.* 1988;7:525–26.

95. Stern, MN, Brown, EW, McCurdy, D, Lehman, TJ. Confusion of a poststreptococcal syndrome complicated by uveitis with mucocutaneous lymph node syndrome. *Annals of Ophthalmology.* 1985;17:259–61.

96. Avner, JR, Shaw, KN, Chin, AJ. Atypical presentation of Kawasaki disease with early development of giant coronary artery aneurysms. *Journal of Pediatrics.* 1989;114:605–6.

97. Canter, CE, Bower, RJ, Strauss, AW. Atypical Kawasaki disease with aortic aneurysm. Pediatrics. 1981;68:885–88.

98. Cloney, DL, Teja, K, Lohr, JA. Fatal case of atypical Kawasaki syndrome. *Pediatric Infectious Disease Journal.* 1987;6:297–99.

99. Melish, ME, Hicks, RV. Kawasaki syndrome: clinical features. Pathophysiology, etiology and therapy. *Journal of Rheumatology,* Supplement. 1990;24:2–10.

100. Bauman, C, Cron, RQ, Sherry, DD, Francis, JS. Reiter syndrome initially misdiagnosed as Kawasaki disease. *Journal of Pediatrics.* 1996;128:366–69.

101. Sundel, RP, Newburger, JW, McGill, T, Cleveland, SS, Miller, WW, et al. Sensorineural hearing loss associated with Kawasaki disease. *Journal of Pediatrics.* 1990;117:371–77.

102. Magilavy, DB, Speert, DP, Silver, TM, Sullivan, DB. Mucocutaneous lymph node syndrome: report of two cases complicated by gallbladder hydrops and diagnosed by ultrasound. *Pediatrics.* 1978;61:699–702.

103. Krensky, AM. Mucocutaneous lymph node syndrome and hydropic gallbladders letter. *Pediatrics.* 1980;66:814.

104. Gururaj, AK, Arrifin, WA, Quah, BS. Hydrops of the gall bladder associated with Kawasaki syndrome. *Journal of the Singapore Paediatric Society.* 1989;31:93–96.

105. Bader-Meunier, B, Hadchouel, M, Fabre, M, Arnoud, MD, Dommergues, JP. Intrahepatic bile duct damage in children with Kawasaki disease. *Journal of Pediatrics.* 1992;120:750–752.

106. Choi, YS, Sharma, B. Gallbladder hydrops in mucocutaneous lymph node syndrome. *Southern Medical Journal.* 1989;82:397–98.

107. Slovis, TL, Hight, DW, Philippart, AI, Dubois, RS. Sonography in the diagnosis and management of hydrops of the gallbladder in children with mucocutaneous lymph node syndrome. *Pediatrics.* 1980;65:789–94.

108. Salcedo, JR, Greenberg, L, Kapur, S. Renal histology of mucocutaneous lymph node syndrome (Kawasaki disease). *Clinical Nephrology.* 1988;29:47–51.

109. Kato, H, Sugimura, T, Akagi, T, Sato, N, Hashino, K, Maeno, Y, et al. Long-term consequences of Kawasaki disease. A 10- to 21-year follow-up study of 594 patients. *Circulation.* 1996;94:1379–85.

110. Fujiwara, H, Hamashima, Y. Pathology of the heart in Kawasaki disease. *Pediatrics.* 1978;61:100–107.

111. Akagi, T, Rose, V, Benson, LN, Newman, A, Freedom, RM. Outcome of coronary artery aneurysms after Kawasaki disease. *Journal of Pediatrics.* 1992;121:689–94.

112. Habon, T, Toth, K, Keltai, M, Lengyel, M, Palik, I. An adult case of Kawasaki disease with multiplex coronary aneurysms and myocardial infarction: the role of transesophageal echocardiography. *Clinical Cardiology.* 1998;21:529–32.

113. Hirose, K, Nakamura, Y, Yanagawa, H. Cardiac sequelae of Kawasaki disease in Japan over 10 years. *Acta Paediatrica Japonica.* 1995;37:667–71.

114. Capannari, TE, Daniels, SR, Meyer, RA, Schwartz, DC, Kaplan, S. Sensitivity, specificity and predictive value of two-dimensional echocardiography in detecting coronary artery aneurysms in patients with Kawasaki disease. *Journal of the American College of Cardiology.* 1986;7:355–60.

115. de Zorzi, A, Colan, SD, Gauvreau, K, Baker, AL, Sundel, RP, Newburger, JW. Coronary artery dimensions may be misclassified as normal in Kawasaki disease. *Journal of Pediatrics.* 1998;133:254–58.

116. Frey, EE, Matherne, GP, Mahoney, LT, Sato, Y, Stanford, W, Smith, WL. Coronary artery aneurysms due to Kawasaki disease: diagnosis with ultrafast CT. *Radiology.* 1988;167:725–26.

117. Nakamura, Y, Fujita, Y, Nagai, M, Yanagawa, H, Imada, Y, Okawa, S, et al. Cardiac sequelae of Kawasaki disease in Japan: statistical analysis. *Pediatrics.* 1991;88:1144–47.

118. Brevard, SB, Smith, VC. Presumed Kawasaki disease resulting in multiple coronary artery aneurysms in an adult. *Annals of Thoracic Surgery.* 1990;50:291–92.

119. Kato, H, Inoue, O, Kawasaki, T, Fujiwara, H, Watanabe, T, Toshima, H. Adult coronary artery disease probably due to childhood Kawasaki disease. *Lancet.* 1992;340:1127–29.

120. Furukawa, S, Matsubara, T, Yone, K, Hirano, Y, Okumura, K, Yabuta, K. Kawasaki disease differs from anaphylactoid purpura and measles with regard to tumour necrosis factor-alpha and interleukin 6 in serum. *European Journal of Pediatrics.* 1992;151:44–47.

121. Onouchi, Z, Hamaoka, K, Kamiya, Y, Hayashi, S, Ohmochi, Y, Sakata, K, et al. Transformation of coronary artery aneurysm to obstructive lesion and the role of collateral vessels in myocardial perfusion in patients with Kawasaki disease. *Journal of the American College of Cardiology.* 1993;21:158–62.

122. Rosenfeld, EA, Corydon, KE, Shulman, ST. Kawasaki disease in infants less than one year of age. *Journal of Pediatrics.* 1995;126:524–29.

123. Nakamura, Y, Oki, I, Tanihara, S, Ojima, T, Yanagawa, H. Cardiac sequelae in recurrent cases of Kawasaki disease: a comparison between the initial episode of the disease and a recurrence in the same patients. *Pediatrics.* 1998;102:E66.

124. Nakamura, Y, Yanagawa, H, Kawasaki, T. Mortality among children with Kawasaki disease in Japan. *New England Journal of Medicine.* 1992;326:1246–49.

125. Nakamura, Y, Yanagawa, H, Kato, H, Kawasaki, T. Mortality rates for patients with a history of Kawasaki disease in Japan. Kawasaki Disease Follow-up Group. *Journal of Pediatrics.* 1996;128:75–81.

126. Sugimura, T, Kato, H, Inoue, O, Takagi, J, Fukuda, T, Sato, N. Vasodilatory response of the coronary arteries after Kawasaki disease: evaluation by intracoronary injection of isosorbide dinitrate. *Journal of Pediatrics*. 1992;121:684–88.

127. Suzuki, A, Yamagishi, M, Kimura, K, Sugiyama, H, Arakaki, Y, Kamiya, T, et al. Functional behavior and morphology of the coronary artery wall in patients with Kawasaki disease assessed by intravascular ultrasound. *Journal of the American College of Cardiology*. 1996;27:291–96.

128. Yamakawa, R, Ishii, M, Sugimura, T, Akagi, T, Eto, G, Iemura, M, et al. Coronary endothelial dysfunction after Kawasaki disease: evaluation by intracoronary injection of acetylcholine. *Journal of the American College of Cardiology*. 1998;31:1074–80.

129. Hamaoka, K, Onouchi, Z, Kamiya, Y, Sakata, K. Evaluation of coronary flow velocity dynamics and flow reserve in patients with Kawasaki disease by means of a Doppler guide wire. *Journal of the American College of Cardiology*. 1998;31:833–40.

130. Noto, N, Ayusawa, M, Karasawa, K, Yamaguchi, H, Sumitomo, N, Okada, T, et al. Dobutamine stress echocardiography for detection of coronary artery stenosis in children with Kawasaki disease. *Journal of the American College of Cardiology*. 1996;27:1251–56.

131. Ogawa, S, Fukazawa, R, Ohkubo, T, Zhang, J, Takechi, N, Kuramochi, Y, et al. Silent myocardial ischemia in Kawasaki disease: evaluation of percutaneous transluminal coronary angioplasty by dobutamine stress testing. *Circulation*. 1997;96:3384–89.

132. Pahl, E, Sehgal, R, Chrystof, D, Neches, WH, Webb, CL, Duffy, CE, et al. Feasibility of exercise stress echocardiography for the follow-up of children with coronary involvement secondary to Kawasaki disease. *Circulation*. 1995;91:122–28.

133. Paridon, SM, Galioto, FM, Vincent, JA, Tomassoni, TL, Sullivan, NM, Bricker, et al. Exercise capacity and incidence of myocardial perfusion defects after Kawasaki disease in children and adolescents. *Journal of the American College of Cardiology*. 1995;25:1420–1424.

134. Muzik, O, Paridon, SM, Singh, TP, Morrow, WR, Dayanikli, F, Di Carli, MF. Quantification of myocardial blood flow and flow reserve in children with a history of Kawasaki disease and normal coronary arteries using positron emission tomography. *Journal of the American College of Cardiology*. 1996;28:757–62.

135. Sugimura, T, Kato, H, Inoue, O, Fukuda, T, Sato, N, Ishii, M, et al. Intravascular ultrasound of coronary arteries in children. Assessment of the wall morphology and the lumen after Kawasaki disease. *Circulation*. 1994;89:258–65.

136. Allen, SW, Shaffer, EM, Harrigan, LA, Wolfe, RR, Glode, MP, Wiggins, JW. Maximal voluntary work and cardiorespiratory fitness in patients who have had Kawasaki syndrome. *Journal of Pediatrics*. 1992;121:221–25.

137. Kuribayashi, S, Ootaki, M, Tsuji, M, Matsuyama, S, Iwasaki, H, Oota, T. Coronary angiographic abnormalities in mucocutaneous lymph node syndrome: acute findings and long-term follow-up. *Radiology*. 1989;172:629–33.

138. Naoe, S, Takahashi, K, Masuda, H, Tanaka, N. Kawasaki disease. With particular emphasis on arterial lesions. *Acta Pathologica Japonica*. 1991;41:785–97.

139. Newburger, JW, Burns, JC, Beiser, AS, Loscalzo, J. Altered lipid profile after Kawasaki syndrome. *Circulation*. 1991;84:625–31.

140. Salo, E, Pesonen, E, Viikari, J. Serum cholesterol levels during and after Kawasaki disease. *Journal of Pediatrics*. 1991;119:557–61.

141. Kobayashi, T, Sone, K, Shinohara, M, Kosuda, T. Images in cardiovascular medicine. Giant coronary aneurysm of Kawasaki disease developing during postacute phase. *Circulation*. 1998;98:92–93.

142. Anonymous. Management of Kawasaki syndrome: a consensus statement prepared by North American participants of the Third International Kawasaki Disease Symposium, Tokyo, Japan, December, 1988. *Pediatric Infectious Disease Journal*. 1989;8:663–67.

143. Dajani, AS, Taubert, KA, Takahashi, M, Bierman, FZ, Freed, MD, Ferrieri, P, et al. Guidelines for long-term management of patients with Kawasaki disease. Report from the Committee on Rheumatic Fever, Endocarditis, and Kawasaki Disease, Council on Cardiovascular Disease in the Young, American Heart Association. *Circulation*. 1994;89:916–22.

144. Furusho, K, Sato, K, Soeda, T, Matsumoto, H, Okabe, T, Hirota, T, et al. High-dose intravenous gammaglobulin for Kawasaki disease letter. *Lancet*. 1983;2:1359.

145. Rowley, AH, Duffy, CE, Shulman, ST. Prevention of giant coronary artery aneurysms in Kawasaki disease by intravenous gamma globulin therapy. *Journal of Pediatrics.* 1988;113:290–294.

146. Coe, JY, McKendrick, R, Duncan, NF. Intravenous gamma globulin to prevent giant coronary artery aneurysm in Kawasaki disease [letter]. *Journal of Pediatrics.* 1989;114:1065–66.

147. Shulman, ST. IVGG therapy in Kawasaki disease: mechanism(s) of action. *Clinical Immunology & Immunopathology.* 1989;53:S141–S146.

148. Koike, R. The effect of immunoglobulin on immune complexes in patients with Kawasaki disease (MCLS). *Acta Paediatrica Japonica.* 1991;33:300–309.

149. Lekova, ES, Joffe, L, Glode, MP. Antigenic recognition by intravenous gamma-globulin of selected bacteria isolated from throats of patients with Kawasaki syndrome. *Pediatric Infectious Disease Journal.* 1990;9:620–623.

150. Mason, W, Jordan, S, Sakai, R, Takahashi, M. Lack of effect of gamma-globulin infusion on circulating immune complexes in patients with Kawasaki syndrome. *Pediatric Infectious Disease Journal.* 1988;7:94–99.

151. Furusho, K, Kamiya, T, Nakano, H, Kiyosawa, N, Shinomiya, K, Hayashidera, T, et al. High-dose intravenous gammaglobulin for Kawasaki disease. *Lancet.* 1984;2:1055–58.

152. Barron, KS, Murphy, DJJ, Silverman, ED, Ruttenberg, HD, Wright, GB, Franklin, W, et al. Treatment of Kawasaki syndrome: a comparison of two dosage regimens of intravenously administered immune globulin. *Journal of Pediatrics.* 1990;117:638–44.

153. Engle, MA, Fatica, NS, Bussel, JB, O'Loughlin, JE, Snyder, MS, Lesser, ML. Clinical trial of single-dose intravenous gamma globulin in acute Kawasaki disease. Preliminary report. *American Journal of Diseases of Children.* 1989;143:1300–1304.

154. Klassen, TP, Rowe, PC, Gafni, A. Economic evaluation of intravenous immune globulin therapy for Kawasaki syndrome. *Journal of Pediatrics.* 1993;122:538–42.

155. Newburger, JW, Takahashi, M, Beiser, AS, Burns, JC, Bastian, Chung, KJ, et al. A single intravenous infusion of gamma globulin as compared with four infusions in the treatment of acute Kawasaki syndrome. *New England Journal of Medicine.* 1991;324:1633–39.

156. Durongpisitkul, K, Gururaj, VJ, Park, JM, Martin, CF. The prevention of coronary artery aneurysm in Kawasaki disease: a meta-analysis on the efficacy of aspirin and immunoglobulin treatment. *Pediatrics.* 1995;96:1057–61.

157. Sundel, RP, Burns, JC, Baker, A, Beiser, AS, Newburger, JW. Gamma globulin re-treatment in Kawasaki disease. *Journal of Pediatrics.* 1993;123:657–59.

158. Yanagawa, H, Kawasaki, T, Shigematsu, I. Nationwide survey on Kawasaki disease in Japan. *Pediatrics.* 1987;80:58–62.

159. Kelly, PC, Pearl, WR, Weir, MR. Infantile polyarteritis nodosa with mucocutaneous lymph node syndrome treated with long-term corticosteroids. *Southern Medical Journal.* 1987;80:1045–48.

160. Kato, H, Koike, S, Yokoyama, T. Kawasaki disease: effect of treatment on coronary artery involvement. *Pediatrics.* 1979;63:175–79.

161. Caputo, AE, Roberts, WN, Yee, YS, Posner, MP. Hepatic artery aneurysm in corticosteroid-treated, adult Kawasaki's disease. *Annals of Vascular Surgery.* 1991;5:533–37.

162. Wright, DA, Newburger, JW, Baker, A, Sundel, RP. Treatment of immune globulin-resistant Kawasaki disease with pulsed doses of corticosteroids. *Journal of Pediatrics.* 1996;128:146–49.

163. Rosenfeld, EA, Shulman, ST, Corydon, KE, Mason, W, Takahashi, M, Kuroda, C. Comparative safety and efficacy of two immune globulin products in Kawasaki disease. *Journal of Pediatrics.* 1995;126:1000–1003.

164. Comenzo, RL, Malachowski, ME, Meissner, HC, Fulton, DR, Berkman, EM. Immune hemolysis, disseminated intravascular coagulation, and serum sickness after large doses of immune globulin given intravenously for Kawasaki disease. *Journal of Pediatrics.* 1992;120:926–28.

165. Hashkes, PJ, Lovell, DJ. Vasculitis in systemic lupus erythematosus following intravenous immuno-globulin therapy. *Clinical & Experimental Rheumatology.* 1996;14:673–75.

166. Daniels, SR, Specker, B, Capannari, TE, Schwartz, DC, Burke, MJ, Kaplan, S. Correlates of coronary artery aneurysm formation in patients with Kawasaki disease. *American Journal of Diseases of Children.* 1987;141:205–7.

167. Ichida, F, Fatica, NS, Engle, MA, O'Loughlin, JE, Klein, AA, Snyder, MS, et al. Coronary artery involvement in Kawasaki syndrome in Manhattan, New York: risk factors and role of aspirin. *Pediatrics*. 1987;80:828–35.

168. Newburger, JW, Sanders, SP, Burns, JC, Parness, IA, Beiser, AS, et al. Left ventricular contractility and function in Kawasaki syndrome. Effect of intravenous gamma-globulin. *Circulation*. 1989;79:1237–46.

169. Jacobs, JC. Salicylate treatment of epidemic Kawasaki disease in New York City. *Therapeutic Drug Monitoring*. 1979;1:123–30.

170. Koren, G, Silverman, E, Sundel, R, Edney, P, Newburger, JW, Klein, J, et al. Decreased protein binding of salicylates in Kawasaki disease. *Journal of Pediatrics*. 1991;118:456–59.

171. Matsubara, T, Mason, W, Kashani, IA, Kligerman, M, Burns, JC. Gastrointestinal hemorrhage complicating aspirin therapy in acute Kawasaki disease. *Journal of Pediatrics*. 1996;128:701–3.

172. Saphyakhajon, P, Greene, GR. Do we need high-dose acetylsalicylic acid (ASA) in Kawasaki disease? [letter]. *Journal of Pediatrics*. 1998;133:167.

173. Terai, M, Shulman, ST. Prevalence of coronary artery abnormalities in Kawasaki disease is highly dependent on gamma globulin dose but independent of salicylate dose. *Journal of Pediatrics*. 1997;131:888–93.

174. Landing, BH, Larson, EJ. Pathological features of Kawasaki disease (mucocutaneous lymph node syndrome). *American Journal of Cardiovascular Pathology*. 1987;1:218–29.

175. Herold, BC, Davis, AT, Arroyave, CM, Duffy, E, Pachman, LM, Shulman, ST. Cryoprecipitates in Kawasaki syndrome: association with coronary artery aneurysms. *Pediatric Infectious Disease Journal*. 1988;7:255–57.

176. Li, CR, Yang, XQ, Shen, J, Li, YB, Jiang, LP. Immunoglobulin G subclasses in serum and circulating immune complexes in patients with Kawasaki syndrome. *Pediatric Infectious Disease Journal*. 1990;9:544–47.

177. Lang, BA, Silverman, ED, Laxer, RM, Rose, V, Nelson, DL, Rubin, LA. Serum-soluble interleukin-2 receptor levels in Kawasaki disease. *Journal of Pediatrics*. 1990;116:592–96.

178. Lang, BA, Silverman, ED, Laxer, RM, Lau, AS. Spontaneous tumor necrosis factor production in Kawasaki disease. *Journal of Pediatrics*. 1989;115:939–43.

179. Lin, CY, Lin, CC, Hwang, B, Chiang, B. Serial changes of serum interleukin-6, interleukin-8, and tumor necrosis factor alpha among patients with Kawasaki disease. *Journal of Pediatrics*. 1992;121:924–26.

180. Lin, CY, Lin, CC, Hwang, B, Chiang, BN. The changes of interleukin-2, tumour necrotic factor and gamma-interferon production among patients with Kawasaki disease. *European Journal of Pediatrics*. 1991;150:179–82.

181. Sakata, K, Kita, M, Imanishi, J, Onouchi, Z, Liu, Y, Mitsui, Y. Effect of Kawasaki disease on migration of human umbilical vein endothelial cells. *Pediatric Research*. 1995;38:501–5.

182. Eberhard, BA, Andersson, U, Laxer, RM, Rose, V, Silverman, ED. Evaluation of the cytokine response in Kawasaki disease. *Pediatric Infectious Disease Journal*. 1995;14:199–203.

183. Furukawa, S, Matsubara, T, Umezawa, Y, Okumura, K, Yabuta, K. Serum levels of p60 soluble tumor necrosis factor receptor during acute Kawasaki disease. *Journal of Pediatrics*. 1994;124:721–25.

184. Guzman, J, Fung, M, Petty, RE. Diagnostic value of anti-neutrophil cytoplasmic and anti-endothelial cell antibodies in early Kawasaki disease. *Journal of Pediatrics*. 1994;124:917–20.

185. Fischer, P, Uttenreuther-Fischer, MM, Gaedicke, G. Superantigens in the aetiology of Kawasaki disease [letter]. *Lancet*. 1996;348:202.

186. Choi, IH, Chwae, YJ, Shim, WS, Kim, DS, Kwon, DH, Kim, JD, et al. Clonal expansion of CD8+ T cells in Kawasaki disease. *Journal of Immunology*. 1997;159:481–86.

187. Brosius, CL, Newburger, JW, Burns, JC, Hojnowski-Diaz, P, Zierler, S, Leung, DY. Increased prevalence of atopic dermatitis in Kawasaki disease. *Pediatric Infectious Disease Journal*. 1988;7:863–66.

188. Masuda, K, Takei, S, Nomura, Y, Imanaka, H, Sameshima, K, Yoshinaga, M. Transient low T-cell response to streptococcal pyrogenic exotoxin-C in patients with Kawasaki disease. *Pediatric Research*. 1998;44:27–31.

189. Aladhami, SMS, Arrowsmith, WA, Inglis, J, Madlom, MM. A young child with Kawasaki syndrome and AIDS [letter]. *Lancet*. 1996;347:912–13.

190. Bertotto, A, Spinozzi, F, Radicioni, M, Vaccaro, R. Mantoux test in Kawasaki disease [letter]. *Pediatrics*. 1996;98:161.

191. Bertotto, A, Spinozzi, F, Vagliasindi, C, Radicioni, M, De Rosa, O, Vaccaro, R. Tuberculin skin test reactivity in Kawasaki disease. *Pediatric Research*. 1997;41:560–562.

192. Hsu, YH, Wang, YH, Hsu, WY, Lee, YP. Kawasaki disease characterized by erythema and induration at the Bacillus Calmette-Guerin and purified protein derivative inoculation sites. *Pediatric Infectious Disease Journal*. 1987;6:576–78.

193. Sato, N, Sagawa, K, Sasaguri, Y, Inoue, O, Kato, H. Immunopathology and cytokine detection in the skin lesions of patients with Kawasaki disease. *Journal of Pediatrics*. 1993;122:198–203.

194. Nagata, S, Yamashiro, Y, Maeda, M, Ohtsuka, Y, Yabuta, K. Immunohistochemical studies on small intestinal mucosa in Kawasaki disease. *Pediatric Research*. 1993;33:557–63.

195. Rowley, AH, Eckerley, CA, Jack, HM, Shulman, ST, Baker, SC. IgA plasma cells in vascular tissue of patients with Kawasaki syndrome. *Journal of Immunology*. 1997;159:5946–55.

196. Mills, JA, Michel, BA, Bloch, DA, Calabrese, LH, Hunder, GG, Arend, WP, et al. The American College of Rheumatology 1990 criteria for the classification of Henoch-Schonlein purpura. *Arthritis & Rheumatism*. 1990;33:1114–21.

197. Steward, M, Savage, JB, Bell, B. Long-term renal prognosis of Henoch-Schoenlien purpura in an unselected childhood population. *Eur. J. Pediatr.* 147, 113, 1988.

198. Abdel-Al, YK, Hejazi, Z, Majeed, HA. Henoch Schonlein purpura in Arab children. Analysis of 52 cases. *Tropical & Geographical Medicine*. 1990;42:52–57.

199. Blanco, R, Martinez-Taboada, VM, Rodriguez-Valverde, V, Garcia-Fuentes, M, Gonzalez-Gay, MA. Henoch-Schonlein purpura in adulthood and childhood: two different expressions of the same syndrome. *Arthritis & Rheumatism*. 1997;40:859–64.

200. Atkinson, SR, Barker, DJ. Seasonal distribution of Henoch-Schonlein purpura. *British Journal of Preventive & Social Medicine*. 1976;30:22–25.

201. al-Sheyyab, M, el-Shanti, H, Ajlouni, S, Batieha, A, Daoud, AS. Henoch-Schonlein purpura: clinical experience and contemplations on a streptococcal association. *Journal of Tropical Pediatrics*. 1996;42:200–203.

202. Amoroso, A, Berrino, M, Canale, L, Coppo, R, Cornaglia, M, Guarrera, S, et al. Immunogenetics of Henoch-Schoenlein disease. *European Journal of Immunogenetics*. 1997;24:323–33.

203. Smith, SM, Tung, KS. Incidence of IgA-related nephritides in American Indians in New Mexico. *Human Pathology*. 1985;16:181–84.

204. Pomeranz, A, Korzets, Z, Eliakim, A, Pomeranz, M, Uziel, Y, Wolach, B. Relapsing Henoch-Schonlein purpura associated with a tubo-ovarian abscess due to Morganella morganii. *American Journal of Nephrology*. 1997;17:471–73.

205. Han, BG, Choi, SO, Shin, SJ, Kim, HY, Jung, SH, Lee, KH. A case of Henoch-Schonlein purpura in disseminated tuberculosis. *Korean Journal of Internal Medicine*. 1995;10:54–59.

206. Reinauer, S, Megahed, M, Goerz, G, Ruzicka, T, Borchard, F, Susanto, F, et al. Schonlein-Henoch purpura associated with gastric Helicobacter pylori infection. *Journal of the American Academy of Dermatology*. 1995;33:876–79.

207. Costa, MM, Lisboa, M, Romeu, JC, Caldeira, J, De, QV. Henoch-Schonlein purpura associated with coxsackie-virus B1 infection [letter]. *Clinical Rheumatology*. 1995;14:488–90.

208. Ferguson, PJ, Saulsbury, FT, Dowell, SF, Torok, TJ, Erdman, DD, Anderson, LJ. Prevalence of human parvovirus B19 infection in children with Henoch-Schonlein purpura. *Arthritis & Rheumatism*. 1996;39:880–881.

209. Frankum, B, Katelaris, CH. Hepatitis C infection and Henoch-Schonlein purpura [letter]. *Australian & New Zealand Journal of Medicine*. 1995;25:176.

210. Singh, PS. Henoch Schonlein purpura in adults associated with hepatitis B antigen [letter]. *Journal of the Association of Physicians of India*. 1995;43:73.

211. Chevalier, X, Rostoker, G, Larget-Piet, B, Gherardi, R. Schoenlein-Henoch purpura with necrotizing vasculitis after cocaine snorting [letter]. *Clinical Nephrology*. 1995;43:348–49.

212. Blanco, R, Gonzalez-Gay, MA, Ibanez, D, Alba, C, Perez, LL. Henoch-Schonlein purpura as a clinical presentation of small cell lung cancer. *Clinical & Experimental Rheumatology*. 1997;15:545–47.

213. Chong, SW, Buckley, M. Henoch-Schonlein purpura associated with adenocarcinoma [correction of adenoma] of the stomach [letter]. *Irish Medical Journal*. 1997;90:194–95.

214. Sivak, LE, Virshup, DM. Occurrence of Henoch-Schonlein purpura in a child with Wilms' tumor. *Medical & Pediatric Oncology.* 1995;24:213–14.

215. Ben-Chaim, J, Korat, E, Shenfeld, O, Shelhav, A, Jonas, P, Goldwasser, B. Acute scrotum caused by Henoch-Schonlein purpura, with immediate response to short-term steroid therapy. *Journal of Pediatric Surgery.* 1995;30:1509–10.

216. Mintzer, CO, Nussinovitch, M, Danziger, Y, Mimouni, M, Varsano, I. Scrotal involvement in Henoch-Schonlein purpura in children. *Scandinavian Journal of Urology & Nephrology.* 1998;32:138–39.

217. Zia, UM, Brereton, RJ. Acute scrotum: an unusual presentation of Henoch-Schonlein purpura in children. *Journal of the Royal College of Surgeons of Edinburgh.* 1996;41:420–421.

218. Choong, CK, Beasley, SW. Intra-abdominal manifestations of Henoch-Schonlein purpura. *Journal of Paediatrics & Child Health.* 1998;34:405–9.

219. Lin, SJ, Chao, HC, Huang, JL. Gastrointestinal involvement as the initial manifestation in children with Henoch-Schonlein purpura — clinical analysis of 27 cases. *Chung-Hua Min Kuo Hsiao Erh Ko i Hsueh Hui Tsa Chih.* 1998;39:186–90.

220. Sharieff, GQ, Francis, K, Kuppermann, N. Atypical presentation of Henoch-Schoenlein purpura in two children. *American Journal of Emergency Medicine.* 1997;15:375–77.

221. Bissonnette, R, Dansereau, A, D'Amico, P, Pateneaude, JV, Paradis, J. Perforation of large and small bowel in Henoch-Schonlein purpura. *International Journal of Dermatology.* 1997;36:361–63.

222. Gow, KW, Murphy, JJ, Blair, GK, Magee, JF, Hailey, J. Multiple entero fistulae: an unusual complication of Henoch-Schonlein purpura. *Journal of Pediatric Surgery.* 1996;31:809–11.

223. Chao, SC, Huang, JL. Ileal perforation in Henoch-Schonlein purpura: report of one case. *Chung-Hua Min Kuo Hsiao Erh Ko i Hsueh Hui Tsa Chih.* 1996;37:455–57.

224. Kawasaki, M, Hizawa, K, Aoyagi, K, Kuroki, F, Nakahara, T, Sakamoto, K, et al. Ileitis caused by Henoch-Schonlein purpura. An endoscopic view of the terminal ileum. *Journal of Clinical Gastroenterology.* 1997;25:396–98.

225. Kawasaki, M, Suekane, H, Imagawa, E, Iida, M, Hizawa, K, Aoyagi, K, et al. Duodenal obstruction due to Henoch-Schonlein purpura. AJR. 1997; *American Journal of Roentgenology.* 168:969–70.

226. Lipsett, J, Byard, RW. Small bowel stricture due to vascular compromise: a late complication of Henoch-Schonlein purpura. *Pediatric Pathology & Laboratory Medicine.* 1995;15:333–40.

227. Kano, K, Ozawa, T, Kuwashima, S, Ito, S. Uncommon multisystemic involvement in a case of Henoch-Schonlein purpura. *Acta Paediatrica Japonica.* 1998;40:159–61.

228. Chen, WP, Lin, CY, Cheng, JH, Hwang, BT. Purpura nephritis in Chinese children from northern Taiwan. *Child Nephrology & Urology.* 1988;9:331–36.

229. Andreoli, SP. Chronic glomerulonephritis in childhood. Membranoproliferative glomerulonephritis, Henoch-Schonlein purpura nephritis, and IgA nephropathy. *Pediatric Clinics of North America.* 1995;42:1487–503.

230. Andreoli, SP. Renal manifestations of systemic diseases. *Seminars in Nephrology.* 1998;18:270–279.

231. Coppo, R, Mazzucco, G, Cagnoli, L, Lupo, A, Schena, FP. Long-term prognosis of Henoch-Schonlein nephritis in adults and children. Italian Group of Renal Immunopathology Collaborative Study on Henoch-Schonlein purpura. *Nephrology, Dialysis, Transplantation.* 1997;12:2277–83.

232. Bruce, RG, Bishof, NA, Jackson, EC, Skinker, DM, McRoberts, JW. Bilateral ureteral obstruction associated with Henoch-Schoenlein purpura. *Pediatric Nephrology.* 1997;11:347–49.

233. Garcia-Nieto, V, Claverie-Martin, F. Additional cases of ureteral obstruction associated with Henoch-Schonlein purpura [letter]. *Pediatric Nephrology.* 1998;12:168–69.

234. Costa, BM, Ades, L, Mougenot, B, Akposso, K, Lahlou, A, Haymann, et al. Acute renal failure in Henoch-Schonlein purpura due to interstitial haemorrhage of the kidney. *Nephrology, Dialysis, Transplantation.* 1998;13:2355–57.

235. Tancrede-Bohin, E, Ochonisky, S, Vignon-Pennamen, MD, Flageul, B, Morel, P, Rybojad, M. Schonlein-Henoch purpura in adult patients. Predictive factors for IgA glomerulonephritis in a retrospective study of 57 cases. *Archives of Dermatology.* 1997;133:438–42.

236. Kaku, Y, Nohara, K, Honda, S. Renal involvement in Henoch-Schonlein purpura: a multivariate analysis of prognostic factors. *Kidney International.* 1998;53:1755–59.

237. Kessler, M, Hiesse, C, Hestin, D, Mayeux, D, Boubenider, K, Charpentier, B. Recurrence of immunoglobulin A nephropathy after renal transplantation in the cyclosporine era. *American Journal of Kidney Diseases.* 1996;28:99–104.

238. Meulders, Q, Pirson, Y, Cosyns, JP, Squifflet, JP, van Ypersele, D. Course of Henoch-Schonlein nephritis after renal transplantation. Report on ten patients and review of the literature. *Transplantation.* 1994;58:1179–86.

239. Carter, ER, Guevara, JP, Moffitt, DR. Pulmonary hemorrhage in an adolescent with Henoch-Schonlein purpura. *Western Journal of Medicine.* 1996;164:171–73.

240. Paller, AS, Kelly, K, Sethi, R. Pulmonary hemorrhage: an often fatal complication of Henoch-Schoenlein purpura see comments. *Pediatric Dermatology.* 1997;14:299–302.

241. Woolfenden, AR, Hukin, J, Poskitt, KJ, Connolly, MB. Encephalopathy complicating Henoch-Schonlein purpura: reversible MRI changes. *Pediatric Neurology.* 1998;19:74–77.

242. Ha, TS, Cha, SH. Cerebral vasculitis in Henoch-Schonlein purpura: a case report with sequential magnetic resonance imaging. *Pediatric Nephrology.* 1996;10:634–36.

243. Elinson, P, Foster, KWJ, Kaufman, DB. Magnetic resonance imaging of central nervous system vasculitis. A case report of Henoch-Schonlein purpura. *Acta Paediatrica Scandinavica.* 1990;79:710–713.

244. Ng, CC, Huang, SC, Huang, LT. Henoch-Schonlein purpura with intracerebral hemorrhage: case report. *Pediatric Radiology.* 1996;26:276–77.

245. Goraya, JS, Jayashree, M, Ghosh, D, Singh, S, Singhi, SC, Kumar, L. Guillain-Barre syndrome in a child with Henoch-Schonlein Purpura. *Scandinavian Journal of Rheumatology.* 1998;27:310–312.

246. Crowe, MA, Jonas, PP. Acute hemorrhagic edema of infancy. *Cutis.* 1998;62:65–66.

247. Gonggryp, LA, Todd, G. Acute hemorrhagic edema of childhood (AHE). *Pediatric Dermatology.* 1998;15:91–96.

248. Ince, E, Mumcu, Y, Suskan, E, Yalcinkaya, F, Tumer, N, Cin, S. Infantile acute hemorrhagic edema: a variant of leukocytoclastic vasculitis. *Pediatric Dermatology.* 1995;12:224–27.

249. Dubin, BA, Bronson, DM, Eng, AM. Acute hemorrhagic edema of childhood: an unusual variant of leukocytoclastic vasculitis. *Journal of the American Academy of Dermatology.* 1990;23:347–50.

250. Long, D, Helm, KF. Acute hemorrhagic edema of infancy: Finkelstein's disease. *Cutis.* 1998;61:283–84.

251. Krause, I, Lazarov, A, Rachmel, A, Grunwald, MM, Metzker, A, Garty, BZ, et al. Acute haemorrhagic oedema of infancy, a benign variant of leucocytoclastic vasculitis. *Acta Paediatrica.* 1996;85:114–17.

252. al-Sheyyab, M, el-Shanti, H, Ajlouni, S, Sawalha, D, Daoud, A. The clinical spectrum of Henoch-Schonlein purpura in infants and young children. *European Journal of Pediatrics.* 1995;154:969–72.

253. Saraclar, Y, Tinaztepe, K, Adalioglu, G, Tuncer, A. Acute hemorrhagic edema of infancy (AHEI) — a variant of Henoch-Schonlein purpura or a distinct clinical entity? *Journal of Allergy & Clinical Immunology.* 1990;86:473–83.

254. Goodyer, PR, de Chadarevian, JP, Kaplan, BS. Acute poststreptococcal glomerulonephritis mimicking Henoch-Schonlein purpura. *Journal of Pediatrics.* 1978;93:412–15.

255. Akimoto, S, Ishikawa, O, Tsukada, Y, Yano, S, Miyachi, Y. Microscopic polyangiitis mimicking Henoch-Schonlein purpura followed by severe renal involvement: a diagnostic role for antineutrophil cytoplasmic autoantibody [letter]. *British Journal of Dermatology.* 1997;136:298–99.

256. Baldree, LA, Gaber, LW, McKay, CP. Anti-neutrophil cytoplasmic autoantibodies in a child with pauci-immune necrotizing and crescentic glomerulonephritis. *Pediatric Nephrology.* 1991;5:296–99.

257. Michel, BA, Hunder, GG, Bloch, DA, Calabrese, LH. Hypersensitivity vasculitis and Henoch-Schonlein purpura: a comparison between the two disorders. *Journal of Rheumatology.* 1992;19:721–28.

258. Szer, IS. Henoch-Schonlein purpura: when and how to treat. *Journal of Rheumatology.* 1996;23:1661–65.

259. van den Broek, RW, van Rossum, MA, van Duinen, CM. A new surgical complication related to corticosteroids in a patient with Henoch-Schonlein purpura. *Journal of Pediatric Surgery.* 1995;30:1341–43.

260. Bergstein, J, Leiser, J, Andreoli, SP. Response of crescentic Henoch-Schoenlein purpura nephritis to corticosteroid and azathioprine therapy. *Clinical Nephrology.* 1998;49:9–14.

261. Niaudet, P, Habib, R. Methylprednisolone pulse therapy in the treatment of severe forms of Schonlein-Henoch purpura nephritis. *Pediatric Nephrology.* 1998;12:238–43.

262. Oner, A, Tinaztepe, K, Erdogan, O. The effect of triple therapy on rapidly progressive type of Henoch-Schonlein nephritis. *Pediatric Nephrology.* 1995;9:6–10.

263. Blanco, R, Gonzalez-Gay, MA, Ibanez, D, Sanchez-Andrade, A, Gonzalez-Vela, C. Paradoxical and persistent renal impairment in Henoch-Schonlein purpura after high-dose immunoglobulin therapy [letter]. *Nephron.* 1997;76:247–48.

264. Catalano, C, Fabbian, F, Bordin, V, Di Landro, D. Failure of cyclosporine A in controlling Schoenlein-Henoch purpura [letter]. *Nephrology, Dialysis, Transplantation.* 1998;13:1605–6.

265. Schmaldienst, S, Winkler, S, Breiteneder, S, Horl, WH. Severe nephrotic syndrome in a patient with Schonlein-Henoch purpura: complete remission after cyclosporin A. *Nephrology, Dialysis, Transplantation.* 1997;12:790–792.

266. Hartley, B, Fuller, CC. Juvenile arthritis: a nursing perspective. *Journal of Pediatric Nursing.* 1997;12:100–109.

267. Kato, S, Ebina, K, Naganuma, H, Sato, S, Maisawa, S, Nakagawa, H. Intestinal IgA deposition in Henoch-Schonlein purpura with severe gastro-intestinal manifestations. *European Journal of Pediatrics.* 1996;155:91–95.

268. Casanueva, B, Rodriguez-Valverde, V, Luceno, A. Circulating IgA producing cells in the differential diagnosis of Henoch-Schonlein purpura. *Journal of Rheumatology.* 1988;15:1229–33.

269. Helander, SD, De Castro, FR, Gibson, LE. Henoch-Schonlein purpura: clinicopathologic correlation of cutaneous vascular IgA deposits and the relationship to leukocytoclastic vasculitis. *Acta Dermato-Venereologica.* 1995;75:125–29.

270. Saulsbury, FT. Alterations in the O-linked glycosylation of IgA1 in children with Henoch-Schonlein purpura. *Journal of Rheumatology.* 1997;24:2246–49.

271. Allen, AC, Willis, FR, Beattie, TJ, Feehally, J. Abnormal IgA glycosylation in Henoch-Schonlein purpura restricted to patients with clinical nephritis. *Nephrology, Dialysis, Transplantation.* 1998;13:930–934.

272. Lasseur, C, Allen, AC, Deminiere, C, Aparicio, M, Feehally, J, Combe, C. Henoch-Schonlein purpura with immunoglobulin A nephropathy and abnormalities of immunoglobulin A in a Wiskott-Aldrich syndrome carrier. *American Journal of Kidney Diseases.* 1997;29:285–87.

273. Casonato, A, Pontara, E, Bertomoro, A, Ossi, E, Vincenti, M, Girolami, A, et al. Abnormally large von Willebrand factor multimers in Henoch-Schonlein purpura. *American Journal of Hematology.* 1996;51:7–11.

274. Ates, E, Bakkaloglu, A, Saatci, U, Soylemezoglu, O. von Willebrand factor antigen compared with other factors in vasculitic syndromes. *Archives of Disease in Childhood.* 1994;70:40–43.

275. Belcheva, A, Mishkova, R, Mutafova, E. Correlation of blood histamine levels with immunological indices in patients with Schonlein-Henoch purpura. *Inflammation Research.* 1996;45 Suppl 1:S39–S40.

276. Belcheva, A, Mishkova, R, Manevska, B. Histamine concentrations in gastric mucosa of patients with Schonlein-Henoch purpura. *Inflammation Research.* 1996;45 Suppl 1:S37–S38.

277. Soylemezoglu, O, Sultan, N, Gursel, T, Buyan, N, Hasanoglu, E. Circulating adhesion molecules ICAM-1, E-selectin, and von Willebrand factor in Henoch-Schonlein purpura. *Archives of Disease in Childhood.* 1996;75:507–11.

278. De Mattia, D, Penza, R, Giordano, P, Del Vecchio, GC, Aceto, G, Altomare, M, et al. von Willebrand factor and factor XIII in children with Henoch-Schonlein purpura. *Pediatric Nephrology.* 1995;9:603–5.

279. Lin, JJ, Stewart, CL, Kaskel, FJ, Fine, RN. IgG and IgA classes of anti-neutrophil cytoplasmic autoantibodies in a 13-year-old girl with recurrent Henoch-Schonlein purpura. *Pediatric Nephrology.* 1993;7:143–46.

280. Fujieda, M, Oishi, N, Naruse, K, Hashizume, M, Nishiya, K, Kurashige, T, et al. Soluble thrombomodulin and antibodies to bovine glomerular endothelial cells in patients with Henoch-Schonlein purpura. *Archives of Disease in Childhood.* 1998;78:240–244.

281. Saulsbury, FT, Kirkpatrick, PR, Bolton, WK. IgA antineutrophil cytoplasmic antibody in Henoch-Schonlein purpura. *American Journal of Nephrology.* 1991;11:295–300.

282. Coppo, R, Cirina, P, Amore, A, Sinico, RA, Radice, A, Rollino, C. Properties of circulating IgA molecules in Henoch-Schonlein purpura nephritis with focus on neutrophil cytoplasmic antigen IgA binding (IgA-ANCA): new insight into a debated issue. Italian Group of Renal Immunopathology Collaborative Study on Henoch-Schonlein purpura in adults and in children. *Nephrology, Dialysis, Transplantation.* 1997;12:2269–76.

283. Burden, AD, Tillman, DM, Foley, P, Holme, E. IgA class anticardiolipin antibodies in cutaneous leukocytoclastic vasculitis. *Journal of the American Academy of Dermatology.* 1996;35:411–15.

284. Smith, GC, Davidson, JE, Hughes, DA, Holme, E, Beattie, TJ. Complement activation in Henoch-Schonlein purpura. *Pediatric Nephrology.* 1997;11:477–80.

285. Lhotta, K, Kronenberg, F, Joannidis, M, Feichtinger, H, Konig, P. Wegener's granulomatosis and Henoch-Schonlein purpura in a family with hereditary C4 deficiency. *Advances in Experimental Medicine & Biology.* 1993;336:415–18.

286. Besbas, N, Saatci, U, Ruacan, S, Ozen, S, Sungur, A, Bakkaloglu, A, et al. The role of cytokines in Henoch Schonlein purpura. *Scandinavian Journal of Rheumatology.* 1997;26:456–60.

287. Besbas, N, Erbay, A, Saatci, U, Ozdemir, S, Bakkaloglu, A, Ozen, S, et al. Thrombomodulin, tissue plasminogen activator and plasminogen activator inhibitor-1 in Henoch-Schonlein purpura. *Clinical & Experimental Rheumatology.* 1998;16:95–98.

288. Gattorno, M, Picco, P, Barbano, G, Stalla, F, Sormani, MP, Buoncompagni, A, et al. Differences in tumor necrosis factor-alpha soluble receptor serum concentrations between patients with Henoch-Schonlein purpura and pediatric systemic lupus erythematosus: pathogenetic implications. *Journal of Rheumatology.* 1998;25:361–65.

289. Saulsbury, FT. Increased serum IgD concentrations in children with Henoch-Schonlein purpura. *British Journal of Rheumatology.* 1998;37:570–572.

290. Pall, AA, Howie, AJ, Adu, D, Richards, GM, Inward, CD, Milford, DV, et al. Glomerular vascular cell adhesion molecule-1 expression in renal vasculitis. *Journal of Clinical Pathology.* 1996;49:238–42.

291. Liu, ZH, Cheng, ZH, Yu, YS, Tang, Z, Li, LS. Interleukin-1 receptor antagonist allele: is it a genetic link between Henoch-Schonlein nephritis and IgA nephropathy? *Kidney International.* 1997;51:1938–42.

292. Namgoong, MK, Lim, BK, Kim, JS. Eosinophil cationic protein in Henoch-Schonlein purpura and in IgA nephropathy. *Pediatric Nephrology.* 1997;11:703–6.

293. Moja, P, Quesnel, A, Resseguier, V, Lambert, C, Freycon, F, Berthoux, F, et al. Is there IgA from gut mucosal origin in the serum of children with Henoch-Schonlein purpura? *Clinical Immunology & Immunopathology.* 1998;86:290–297.

294. Davin, JC, Li, VM, Mahieu, P. No pathogenic role of enhanced plasma IgA binding capacity to fibronectin and IgA-fibronectin aggregates in Henoch-Schonlein purpura [letter]. *Nephron.* 1996;74:435–36.

295. Magilavy, DB, Petty, RE, Cassidy, JT, Sullivan, DB. A syndrome of childhood polyarteritis. *Journal of Pediatrics.* 1977;91:25–30.

296. Maeda, M, Kobayashi, M, Okamoto, S, Fuse, T, Matsuyama, T, Watanabe, N, et al. Clinical observation of 14 cases of childhood polyarteritis nodosa in Japan. *Acta Paediatrica Japonica.* 1997;39:277–79.

297. Duffy, J, Lidsky, MD, Sharp, JT, Davis, JS, Person, DA, Hollinger, FB, et al. Polyarthritis, polyarteritis and hepatitis B. *Medicine.* 1976;55:19–37.

298. Guillevin, L, Lhote, F, Cohen, P, Sauvaget, F, Jarrousse, B, Lortholary, O, et al. Polyarteritis nodosa related to hepatitis B virus. A prospective study with long-term observation of 41 patients. *Medicine.* 1995;74:238–53.

299. Fink, CW. The role of the streptococcus in poststreptococcal reactive arthritis and childhood polyarteritis nodosa. *Journal of Rheumatology, Supplement.* 1991;29:14–20.

300. Ozen, S, Saatci, U, Balkanci, F, Besbas, N, Bakkaloglu, A, Tacal, T. Familial Mediterranean fever and polyarteritis nodosa. *Scandinavian Journal of Rheumatology.* 1992;21:312–13.

301. Holt, S, Jackson P. Ruptured coronary aneurysm and valvulitis in an infant with polyarteritis nodosa. *Journal of Pathology.* 1975;117:83–87.

302. Ozen, S, Besbas, N, Saatci, U, Bakkaloglu, A. Diagnostic criteria for polyarteritis nodosa in childhood. *Journal of Pediatrics.* 1992;120:206–9.

303. Albornoz, MA, Benedetto, AV, Korman, M, McFall, S, Tourtellotte, CD, Myers, et al. Relapsing cutaneous polyarteritis nodosa associated with streptococcal infections. *International Journal of Dermatology.* 1998;37:664–66.

304. Blau, EB, Morris, RF, Yunis, EJ. Polyarteritis nodosa in older children. *Pediatrics.* 1977;60:227–34.

305. David, J, Ansell, BM, Woo, P. Polyarteritis nodosa associated with streptococcus. *Archives of Disease in Childhood.* 1993;69:685–88.

306. Mader, R, Schaffer, I, Schonfeld, S. Recurrent poststreptococcal cutaneous polyarteritis nodosa. *Israel Journal of Medical Sciences.* 1988;24:269–70.
307. Till, SH, Amos, RS. Long-term follow-up of juvenile-onset cutaneous polyarteritis nodosa associated with streptococcal infection. *British Journal of Rheumatology.* 1997;36:909–11.
308. Stone, MS, Olson, RR, Weismann, DN, Giller, RH, Goeken, JA. Cutaneous vasculitis in the newborn of a mother with cutaneous polyarteritis nodosa. *Journal of the American Academy of Dermatology.* 1993;28:101–5.
309. Chochrad, D, Langhendries, JP, Stolear, JC, Godin, J. Isotretinoin-induced vasculitis imitating polyarteritis nodosa, with perinuclear antineutrophil cytoplasmic antibody in titers correlated with clinical symptoms. *Revue Du Rhumatisme,* English Edition. 1997;64:129–31.
310. Frayha, RA. Trichinosis-related polyarteritis nodosa. *American Journal of Medicine.* 1981;71:307–12.
311. Kahn, EI, Daum, F, Aiges, HW, Silverberg, M. Cutaneous polyarteritis nodosa associated with Crohn's disease. *Diseases of the Colon & Rectum.* 1980;23:258–62.
312. Verbov, J, Stansfeld, AG. Cutaneous polyarteritis nodosa and Crohn's disease. *Transactions of the St Johns Hospital Dermatological Society.* 1972;58:261–68.
313. Silverman, MH. Polyarteritis nodosa associated with ulcerative colitis. *Journal of Rheumatology.* 1984;11:377–79.
314. Volk, DM, Owen, LG. Cutaneous polyarteritis nodosa in a patient with ulcerative colitis. *Journal of Pediatric Gastroenterology & Nutrition.* 1986;5:970–972.
315. Glikson, M, Galun, E, Schlesinger, M, Cohen, D, Haskell, L, Rubinow, A, et al. Polyarteritis nodosa and familial Mediterranean fever: a report of two cases and review of the literature. *Journal of Rheumatology.* 1989;16:536–39.
316. Kocak, H, Cakar, N, Hekimoglu, B, Atakan, C, Akkok, N, Unal, S. The coexistence of familial Mediterranean fever and polyarteritis nodosa; report of a case. *Pediatric Nephrology.* 1996;10:631–33.
317. Ozdogan, H, Arisoy, N, Kasapcapur, O, Sever, L, Caliskan, S, Tuzuner, N, et al. Vasculitis in familial Mediterranean fever. *Journal of Rheumatology.* 1997;24:323–27.
318. Tinaztepe, K, Gucer, S, Bakkaloglu, A, Tinaztepe, B. Familial Mediterranean fever and polyarteritis nodosa: experience of five paediatric cases. A causal relationship or coincidence? [letter]. *European Journal of Pediatrics.* 1997;156:505–6.
319. Gunal, N, Kara, N, Cakar, N, Kocak, H, Kahramanyol, O, Cetinkaya, E. Cardiac involvement in childhood polyarteritis nodosa. *International Journal of Cardiology.* 1997;60:257–62.
320. Ettlinger, RE, Nelson, AM, Burke, EC, Lie, JT. Polyarteritis nodosa in childhood a clinical pathologic study. *Arthritis & Rheumatism.* 1979;22:820–825.
321. Matsumoto, T, Homma, S, Okada, M, Kuwabara, N, Kira, S, Hoshi, T, et al. The lung in polyarteritis nodosa: a pathologic study of ten cases. *Human Pathology.* 1993;24:717–24.
322. Almgren, B, Eriksson, I, Foucard, T, Lorelius, LE, Olsen, L. Multiple aneurysms of visceral arteries in a child with polyarteritis nodosa. *Journal of Pediatric Surgery.* 1980;15:347–48.
323. Lightman, HI, Valderrama, E, Ilowite, NT. Cutaneous polyarteritis nodosa and thromboses of the superior and inferior venae cavae. *Journal of Rheumatology.* 1988;15:113–16.
324. Engel, DG, Gospe, SMJ, Tracy, KA, Ellis, WG, Lie, JT. Fatal infantile polyarteritis nodosa with predominant central nervous system involvement. *Stroke.* 1995;26:699–701.
325. Buchanan, N, Berkowitz, F, Gold, C, Freinkel, AL, Briede, W. Granulomatous glomerulonephritis and fulminant polyarteritis nodosa in a child. *South African Medical Journal.* 1976;50:1057–59.
326. Gundogdu, HZ, Kale, G, Tanyel, FC, Buyukpamukcu, N, Hicsonmez, A. Intestinal perforation as an initial presentation of polyarteritis nodosa in an 8-year-old boy. *Journal of Pediatric Surgery.* 1993;28:632–34.
327. Lie, JT. Retroperitoneal polyarteritis nodosa presenting as ureteral obstruction. *Journal of Rheumatology.* 1992;19:1628–31.
328. Kumar, L, Thapa, BR, Sarkar, B, Walia, BN. Benign cutaneous polyarteritis nodosa in children below 10 years of age — a clinical experience. *Annals of the Rheumatic Diseases.* 1995;54:134–36.
329. Chen, KR. Cutaneous polyarteritis nodosa: a clinical and histopathological study of 20 cases. *Journal of Dermatology.* 1989;16:429–42.

330. Guillevin, L, Lhote, F, Cohen, P, Jarrousse, B, Lortholary, O, Genereau, T, et al. Corticosteroids plus pulse cyclophosphamide and plasma exchanges versus corticosteroids plus pulse cyclophosphamide alone in the treatment of polyarteritis nodosa and Churg-Strauss syndrome patients with factors predicting poor prognosis. A prospective, randomized trial in 62 patients. *Arthritis & Rheumatism.* 1995;38:1638–45.

331. Uziel, Y, Silverman, ED. Intravenous immunoglobulin therapy in a child with cutaneous polyarteritis nodosa. *Clinical & Experimental Rheumatology.* 1998;16:187–89.

332. Jorizzo, JL, White, WL, Wise, CM, Zanolli, MD, Sherertz, EF. Low-dose weekly methotrexate for unusual neutrophilic vascular reactions: cutaneous polyarteritis nodosa and Behcet's disease. *Journal of the American Academy of Dermatology.* 1991;24:973–78.

333. Cotch, MF, Hoffman, GS, Yerg, DE, Kaufman, GI, Targonski, P, Kaslow, RA. The epidemiology of Wegener's granulomatosis. Estimates of the five-year period prevalence, annual mortality, and geographic disease distribution from population-based data sources. *Arthritis & Rheumatism.* 1996;39:87–92.

334. Hoffman, GS, Kerr, GS, Leavitt, RY, Hallahan, CW, Lebovics, RS, Travis, WD, et al. Wegener granulomatosis: an analysis of 158 patients. *Annals of Internal Medicine.* 1992;116:488–98.

335. Halstead, LA, Karmody, CS, Wolff, SM. Presentation of Wegener's granulomatosis in young patients. *Otolaryngology — Head & Neck Surgery.* 1986;94:368–71.

336. Orlowski, JP, Clough, JD, Dyment, PG. Wegener's granulomatosis in the pediatric age group. *Pediatrics.* 1978;61:83–90.

337. Rottem, M, Fauci, AS, Hallahan, CW, Kerr, GS, Lebovics, R, Leavitt, RY, et al. Wegener granulomatosis in children and adolescents: clinical presentation and outcome. *Journal of Pediatrics.* 1993;122:26–31.

338. Morris, CJ, Byrd, RP, Roy, TM. Wegener's granulomatosis presenting as subglottic stenosis. *Journal of the Kentucky Medical Association.* 1990;88:547–50.

339. Allen, JC, France, TD. Pseudotumor as the presenting sign of Wegener's granulomatosis in a child. *Journal of Pediatric Ophthalmology.* 1977;14:158–59.

340. Parelhoff, ES, Chavis, RM, Friendly, DS. Wegener's granulomatosis presenting as orbital pseudotumor in children. *Journal of Pediatric Ophthalmology & Strabismus.* 1985;22:100–104.

341. Leavitt, JA, Butrus, SI. Wegener's granulomatosis presenting as dacryoadenitis. *Cornea.* 1991;10:542–45.

342. Sinnassamy, P, O'Regan, S. Wegener's granulomatosis in a seven-year-old child. *International Journal of Pediatric Nephrology.* 1984;5:227–28.

343. Matt, BH. Wegener's granulomatosis, acute laryngotracheal airway obstruction and death in a 17-year-old female: case report and review of the literature. *International Journal of Pediatric Otorhinolaryngology.* 1996;37:163–72.

344. Barksdale, SK, Hallahan, CW, Kerr, GS, Fauci, AS, Stern, JB, Travis, WD. Cutaneous pathology in Wegener's granulomatosis. A clinicopathologic study of 75 biopsies in 46 patients. *American Journal of Surgical Pathology.* 1995;19:161–72.

345. Chyu, JY, Hagstrom, WJ, Soltani, K, Faibisoff, B, Whitney, DH. Wegener's granulomatosis in childhood: cutaneous manifestations as the presenting signs. *Journal of the American Academy of Dermatology.* 1984;10:341–46.

346. Stein, SL, Miller, LC, Konnikov, N. Wegener's granulomatosis: case report and literature review. *Pediatric Dermatology.* 1998;15:352–56.

347. von Scheven, E, Lee, C, Berg, BO. Pediatric Wegener's granulomatosis complicated by central nervous system vasculitis. *Pediatric Neurology.* 1998;19:317–19.

348. Hall, SL, Miller, LC, Duggan, E, Mauer, SM, Beatty, EC, Hellerstein, S. Wegener granulomatosis in pediatric patients. *Journal of Pediatrics.* 1985;106:739–44.

349. May, KP, West, SG. Henoch-Schonlein purpura followed by Wegener's granulomatosis. *Clinical Pediatrics.* 1993;32:555–57.

350. Freed, GL. Wegener's granulomatosis presenting as fever of unknown origin. *Clinical Pediatrics.* 1994;33:162–65.

351. Hansen, LP, Jacobsen, J, Skytte, H. Wegener's granulomatosis in a child. *European Journal of Respiratory Diseases.* 1983;64:620–624.

352. Bullen, CL, Liesegang, TJ, McDonald, TJ, DeRemee, RA. Ocular complications of Wegener's granulomatosis. *Ophthalmology.* 1983;90:279–90.

353. Sacks, RD, Stock, EL, Crawford, SE, Greenwald, MJ, O'Grady, RB. Scleritis and Wegener's granulomatosis in children. *American Journal of Ophthalmology.* 1991;111:430–433.

354. Bambery, P, Sakhuja, V, Behera, D, Deodhar, SD. Pleural effusions in Wegener's granulomatosis: report of five patients and a brief review of the literature. *Scandinavian Journal of Rheumatology.* 1991;20:445–47.

355. Cohen, SR, Landing, BH, King, BK, Isaacs, H. Wegener's granulomatosis causing laryngeal and tracheobronchial obstruction in an adolescent girl. *Annals of Otology, Rhinology, & Laryngology,* Supplement. 1978;87:15–19.

356. Sokol, RJ, Farrell, MK, McAdams, AJ. An unusual presentation of Wegener's granulomatosis mimicking inflammatory bowel disease. *Gastroenterology.* 1984;87:426–32.

357. Wedderburn, LR, Kwan, JT, Thompson, PW, Rudge, SR. Juvenile chronic arthritis and Wegener's granulomatosis. *British Journal of Rheumatology.* 1992;31:121–23.

358. Wong, SN, Shah, V, Dillon, MJ. Antineutrophil cytoplasmic antibodies in Wegener's granulomatosis. *Archives of Disease in Childhood.* 1998;79:246–50.

359. Andrassy, K, Koderisch, J, Rufer, M, Erb, A, Waldherr, R, Ritz, E. Detection and clinical implication of anti-neutrophil cytoplasm antibodies in Wegener's granulomatosis and rapidly progressive glomerulonephritis. *Clinical Nephrology.* 1989;32:159–67.

360. McHugh, K, Manson, D, Eberhard, BA, Shore, A, Laxer, RM. Wegener's granulomatosis in childhood. *Pediatric Radiology.* 1991;21:552–55.

361. Wadsworth, DT, Siegel, MJ, Day, DL. Wegener's granulomatosis in children: chest radiographic manifestations. *American Journal of Roentgenology.* 1994;163:901–4.

362. Andrassy, K, Erb, A, Koderisch, J, Waldherr, R, Ritz, E. Wegener's granulomatosis with renal involvement: patient survival and correlations between initial renal function, renal histology, therapy and renal outcome. *Clinical Nephrology.* 1991;35:139–47.

363. Baliga, R, Chang, CH, Bidani, AK, Perrin, EV, Fleischmann, LE. A case of generalized Wegener's granulomatosis in childhood: successful therapy with cyclophosphamide. *Pediatrics.* 1978;61:286–90.

364. Dabbagh, S, Chevalier, RL, Sturgill, BC. Prolonged anuria and aortic insufficiency in a child with Wegener's granulomatosis. *Clinical Nephrology.* 1982;17:155–59.

365. Guillevin, L, Cordier, JF, Lhote, F, Cohen, P, Jarrousse, B, Royer, I, et al. A prospective, multicenter, randomized trial comparing steroids and pulse cyclophosphamide versus steroids and oral cyclophosphamide in the treatment of generalized Wegener's granulomatosis. *Arthritis & Rheumatism.* 1997;40:2187–98.

366. Gottlieb, BS, Miller, LC, Ilowite, NT. Methotrexate treatment of Wegener granulomatosis in children. *Journal of Pediatrics.* 1996;129:604–7.

367. Backman, A, Grahne, B, Holopainen, E, Leisti, J, Paavolainen, M. Wegener's granulomatosis in childhood. A clinical report based on three cases. *International Journal of Pediatric Otorhinolaryngology.* 1979;1:145–49.

368. Adlakha, A, Rao, K, Adlakha, K, Ryu, JH. A case of pediatric Wegener's granulomatosis with recurrent venous thromboses treated with intravenous immunoglobulin and laryngotracheoplasty. *Pediatric Pulmonology.* 1995;20:265–68.

369. Lupi-Herrera, E, Sanchez-Torres, G, Marcushamer, J, Mispireta, J, Horwitz, S, Vela, JE. Takayasu's arteritis. Clinical study of 107 cases. *American Heart Journal.* 1977;93:94–103.

370. Morales, E, Pineda, C, Martinez-Lavin, M. Takayasu's arteritis in children. *Journal of Rheumatology.* 1991;18:1081–84.

371. Zheng, D, Fan, D, Liu, L. Takayasu arteritis in China: a report of 530 cases. *Heart & Vessels,* Supplement. 1992;7:32–36.

372. Hahn, D, Thomson, PD, Kala, U, Beale, PG, Levin, SE. A review of Takayasu's arteritis in children in Gauteng, South Africa. *Pediatric Nephrology.* 1998;12:668–75.

373. Hong, CY, Yun, YS, Choi, JY, Sul, JH, Lee, KS, Cha, SH, et al. Takayasu arteritis in Korean children: clinical report of seventy cases. *Heart & Vessels,* Supplement. 1992;7:91–96.

374. Golding, RL, Perri, G, Cremin, BJ. The arteriographic manifestations of Takayasu's arteritis in children. *Pediatric Radiology.* 1977;5:224–30.

375. Milner, LS, Jacobs, DW, Thomson, PD, Kala, UK, Franklin, J, Beale, P, et al. Management of severe hypertension in childhood Takayasu's arteritis. *Pediatric Nephrology.* 1991;5:38–41.
376. Tsai, MJ, Lin, SC, Wang, JK, Chou, CC, Chiang, BL. A patient with familial Takayasu's arteritis presenting with fever of unknown origin. *Journal of the Formosan Medical Association.* 1998;97:351–53.
377. Vaz, RM, Formanek, AG, Roach, ES. Takayasu's arteritis. Protean manifestations. *Journal of Adolescent Health Care.* 1988;9:414–17.
378. Wiggelinkhuizen, J, Cremin, BJ. Takayasu arteritis and renovascular hypertension in childhood. *Pediatrics.* 1978;62:209–17.
379. Sharma, S, Rajani, M, Shrivastava, S, Kaul, U, Kamalakar, T, Talwar, KK, et al. Non-specific aorto-arteritis (Takayasu's disease) in children. *British Journal of Radiology.* 1991;64:690–698.
380. Meyers, KE, Thomson, PD, Beale, PG, Morrison, RC, Kala, UK, Jacobs, DW, et al. Gallium scintigraphy in the diagnosis and total lymphoid irradiation of Takayasu's arteritis. *South African Medical Journal.* 1994;84:685–88.
381. Miller, JH, Gunarta, H, Stanley, P. Gallium scintigraphic demonstration of arteritis in Takayasu disease. *Clinical Nuclear Medicine.* 1996;21:882–83.
382. Moore, JW, Reardon, MJ, Cooley, DA, Vargo, TA. Severe Takayasu's arteritis of the pulmonary arteries: report of a case with successful surgical treatment. *Journal of the American College of Cardiology.* 1985;5:369–73.
383. Haas, A, Stiehm, ER. Takayasu's arteritis presenting as pulmonary hypertension. *American Journal of Diseases of Children.* 1986;140:372–74.
384. Said, SA, Koetsveld-Baart, JC, Den Hollander, JC. Takayasu's arteritis: a rare cause of cardiac death in a Caucasian teenage female patient. *Netherlands Journal of Medicine.* 1997;51:182–86.
385. Basso, C, Baracca, E, Zonzin, P, Thiene, G. Sudden cardiac arrest in a teenager as first manifestation of Takayasu's disease. *International Journal of Cardiology.* 1994;43:87–89.
386. Lee, HY, Rao, PS. Percutaneous transluminal coronary angioplasty in Takayasu's arteritis. *American Heart Journal.* 1996;132:1084–86.
387. Kaditis, AG, Nelson, AM, Driscoll, DJ. Takayasu's arteritis presenting with unilateral digital clubbing. *Journal of Rheumatology.* 1995;22:2346–48.
388. Kohrman, MH, Huttenlocher, PR. Takayasu arteritis: a treatable cause of stroke in infancy. *Pediatric Neurology.* 1986;2:154–58.
389. Saxe, PA, Altman, RD. Takayasu's arteritis syndrome associated with systemic lupus erythematosus. *Seminars in Arthritis & Rheumatism.* 1992;21:295–305.
390. Hall, S, Nelson, AM. Takayasu's arteritis and juvenile rheumatoid arthritis. *Journal of Rheumatology.* 1986;13:431–33.
391. Hayes, MM, Gwata, T, Gelfand, M. Takayasu's disease in association with probable Still's syndrome in a nine-year-old African male. *Central African Journal of Medicine.* 1978;24:144–48.
392. Rossor, E. Takayasu's arteritis as a differential diagnosis of systemic juvenile chronic arthritis. *Archives of Disease in Childhood.* 1979;54:798–800.
393. Hilario, MO, Terreri, MT, Prismich, G, Len, C, Kihara, EN, Goldenberg, J, et al. Association of ankylosing spondylitis, Crohn's disease and Takayasu's arteritis in a child. *Clinical & Experimental Rheumatology.* 1998;16:92–94.
394. Owyang, C, Miller, LJ, Lie, JT, Fleming, CR. Takayasu's arteritis in Crohn's disease. *Gastroenterology.* 1979;76:825–28.
395. Sato, R, Sato, Y, Ishikawa, H, Oshima, Y, Suzuki, T, Watanabe, S, et al. Takayasu's disease associated with ulcerative colitis. *Internal Medicine.* 1994;33:759–63.
396. Zilleruelo, GE, Ferrer, P, Garcia, OL, Moore, M, Pardo, V, Strauss, J. Takayasu's arteritis associated with glomerulonephritis. A case report. *American Journal of Diseases of Children.* 1978;132:1009–13.
397. Hellmann, DB, Hardy, K, Lindenfeld, S, Ring, E. Takayasu's arteritis associated with crescentic glomerulonephritis. *Arthritis & Rheumatism.* 1987;30:451–54.
398. Sousa, AE, Lucas, M, Tavora, I, Victorino, RM. Takayasu's disease presenting as a nephrotic syndrome due to amyloidosis. *Postgraduate Medical Journal.* 1993;69:488–89.
399. Beale, PG, Meyers, KE, Thomson, PD. Management of renal hypertension in children with Takayasu's arteritis using renal autografting or allograft transplantation in selected circumstances and total lymphoid irradiation. *Journal of Pediatric Surgery.* 1992;27:836–39.

400. Noy, J, Lemermeyer, G, Mullen, JC, Harley, FL. Splenorenal arterial bypass in a child with Takayasu's disease: a case report. *Canadian Journal of Surgery.* 1996;39:243–46.

401. Shetty, AK, Stopa, AR, Gedalia, A. Low-dose methotrexate as a steroid-sparing agent in a child with Takayasu's arteritis. *Clinical & Experimental Rheumatology.* 1998;16:335–36.

402. Rydel, JJ, Rodby, RA. An 18-year-old man with Goodpasture's syndrome and ANCA-negative central nervous system vasculitis. *American Journal of Kidney Diseases.* 1998;31:345–49.

403. Strole, WE, Jr., Clark, WH, Jr., Isselbacher, KJ. Progressive arterial occlusive disease (Kohlmeier-Degos). A frequently fatal cutaneosystemic disorder. *New England Journal of Medicine.* 1967;276:195–201.

404. Korppi, M, Tenhola, S, Hollmen, A. Mucha-Habermann disease: a diagnostic possibility for prolonged fever associated with systemic and skin symptoms. *Acta Paediatrica.* 1993;82:627–29.

405. Frayha, RA. Churg-Strauss syndrome in a child [letter]. *Journal of Rheumatology.* 1982;9:807–9.

406. Wishnick, MM, Valensi, Q, Doyle, EF, Balian, A, Genieser, NB, Chrousos, G. Churg-Strauss syndrome. Development of cardiomyopathy during corticosteroid treatment. *American Journal of Diseases of Children.* 1982;136:339–44.

407. Augarten, A, Yahav, Y, Szeinberg, A, Fradkin, A, Gazit, E, Laufer, J. HLA-B5 in the diagnosis of Behcet's disease. *Journal of Medicine.* 1995;26:133–38.

408. Lehman, TJ, Allen, JB, Plotz, PH, Wilder, RL. Polyarthritis in rats following the systemic injection of Lactobacillus casei cell walls in aqueous suspension. *Arthritis & Rheumatism.* 1983;26:1259–65.

28 Pulmonary Hypertension

Simon P. Wharton and Tim W. Higenbottam

CONTENTS

I. INTRODUCTION

Pulmonary hypertension (PH) is a disorder characterized by abnormally high pressure in the pulmonary circulation and increased pulmonary vascular resistance. It was first documented in 1865 by the Austrian physician Dr. J. Klob under the term "endarteritis pulmonalis deformans."[1] The modern study of the disorder began with Dr. D. T. Dresdale's description of primary pulmonary hypertension in 1951.[2] Since then there has been a growing understanding of the pathophysiology of this disorder, but PH is still not completely understood.

II. EPIDEMIOLOGY

Pulmonary hypertension can occur either as an unexplained disease or as a complication of a wide range of respiratory and cardiac diseases. In the setting of connective tissue disease, PH can be primary (pre-capillary), secondary to parenchymal lung disease (chronic-hypoxia induced), or secondary to chronic thrombo-embolic disease (Table 28.1).

A. PULMONARY ARTERIAL HYPERTENSION

Primary pulmonary hypertension (PPH) is an example of pulmonary arterial hypertension. It has an annual incidence of 2 to 3 in 1 million people. It is defined as a mean pulmonary artery pressure of greater than 25 mmHg at rest or greater than 30 mmHg during exercise in the absence of left-sided cardiac valvular disease, myocardial disease, congenital heart disease, or clinically important respiratory, connective-tissue, or chronic thrombo-embolic diseases.[3] The pathogenic mechanism of PPH is unknown but, characteristically, the disease process is maximal in the small precapillary pulmonary arteries. Marked intimal thickening through proliferation of the fibroblast and smooth muscle cells leads to obliteration and narrowing of the lumen. The same precapillary pulmonary

TABLE 28.1
A Possible Classification for Pulmonary Hypertension Based on Anatomic
Localization of the Disease, Together with Associated Diseases

Pulmonary Arterial Hypertension
- Unexplained or primary
- Familial PH
- Congenital heart disease and atrial septal defect
- Autoimmune-induced PH (scleroderma myositis, systemic lupus erythematosus, Sjögren's syndrome)
- Portal hypertension- (chronic liver disease-) associated
- Drug-induced PPH (e.g., fenfluramine and aminorex)
- HIV infection

Pulmonary Venous Hypertension
- Left ventricular failure
- Left-sided valvular heart disease
- Pulmonary veno-occlusive disease
- Pulmonary capillary hemangiomatosis

Hypoxic-Induced Pulmonary Hypertension
- Parenchymal lung disease
- Alveolar hypoventilation syndromes (e.g., sleep apnea syndrome)
- Chronic obstructive pulmonary disease (COPD)
- Neuromuscular disorders
- High-altitude pulmonary edema (HAPE)

Chronic Thrombo-Embolic Pulmonary Hypertension
- External vascular compression

hypertension is also seen associated with connective diseases, particularly scleroderma. A similar disease distribution has been found in patients with portal hypertension,[4] infection with human immunodeficiency virus (HIV),[5] and with cocaine abuse.[6] Although precapillary pulmonary hypertension affects both men and women of all ages, races, and ethnicities, the incidence is highest in women between the ages of 21 and 40.[3]

In the setting of connective tissue disease, PH can also occur secondary to interstitial lung disease and thrombo-embolic disease. In these cases the proximal arteries to the level of the segmental arteries are affected, being obstructed with thrombus.

III. SYMPTOMS AND PROGNOSIS OF PULMONARY HYPERTENSION

PH is a progressive disease characterized by structural changes to the large and small pulmonary blood vessel walls. These changes are frequently associated with *in situ* thrombosis of small arteries. Obliteration and narrowing of the vessels results from these changes. This leads to a rise in the resistance to pulmonary blood flow. This ultimately leads to hypertrophy and dilatation of the right ventricle, progressing to right ventricular failure, and death.[7] Fatigue, accompanied by dyspnoea, is a common early symptom of PH. Late clinical symptoms include angina, syncope, and edema. Symptoms of Raynaud's syndrome have been observed in 10% of female patients with PPH. Cardiopulmonary exercise tests usually show a pattern of altered cardiac function, in which maximal oxygen consumption is reduced and the alveolar-arterial oxygen gradient increased. Pulmonary hemodynamics are also significantly altered, with pulmonary artery pressure three or more times above normal, right arterial pressure increased, and cardiac output depressed.[3]

Currently available therapies (calcium channel blockers, oxygen, diuretics, digoxin, and anti-coagulants) can bring symptomatic relief to some patients. The prognosis of PH remains poor, with a mean survival rate of less than three years from the date of diagnosis.[8]

IV. PATIENTS WITH SYSTEMIC SCLEROSIS OR SCLERODERMA

Systemic sclerosis (SSc) is a multisystem disorder of unidentified cause in which various organs become fibrosed. The most widely used classification of SSc defines two subsets based on the extent of skin involvement together with a number of reliable clinical, laboratory, and natural history associations. Over 60% of patients with SSc are defined as having limited cutaneous SSc (lcSSc), where visceral involvement is a late event and tends to occur 10 to 30 years after onset of Raynaud's disease. Patients with lcSSc often exhibit features of the CREST syndrome. However, the term lcSSc is more appropriate than CREST since cutaneous manifestations often extend beyond scle-rodactyly, and calcinosis may be present only at a late stage or observable only radiologically. The remaining 40% of patients are defined as having diffuse cutaneous SSc (dcSSc). This is the more serious form of the disease, with more rapid onset, and organ failure frequently presenting within five years of the first symptoms. The features of lcSSc and dcSSc are outlined in Table 28.2.

Within each subset of SSc there is great variability in the pace of the disease. Some patients with dcSSc develop extensive internal organ complications after two to four years. Others have widespread skin disease but more limited interstitial lung disease. Some patients with lcSSc may never develop clinically apparent PH or mid-gut disease, whereas others develop this complication typically late in the disease course, but occasionally as early as five to seven years after diagnosis. Thus, not only is there heterogeneity of the disease, but differential rates of progression within each subset.

In patients with SSc or scleroderma, PH can be a fatal complication. PH can affect 8 to 10% of patients with dcSSc, and up to 50% of patients with lcSSc. In patients with dcSSc, PH occurs secondary to advanced interstitial lung disease. By contrast, in lcSSc, primary PH can occur in the absence of pulmonary fibrosis. The most lethal organ complication of systemic sclerosis is isolated pulmonary hypertension (IPHT),[9] which is associated with a much poorer prognosis than the PH that occurs secondary to pulmonary fibrosis.

The recognition that PH occurs early in the course of SSc, accelerates rapidly, and is associated with a high mortality even at moderately high levels of pulmonary artery pressure ($\geq$30 mmHg) provides an opportunity to study the pathophysiology of early-stage PH in a discrete patient population. It also offers the possibility to develop treatment strategies that, at the very least, may help to stabilize or attenuate the progression of PH in its early stages.

TABLE 28.2
Features of Diffuse and Limited Cutaneous Systemic Sclerosis

Diffuse	Limited
• Onset of skin changes (puffiness or hidebound) within one year of onset of Raynaud's disease	• Raynaud's disease for years (occasionally decades)
• Truncal and acral skin involvement	• Skin involvement limited to hands, face, feet, and forearms (acral)
• Presence of tendon friction rubs	• Signification (10 to 15%) late incidence of PH, with or without interstitial lung disease, skin calcification, telangiectasiae, and gastric intestinal involvement
• Early and significant incidence of interstitial lung disease, oliguric renal failure, diffuse gastrointestinal disease, and myocardial involvement	• High incidence of ACA (70 to 80%)
• Nailfold capillary involvement and dropout	• Dilated nailfold capillary loops, usually without capillary dropout
• Antitopoisomerase-I (Scl-70) antibodies (30% of patients)	

V. PHYSIOLOGY OF PULMONARY HYPERTENSION

It is becoming increasingly clear that the vascular endothelium plays a central role in the pathogenesis of PH, the key pathogenic features of which are vasoconstriction, pulmonary vascular remodeling, and *in situ* thrombotic lesions. Voelkel and Tuder[10] put forward the hypothesis that PH is an endothelial cell-driven disease in which the cells switch to a hypertensive phenotype. This phenotype is characterized by an enhanced capacity for proliferation, secretion of matrix proteins, and development of a procoagulant surface. The vascular endothelium synthesizes a number of eicanosoids, including the potent vasodilator prostacyclin I_2 (PGI_2). PGI_2 is the primary metabolite of arachidonic acid metabolism and is derived from the conversion of PGH_2 (prostaglandin H_2) by prostacyclin synthase via the cyclo-oxygenase pathway. In addition to its vasodilatory effects, PGI_2 potently inhibits platelet aggregation, vascular smooth muscle cell proliferation, and leucocyte adherence to the vascular wall, and maintains vascular tone and vessel patency.[11,12] In addition to the synthesis of eicosanoids, the vascular endothelium also synthesizes nitric oxide and endothelin, and metabolizes many substances produced elsewhere in the body, e.g., eicosanoids and vasoactive amines including noradrenaline, serotonin, and angiotensin.[13] This is particularly important since the lung receives the total cardiac output of the right ventricle and is therefore exposed to high levels of these agents, and since any alteration to endothelial function could seriously compromise the metabolism of these potent vasoactive agents.

Diminished synthesis of PGI_2 has been implicated in the pathogenesis of PH. Immuno-histochemical analysis of lung tissue from patients with primary and secondary PH has shown a marked absence of prostacyclin synthase (PGI_2-S) in the plexiform lesions. There is also a striking reduction of the PGI_2-S gene transcript and protein in the patent precapillary arteries in the lungs of PH patients compared with healthy patients (Voelkel, N.F., et al. In press). These findings have been confirmed by Western blot analyses of normal human lung tissue and lung tissue from patients with end-stage primary and secondary PH. The defect in prostacyclin synthase expression observed in patients with both PPH and SPH may be an acquired trait, and may be an important part of the hypertensive pulmonary vascular phenotype. Decreased synthesis of PGI_2 is also likely to promote cell growth and so contribute to vascular remodeling. The decreased expression of prostacyclin synthase in the lung tissue of patients with PH is in marked contrast to the overexpression of endothelial nitric oxide synthase, itself a likely potential marker of pulmonary vascular remodeling (Voelkel, N.F., et al. In press).

The importance of prostacyclin synthase in the pathogenesis of PH has been explored in animal models. In these models, the hemodynamic effects of overexpression of prostacyclin synthase on lung tissue have been studied by adenovirus transfection of the PGI_2-S gene into rats. These experiments have shown that 5 days after the installation of the viral construct into rat lungs, there is an abundance of prostacyclin synthase in the lungs in comparison with control animals. Subsequent tests of vasoconstriction, after transfection and perfusion of lung tissue under *ex-vivo* conditions, show that both the angiotensin and hypoxia-induced vasoconstriction responses are blunted in the transfected animals compared with control animals given inactive virus.

Studies in transgenic mice that have a prostacyclin synthase construct built on a surfactant-protein C promoter, which ensures that overexpression of the transgene occurs only in the surfactant-producing lung cells, have shown that when exposed to chronic hypoxia the transgene-positive animals develop less pulmonary hypertension than transgene-negative animals. In transgene-positive animals, levels of PGI_2 in the lung are twice those of the transgene-negative animals (Voelkel, N.F., et al. In press). Interestingly, right-ventricular systolic pressure and right-ventricular mass, an index of right hypertrophy, are significantly lower in the transgene-positive animals, suggesting that overexpression of prostacyclin synthase may protect against the development of pulmonary hypertension.

A. Vascular Endothelial Growth Factor

There is evidence to show that when prostacyclin synthase is absent from plexiform pulmonary lesions of patients with PH, the gene encoding vascular endothelial growth factor (VEGF) is highly expressed. VEGF is present in alveolar and bronchial epithelial cells as well as vascular smooth muscle cells and macrophages. It is known to both promote endothelial cell proliferation and enhance vascular permeability. Thus, VEGF may be important in the development of PH.[14,15] The VEGF receptor, which drives endothelial cell proliferation, is also highly expressed in cells deficient in PGI_2-S. Tuder et al.[14] have shown that hypoxia not only increases synthesis of VEGF but also upregulates VEGF receptor expression.

B. Endothelin-1 (ET-1) in Patients with Pulmonary Hypertension

Endothelins are endothelium-derived peptides with potent vasoconstricting properties. Endothelin-1 (Et-1) is the principal endothelin produced by the endothelium. It mediates transient vasodilation followed by profound and sustained vasoconstriction, as well as inducing smooth muscle cell proliferation. To exert their biological effects, endothelins activate specific receptors present on endothelial cells, ET (B) or vascular smooth muscle cells, ET (A), and ET (B). Both hypoxia[16] and ischemia[17] appear to stimulate the production of Et-1, whereas nitric oxide inhibits the synthesis of Et-1.[18]

Endothelins have been implicated in moderate to severe essential hypertension, cardiac hypertrophy, atherogenesis, and vasospasm accompanying stroke or subarachnoid hemorrhage.[19] Evidence that endothelin expression is enhanced in both neonatal PH and primary PH has led to suggestions that endothelin may also have a pathophysiological role to play in the development of PH.[20]

It has been suggested that elevations in plasma Et-1 activity in patients with left-to-right shunts may be related to increased pulmonary blood flow.[21] To date there has been no independent confirmation of this finding. On the contrary, no direct positive correlation has been found between increased pulmonary blood flow and increased plasma levels of Et-1 in patients with normal pulmonary vascular resistance.[22] Therefore, it is thought that some other factor must contribute toward increased pulmonary resistance in such patients. Interestingly, Et-1 receptor density appears to be increased in patients with high pulmonary resistance and low pulmonary flow compared with patients who have low pulmonary resistance and high pulmonary flow.

C. Nitric Oxide Synthase in Patients with Pulmonary Hypertension

Endothelium-derived NO is released following an enzymatic reaction involving NO synthases, which are products of several genes. In man and some mammals, continuous release of nitric oxide is an important physiological determinant of pulmonary vascular tone[23] and appears to regulate the distribution of pulmonary flow.[24] There is also evidence that, in humans with PH, NO release is impaired in pulmonary arteries.[25] Interestingly, chronic inhaled NO appears to protect against the development of PH.[26,27] Attention is now directed toward the plexogenic lesions where NO synthase activity is high while PGI_2 is low or absent (Voelkel, N.J. Personal communication.). The function and hemodynamic importance of the plexogenic lesion is still speculative and may represent both an attempt to revascularize the arterial bed and an end-stage product of remodeling. Since this lesion is unique to severe PH, it makes a particularly inviting target for further study.

D. Noradrenaline

Another recent finding, which may have important implications for the pathophysiology of PH, is the discovery that circulating levels of noradrenaline are markedly increased in patients with PH in comparison with normal control subjects, and compared with patients with atrial and ventricular septal defects without pulmonary hypertension. The pulmonary (RP) to systemic (RS) vascular resistance ratio also appears significantly higher in patients with PH, and increases in parallel with levels of noradrenaline.

It has been suggested that noradrenaline, as well as angiotensin II, may act as a mediator of the prostacyclin cessation syndrome; this condition arises following abrupt cessation of chronic prostacyclin therapy and is characterized by a severe dyspnoea of unknown origin together with a marked rebound in both mean systemic arterial pressure (30%), systemic vascular resistance (60%), and pulmonary vascular resistance (>20%).[28]

REFERENCES

1. Klob, J. Endarteritis pulmonalis deformans. *Wochenblatt der Zeitschrift der k.k. Gesellschaft der Aerzte in Wien* 1865; 21: 357–361.
2. Dresdale, DT, Schultz, M, Michtom, RJ. Primary pulmonary hypertension. 1. Clinical and hemodynamic study. *Am. J. Med.,* 1951; 11: 686–705.
3. Rich, S, Dantzker, DR, Ayres, SM, Bergofsky, EH, Brundage, BH, Detre, KM, Fishman, AP, Goldring, RM, Groves, BM, Koerner, SK, Levy, PS, Reid, LM, Vreim, CE, Williams, GW. Primary pulmonary hypertension: A national prospective study. *Ann. Intern. Med.,* 1987; 107: 216–223.
4. Hadengue, A, Benhayoun, MK, Lebrec, D, Benhamou, JP. Pulmonary hypertension complicating portal hypertension: prevalence and relation to splanchnic hemodynamics. *Gastroenterology,* 1991; 100: 520–528.
5. Legoux, B, Piette, AM, Bouchet, PE, Laudau, JF, Gepner, P, Chapman, AM. Pulmonary hypertension and HIV infection. *Am. J. Med.,* 1990; 89: 122.
6. Collins, E, Hardwich, H, Jeffery, H. Perinatal cocaine intoxication. *Med. J. Aust.,* 1989; 150: 331–332.
7. Rubin, LJ. Primary pulmonary hypertension. *Chest,* 1993; 104: 236–250.
8. D'Alonzo, GE, Barst, RJ, Ayres, SM, Bergofsky, EH, Brundage, BH, Detre, KM, Fishman, AP, Goldring, RM, Groves, BM, Kernis, JT, Levy, PS, Pietra, GG, Reid, LM, Reeves, RT, Ruch, S, Vrein, CE, Williams, GW, Wu, M. Survival in patients with primary pulmonary hypertension. Results from a national prospective registry. *Ann. Intern. Med.,* 1991; 115: 343–349.
9. Lee, P, Langevitz, P, Alderdice, CA, Aubrey, M, Baer, PA, Baron, M, Buskila, D, Dutz, JP, Khostanteen, I, Piper, S, Ramsden, M, Rosenbach, TO, Sukenik, S, Wilkinson, S, Keystone, EC. Mortality in systemic sclerosis (scleroderma). *Q. J. Med.,* 1992; 82: 139–148.
10. Voelkel, NF, Tuder, RM. Cellular and molecular mechanisms in the pathogenesis of severe pulmonary hypertension. *Eur. Respir. J.,* 1995; 8: 2129–2138.
11. Moncada, S, Vane, JR. Arachidonic acid metabolites and the interactions between platelets and blood vessel walls. *N. Engl. J. Med.,* 1979; 300: 1142–1147.
12. Hyman, AL, Kadowitz, PJ. Pulmonary vasodilator activity of prostacyclin in the cat. *Circ. Res.,* 1979; 45: 404–409.
13. Catravas, JD, Gillis, CN. Single-pass removal of [^{14}C]-5-hydroxytryptamine and [^{3}H]-norepinephrine by rabbit lung, *in vivo*: Kinetics and sites of removal. *J. Pharmacol. Exp. Ther.,* 1983; 224: 28–33.
14. Tuder, RM, Voelkel, NF. Vascular endothelial growth factor (VEGF) induction in primary pulmonary hypertension. *J. Cell. Biochem.,* 1994; 18A: 330.
15. Voelkel, NF, Hoeper, M, Maloney, J, Tuder, RM. Vascular endothelial growth factor in pulmonary hypertension. *Ann. N.Y. Acad. Sci.,* 1996; 796: 186–193.
16. Kourembanas, S, Marsden, PA, McQuillan, LP, Fuller, DV. Hypoxia induces endothelin gene expression and secretion in cultured human endothelium. *J. Clin. Invest.,* 1991; 88: 1054–1057.
17. Ziv, I, Fleminger, G, Djaldetti, R, Achiran, A, Melamcel, E, Sokolovsky, M. Increased plasma endothelin-1 in acute ischemic stroke. *Stroke,* 1992; 23: 1014–1016.
18. Boulanger, C, Luscher, TF. Release of endothelin from the porcine aorta. Inhibition by endothelium-derived nitric oxide. *J. Clin. Invest.,* 1990; 85: 587–590.
19. Schiffrin, EL, Intengan, HD, Thibault, G, Touyz, RM. Clinical significance of endothelin in cardiovascular disease. *Curr. Opin. Cardiol.,* 1997; 12: 354–367.

20. Giaid, A, Yanagisawa, M, Langleben, D, Michel, RP, Levy, R, Shennib, H, Kimura, S, Masaki, T, Duguid, WP, Stewart, DJ. Expression of endothelin-1 in the lungs of patients with pulmonary hypertension. *N. Engl. J. Med.,* 1993; 328: 1732–1739.

21. Vincent, JA, Ross, RD, Kassals, J, Hzu, JM, Pinky, WW. Relation of elevated plasma endothelin in congenital heart disease to increased pulmonary blood flow. *Am. J. Cardiol.,* 1993; 71: 1204–1207.

22. Gorenflo, M, Gross, P, Bodey, A, Schmitz, L, Brockmeier, K, Berger, F, Bein, G, Lange, PE. Plasma endothelin-1 in patients with left-to-right shunt. *Am. Heart J.,* 1995; 130: 537–542.

23. Cremona, G, Wood, AM, Hall, LW, Bower, EA, Higenbottam, TW. Effects of inhibitors of nitric oxide release and action on vascular tone in isolated lungs of pigs, sheep, dogs and man. *J. Physiol. Lond.,* 1994; 481:185–195.

24. Cremona, G, Higenbottam, TW, Takao, M, Bower, BA, Hall, LW. Nature and site of action of endogenous nitric oxide in the vasculature of isolated pig lungs. *J. Appl. Physiol.,* 1997; 82: 23–31.

25. Giaid, A, Saleh, D. Reduced expression of endothelial nitric oxide synthase in the lungs of patients with pulmonary hypertension. *N. Engl. J. Med.,* 1995; 333: 214–221.

26. Kouyoumdjian, C, Adnot, S, Levam, M, Eddahibi, S, Bousbaa, H, Raffestin, B. Continuous inhalation of nitric oxide protects against the development of pulmonary hypertension in chronically hypoxic rats. *J. Clin. Invest.,* 1994; 94: 578–584.

27. Roos, CM, Frank, DU, Xue, C, Johns, RA, Rich, GF. Chronic inhaled nitric oxide: effects on pulmonary vascular endothelial function and pathology in rats. *J. Appl. Physiol.,* 1996; 80: 252–268.

28. Cuiper, LL, Price, PV, Christman, BW. Systemic and pulmonary hypertension after abrupt cessation of prostacyclin: role of thromboxane A2. *J. Appl. Physiol.,* 1996; 80: 191–197.

29 Renal Vasculitis

Michael Samarkos, Sozos Loizou, and Kevin A. Davies

CONTENTS

0-8493-1335-X/01/$0.00+$.50
© 2001 by CRC Press LLC

I. INTRODUCTION

Systemic vasculitides comprise a large group of disorders involving blood vessels of varying size, from capillaries to the aorta. They are characterized by inflammatory changes of the involved vessels, and the clinical syndromes associated with the vasculitides can be diverse in presentation and evolution. Because of their nonspecific clinical and laboratory features, the diagnosis of systemic vasculitides can be difficult. Distinction between different vasculitides is not always easy, as specific classification criteria for vasculitis are still under discussion. Necrotizing and granulomatous vasculitides, Takayasu's arteritis, giant cell arteritis, and Behçet's disease are discussed in other chapters. We will therefore limit our discussion to the renal involvement encountered in the different vasculitic syndromes.

The kidney can be affected by various types of systemic vasculitis, but is more frequently affected in certain forms of primary systemic vasculitis, i.e., polyarteritis nodosa, microscopic polyarteritis, the Churg-Strauss syndrome, and Wegener's granulomatosis. Other primary vasculitides which can affect the kidney are giant cell arteritis, Takayasu's arteritis, Behçet's disease, and relapsing polychondritis. The patterns of kidney involvement in vasculitis are either necrotizing and crescentic glomerulonephritis, or arteritis of medium-sized renal vessels. Both patterns may cause renal failure. The secondary vasculitides which can involve the kidney, e.g., lupus nephritis, cryoglobulinemia, and Henoch-Schöenlein purpura, will not be discussed here.

II. POLYARTERITIS NODOSA

A. General Considerations

Polyarteritis nodosa (PAN) is a form of necrotizing arteritis of small- and medium-sized muscular arteries with multiple organ involvement. The most commonly involved organs are the skin, joints, kidneys, peripheral nerves, and gut.[1-3] The severity of disease varies from a mild form to a progressive, fulminant disease.[4,5] Although PAN is a primary vasculitis, an association between PAN and hepatitis B virus infection (HBV) as well as with hepatitis C virus (HCV) and human immunodeficiency virus (HIV) infections has been well documented.[6-10] An association has also been noted between polyarteritis nodosa and Familial Mediterranean Fever.[11] In 1990 the American College of Rheumatology established classification criteria for PAN, the main goal of which was to help in the classification of patients for clinical studies, not to serve as diagnostic criteria.[12] The ACR criteria did not make any distinction between "classic" PAN (c-PAN) and microscopic polyangiitis (MPA), which was classified as belonging to the PAN group of vasculitides. In 1994 the Chapel Hill International Consensus Conference (CCHC) attempted to establish a nomenclature for the most common forms of noninfectious systemic vasculitides.[13] One major change was the attempt to distinguish c-PAN from MPA. According to this consensus, "classic" polyarteritis nodosa was defined as a necrotizing inflammation of medium-sized or small arteries, without any evidence of glomerulonephritis or vasculitis in arterioles, capillaries, or venules. The term "microscopic polyangiitis" was used to describe the cases previously defined as polyarteritis nodosa in which there was involvement of arterioles, venules or capillaries, or glomerulonephritis.[13] Hence, polyarteritis nodosa and microscopic polyangiitis could be differentiated by the presence or absence of small-vessel involvement. Since glomerulonephritis is a common form of small-vessel involvement, it became an important feature distinguishing MPA from c-PAN. The CHCC proposals were criticized for being "not dissimilar" to earlier classification schemes.[14] Furthermore, some researchers disagreed with the redefinition of polyarteritis nodosa and microscopic polyangiitis on the grounds that it gave MPA too important a place in the vasculitides.[15] Indeed, using CHCC nomenclature, c-PAN is a rare disorder.[16,17] In a series of 130 patients with systemic vasculitis in the U.K., there were eight patients who met both the ACR criteria for PAN and the CHCC criteria for MPA, while none of the patients met the CHCC criteria for c-PAN.[16] In a similar cohort of patients in

France, no patient meeting the CHCC criteria for PAN was found.[17] The suggestion was put forward that MPA should not be considered synonymous to the microscopic form of polyarteritis nodosa as described by Dawson, but as a different disease entity.[14] Although the CHCC nomenclature is now widely accepted, some authors still believe that it is necessary for MPA to be more clearly defined on the basis of criteria which are not exclusively histological, e.g., clinical manifestations (lung and kidney involvement), biologic markers (antineutrophil cytoplasm autoantibodies (ANCA), hepatitis B and C virus antibodies), and angiographic data.[18]

B. Epidemiology

PAN is a rare disease which affects men and women equally in all racial groups.[2] The highest incidence is seen at 40 to 60 years of age.[3,19,20] There are few published estimates of the exact incidence of PAN, and most of these studies were conducted before the CHCC.[4,7,16,21-23] Hence, a number of patients who would now be classified as having MPA were included. The annual incidence of PAN in the pre-CHCC studies ranged from 2.0 to 9.0 million,[4,21-23] while in two studies published in 1995, no patient with c-PAN was found using the CHCC criteria, and the incidence was estimated to be less than 1.5 million.[16,17,19] In contrast, a third study conducted in Kuwait in 1997 reported an annual incidence of 16 million; the authors attributed this finding to their aggressive diagnostic methodology and the prospective design of their study.[24] Since c-PAN is associated with HBV infection, the incidence of c-PAN is greater in populations in which HBV infection is more frequent.[7] Some authors have suggested that the decline in the incidence of PAN is in part due to the development of vaccines against HBV and the more effective screening of blood donors.[3] It is noteworthy that familial cases of PAN have also been reported.[25]

C. Clinical Features

Most patients with PAN present with constitutional symptoms such as malaise, weight loss, and fever.[1,2,4,5,20,26-29] General symptoms are usually associated with symptoms of specific organ involvement, and besides the kidneys, the skin, joints, nerves, and gut are often involved. Skin involvement includes a purpuric rash, livedo reticularis, ischemia of the distal digits, and ulcerations.[30] Around 50% of PAN patients present with arthritis or arthralgia,[1,2] and 50 to 70% can have peripheral neuropathy which can produce mononeuritis multiplex, but central nervous system involvement is rare.[31] Gastrointestinal involvement is one of the more serious manifestations of PAN; it presents with abdominal pain, ischemia or perforation of the small bowel, gastrointestinal tract bleeding, and gallbladder or appendix vasculitis.[32-34] Orchitis is one of the ACR classification criteria for PAN.[12] Other organs such as the heart, breast, uterus, and eyes are less frequently involved.[20]

D. Renal Involvement

In older reports renal involvement was noted in 63 to 76% of patients with PAN,[1,22,28] whereas in three more recent prospective studies, which included patients with PAN and Churg-Strauss syndrome (CCS), kidney involvement occurred in only 26, 36%, and 44%, respectively.[2,5,29] It has to be noted that in all the above reports, c-PAN and MPA were investigated together. Two reports, however, studied patients with classic PAN separately from patients with MPA. In the first of these, at least 14 of 16 (87.5%) patients had either hematuria or creatinine clearance less than 50 ml.min, while in a second, smaller study, 2 of 5 (40%) patients had proteinuria or raised serum creatinine.[24,35]

In classic PAN, renal involvement is seldom a prominent manifestation, and damage to other organs is more likely to dominate the clinical picture.[26] A few cases of c-PAN have been reported that present only with kidney involvement.[36] The underlying mechanism for renal damage is arteritis of medium-sized renal arteries, resulting in renal ischemia, which in the more severe cases may lead to renal infarction. Renal involvement in c-PAN may present with loin pain, gross or microscopic hematuria, moderate proteinuria, slowly progressive renal insufficiency, and hypertension.

During the acute phase of the disease there may be oliguria or anuria, although acute renal failure is uncommon.[37] This complication has been reported after angiography,[38] following treatment with angiotensin-converting enzyme inhibitors,[39] and in association with other aggravating conditions such as multiple myeloma.[40] In some cases renal infarction is clinically silent, and renal failure develops over the course of months or years.[3] Slowly progressive renal insufficiency finally develops in approximately 30% of patients. Proteinuria is usually minimal to moderate and the urine sediment presents very few abnormalities; findings are probably due to glomerular ischemic changes rather than to true glomerulonephritis.[26] Rupture of renal artery aneurysms is responsible for the renal or perirenal hematomas, which are an uncommon finding but a well-described manifestation of PAN.[41,42] There are also a few case reports of spontaneous kidney rupture in patients with PAN,[43] as well as of papillary necrosis due to calyceal artery involvement.[44] A rarer complication is bilateral renal artery dissection.[45] Hypertension is common, although in different reports its frequency varies from 25 to 71%,[1,2,4,29,46] and it is usually renin-mediated, with concomitant secondary hyperaldosteronism.[47,48] Immunohistochemical studies have shown hyperplasia of the renin-producing cells in the ischemic areas of the renal cortex, as well as alterations in their distribution. These changes are similar to those found in renal artery stenosis. In rare cases hypertension may be due to ischemia secondary to compression from perinephric hematoma.[49] Ureteral involvement with unilateral or bilateral stenosis has been described, and is usualy due to periureteric vasculitis and fibrosis.[50,51]

E. PATHOLOGY

Classic polyarteritis nodosa is a necrotizing vasculitis, which, according to CHCC proposals, does not involve vessels smaller than arteries.[13] The arteritis of c-PAN is irregular in distribution and the lesions are segmental, showing a predilection for vessel bifurcation.[20] In the kidney, vessels which range in size from interlobar and arcuate to interlobular are involved.[26] The acute arterial lesions of PAN are focal segmental inflammatory lesions, where fibrinoid necrosis and a mural and perivascular pleomorphic infiltrate are common. Early lesions consist mainly of neutrophils, while mononuclear leukocytes predominate in older lesions. Variable numbers of lymphocytes and esinophils are also present, and leucocytoclasia is frequent in acute lesions, but granulomas are absent.[52] If there is sufficient tissue taken at biopsy, one can find lesions at different stages of progression and healing. The normal architecture of the vessel is disrupted, and elastic lamina destruction and erosion of the inflammation into the perivascular tissues leads to aneurysm formation, thrombosis, or rupture of the vessel with hemorrhage. Acute lesions evolve into sclerotic, fibrous tissue, and formed thrombi are recanalized. Occasionally, chronic arterial stenosis may follow, and the chronic ischemia results in zones of atrophy alternating with zones of compensatory hyperptrophy, leading to a macroscopically irregular appearance of the renal cortex.[26] No changes are observed in the glomeruli except for the ischemic collapse of tufts. Hyperplasia of the juxtaglomerular apparatus may also be present, as well as hypertensive changes in the afferent arterioles.[26]

Tubulointerstitial changes have been described in patients with PAN, and consist of interstitial inflammatory infiltrate composed predominantly of lymphocytes and tubulitis.[53] The necrotizing arterial lesions of c-PAN, per se, are difficult to distinguish histologically from those seen in MPA, Wegener's granulomatosis (WG), or in CSS. Microscopic polyangiitis will manifest as glomerulonephritis or pulmonary capillaritis. A necrotizing granulomatous inflammation of the respiratory tract will be present in WG, while the CSS will be associated with eosinophilia and asthma.[52] Additionally, an uneven distribution of the pathological changes, i.e., areas of active arteritis alternating with fibrotic areas accompanied by disruption of the elastic lamina, is suggestive of c-PAN.

F. LABORATORY FINDINGS AND DIAGNOSIS

There are no laboratory tests specific for c-PAN per se. The most common findings are indicative of chronic inflammation, and these are usually an increased erythrocyte sedimentation rate (ESR), elevated C-reactive protein (CRP), and raised fibrinogen and complement components, as well as

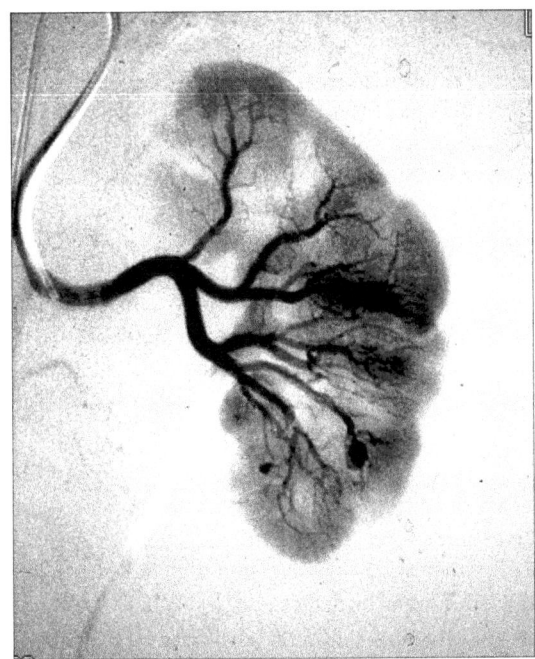

FIGURE 29.1 Selective digital subtraction renal angiogram showing typical appearance of classic polyarteritis nodosa (c-PAN) with aneurysm formation.

normochromic anemia and leukocytosis. When c-PAN is associated with a viral disease such as HBV, HCV, HIV, or parvovirus B19 infection, serological findings of the corresponding infection may be seen. Surface HBV antigen (HBsAg) is found in 7 to 36% of patients.[6] Antineutrophil cytoplasmic antibodies (ANCA) are detected by indirect immunofluoresence (IIF), and three patterns are recognized in ethanol-fixed specimens: a perinuclear type, (p-ANCA); a cytoplasmic type, (c-ANCA); and an atypical type, (X-ANCA). Antineutrophil cytoplasmic antibodies are detected in 10 to 20% of patients with c-PAN, and are more frequently p-ANCA. The different IIF patterns correspond roughly to different antigenic specificities which can be detected by ELISA. Cytoplasmic ANCA IIF pattern in most cases can be attributed to antibodies against proteinase 3 (anti-PR3), while p-ANCA pattern can be due to antibodies against myeloperoxidase (anti-MPO), and less frequently to elastase,or lactoferrin.[3,15,26,54-62] In a large study of 62 patients, 11% of patients with HBV-associated c-PAN were positive for ANCA, in contrast to non-HBV-related PAN (including c-PAN and MPA) where the incidence of ANCA was 27%.[54,63] Antinuclear and antibodies against native DNA are uncommon (<10%), while antismooth muscle antibodies were reported in 10% of patients in the study of Serra et al. Rheumatoid factor is frequently (39%) found.[64,65]

   In c-PAN, a patient's renal angiography may demonstrate the presence of arterial stenosis (narrowing or tapering of arteries) and microaneurysms, which are usually located at the level of interlobar down to arcuate arteries (Figure 29.1).[46,66-70] They are saccular or fusiform, and their size ranges from 1 to 5 mm.[3] The presence of microaneurysms, is usually associated with more severe disease and can regress with treatment.[71-73] Microaneurysms however, are not specific for c-PAN, as they can also be seen in other conditions, such as MPA, severe hypertension, and rheumatoid arthritis.[74-77]

   In cases where the clinical picture is suggestive of c-PAN but without focal signs or symptoms, visceral angiography (renal, mesenteric, or hepatic) is currently preferred over nondirected biopsies. In this setting the presence of angiographic abnormalities constitutes strong diagnostic evidence for c-PAN.[4,26,78,79] In a study by Guillevin et al. in 1992, angiography suggested the diagnosis of vasculitis in 39% of patients;[29] this same group considered the presence of microaneurysms characteristic of c-PAN and suggested that the presence of microaneurysms should exclude the diagnosis of MPA, a suggestion which is not in agreement with the CHCC proposals.[3]

The strongest evidence for the diagnosis of c-PAN is offered by tissue biopsies; the most common sites for biopsy in suspected cases of c-PAN are the skin and skeletal muscle, sural nerve, kidney, liver, and testis. Nondirected biopsies have a low yield, and therefore biopsies are best taken from affected organs.[26] When renal involvement is suspected, renal angiography prior to biopsy may be of help, as the presence of intrarenal arterial aneurysms increases the risk of postbiopsy bleeding.[80]

Other imaging methods, which have an ancillary role but can help in diagnosing c-PAN or some of its associated complications, are ultrasonography, renal radionuclide scanning, excretory urography, computerized tomography, magnetic resonance imaging , and Gallium-67 imaging.[51,81,82] Most of these tests, however, have low specificity and are expensive. Some authors consider renal radionuclide scan as an effective screening test for renal vascular insufficiency.[26]

G. Course and Prognosis

The clinical course of c-PAN is not uniform because of the large variations in organ involvement. Balow and Fauci described three groups of patients according to the course of the disease.[26] The first group consists of approximately 25% of patients who have a rapidly progressive course and multiple organ involvement resulting in high mortality, especially during the first three to six months after diagnosis.[4] The second group includes about 50% of patients with c-PAN who have a moderately severe disease with marked fluctuations in disease activity. The third group consist of a small number of patients who have an initial episode of vasculitis followed by long-term remission of disease, irrespective of whether they had been treated.

The mean survival for patients with c-PAN has changed dramatically with the use of corticosteroids and immunosuppressive treatment. The five-year survival rate has increased from 10% for untreated patients,[27] to 55 to 76% for patients treated with corticosteroids,[1] and to 64 to 80% for patients treated with a combination of corticosteroids and immunosuppressive drugs or cyclophosphamide.[28,83] In most studies the addition of plasma exchange has not significantly improved the survival rate[84] except in patients with c-PAN associated with HBV infection.[6] The overall five-year survival rate for c-PAN quoted in most studies is around 60%.[1,2,4,5]

In a number of different studies several disease markers have been reported to have an adverse effect on prognosis of c-PAN, and these include renal involvement, hypertension, cardiac involvement, gastrointestinal involvement, peripheral nervous system involvement, and age at onset of the condition.[1,2,4,5,85] Guillevin et al. developed a prognostic scoring system for c-PAN, MPA, and CSS based on five clinical and laboratory parameters.[85]

III. MICROSCOPIC POLYANGIITIS

A. General Considerations

Although a microscopic form of PAN with renal involvement characterized by segmental crescentic glomerulonephritis was described as early as 1948,[86] microscopic PAN was not classified as a distinct form of vasculitis in most vasculitis classification schemes until the CHCC.[13] The CHCC proposed the term "microscopic polyangiitis" (MPA), which was defined as a necrotizing vasculitis affecting small vessels (i.e., capillaries, venules, or arterioles), with a few or no immune deposits (pauci-immune), but without granuloma formation, and which was almost invariably associated with glomerulonephritis. It has also been noted that small and medium-sized arteries can also be involved. The term "polyangiitis" was preferred over "polyarteritis" to describe patients in which only small vessels were involved.[13] The CHCC did not manage to completely solve the problem of distinguishing between c-PAN and MPA, although in most patients these two conditions can be differentiated on the basis of the CCHC criteria.[20]

B. Epidemiology

Microscopic polyangiitis is a rare disorder. The male-to-female ratio ranges from 1 to 1.8[65,87-90] and the age of onset is usually 50 to 60 years old.[65,87] It should be noted that in most of the above reports, patients with c-PAN and MPA were studied as one group. Only a few studies deal with the epidemiology of MPA per se. The annual incidence of MPA in a particular area of the United Kingdom (Leicester) using the Fauci classification[91] increased from 0.5 million to 3.3 million following the introduction of ANCA testing.[92] Another study from the U.K. using the CHCC nomenclature estimated the annual incidence of MPA to be 3.6 million,[16] while a more recent study from Kuwait found an annual incidence of 29 million.[24]

C. Clinical Features

Constitutional symptoms are present at diagnosis in 56 to 76% of patients with MPA,[65,87-90] and symptoms might have been present up to two years before a diagnosis is made.[89] The clinical manifestations of MPA are similar to those of c-PAN, the main difference being that renal involvement is almost invariably present in MPA in the form of glomerulonephritis, while in c-PAN renal involvement is not as frequent and usually takes the form of renal vessel vasculitis. Another important difference is that peripheral neuropathy is less common in MPA (14 to 19%) than in c-PAN (50 to 70%).[65,87-89] In contrast, pulmonary involvement, presenting as lung hemorrhage, dyspnea, lung infiltrates, pleural effusions, or interstitial fibrosis, is a relatively frequent finding in MPA (25 to 55%) while it is rather uncommon in c-PAN.[80]

D. Renal Involvement

The vast majority of MPA patients present renal involvement during the course of the disease. It has to be noted that most series are reported by nephrologists, so there might be a bias towards overestimating the incidence of renal disease in MPA.[80] Renal disease at presentation occurred in 17 to 36% of patients,[65,87] while a recent study of 85 patients with MPA, who were followed for up to 15 years, reported that renal manifestations developed in 78.8%.[90] The usual form of renal involvement in MPA is rapidly progressive glomerulonephritis, although in some cases renal function may decline slowly.[26] Renal involvement may range from asymptomatic renal impairment, hematuria, and proteinuria, to rapidly progressive renal failure. Hematuria occurs in 64 to 100% of patients in the various patients' series, and is usually microscopic rather than gross hematuria. Proteinuria is found in 80 to 90% of patients, while nephrotic range proteinuria has been reported in 9 to 41% of patients.[65,87,89,90] Abnormal urinary sediment is also a very common finding. Functional renal impairment at presentation occurred in 13 to 17%, but finally developed in 70 to 100% of patients. Guillevin et al. reported that patients with MPA had mean serum creatinine 230 µmol/l (range 51 to 1500 µmol/l) at presentation. Adu et al. found that 55% of patients had serum creatinine over 500 µmol/l at diagnosis, and Savage et al. reported a mean serum creatinine of 574 µmol/l (range 147 to 1405 µmol/l) at the time of referral. In these three studies dialysis was required in 12%, 46%, and 23% of patients, respectively.[87,89,90] Hypertension is not as common in MPA as is in c-PAN, and occurs in 20 to 35% of patients, possibly because the glomerular involvement is focal and segmental and renal ischemia is infrequent.[65,87-90] As renal artery involvement and the presence of aneurysms are uncommon, renal infarction and renal or perirenal hematomas are very rare in MPA.

E. Pathology

The extrarenal pathology of MPA is similar to that of c-PAN, although MPA has a predilection for smaller vessels and frequently involves alveolar capillaries.[88,93]

Microscopic polyangiitis is characterized by a focal and segmental glomerulonephritis, which is found in 80 to 100% of renal biopsies (Figure 29.2).[80] There is segmental fibrinoid necrosis, and

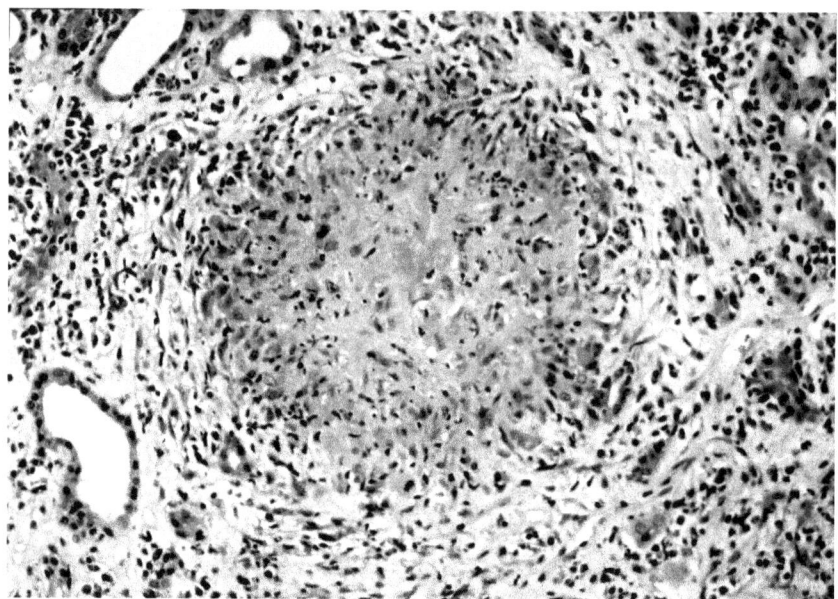

FIGURE 29.2 Severe nephritis causing complete glomerular destruction in a patient with microscopic polyarteritis.

prominent crescents which are found in more than 60% of glomeruli. Crescents are formed by rupture of the glomerular capillaries, which leads to fibrin exudation, epithelial cell proliferation, and monocyte accumulation. Adhesions to the Bowman's capsule are frequent, and there may also be disruption of glomerular basement membrane and of Bowman's capsule. Numerous neutrophils may infiltrate within and around necrotic glomerular segments, although nonnecrotic segments are only modestly hypercellular.[26,52] Granulomas are absent in MPA, although epithelial cells have been described in association with glomeruli.[87] It has been suggested that the glomerular lesions of MPA tend to be of similar age,[88] but some authors suggest that they may be of mixed types and at different stages, and that acute necrotic lesions may coexist with healed sclerotic ones.[26,52] Glomerulonephritis in MPA is, by definition, pauci-immune, and therefore no or scanty immune deposits, usually of immunoglobulin and complement, are found in the glomeruli, either immunohistochemically or by electron microscopy.[52]

Tubulointerstitial changes are a common finding in MPA with an interstitial infiltrate consisting of mixed inflammatory cells, usually lymphocytes, monocytes, and plasma cells. Occasionally, esinophils and epitheloid and giant cells may be found.[53,80] The tubular changes of MPA consist of vacuolization, degeneration, and atrophy, possibly due to tubular ischemia caused by small-vessel vasculitis; in a significant number of cases there is also fragmentation of the tubular basement membrane (tubulorrhexis).[53] Although it is believed that interstitial changes are generally proportional to the glomerular damage, Adu et al. found that interstitial damage reflects renal functional impairment better than glomerular damage.[53,80,89]

Vasculitis of the renal vessels is found in 19 to 34% of cases and usually affects subarcuate lobular arteries and arterioles.[15,80] The vasculitic lesions are similar to those of Wegener's granulomatosis and Churg-Strauss syndrome, and they consist of segmental fibrinoid necrosis, with mural and perivascular infiltrates of neutrophils or monocytes.[52]

Microaneurysms are not commonly found in MPA. Savage et al. did not find aneurysms in any of their 34 patients, while Adu et al. and Guillevin et al. described microaneurysms in 3 of 11 (27%) and 3 of 30 (10%) of their patients, respectively.[87,89,90] A recent study using histological techniques to study the three-dimensional morphology of vessels reported that microaneurysms

(<1mm) were frequent in patients with MPA. Microaneurysms in MPA were sausage-shaped, suggesting a necrotizing panangiitis involving the entire circumference of the vessel. In contrast, in c-PAN the aneurysms are usually saccular, possibly suggesting vasculitic involvement of only a part of the vessel circumference.[94,95]

F. Laboratory Findings and Diagnosis

Laboratory findings in MPA are nonspecific, are very similar to those seen in c-PAN, and reflect the chronic inflammation. Interestingly, esinophilia was reported in 14% of patients studied by Adu et al., and in 25% of patients studied by Ronco et al., although in both studies c-PAN and MPA were not separated.[64,89] Laboratory findings relevant to renal involvement have already been discussed. Serological findings of HBV or HCV infection are rare in MPA, in contrast with c-PAN. Guillevin et al. found HbeAg in only 2 of 85, anti-HCV in 1 of 85 patients, and considered this a coincidental finding.[90]

The most important laboratory feature of MPA is the frequent detection of ANCA, in contrast with c-PAN in which ANCA are uncommon or rare.[15,57] Antineutrophil cytoplasmic antibodies were detected in 25 of 33 (75%), 22 of 43 (51%), and 38 of 51 (74.5%) of patients with MPA reported by Hauschild et al., Davenport et al., and Guillevin et al., respectively.[90,96,97] The ANCA were perinuclear in 60% of patients in the series of Hauschild et al., in 28% of patients studied by Davenport et al., and in 65% in the report by Guillevin et al. Antibodies against myeloperoxidase are more frequent than anti-PR3 in patients with MPA.[80,90] On the other hand, Geffriaud-Ricouard et al. reported that 26 of 45 (57%) anti-MPO-positive patients and 15 of 38 (39%) anti-PR3-positive patients had MPA.[98] The specificity and sensitivity of any pattern of positive ANCA for MPA is 80% and 51%, respectively, but the positive predictive value is only 12%.[96] The value of ANCA in diagnosis of MPA cannot be overestimated. They are very useful, especially in differentiating c-PAN from MPA, and their presence should exclude c-PAN. Alone, however, they cannot distinguish MPA from WG or other forms of necrotizing systemic vasculitis.[80] Other immunological abnormalities found in MPA are the presence of rheumatoid factor (RF) in 23–50%, and of antinuclear antibodies (ANA) in 17–33%.[80,90]

As vasculitis of the renal vessels is not common in MPA, the relevant angiographic findings are also relatively uncommon. When renal vessels are involved, however, the findings are similar to those of c-PAN. The role of renal biopsy in MPA is crucial from a diagnostic and prognostic point of view. Rapidly progressive glomerulonephritis (RPGN) is very important in the definition of MPA, and its presence favors a diagnosis of MPA or WG. Clinically, RPGN may rapidly progress to renal failure, therefore the institution of the appropriate treatment as soon as possible is mandatory.[80]

Guillevin at al. studied the value of clinical, immunological, radiological, and pathological characteristics differentiating MPA from c-PAN and CCS. They found that ANCA positivity, glomerulonephritis, and skin involvement were significantly more frequent in patients with normal angiograms, while hypertension, renal vascular involvement, and HBV antigenemia were more frequent in patients with abnormal angiograms. The authors suggested that ANCA and angiographic findings should be considered when attempting to differentiate MPA from c-PAN because small vessel involvement by itself is not a sufficient criterion.[99]

G. Course and Prognosis

The clinical course of MPA is variable. Renal disease is almost always present, and about two-thirds of patients will develop progressive renal insufficiency, half of these going on to end-stage renal failure.[26] A fulminant form of MPA with poor prognosis is recognized, usually presenting as pulmonary-renal failure, and requiring intensive treatment with respiratory support and hemodialysis. Another form with a bad prognosis is the so-called smouldering vasculitis described by Serra et al. in which patients follow a chronically active course.[65] A chronic relapsing form is common, with the relapse rate ranging from 25.4 to 35.3%, and the median time to relapse being between 24 and 43 months.[87,90,100] Interestingly, it has been reported that in MPA kidneys were involved less during relapses.[100] The overall five-year survival of MPA reported by Savage et al. was 65%, and the renal survival was 55%; in the most recent study, published by Guillevin in 1999, a survival of 67.1% during a follow up period of 70 ± 60 months was reported.[87,90] In other reports in which not only MPA but all ANCA-associated glomerulonephritides were studied, the survival rate ranged from 61 to 77% at five years.[101-103] Factors that may adversely affect prognosis are age, renal insufficiency, proteinuria, and hypertension.[80,87,90,103]

IV. CHURG-STRAUSS SYNDROME

A. GENERAL CONSIDERATIONS

Churg-Strauss syndrome, or allergic granulomatosis and angiitis, is characterized by systemic small-vessel vasculitis with extravascular granulomas and hypereosinophilia in patients with a history of asthma and atopic allergies. The three major histological criteria in the original description of the syndrome were necrotizing vasculitis, extravascular granulomas, and tissue infiltration by eosinophils.[104] However, in a review of 154 patients with CSS by Lanham et al., it was recognized that the above criteria are met in only a minority of patients, and are not pathognomonic of the condition. This group suggested a clinical definition based on a history of asthma, eosinophilia, and vasculitis affecting at least two extrapulmonary sites.[105] The ACR has also established classification criteria for CSS.[106]

B. EPIDEMIOLOGY

The Churg-Strauss syndrome is rare, with an annual incidence ranging from 2.4 million to 4.0 million.[19,23] In France, CSS accounts for about 20% of vasculitides.[80] It is slightly more frequent in males (55 to 65%), and the age at onset varies from 15 to 70 years, with a mean of about 38.[105]

C. RENAL INVOLVEMENT

The frequency of renal involvement in CSS is not exactly known. In the initial report by Churg and Strauss, 8 of 13 patients had histologically proven renal disease,[104] while in another large series from the Mayo Clinic, renal involvement was not a prominent characteristic, and only 1 of 30 patients had renal failure.[107] In the review by Lanham et al., renal disease was generally benign; 42% of patients had mild or moderate renal disease, and only 10% had renal failure.[105] In contrast, in the study by Clutterbuck et al., renal disease was not only more frequent, with 16 of 19 (84%) patients having renal disease, but also more severe than previously thought. Renal function was impaired in 14 of 19 (73.6%) patients, 4 of 19 (21%) had serum creatinine over 500 μmol/l, and two required dialysis at presentation.[108] Glutterburg et al. recognized that these differences might be due in part to referral bias.

Clinically, renal disease presents with microscopic hematuria, granular or red cell casts, proteinuria or nephrotic syndrome, and impaired renal function. Acute renal failure is uncommon in CSS,[109,110] and a case of ureteral involvement with bilateral stenosis has been reported.[111] Moderate hypertension was found in 37% of patients in the study by Clutterbuck et al., but was not related to renal involvement.[108]

D. LABORATORY FINDINGS

Laboratory features characterizing CSS are eosinophilia, elevated serum IgE levels, and the presence of p-ANCA. Eosinophilia is constant and is usually >10⁹/l, while the mean peak eosinophil count is 12.9×10^9/l.[105] Antineutrophil cytoplasmic antibodies are detected in over 60% of patients with

CSS, and they are usually anti-MPO ANCA.[54,112-114] They are very useful in the diagnosis of CSS, but it is not clear if they should be used to monitor disease activity.[80] Elevated serum IgE levels are found in about 75% of patients, while HbsAg is negative in almost all patients.[80] Renal angiography is almost always normal, although Clutterbuck et al detected small aneurysms in two of their patients.[108]

E. PATHOLOGY

The Churg-Strauss syndrome is characterized by necrotizing vasculitis, extravascular necrotizing granulomas, and eosinophilic infiltrates. Vasculitis involves arteries and veins and is characterized by granulomatous inflammation or giant-cell infiltration of vessel walls.[80] Fibrinoid necrosis and eosinophilic and histiocytic infiltrates are occasionally found. Extravascular granulomas and necrotizing vasculitis are rare in the kidney, and eosinophil infiltrates are uncommon. The most common histological finding in the kidney is focal segmental glomerulonephritis, usually necrotizing and with crescents. The glomerulonephritis of CSS may be pathologically identical to that of patients with MPA or Wegener's granulomatosis.[52] Eosinophilic interstitial nephritis was reported in 3 of 13 patients of Clutterbuck et al.[108]

F. COURSE AND PROGNOSIS

Although relatively recent data suggest that renal disease in CSS is not as benign as it was initially thought, its prognosis is better than that of other vasculitides. Chumbley reported an overall five-year survival of 62%, but renal disease was not among the most frequent causes of death.[107] In the series of Clutterbuck, renal function improved in 14 of 16 patients, and only one patient died from cardiac causes.[108] Using the ACR criteria, Churg-Strauss syndrome has lower morbidity and relapse rate and a lower, but not significantly so, mortality in comparison with PAN. The relapse rate was 42% and the mean number of relapses was 1.4 for an average follow-up period of eight years.[115]

V. WEGENER'S GRANULOMATOSIS

A. GENERAL CONSIDERATIONS

Wegener's granulomatosis (WG) is a disease of unknown etiology characterized by necrotizing granulomatous inflammation of the upper and lower respiratory tract, small and medium-sized systemic vasculitis, and necrotizing glomerulonephritis. WG was first described by H. Klinger in 1931 as a variant of periarteritis nodosa,[116] but was named after F. Wegener, who described three similar cases in 1936 and 1939.[117] Since then, the features of WG have been well delineated, classification criteria and disease definitions have been established,[13,118] and the diagnosis has become easier with the introduction of ANCA testing.[119,120]

B. EPIDEMIOLOGY

The annual incidence of WG has been estimated to be between 0.5 and 8.5 million,[22,23,121,122] and the prevalence around 3.0 100,000.[123] It affects men and women with equal frequency, 97% of patients are white, and the mean age at diagnosis is 40 to 45 years (range 9 to 78 years).[118,124,125]

C. CLINICAL FEATURES

The spectrum of clinical manifestations of WG is wide. At the one end of the spectrum is an indolent granulomatous lesion, usually of the upper respiratory tract, presenting with sinusitis, nasal disease, otitis media, hearing loss, and subglottic stenosis.[119] At the other end is the potentially fatal vasculitic pulmonary-renal syndrome, with alveolar hemorrhage due to lung capillaritis and renal failure due to rapidly progressive glomerulonephritis. In the majority of patients, WG follows a course between these two extremes, with initially local and later generalized manifestations, but in a chronic time pattern.[120] Constitutional symptoms usually accompany the transition from the local to the generalized phase, although fever is present in 25 to 34% and weight loss in 15% of patients at onset.[124,125] In the common form of the disease there is ear, nose, and throat involvement (75 to 90% of patients); lung involvement (80 to 94% of patients); kidney involvement (77 to 85%); and eye disease (30 to 50% of patients).[119,120,124-126] The variability in the clinical presentation led to the development of the ELK concept (E for symptoms from the upper respiratory tract, L for lung, and K for kidney involvement) as a semiquantitative measure of disease extent.[119,120,127]

D. Renal Involvement

According to the presence or not of renal disease, WG can be divided into classical or "renal," or in limited or "non-renal" form. These two forms of the disease differ in presentation as well as in outcome. Cutaneous and pulmonary disease and hematologic abnormalities are more frequent in the classic form, while ENT manifestations are more frequent in the limited form. Limited WG is generally milder and runs a longer course, consequently it may go undiagnosed for a long time. Additionally, limited WG may change toward classic WG with renal involvement.[128,129] Because of the above factors, it is difficult to accurately estimate the frequency of renal involvement in WG. In the larger published series the frequency of renal involvement (i.e., abnormal urine sediment or pathologic findings on renal biopsy) in WG ranges from 11 to 18% at presentation, and from 77 to 85% during the course of the disease.[124,125] Interestingly, other, smaller studies report a frequency of renal disease at presentation between 35 and 60%.[126,128,130] Renal disease early in the course of WG usually presents as asymptomatic renal biopsy abnormalities.[124,125,131] Extrarenal manifestations usually precede renal disease, although in some cases renal disease is the first presenting feature of WG.[132] In almost all cases renal involvement in WG presents as glomerulonephritis of variable severity. Asymptomatic or mild renal disease in WG may progress to fulminant glomerulonephritis and end-stage renal failure within days or weeks; therefore, it is necessary for the physician to look carefully for evidence of renal disease.[119] Microscopic urinalysis is a very useful tool in the evaluation and follow-up of renal involvement in patients with WG. The presence of red blood cell casts has a very high positive predictive value for glomerulonephritis.[119] A recent study suggested that the level of red blood cells in urine is a reliable marker of renal disease activity in WG, and is more sensitive than other disease markers such as C-reactive protein and erythrocyte sedimentation rate.[133]

    A minority of patients (8%) with WG will have vasculitis of the renal vessels, usually of the interlobular arteries, the medullary vasa recta, or branches of the spiral arteries.[52,125,126,134] A study of 23 patients with WG found that 5 of them (21.5%) had papillary necrosis because of necrotizing vasculitis of the renal vessels.[135] In rare cases, renal involvement in WG may present as perinephric hematoma after rupture of renal artery aneurysms, ureteral obstruction due to vasculitis of the periureteral vessels, or as a renal mass due to cystic dilatation of the renal tubules or to large necrotizing granulomas.[125,136,137]

E. Pathology

The most characteristic histological feature of WG is the presence of necrotizing granulomatous inflammation, but this finding is usually not found in the kidney.[52] Renal disease in WG is almost always a pauci-immune, necrotizing, and crescentic glomerulonephritis (Figure 29.3). The distribution of the lesions is focal segmental and there are extracapillary cellular crescents; glomerular mesangial and/or endocapillary hypercellularity are generally absent.[138] In some cases there may be partial rupture of Bowman's capsule resulting in periglomerular extension of a cellular infiltrate consisting of lymphocytes, plasma cells, and mononuclear and polymorphonuclear leucocytes.[138]

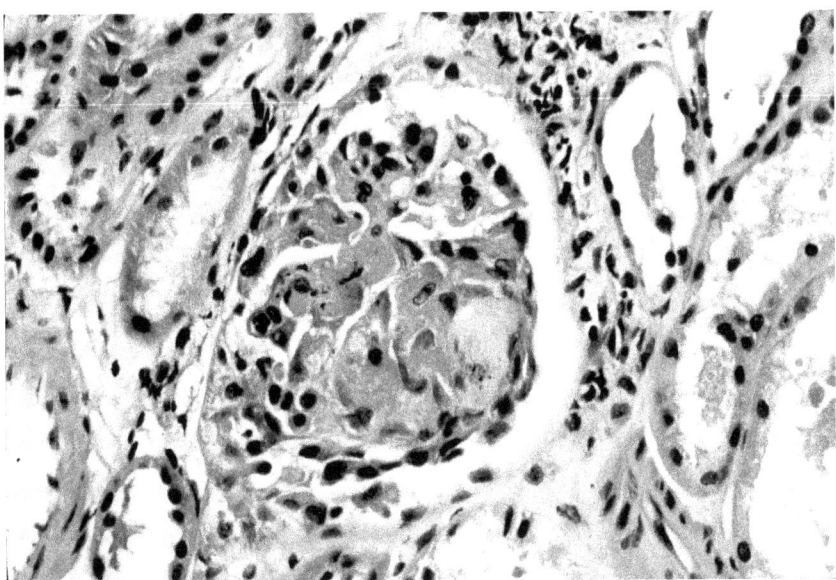

FIGURE 29.3 Proliferative nephritis with crescent formation in severe Wegener's granulomatosis affecting the kidney.

Immunofluorescence studies have shown nonspecific deposition of immune complexes containing C3, IgM, IgG, and IgA in the mesangium, while electron microscopy failed to demonstrate significant deposits.[26,64,124,131] Histologically, the glomerulonephritis of WG is almost identical to that found in MPA, and is compatible with WG rather than diagnostic of WG.[52,139] Antonovych et al. compared renal histology in PAN and WG and reported that extracapillary glomerulonephritis, with Bowman's capsule breaks and periglomerular infiltrate, are characteristic of WG, while fibrinoid necrosis of glomerular tufts predominated in PAN.[140] Another study reported that kidney biopsies from patients with anti-PR3 antibodies, which are characteristic of WG, have a higher activity and a lower chronicity index than biopsies from patients with anti-MPO antibodies, which are found in other types of vasculitis and in only a minority of WG patients.[141]

The so-called granulomatous glomerulonephritis, which is characterized by the presence of a periglomerular zone of macrophage-like cells with or without multinucleated giant cells, is found in only a minority of patients with WG.[129,142,143] This granulomatous reaction is usually found around glomeruli in which Bowman's capsule is destroyed,[142] and it is not specific for WG as it can also be found in conditions such as the PAN group of vasculitides and sarcoidosis.[86,95,144] The presence of multinucleated giant cells distinguishes granulomatous glomerulonephritis from the abovementioned nonspecific inflammatory periglomerular infiltrates. Granulomatous changes have been rarely observed in the interstitial space, and may rarely develop to large renal masses.[125,126,137]

Segmental necrotizing vasculitis of the renal vessels (spiral arteries, medullary vasa recta, and preglomerular arterioles) is uncommon, and is characterized by fibrinoid necrosis of the inner half of the vessel wall.[125,126,138,142]

F. LABORATORY FINDINGS AND DIAGNOSIS

The diagnosis of WG is based on a combination of clinical features and histological and laboratory findings.[26,118] The introduction of ANCA testing using indirect immunofluoresence has facilitated the diagnosis of WG.[145,146] The specificity of c-ANCA for WG ranges from 88 to 100% (pooled specificity 98%), and the sensitivity varies from 34 to 92% (pooled sensitivity 66%).[147-150] The diagnostic utility of c-ANCA testing depends on the prevalence of WG in the population tested, and it is less when the prevalence is either too low or too high.[147,151,152] Detection of anti-PR3 antibodies by ELISA generally correlates well with c-ANCA testing in terms of positivity, but only poorly in quantitative terms.[62] The combination of c-ANCA and anti-PR3 testing, however, has significantly increased sensitivity and specificity in comparison with c-ANCA alone.[153] Testing for p-ANCA has limited value in the diagnosis of WG as they can be frequently detected in conditions such as other vasculitides, Goodpasture disease, Sjøgren's syndrome, and rheumatoid arthritis.[62] A recent study reported that the sensitivity of p-ANCA for WG was only 21%.[153] Similarly, detection of anti-MPO is not useful in the diagnosis of WG.

ANCA may be useful as markers for disease monitoring, although this issue remains controversial.[154] A number of studies have reported that c-ANCA titers are higher in active WG,[145] or that they rise before relapses,[127,146,155-157] and they even suggested treatment based on c-ANCA titers.[155] On the other hand, some studies failed to fully confirm these findings.[158,159] Some authors suggest that rises in c-ANCA titers should raise suspicion of ensuing relapse in patients with WG who may therefore need more aggressive treatment.[152]

Elevated acute phase reactants, especially CRP, increased ESR, and anemia of chronic disease, are common in WG as they are in all forms of systemic vasculitis.[152] As far as renal disease is concerned, the value of microscopic urine examination is very high, as the presence of red blood cells and casts signifies renal involvement.[119] Angiographic abnormalities (stenosis or aneurysms) of the renal vessels are not common in WG and do not contribute to the diagnosis.[160]

G. Course and Prognosis

It has already been mentioned that WG can present as a limited or a generalized form or have an intermediate course.[120] The prognosis of WG was initially considered very poor with 80% two-year mortality, and the advent of corticosteroids little improved the prognosis.[26] The introduction of immunosuppresive drugs, and especially cyclophosphamide, improved the prognosis significantly. In a large NIH study, 91% of patients achieved partial remission or were improved, and 75% achieved complete remission when treated with a combination of corticosteroids and immunosuppressive drugs. Chronic renal insufficiency developed in 42% of patients, 11% of patients required dialysis, while 5% had to undergo renal transplantation.[125] Renal disease was the cause of death in about 25% of cases in which death could at least partially be attributed to WG.[125]

VI. BEHÇET'S DISEASE

Behçet's disease is a systemic vasculitis affecting both arteries and veins of all sizes. It is clinically characterized by mucocutaneous, occular, and musculoskeletal involvement. Its annual incidence is unknown, and its prevalence ranges from 10 to 100,000 in Japan to 300 to 100,000 in Turkey. Males and females are affected at the same rate, but males usually have more severe disease.[161]

The clinical spectrum of Behçet's disease includes recurrent aphthous stomatitis, genital ulcers, uveitis, various types of skin lesions, thrombophlebitis, arthritis, neuropsychiatric symptoms, and, more rarely, pulmonary and gastrointestinal involvement.

The frequency of renal disease in Behçet's disease is not exactly known, but it is not as rare as it was once thought to be. In a study of 77 patients with Behçet's disease, approximately one third (25 of 77) finally developed some form of renal involvement, usually presenting as proteinuria and/or microscopic hematuria. These abnormalities were intermittent and the renal disease was mild, although no renal biopsies were done.[162] In a more recent study, renal disease was reported in only 9 of 120 patients (7.5%), and it was generally mild.[163] Most reports of renal involvement, though, are case reports. Glomerulonephritis in patients with Behçet's disease can be focal proliferative,[162,164] diffuse proliferative,[165,166] crescentic,[167-169] or mesangial proliferative,[163] and its course can be chronic or rapidly progressive.[166,167,170] Nephrotic syndrome in Behçet's disease has been described in association with secondary AA amyloidosis,[163,171-173] or as a manifestation of membranous nephropathy or minimal change disease.[174,175] Finally, IgA nephropathy has been reported in Behçet's disease.[176-178] Histologically, the glomerular lesions can be differentiated from those of other vasculitides by the presence of subendothelial, mesangial, and capillary immune deposits, which can be IgG, IgM, IgA, complement, or fibrinogen.[.26,165,168,176,179] It is noteworthy that in a small series of patients, interstitial fibrosis and inflammation with tubular atrophy were reported, but they were attributed to the cyclosporine these patients were receiving, and not to Behçet's disease per se.[180] Microaneurysms of the renal vessels with renal infarction[181] and renal vein thrombosis have been reported in rare cases.[175]

The course of renal involvement in Behçet's disease is variable, ranging from acute renal failure to spontaneous remission.[168,170] The response to treatment is difficult to estimate, as spontaneous remissions are common.[161]

VII. TAKAYASU'S ARTERITIS

Takayasu's arteritis is a chronic inflammatory disease characterized by giant-cell vasculitis involving the aorta and its major branches.[182,183] It is a rare disease, and its annual incidence in European and American populations ranges from 1.2 to 2.6 per million,[184,185] while it is much more frequent in Japan, China, and Southeast Asia.[186] The disease usually (70 to 90%) affects women of reproductive age.[183]

The clinical features of Takayasu's arteritis include constitutional symptoms, decreased peripheral pulses, claudication, bruits, and hypertension. Abnormal angiograms are characteristic and are included in the ACR classification criteria for the disease.[187]

Renal involvement in Takayasu's arteritis is usually due to renal artery stenosis, and renal angiography demonstrates main renal artery stenosis or occlusion resulting in renal infarcts in about 65 to 75% of patients.[187,188] Hypertension is found in 33 to 76% of patients and is usually but not always associated with renal artery stenosis.[182] As is the case in c-PAN, concomitant use of angiotensin-converting enzyme inhibitors may precipitate ischemic complications.[189,190] Glomerular disease is rather uncommon is Takayasu's arteritis and the literature consists of case reports. Different forms of glomerulonephritis have been reported such as focal and segmental, crescentic, proliferative, membranoproliferative, and mesangial.[191-196] Occasionally, mesangial immune or hyaline deposits and microaneurysms in the glomeruli have been described.[196] In a small number of patients nephrotic syndrome has been described associated with amyloidosis[197-199] or with membranoproliferative glomerulonephritis.[200] There is also a case report of IgA nephropathy.[201]

Pathologically, Takayasu's arteritis is a focal panarteritis with, initially, an inflammatory and subsequently a sclerotic phase. The typical changes of the initial phase are thickening of the intima due to mucopolysaccharide accumulation, with granuloma formation, multinucleated giant cells, and mononuclear infiltration.[52] In later stages degeneration of the elastic lamina of the media, adventitial fibrosis, and neovascularization are present.[182,183] Arteries of the renal parenchyma are rarely involved.

Renal involvement in Takayasu's arteritis can lead to renal failure, although this is not among the leading causes of mortality. Glomerulonephritis is generally mild, while hypertension may be a marker of severe disease.[182]

VIII. TEMPORAL ARTERITIS

Temporal arteritis is a giant-cell arteritis associated with polymyalgia rheumatica, and occuring in people older than 50 years.[202,203] It is more common than other vasculitides, and the annual incidence of biopsy positive cases is 9.3 per 100,000 in the general population, and 17 to 28.6 in people over 50 years of age.[204,205] It almost always affects whites, and the female/male ratio is 3 to 4:1.[203]

Clinically, temporal arteritis is characterized by headaches, fatigue, fever, jaw claudication, loss of vision, arthralgias, and aortic arch syndrome. Skin and lungs are rarely involved.[206]

Renal involvement is unusual in temporal arteritis and is usually not mentioned in reviews,[202,203] although in a study of 248 patients, approximately 10% were found to have renal involvement presenting as microscopic hematuria, proteinuria (usually minimal), and red blood cell casts.[207] Unfortunately, in the above study renal involvement was not documented by biopsy, although evidence of vasculitis of renal parenchymal arteries was found at autopsy with the characteristic lesions of temporal arteritis.[207] In a small number of patients renal involvement was well documented, although not in the context of a large series, but as isolated case reports. In some patients there is widespread vasculitis of the renal arteries and arterioles, while in others there is glomerular disease such as focal glomerulonephritis or membranous glomerulopathy.[208-211] Glomerulonephritis can be necrotizing or not, and with or without crescents.[209,210] In some cases of temporal arteritis, glomerulonephritis was similar to that of microsopic polyangiitis, and it was thought that there might be an overlap syndrome.[212] Clinically, progressive renal failure and nephrotic syndrome have been reported.[209-211,213,214] Temporal arteritis in association with amyloidosis and nephrotic syndrome has also been described.[215]

When renal arteries are involved the lesions are histologically similar to those of temporal arteritis, i.e., multinucleated giant cells and monocytes within the inflamed vascular segments, and occasionally fibrinoid necrosis.[52] Glomerular involvement has no typical features and is indistinguishable from those in other forms of vasculitis.

IX. RELAPSING POLYCHONDRITIS

Relapsing polychondritis is an autoimmune disease characterized by inflammatory involvement of the cartilaginous structures of the body (e.g., ears, nose, bronchial cartilage, etc.). It is a rare disease, with annual incidence 3.5 cases per million, affecting both sexes and all racial groups.[216]

Clinical features include auricular and nasal chondritis, hearing loss, arthritis, scleritis or episcleritis, and laryngotracheal and bronchial symptoms. In about 30% of cases it may be associated with other autoimmune diseases such as systemic vasculitic syndromes, systemic lupus erythematosus, and rheumatoid arthritis.[216]

Renal involvement is not uncommon. In two large series renal involvement was found in 22% and 6.5% of patients, although renal functional impairment was noted in less than half of these patients.[217,218] The true frequency of renal disease might be lower, as a referral bias was recognized.[217] Renal involvement was not histologically confirmed in all cases, but where renal biopsy was performed segmental necrotizing glomerulonephritis with or without crescents, glomerulosclerosis, interstitial cellular infiltrates, interstitial fibrosis, and active tubulitis were noted in different cases, while renal arteritis or arteriolitis were not found.[217,219-221] Two cases of relapsing polychondritis with IgA nephropathy have also been reported.[222] Immunofluorescence microscopy showed faint imunoglobulin deposition in the capillary wall, the mesangium, and the tubular basement membrane. Electron microscopy studies revealed subendothelial or mesangial deposits of IgG, IgM, or C3.[216,217] Patients with renal involvement were generally older, and systemic vasculitis and arthritis were more frequent. Additionally, renal involvement was associated with more severe disease and a poorer prognosis.[217]

REFERENCES

1. Cohen, R. D., Conn, D. L., and Ilstrup, D. M., Clinical features, prognosis, and response to treatment in polyarteritis, *Mayo Clinic Proceedings,* 55, 146, 1980.

2. Guillevin, L., Le Thi, H., Godeau, P., Jais, P., and Wechsler, B., Clinical findings and prognosis of polyarteritis nodosa and Churg-Strauss angiitis: a study in 165 patients, *British Journal of Rheumatology,* 27, 258, 1988.

3. Lhote, F. and Guillevin, L., Polyarteritis nodosa, microscopic polyangiitis, and Churg-Strauss syndrome. Clinical aspects and treatment, *Rheumatic Diseases Clinics of North America,* 21, 911, 1995.

4. Sack, M., Cassidy, J. T., and Bole, G. G., Prognostic factors in polyarteritis, *Journal of Rheumatology,* 2, 411, 1975.

5. Fortin, P. R., Larson, M. G., Watters, A. K., Yeadon, C. A., Choquette, D., and Esdaile, J. M., Prognostic factors in systemic necrotizing vasculitis of the polyarteritis nodosa group — a review of 45 cases, *Journal of Rheumatology,* 22, 78, 1995.

6. Guillevin, L., Lhote, F., Cohen, P., Sauvaget, F., Jarrousse, B., Lortholary, O., Noel, L. H., and Trepo, C., Polyarteritis nodosa related to hepatitis B virus. A prospective study with long-term observation of 41 patients, *Medicine* (Baltimore), 74, 238, 1995.

7. McMahon, B. J., Heyward, W. L., Templin, D. W., Clement, D., and Lanier, A. P., Hepatitis B-associated polyarteritis nodosa in Alaskan Eskimos: clinical and epidemiologic features and long-term follow-up, *Hepatology,* 9, 97, 1989.

8. Johnson, R. J. and Couser, W. G., Hepatitis B infection and renal disease: clinical, immunopathogenetic and therapeutic considerations, *Kidney International,* 37, 663, 1990.

9. Quint, L., Deny, P., Guillevin, L., Granger, B., Jarrousse, B., Lhote, F., and Scavizzi, M., Hepatitis C virus in patients with polyarteritis nodosa. Prevalence in 38 patients, *Clinical and Experimental Rheumatology,* 9, 253, 1991.

10. Font, C., Miro, O., Pedrol, E., Masanes, F., Coll-Vinent, B., Casademont, J., Cid, M. C., and Grau, J. M., Polyarteritis nodosa in human immunodeficiency virus infection: report of four cases and review of the literature, *British Journal of Rheumatology,* 35, 796, 1996.

11. Ozen, S., Saatci, U., Balkanci, F., Besbas, N., Bakkaloglu, A., and Tacal, T., Familial Mediterranean fever and polyarteritis nodosa, *Scandinavian Journal of Rheumatology,* 21, 312, 1992.

12. Sachs, D., Langevitz, P., Morag, B., and Pras, M., Polyarteritis nodosa and familial Mediterranean fever, *British Journal of Rheumatology,* 26, 139, 1987.

13. Lightfoot, R. W. J., Michel, B. A., Bloch, D. A., Hunder, G. G., Zvaifler, N. J., McShane, D. J., Arend, W. P., Calabrese, L. H., Leavitt, R. Y., and Lie, J. T., The American College of Rheumatology 1990 criteria for the classification of polyarteritis nodosa, *Arthritis and Rheumatism,* 33, 1088, 1990.

14. Jennette, J. C., Falk, R. J., Andrassy, K., Bacon, P. A., Churg, J., Gross, W. L., Hagen, E. C., Hoffman, G. S., Hunder, G. G., Kallenberg, C. G., MacCluskey, R. T., Sinico, A., Rees, A. J., Van Es, L. A., Waldherr, R., and Wiik, A., Nomenclature of systemic vasculitis, *Arthritis and Rheumatism,* 37, 187, 1994.

15. Lie, J. T., Nomenclature and classification of vasculitis: Plus ca change, plus c'est la meme chose, *Arthritis and Rheumatism,* 37, 181, 1994.

16. Guillevin, L. and Lhote, F., Distinguishing polyarteritis nodosa from microscopic polyangiitis and implications for treatment, *Current Opinion in Rheumatology,* 7, 20, 1995.

17. Watts, R. A., Jolliffe, V. A., Carruthers, D. M., Lockwood, M., and Scott, D. G., Effect of classification on the incidence of polyarteritis nodosa and microscopic polyangiitis, *Arthritis and Rheumatism,* 39, 1208, 1996.

18. Jolliffe, V. A., Watts, R. A., and Scott, D. G., Has polyarteritis nodosa (PAN) been classified out of existence? *Clinical and Experimental Immunology,* 101[Suppl. 1], 64, 1995.

19. Guillevin, L. and Lhote, F., Polyarteritis nodosa and microscopic polyangiitis, *Clinical and Experimental Immunology,* 101[Suppl. 1], 22, 1995.

20. Watts, R. A., Carruthers, D. M., and Scott, D. G., Epidemiology of systemic vasculitis: changing incidence or definition? *Seminars in Arthritis and Rheumatism,* 25, 28, 1995.

21. Valente, R. M., Hall, S., O'Duffy, J. D., and Conn, D. L., Vasculitis and related disorders, in *Textbook of Rheumatology,* 5th edition, Kelley, K. M., Harris, E. D. Jr, Ruddy, S., and Sledge, C. B., Eds, W.B. Saunders Company, Philadelphia, 1997.

22. Kurland, L. T., Hauser, W. A., Ferguson, R. H., and Holley, K. E., Epidemiologic features of diffuse connective tissue disorders in Rochester, Minn., 1951 through 1967, with special reference to systemic lupus erythematosus, *Mayo Clinics Proceedings,* 44, 649, 1969.

23. Scott, D. G., Bacon, P. A., Elliott, P. J., Tribe, C. R., and Wallington, T. B., Systemic vasculitis in a district general hospital 1972-1980: clinical and laboratory features, classification and prognosis of 80 cases, *Quarterly Journal of Medicine,* 51, 292, 1982.

24. Kurland, L. T., Chuang, T. Y., and Hunder, G. G., The epidemiology of systemic arteritis, in *The Epidemiology of the Rheumatic Diseases,* Lawrence, R. C. and Shulman, L. E., Eds, Gower, New York, 1984.

25. el-Reshaid, K., Kapoor, M. M., el-Reshaid, W., Madda, J. P., and Varro, J., The spectrum of renal disease associated with microscopic polyangiitis and classic polyarteritis nodosa in Kuwait, *Nephrology Dialysis Transplantation,* 12, 1874, 1997.

26. Mason, J. C., Cowie, M. R., Davies, K. A., Schofield, J. B., Cambridge, J., Jackson, J., So, A., Allard, S. A., and Walport, M. J., Familial polyarteritis nodosa, *Arthritis and Rheumatism,* 37, 1249, 1994.

27. Balow, J. E. and Fauci, A. S., Vasculitic Diseases of the Kidney, in *Diseases of the Kidney,* 6th edition, Schrier, R. W. and Grace, W. J., Eds, Little Brown, Boston, 1997.

28. Frohnert, P. P. and Sheps, S. G., Long-term follow-up study of periarteritis nodosa, *American Journal of Medicine,* 43, 8, 1967.

29. Leib, E. S., Restivo, C., and Paulus, H. E., Immunosuppressive and corticosteroid therapy of polyarteritis nodosa, *American Journal of Medicine,* 67, 941, 1979.

30. Guillevin, L., Lhote, F., Jarrousse, B., and Fain, O., Treatment of polyarteritis nodosa and Churg-Strauss syndrome. A meta-analysis of 3 prospective controlled trials including 182 patients over 12 years, *Annalles de Médecine Interne* (Paris), 143, 405, 1992.

31. Thomas, R. H. and Black, M. M., The wide clinical spectrum of polyarteritis nodosa with cutaneous involvement, *Clinical and Experimental Dermatology,* 8, 47, 1983.

32. Guillevin, L., Lhote, F., and Gherardi, R., Polyarteritis nodosa, microscopic polyangiitis, and Churg-Strauss syndrome: clinical aspects, neurologic manifestations, and treatment, *Neurölögy Clinics,* 15, 865, 1997.

33. Guillevin, L., Lhote, F., Gallais, V., Jarrousse, B., Royer, I., Gayraud, M., and Benichou, J., Gastrointestinal tract involvement in polyarteritis nodosa and Churg-Strauss syndrome, *Annalles de Médecine Interne* (Paris), 146, 260, 1995.

34. Cabal, E. and Holtz, S., Polyarteritis as a cause of intestinal hemorrhage, *Gastroenterology,* 61, 99, 1971.

35. Chen, K. T., Gallbladder vasculitis, *Journal of Clinical Gastroenterology,* 11, 537, 1989.

36. Kirkland, G. S., Savige, J., Wilson, D., Heale, W., Sinclair, R. A., and Hope, R. N., Classical polyarteritis nodosa and microscopic polyarteritis with medium vessel involvement — a comparison of the clinical and laboratory features, *Clinical Nephrology,* 47, 176, 1997.

37. Gorriz, J. L., Sancho, A., Ferrer, R., Alcoy, E., Crespo, J. F., Palmero, J., and Pallardo, L. M., Renal-limited polyarteritis nodosa presenting with loin pain and haematuria, *Nephrology Dialysis Transplantation,* 12, 2737, 1997.

38. Ladefoged, J., Nielsen, B., Raaschou, F., and Sorensen, A. W., Acute anuria due to polyarteritis nodosa, *American Journal of Medicine,* 46, 827, 1969.

39. Kaur, J. S., Goldberg, J. P., and Schrier, R. W., Acute renal failure following arteriography in a patient with polyarteritis nodosa, *JAMA,* 247, 833, 1982.

40. Wang, A. Y., Lai, K. N., Li, P. K., Leung, C. B., and Lui, S. F., Acute renal failure induced by angiotensin converting enzyme inhibitor in a patient with polyarteritis nodosa, *Renal Failure,* 18, 293, 1996.

41. Williams, A. J., Newland, A. C., and Marsh, F. P., Acute renal failure with polyarteritis nodosa and multiple myeloma, *Postgraduate Medical Journal,* 61, 445, 1985.

42. Schlesinger, M., Oren, S., Fano, M., and Viskoper, J. R., Perirenal and renal subcapsular haematoma as presenting symptoms of polyarteritis nodosa, *Postgraduate Medical Journal,* 65, 681, 1989.

43. Peterson, C. J., Willerson, J. T., Doppman, J. L., and Decker, J. L., Polyarteritis nodosa with bilateral renal artery aneurysms and perirenal haematomas: angiographic and nephrotomographic features, *British Journal of Radiology,* 43, 62, 1970.

44. Romijn, J. A., Blaauwgeers, J. L., van Lieshout, J. J., Vijverberg, P. L., Reekers, J. A., and Krediet, R. T., Bilateral kidney rupture with severe retroperitoneal bleeding in polyarteritis nodosa, *Netherlands Journal of Medicine,* 35, 260, 1989.

45. Heaton, J. M. and Bourke, E., Papillary necrosis associated with calyceal arteritis, *Nephron,* 16, 57, 1976.
46. Hekali, P. E., Pajari, R. I., Kivisaari, M. L., Haapanen, E. J., and Leirisalo, M., Bilateral renal artery dissections: unusual complication of polyarteritis nodosa, *European Journal of Radiology,* 4, 6, 1984.
47. White, R. H. and Schambelan, M., Hypertension, hyperreninemia, and secondary hyperaldosteronism in systemic necrotizing vasculitis, *Annals of Internal Medicine,* 92, 199, 1980.
48. Pickering, T. G., Lockshin, M. D., and Eisenmenger, W. J., Renin-dependent hypertension in polyarteritis nodosa, *British Medical Journal* (Clinical Research Edition), 282, 1758, 1981.
49. Pintar, T. J. and Zimmerman, S., Hyperreninemic hypertension secondary to a subcapsular perinephric hematoma in a patient with polyarteritis nodosa, *American Journal of Kidney Diseases,* 32, 503, 1998.
50. Azar, N., Guillevin, L., Huong, D. L., Herreman, G., Meyrier, A., and Godeau, P., Symptomatic urogenital manifestations of polyarteritis nodosa and Churg-Strauss angiitis: analysis of 8 of 165 patients, *Journal of Urology,* 142, 136, 1989.
51. Glanz, I. and Grunebaum, M., Ureteral changes in polyarteritis nodosa as seen during excretory urography, *Journal of Urology,* 116, 731, 1976.
52. Jennette, J. C. and Falk, R. J., The pathology of vasculitis involving the kidney, *American Journal of Kidney Diseases,* 24, 130, 1994.
53. Akikusa, B., Irabu, N., Matsumura, R., and Tsuchida, H., Tubulointerstitial changes in systemic vasculitic disorders: a quantitative study of 18 biopsy cases, *American Journal of Kidney Diseases,* 16, 481, 1990.
54. Guillevin, L., Visser, H., Noel, L. H., Pourrat, J., Vernier, I., Gayraud, M., Oksman, F., and Lesavre, P., Antineutrophil cytoplasm antibodies in systemic polyarteritis nodosa with and without hepatitis B virus infection and Churg-Strauss syndrome — 62 patients, *Journal of Rheumatology,* 20, 1345, 1993.
55. Guillevin, L., Lhote, F., Brauner, M., and Casassus, P., Antineutrophil cytoplasmic antibodies and abnormal angiograms in polyarteritis nodosa and Churg-Strauss syndrome: indications for the diagnosis of microscopic polyangiitis, *Annalles de Médecine Interne* (Paris), 146, 548, 1995.
56. Baranger, T. A., Audrain, M. A., Testa, A., Besnier, D., Guillevin, L., and Esnault, V. L., Anti-neutrophil cytoplasm antibodies in patients with ACR criteria for polyarteritis nodosa: help for systemic vasculitis classification?, *Autoimmunity,* 20, 33, 1995.
57. Cohen, T. J., Limburg, P. C., Elema, J. D., Huitema, M. G., Horst, G., The, T. H., and Kallenberg, C. G., Detection of autoantibodies against myeloid lysosomal enzymes: a useful adjunct to classification of patients with biopsy-proven necrotizing arteritis, *American Journal of Medicine,* 91, 59, 1991.
58. Kallenberg, C. G., Brouwer, E., Weening, J. J., and Cohen Tervaert, J. W., Anti-neutrophil cytoplasmic antibodies: Current diagnostic and pathophysiologic potential, *Kidney International,* 46, 1, 1994.
59. Cohen, T. J., Goldschmeding, R., Elema, J. D., Limburg, P. C., van der Giessen, M., Huitema, M. G., Koolen, M. I., Hene, R. J., The, T. H., and van der Hem, G. K., Association of autoantibodies to myeloperoxidase with different forms of vasculitis, *Arthritis and Rheumatism,* 33, 1264, 1990.
60. Hauschild, S., Schmitt, W. H., Csernok, E., Flesch, B., Rautmann, A., and Gross, W. L., ANCA in Wegener's granulomatosis and related vasculitides, in *Abstract Book of the 4th International Workshop on ANCA,* Gross, W. L., Ed, Plenum, London, 1992.
61. Hoffman, G. S. and Specks, U., Antineutrophil cytoplasmic antibodies, *Arthritis and Rheumatism,* 41, 1521, 1998.
62. Gross, W. L., Antineutrophil cytoplasmic autoantibody testing in vasculitides, *Rheumatic Diseases Clinics of North America,* 21, 987, 1995.
63. Guillevin, L., Visser, H., Oksman, F., and Pourrat, J., Antineutrophil cytoplasmic antibodies in polyarteritis nodosa related to hepatitis B virus, *Arthritis and Rheumatism,* 33, 1871, 1990.
64. Ronco, P., Verroust, P., Mignon, F., Kourilsky, O., Vanhille, P., Meyrier, A., Mery, J. P., and Morel-Maroger, L., Immunopathological studies of polyarteritis nodosa and Wegener's granulomatosis: a report of 43 patients with 51 renal biopsies, *Quarterly Journal of Medicine,* 52, 212, 1983.
65. Serra, A., Cameron, J. S., Turner, D. R., Hartley, B., Ogg, C. S., Neild, G. H., Williams, D. G., Taube, C. B., Brown, C. B., and Hicks, J. A., Vasculitis affecting the kidney: presentation, histopathology, and long-term outcome, *Quarterly Journal of Medicine,* 53, 181, 1984.
66. Bron, K. M., Strott, C. A., and Shapiro, P. A., The diagnostic value of angiographic observations in polyarteritis nodosa. A case of multiple aneurysms in the visceral organs, *Archives of Internal Medicine,* 116, 450, 1965.

67. Fleming, R. J. and Stern, L. Z., Multiple intraparenchymal renal aneurysms in polyarteritis nodosa, *Radiology,* 84, 100, 1965.

68. Vazquez, J. J., San Martin, P., Barbado, F. J., Gil, A., Guerra, J., Arnalich, F., Garcia, P. J., and Sanchez, M. F., Angiographic findings in systemic necrotizing vasculitis, *Angiology,* 32, 773, 1981.

69. Dornfeld, L., Lecky, J. W., and Peter, J. B., Polyarteritis and intrarenal renal artery aneurysms, *JAMA,* 215, 1950, 1971.

70. Travers, R. L., Allison, D. J., Brettle, R. P., and Hughes, G. R., Polyarteritis nodosa: a clinical and angiographic analysis of 17 cases, *Seminars in Arthritis and Rheumatism,* 8, 184, 1979.

71. Ewald, E. A., Griffin, D., and McCune, W. J., Correlation of angiographic abnormalities with disease manifestations and disease severity in polyarteritis nodosa, *Journal of Rheumatology,* 14, 952, 1987.

72. Darras-Joly, C., Lortholary, O., Cohen, P., Brauner, M., and Guillevin, L., Regressing microaneurysms in 5 cases of hepatitis B virus related polyarteritis nodosa, *Journal of Rheumatology,* 22, 876, 1995.

73. Guillevin, L., Merrouche, Y., and Ruel, M., Regressing aneurysms in polyarteritis nodosa related to hepatitis B virus., *European Journal of Internal Medicine,* 1, 267, 1990.

74. Hekali, P., Kajander, H., Pajari, R., Stenman, S., and Somer, T., Diagnostic significance of angiographically observed visceral aneurysms with regard to polyarteritis nodosa, *Acta Radiologica.,* 32, 143, 1991.

75. Smith, J. N. and Hinman, F. J., Intrarenal arterial aneurysms, *Journal of Urology,* 97, 990, 1967.

76. Easterbrook, J. S., Renal and hepatic microaneurysms: report of a new entity simulating polyarteritis nodosa, *Radiology,* 137, 629, 1980.

77. Longstreth, P. L. and Korobkin, M., Intrarenal arterial aneurysms, *CRC, Critical Reviews in Clinical Radiology and Nuclear Medicine,* 8, 129, 1976.

78. Albert, D. A., Silverstein, M. D., Paunicka, K., Reddy, G., Chang, R. W., and Derus, C., The diagnosis of polyarteritis nodosa. II. Empirical verification of a decision analysis model, *Arthritis and Rheumatism,* 31, 1128, 1988.

79. Fisher, R. G., Graham, D. Y., Granmayeh, M., and Trabanino, J. G., Polyarteritis nodosa and hepatitis-B surface antigen: role of angiography in diagnosis, *American Journal of Roentgenology,* 129, 77, 1977.

80. Lhote, F., Cohen, P., and Guillevin, L., Polyarteritis nodosa, microscopic polyangiitis and Churg-Strauss syndrome, *Lupus,* 7, 238, 1998.

81. Pope, T. L. J., Buschi, A. J., Moore, T. S., Williamson, B. R., and Brenbridge, A. N., CT features of renal polyarteritis nodosa, *American Journal of Roentgenology,* 136, 986, 1981.

82. Alexander, J. E., Seibert, J. J., and Lowe, B. A., Cutaneous uptake of gallium-67 in polyarteritis nodosa, *Clinical Nuclear Medicine,* 12, 883, 1987.

83. Fauci, A. S., Katz, P., Haynes, B. F., and Wolff, S. M., Cyclophosphamide therapy of severe systemic necrotizing vasculitis, *New England Journal of Medicine,* 301, 235, 1979.

84. Guillevin, L., Fain, O., Lhote, F., Jarrousse, B., Le Thi, H., Bussel, A., and Leon, A., Lack of superiority of steroids plus plasma exchange to steroids alone in the treatment of polyarteritis nodosa and Churg-Strauss syndrome. A prospective, randomized trial in 78 patients, *Arthritis and Rheumatism,* 35, 208, 1992.

85. Guillevin, L., Lhote, F., Gayraud, M., Cohen, P., Jarrousse, B., Lortholary, O., Thibult, N., and Casassus, P., Prognostic factors in polyarteritis nodosa and Churg-Strauss syndrome. A prospective study in 342 patients, *Medicine* (Baltimore), 75, 17, 1996.

86. Davson, J., Ball, J., and Platt, R., The kidney in periarteritis nodosa., *Quarterly Journal of Medicine,* 17, 175, 1948.

87. Savage, C. O., Winearls, C. G., Evans, D. J., Rees, A. J., and Lockwood, C. M., Microscopic polyarteritis: presentation, pathology and prognosis., *Quarterly Journal of Medicine,* 56, 467, 1985.

88. D'Agati, V., Chander, P., Nash, M., and Mancilla-Jimenez, R., Idiopathic microscopic polyarteritis nodosa: ultrastructural observations on the renal vascular and glomerular lesions, *American Journal of Kidney Diseases,* 7, 95, 1986.

89. Adu, D., Howie, A. J., Scott, D. G., Bacon, P. A., McGonigle, R. J., and Micheal, J., Polyarteritis and the kidney, *Quarterly Journal of Medicine,* 62, 221, 1987.

90. Guillevin, L., Durand-Gasselin, B., Cevallos, R., Gayraud, M., Lhote, F., Callard, P., Amouroux, J., Casassus, P., and Jarrousse, B., Microscopic polyangiitis. Clinical and laboratory findings in 85 patients., *Arthritis and Rheumatism,* 42, 421, 1999.

91. Fauci, A. S., Haynes, B., and Katz, P., The spectrum of vasculitis: clinical, pathologic, immunologic and therapeutic considerations, *Annals of Internal Medicine,* 89, 660, 1978.

92. Andrews, M., Edmunds, M., Campbell, A., Walls, J., and Feehally, J., Systemic vasculitis in the 1980s — is there an increasing incidence of Wegener's granulomatosis and microscopic polyarteritis? *Journal of the Royal College of Physicians* (London), 24, 284, 1990.

93. Croker, B. P., Lee, T., and Gunnells, J. C., Clinical and pathologic features of polyarteritis nodosa and its renal-limited variant: primary crescentic and necrotizing glomerulonephritis, *Human Pathology,* 18, 38, 1987.

94. Inoue, M., Akikusa, B., Masuda, Y., and Kondo, Y., Demonstration of microaneurysms at the interlobular arteries of the kidneys in microscopic polyangiitis: a three-dimensional study, *Human Pathology,* 29, 223, 1998.

95. Heptinstall, R. H., Polyarteritis nodosa, Wegener's syndrome, and other forms of vasculitis., in *Pathology of the Kidney*, 4th edition, Heptinstall, R. H., Ed, Little Brown, Boston, 1992.

96. Davenport, A., Lock, R. J., Wallington, T. B., and Feest, T. G., Clinical significance of anti-neutrophil cytoplasm antibodies detected by a standardized indirect immunofluorescence assay, *Quarterly Journal of Medicine,* 87, 291, 1994.

97. Hauschild, S., Schmitt, W. H., Csernok, E., and Gross, W. L., ANCA in systemic vasculitides, collagen vascular disorders and inflammatory bowel diseases, in *ANCA-Associated Vasculitis*, Gross, W. L., Ed., Plenum, New York, 1993.

98. Geffriaud-Ricouard, C., Noel, L. H., Chauveau, D., Houhou, S., Grunfeld, J. P., and Lesavre, P., Clinical spectrum associated with ANCA of defined antigen specificities in 98 selected patients, *Clinical Nephrology,* 39, 125, 1993.

99. Guillevin, L., Lhote, F., Amouroux, J., Gherardi, R., Callard, P., and Casassus, P., Antineutrophil cytoplasmic antibodies, abnormal angiograms and pathological findings in polyarteritis nodosa and Churg-Strauss syndrome: indications for the classification of vasculitides of the Polyarteritis Nodosa Group, *British Journal of Rheumatology,* 35, 958, 1996.

100. Gordon, M., Luqmani, R. A., Adu, D., Greaves, I., Richards, N., Michael, J., Emery, P., Howie, A. J., and Bacon, P. A., Relapses in patients with a systemic vasculitis, *Quarterly Journal of Medicine,* 86, 779, 1993.

101. Falk, R. J., Hogan, S., Carey, T. S., and Jennette, J. C., Clinical course of anti-neutrophil cytoplasmic autoantibody-associated glomerulonephritis and systemic vasculitis. The Glomerular Disease Collaborative Network, *Annals of Internal Medicine,* 113, 656, 1990.

102. Fuiano, G., Cameron, J. S., Raftery, M., Hartley, B. H., Williams, D. G., and Ogg, C. S., Improved prognosis of renal microscopic polyarteritis in recent years, *Nephrology Dialysis Transplantation,* 3, 383, 1988.

103. Wilkowski, M. J., Velosa, J. A., Holley, K. E., Offord, K. P., Chu, C. P., Torres, V. E., McCarthy, J. T., Donadio, J. V. J., and Wagoner, R. D., Risk factors in idiopathic renal vasculitis and glomerulonephritis, *Kidney International,* 36, 1133, 1989.

104. Churg, J. and Strauss, L., Allergic granulomatosis, allergic rhinitis and periarteritis nodosa, *American Journal of Pathology,* 27, 277, 1951.

105. Lanham, J. G., Elkon, K. B., Pusey, C. D., and Hughes, G. R., Systemic vasculitis with asthma and eosinophilia: a clinical approach to the Churg-Strauss syndrome, *Medicine* (Baltimore), 63, 65, 1984.

106. Masi, A. T., Hunder, G. G., Lie, J. T., Michel, B. A., Bloch, D. A., Arend, W. P., Calabrese, L. H., Edworthy, S. M., Fauci, A. S., and Leavitt, R. Y., The American College of Rheumatology 1990 criteria for the classification of Churg-Strauss syndrome (allergic granulomatosis and angiitis), *Arthritis and Rheumatism,* 33, 1094, 1990.

107. Chumbley, L. C., Harrison, E. G. J., and DeRemee, R. A., Allergic granulomatosis and angiitis (Churg-Strauss syndrome). Report and analysis of 30 cases, *Mayo Clinic Proceedings,* 52, 477, 1977.

108. Clutterbuck, E. J., Evans, D. J., and Pusey, C. D., Renal involvement in Churg-Strauss syndrome, *Nephrology Dialysis Transplantation,* 5, 161, 1990.

109. Jennette, J. C., Antineutrophil cytoplasmic autoantibody-associated diseases: a pathologist's perspective, *American Journal of Kidney Diseases,* 18, 164, 1991.

110. Davenport, A., McDicken, I., and Goldsmith, H. J., Reversible acute renal failure due to Churg-Strauss syndrome, *Postgraduate Medical Journal,* 64, 713, 1988.

111. Cortellini, P., Manganelli, P., Poletti, F., Sacchini, P., Ambanelli, U., and Bezzi, E., Ureteral involvement in the Churg-Strauss syndrome: a case report, *Journal of Urology,* 140, 1016, 1988.

112. Cohen, T. J., Elema, J. D., and Kallenberg, C. G., Clinical and histopathological association of 29kD-ANCA and MPO-ANCA, *APMIS Supplement,* 19, 35, 1990.

113. Gaskin, G., Ryan, J., and Rees, A. J., Anti-myeloperoxidase antibodies in vasculitis: relationship to ANCA and clinical diagnosis, *APMIS* Supplement, 19, 33, 1990.

114. O'Donoghue, D. J., Nusbaum, P., and Halbwachs-Mecarelli, L., Anti-neutrophil cytoplasmic antibodies associated with polyarteritis nodosa, Churg-Strauss syndrome and HIV related systemic vasculitis, *American Journal of Kidney Diseases*, 18, 208, 1991.

115. Abu-Shakra, M., Smythe, H., Lewtas, J., Badley, E., Weber, D., and Keystone, E., Outcome of polyarteritis nodosa and Churg-Strauss syndrome. An analysis of 25 patients, *Arthritis and Rheumatism*, 37, 1798, 1994.

116. Klinger, H., Grenzformen der periarteritis nodosa, *Frankfurter Zeitschrift fur Pathologie (Frankfurt. Ztschr. Pathol.)*, 42, 455, 1931.

117. Wegener, F., Uber eine generalisierte, septische of gefaberkrankungen., *Verhandlungen der Deurchen Gesellschaft fur Pathologie (Verh. Dtsch. Ges. Pathol).*, 29, 202, 1936.

118. Leavitt, R. Y., Fauci, A. S., Bloch, D. A., Michel, B. A., Hunder, G. G., Arend, W. P., Calabrese, L. H., Fries, J. F., Lie, J. T., and Lightfoot, R. W. J., The American College of Rheumatology 1990 criteria for the classification of Wegener's granulomatosis, *Arthritis and Rheumatism*, 33, 1101, 1990.

119. Duna, G. F., Galperin, C., and Hoffman, G. S., Wegener's granulomatosis, *Rheumatic Diseases Clinics of North America*, 21, 949, 1995.

120. Gross, W. L., Systemic necrotizing vasculitis, *Bailliere's Clinical Rheumatology*, 11, 259, 1997.

121. Carruthers, D. M., Watts, R. A., Symmons, D. P., and Scott, D. G., Wegener's granulomatosis — increased incidence or increased recognition?, *British Journal of Rheumatology*, 35, 142, 1996.

122. Andrews, M., Edmunds, M., Campbell, A., Walls, J., and Feehally, J., Systemic vasculitis in the 1980s — is there an increasing incidence of Wegener's granulomatosis and microscopic polyarteritis?, *Journal of the Royal College of Physicians* (London), 24, 284, 1990.

123. Cotch, M. F., Hoffman, G. S., Yerg, D. E., Kaufman, G. I., Targonski, P., and Kaslow, R. A., The epidemiology of Wegener's granulomatosis. Estimates of the five-year period prevalence, annual mortality, and geographic disease distribution from population-based data sources, *Arthritis and Rheumatism*, 39, 87, 1996.

124. Fauci, A. S., Haynes, B. F., Katz, P., and Wolff, S. M., Wegener's Granulomatosis: Prospective clinical and therapeutic experience with 85 patients for 21 years, *Annals of Internal Medicine*, 98, 76, 1983.

125. Hoffman, G. S., Kerr, G. S., Leavitt, R. Y., Hallahan, C. W., Lebovics, R. S., Travis, W. D., Rottem, M., and Fauci, A. S., Wegener granulomatosis: an analysis of 158 patients, *Annals of Internal Medicine*, 116, 488, 1992.

126. Anderson, G., Coles, E. T., Crane, M., Douglas, A. C., Gibbs, A. R., Geddes, D. M., Peel, E. T., and Wood, J. B., Wegener's granuloma. A series of 265 British cases seen between 1975 and 1985. A report by a sub-committee of the British Thoracic Society Research Committee, *Quarterly Journal of Medicine*, 83, 427, 1992.

127. Nolle, B., Specks, U., Ludemann, J., Rohrbach, M. S., DeRemee, R. A., and Gross, W. L., Anticytoplasmic autoantibodies: their immunodiagnostic value in Wegener granulomatosis, *Annals of Internal Medicine*, 111, 28, 1989.

128. Luqmani, R. A., Bacon, P. A., Beaman, M., Scott, D. G., Emery, P., Lee, S. J., Howie, A. J., Richards, N., Michael, J., and Adu, D., Classical versus non-renal Wegener's granulomatosis, *Quarterly Journal of Medicine*, 87, 161, 1994.

129. Bajema, I. M., Hagen, E. C., van der Woude, F. J., and Bruijn, J. A., Wegener's granulomatosis: a meta-analysis of 349 literary case reports, *Journal of Laboratory Clinical Medicine*, 129, 17, 1997.

130. Romas, E., Murphy, B. F., d'Apice, A. J., Kennedy, J. T., and Niall, J. F., Wegener's granulomatosis: clinical features and prognosis in 37 patients, *Australia and New Zealand Journal of Medicine*, 23, 168, 1993.

131. Horn, R. G., Fauci, A. S., Rosenthal, A. S., and Wolff, S. M., Renal biopsy pathology in Wegener's granulomatosis, *American Journal of Pathology*, 74, 423, 1974.

132. Anderson, C. L. and Stavrides, A., Rapidly progressive renal failure as the primary manifestation of Wegener's granulomatosis, *American Journal of Medical Science*, 275, 109, 1978.

133. Fujita, T., Ohi, H., Endo, M., Ohsawa, I., and Kanmatsuse, K., Level of red blood cells in the urinary sediment reflects the degree of renal activity in Wegener's granulomatosis, *Clinical Nephrology*, 50, 284, 1998.

134. Novak, R. F., Christiansen, R. G., and Sorensen, E. T., The acute vasculitis of Wegener's granulomatosis in renal biopsies, *American Journal of Clinical Pathology,* 78, 367, 1982.

135. Watanabe, T., Nagafuchi, Y., Yoshikawa, Y., and Toyoshima, H., Renal papillary necrosis associated with Wegener's granulomatosis, *Human Pathology,* 14, 551, 1983.

136. Baker, S. B. and Robinson, D. R., Unusual renal manifestations of Wegener's granulomatosis. Report of two cases, *American Journal of Medicine,* 64, 883, 1978.

137. Boubenider, S. A., Akhtar, M., and Nyman, R., Wegener's granulomatosis limited to the kidney as a masslike lesion, *Nephron,* 68, 500, 1994.

138. Grotz, W., Wanner, C., Keller, E., Bohler, J., Peter, H. H., Rohrbach, R., and Schollmeyer, P., Crescentic glomerulonephritis in Wegener's granulomatosis: morphology, therapy, outcome, *Clinical Nephrology,* 35, 243, 1991.

139. Weiss, M. A. and Crissman, J. D., Renal biopsy findings in Wegener's granulomatosis: segmental necrotizing glomerulonephritis with glomerular thrombosis, *Human Pathology,* 15, 943, 1984.

140. Antonovych, T. T., Sabnis, S. G., Tuur, S. M., Sesterhenn, I. A., and Balow, J. E., Morphologic differences between polyarteritis and Wegener's granulomatosis using light, electron and immunohistochemical techniques, *Modern Pathology,* 2, 349, 1989.

141. Franssen, C. F., Gans, R. O., Arends, B., Hageluken, C., ter Wee, P. M., Gerlag, P. G., and Hoorntje, S. J., Differences between anti-myeloperoxidase- and anti-proteinase 3-associated renal disease, *Kidney International,* 47, 193, 1995.

142. Bhathena, D. B., Migdal, S. D., Julian, B. A., McMorrow, R. G., and Baehler, R. W., Morphologic and immunohistochemical observations in granulomatous glomerulonephritis., *American Journal of Pathology,* 126, 581, 1987.

143. Watanabe, T., Yoshikawa, Y., and Toyoshima, H., Morphological and clinical features of the kidney in Wegener's granulomatosis. A survey of 28 autopsies in Japan, *Nippon Jinzo Gakkai Shi,* 23, 921, 1981.

144. Bajema, I. M., Hagen, E. C., Ferrario, F., Waldherr, R., Noel, L. H., Hermans, J., van der Woude, F. J., and Bruijn, J. A., Renal granulomas in systemic vasculitis. EC/BCR Project for ANCA-Assay Standardization, *Clinical Nephrology,* 48, 16, 1997.

145. van der Woude, F. J., Rasmussen, N., Lobatto, S., Wiik, A., Permin, H., Van Es, L. A., van der Giessen, M., van der Hem, G. K., and The, T. H., Autoantibodies against neutrophils and monocytes: tool for diagnosis and marker of disease activity in Wegener's granulomatosis, *Lancet,* 1, 425, 1985.

146. Cohen, T. J., van der Woude, F. J., Fauci, A. S., Ambrus, J. L., Velosa, J., Keane, W. F., Meijer, S., van der Giessen, M., van der Hem, G. K., and The, T. H., Association between active Wegener's granulomatosis and anticytoplasmic antibodies, *Archives of Internal Medicine,* 149, 2461, 1989.

147. Rao, J. K., Weinberger, M., Oddone, E. Z., Allen, N. B., Landsman, P., and Feussner, J. R., The role of antineutrophil cytoplasmic antibody (c-ANCA) testing in the diagnosis of Wegener granulomatosis. A literature review and meta-analysis, *Annals of Internal Medicine,* 123, 925, 1995.

148. Venning, M. C., Quinn, A., Broomhead, V., and Bird, A. G., Antibodies directed against neutrophils (C-ANCA and P-ANCA) are of distinct diagnostic value in systemic vasculitis, *Quarterly Journal of Medicine,* 77, 1287, 1990.

149. Bosch, X., Mirapeix, E., Font, J., Cervera, R., Ingelmo, M., Khamashta, M. A., Revert, L., Hughes, G. R., and Urbano-Marquez, A., Anti-myeloperoxidase autoantibodies in patients with necrotizing glomerular and alveolar capillaritis, *American Journal of Kidney Diseases,* 20, 231, 1992.

150. Bindi, P., Mougenot, B., Mentre, F., Noel, L. H., Peraldi, M. N., Vanhille, P., Lesavre, P., Mignon, F., and Ronco, P. M., Necrotizing crescentic glomerulonephritis without significant immune deposits: a clinical and serological study, *Quarterly Journal of Medicine,* 86, 55, 1993.

151. Specks, U. and Homburger, H. A., Anti-neutrophil cytoplasmic antibodies., *Mayo Clinic Proceedings,* 69, 1197, 1994.

152. Kallenberg, C. G., Laboratory findings in the vasculitides., *Bailliere's Clinical Rheumatology,* 11, 395, 1997.

153. Hagen, E. C., Daha, M. R., Hermans, J., Andrassy, K., Csernok, E., Gaskin, G., Lesavre, P., Ludemann, J., Rasmussen, N., Sinico, R. A., Wiik, A., and van der Woude, F. J., Diagnostic value of standardized assays for anti-neutrophil cytoplasmic antibodies in idiopathic systemic vasculitis. EC/BCR Project for ANCA Assay Standardization, *Kidney International,* 53, 743, 1998.

154. Bajema, I. M. and Hagen, E. C., Evolving concepts about the role of antineutrophil cytoplasm autoantibodies in systemic vasculitides, *Current Opinion in Rheumatology*, 11, 34, 1999.

155. Cohen Tervaert, J. W., Huitema, M. G., Hene, R. J., Sluiter, W. J., The, T. H., van der Hem, G. K., and Kallenberg, C. G., Prevention of relapses in Wegener's granulomatosis by treatment based on antineutrophil cytoplasmic antibody titre., *Lancet,* 336, 709, 1990.

156. De'Oliviera, J., Gaskin, G., Dash, A., Rees, A. J., and Pusey, C. D., Relationship between disease activity and anti-neutrophil cytoplasmic antibody concentration in long-term management of systemic vasculitis, *American Journal of Kidney Diseases,* 25, 380, 1995.

157. Jayne, D. R., Gaskin, G., Pusey, C. D., and Lockwood, C. M., ANCA and predicting relapse in systemic vasculitis, *Quarterly Journal of Medicine,* 88, 127, 1995.

158. Kerr, G. S., Fleisher, T. A., Hallahan, C. W., Leavitt, R. Y., Fauci, A. S., and Hoffman, G. S., Limited prognostic value of changes in antineutrophil cytoplasmic antibody titer in patients with Wegener's granulomatosis, *Arthritis and Rheumatism,* 36, 365, 1993.

159. Davenport, A., "False positive" perinuclear and cytoplasmic anti-neutrophil cytoplasmic antibody results leading to misdiagnosis of Wegener's granulomatosis and/or microscopic polyarteritis, *Clinical Nephrology,* 37, 124, 1992.

160. Moutsopoulos, H. M., Avgerinos, P. C., Tsampoulas, C. G., and Katsiotis, P. A., Selective renal angiography in Wegener's granulomatosis, *Annals of Rheumatic Diseases,* 42, 192, 1983.

161. Yazici, H., Behcet's syndrome, in *Rheumatology*, Klippel, J. H. and Dieppe P. A., Eds, Mosby, St Louis, 1994.

162. Rosenthal, T., Weiss, P., and Gafni, J., Renal involvement in Behcet's syndrome, *Archives of Internal Medicine,* 138, 1122, 1978.

163. El Ramahi, K. M., Al Dalaan, A., Al Shaikh, A., Al Meshari, K., and Akhtar, M., Renal involvement in Behcet's disease: review of 9 cases, *Journal of Rheumatology,* 25, 2254, 1998.

164. Kansu, E., Deglin, S., Cantor, R. I., Burke, J. F. J., Cho, S. Y., and Cathart, R. T., The expanding spectrum of Behcet syndrome: a case with renal involvement, *JAMA,* 237, 1855, 1977.

165. Hamuryudan, V., Yurdakul, S., Kural, A. R., Ince, U., and Yazici, H., Diffuse proliferative glomerulonephritis in Behcet's syndrome, *British Journal of Rheumatology,* 30, 63, 1991.

166. Olsson, P. J., Gaffney, E., Alexander, R. W., Mars, D. R., and Fuller, T. J., Proliferative glomerulonephritis with crescent formation in Behcet's syndrome, *Archives of Internal Medicine,* 140, 713, 1980.

167. Tietjen, D. P. and Moore, W. J., Treatment of rapidly progressive glomerulonephritis due to Behcet's syndrome with intravenous cyclophosphamide, *Nephron,* 55, 69, 1990.

168. Donnelly, S., Jothy, S., and Barre, P., Crescentic glomerulonephritis in Behcet's syndrome — results of therapy and review of the literature, *Clinical Nephrology,* 31, 213, 1989.

169. Landwehr, D. M., Cooke, C. L., and Rodriguez, G. E., Rapidly progressive glomerulonephritis in Behcet's syndrome, *JAMA,* 244, 1709, 1980.

170. Bemelman, F. J., Krediet, R. T., Schipper, M. E., and Arisz, L., Renal involvement in Behcet's syndrome. Report of a case and a review of the literature, *Netherlands Journal of Medicine,* 34, 148, 1989.

171. Tasdemir, I., Sivri, B., Turgan, C., Emri, S., Yasavul, U., and Caglar, S., The expanding spectrum of a disease. Behcet's disease associated with amyloidosis, *Nephron,* 52, 154, 1989.

172. Peces, R., Riesgo, I., Ortego, F., Velasco, J., and Alvarez, G. J., Amyloidosis in Behcet's disease, *Nephron,* 36, 114, 1984.

173. Dilsen, N., Konice, M., Aral, O., Erbengi, T., Uysal, V., Kocak, N., and Ozdogan, E., Behcet's disease associated with amyloidosis in Turkey and in the world, *Annals of Rheumatic Diseases,* 47, 157, 1988.

174. Miura, M., Tomino, Y., Suga, T., Endoh, M., Nomoto, Y., Sakai, H., Furuya, K., and Kobayashi, Y., A case of Behcet's disease associated with membranous nephropathy, *Tokai Journal of Experimental and Clinical Medicine,* 9, 231, 1984.

175. Malik, G. H., Sirwal, I. A., and Pandit, K. A., Behcet's syndrome associated with minimal change glomerulonephritis and renal vein thrombosis, *Nephron,* 52, 87, 1989.

176. Akutsu, Y., Itami, N., Tanaka, M., Kusunoki, Y., Tochimaru, H., and Takekoshi, Y., IgA nephritis in Behcet's disease: case report and review of the literature, *Clinical Nephrology,* 34, 52, 1990.

177. Yver, L., Blanchier, D., Aouragh, F., Turpin, Y., Chaubert, N., Laregue, M., Goujon, J. M., and Touchard, G., Renal involvement in Behcet's disease. Case report and review of the literature, *Nephron,* 73, 689, 1996.

178. Hemmen, T., Perez-Canto, A., Distler, A., Offermann, G., and Braun, J., IgA nephropathy in a patient with Behcet's syndrome — case report and review of literature, *British Journal of Rheumatology,* 36, 696, 1997.
179. Herreman, G., Beaufils, H., Godeau, P., Cassou, B., Wechsler, B., Boujeau, J., and Chomette, G., Behcet's syndrome and renal involvement: a histological and immunofluorescent study of eleven renal biopsies, *American Journal of Medical Science,* 284, 10, 1982.
180. Svenson, K., Bohman, S. O., and Hallgren, R., Renal interstitial fibrosis and vascular changes. Occurrence in patients with autoimmune diseases treated with cyclosporine, *Archives of Internal Medicine,* 146, 2007, 1986.
181. Fukuda, T., Hayashi, K., Sakamoto, I., and Mori, M., Acute renal infarction caused by Behcet's disease, *Abdominal Imaging,* 20, 264, 1995.
182. Kerr, G. S., Takayasu's arteritis, *Rheum. Dis. Clin. North Am.,* 21, 1041, 1995.
183. Wilke, W. S., Large vessel vasculitis, *Bailliere's Clinical Rheumatology,* 11, 287, 1997.
184. Hall, S., Barr, W., Lie, J. T., Stanson, A. W., Kazmier, F. J., and Hunder, G. G., Takayasu's arteritis: A study of 32 North American patients, *Medicine* (Baltimore), 64, 89, 1985.
185. Waern, A. U., Anderson, P., and Hemmingsson, A., Takayasu arteritis: a hospital-region based study on occurrence treatment and prognosis, *Angiology,* 34, 311, 1983.
186. Koide, K., Takayasu arteritis in Japan, *Heart and Vessels,* 7, 48, 1992.
187. Arend, W. P., Michel, B. A., Bloch, D. A., Hunder, G. G., Calabrese, L. H., Edworthy, S. M., Fauci, A. S., Leavitt, R. Y., Lie, J. T., and Lightfoot, R. W. J., The American College of Rheumatology 1990 criteria for the classification of Takayasu arteritis, *Arthritis and Rheumatism,* 33, 1129, 1990.
188. Lupi-Herrera, E., Sanchez-Torres, G., Marcushamer, J., Mispireta, J., Horwitz, S., and Espino Vela, J., Takayasu's arteritis. Clinical study of 107 cases, *American Heart Journal,* 93, 94, 1977.
189. Rapoport, M., Averbukh, Z., Chaim, S., Klinovski, E., Modai, D., and Gilboa, Y., Takayasu aortitis simulating bilateral renal-artery stenoses in patients treated with ACE inhibitors, *Clinical Nephrology,* 36, 156, 1991.
190. Huddle, K. R., Doodha, M. I., and Mackenzie, M., Captopril in the treatment of renovascular hypertension secondary to Takayasu's arteritis. A case report, *South Africa Medical Journal,* 69, 58, 1986.
191. Zilleruelo, G. E., Ferrer, P., Garcia, O. L., Moore, M., Pardo, V., and Strauss, J., Takayasu's arteritis associated with glomerulonephritis. A case report, *American Journal of Diseases of Children,* 132, 1009, 1978.
192. Hellmann, D. B., Hardy, K., Lindenfeld, S., and Ring, E., Takayasu's arteritis associated with crescentic glomerulonephritis, *Arthritis and Rheumatism,* 30, 451, 1987.
193. Takagi, M., Ikeda, T., Kimura, K., Saito, Y., Ishii, M., Takeda, T., and Murao, S., Renal histological studies in patients with Takayasu's arteritis. Report of 3 cases, *Nephron,* 36, 68, 1984.
194. Yoshikawa, Y., Truong, L. D., Mattioli, C. A., and Lederer, E., Membranoproliferative glomerulonephritis in Takayasu's arteritis, *American Journal of Nephrology,* 8, 240, 1988.
195. Greene, N. B., Baughman, R. P., and Kim, C. K., Takayasu's arteritis associated with interstitial lung disease and glomerulonephritis, *Chest,* 89, 605, 1986.
196. Yoshimura, M., Kida, H., Saito, Y., Yokoyama, H., Tomosugi, N., Abe, T., and Hattori, N., Peculiar glomerular lesions in Takayasu's arteritis, *Clinical Nephrology,* 24, 120, 1985.
197. Dash, S. C., Sharma, R. K., Malhotra, K. K., and Bhuyan, U. N., Renal amyloidosis and non-specific aorto-arteritis — a hitherto undescribed association, *Postgrauate Medical Journal,* 60, 626, 1984.
198. Graham, A. N., Delahunt, B., Renouf, J. J., and Austad, W. I., Takayasu's disease associated with generalised amyloidosis, *Australia and New Zealand Journal of Medicine,* 15, 343, 1985.
199. Sousa, A. E., Lucas, M., Tavora, I., and Victorino, R. M., Takayasu's disease presenting as a nephrotic syndrome due to amyloidosis, *Postgraduate Medical Journal,* 69, 488, 1993.
200. Koumi, S., Endo, T., Okumura, H., Yoneyama, K., Fukuda, Y., and Masugi, Y., A case of Takayasu's arteritis associated with membranoproliferative glomerulonephritis and nephrotic syndrome, *Nephron,* 54, 344, 1990.
201. Cavatorta, F., Campisi, S., Trabassi, E., Zollo, A., and Salvidio, G., IgA nephropathy associated with Takayasu's arteritis: report of a case and review of the literature, *American Journal of Nephrology,* 15, 165, 1995.
202. Nordborg, E., Nordborg, C., Malmvall, B., Andersson, R., and Bengtsson, B. A., Giant cell arteritis, *Rheumatic Diseases Clinics of North America,* 21, 1013, 1995.

203. Wilke, W. S., Large vessel vasculitis, *Bailliere's Clinical Rheumatology,* 11, 285, 1997.
204. Nordborg, E. and Bengtsson, B. A., Epidemiology of biopsy-proven giant cell arteritis, *Journal of Internal Medicine,* 227, 233, 1990.
205. Machado, E. B., Mitchet, C. J., Ballard, D. J., Hunder, G. G., Beard, C. M., Chu, C. P., and O'Fallon, W. M., Trends in incidence and clinical presentation of temporal arteritis in Olmsted County, Minnesota, 1950-1985, *Arthritis and Rheumatism,* 31, 745, 1988.
206. Hunder, G. G., Bloch, D. A., Michel, B. A., Stevens, M. B., Arend, W. P., Calabrese, L. H., Edworthy, S. M., Fauci, A. S., Leavitt, R. Y., and Lie, J. T., The American College of Rheumatology 1990 criteria for the classification of giant cell arteritis, *Arthritis and Rheumatism,* 33, 1122, 1990.
207. Klein, R. G., Hunder, G. G., Stanson, A. W., and Sheps, S. G., Large artery involvement in giant cell (temporal) arteritis, *Annals of Internal Medicine,* 83, 806, 1975.
208. Elling, H. and Kristensen, I. B., Fatal renal failure in polymyalgia rheumatica caused by disseminated giant cell arteritis, *Scandinavian Journal of Rheumatology,* 9, 206, 1980.
209. Pascual, J., Quereda, C., Liano, F., Garcia-Villanueva, M. J., Mampaso, F., and Ortuno, J., End-stage renal disease after necrotising glomerulonephritis in an elderly patient with temporal arteritis, *Nephron,* 66, 236, 1994.
210. Canton, C. G., Bernis, C., Paraiso, V., Barril, G., Garcia, A., Osorio, C., Rincon, B., and Traver, J. A., Renal failure in temporal arteritis, *American Journal of Nephrology,* 12, 380, 1992.
211. Truong, L., Kopelman, R. G., Williams, G. S., and Pirani, C. L., Temporal arteritis and renal disease. Case report and review of the literature, *American Journal of Medicine,* 78, 171, 1985.
212. O'Neill, W. M. J., Hammar, S. P., and Bloomer, A., Giant cell arteritis with visceral angiitis, *Archives of Internal Medicine,* 136, 1157, 1976.
213. Lenz, T., Schmidt, R., Scherberich, J. E., and Grone, H. J., Renal failure in giant cell vasculitis, *American Journal of Kidney Diseases,* 31, 1044, 1998.
214. Sonnenblick, M. and Slotki, I. N., Nephrotic syndrome in temporal arteritis, *British Journal of Clinical Practice,* 43, 420, 1989.
215. Monteagudo, M., Vidal, G., Andreu, J., Oristrell, J., Tolosa, C., Larrosa, M., Casanovas, A., and Almirall, J., Giant cell arteritis and secondary renal amyloidosis: report of 2 cases, *Journal of Rheumatology,* 24, 605, 1997.
216. Luthra, H. S. and Michet, C. J., Relapsing polychondritis, in *Rheumatology,* Klippel, J. H. and Dieppe, P. A., Eds, Mosby, St Louis, 1994.
217. Chang-Miller, A., Okamura, M., Torres, V. E., Michet, C. J., Wagoner, R. D., Donadio, J. V. J., Offord, K. P., and Holley, K. E., Renal involvement in relapsing polychondritis, *Medicine* (Baltimore), 66, 202, 1987.
218. Zeuner, M., Straub, R. H., Rauh, G., Albert, E. D., Scholmerich, J., and Lang, B., Relapsing polychondritis: clinical and immunogenetic analysis of 62 patients, *Journal of Rheumatology,* 24, 96, 1997.
219. Espinoza, L. R., Richman, A., Bocanegra, T., Pina, I., Vasey, F. B., Rifkin, S. I., and Germain, B. F., Immune complex-mediated renal involvement in relapsing polychondritis, *American Journal of Medicine,* 71, 181, 1981.
220. Ruhlen, J. L., Huston, K. A., and Wood, W. G., Relapsing polychondritis with glomerulonephritis. Improvement with prednisone and cyclophosphamide, *JAMA,* 245, 847, 1981.
221. Neild, G. H., Cameron, J. S., Lessof, M. H., Ogg, C. S., and Turner, D. R., Relapsing polychondritis with crescentic glomerulonephritis, *British Medical Journal,* 1, 743, 1978.
222. Dalal, B. I., Wallace, A. C., and Slinger, R. P., IgA nephropathy in relapsing polychondritis, *Pathology,* 20, 85, 1988.

30 Skin Manifestations of Vasculitis

Camille Francès, Pierre-André Bécherel, and Jean-Charles Piette

CONTENTS

I. DERMATOLOGIC MANIFESTATIONS

Dermatologic manifestations are frequently observed in almost all systemic vasculitis. Some of them correspond to a skin localization of the systemic vasculitis, while others result from a distinct pathologic process. As histologic examination of dermatologic lesions is easy to obtain, the former is often used to confirm the diagnosis of vasculitis. However, their contribution to the determination of the type of vasculitis is far from guaranteed. Indeed, clinical and pathologic dermatologic manifestations are not specific for a peculiar category of vasculitis. Furthermore, there is no constant relationship between skin vasculitis and systemic vasculitis, such as when the skin vasculitis is induced by drugs or by a transient viral infection.

A. Dermatologic Manifestations of Vasculitis

1. Clinical Manifestations

Skin vasculitis manifests clinically by a spectrum of lesions including erythema, purpura, papules, pustules, nodules, livedo, necrosis, ulcerations, and bullae. These various lesions are often associated, giving a pleomorphic appearance to the eruption.

Palpable purpura is unquestionably the most frequent manifestation. Lesions usually begin as tiny red macules that later become papules and plaques ranging from several millimeters to centimeters. The larger lesions are more ecchymotic than purpuric. The color may evolve from red or purple to brownish yellow when the extravasated blood is degraded. They are prominently localized on legs, ankles, and feet, but may also occur everywhere else, especially after local pressure.

Urticarial vasculitis is characterized by the presence of wheals, which persist for two to three days, unlike ordinary urticaria that clears within 24 hours. Pruritus is less intense. Lesions may evolve into purpuric lesions. They are mainly localized on the trunk and limbs. Other neither nonpurpuric nor urticarial papules may also correspond to a skin vasculitis especially papules on the extensor surfaces of the extremities. Some of them have a chronic evolution, such as erythema elevatum diutinum.

Pustular vasculitis is usually nonfollicular and underlined by erythema. Other frequently observed pustular lesions result from secondary infection of necrotic areas.

Nodular lesions due to vasculitis are typically hot, tender, red, and small-sized; they may be surrounded by livedo reticularis. As the livedo, they are mainly localized on the lower limbs (legs, soles of the feet) but are also frequently observed on other sites such as the dorsal face of the upper limbs or, more rarely, on the trunk. They may occur in groups along the course of superficial arteries.

Livedo reticularis is a reddish-blue mottling of the skin in a "fishnet" reticular pattern. When associated with vasculitis, it is persistent, although some fluctuations in intensity and extension may be observed, especially with variations of temperature. The fishnet reticular pattern is typically irregular with broken circles. On careful examination, some infiltrated areas are usually detected.

Necrosis results from the obstruction of dermal vessels. Its extension and depth are highly variable depending on the number of involved vessels. Localized purpuric and necrotic lesions turn into vesicles and sometimes into pustules when infected. When necrosis is extensive, a black necrotic plaque with an active purpuric border and bullous lesions follows painful purpura. After removal of necrotic tissue, ulcerations of various sizes are usually present.

2. Histopathology and Clinicopathologic Correlation

The histopathological hallmark of purpuric lesions is leukocytoclastic vasculitis of the small dermal vessels. Postcapillary venules are preferentially involved. Vascular alterations and dermal cellular infiltrates characterize leukocytoclastic vasculitis. Vascular alterations consist of endothelial cell swelling, activation of nuclei, wrinkling of nuclear membranes, wall necrosis with deposition of fibrinoid material, and sometimes thrombosis. The fibrinoid material consists predominantly of fibrin, but also contains necrotic endothelial cells and deposited immunoreactants (immunoglobulins and/or complement proteins). Infiltrates vary in intensity and are usually perivascular in location, but at times are dispersed widely. They are mainly composed of neutrophils showing fragmentation of nuclei (karyorrhexis or leukocytoclasia). In other cases or in the later phase, lymphocytes and monocytes may predominate in the infiltrates. In some patients, especially those with immune complex-mediated vasculitis with extensive complement activation, dermal small-vessel vasculitis causes focal edema with resultant urticaria.

Nodular forms of vasculitis result from wall inflammation of the blood vessels located at the junction of dermis/subcutis, or in the subcutis. When arterioles are involved the pathologic features are similar to those observed in cutaneous polyarteritis nodosa. Endothelial swelling and fibrinoid necrosis of the media are often severe, sometimes with thrombosis. Infiltration of the vessel wall with neutrophils is usual in the acute phase, whereas leukocytoclasis is less frequently seen. In some cases the infiltrate is granulomatous. In the healing stage, the vessel wall is invaded by granulation tissue and replaced by a fibrous scar. Persistent proliferation of capillaries occurs. Rarely, nodules are the clinical manifestations of a leukocytoclastic vasculitis affecting the small vessels of the subcutis.

In brief, palpable purpura and papular lesions such as urticaria correspond to a leukocytoclastic or to a lymphocytic vasculitis of the small vessels of the dermis. Nodules correspond to vasculitis of arterioles or small vessels located at the dermis/subcutis junction or in the subcutis. Necrosis and livedo are observed when either small or larger vessels or both are involved.

B. OTHER DERMATOLOGIC MANIFESTATIONS ASSOCIATED WITH SYSTEMIC VASCULITIS

1. Extravascular Necrotizing Granuloma

Initially described by Churg and Strauss in 1951[1] as a manifestation of allergic angiitis (Churg-Strauss syndrome), the extravascular granuloma has been further reported in a large variety of other systemic vasculitis and connective tissue diseases.[2] However, it is mainly observed in Churg-Strauss syndrome and Wegener's granulomatosis. Clinically, papular or nodular lesions vary in size from 2 mm to 2 cm or more. They also vary in color from red to violaceous. Central crusting and/or ulceration are frequent. Rarely, other clinical aspects are observed such as vesicles, pustules, arciform plaques, or an indurated mass. Localization of lesions are the extensor surfaces of the elbows, the digits, where they are usually multiple and often symmetrical, and, less frequently, the buttocks, scalp, extensor surfaces of knees, hands, the dorsum of foot, neck, forehead, and ear. Histological features include endothelial necrosis and edema, fibrinoid necrosis of the collagen, and granulomas containing eosinophils, histiocytes, and lymphocytes. The center of the granuloma consists of basophilic fibrillar necrosis in which bands (sometimes linear) of destroyed tissue are interspersed with polymorphonuclear leukocytes and leukocytoclastic debris. This necrotic area is surrounded by a granulomatous mass predominantly made of histiocytes, often in palisading array. Decrease or absence of elastic fibers is observed in foci of degenerated collagen. No strict relationship was noted between the clinical appearance of clinical lesions, the histologic features, and the associated systemic disease, even when it was especially noted in Churg-Strauss syndrome and Wegener's granulomatosis. However, tissue eosinophilia is more frequently reported in patients with Churg-Strauss syndrome.

2. Panniculitis

Cutaneous eruption consists of recurrent crops of erythematous, edematous, and tender subcutaneous nodules. The nodules are usually 1 to 2 cm in size but may be much larger. In lobular panniculitis, lesions are usually symmetrical in distribution and occur often on the thighs and lower legs. They usually regress spontaneously, leaving hypopigmented and atrophic scars due to fat necrosis. Occasionally, they may suppurate. In septal panniculitis, nodular lesions are located primarily over the extensor surfaces of the lower limbs. They regress spontaneously without atrophic scar. Lobular infiltrates of lymphocytes, plasma cells, and histiocytes with fat necrosis are observed in lobular panniculitis, while infiltrates of septal panniculitis are observed in the septa where they affect perivascular distribution.

3. Pyoderma Gangrenosum

Pyoderma gangrenosum lesions usually start as deep-seated, painful nodules or as superficial hemorrhagic pustules, either *de novo* or after a slight trauma. They further break down and ulcerate, discharging a purulent and hemorrhagic exudate. The ulcers increase in size to 10 cm or more, spreading, partially receding, or remaining indolent for long periods. The irregular edges are raised, red or purplish, undermined, soggy, and often perforated. The predilection sites are the lower extremities, buttocks, and abdomen, but any area of the body may be involved. Lesions are usually solitary but may arise in clusters, which then coalesce to form polycyclic irregular ulcerations. When healing occurs, it leaves an atrophic and often cribriform scar. The histopathologic features consist of large, sterile abscess formation in which thrombosis of small- and medium-sized vessels, hemorrhage, and necrosis are present. Polymorph neutrophils are numerous but epithelioid; giant and mononuclear cells are also seen mainly in more chronic forms. Leukocytoclastic or lymphocytic vasculitis may be observed, especially in the advancing border of the lesions. These changes are not pathognomonic and the diagnosis is essentially based on the clinical aspect.

4. Granuloma

Granulomatous lesions without vasculitis or central necrosis may be observed in systemic vasculitis, especially in Wegener's granulomatosis. Their clinical aspects are highly variable ranging from papules, nodules, subcutaneous infiltration, and pseudo-tumor to chronic ulcers. Any site of the body may be involved: breast, scrotum, face, or gingivae. Nonvasculitis granulomatous diseases have to be considered in the differential diagnosis including sarcoidosis, Crohn's disease, primary biliary cirrhosis, mycobacterium infections, and foreign bodies granulomas.

5. Superficial Thrombophlebitis

Thrombophlebitis of a superficial vein is clinically evident in most cases due to the presence of painful induration along the vein with redness and increased heat. Sometimes, the clinical aspect is a nonspecific red nodule and diagnosis is only confirmed by histological examination of a deep skin biopsy. Such lesions are essentially observed in thromboangiitis obliterans, Behçet's disease, Crohn's disease, and relapsing polychondritis.

6. Gangrenes

Gangrenes resulting from arterial occlusion may be observed in all vasculitis involving medium-sized or large-sized arteries. Clinically, gangrene is initially characterized by a sharply demarcated blue-black color of the extremities. The main differential diagnosis is thrombosis without inflammation of the vessel walls and emboli. Angiography visualizes occlusion or stenosis of arteries and does not help to distinguish between these different pathologic processes. The presence of other skin lesions with histologically proven vasculitis is in favor of vasculitis, although thrombosis, vasculitis, and emboli may be associated, such as in cholesterol crystals embolism.

7. Raynaud's Phenomenon

Bilateral Raynaud's phenomenon occurs in 5 to 30% of the normal population.[3,4] It is classically associated with many forms of vasculitis. However, its prevalence in vasculitis is unknown and its diagnostic value is very low. In contrast, unilateral Raynaud's phenomenon suggests an obstructive arterial disease and is mainly observed in Takayasu's arteritis.

II. DERMATOLOGIC FINDINGS IN SYSTEMIC VASCULITIS

A. HENOCH-SCHÖNLEIN PURPURA

The association of purpuric lesions with arthritis, gastrointestinal symptoms and, IgA nephritis is regarded as a distinctive entity among the group of angiitis and called Henoch-Schönlein purpura. Synonyms for this illness are anaphylactoid purpura, allergic purpura, and hemorrhagic capillary toxicosis. This type of vasculitis occurs predominantly in children, although all ages are represented. There is no definite seasonal pattern, but higher incidences in the winter and lower incidences in the summer have been recorded.

Skin lesions begin as a crop of red macules, some of which may resolve in the early stage, while others become papular, urticarial, or purpuric. In some cases the characteristic urticarial component of the rash is lacking and purpura is the only symptom. When the inflammation and exudation are severe with involvement of all superficial vessels, hemorrhagic vesicles, bullae, necrosis, and ulcers may develop. The sites of predilection are the extensor surfaces of the limbs, the buttocks, back, and, occasionally, the face. Rarely, oral mucosa is involved. Lesions occur in successive waves that resolve spontaneously.

Infantile acute hemorrhagic edema is characterized by the following features: febrile onset in children younger than two years of age; edema of the scalp, hands, feet, and periorbital tissues before the development of purpura; and lack of renal and gastrointestinal involvement. Recovery is expected within three weeks. This edema probably results from an increased capillary permeability due to the underlying vasculitis. This entity is considered by some as a distinct clinical entity, especially because of its better prognosis. It is believed by others to be a variant of Henoch-Schönlein purpura.[5,7]

Histologically, the early changes are essentially those of leukocytoclastic vasculitis with extravasation of erythrocytes. In the later stages, mononuclear cells may predominate. The superficial dermal vessels are quite exclusively involved. The frequency of dermal IgA vessel deposits varies depending on the series. These IgA deposits are sometimes included in the diagnosis criteria of dermatologic series and then present in 100% of cases.[8] On the contrary, these deposits are reported in only 50% of cases of nephrologic series, while IgA nephropathy is a constant finding.[9] These dermal IgA deposits are not specific for Henoch-Schönlein purpura. Indeed, they may be encountered in a large variety of cutaneous vasculitis.[10] In the recent French series of IgA skin vasculitis, 25% had another identified cause of vasculitis (Tancrede-Bohin, Piette).[8]

B. Essential Cryoglobulinemic Vasculitis

Cutaneous manifestations occur in 60 to 100% of patients with symptomatic cryoglobulinemia. They are a frequent presenting complaint.[11,12] Arthralgias and fatigue often accompany them. The disease has a tendency to wax and wane. There is a predominance of women with a sex ratio W/M of about 1.3/1. The average age of onset is about 50 years. The interval between the first cutaneous manifestation and diagnosis of cryoglobulinemia varies from 0 to 10 years, and was as long as 37 years in one case.[13]

Palpable purpura of the lower extremities is the main manifestation, present in up to 92% of patients.[14] Localization of the lesions on the head and mucosal surfaces (ears, nose, mouth) are observed more commonly in type I cryoglobulinemia. Seasonal triggering of the lesions is frequently reported.[14] Postinflammatory hyperpigmentation is noted in 40% and can retrospectively evoke the diagnosis. Infarction, hemorrhagic crusts, and ulcers are present in 10 to 25% of patients. Widespread necrotic areas are relatively more common in type I cryoglobulinemia than in other types. Histologically, purpura corresponds to a leukocytoclastic vasculitis of the small dermal vessels. Direct immunofluorescence studies have sometimes shown IgM, IgG, and C3 deposits in patients with acute vasculitis. In type I cryoglobulinemia, thrombosis is the main histological feature sometimes associated with vasculitis.

As HCV infection is the leading recognized cause of essential mixed cryoglobulinemia (especially type II), the influence of this infection on clinical presentation has been studied. Globally, the clinical and histologic aspects of purpura are not different regarding the presence of HCV infection. Nevertheless, in one series, necrotizing vasculitis was found to be a marker of chronic active hepatitis.[15] A correlation between the intensity of the cutaneous manifestations and the cryoglobulin levels has been observed.[16] Whether HCV is responsible for purpura by replicating inside the skin or via the cryoglobulin remains a matter of debate. Other cutaneous manifestations which could be related to the cryoglobulinemia, such as Raynaud's phenomenon, livedo reticularis, acral cyanosis, erythematous nodules, chronic nonhealing wounds, and cold urticaria are present in up to 50% of cases.[17]

C. POLYARTERITIS NODOSA

According to the names and definitions adopted by the Chapel Hill Consensus Conference on the Nomenclature of Systemic Vasculitis, classic polyarteritis nodosa (PAN) is characterized by a necrotizing inflammation of medium-sized or small arteries without glomerulonephritis or vasculitis in arterioles, capillaries, or venules.[18] Theoretically, the skin hallmarks of PAN are nodules. These cutaneous or subcutaneous nodules occur in groups along the course of superficial arteries. They measure 5 to 15 mm in diameter and are mainly localized on the lower legs, especially around the knees and on the feet (sometimes on the forearms). Livedo reticularis may precede or follow the onset of nodules; sometimes livedo and nodules occur together. Livedo reticularis in polyarteritis nodosa is typically suspended, localized on the lower limbs, the dorsal face of the upper limbs, and, rarely, on the trunk. The fishnet reticular pattern is irregular with broken circles, and some infiltrated areas are usually detected on careful examination. Painful ulcerations are frequently associated with tender indurated plaques resulting from the coalescence of nodules. Local rupture of superficial arteries may give rise to local intracutaneous hematoma or ecchymosis. Peripheral embolization of thrombi may cause infarction of the extremities (toes, fingers) or of skin areas. These clinical features are characteristic of cutaneous PAN, which, by definition, only affects small arteries of the skin. These chronic, benign, limited cutaneous forms of PAN are in fact frequently associated with arthralgias and sensitive neuropathy without motor deficiency. Systemic disease may rarely develop in such patients after 1 to 20 years.[19-21] So the spectrum of the disease is continuous, ranging from chronic cutaneous forms to acute systemic PAN, as is also encountered in lupus erythematosus. The transition from one end of the spectrum to the other is uncommon. Skin lesions occur in 15 to 60% of patients with systemic PAN;[22,23] they are less frequently observed in patients older than 65 years.[24] Although this systemic disease mainly affects the medium-sized arteries of the kidney, liver, heart, and gastrointestinal tract, the most common cutaneous finding is palpable purpura corresponding to small-vessel vasculitis.[25] Nodules (8 to 27%), ulcerations, and livedo are less frequent.[26] Other manifestations have been reported such as urticaria, transient erythema, superficial thrombophlebitis, Raynaud's phenomenon, and splinter hemorrhages. Localized edema is usually associated with underlying muscular involvement, and may precede the onset of peripheral neuropathy.

D. MICROSCOPIC POLYANGIITIS

The microscopic form of polyarteritis nodosa, now called microscopic polyangiitis (MPA), is defined as a systemic necrotizing vasculitis that clinically and histologically affects small-sized vessels (i.e., capillaries, venules, or arterioles) without granulomas. MPA is associated with segmental necrotizing glomerulonephritis and antineutrophil cytoplasm antibodies of the myeloperoxidase type. This systemic vasculitis does not differ significantly from the hypersensitivity vasculitis described by Zeek in 1948.[27] In fact, MPA is frequently difficult to distinguish from PAN, and in most series reported in the literature MPA was not identified as a separate entity. Thus, skin lesions of MPA have only been described in dermatological case reports.

Dermatologic manifestations occur in 30 to 58% of patients.[28,29] Purpuric lesions of the lower limbs are the most frequent skin manifestations. Other lesions have been reported such as mouth ulcers, vesicles, necrosis, ulcerations, nodules, splinter hemorrhages, and facial edema.[30] Leukocytoclastic vasculitis of dermal small vessels is usually observed. Sometimes, arterioles or smaller vessels of the deep dermis and subcutis are also involved by the vasculitis, which explains the nodular appearance of skin lesions. In one case vasculitis was associated with an eosinophilic panniculitis.[29] All these lesions disappear rapidly with treatment of MPA, but relapses are frequent. According to Gordon, the clinical manifestations at relapse are usually less severe than at initial presentation, with skin lesions and arthralgias as the main features.[31]

E. CHURG-STRAUSS SYNDROME

In 1951, Churg and Strauss defined allergic granulomatosis as a distinct entity occurring in adult patients with asthma and associated with fever, eosinophilia, multisystemic vasculitis, and extravascular granuloma.[1] Cutaneous lesions have been observed in 40 to 70% of cases, depending on the series.[2,32] They are rarely (6%) the presenting manifestations.[32] Palpable purpura on the lower extremities is the most frequently observed dermatologic manifestation; it is frequently necrotic. Cutaneous nodules or papules are also very frequent, localized on the lower limbs or on the extensor side of the elbows, the fingers, the scalp, and the breast. Lesions of the digits are usually multiple, often symmetrical, and most commonly localized at the distal interphalangeal joint. These nodules or papules of the upper limbs frequently have central crusting or ulceration. Their consistency is usually firm. A pustular or vesicular component is rarely noted. Various other dermatologic lesions have been reported: maculo-papules resembling erythema multiforme, ulcerations, livedo reticularis, patchy and migratory urticarial rashes, nailfold infarctions with splinter hemorrhages, and facial edema.[33]

Histologically, purpuric lesions usually correspond to leukocytoclastic or necrotizing vasculitis. Vasculitis affects not only small and medium-sized arteries, but also veins, which explains the frequency of skin necrosis. The inflammatory infiltrate is sometimes rich in eosinophils.[34] Nodules correspond to granulomatous vasculitis or necrotizing vasculitis of arterioles in the deep dermis or the subcutis (similar to those observed in PAN), or to extravascular granuloma. In fact, extravascular granuloma correlates with papules and nodules on the extensor surfaces of the elbows in the majority of patients. Nonspecific granulomata without necrosis may also be observed in the dermis or the subcutis. Finally, histologic findings of cutaneous lesions are often disappointing, as typical granuloma and eosinophilia are not detected in more than half of the patients with skin lesions. Skin lesions disappear rapidly under systemic steroid treatment, but additional immunosuppressive medications are often used to control the disease.[35,36]

F. WEGENER'S GRANULOMATOSIS

Wegener's granulomatosis is characterized by involvement of the upper airway, lung, and kidneys, although almost any organ may be affected. Skin lesions occur in 14 to 77% of cases, depending on the series.[37-39] They are noted at the initial presentation in about 10% of cases, exceptionally alone.[39,40] Palpable purpura of the lower extremities is undoubtedly the most frequently observed cutaneous lesion. Necrotic papules of the extensor surface of the limbs are less frequent but more suggestive of Wegener's granulomatosis. Exceptionally, they have the clinical features of erythema elevatum diutinum associated with IgA paraproteinemia. Nodules are quite frequent, mainly localized on the limbs. Extensive and painful cutaneous ulcerations may precede other systemic manifestations from some weeks to several years.[41] These ulcers are sometimes described as "pyoderma gangrenosum-like lesions," especially when resulting from the breakdown of painful nodules or pustules after a localized trauma. However, they usually lack the typical raised, tender, undermined border of pyoderma gangrenosum. Sometimes numerous, they are localized on the limbs, trunk, face (preauricular area), breasts, and perineum. On breasts, lesions may mimic adenocarcinoma with possible nipple retraction and galactorhea. Digital gangrenes are occasionally reported.[42] Florid xanthelasma is associated with longstanding granulomatous orbital and periorbital infiltration.[40,43] In contrast to PAN, livedo reticularis is unusual in Wegener's granulomatosis.

The frequency of oral manifestations is difficult to estimate from literature, as they are often included in ear-nose-throat symptoms and not described separately. Oral ulcers are sometimes reported independently of other oral manifestations. They are undoubtedly frequent, present in 10 to 50% of cases.[40,44-46] Contrary to aphthae, they are persistent and not recurrent. Their number and localization are highly variable. Hyperplastic gingivitis is rarely mentioned in the largest series. However, well-documented case reports have been published.[44] The gingiva is generally described as granular and red to purple with many petechiae. The entire gingiva and peri-odontium may be involved, resulting in tooth mobility and loss. Significant, although incomplete, improvement can be observed with empiric antimicrobial therapy. Genital ulcers are uncommon, although penile necrosis has been described.[47]

Purpuric papules correspond to leukocytoclastic vasculitis of small vessels; necrotic and purpuric lesions could result from necrotizing vasculitis of superficial and/or deep dermal and subcutaneous vessels. Other lesions are more frequently associated with granulomatous inflammation. Papules or papulonecrotic lesions correspond to leukocytoclastic or granulomatous vasculitis of small vessels or to extravascular granuloma. Nodules correspond to necrotizing or granulomatous vasculitis of medium-sized arterioles, or to extravascular granuloma. All of these lesions may evolve to ulceration with a secondary mixed inflammatory pattern. Histopathologic findings of oral ulcerations are often nonspecific, showing acute and chronic inflammation.[44] In other cases, a granulomatous infiltration is present.[40] Gingival hyperplasia corresponds to a chronic histiocytic inflammation with inconstant vasculitis, necrosis, and giant cells. Pseudoepitheliomatous hyperplasia and microabscesses with polymorphonuclear leukocytes and eosinophils are occasionally encountered.[48]

Whatever the type of clinical or pathological dermatologic lesions, all of them, except xanthelasma, are associated with active systemic disease. They disappear in a few weeks or months after treatment onset and are observed in about 50% of relapses. A significant association of dermatological lesions with articular and renal involvement was reported in one series.[40]

Since 1966, limited, i.e., without kidney involvement, and subacute forms of Wegener's granulomatosis have been individualized.[49-51] In our experience, the most frequently observed skin lesions in these forms are nodules with histologically a granulomatous infiltration or granulomatous vasculitis.

G. Behçet's Disease

In 1937, a Turkish dermatologist, Hulusi Behçet, described an entity associating oral aphthosis, genital aphthosis, and ocular inflammation. Since then, various other manifestations have been related to this disease, known as Behçet's disease. Dermatologic lesions are a cornerstone for the diagnosis.[52]

Complex aphthosis is the mucosal hallmark of this disease. Oral aphthae occur as the first manifestation in 25 to 75% of cases.[53] They are usually undistinguishable from ordinary aphthae. They form a painful ulceration 0.5 to 3 cm in diameter, shallow or deep, and have a yellow fibrinous base surrounded by erythema. Patients may have single or multiple ulcers which heal spontaneously without scarring after one to four weeks. Ulcers may also be herpetiform, with pinpoint lesions occurring in coalescing clusters. The usual affected sites are lips, gums, cheeks, and tongue and, less frequently, pharynx and palate. The frequency of the aphthae recurrence is highly variable. In the diagnostic criteria of the International Study Group on Behçet's disease, at least three recurrences a year are required.[52] Pathologic features are usually nonspecific, with rarely a lymphocytic or leukocytoclastic vasculitis.[54] Genital aphthae are present in 60 to 80% of cases. They are similar to oral aphthae but do not usually recur as often. In men, they are mainly localized on the scrotum with a permanent residual scar of great diagnostic value, and more rarely on the sheath or meatus. In women, the vulva is predominantly involved; aphthae resolve without scars. Ocular or perineal aphthae are rarely reported.[53]

Pseudo-folliculitis is the most frequent skin lesion, observed in 39 to 60% of cases.[55,56] It presents as nonfollicular erythematous papules which become pustular and may secondly resolve or ulcerate. They are mainly localized on the trunk, lower limbs, buttocks, and genitalia, but may occur on all parts of the body, even on palms and soles.[57] Histologically, there is an amicrobial neutrophilic infiltration with a lymphocytic infiltrate, and sometimes a leukocytoclastic vasculitis.[58-59] A nonbacterial folliculitis is also observed that is histologically undistinguishable from a bacterial folliculitis. Cutaneous aphthae are less frequent, mainly observed in the folds. Nodules are present in 30 to 40% of cases. Sometimes they look like erythema nodosum, localized on the anterior face of the lower limbs. They show histologically a septal or lobular panniculitis infiltration composed of lymphocytes, histiocytes, and neutrophils and, rarely, a lymphocytic or a leukocytoclastic vasculitis.[60,61] Sometimes these nodules correspond to a superficial thrombophlebitis.[62] In a few patients, tender erythematous papules and plaques resembling those of Sweet's syndrome may be present on the face and neck.[63] Pyoderma gangrenosum-like lesions have also been reported in some cases.[64,65] The association with gastrointestinal involvement raises the difficult problem of the differential diagnosis with distinct inflammatory enterocolitis. Other manifestations have been occasionally described: livedo reticularis, purpuric lesions, and erythema multiforme-like lesions.[66]

The pathergy test is an induced cutaneous reaction resembling pseudo-folliculitis. When a needle pricks the skin or injects saline, an erythematous papule or pustule develops within 24 to 48 hours. Pathergy is a characteristic response in Turkish, Israeli, French, and Japanese patients with Behçet's disease, but is uncommon in North American and British patients.[67,68] The use of needles of large diameter with blunt points seems to increase the sensitivity of this test.[69] Histologically, a lymphocytic and neutrophilic dermal infiltration has been observed in the first 24 hours. Vasculitis is rare.[70] Vessel-wall immunoglobulins and/or complement deposits may be objectivated using direct immunofluorescence techniques.[71]

H. TAKAYASU'S ARTERITIS

Takayasu's arteritis is a rare, chronic inflammatory arteriopathy of unknown origin that predominantly affects the aorta, its main branches, and the pulmonary arteries. Histologically, the disease is characterized by inflammation of the media and adventitial layers of the large vessel-walls, resulting in vascular stenosis and/or aneurysm formation. Two stages have been distinguished which may overlap: a systemic inflammatory stage followed by an occlusive one.

Cutaneous manifestations have been reported in 2.8 to 28% of patients.[72] Some of them are directly related to large vessel occlusions such as unilateral Raynaud's phenomenon, digital gangrenes, or unilateral digital clubbing.[73,74] Other skin manifestations are thought to be related to the systemic vasculitis, i.e., ulcerated or nonulcerated nodules of the lower limbs, pyoderma gangrenosum,[75] livedo reticularis,[76,77] papular or papulonecrotic lesions,[78] superficial thrombophlebitis, and Sweet's lesions.[79] Various manifestations are occasionally reported without evident relationship with Takayasu's arteritis: urticaria, angioedema, erythema multiforme, erythematous eruptions, and " dermatitis."[76,77,80] The prevalence of these different skin lesions greatly varies between Asian and European countries.

In Northern America and Europe, acute or subacute inflammatory nodules are the most commonly observed skin lesions. Erythema induratum corresponds to ulcerated subacute nodular lesions. The histological features of these nodules are variable. They may correspond to granulomatous or necrotizing vasculitis of small-sized or medium-sized arterioles of the dermis or subcutis, extravascular granuloma, or septal or lobular panniculitis.[73,76] Usually there is no correlation between the localization of the nodules and any involvement of large vessels revealed by angiography.[75] Furthermore, these nodules can occur at any stage of the disease. Tuberculoid infiltration has been reported in biopsies from papular or papulonecrotic lesions, raising the problem of the possible infectious origin of TA. Such lesions mainly occur at the occlusive stage of the disease.

In Japan, pyoderma gangrenosum-like lesions are frequent, especially at the occlusive stage;[75] this type of lesion has also been reported in patients from northern Africa.[81]

The relationship between dermatologic manifestations and Takayasu's arteritis is established on the lack of other etiology for skin lesions and on a parallel course of skin lesions and large vessel vasculitis. Whatever the stage of the disease, the recurrence of skin lesions is strongly suggestive of a persistant activity of Takayasu's arteritis.[82]

I. Giant-Cell Arteritis

Giant-cell arteritis (GCA) is a systemic vasculitis which predominantly affects small- to medium-sized cranial arteries in elderly patients. Dermatologic manifestations are mainly observed in the late stages of the disease. Nowadays, they tend to be rare due to an early diagnosis.

Classically, the scalp and temples are tender and red, with tender nodules palpable over the temporal, occipital, or facial arteries. Pulsations in these arteries are diminished or absent. Exceptionally, multiple scalp aneurysms have been reported.[83]

The majority of other dermatologic lesions are the consequence of ischemia related to cranial artery occlusion and are localized, especially on the tongue and the scalp. Glossitis occurs in 10% of patients, and may sometimes reveal the disease.[84-86] The tongue has a red, raw-beef color and becomes blistered, desquamated, or gangrenous. Necrosis may occur and usually affects the anterior two-thirds. Bullae, ulcers, or massive necrosis may be present on the scalp. Those patients with scalp necrosis constitute a subgroup of severe GCA with older age of onset and frequent serious complications such as visual loss, gangrene of the tongue, or nasal septum necrosis. The mean interval between the onset of symptoms of GCA and scalp necrosis is three months. Under treatment, scalp healing is complete or satisfactory in 75% of cases.[87] In other cases, skin grafts provide satisfactory results. Less severe chronic ischemia of the scalp leads to thinning or loss of hair. Ischemic skin lesions of the neck or the cheeks are occasionally reported.[88] Rarely, vessels of the lower or upper limbs are involved by the vasculitis, leading to ischemic ulcerations or distal gangrene.[89,90] Skin biopsies of the borders of ulcerations or necrotic tissues are rarely contributive since granulomatous vasculitis has been shown in only 2 of 24 biopsies from patients with scalp necrosis.[87] Other dermatologic manifestations have been mentioned in case reports: nodules of the lower limbs with granulomatous vasculitis in the subcutis or septal panniculitis, and butterfly rash with transient edema.[91,92] Purpura due to vasculitis is exceptional in GCA. In contrast, senile purpura is frequent on exposed skin areas in elderly patients, especially when treated with corticosteroids.

In conclusion, dermatologic lesions are frequent in many systemic vasculitis. The most usual cutaneous lesion is palpable purpura, which allows confirmation of the vasculitis on pathological grounds, but is not contributive to determine its type. A histological examination of all other skin lesions is necessary. There is no correlation between the size of involved vessels and the type of the perivascular infiltrate observed in the skin.

REFERENCES

1. Churg, J., Strauss, L., Allergic granulomatosis, allergic angiitis and periarteritis nodosa, *Am. J. Pathol.*, 27, 277, 1951.
2. Crotty, C. P., Deremee, R. A., Winkelmann, R. K., Cutaneous clinicopathologic correlation of allergic granulomatosis, *J. Am. Acad. Dermatol.*, 5, 571, 1981.
3. Maricq, H. R., Prevalence of Raynaud's phenomenon in the general population, *J. Chronic Dis.*, 39, 423, 1986.
4. Olsen, N., Nielsen, S. L., Prevalence of primary Raynaud's phenomenon in young females, *Scand. J. Clin. Lab. Invest.*, 37, 71, 1977.
5. Nussinovitch, M., Prais, D., Finkelstein, Y., Varsano, I., Cutaneous manifestations of Henoch-Schonlein purpura in young children, *Pediatric Dermatology*, 15, 426, 1998.

6. Legrain, V., Lejean, S., Taieb, A., Infantile acute hemorrhagic edema of the skin: study of ten cases, *J. Am. Acad. Dermatol.*, 24, 17, 1991.

7. Saraclair, Y., Tinaztepe, K., Adalioglou, G., Tunger, A., Acute hemorrhagic edema of infancy (AHEI)-a variant of Henoch-Schonlein purpura or a distinct clinical entity, *J. Allergy Clin. Immunol.*, 86, 473, 1990.

8. Tancrede-Bohin, E., Ochonisky, S., Vignon-Pennamen, M. D., Flageul, B., Morel, P., Rybojad M., Schönlein-Henoch purpura in adults patients, *Arch. Dermatol.*, 133, 438, 1997.

9. Beaufils, H., Baumelou, A., *Traité de Médecine*, Godeau, P., Herson, S., Piette, J. C., editors, Masson, Paris, 1996.

10. Piette W. W., What is Schönlein-Henoch purpura and why should we care?, *Arch. Dermatol.*, 133, 515, 1997.

11. Brouet, J. C., Clauvel, J. P., Danon, F., Klein, M., Seligmann, M., Biological and clinical significance of cryoglobulins: a report of 86 cases, *Am. J. Med.*, 57, 775, 1974.

12. Gorevic, P. D., Kassab, H. J., Levoy, L., Mixed cryoglobulinemia: clinical aspects and long term follow-up of 40 patients, *Am. J. Med.*, 69, 287, 1980.

13. Davies, M., Su, W. P. D., Cryoglobulonemia: recent findings in cutaneous and extracutaneous manifestations, *Int. J. Dermatol.*, 4, 240, 1996.

14. Lotti, T., Comacchi, M., Ghersetich, I., Jorizzo, J. L., Cutaneous necrotizing vasculitis, *Int. J. Dermatol.*, 35, 457, 1996.

15. Daoud, M. S., Rokea, A. A., Gibson, L. E., Chronic hepatitis C, cryoglobulinemia, and cutaneous necrotizing vasculitis, *J. Am. Acad. Dermatol.*, 34, 219, 1996.

16. Dupin, N., Chosidow, O., Lunel, F., Cacoub, P., Musset, L., Cresta, P., Frangeul, L., Piette, J. C., Godeau, P., Opolon, P., Francès, C., Essential mixed cryoglobulinemia: a comparative study of dermatologic manifestations in patients infected or noninfected with hepatitis C virus, *Arch. Dermatol.*, 131, 1124, 1995.

17. Cohen, S. J., Pittlekow, M. R., Su, W. D. P., Cutaneous manifestations of cryoglobulinemia: clinical and histopathologic study of 72 patients, *J. Am. Acad. Dermatol.*, 25, 21, 1991.

18. Jennette, J. C., Falk, R. J., Andrassy, K., Nomenclature of systemic vasculitides. Proposal of an international consensus conference, *Arthritis Rheum.*, 37, 187, 1994.

19. Diaz-Perez J. L., Winkelmann, R. K., Cutaneous periarteritis nodosa. A study of 33 cases, *Major. Probl. Dermatol.*, 10, 273, 1980.

20. Minkowitz, G., Smoller, B. R., Mcnutt N. S., Benign cutaneous periarteritis nodosa. Relationship to systemic periarteritis nodosa and to hepatitis B infection, *Arch. Dermatol.*, 127, 1520, 1991.

21. Daoud, M. S., Hutton, K. P., Gibson, L. E., Cutaneous periarteritis nodosa: a clinicopathological study of 79 cases, *Br. J. Dermatol.*, 136, 706, 1997.

22. Guillevin, L., Fechner, J., Godeau, P., Bletry, O., Wechsler, B., Herreman, G., Herson, S., Périartérite noueuse: étude clinique et thérapeutique de 126 malades étudiés en 23 ans, *Ann. Med. Interne* (Paris), 136, 6, 1985.

23. Thomas, R. H. M., Black, M. M., The wide clinical spectrum of cutaneous periarteritis nodosa with cutaneous involvement, *Clin. Exp. Dermatol.*, 8, 47, 1983.

24. Puisieux, F., Woestland, H., Hachulla, E., Hatron, Y., Dewailly, P., Devulder, B., Symptomatologie clinique et pronostic de la périartérite noueuse du sujet âgé. Etude rétrospective de 25 périartérites noueuses de l'adulte jeune et de 22 périartérites noueuses du sujet âgé, *Rev. Med. Interne* (Paris), 18, 195, 1997.

25. Cohen, R. D., Conn, D. L., Ilstrup, D. M., Clinical features, prognosis and response to treatment in polyarteritis, *Mayo Clin. Proc.*, 55, 146, 1980.

26. Leib, E. S., Restivo, C., Paulus, H. E., Immunosuppressive and corticosteroid therapy of polyarteritis nodosa, *Am. J. Med.*, 67, 94, 1979.

27. Zeek, P. M., Smith, C. C., Weeter J. C., Studies on periarteritis nodosa. The differentiation between the vascular lesions of periarteritis nodosa and hypersensitivity, *Am. J. Pathol.*, 24, 889, 1948.

28. Penas, P. F., Porras, I. J., Fraga, J., Bernis, C., Sarria, C., Dauden, E., Microscopic polyangiitis. A systemic vasculitis with p-ANCA, *Br. J. Dermatol.*, 134, 54, 1996.

29. Lhote, F., Cohen, P., Genereau, T., Gayraud, M., Guillevin, L., Microscopic polyangiitis: clinical aspects and treatment, *Ann. Med. Interne* (Paris), 147, 165, 1996.

30. Homas, P. B., David-Bajar, K. M., Fitzpatrick, J. E., West, S. G., Tribelhorn, D. R., Microscopic polyarteritis. Report of a case with cutaneous involvement and antimyeloperoxidase antibodies, *Arch. Dermatol.*, 128, 1223, 1992.

31. Gordon, M., Luqmani, R. A., Adu, D., Greaves, I., Richards, N., Michael, J., Emery, P., Howie, A. J., Bacon, P. A., Relapses patients with a systemic vasculitis, *Q. J. Med.*, 86, 779, 1993.

32. Davis, M. P. D., Daoud, M. S., Moevoy, M. T., Su, W. P. D., Cutaneous manifestations of Churg-Strauss syndrome: a clinicopathologic correlation, *J. Am. Acad. Dermatol.*, 37, 199, 1997.

33. Schwarz, R. A., Churg, J., Churg-Strauss syndrome, *Br. J. Dermatol.*, 127, 199, 1992. Chen, K. R., Eosinophilic vasculitis in connective disease, *J. Am. Acad. Dermatol.*, 35, 173, 1996.

34. Guillevin, L., Cohen, P., Gayraud, M., Lhote, F., Jarousse, B., Casassus, P., Churg-Strauss syndrome. Clinical study and long term follow-up of 96 patients, *Medicine*, 78, 26, 1999.

35. Guillevin, L., Fain, O., Lhote, F., Lack of superiority of steroids plus plasma exchanges to steroids alone in the treatment of polyarteritis nodosa and Churg-Strauss syndrome: a prospective, randomized trial in 78 patients, *Arthritis Rheum.*, 35, 208, 1992.

36. Finan, M. C., Winkelman, R. K., The cutaneous extravascular necrotizing granuloma and systemic diseases, *Medicine,* 62, 142, 1983.

37. Daoud, M. S., Gibson, L. E., De Remee, R. A., Specks, U., El-Azhari, R. A., Su, W. P. D., Cutaneous Wegener granulomatosis: clinical, histopathologic and immunopathologic findings of thirty patients, *J. Am. Acad. Dermatol.*, 31, 605, 1994.

38. Brandwein, S., Esdaile, J., Danoff, D., Tannenbaum, H., Wegener granulomatosis. Clinical features and outcome in 13 patients, *Arch. Intern. Med.*, 143, 476, 1983.

39. Hoffman, G. S., Kerr, G. S., Leavitt, R. Y., Hallahan, C. W., Wegener granulomatosis: an analysis of 158 patients, *Ann. Intern. Med.*, 116, 488, 1992.

40. Frances, C., Du, L. T., Piette, J. C., Saada, V., Boisnic, S., Wechsler, B., Bletry, O., Godeau, P., Wegener's granulomatosis. Dermatological manifestations in 75 cases with clinicopathologic correlation, *Arch Dermatol.*, 130, 86, 1994.

41. Hanfield-Jones, S. E., Parker, S. C., Fenton, D. A., Nexton, J. A., Greaves, M. W., Wegener's granulomatosis presenting as pyoderma gangrenosum, *Clin. Exp. Dermatol.*, 17, 197, 1992.

42. Handa, R., Wali, J. P., Wegener's granulomatosis with gangrena of toes, *Scand. J. Rheumatol.*, 25, 103, 1996.

43. Tullo, A. B., Durrington, P., Graham, E., Holt, L. P., Easty, D. L., Bonsher, R., Florid xanthelasma (yellow lids) in orbital Wegener's granulomatosis, *Br. J. Dermatol.*, 79, 453, 1995.

44. Patten, S. F., Tomecki, K. J., Wegener's granulomatosis: cutaneous and oral mucosal disease, *J. Am. Acad. Dermatol.,* 28, 710, 1993.

45. D'cruz, D. P., Baguley, E., Asherson, R. A., Hughes, G. R. V., Ear, nose, and throat symptoms in subacute Wegener's granulomatosis, *Br. Med. J.*, 299, 419, 1989.

46. Mc Donald, T. J., De Remee, R. A., Wegener granulomatosis, *Laryngoscope*, 93, 220, 1983.

47. Matsuda, S., Mitsukawa, S., Ishii, N., Shirai, M., A case of Wegener's granulomatosis with necrosis of the penis, *Tohoku J. Exp. Med.*, 118, 145, 1976.

48. Handlers, P., Waterman, J., Abrams, A. M., Melrose, R. J., Oral features of Wegener's granulomatosis, *Arch. Otolaryngol.,* 111, 267, 1985.

49. Carrington, C. B., Liebow, A. A., Limited forms of angiitis and granulomatosis of Wegener's type, *Am. J. Med.*, 41, 497, 1966.

50. Gibson, L. E., Daoud, M. S., Muller, S. A., Perry, A. O., Malignant pyoderma revisited, *Mayo Clin. Proc.*, 72, 734, 1997.

51. Trueb, R. M., Pericin, M., Kohler, E., Barandun, J., Burg, G., Necrotizing granulomatosis of the breast, *Br. J. Dermatol.*, 137, 799, 1997.

52. International Study group for Behçet's disease, Criteria for diagnosis of Behçet's disease, *Lancet,* 335, 1078, 1990.

53. Chams, C., Mansoori, P., Shahram, F., Akbarian, M., Gharibdoost, F., Davatchi, F., Iconography of mucocutaneous lesions of Behçet's disease, in *Behçet's Disease*, Wechsler, B., and Godeau, P., Eds., Elsevier Science Publishers BV, Amsterdam, 1993.

54. Mangelsdorf, H. C., White, W. L., Jorizzo, J. L., Behçet's disease, Report of 25 patients from the United States with prominent mucocutaneous involvement, *J. Am. Acad. Dermatol.*, 34, 745, 1996.

55. Arbeesfeld, S. J., Kurban, A. K., Behçet's disease. New perspectives on an enigmatic syndrome, *J. Am. Acad. Dermatol.,* 19, 767, 1988.

56. Homma, T., Saito, T., Fujioka, Y., Intraepithelial atypical lymphocytes in oral lesions of Behçet's syndrome, *Arch. Dermatol.,* 117, 83, 1981.

57. Alpsoy, E., Aktekin, M., Er, H., Durusoy, C., Yilmaz, E., A randomized, controlled and blinded study of papulopustular lesions in Turkish Behcet's patients, *Int. J. Dermatol.,* 37, 839, 1998.

58. Ergun, T., Gurbuz, O., Dogusoy, G., Mat, C., Yazici, H., Histopathologic features of the spontaneous pustular lesions of Behcet's disease, *Int. J. Dermatol.,* 37, 194, 1998.

59. Magro, C. M., Crowson, A. M., Sterile neutrophilic folliculitis with perifollicular vasculopathy: a distinctive cutaneous reaction pattern reflecting systemic disease, *J. Cut. Pathol.,* 25, 215, 1998.

60. Chen, K. R., Kawahara, Y., Miyakawa, S., Nishikawa, T., Cutaneous vasculitis in Behçet's disease: a clinical and histological studies in 20 patients, *J. Am. Acad. Dermatol.,* 36, 689, 1997.

61. Ghate, J. V., Jorizzo, J. L., Behçet's disease and complex aphthosis, *J. Am. Acad. Dermatol.,* 40, 1, 1999.

62. Senturk, T., Aydintug, O., Kuzu, I., Tokgoz, G., Gurler, A., Tulunay, O., Adhesion molecule expression in erythema nodosum-like lesions in Behçet's disease. A histopathological and immunohistochemical study, *Rheumatol. Int.,* 18, 51, 1998.

63. Lee, E. S., Lee, S. H., Bang, D., Lee, S., Sweet's syndrome-like skin lesions in Behçet's syndrome: an additional cutaneous manifestation, in *Behçet's Disease: Basic and Clinical Aspects,* O'Duffy, J. D. and Kokmen, E., Eds., Marcel Dekker, Inc, New York, 1991.

64. Rustin, M. H. A., Gilkes, J. J. H., Robinson, T. W. E., Pyoderma gangrenosum associated with Behçet's disease; treatment with thalidomide, *Arch. Dermatol.,* 23, 941, 1990.

65. Armas, J. B., Davies, J., Davis, M., Lovell, C., Mchugh, N., Atypical Behçet's disease with peripheral erosive arthropathy and pyoderma gangrenosum, *Clin. Exp. Dermatol.,* 10, 177, 1992.

66. Cantini, F., Salvarini, C., Niccoli, L., Sene, S. I. C., Truglia, M. C., Padula, A., Olivieri, I., Behçet's disease with unusual cutaneous lesions, *J. Rheumatol.,* 25, 2469, 1998.

67. Friedman-Birnbaum, R., Bergman, R., Aizen, E., Sensitivity and specificity of pathergy test results in Israeli patients with Behçet's disease, *Cutis,* 45, 261, 1990.

68. Gilhar, A., Winterstein, G., Turani, H., Landau, J., Etzioni, A., Skin hyperreactivity response (pathergy) in Behçet's disease, *J. Am. Acad. Dermatol.,* 21, 547, 1989.

69. Dilsen, N., Koniçe, M., Aral, O., Inanç, M., Gül, A., Comparative study of the skin pathergy test with blunt and sharp needles in Behçet's disease comfirmed specificity but decreased sensitivity with sharp needles, *Ann. Rheum. Dis.,* 52, 823, 1993.

70. Ergun, T., Gurbuz, O., Harvell, J., Jorizzo, J., White, W., The histopathology of pathergy: a chronologic study of skin hyperreactivity in Behcet's disease, *Int. J. Dermatol.,* 37, 929, 1998.

71. Wechsler, J., Wechsler, B., Revuz, J., Godeau, P., Skin hyperreactivity response (pathergy) in Behçet's disease. Useful of direct immunofluorescence, *J. Am. Acad. Dermatol.,* 23, 329, 1990.

72. Shelhamer, J. H., Vockman, D. J., Parrillo, J. E., Takayasu's arteritis and its therapy, *Ann. Intern. Med.,* 103, 121, 1985.

73. Francès, C., Boisnic, S., Blétry, O., Cutaneous manifestations of Takayasu arteritis, *Dermatologica,* 181, 266, 1990.

74. Kaditis, A. G., Nelson, A. M., Driscoll, D. J., Takayasu's arteritis presenting with unilateral digital clubbing, *J. Rheumatol.,* 22, 2346, 1995.

75. Hidano, A., Watanabe, K., Pyoderma gangrenosum et cardiovasculopathies en particulier artérite de takayasu, *Ann. Dermatol. Venereol.,* 108, 13, 1981.

76. Perniciaro, C. V., Winkelmann, R. K., Hunder, G. G., Cutaneous manifestations of Takayasu arteritis. A clinicopathologic correlation, *J. Am. Acad. Dermatol.,* 17, 998, 1987.

77. Mousa, A. R. M., Marafie, A. A., Dajani, A., Cutaneous necrotizing vasculitis complicating Takayasu arteritis with a review of cutaneous manifestations, *J. Rheumatol.,* 12, 607, 1985.

78. Amblard, P., Reymond, J. L., Beani, J. C., Perillat, Y., Association maladie de Takayasu et tuberculides papulonecrotiques, *Nouv. Dermatol.,* 6, 502, 1987.

79. Nakayama, H., Shimao, S., Hamamoto, T., Munemura, C., Nakai, A., Neutrophilic dermatosis of the face associated with aortitis syndrome and Hashimoto's thyroiditis, *Acta Dermatol. Venereol.,* 73, 380, 1993.

80. Werfel, T., Kuipers, J. G., Zeidler, H., Kapp, A., Kiehl, P., Cutaneous manifestations of Takayasu arteritis, *Acta Derm. Venereol.,* 76, 496, 1996.

81. Land, A., Bard, R., Rossi, P., Takayasu's arteritis: a worldwide entity, *NY State J. Med.*, 76, 1477, 1976.

82. Ryan, J. T., *Textbook of Dermatology,* Blackwell Scientific Publications, Rook, A., Wilkinson, D. S., Ebling, F. J. G., editors, Oxford, 1992.

83. Yoshimoto, T., Kobayashi, H., Murai, H., Echizenya, K., Satoh, M., Multiple scalp aneurysms caused by atypical temporal arteritis: case report, *Neurol. Med. Chir.* (Tokyo), 38, 405, 1998.

84. Kinmont, P. D. C., Mc Callum, D. I., Skin manifestations of giant cell arteritis, *Br. J. Dermatol.,* 76, 299, 1964.

85. Ekenstam, E., Callen, J. P., Cutaneous leukocytoclastic vasculitis: clinical and laboratory features of 82 patients seen in private practice, *Arch. Dermatol.*, 120, 484, 1984.

86. Lotti, T., Ghersetich, I., Comacchi, C., Jorizzo, J. L., Cutaneous small vessel vasculitis, *J. Am. Acad. Dermatol.*, 39, 667, 1998.

87. Currey, J., Scalp necrosis in giant cell arteritis and review of the literature, *Br. J. Rheumatol.*, 36, 814, 1997.

88. Hansen, B. L., Junker, P., Giant cell arteritis presenting with ischaemic skin lesions of the neck, *Br. J. Rheumatol.*, 34, 1182, 1995.

89. Greene, G. M., Lain, D., Sherwin, R. M., Wilson, J. E., McManus, B. M., Giant cell arteritis of the legs. Clinical isolation of severe disease with gangrene and amputations, *Am. J. Med.*, 81, 727, 1986.

90. DeGennes, C., Le Thi Huong, D., Wechsler, B., Bercy, J., Foncin, J. F., Piette, J. C., Godeau, P., Temporal arteritis revealed by upper limb gangrene, *J. Rheumatol.*, 16, 130, 1989.

91. Goldberg, J. W., Lee, M. L., Sajjad, S. M., Giant cell arteritis of the skin simulating erythema nodosum, *Ann. Rheum. Dis.*, 46, 706, 1987.

92. Barriere, H., Barrier, J., Dreno, B., Renaut, J. J., Erythema nodosum disclosing Horton's disease (three cases), *Ann. Dermatol. Venereol.*, 114, 71, 1987.

Section III

Treatment

31 Pharmacological Treatments for Thrombotic Diseases

*Joan-Carles Reverter, Dolors Tàssies,
and Gerard Espinosa*

CONTENTS

There are several groups of pharmacological treatments for the hemostasis-related complications of vascular diseases. In this chapter we will describe the most important of these treatments considered in the following categories: heparin and low-molecular-weight heparins, oral anticoagulants, antiplatelet agents, fibrinolytics, and eicosanoids. We will give an overview of the general characteristics of these treatments referred as the medical therapy of vascular diseases in the appropriate chapters of this book.

I. HEPARIN AND LOW-MOLECULAR-WEIGHT HEPARINS

Heparin and its derivative low-molecular-weight heparins are the anticoagulants of choice when a rapid anticoagulation effect is required.[1] Heparin is a physiological anticoagulant introduced early in clinical human therapeutics.[1] It is usually employed only in the initial phases of treatment or during in-hospital settings due to its pharmacodynamic characteristics that require frequent dose monitoring. When long-term treatments are required, heparin is usually replaced by oral anticoagulants, antiplatelet agents, or low-molecular-weight heparins.[1]

A. CHEMICAL STRUCTURE

Heparins are defined as a family of glycosaminoglycans of natural origin, with a mean molecular weight of 10 to 15 KDa[2-5] composed of a mixture of chains with a wide range of molecular weights (5 to 30 KDa). Natural heparin (also known as unfractionated heparin) is composed of chains of alternating molecules of D-glucosamine and uronic acid with a variable number of sulphate residues.[2-5] Heparin is synthesized by tissular mast cells and is mainly obtained from the intestinal or the pulmonary mucosae, but is widely distributed in other organs such as the liver or the skin.[2] Commercial heparins are usually obtained from porcine or bovine intestinal mucosae.

Low-molecular-weight heparins are derived from unfractionated heparin. They are a heterogeneous family of glycosaminoglycans obtained after industrial manipulation of natural heparin. To obtain low-molecular-weight heparins, heparin is gel-filtrated or extracted with solvents, and then glycosaminoglycans are chemically or enzymatically depolymerized to obtain molecular mixtures of chains ranging from 5 to 30 monosaccharides, with a molecular weight ranging from 1.5 to 9 KDa.[2]

B. Mechanisms of Action

The anticoagulant effect of heparins (unfractionated heparin or low-molecular-weight-heparins) is mediated largely through their interaction with antithrombin III. Heparin, through a pentasaccharide sequence, binds to the lysine residues on antithrombin III, inducing a conformational change in its active site.[2-5] This change accelerates the ability of antithrombin III to inactivate the activated coagulation factors, mainly thrombin (factor IIa) and factor Xa.[2-6] Once the complex antithrombin III/activated factor is formed, heparin is liberated and is then capable of reinitiating the process.[2] Approximately 30 to 50% of heparin chains have the pentasaccharide sequence. Heparin chains without the pentasaccharide sequence, but longer than 24 monosaccharides, can catalyze the inactivation of thrombin by the heparin cofactor II.[5] Moreover, heparin promotes the release of the tissue factor pathway inhibitor from its cellular membranes pool, contributing to the anticoagulant effect through the inhibition of factor VIIa/tissue factor complexes.[5]

Factor Xa and thrombin are inhibited by antithrombin III/heparin in a different degree, explaining some of the differences between unfractionated heparin and low-molecular-weight-heparins.[2,3,5] Since a minimum chain length of 18 saccharides (including the pentasaccharide sequence) is required for heparin/antithrombin III/activated factor ternary complex formation, heparin molecules containing fewer than 18 monosaccharides are unable to accelerate the inactivation of thrombin, but retain the ability to catalyze the inhibition of factor Xa that does not need the simultaneous binding of heparin to Xa and antithrombin III.[2,3,5] Then, low-molecular-weight-heparins may catalyze factor Xa inhibition more efficiently than the thrombin inhibition.[2,3,5] The lower the molecular weight of heparin, the lower the capability of catalyzing the neutralization of thrombin.

In addition to the anticoagulant effect, heparin has other actions such as platelet function inhibition, increase of vascular wall permeability (more evident for unfractionated heparin), and inhibition of smooth muscle cell proliferation.[2,4,5]

C. Pharmacodynamics

Unfractionated heparin and low-molecular-weight heparins have different biodisponibilities, protein binding capacities, and excretion and neutralization properties.[2,5,7-10] Unfractionated heparin is eliminated by two mechanisms: a saturable mechanism (supported by macrophages and endothelial cells) and a nonsaturable mechanism (renal excretion).[2,5] In the nonsaturable mechanism the amount of heparin eliminated is always proportional to the doses of heparin administered.[2,5,9] In the saturable mechanism the amount of heparin eliminated achieves a maximum at high doses.[7,9] Low doses of unfractionated heparin are eliminated mainly by the saturable mechanism, while higher doses are eliminated by the nonsaturable mechanism.[2,5] On the other hand, low-molecular-weight heparins that show lower affinity for the endothelial cells than unfractionated heparin are mainly eliminated by the nonsaturable mechanism, either at low or high doses.[2,5] Thus, after intravenous administration of low-molecular-weight heparins the disappearance of the inhibitory activity of factor Xa shows a half-life of 2 to 4 hours, while in unfractionated heparin the half-life is 45 to 60 minutes.[5,9]

The subcutaneous biodisponibility of unfractionated heparin is around 30%, while for low-molecular-weight heparins it is nearly 100%.[7] The excellent subcutaneous biodisponibility and the long half-life of low-molecular-weight heparins have allowed the introduction of treatment schedules with subcutaneous administration once or twice a day, and low-molecular-weight heparins are administered almost exclusively subcutaneously.

Renal failure modifies the excretion of unfractionated heparin and low-molecular-weight heparins to different extents.[9] The pharmacokinetics of unfractionated heparin are only modified by renal insufficiency at higher doses.[9] However, the excretion of low-molecular-weight heparins in renal insufficiency is substantially reduced and the half-life prolonged either at low or high doses,[2] having greater potential risk of accumulation than unfractionated heparin in kidney diseases.[2]

Unfractionated heparin is able to bind to some plasma proteins such as histidine-rich glyco-protein, fibronectin, vitronectin, lipoproteins, and von Willebrand factor; low-molecular-weight heparins only bind to vitronectin.[2,5,10] As protein binding contributes to the neutralization of the anticoagulant action of heparins,[2,10] the reduced nonspecific binding to plasma proteins of low-molecular-weight heparins is associated with an improvement of the predictability of their dose-response relationship.

The effect of unfractionated heparin and low-molecular-weight heparins on platelet function is under discussion.[5,11,12] Platelet factor 4 contained in platelet alpha granules and released during the coagulation process is a potent inhibitor of unfractionated heparin but inhibits to a lesser extent low-molecular-weight heparins.[13] In addition, factor Xa bound to platelet surfaces is not accessible to unfractionated heparin but can be inhibited by low-molecular-weight heparins.[4,14] Therefore, low-molecular-weight-heparins may be more efficient anticoagulants than unfractionated heparin in the presence of a high number of platelets.

The anticoagulant effect of unfractionated heparin is usually monitored by the activated partial thromboplastin test (or APTT) that is sensitive to the inhibitory effects of heparin in factor Xa, factor IXa, and thrombin.[1] However, the correlation between APTT and heparin concentration is not very good because APTT only reflects 40% of the actual variation of plasma heparin levels, but it continues to be the most useful test for monitoring unfractionated heparin.[1] The recommended therapeutic range of APTT derives from an original study performed in rabbits[15] which demonstrated prevention of thrombus extent when APTT ratios were above 1.5 (equivalent to 0.2 U/mL of heparin or 0.3 U/mL of anti-factor Xa activity). However, different commercially available APTT reagents have different responsiveness to similar doses of heparin, and technical variables such as the type of clot detection method, patients' characteristics, or the level of factor VIII can cause great variability.[1] For these reasons, the therapeutic range of unfractionated heparin needs to be recali-brated in each laboratory in order to be equivalent to 0.2 to 0.4 U/mL of heparin, or 0.3 to 0.6 U/mL of anti-factor Xa activity.[1]

Low-molecular-weight heparins, due to their very good biodisponibility and predictable effect, do not need laboratory monitorization.[16,17] Only in high-risk patients, such as renal insufficiency patients or pregnant women, low-molecular-weight heparins should be monitored using anti-factor Xa plasma levels (therapeutic range 0.3 to 0.7 U/mL).[16]

D. Clinical Uses

Heparin is a very effective drug and is indicated for the following clinical uses: prevention of venous thromboembolism during surgery or immobilization, prevention of thrombosis in patients under cardiac bypass or hemodialysis, prevention of thrombosis in patients who have vascular surgery, prevention of thrombosis during and after coronary angioplasty, prevention of thrombosis in patients with coronary stents, prevention of systemic embolism in patients with mechanical heart valves in whom warfarin needs to be temporarily discontinued, treatment of venous thromboem-bolism, and early treatment of patients with unstable angina or myocardial infarction. Low-molec-ular-weight heparins can be used for most of the indications of unfractionated heparin, and have advantages over unfractionated heparin in some of them.

1. Prevention of Venous Thromboembolism during Surgery or Immobilization

Unfractionated heparin and low-molecular-weight heparins are frequently used in the prevention of venous thromboembolism in immobilized patients (by surgical or medical causes) and during surgery. In most of these situations low-molecular-weight heparins have replaced unfractionated heparin due to their easy administration and better results.[17] In the following section we will analyze the use of unfractionated heparin and low-molecular-weight heparins in prevention of venous thromboembolism during general surgery, during orthopedic surgery, and in patients immobilized for medical causes.

a. Prevention of venous thromboembolism during general surgery

Deep venous thrombosis is frequent in patients undergoing general surgery, ranging from 0.5% in low-risk patients to more than 20% in high-risk patients (older than 40 years and previous thrombosis, open urological surgery, and gynecological or oncological surgery).[18] Several studies have demonstrated that low doses of unfractionated heparin are useful in preventing thromboembolic disease in surgery patients with moderate or high thrombotic risk.[2,3,5,18] Low-molecular-weight heparins have been recently introduced in this indication and they present a slightly better efficacy and lower risk of bleeding than unfractionated heparin.[2,3,5,18] These facts, together with the possibility of the administration of low-molecular-weight heparins once a day subcutaneously, explain the extension of their use in this indication. Unfractionated heparin and low-molecular-weight heparins prophylaxis needs to be started before the surgical procedure.[18]

b. Prevention of venous thromboembolism during orthopedic surgery

In orthopedic surgery (major knee or hip surgery) thrombotic risk is very high, up to 40% without prophylaxis.[18] Unfractionated heparin has been demonstrated to be useful in these patients, but the results obtained with low-molecular-weight heparins are better.[19,20] Low-molecular-weight heparins treatment shows a lower prevalence of thrombosis[2,20] and a lower bleeding risk.[2,18-20] As in general surgery, unfractionated heparin or low-molecular-weight heparins have to be started before the orthopedic surgery,[2,18] but low-molecular-weight heparins have been demonstrated to be effective, although less so than in the regular schedule, starting early in the postsurgical period (12 to 24 hours after surgery).[18]

c. Prevention of venous thromboembolism in patients immobilized for medical causes

Thromboembolism is a frequent complication of paraplegia (approximately 40% of cases in the first two weeks).[2] Both unfractionated heparin and low-molecular-weight heparins are useful in the prevention of venous thromboembolism in paraplegic patients.[2,21] However, too few patients have been treated with low-molecular-weight heparins to be compared with patients treated with unfractionated heparin.[2,21]

Patients immobilized for medical causes such as myocardial infarction, cardiac insufficiency, or ischemic stroke, or older patients frequently suffer venous thromboembolism. Both unfractionated heparin and low-molecular-weight heparins have been demonstrated to be useful without increasing the risk of bleeding.[2,22-24] Low-molecular-weight heparins seem to be slightly more effective in these patients.[22-24]

2. Prevention of Thrombosis in Patients under Cardiac Bypass or Hemodialysis

Unfractionated heparin is the standard drug for preventing cardiopulmonary bypass or hemodialysis circuit occlusion during the procedures.[1,6] In the last few years several low-molecular-weight heparins assayed in these indications have been useful.[6] However, low-molecular-weight heparins neutralization by protamine after surgery is more difficult than unfractionated heparin neutralization.

3. Prevention of Thrombosis in Patients Who Have Vascular Surgery

Low-molecular-weight heparins have been used to prevent femoropopliteal bypass occlusion, showing better results than aspirin plus dipyridamole.[25]

4. Prevention of Thrombosis during and after Coronary Angioplasty

Unfractionated heparin is used at high doses during coronary angioplasty in association with antiplatelet agents.[1] Several studies have evaluated low-molecular-weight heparins in coronary angioplasty, but their results have not improved upon those obtained with unfractionated heparin.[2,26]

5. Prevention of Thrombosis in Patients with Coronary Stents

Unfractionated heparin is usually employed at high doses during the stent deployment procedure without routine postprocedural use.[27] However, postprocedural aspirin and ticlopidine have shown better results in stent thrombosis prevention than unfractionated heparin or warfarin.[28]

6. Prevention of Systemic Embolism in Patients with Mechanical Heart Valves

Unfractionated heparin is used in prevention of systemic embolism in patients with mechanical heart valves in whom warfarin needs to be temporarily discontinued.[1] Low-molecular-weight heparins have been used off-label for these patients, but there are no data to support this use.[17]

7. Treatment of Venous Thromboembolism

During the last 50 years unfractionated heparin has been chosen as the standard initial treatment of deep venous thrombosis.[17] However, in the last few years, low-molecular-weight heparins have demonstrated in several double-blind studies to be most effective and to have less bleeding complications than unfractionated heparin in the treatment of thromboembolic disease,[2,16,29-34] and there is a reduction in overall mortality.[35] In addition, low-molecular-weight heparins can be administered subcutaneously (some of them once daily), do not require monitorization,[30,36,37] and then can be administered in an out-hospital setting,[36,37] reducing sanitary costs.[38,39] In the treatment of venous thromboembolism, unfractionated heparin or low-molecular-weight heparins should be maintained at least five days before, and then be replaced by warfarin therapy.[1]

8. Early Treatment of Patients with Unstable Angina or Myocardial Infarction

Standard treatment of acute unstable angina includes unfractionated heparin plus aspirin, but low-molecular-weight heparins have recently been shown to be useful in this indication. It is not known if they are better than unfractionated heparin.[1,2,40-44]

In the treatment of myocardial infarction, unfractionated heparin can be used without thrombolytic therapy, reducing reinfarction, death rates and mural thrombosis in comparison to untreated patients[1] or as adjunctive therapy to thrombolysis.[1]

E. COMPLICATIONS

Unfractionated heparin and low-molecular-weight heparins have essentially the same complications, although some of them are less prevalent in low-molecular-weight heparins. The main complications are the following:

1. Bleeding

Bleeding is the major complication of heparin treatment.[2,4,6] Bleeding risk is modified by heparin dose, individual response, or concomitant administration of anti-platelet agents.[1,18] Low-molecular-weight heparins have a lower prevalence of bleeding than unfractionated heparin.[2,5,6] Bleeding risk is more related *in vivo* with the anti-thrombin activity than with the anti-Xa activity.[6]

Protamine (sulphate or chlorhidrate) neutralizes unfractionated heparin and, to a lesser extent, low-molecular-weight heparins, and may be used in serious bleeding.[8] Each milligram of protamine neutralizes approximately 100 U of heparin. After protamine neutralization, about 30% of the initial anti-Xa activity of low-molecular-weight heparins remains, although anti-thrombin activity is fully neutralized.[8] Moreover, a rebound effect of low-molecular-weight heparins can be seen three hours after protamine administration due to the absorption of low-molecular-weight heparins from subcutaneous tissue.[6]

2. Thrombocytopenia

Heparin-induced thrombocytopenia is a sometimes severe and relatively unusual complication of heparin treatment.[6,45] This entity is more prevalent when heparin from bovine origin is used.[45] The severity of this complication is associated to arterial or venous thrombosis occurring in a small proportion of patients that produces severe clinical consequences.[6,45] Heparin causes thrombocytopenia by an immune mechanism. In this entity, antibodies directed mainly to heparin/platelet factor 4 complexes on the platelet surface are present.[2,5,45] These antibodies are able to activate platelets through the Fc-gamma-RIIA receptor and, in this way, cause thrombosis.[5,45] The lower affinity of low-molecular-weight heparins for platelet factor 4 may explain the lower prevalence of thrombocytopenia when low-molecular-weight heparins are used.[2] Nevertheless, *in vitro* tests demonstrate cross-reactivity of low-molecular-weight heparins with unfractionated heparin in patients with heparin-induced thrombocytopenia.[6,45] Thus, to continue anticoagulation in patients with heparin-induced thrombocytopenia, the use of heparinoids, peptides with anti-thrombin activity, or hirudin is recommended.[3,45]

3. Osteoporosis

Prolonged heparin treatment may produce osteoporosis.[45] The actual prevalence of this complication is not well known. Heparin-associated osteoporosis is caused by both decreased bone synthesis and increased bone destruction, and is associated with the heparin doses and the duration of treatment.[45] Low-molecular-weight heparins seem to produce less osteoporosis than unfractionated heparin.[45]

4. Skin Lesions

The most frequent skin lesions during heparin treatment are ecchymoses at the sites of heparin injection.[45,46] Skin necrosis is the most serious dermal complication caused by heparin.[45,46] Hypersensitivity reactions to heparin are rare, but may include generalized urticaria, edema, rhinitis, and cyanosis.[45]

5. Hypoaldosteronism

Hypoaldosteronism is a rare complication of unfractionated heparin treatment and is less frequent with the use of low-molecular-weight heparins.[6] Hypoaldosteronism due to heparin treatment usually has no clinical significance, but it may occasionally produce hyperkalemia.[6] Hypoaldosteronism reverts to normal when heparin treatment is discontinued.

6. Hypertrasaminansemia

Increased transaminase levels occur in almost 60% of patients treated with unfractionated heparin,[6] and low-molecular-weight heparins may also produce increased liver enzyme levels. Hypertransaminasemia is not accompanied by liver function impairment, and transaminase levels usually return to normal after discontinuation of treatment.[6]

7. Eosinophilia

Eosinophilia occurs in around 10% of patients treated with heparin, either unfractionated heparin or low-molecular-weight heparins.[45,47] It has been attributed to cellular activation and cytokine release.[45]

II. ORAL ANTICOAGULANT DRUGS

Oral anticoagulant drugs interfere with vitamin K metabolism, causing a decrease in the biological coagulation pathways. They have been widely used in the treatment of thrombosis since the first decades of this century.[48] Oral anticoagulants are the drugs commonly used in the chronic treatment or prevention of thrombotic diseases.[48,49] Warfarin is the compound most widely used in the Anglo-Saxon countries, and most of the medical literature refers to it. However, other oral anticoagulants such as acenocumarol are used in several countries. In this chapter we will refer preferentially to warfarin, although most of the comments, excluding some of pharmacodynamical properties, may be generalized to the remainder of the oral anticoagulants.

A. CHEMICAL STRUCTURE

Oral anticoagulants have a chemical structure similar to vitamin K. Most of the oral anticoagulants have a common coumadin nucleus and constitute the coumadin family. Oral anticoagulants may have two coumadin nuclei (as dicumarol or the ethyl biscumacetate), or only one coumadin nucleus together with an aromatic cycle (as warfarin or acenocumarol). Warfarin is a 4-hydroxycoumadin compound.[49,50] The other family of oral anticoagulants is less frequently employed and has a different nucleus composed by an indanodione (as phenynidione).

Warfarin sodium is a racemic mixture of optical isomers (R- and S-) with different metabolic characteristics.[49] In warfarin, both S- and R- isomers have approximately the same concentration.[49] S-warfarin is five times more potent than R-warfarin as a vitamin K antagonist.[51,52]

B. VITAMIN K AND ORAL ANTICOAGULANT DRUGS: MECHANISM OF ACTION

Vitamin K participates in the posttranscriptional process of synthesis of the amino terminal region of several proteins, acting as a cofactor in the gamma-carboxylation of glutamic acid.[49,53-56] Vitamin K-dependent gamma carboxylation is catalyzed by the enzyme gamma-glutamyl-carboxylase, also named vitamin K-2,3 epoxidase.[53,56] Thus, by the action of this enzyme, and when vitamin K is present, glutamic residue changes to gamma-carboxyl-glutamic residue.[49,53-55] Gamma-glutamyl-carboxylase function requires reduced vitamin K (vitamin KH_2), O_2, and CO_2.[56] During this reaction, vitamin KH_2 is oxidized to vitamin K-2,3 epoxide.[56] Vitamin K-2,3 epoxide is subsequently recycled to vitamin K by the enzyme vitamin K-2,3 epoxide reductase.[53,56] Afterwards, vitamin K may be reduced again to vitamin KH_2 by the action of vitamin K reductase.[56] Thus, recycling of vitamin K prevents a rapid depletion during protein synthesis.

Oral anticoagulants are vitamin K antagonists that produce inhibition of vitamin K-2,3 epoxide reductase and possibly inhibition of vitamin K reductase.[49,57] This inhibition produces the depletion of vitamin KH_2 and reduces the gamma-carboxylation of vitamin K-dependent proteins.[49] Oral anticoagulants interfere with vitamin K action, but not with vitamin K absorption.[49] Thus, oral anticoagulant treatment does not affect the vitamin K amount, but affects its function.[49,58]

Vitamin K-dependent gamma-carboxylation of glutamic acid is necessary for the synthesis of the amino-terminal region of several proteins, the so-called vitamin K-dependent proteins.[53] Some of the vitamin K-dependent proteins are involved in hemostasis and, recently, it has been demonstrated that others are involved in metabolic processes such as osteogenesis.[59] Vitamin K-dependent proteins involved in hemostasis are coagulation factors II, VII, IX, and X; proteins C and S,[59] related to plasmatic coagulation regulation; and protein Z.[58] All of these proteins have a very similar amino-terminal end.[55] In addition to the hemostasis-related protein, the more important vitamin K-dependent proteins are those related to bone metabolism.[59,60] These vitamin K-dependent bone proteins are osteocalcin or "bone gamma-carboxyglutamate protein" (BGP), and the matrix protein Gla (gamma-carboxyl-glutamic).[59,61]

Vitamin K-dependent gamma-carboxylation produces the carboxylation of 9 to 15 glutamic residues of the first 45 residues located in he amino-terminal region of these proteins.[56] Gamma-carboxylation permits these coagulation proteins to have conformational changes when calcium ions are present.[53] These conformational changes are essential for the calcium-dependent binding of vitamin K-dependent proteins to its cofactors on the phospholipidic surfaces in order to exert their biological function.[53] Thus, the reduction of gamma-carboxyl-glutamic residues from the normal number of 10 to 13 in the prothrombin molecule to 9 reduces its coagulant function in 70%, and the reduction to 6 or fewer gamma-carboxyl residues reduces coagulant function to less than 5%.[51,62] Thereby, warfarin administration produces a loss of function of vitamin K-dependent coagulation factors.[49,50]

The physiological function of bone vitamin K-dependent proteins is not well known.[59,61] Plasma osteocalcin levels may reflect bone osteoblastic activity,[61] and the presence of osteocalcin with a normal number of gamma-carboxyl-glutamic residues is essential to maintain mature bone in good conditions.[59,61]

C. PHARMACODYNAMICS

Although warfarin can be administered by injection, it is usually given orally.[48-50] Warfarin is rapidly and completely absorbed in the intestinal tract and is metabolized and excreted with a mean half-life of approximately 40 hours.[49,50] Warfarin circulates bound to plasma proteins, mainly to albumin.[51] The two isomers (R- and S-) of warfarin are metabolically transformed by different pathways.[49-51] R-warfarin is metabolized primarily by reduction into warfarin alcohols and eliminated by urine, and S-warfarin is metabolized by oxidation to 7-hydroxy-warfarin and eliminated by bile.[49,51]

The reduction of the activity of the vitamin K-dependent coagulation factors at the onset of treatment with warfarin depends on the half-life of these factors.[51] For this reason, the first factor that decreases is factor VII.[58] Protein C, which has an anticoagulant effect, has a half-life similar to that of factor VII.[58] This may produce a pro-thrombotic situation when warfarin treatment is initiated, producing "warfarin-induced skin necrosis."[50,58].

Warfarin has numerous pharmacological interactions.[49,51] The most important of these interactions are reflected in Table 31.1, although the list is not exhaustive.[51] Drugs can interfere with the metabolism of warfarin by reducing its absorption from the intestine (as cholestiramine) or by modifying its metabolic clearance by stereoselective or nonselective pathways.[51] Inhibition of the metabolism of S-warfarin is clinically more important than inhibition of that of R-warfarin because of the greater potency of the s-isomer.[51,52] S-warfarin metabolism is inhibited by drugs such as phenylbutazone, sulfinpyrazolone, or metronidazole.[51] R-warfarin metabolism is inhibited by drugs such as omeprazole or cimetidine.[51] Other drugs (like amiodarone) can inhibit both the S- and R-warfarin pathways.[51] Drugs such as barbiturates, rifampicin, or carbamacepine can induce increased metabolic clearance of warfarin by inducing the activity of hepatic oxydases.[51,63] In addition, patients receiving warfarin treatment are sensitive to the fluctuations in the levels of dietary vitamin K intake.[51] Hepatic dysfunction also potentiates the warfarin effect due to the impaired synthesis of coagulation factors.[49,51] For all of these reasons the dose-effect of warfarin differs to a great extent between individuals due to differences in absorption, metabolism, or its effect on the hemostatic factors.[51] Thus, an accurate monitorization is required.[51]

Prothrombin time is used to evaluate the therapeutic effect of oral anticoagulants.[49] However, prothrombin time must be normalized and expressed as INR (International Normalized Ratio).[49,50] INR is calculated by the following formula: INR = (patient time/controls time)^{ISI} where patient time is the prothrombin time of the propositus expressed in seconds, controls time is the geometrical

TABLE 31.1
Main Drug Interactions with Warfarin Metabolism

Warfarin Potentiation	Warfarin Inhibition
Acetylsalicylic acid	Barbiturates
Alcohol	Carbamazepine
Amiodarone	Cholestyramine
Anabolic steroids	Chlordiacepoxide
Cefamandole	Griseofulvin
Chloral hydrate	Mercaptopurine
Chlorpromacin	Nafcillin
Claritromicin	Rifampicin
Clofibrate	Sucralfate
Cimetidine	Azathioprine
Cotrimoxazole	Vitamin K
Disulfiram	
Erythromicin	
Fluconazole	
Indomethacin	
Isoniazid	
Itrakonazole	
Ketoconazole	
Metronidazole	
Miconazole	
Moxalactam	
Omeprazole	
Paroxetine	
Phenylbutazone	
Phenytoin	
Piroxicam	
Propafenone	
Sulfonamides	
Sulfynpyrazolone	
Sulindac	
Tamoxifen	
Tetracyclines	
Thyroid hormones	
Venlafaxin	

mean of the prothrombin time of at least 20 normal individuals, and ISI is the international sensibility index of the thromboplastin batch used, identifying the sensitivity of thromboplastin to the alterations induced by warfarin.[49,50] Recommendations of the level of anticoagulation with oral anticoagulants (to obtain the maximal antithrombotic effect with the minimal hemorrhagic risk) are expressed in INR units. For example, for deep vein thromboses, an INR range from 2.0 to 3.0 is recommended.[49-51]

D. CLINICAL USES

Oral anticoagulants have demonstrated usefulness as antithrombotic agents. At the present warfarin has the following clinical uses: prevention and treatment of venous thromboembolism, prevention of systemic embolism in patients with tissue or mechanical prosthetic heart valves, prevention of systemic embolism in atrial fibrillation, prevention of systemic embolism in patients with mitral stenosis, prevention of myocardial infarction in patients with peripheral arterial disease, prevention of stroke or recurrent infarction in patients with acute myocardial infarction, and prevention of myocardial infarction in high-risk patients.[51]

1. Prevention of Venous Thromboembolism

Warfarin can be used in preventing venous thrombosis after hip surgery or gynecological surgery.[49-51] Warfarin is effective if the treatment is started before surgery or on the first postoperative day,[49,51] and the targeted INR is 2.0–3.0.[51] The risk of bleeding is small, but this treatment is much more complicated than the use of low-molecular-weight heparins, and these are now preferred.[51]

2. Treatment of Venous Thromboembolism

In venous thrombosis, treatment with warfarin needs to be continued for at least three months after the initial heparin therapy.[49-51,64] However, the following factors need to be considered in order to determine treatment duration:[51,64] idiopathic versus secondary thrombosis with reversible cause, proximal versus calf-vein thrombosis, recurrent thromboembolism versus first episode, and presence versus absence of laboratory-detectable thrombophilia. Longer treatment (from six months to permanent anticoagulation) should be considered in idiopathic thrombosis, proximal thrombosis, recurrent thromboembolism, or thrombophilia.[51,64] The target INR for treatment of venous thromboembolism is 2.0–3.0.[49-51]

3. Prevention of Systemic Embolism in Patients with Tissue or Mechanical Prosthetic Heart Valves

For ethical reasons, there are no randomized studies comparing warfarin and placebo in patients with prosthetic heart valves, but historical series indicate the efficacy of warfarin.[51] In the last few years most of the studies in these patients have focused on the intensity of anticoagulation. In seems that the older warfarin regimens with very high anticoagulation levels can be replaced by less intense warfarin treatments without increasing embolic events, but reducing bleeding.[49-51] As an example, the guidelines developed by the European Society of Cardiology recommended INR ranging from 3.0 to 4.5 for first-generation valves, INR ranging from 3.0 to 3.5 for second-generation mitral valves, and INR ranging from 2.5 to 3.0 for second-generation valves in aortic position.[65]

4. Prevention of Systemic Embolism in Atrial Fibrillation

Several studies including a placebo group or an aspirin-treated group have demonstrated that warfarin significantly reduces systemic embolism (mainly stroke) in patients with atrial fibrillation.[49-51] The recommended INR in this situation ranges from 2.0 to 3.0.[51] Warfarin is also used in patients who undergo direct cardioversion.[51] In this case the INR target is the same, and the treatment needs to be continued for at least four weeks after cardioversion.

5. Prevention of Systemic Embolism in Patients with Mitral Stenosis

Although no randomized studies are available, warfarin is used to prevent systemic embolism in patients with mitral stenosis.[49,51] In this situation a target INR range from 2.0 to 3.0 is recommended.[51]

6. Prevention of Myocardial Infarction in Patients with Peripheral Arterial Disease

Evidence exists of the utility of warfarin in preventing myocardial infarction in patients with peripheral arterial disease[51] in a randomized trial using high-intensity oral anticoagulant treatment (INR from 2.5 to 4.5) in comparison with an untreated group.

7. Prevention of Stroke or Recurrent Infarction in Patients with Acute Myocardial Infarction

Warfarin at target INR of 2.0 to 3.0 has been demonstrated effective in preventing stroke and venous thromboembolism in patients suffering acute myocardial infarction.[49-51] More recently, it has been reported that warfarin at INR ranging from 3.0 to 4.5 is effective in preventing stroke, death, or recurrent infarction in patients with acute myocardial infarction.[51]

8. Prevention of Myocardial Infarction in High-Risk Patients

In patients with high risk of ischemic heart disease, the "Thrombosis Prevention Trial"[66] demonstrated that low-degree anticoagulation (target INR 1.3 to 1.8) was effective in preventing an acute ischemic myocardial events, and that the combination of low-intensity warfarin and low-dose aspirin was more effective than warfarin or aspirin alone, but there was an increased bleeding risk.[51,66]

E. COMPLICATIONS

Oral anticoagulant treatment has several complications. Warfarin treatment requires a periodic laboratory control, has pharmacological interactions that limit the therapeutic options, and, during treatment, complications may occur. The more frequent complication is bleeding, although other complications such as warfarin embryopathy, skin necrosis, purple toe syndrome, or tracheobronchial calcifications may occur.

1. Bleeding

Bleeding during oral anticoagulant treatment may be due to an excess of warfarin dose, to local causes, or to alterations of other hemostatic components, mainly platelets.[49] An excess of anticoagulant dose may be due to dietary causes, to the accidental ingestion of warfarin, or to pharmacological interactions.[49,51] Local lesions may be the main cause of bleeding, and the oral anticoagulants only increase or prolong the bleeding.[49] On the other hand, platelet alterations may be caused by an accompanying thrombocytopenia or by the administration of inhibitors of platelet function such as aspirin.[67]

The prevalence of bleeding during warfarin treatment varies between 5 and 40% depending on the treatment intensity,[68-70] and on the cause of anticoagulation.[71,72] From 5 to 30% of bleeding episodes are life-threatening or require transfusion.[71,72] Minor bleeding includes cutaneous or subcutaneous hematomas, gingivorrhages, epistaxis, uterine bleeding, or hematuria.[73] Major bleeding episodes occur in the central nervous system, digestive tract, or retroperitoneum.[71,73] Patients requiring a higher level of anticoagulation, patients with vascular cerebral lesions, and patients suffering deep vein thrombosis or ischemic heart disease are more prone to bleed. Older age is a controversial factor,[74-76] and arterial hypertension has been related to hemorrhagic stroke.[76-79] Moreover, severe anemia, renal failure, or a recent myocardial infarction are risk factors for bleeding during warfarin treatment.[72,75,76,79] During pregnancy, the bleeding risk is higher in the third trimester.[80]

For minor bleeding episodes, the temporal suppression of treatment or diminishing the dose is usually sufficient, but severe bleeding episodes may require blood transfusion or vitamin K_1 administration that exerts its action in 8 to 12 hours.[51]

2. Warfarin Embryopathy

Oral anticoagulants may produce fetal malformations called warfarin embryopathy.[80-83] Warfarin embryopathy is caused in the first trimester of gestation by the interference of warfarin with the fetal bone metabolism. This inhibition is due to the inhibition of vitamin K-dependent fetal or placental proteins. The prevalence of warfarin-induced fetal malformations range from 1 to 5% of pregnancies exposed to warfarin in the first three months.[80-83] In this syndrome, newborns may have malformations due to irregular calcifications, usually caused by isolated nasal hypoplasia to condrodisplasia punctata.[80-83] In addition, newborns may have kyphosis, scoliosis, microcephaly, hypertelorism, and bracchidactilia.[80-83] In some cases bone manifestations may be associated with microftalmia, optical atrophia, ductus arteriosus persistence, or macroglossia.[80-83] Warfarin treatment may be avoided during the first trimester of gestation and substituted by heparin or low-molecular-weight heparin treatment.[80,81]

3. Warfarin-Induced Skin Necrosis

Skin necrosis is a rare but severe complication of oral anticoagulant treatment.[84] It is characterized by cutaneous violaceous plaques that may evolve to skin and subcutaneous tissue necrosis. Skin necrosis appears between the third and eighth day of the warfarin treatment, and in 75% of cases the affected person is a woman.[84] Usually, the breasts, ankles, and gluteus are the most affected areas. Skin necrosis is produced by thrombosis of capillary and venules of the subcutaneous fat tissue, and has been associated with protein S,[84,85] protein C deficiency,[84,86,87] and, occasionally, with antithrombin III deficiency[88] or with lupus anticoagulant.[89] Skin necrosis has been associated with the rapid onset of anticoagulation, which produces a rapid decrease of protein C levels before the diminution of factor VII.[49,84,86,87] Preventive measures include a slow start of warfarin treatment, or the combination of warfarin with heparin at the onset of treatment.[84,86]

4. Purple Toe Syndrome

Purple toe syndrome consists of one or more cyanotic, painful, and cold areas on the toes.[90] This syndrome is produced by cholesterol microemboli.[90,91] Because warfarin avoids thrombi formation over the atherosclerotic plaques, warfarin treatment facilitates the liberation of cholesterol microemboli from the arteriosclerotic lesions.[90,91] When this complication appears, warfarin treatment must be discontinued.

5. Tracheobronchial Calcifications

Tracheobronchial calcifications are a radiological finding with no clinical significance. They are found in children treated with warfarin for a prolonged time,[92] but sometimes they can also be found in adults.[93]

III. ANTIPLATELET AGENTS

Aspirin is the most widely used antithrombotic agent based on numerous basic and clinical studies.[94,95] Aspirin has proven its utility in the prevention and treatment of acute arterial thrombosis and in other entities. More recently, several other drugs corresponding to different pharmacological families have been introduced in the human clinic as antiplatelet agents, but aspirin continues to be the reference drug.[94,96]

A. CHEMICAL STRUCTURE

There are three different types of antiplatelet agents based on their mechanism of action, but with different chemical structure:[94,96] cyclo-oxygenase inhibitors, thienopyridines, and anti-glycoprotein IIb/IIIa agents.

1. Cyclo-Oxygenase Inhibitors and Dipyridamole

Aspirin is the most important of the cyclo-oxygenase inhibitors used as antiplatelet agents. Aspirin is acetylsalicylic acid and acts in the hemostasis as an irreversible inhibitor of cyclo-oxygenase.[94,96,97]

It was initially introduced in clinic by its analgesic/antipyretic and antirrheumatic effect.[96] In this chapter we will focus on its antithrombotic function.

Reversible cyclo-oxygenase inhibitors tested as antiplatelet agents are sulfinpyrazolone, indobufen, and triflusal. Sulfinpyrazolone is structurally related to phenylbutazone, and triflusal is a salicylic acid derivative.[94] These reversible inhibitors of cyclo-oxygenase have been employed in clinical trials but are not approved as antiplatelet drugs.[94]

Related with the cyclo-oxygenase inhibitors it can be cited dipyridamole, although it acts by a different mechanism.[98] Dipyridamole is a pyrimidopyrimidine derivative.[96,98]

2. Thienopyridines

Recently, two related drugs from the thienopyridine family were introduced as antiplatelet agents. These drugs are ticlopidine and clopidogrel, which have related chemical structures[94,96] differing only by carboxymethyl group.

3. Anti-Glycoprotein IIb/IIIa Agents

There are two groups of anti-glycoprotein IIb/IIIa agents. The first group is composed of non-competitive inhibitors, and the representative agent is abciximax.[99] The second group is integrated by competitive inhibitors such as tirofiban, eptifibatide, and lamifiban.[94] Abciximab is a mouse/human chimeric Fab antibody created from the monoclonal antibody 7E3 and directed against the glycoprotein IIb/IIIa.[99-101] Tirofiban is a nonpeptide derivative of tyrosine,[102] eptifibatide is a disulphide-linked cyclic heptapeptide,[103] and lamifiban is also a nonpeptide compound.[104] The most assayed of the anti-glycoprotein IIb/IIIa agents is abciximab.

B. MECHANISMS OF ACTION

In this section we will discuss the mechanisms of action of the three families of antiplatelet agents.

1. Cyclo-Oxygenase Inhibitors and Dipyridamole

Cyclo-oxygenase inhibitors act on the eicosanoid synthesis pathway, inhibiting prostaglandin formation from the arachidonate substrate.[97,105,106] This biological pathway is described in more detail in the eicosanoid and prostaglandin derivatives section (Section V) of this chapter.

Aspirin acetylates prostaglandin H-synthase and irreversibly inhibits its cyclo-oxygenase activity.[97,105,106] Prostaglandin H-synthase has two activities in the synthesis of prostaglandin H: first oxygenates and cycles arachidonic acid to prostaglandin G through its cyclo-oxygenase activity, and then reduces prostaglandin G to prostaglandin H through its peroxidase component.[96] Aspirin inhibits cyclo-oxygenase in a highly selective manner without affecting the remainder of the enzymatic activities of the prostaglandin synthesis pathway.[97,105,106] Acetylation of cyclo-oxygenase is produced at the serine 529, producing a covalent O-acetyl bond that resists intracellular hydrolysis.[96] Of the two isoforms of cyclo-oxygenase (or COX) named COX-1 and COX-2,[107] aspirin is a relatively selective inhibitor of COX-1.[94] COX-1 is constitutively present in platelets, endothelial cells, and most other cell types; COX-2 is usually undetectable, but is expressed rapidly in response to inflammatory stimuli.[107] The action of aspirin on cyclo-oxygenase causes inhibition of platelets and endothelial cells in the formation of thromboxane A_2 and prostacyclin, respectively.[96,108] Thromboxane A_2 and prostacyclin have opposite actions on platelet aggregation and vascular tone. Thromboxane A_2 produces platelet aggregation and vasoconstriction, while prostacyclin inhibits platelet aggregation and causes vasodilatation.[108] Aspirin inhibits both platelet and endothelial cyclo-oxygenase, but inhibition in platelets cannot be repaired by the platelet during its lifetime due to the anucleated condition of platelets lacking biosynthetic mechanisms.[96] Cyclo-oxygenase inhibitors sulfinpyrazolone, indobufen, and triflusal have the same mechanism of action, but in a reversible way.[109]

The mechanism of action of dipyridamole is not well known. It has been attributed to the inhibition of platelet cyclic acid nucleotide phosphosdiesterase.[98] The inhibition of this enzyme causes cyclic AMP accumulation and, in this way, blocks adenosine uptake which acts at A_2 receptors for adenosine to stimulate platelet adenylyl cyclase.[98] In addition, it has been suggested that dipyridamole may directly stimulate prostacyclin synthesis or protect prostaglandin against degradation.[98]

2. Thienopyridines

Ticlopidine and clopidogrel selectively inhibit ADP-induced platelet aggregation without interfering in arachidonate metabolism.[110,111] The mechanism of action of both thienopyridine drugs seems to be the inhibition of the ADP receptor itself, or components closely related to them.[110,111] Ticlopidine and clopidogrel can also inhibit collagen and thrombin aggregation, but these effects seem to be related to the inhibition of the ADP-mediated amplification of the aggregation response induced by these agonists.[110,111]

3. Anti-Glycoprotein IIb/IIIa Agents

Both competitive and noncompetitive anti-glycoprotein IIb/IIIa agents act through the inhibition of the integrin IIb/IIIa.[94,96] Glycoprotein IIb/IIIa ($alpha_{IIb}/beta_3$) is the final common pathway of platelet aggregation. Blocking glycoprotein IIb/IIIa platelets acquire a functional thrombasthenic phenotype, inhibiting platelet aggregation to a important extent.[100,101] Abciximax also causes decreased thrombin generation, probably due to its potent inhibition of platelet aggregation.[112] In addition, abciximax is unique of the anti-IIb/IIIa agents as it also blocks the $alpha_V/beta_3$ receptor, but the role of $alpha_V/beta_3$ receptor blockade in abciximab's effects is not well known.[100,112]

C. PHARMACODYNAMICS

The main characteristics of pharmacodynamics of the antiplatelet agents are the following:

1. Cyclo-Oxygenase Inhibitors and Dipyridamole

Aspirin is absorbed in the stomach and upper intestine.[94,113] Peak plasma levels are detected 30 to 40 minutes after aspirin ingestion, and platelet inhibition can be observed by 60 minutes.[94,113] Enteric-coated tablets need three to four hours to reach peak plasma levels.[94] Oral bioavailability is around 50%, but it is lower with enteric-coated tablets.[94,113] Aspirin's half-life is 20 minutes, but its effect on platelets persists during the platelets' lifetime (approximately ten days) because of the inability of platelets to repair the acetylated enzyme.[96]

The reversible cyclo-oxygenase inhibitors sulfinpyrazolone, indobufen, and triflusal are administered orally.[109] Sulfinpyrazone is a weak cyclo-oxygenase inhibitor, while indobufen is a very potent inhibitor.[94] Triflusal acts on cyclo-oxygenase through an active metabolite, 2-hydroxy-4-trifluoromethyl-benzoic acid.[114] Triflusal metabolite has a half-life of two days, much longer than the other reversible cyclo-oxygenase inhibitors.[114]

Oral absorption of dipyridamole is quite variable, and the biodisponibility of the drug is low.[94] Dipyridamole is eliminated by the bile as a glucuronide conjugate.[94]

2. Thienopyridines

The bioavailability of ticlopidine after an oral dose is up to 90%.[110] Peak plasma concentration is obtained one to three hours after oral dose administration. Drug accumulation causes three-fold plasma levels after three weeks of treatment.[110] Ticlopidine circulates reversibly bound to plasma proteins, primary albumin. Ticlopidine metabolism produces several metabolites including a 2-keto derivate more active than the parent compound.[110] The half-life of the drug ranges from 24 to 36 hours.[110] The antiplatelet effect of ticlopidine is relatively slow and is not recommended when a very rapid onset of antiplatelet effect is required.[94]

Clopidogrel is not detected unchanged in plasma after oral doses.[94,111] Clopidogrel, as ticlopidine, needs to be transformed into a metabolite in order to exert its action.[111] The main metabolite of clopidogrel is its carboxylic acid derivative.[111]

3. Anti-Glycoprotein IIb/IIIa Agents

Abciximax is administered intravenously.[99,100] After injection, free plasma concentration decreases rapidly due to its binding to circulating platelets.[100] The peak effect on receptor blockade is seen around two hours after abciximab administration.[99] The use of a chimeric mouse/human Fab fragment decreases the immunogenicity-associated problems that can be due to the use of a murine monoclonal antibody.[100]

Competitive inhibitors are used by intravenous injection.[102-104] Tirofiban has a half-life of 1.6 hours, and bleeding time returns to the normal range four hours after the end of the therapy.[94,102] Eptifibatide has a shorter effect on platelets, returning to normal values in the first four hours after stopping treatment.[94,103] Lamifiban has a half-life of 40 minutes.[94,104]

D. Clinical Uses

Antiplatelet agents are widely used in the treatment and prevention of arterial atherothrombosis.[94-96] In fact, aspirin is the antithrombotic drug most used in human clinics.[95] Together with aspirin's utility in arterial vascular disease, other indications for antiplatelet agents have been assayed. The most important of these indications are prevention of systemic embolism in atrial fibrillation, prevention of deep venous thrombosis, and treatment and prevention of placental insufficiency.[94]

1. Prevention and Treatment of Arterial Atherothrombosis

Aspirin is a safe and effective drug in the prevention and treatment of thrombotic complications of arteriosclerosis.[94,95] Aspirin has demonstrated its utility in primary and secondary prevention of acute myocardial infarction,[94,115] treatment of patients with unstable angina or myocardial infarction,[94,116] prevention of reocclusion in coronary angioplasty, prevention of reocclusion in patients with coronary stents, prevention of femoropopliteal bypass occlusion, and treatment and primary and secondary prevention of stroke.[94,117] Aspirin's effect on coronary disease is more beneficial than in patients with cerebrovascular disease. Aspirin should be administered to virtually all patients with clinical suspicion of myocardial infarction.[118] The degree of efficacy of this preventive measure is greater in patients with more vascular risk factors.[95]

Reversible cyclo-oxygenase inhibitors such as sulfinpyrazolone, indobufen, and triflusal have been used in several trials. No advantages vs. standard treatment with aspirin were demonstrated.[94,109]

Dipyridamole has been used alone or in combination with aspirin in stroke prevention trials.[94,98] The results of these studies showed a very low risk of complications due to dipyridamole treatment, but its efficacy remains controversial.[94,96]

Ticlopidine has been evaluated in patients with stroke, transient cerebral ischemia, unstable angina, intermittent claudication, and after aortocoronary bypass.[94,96,110,119,120] Ticlopidine is more effective than aspirin in reducing stroke or in unstable angina,[121] and more effective than placebo in patients with intermittent claudication or after aortocoronary bypass.[94,119] Ticlopidine in combination with aspirin is effective in the prevention of reocclusion in patients with coronary stents.[122]

Clopidogrel has been demonstrated more potent than aspirin in preventing arterial ischemic events in high-risk patients, those who have suffered a recent stroke or myocardial infarction, or those with symptomatic peripheral arterial disease.[40,96,123]

Abciximax inhibits platelet aggregation to a greater extent than aspirin.[101] Abciximab has proven useful in reducing the incidence of ischemic events in patients undergoing percutaneous transluminal coronary angioplasty.[94,96,100,124,125]

The recently introduced competitive inhibitors tirofiban, eptifibatide, and lamifiban have been assayed in the prevention of the reocclusion in patients undergoing coronary angioplasty.[102-104] The results of the initial trials suggest that they may be useful in this situation, but more data are needed.[94]

2. Prevention of Systemic Embolism in Atrial Fibrillation

Aspirin is employed in systemic embolism in atrial fibrillation.[94,126,127] However, warfarin is more effective than aspirin in preventing embolism, and is the drug of choice in high-risk patients.[94,126,127] Aspirin is a safer and cheaper treatment than warfarin and can be used in low-risk patients with atrial fibrillation.[94] Aspirin can be also used in combination with warfarin in prevention systemic embolism in very high-risk patients with mechanical heart valves in whom warfarin alone has failed.[96]

3. Prevention of Deep Venous Thrombosis

Although the effectiveness of aspirin in preventing arterial thrombotic disease is beyond any doubt, its effect in the prevention of venous thrombosis is controversial.[94,128] On balance, it is likely that aspirin produces a modest reduction in the risk of postoperative venous thrombosis, but it seems to be less beneficial than other prophylaxis treatments such as warfarin, unfractionated heparin, or low-molecular-weight heparins.[94,128]

4. Treatment and Prevention of Placental Insufficiency

Aspirin has been used in the treatment of preeclampsia, which is attributed to constriction or thrombosis of small placental arterioles, but several large trials have not demonstrated a beneficial effect on perinatal outcomes.[94,129,130] However, no adverse consequences were identified with the use of aspirin for several months during pregnancy.[94,129,130] At present, aspirin is only employed in the prevention of fetal losses in women with the antiphospholipid syndrome and previous fetal miscarriages.

E. COMPLICATIONS

Antiplatelet agents use can produce several clinical complications.

1. Cyclo-Oxygenase Inhibitors and Dipyridamole

Aspirin does not usually cause generalized bleeding unless the patient has an underlying hemostatic defect, such as hemophilia or related diseases, uremia, liver diseases, or treatment with oral antico-agulants or heparin.[94] In these cases, bleeding tendency is mainly independent on the aspirin dose.[94]

Aspirin-induced gastrointestinal toxicity is frequent. It appears to be dose-related but it can appear at doses as low as 30 mg/day.[131] Clinical manifestations of aspirin-induced gastrointestinal toxicity range from abdominal discomfort to severe gastrointestinal bleeding.[94,131] It seems that aspirin-induced gastrointestinal toxicity is related to the aspirin activity inhibiting cyclo-oxygenase of the gastric mucosae lining cells.[131] Even at low doses aspirin can cause severe gastrointestinal toxicity. In the presence of gastric mucosal erosions, due to other non-steroidal anti-inflammatory drugs or to the presence of *Helicobacter pylori* infection, aspirin may cause gastrointestinal bleeding.[132] Enteric-coated or buffered aspirin tablets introduced to reduce the risk of aspirin-induced gastrointestinal toxicity seemed not to have this beneficial effect in a multicenter study.[133]

In several patients aspirin treatment can cause bronchospasm that can be severe.[96] This effect is not dose-dependent. The effect of aspirin impairing blood pressure control in patients with hypertension or increasing the risk of renal disease is controversial.[94,96] However, at the low doses when used as an antithrombotic agent these complications are not present. The reversible cyclo-oxygenase inhibitors sulfinpyrazolone, indobufen, and triflusal have essentially the same complications as aspirin.[94]

The toxicity of dipyridamole is very low. The risk of bleeding in dipyridamole-treated patients is not different from the risk observed in controls.[98,132] The most frequent complication in dipyridamole treatment is headache.[132]

2. Thienopyridines

Both ticlopidine and clopidogrel increase the risk of bleeding, especially if the additive effect of aspirin or other underlying hemostasis defects are present.[96,120] The most severe complication of ticlopidine is the development of neutropenia, which can occur in more than 2% of treated patients.[120] This complication can be severe and motivates treatment discontinuation. Ticlopidine has also been occasionally associated to thrombocytopenia,[120] aplastic anemia,[134] and thrombotic thrombocytopenic purpura.[135] Another complication of ticlopidine treatment is the development of hypercholesterolemia.[120] Clopidogrel treatment may cause cutaneous rash or diarrhea that can be severe.[94,123] Clopidogrel does not cause neutropenia[92,123] but can cause thrombotic thrombocytopenic purpura.

3. Anti-Glycoprotein IIb/IIIa Agents

Anti-glycoprotein IIb/IIIa agents may cause bleeding.[94] In abciximab treatment the prevalence of bleeding is associated to the dose of heparin concomitantly administered.[124,125] The reduction of the dose of heparin greatly reduces abciximab-induced bleeding tendency.[125]

In addition to the bleeding risk, abciximab can cause thrombocytopenia.[124,125] It appears in nearly 2% of treated patients, and appears rapidly after drug administration. Abciximab-induced thrombocytopenia is reversible, with recovery over several days.[124,125] Although the use of a chimeric mouse/human Fab fragment theoretically reduces immunogenicity-associated problems, approximately 6% of treated patients develop antibodies to the variable regions of the antibody.[100,124] There is little data about the risk of anaphylaxis and immunological neutralization of abciximab in the case of reinfusion.[94]

The main complication of the competitive inhibitors tirofiban, eptifibatide, and lamifiban is bleeding, in the same way as abciximab.[94,102-104]

Tirofiban can cause severe but reversible thrombocytopenia in a small percentage of patients.[94,136] Thrombocytopenia is due to the development of antibodies against conformational changes of the glycoprotein IIb/IIIa receptor induced by the binding of tirofiban. At the present, there are no data available about the safety of tirofiban reinfusion. Eptifibatide has not been associated with thrombocytopenia, and no data about its safety in reinfusion are currently available.[94,103] Finally, there are no data about the risk of thrombocytopenia or safety in reinfusion with the use of lamifiban.

IV. FIBRINOLYTIC AGENTS

Fibrinolytic agents are drugs that dissolve thrombi by activating an inactive plasma enzyme, plasminogen, to the active agent, plasmin.[137] Plasmin degrades fibrin to soluble peptides, and fibrinolytic treatment hypothesis is that early recanalization prevents cell death, reduces infarct size, and preserves organ function.

A. Chemical Structure

The first fibrinolytic drug introduced in clinical use was streptokinase, a highly purified protein with a molecular weight of 47 KDa.[138] Streptokinase derives from group C, beta-hemolytic streptococci.[139,140]

Two-chain urokinase-type plasminogen activator (or urokinase) is a protein of 34 KDa.[138] Urokinase was initially purified from human urine, but is currently derived from human fetal kidney cells grown in culture, and clinical investigation of recombinant products is proceeding.[138-140] One of these derivatives of urokinase with theoretical advantages, the recombinant single-chain urokinase-type plasminogen activator (single chain urokinase or scu-PA or pro-urokinase), has been introduced in clinical trials.[137]

Recombinant tissue-type plasminogen activator (rt-PA or alteplase) is a fibrinolysis activator obtained by recombinant technologies from human cells.[138,139] Recombinant tissue-type plasminogen activator is a protein with a molecular weight of 56 KDa. Two variants of recombinant tissue-type plasminogen activator have been recently introduced in clinical trials: reteplase and TNK-rt-PA. Reteplase is a single-chain non-glycosilated deletion variant consisting only in the kringle 2 and the proteinase domain of human tissue-type plasminogen activator.[141] TNK-rt-PA consist in a replacement of Asn^{117} with Gln deleting the glycosylation site in kringle 1, whereas substitution of Thr^{103} with Asn reintroduces a glycosylation locus in the same kringle but in a different locus.[142] These modifications substantially decrease plasma clearance rate and decrease inhibition by type 1 plasminogen activator inhibitor (or PAI-1).

Anisoylated plasminogen-streptokinase activator complex (anistreplase or APSAC) is a complex formed by single-chain tissue-type plasminogen activator and single-chain streptokinase.[138,143] This complex has been made inactive by acylation of the catalytic center of the plasmin portion.[143,144] This product activates after injection, sustaining fibrinolytic activity.[143,144]

Staphylokinase is a recently introduced drug. It consists of a nonenzymatic protein produced by some strains of *Staphylococcus aureus*.[137]

B. MECHANISMS OF ACTION

Physiological fibrinolysis is regulated by specific molecular interactions among its main components fibrin, plasminogen, plasminogen activators, and the fibrinolysis inhibitors such as type 1 plasminogen activator inhibitor or alpha-2-antiplasmin.[145] The end point of the physiological fibrinolysis pathway is the formation of plasmin. Plasmin is a proteolytic enzyme that degrades the fibrin clot forming soluble fibrin degradation fragments.[145] Plasmin is generated from an inactive pro-enzyme, plasminogen, when it is activated by several activators. The most important of these plasminogen activators is the tissue-type plasminogen activator synthesized in endothelial cells. Another physiological plasminogen activator is urokinase, which exerts its action preferentially in the urinary tract. There are also several inhibitors of the plasminogen activators. The most important of them is the type 1 plasminogen activator inhibitor present in endothelial cells and platelets. Plasminogen is primarily activated at the fibrin surface and regulates thrombi extension.[146] However, in some cases, or after the use of no-fibrin-specific fibrinolytic agents, plasmin can be generated in plasma and then exert its action on fibrinogen causing a decrease in this protein. In plasma, plasmin is rapidly inactivated by alpha-2-antiplasmin, and also, but to a much lesser extent, by alpha-2-macroglobulin.[145] Plasmin formed on the fibrin surface is only slowly inactivated by alpha-2-antiplasmin, whereas once liberated to the clot or generated in plasma, plasmin is rapidly cleared.[145,146] This plasmin-inhibitory process tends to limit fibrinolysis to the thrombus area, preventing excessive alpha-2-antiplasmin depletion or fibrinogen degradation in plasma.[145] Fibrinolytic agents modulate physiological fibrinolysis.

Streptokinase combines noncovalently with plasminogen to form a complex that activates adjacent plasminogen to plasmin.[138]

Urokinase is a direct endogenous plasminogen activator. It activates plasminogen to plasmin in a no fibrin-specific way.[138] Single-chain urokinase also directly activates plasminogen to plasmin, but is more fibrin-specific than urokinase.

Recombinant tissue-type plasminogen activator converts plasminogen to plasmin directly by enzymatic cleavage of a single Arg^{561}-Val^{562} peptide bond.[146] This enzymatic action is much more efficient in the presence of fibrin.[137] Kinetic data supports that fibrin provides a surface in which recombinant tissue-type plasminogen activator and plasminogen absorb in a sequential way, yielding a cyclic ternary complex.[146] However, fibrin specificity is relative, and sometimes systemic fibrinogenolysis may occur after the administration of recombinant tissue-type plasminogen activator.[147]

Both reteplase and TNK-rt-PA have essentially the same mechanism of action as recombinant tissue-type plasminogen activator.[141,142]

Anisoylated plasminogen-streptokinase activator complex acts combining both streptokinase and tissue-type plasminogen activator activities after its spontaneous activation, which occurs after injection.[143,144]

Staphylokinase is not an enzyme but it forms a 1:1 stoichiometric complex with plasminogen or plasmin that activates other plasminogen molecules.[148] It needs the presence of at least trace amounts of plasmin to efficiently activate plasminogen.[148] Staphylokinase is highly fibrin-selective. Plasmin/staphylokinase complexes are protected against alpha-2-antiplasmin inhibition.[148]

C. CLINICAL USES

Fibrinolytic agents are used for arterial or venous thrombolysis. Arterial thrombolysis includes acute treatment of myocardial infarction, peripheral arterial emboli, and stroke.[137] Its use in myocardial infarction is the most important of these indications.[137] Venous thrombolysis includes acute treatment of pulmonary embolism, deep venous thrombosis, and clearing acutely occluded arteriovenous fistulas.[138,139]

1. Arterial Thrombolysis

In myocardial infarction, several studies have demonstrated that endovenous fibrinolytic agents significantly reduce mortality.[137] An overview of the studies performed between 1959 and 1979 demonstrated a 22% of reduction of mortality.[149] Most large and well-designed studies have demonstrated the beneficial effect of streptokinase,[150,151] APSAC,[151,152] and recombinant tissue-type plasminogen activator.[151,153] The most recent clinical trials have compared the effects of different fibrinolytic agents, different doses, or different adjuvant therapies.[137,151,154-159] Recent recommendations of the ACCP Consensus Conference[137] indicate recombinant tissue-type plasminogen activator in patients who meet all the following criteria: treatment started before 6 hours of the onset of symptoms, less than 75 years of age, and myocardial infarction anterior or inferior with a poor prognosis. For the remainder of patients treated before 6 hours of the onset of the symptoms, APSAC, reteplase, or streptokinase are reasonable alternatives. For patients treated after 6 hours of the onset of the myocardial infarction, streptokinase is the drug of choice because it is the least expensive. APSAC, reteplase, or recombinant tissue-type plasminogen activator can also be used to reduce mortality.

As adjuvant therapy in arterial thrombolysis, all of the fibrin-selective agents need the concomitant administration of heparin to prevent immediate rethrombosis.[137] Aspirin is strongly recommended in all patients with myocardial infarction, whether or not they are receiving thrombolytic treatment, with the first dose starting as soon as possible after clinical symptoms.[118,137]

2. Venous Thrombolysis

Three drugs are currently approved for use in venous thrombolysis.[139] These are streptokinase, urokinase, and recombinant tissue-type plasminogen activator. All the three have been demonstrated to be effective and safe in the treatment of pulmonary embolism.[138,139] Unlike in myocardial infraction, heparin is not infused during pulmonary embolism thrombolysis, but heparin is started after termination of fibrinolytic infusion.[139] Several reports have demonstrated that fibrinolytics can be useful in cases of deep venous thrombosis and in clearing acutely occluded arteriovenous fistulas.[138]

D. COMPLICATIONS

Bleeding and allergic reactions are the major adverse effects of fibrinolytic therapy. Hypotension can also appear during thrombolytic treatment,[154] whereas arrhythmias reported as frequent in early trials have not been confirmed in the most recent studies.[137]

1. Bleeding

Fibrinolytic agents produce their benefit by lysing coronary or other territories' thrombi. However, they are not selective in their territory of action, and bleeding can occur in other territories where hemostasis is required. Hemostasis impairment is not only due to the clot lysis or to the possible hyfibrinogenemia. Fibrinolytic agents can also cause the decrease in plasma factors V and VIII levels, and the fibrinogen and fibrin degradation products have anticoagulant properties and produce platelet dysfunction.[160] The rates of major bleeding and intracerebral bleeding among the different fibrinolytic treatments are controversial but they seem related to their combination with the different adjuvant heparin treatments.[137,151,154,156-159]

2. Allergic Reactions

Streptokinase as a microbial protein is antigenic. Humans can develop antibodies against this protein, and these antibodies inactivate the administered drug.[137] Within three or four days of streptokinase administration the levels of neutralizing antibodies rise and the titer of antibodies achieve values able to neutralize usual streptokinase doses for up to one year.[137] Severe allergic reactions can occur, but anaphylaxis is rare with the new, more purified preparations.[137,154] APSAC has a potential risk similar to streptokinase of allergic reactions and anaphylactic shock.[152]

3. Hypotension

Hypotension is often observed during the administration of streptokinase.[137] It has been attributed to the increased plasmenemia which leads to bradykyn release from kallicrein, from activation of complement, and to endothelial prostacyclin secretion.[161] Hypotension can also be observed in APSAC treatment, and with a lower prevalence in recombinant tissue-type plasminogen activator.[154]

V. EICOSANOIDS AND PROSTAGLANDIN DERIVATIVES

Eicosanoids, which are formed from certain polyunsatured fatty acids (mainly arachidonic acid), include prostaglandins, prostacyclin, thromboxane A2, and leukotrienes. Eicosanoids are extremely prevalent and are present in almost every tissue and body fluid. Their production increases in response to diverse stimuli, and they produce a broad spectrum of biological effects. These lipids contribute to a number of physiological and pathological events, such as inflammation, smooth muscle tone, hemostasis, thrombosis, parturition, and gastrointestinal secretion. Several drugs, most notably nonsteroidal antiinflammatory drugs, owe their therapeutic effects to the blockade of eicosanoids formation.

A. CHEMICAL STRUCTURE AND BIOSYNTHESIS

Prostaglandins, leukotrienes, and related compounds are called eicosanoids because they are derived from 20-carbon essential fatty acids that contain three, four, or five double bonds; 8,11,14-eicosa-trienoic acid; 5,8,11,14-eicosatetraenoic acid; and 5,8,11,14,17-eicosapentaenoic acid. In humans, arachinodate is the most important precursor of eicosanoids, and it is derived from dietary constituents. Dietary arachidonate is sterified to the phospholipids of cell membranes or other complex lipids.[162] Since the concentration of free arachidonate in the cell is very low, the biosynthesis of eicosanoids depends primarily upon its availability to the eicosanoid-synthesizing enzymes. The availability of arachidonate results from its release from the cellular stores of lipids by acyl hydro-lases, mostly phospholipase A_2, and, in platelets, diacylglycerol lipase.[163] Hormones, autacoids, and other substances increase eicosanoids biosynthesis by interacting with plasma membrane-bound receptors. This results in the direct activation of phospholipases (C and/or A_2) with the release of arachidonate.[162] Once released, a portion of arachidonate is metabolized to oxygenated products by several enzyme systems, including cyclo-oxygenases, lipo-oxygenases, or cytochrome P450.[162]

1. Products of Cyclo-Oxygenases

The first enzymatic activity in this synthetic pathway is prostaglandin endoperoxide synthase, also called fatty acid cyclo-oxygenase, that forms part of the prostaglandin H synthetase.[162] There are two isoforms of this enzyme, cyclo-oxygenase-1 (COX-1) and cyclo-oxygenase-2 (COX-2).[162] The cyclo-oxygenases oxygenate and cycle the unesterified precursor fatty acid to form the cyclic endoperoxide prostaglandin G, and then the second component of the prostaglandin H synthetase converts prostaglandin G to prostaglandin H. Both prostaglandin G and H are unstable, but they can be transformed into a variety of products, including prostaglandin I; thromboxane A_2; and prostaglandins E, F, and D. The endoperoxide prostaglandin H_2 is also metabolized into two unstable and highly active compounds: thromboxane A_2 formed by thromboxane synthase, and prostaglandin I_2 (also called prostacyclin) formed by prostacyclin synthase.[164] Thromboxane A_2 breaks down nonenzymatically into the stable but inactive thromboxane B_2, and prostacyclin is hydrolyzed nonenzymatically to the inactive 6-keto-prostaglandin$_{1\alpha}$.

2. Products of Lipo-Oxygenases

Lipo-oxygenases are cytosolic enzymes that catalyze the oxygenation of polyenic fatty acids to lipid hydroperoxides. Arachidonate is metabolized to a number of metabolites with the hydroperoxy group in different positions. These metabolites are called hydro-peroxy-eicosa-tetramoic acids (HPETEs). HPETEs are unstable intermediates, analogous to prostaglandin G or H, and are further metabolized. All HPETEs may be converted to their corresponding hydroxy fatty acid (HETE), either by a peroxydase or nonenzymatically.[164] The 5-lipo-oxygenase is the most important of these enzymes since it leads to the synthesis of the leukotrienes. Arachidonic acid is the precursor of the four series of leukotrienes.[164] When cells are activated and intracellular Ca^{2+} increases, 5-lipo-oxygenase binds to a 5-lipo-oxygenase-activating protein. This binding activates the enzyme, resulting in its increased synthesis of 5-HPETE and leukotrienes. Leukotriene A synthase is associated with 5-lipo-oxygenase and promotes the rearrangement of 5-HPETE to an unstable 5,6-epoxide, leukotriene A_4. Leukotriene A_4 may be transformed by leukotriene A hydrolase to leukot-riene B_4; alternatively, it may be conjugated with glutathione by leukotriene C_4 synthase to form leukotriene C_4. Leukotriene D_4 is produced by the removal of glutamic acid from leukotriene C_4, and leukotriene E_4 results from the subsequent cleavage of glycine; the reincorporation of glutamic acid yields leukotriene F_4.

3. Products of Cytochrome P450

Arachidonate can be metabolized by enzymes that contain cytochrome P450. While these metab-olites have vascular, endocrine, renal, and ocular effects, the physiological importance of this pathway remains to be clarified.

B. Biological Function and Mechanisms of Action

The biological effects of eicosanoids cover a broad spectrum of biological functions. In the present review we will only refer to their actions that are thought to be the most important for their pharmacological use in vascular diseases: platelet function and vascular smooth muscle tone.

TABLE 31.2
Prostaglandin Receptors Effect on Platelet Aggregation and on Smooth Muscle Tone

Prostaglandin Receptor Subtype	Platelet Aggregation	Smooth Muscle Tone	Natural Agonist
DP	–		PGD_2
EP_1		+	$PGE, PGF_{2\alpha}$
EP_2		–	PGE
EP_3	+/–	+	PGE
FP		+	$PGF_{2\alpha}$
IP	–	–	PGI_2
TP	+	+	TXA_2, PGH_2

Note: PG: Prostaglandin. TX: Thromboxane.

The diversity of the effects of prostanoids is explained by the existence of a number of distinct receptors that mediate their actions.[165] Prostaglandin receptors are named for the natural prostaglandin for which they have the greatest apparent affinity and have been divided into five main types, designated DP (prostaglandin D), FP (prostaglandin F), IP (prostaglandin I_2), TP (thromboxane A_2), and EP (prostaglandin E).[165] The EP receptors have been further subdivided into EP_1 (smooth muscle contraction), EP_2 (smooth muscle relaxation), EP_3, and EP_4, based on physiological and molecular cloning information. Table 31.2 indicates the effects of prostaglandins on smooth muscle tone and platelet aggregation when the various prostaglandin receptors are stimulated. In addition, three distinct receptors for leukotrienes (leukotriene B_4, C_4 and D_4/E_4) also have been identified in different tissues, and all of them appear to activate phospholipase C.

1. Vascular Smooth Muscle Tone

Eicosanoids have different activities on vascular smooth muscle tone. Some of them act as vasoconstrictors, and others as vasodilators.

a. Prostaglandins

In most species (including humans) and in most vascular beds, the prostaglandins E are potent vasodilators. This dilatation involves arterioles, precapillary sphincters, and postcapillary venules, but not large veins. However, prostaglandins E are not universally vasodilatory, and vasoconstrictory effects have been noted at selected sites. Prostaglandin D_2 can cause both vasodilation and vasoconstriction. In most vascular beds, including the mesenteric, coronary, and renal, prostaglandin D_2 causes vasodilation at lower concentrations than vasoconstriction. However, in pulmonary circulation, prostaglandin D_2 causes only vasoconstriction. Systemic blood pressure generally falls in response to prostaglandins E, and blood flow to most organs, including the heart, mesentery, and kidney, increases. Cardiac output is generally increased by prostaglandins of the E and F prostaglandin series.[165]

Prostaglandins endoperoxides have variable effects in vascular beds. Their major effects are a result of intrinsic vasoconstrictor conversion to a prostaglandin that is a vasodilator (probably prostaglandin I_2). Intravenous administration of prostaglandin I_2 causes prominent hypotension, and this effect is accompanied by a reflex increase in heart rate.

b. Thromboxane A_2

Thomboxane A_2 is a potent vasoconstrictor. It contracts vascular smooth muscle *in vitro,* and is a vasoconstrictor in the whole animal and in isolated vascular beds.[165]

c. Leukotrienes

In humans, leukotriene C_4 and D_4 cause hypotension. This may result, in part, from a decrease in intravascular volume and in cardiac contractility that is secondary to a marked leukotriene-induced reduction in coronary blood flow.

2. Platelet Function

The effect of eicosanoids on platelet function is variable. Some of them are pro-aggregant agents, and others are platelet function inhibitors.

a. Prostaglandins

Prostaglandins and related products modulate platelet function. Prostaglandin I_2 inhibits the aggregation of human platelets *in vitro* at concentrations between 1 and 10 nmol/L. In addition, prostaglandin I_2 is synthesized by the vascular endothelium and contributes to the antithrombotic properties of the intact vascular wall.[166]

b. Thromboxane A_2

Thromboxane A_2 is a major product of the arachidonate metabolism in platelets and, as a powerful inducer of platelet aggregation and platelet release reaction, is a physiological mediator of platelet aggregation.[166]

c. Leukotrienes

Leukotriene B_4 is a potent chemotactic agent for polymorphonuclear leukocytes, eosinophils, and monocytes. At higher concentrations it promotes degranulation and the generation of superoxide. Leukotriene B_4 also promotes adhesion of neutrophils to vascular endothelial cells and their transendothelial migration. By these mechanisms leukotriene B_4 can contribute to the process of thrombogenesis.

C. CLINICAL USES

Eicosanois and related compounds have been used in vascular diseases as part of the treatment of two clinical manifestations: Raynaud's phenomenon and pulmonary hypertension. In addition, several antiplatelet agents, such as aspirin or others, exert their action via eicosanoid synthesis inhibition or eicosanoid receptor inhibition.

1. Raynaud's Phenomenon

Prostacyclin and its analogue iloprost have been used in several studies on Raynaud's phenomenon. Zachariaea et al.[167] reported the efficacy of iloprost in blocking imminent gangrene and in healing ischemic ulcers in patients with systemic sclerosis. A large double-blind, placebo-controlled parallel study in patients with scleroderma found that the mean weekly attack rate fell by 39%.[168] Another iloprost study compared low dose (0.5 ng/kg/min) to standard maximal dose (2 ng/kg/min) and found that both the high- and low-dose iloprost resulted in a reduction in the severity of Raynaud's phenomenon. Oral iloprost was studied in 103 patients with systemic sclerosis, comparing two different doses and placebo, and both doses of oral iloprost twice daily were shown to be effective.[169] Another prostacyclin oral analogue, beraprost, has shown controversial results.[170,171] In an open study,[170] after 12 weeks of treatment of secondary Raynaud's phenomenon, a significant reduction of the duration and incidence of Raynaud's phenomenon was seen. However, in a double-blind, placebo-controlled study in primary Raynaud's phenomenon patients, the beraprost treatment was not statistically more beneficial than placebo.[171] Finally, another related drug, cicaprost, demonstrated improvement in the severity of Raynaud's phenomenon in a double-blind, placebo-controlled study.[172]

2. Pulmonary Hypertension

The most exciting recent advance in the treatment of pulmonary hypertension is the use of prostacyclin. In patients with primary pulmonary hypertension, continuous infusion of prostacyclin resulted in improved symptoms and a decline of pulmonary artery pressure by more than 10 mm Hg in more than 60% of patients.[173] However, the drug is not approved for use in secondary forms of pulmonary hypertension such as scleroderma-related pulmonary hypertension. In a study in systemic lupus erythematosus-related pulmonary hypertension, short-term continuous infusion of prostaglandin I_2 and E_1 supplementing pulse cyclophosphamide produced satisfactory results.[174] This was in a 48-month experience of the use of monthly low-dose infusion of iloprost in a SLE patient with pulmonary hypertension.[175] In another study, in twelve patients with severe pulmonary hypertension and connective tissue diseases treated with continuous infusion of prostacyclin, a significant improvement was demonstrated in pulmonary artery pressure, cardiac index, and mixed venous oxygen saturation.[176] More recently, continuous infusion of prostacyclin in patients with severe pulmonary hypertension secondary to connective tissue diseases (six with CREST syndrome, five with SLE, three with mixed connective tissue disease, two with systemic sclerosis, and one with primary Sjogren's syndrome) demonstrated significant improvements in mean pulmonary artery pressure and exercise tolerance.[177]

REFERENCES

1. Hirsh, J., Warkentin, T. E., Rashke, R., Granger, C., Ohman, E. M., Dalen, J. E., Heparin and low-molecular-weight heparin: mechanisms of action, pharmacokinetics, dosing considerations, monitoring, efficacy, and safety, *Chest*, 114 (Suppl.), 489, 1998.
2. Weitz, J. I., Low-Molecular Weight Heparins, *N. Engl. J. Med.*, 337, 688, 1997.
3. Pineo, G. F., Hull, R. D., Unfractionated and Low-Molecular-Weight Heparin: Comparisons and current recommendations, *Med. Clin. North Am.*, 82, 587, 1998.
4. Hirsh, J., Levine M. N., Low molecular weight heparin, *Blood*, 79, 1, 1992.
5. Rosenberg, R. D., Biochemistry and pharmacology of Low Molecular Weight Heparin, *Semin. Hematol.*, 34 (Suppl. 4), 2, 1997.
6. Kessler, C. M., Low Molecular Weight Heparins: Practical considerations, *Semin. Hematol.*, 34 (Suppl. 4), 35, 1997.
7. Bara, L., Billaud, E., Gramond, G., Kher, A., Samama, M., Comparative pharmacokinetics of a low molecular weight heparin (PK 10 169) and unfractionated heparin after intravenous and subcutaneous administration, *Thromb. Res.*, 39, 631, 1985.
8. Gram, J., Mercker, S., Brühn, H. D., Does Protamine chloride neutralize low molecular weight heparin sufficiently? *J. Cardiothor. Anesth.*, 3, 659, 1989.
9. Frydman, A., Low-molecular-weight heparins: An overview of their pharmacodynamics, pharmacokinetics and metabolism in humans, *Haemostasis*, 26 (Suppl. 2), 24, 1996.
10. Young, E., Wells, P., Holloway, S., Weitz, J., Hirsh, J., *Ex-vivo* and *in-vivo* evidence that low molecular weight heparins exibit less binding to plasma proteins than unfractionated heparin, *Thromb. Haemost.*, 71, 300, 1994.
11. Krupinski, K., Basic-Micic, M., Lindhoff, E., Breddin, H. K., Inhibition of coagulation and platelet adhesion to extracellular matrix by unfractionated heparin and a low molecular weight heparin, *Blut*, 61, 289, 1990.
12. Serra, A., Esteve, J., Reverter, J. C., Lozano, M., Escolar, G., Ordinas, A., Differential effect of a low-molecular-weight heparin (Dalteparin) and unfractionated heparin on platelet interaction with the subendothelium under flow conditions, *Thromb. Res.*, 87, 405, 1997.
13. Lane, D. A., Pejler, G., Flynn, A. M., Thompson, E. A., Lindahl, U., Neutralization of heparin-related saccharides by histidine-rich glycoprotein and platelet factor 4, *J. Biol. Chem.*, 261, 3980, 1986.
14. Teitel, J. M., Rosenberg, R. D., Protection of factor Xa from neutralization by the heparin-antithrombin complex, *J. Clin. Invest.*, 71, 1383, 1983.

15. Chiu, H. M., Hirsh, J., Young, W. L., Regoeczi, E., Gent, M., Relationship between anticoagulant and antithrombotic effects of heparin, *Blood*, 49, 171, 1987.

16. Hirsh, J., Comparison of the relative efficacy and safety of low molecular weight heparin and unfractionated heparin for the treatment of deep venous thrombosis, *Semin. Hematol.*, 34 (Suppl. 4), 20, 1997.

17. Aguilar, D., Goldhaber, S. Z., Clinical uses of low-molecular-weight heparins, *Chest*, 115, 1418, 1999.

18. Kakkar, V. V., Low Molecular Weight Heparins: Prophylaxis on venous thromboembolism in surgical patients, *Semin. Hematol.*, 34 (Suppl. 4), 9, 1997.

19. Nurmohamed, M. T., Rosendaal, F. R., Buller, H. R., Dekker, E., Hommes, D. W., Vanderbrouke, J. P., Briet, E., Low-molecular-weight heparin versus standard heparin in general and orthopaedic surgery: a meta-analysis, *Lancet*, 340, 152, 1992.

20. Imperiale, T. F., Speroff, T., A meta-analysis of methods to prevent venous thromboembolism following total hip repleacement, *JAMA*, 271, 1780, 1994.

21. Green, D., Prophylaxis of thromboembolism in spinal cord-injuried patients, *Chest*, 102 (Suppl.), 649, 1994.

22. Bergmann, J. F., Elkharrat, D., Prevention of venous thromboembolic risk in non-surgical patients, *Haemostasis*, 26 (Suppl. 2), 16, 1996.

23. Halkin, H., Goldberg, J., Modan, M., Modan, B., Reduction of mortality in general medical in-patients by low-dose heparin prophylaxis, *Ann. Intern. Med.*, 96, 561, 1982.

24. Dahan, R., Houlbert, D., Caulin, C., Cuzin, E., Viltart, C., Woler, M., Segrestaa, J. M., Prevention of deep thrombosis in elderly medical in-patients by a low molecular weight heparin: A randomized double-blind trial, *Haemostasis*, 16, 159, 1986.

25. Edmonson, R. A., Cohen, A. T., Das, S. K., Wagner, M. B., Kakkar, V. V., Low molecular weight heparin versus aspirin and dipyridamole after femoro-popliteal by pass engrafting, *Lancet*, 344, 914, 1994.

26. Faxon, D. P., Spiro, T. E., Minor, S., Coté, G., Douglas, J., Gottlieb, R., Califf, R., Dorosti, K., Topol, E., Gordon J. B., for the ERA Investigators, Low molecular weight heparin in prevention of restenosis after angioplasty: Results of enoxiparin restenosis (ERA) trial, *Circulation*, 90, 908, 1994.

27. Pepine, C. J., Holmes, D. R. Jr., Coronary artery stents, *J. Am. Coll. Cardiol.*, 28, 782, 1996.

28. Ferguson, J. J., Fox, R., Meeting highlights, *Circulation*, 95, 761, 1997.

29. Siragusa, S., Cosmi, B., Piovella, F., Hirsh, J., Ginsberg, J. S., Low-molecular-weight heparin in the treatment of patients with acute venous thromboembolism: Results of a meta-analysis, *Am. J. Med.*, 100, 269, 1996.

30. Harenberg, J., Schmitz-Huebner, U., Breddin, K. H., Haas, S., Heinrich, F., Heinrichs, C., Kienast, J., Roebruck, P., Theiss, W., Treatment of deep vein thrombosis with low-molecular-weight heparins: A Consensus Statement of the Gesellschaf für Thrombose-und Hämostaseforschung (GTH), *Semin. Thromb. Hemost.*, 23, 91, 1997.

31. Lensing, A. W., Prins, M. H., Davidson, B. L., Hirsh, J., Treatment of deep venous thrombosis with low-molecular weight heparins: A meta-analysis, *Arch. Intern. Med.*, 155, 601, 1995.

32. Turkstra, F., Koopman, M. M. W., Büller, H., The treatment of deep venous thrombosis and pulmonary embolism, *Thromb. Haemost.*, 78, 489, 1997.

33. Hull, R. D., Raskob, G. E., Pineo, G. F., Green, D., Trowbridge, A. A., Elliott, C. G., Lerner, R. G., Hall, J., Sparling, T., Brettell, H. R., Subcutaneous low-molecular-weight heparin compared with continuous intravenous heparin in the initial treatment of proximal-vein thrombosis, *New Engl. J. Med.*, 326, 975, 1992.

34. Hyers, T. M., Hull, R. D., Weg, J. G., Antithrombotic therapy for venous thromboembolic disease, *Chest*, 108 (Suppl.), 335, 1995.

35. Dolovich, L., Ginsberg, S., Low molecular weight heparin in the treatment of thromboembolism: an updated meta-analysis, *Vessels*, 3, 4, 1997.

36. The Columbus Investigators, Low-molecular-weight heparin in the treatment of patients with venous thromboembolism, *N. Engl. J. Med.*, 337, 657, 1997.

37. Simonneau, G., Sors, H., Charbonnier, B., Page, Y., Laaban, J. P., Azarian, R., Laurent, M., Hirsh, J. L., Ferrari, E., Bosson J. L., Mottier, D., Beau, B., for the THÉSÉE Study Group, A comparison of low-molecular-weight heparin with unfractionated heparin for acute pulmonary embolism, *N. Engl. J. Med.*, 337, 663, 1997.

38. van der Belt, A. G. M., Bossuyt, P. M. M., Prins, M. H., Gallus, A. S., Büller, H. S., for the TASMAN Study Group, Replacing inpatient care by outpatient care in the treatment of deep venous thrombosis: an economic evaluation, *Thromb. Haemost.*, 79, 259, 1998.

39. Lindmarker, P., Holmström, M., Use of low molecular weight heparin (dalteparin), once daily, for the treatment of deep vein thrombosis: A feasibility and health economic study in an outpatient setting, *J. Intern. Med.*, 240, 395, 1996.

40. Fragmin during Inestability in Coronary Artery Disease (FRISC) Study Group, Low-molecular-weight heparin during inestability in coronary artery disease, *Lancet*, 347, 561, 1996.

41. Cohen, M., Demers, C., Gurfinkel, E. P., Turpie, A. G. G., Fromell, G. J., Goodman, S., Langer, A., Califf, R. M., Fox, K. A., Premmereur, J., Bingozi, F., A comparison of low-molecular-weight heparin with unfractionated heparin for unstable coronary artery disease. Efficacy and Safety of Subcutaneous Enoxiparin in Non-Q Wave Coronary Events Study Group, *N. Engl. J. Med.*, 337, 447, 1997.

42. The Thrombolysis in Miocardial Infarction (TIMI) 11A Trial Investigators, Dose ranging trial of enoxiparin for unstable angina: Results of TIMI 11A, *J. Am. Coll. Cardiol.*, 29, 1474, 1997.

43. Gurfinkel, E. P., Manos, E. J., Mejail, R. I., Cerda, M. A., Duronto, E. A., García, C. N., Daroca, A. M., Mautner, B., Low molecular weight heparin versus regular heparin or aspirin in the treatment of unstable angina and silent ischemia, *J. Am. Coll. Cardiol.*, 26, 313, 1995.

44. Chesebro, J. H., Treatment of arterial thrombosis with low molecular weight heparins, *Semin. Hematol.*, 34 (Suppl. 4), 26, 1997.

45. Walenga, J. M., Bick, R. L., Heparin-induced thrombocytopenia, paradoxical thromboembolism, and other side-effects of heparin therapy, *Med. Clin. North Am.*, 82, 635, 1998.

46. Kumar, P. D., Heparin-induced skin necrosis, *N. Engl. Med. J.*, 336, 588, 1997.

47. Giustolisi, R., Gugliemo, P., di Raimondo, F., Cacciola, E., Stagno, F., Hypereosinophilia and subcutaneous heparin, *N. Engl. J. Med.*, 342, 1371, 1993.

48. Triplett, D. A., Current recommendations for Warfarin therapy, *Med. Clin. North Am.*, 82, 601, 1998.

49. Hirsh, J., Oral anticoagulant drugs, *N. Eng. J. Med.*, 324, 1865, 1991.

50. Hirsh, J., Dalen, J. E., Deykin, D., Poller, L., Bussey, H., Oral anticoagulants. Mechanism of action, clinical effectiveness, and optimal therapeutic range, *Chest*, 108 (Suppl.), 231, 1995.

51. Hirsh, J., Dalen, J. E., Anderson, D. R., Poller, L., Bussey, H., Ansell, J., Deykin, D., Brandt, J. T., Oral anticoagulants. Mechanism of action, clinical effectiveness, and optimal therapeutic range, *Chest*, 114 (Suppl.), 445, 1998.

52. O'Relly, R. A., Studies on the optical enantiomorphs of warfarin in man, *Clin. Pharmacol. Ther.*, 16, 348, 1974.

53. Dowd, P., Ham, S. W., Naganathan, S., Hershline, R., The mechanisms of action of vitamin K, *Annu. Rev. Nutr.*, 15, 419, 1995.

54. Fasco, M. J., Hildebrandt, E. F., Suttie, J. W., Evidence that warfarin anticoagulant action involves two distinct reductase activities, *J. Biol. Chem.*, 257, 11210, 1982.

55. Suttie, J. W., Synthesis of vitamin K-dependent proteins, *FASEB J*, 7, 445, 1993.

56. Suttie, J. W., Vitamin K, in *Present Knowledge in Nutrition*, Ziegler, E. E., Filer, L. J., Eds., ILSI Press, Washington, 1996.

57. Hildebrandt, E. F., Suttie, J. W., Mechanism of coumarin action: sensitivity of vitamin K metabolizing enzymes of normal and warfarin-resistant rat liver, *Biochemistry*, 21, 2406, 1982.

58. Stirling, Y., Warfarin-induced changes in procoagulant and anticoagulant proteins, *Blood Coag. Fibrinolysis*, 6, 361, 1995.

59. Shearer, M. J., Vitamin K, *Lancet*, 345, 229, 1995.

60. Shearer, M. J., Bach, A., Kohlmeier, M., Chemistry, nutritional sources, tissue distribution and metabolism of vitamin K with special reference to bone health, *J. Nutr.*, 126 (Suppl.), 1181, 1996.

61. Booth, S. L., Skeletal functions of vitamin K-dependent proteins: not just for clotting anymore, *Nutr. Rev.*, 55, 282, 1997.

62. Stenflo, J., Ferlund, P., Egan, W., Roepstorff, P., Vitamin K-dependent modifications of glutamic acid residues in prothrombin, *Proc. Natl. Acad. Sci. U.S.A.*, 71, 2730, 1974.

63. Cropp, J. S., Bussey, H. I., A review of enzyme induction of warfarin metabolism with recommendations for patient management, *Pharmacotherapy*, 17, 917, 1997.

64. Hirsh, J., The optimal duration of anticoagulant therapy for venous thrombosis, *N. Engl. J. Med.*, 332, 1710, 1995.

65. Gohlke-Barwolf, C., Acar, J., Oakley, C., Butchart, D., Bodnar, E., Hall, R., Dalehaye, J. P., Horstkotte, D., Kremer, R., Guidelines for prevention of thromboembolism events in valvular heart disease, *Eur. J. Heart*, 16, 1320, 1995.
66. The Medical Research Council's General Practice Research Framework, Thrombosis Prevention Trial: randomised trial of low-intensity oral anticoagulation with warfarin and low-dose aspirin in the primary prevention of ischaemic heart disease in men at increased risk, *Lancet*, 351, 233, 1998.
67. Chesebro, J. H., Fuster, V., Elveback, L. R., McGoon D. C., Pluth, J. R., Puga, F. J., Wallace, R. B., Danielson, G. K., Orszulak, T. A., Piehler, J. M., Schaff, H. V., Trial of combined warfarin plus dipyridamole or aspirin therapy in prosthetic heart valve replacement: danger of aspirin compared with dipyridamole, *Am. J. Cardiol.*, 51, 1537, 1983.
68. Hull, R., Hirsh, J., Jay, R., Carter, C., England, C., Gent, M., Turpie, A. G., McLoughlin, G., Dodd, P., Thomas, M., Raskob, G., Ockelford, P., Different intensities of oral anticoagulant therapy in the treatment of proximal-vein thrombosis, *N. Engl. J. Med.*, 307, 1676, 1982.
69. Saour, J. N., Sieck, J. O., Mamo, L. A., Gallus, A. S., Trial of different intensities of anticoagulation in patients with prosthetic heart valves, *N. Engl. J. Med.*, 322, 428, 1990.
70. Altman, R., Rouvier, J., Gurfinkel, E., Comparison of two levels of anticoagulant therapy in patients with substitute heart valves, *J. Thorac. Cardiovasc. Surg.*, 101, 427, 1991.
71. Levine, M. N., Raskob, G., Hirsh, J., Hemorrhagic complications of long-term anticoagulant therapy, *Chest*, 95 (Suppl.), 26, 1989.
72. Levine, M. N., Hirsh, J., Landefeld, S., Raskob, G., Hemorrhagic complications of anticoagulant treatment, *Chest*, 102 (Suppl.), 352, 1992.
73. Levine, M. N., Hirsh, J., Hemorrhagic complications of anticoagulant therapy, *Semin. Throm. Hemost.*, 12, 39, 1986.
74. Forfar, J. C., A 7-year analysis of hemorrhage in patients on long-term anticoagulant treatment, *Br. Heart J.*, 42, 128, 1979.
75. Fihn, S. D., McDonell, M., Martin, D., Henikoff, J., Vermes, D., Kent, D., White, R. H., Risk factors for complications of chronic anticoagulation. A multicenter study. Warfarin Optimized Outpatient Follow-up Study Group, *Ann. Intern. Med.*, 118, 511, 1993.
76. Landenfeld, C. S., Goldman, L., Bleeding in outpatients treated with warfarin: incidence and prediction by factors known at the start of outpatient therapy, *Am. J. Med.*, 87, 144, 1989.
77. Baker, R. N., An evaluation of anticoagulant therapy in the treatment of cerebrovascular disease: report of the Veterans Administration Cooperative study of atherosclerosis, *Neurology*, 11, 132, 1961.
78. Hill, A. B., Marshall, J., Shaw, D. A., A controlled clinical trial of long-term anticoagulant therapy in cerebrovascular disease, *Q. J. Med.*, 29, 597, 1960.
79. Launbjerg, J., Egeblad, H., Heaf, J., Nielsen, N. H., Fugleholm, A. M., Ladefoged, K., Bleeding complications to oral anticoagulant therapy: multivariate analysis of 1010 treatment years in 551 outpatients, *J. Intern. Med.*, 229, 351, 1991.
80. Ginsberg, J. S., Hirsh, J., Turner, D. C., Levine, M. N., Burrows, R., Risk to the fetus of anticoagulant therapy during pregnancy, *Throm. Haemost.*, 61, 197, 1989.
81. Wong, V., Cheng, C. H., Chan, K. C., Fetal and neonatal outcome of exposure to anticoagulants during pregnancy, *Am. J. Med. Gen.*, 45, 17, 1993.
82. Vitalli, E., Doantelli, F., Quaini, E., Gropelli, G., Pellegrini, A., Pregnancy in patients with mechanical prostetic heart valves: our experience regarding 98 pregnancies in 57 patients, *J. Cardiovasc. Surg.*, 8, 221, 1986.
83. Sareli, P., England, M. J., Berk, M. R., Marcus, R. H., Epstein, M., Driscoll, J., Meyer, T., McIntyre, J., van Gelderen, C., Maternal and fetal sequelae of anticoagulation during pregnancy in patients with mechanical heart valve protheses, *Am. J. Cardiol.*, 63, 1465, 1989.
84. Comp, P. C., Elrod, J. P., Karzenski, S., Warfarin-induced skin necrosis, *Semin. Thromb. Hemost.*, 16, 293, 1990.
85. Grimaudo, V., Gueissaz, F., Hauert, J., Sarraj, A., Kruithof, E. K. O., Bachmann, F., Necrosis of skin induced by coumarin in a patient deficient in protein S, *Br. Med. J.*, 298, 233, 1989.
86. Samama, M., Horellou, M. H., Soria, J., Conard, J., Nicolas, G., Succesful progressive anticoagulation in a severe protein C deficiency and previous skin necrosis at the initiation of oral anticoagulant treatment, *Throm. Haemost.*, 51, 132, 1984.

87. Locht, H., Lindstrom, F. D., Severe skin necrosis following warfarin therapy in a patient with protein C deficiency, *J. Intern. Med.*, 233, 287, 1993.

88. Kiehl, R., Hellstern, P., Wenzel, E., Hereditary antithrombin III deficiency and an atypical localization of coumarin necrosis, *Throm. Res.*, 45, 191, 1987.

89. Moreb, J., Kitchens, C. S., Acquired functional protein S deficiency, cerebral venous thrombosis, and coumarin skin necrosis in association with antiphospholipid syndrome: report of two cases, *Am. J. Med.*, 87, 207, 1989.

90. O'Keeffe, S., Woods, B. O., Breslin, D. J., Tsapatsaris, N. P., Blue toe syndrome. Causes and management, *Arch. Intern. Med.*, 152, 2197, 1992.

91. Moldveen Geronimus, M., Merrian, J. C., Cholesterol embolization: from pathological curiosity to clinical entity, *Circulation*, 35, 946, 1967.

92. Taybi, H., Capitanio, M. A., Tracheobronchial calcification: an observation in three children after mitral valve replacement and Warfarin sodium therapy, *Radiology*, 176, 728, 1990.

93. Moncada, R. M., Venta, L. A., Venta, E. R., Fareed, J., Walenga, J. M., Messmore, H. L., Tracheal and bronchial cartilaginous rings: warfarin sodium-induced calcification, *Radiology*, 184, 437, 1992.

94. Patrono, C., Dalen, J. E., Gent, M., Hirsh, J., Platelet-active drugs. The relationships among dose, effectiveness, and side effects, *Chest*, 114, 470S, 1998.

95. Antiplatelet Trialists' Collaboration. Collaborative overview of randomized trials of antiplatelet therapy: I. Prevention of death, myocardial infraction, and stroke by prolonged antiplatelet therapy in various categories of patients, *Br. Med. J.*, 308, 81, 1994.

96. Calverley, D. C., Roth, G. J., Antiplatelet therapy: Aspirin, ticlopidine/clopidogrel, and anti-integrin agents, *Hematol. Oncol. Clin. North Am.*, 12, 1231, 1998.

97. Roth, G. J., Stanford, N., Majerus, P. W., Acetylation of prostaglandin synthase by aspirin, *Proc. Natl. Acad. Sci. U.S.A.*, 72, 3073, 1975.

98. FitzGerald, G. A., Dipyridamole, *N. Engl. J. Med.*, 316, 1247, 1987.

99. Tcheng, J. E., Ellis, S. G., George, B. S., Kereiakes, D. J., Keiman, N. S., Talley, J. D., Wang, A. L., Weisman, H. F., Califf, R. M., Topol, E. J., Pharmacodynamics of chimeric glycoprotein IIb/IIIa integrin antiplatelet antibody Fab 7E3 in high-risk coronary angioplasty, *Circulation*, 90, 1757, 1994.

100. Coller, B. S., Platelet GPIIb/IIIa antagonists: the first antiintegrin receptor therapeutics, *J. Clin. Invest.*, 99, 1467, 1997.

101. Coller, B. S., Peerschke, E. L., Scudder, L. E., Sullivan, C. A., A murine monoclonal antibody that completely blocks the binding of fibrinogen to platelets produces a thrombasthenic-like state in normal platelets and binds to glycoprotein IIb and/or IIIa, *J. Clin. Invest.*, 72, 325, 1983.

102. Egbertson, M. S., Chang, C. T., Duggan, M. E., Gould, R. J., Halczenko, W., Hartman, G. D., Laswell, W. L., Lynch, J. J. Jr., Lynch R. J., Manno, P. D., Non-peptide fibrinogen receptor anatagonists: II. Optimization of a tyrosine template as a mimic for Arg-Gly-Asp, *J. Med. Chem.*, 37, 2537, 1994.

103. Scarborough, R. M., Naughton, M. A., Teng, W., Rose, J. V., Phillips, D. R., Nannizzi, L., Arfsten, A., Campbell, A. M., Charo, I. F., Design of potent and specific integrin antagonists: peptide antagonists with high specificity for glycoprotein IIb/IIIa, *J. Biol. Chem.*, 268, 1066, 1993.

104. Carteaux, J. P., Steiner, B., Roux, S., Ro 44-9883, a new non-peptidic GPIIb/IIIa antagonist prevents platelet loss in a guinea pig model of extracorporeal circulation, *Thromb. Haemost.*, 70, 817, 1993.

105. Roth, G. J., Majerus, P. W., The mechanism of the effect of aspirin in human platelets: I. Acetylation of a particulate fraction protein, *J. Clin. Invest.*, 56, 624, 1975.

106. Burch, J. W., Stanford, P. W., Majerus, P. W., Inhibition of platelet prostaglandin synthase by oral aspirin, *J. Clin. Invest.*, 61, 314, 1979.

107. Smith, W. L., Garavito, R. M., DeWitt, D. L., Prostaglandin endoperoxide H synthases (cyclooxygenases)-1 and -2, *J. Biol. Chem.*, 271, 33157, 1996.

108. Moncada, S., Vane, J. R., Pharmacology and endogenous roles of prostaglandin endoperoxides, thromboxane-A_2 and prostacyclin, *Pharmacol. Rev.*, 30, 293, 1978.

109. FitzGerald, G. A., Patrono, C., Antiplatelet Drugs, in: *Cardiovascular Thrombosis-Thrombocardiology, Thromboneurology*, Verstraete, M., Fuster, V., Topol, E., Eds., Lippincott-Raven, Philadelphia, 1998.

110. Ito, M. K., Smith, A. R., Lee, M. L., Ticlopidine: a new platelet aggregation inhibitor, *Clin. Pharm.*, 11, 603, 1992.

111. Savi, P., Heilmann, E., Nurden, P., Clopidogrel: an antithrombotic drug acting on the ADP-dependent activation pathway of human platelets, *Clin. Appl. Thromb. Hemost.*, 2, 35, 1996.

112. Reverter, J. C., Bèguin, S., Kessels, H., Kumar, R., Hemker, H. C., Coller, B. S., Inhibition of platelet-mediated, tissue factor-induced thrombin generation by the mouse/human chimeric 7E3 antibody: potential implications for effect of c7E3 Fab treatment on acute thrombosis and "clinical restenosis," *J. Clin. Invest.*, 98, 863, 1996.

113. Pedersen, A. K., FitzGerad, G. A., Dose-related kinetics of aspirin: presystemic acetylation of platelet cyclo-oxygenase, *N. Engl. J. Med.*, 311, 1206, 1984.

114. Ramis, J., Torrent, J., Mis, R., Conte, L., Barbanoj, M. J., Jane, J., Forn, J., Pharmacokinetics of trifusal after single and repeated doses in man, *Int. J. Clin. Pharmacol. Ther. Toxicol.*, 28, 344, 1990.

115. ISIS-2 Collaborative Group. Randomised trial of intravenous streptokinase, oral aspirin, both or neither among 17,187 cases of suspected acute myocardial infarction: ISIS-2, *Lancet*, 2, 349, 1988.

116. The RISC Group. Risk of myocardial infarction and death during treatment with low dose aspirin and intravenous heparin in men with unstable coronary artery disease, *Lancet*, 336, 827, 1990.

117. International Stroke Trial Collaborative Group. The International Stroke Trial (IST): a randomised trial of aspirin, subcutaneous heparin, both, or neither among 19,435 patients with acute ischemic stroke, *Lancet*, 349, 1569, 1997.

118. Hennekens, C. H., Dyken, M. L., Fuster, V., Aspirin as a therapeutic agent in cardiovascular disease, *Circulation*, 96, 2751, 1997.

119. Hass, W. K., Easton, J. D., Adams, H. P., Pryse-Phillips, W., Molony, B. A., Anderson, S., Kamm, B., A randomized trial comparing ticlopidine hydrochloride with aspirin for the prevention of stroke in high-risk patients, *N. Engl. J. Med.*, 321, 501, 1989.

120. FitzGerald, G. A., Ticlopidine in unstable angina: a more expensive aspirin?, *Circulation*, 82, 296, 1990.

121. Balsano, F., Rizzon, P., Violi, F., Scrutinio, D., Cimminiello, C., Aguglia, F., Pasotti, C., Rudelli, G., Antiplatelet treatment with ticlopidine in unstable angina: a controlled multicenter clinical trial, *Circulation*, 82, 17, 1990.

122. More, R. S., Chauhan, A., Antiplatelet rather than anticoagulant therapy with coronary stenting, *Lancet*, 349, 146, 1997.

123. CAPRIE Steering Committee. A randomised, blinded, trial of clopidogrel versus aspirin in patients at risk of ischemic events (CAPRIE), *Lancet*, 348, 1329, 1996.

124. The EPIC Investigators. Use of a monoclonal antibody directed against the platelet glycoprotein IIb/IIIa receptor in high-risk coronary angioplasty, *N. Engl. J. Med.*, 330, 956, 1994.

125. The EPILOG Investigators. Platelet glycoprotein IIb/IIIa receptor blockade and low-dose heparin during percutaneous coronary revascularization, *N. Engl. J. Med.*, 336, 1689, 1997.

126. Petersen, P., Boysan, G., Godtfredsen, J., Andersen, E. D., Andersen, B., Placebo controlled, randomized trial of warfarin and aspirin for prevention of thromboembolic complications in chronic atrial fibrillation: the Copenhagen AFASAK Study, *Lancet*, 1, 175, 1989.

127. EAFT (European Atrial Fibrillation Trial) Study Group. Secondary prevention in nonrheumatic atrial fibrillation after transient ischaemic attack or minor stroke, *Lancet*, 342, 1255, 1993.

128. Powers, P. J., Gent, M., Jay, R. M., Julian, D. H., Turpie, A. G., Levine, M., Hirsh, J., A randomized trial of less intensive post-operative warfarin and aspirin therapy in the prevention of venous thromboembolism after surgery for fractured hip, *Arch. Intern. Med.*, 149, 771, 1989.

129. Golding, J., A randomised trial of low dose aspirin in primiparae in pregnancy. The Jamaica Low-Dose Aspirin Study Group, *Br. J. Obstet. Gynaecol.*, 105, 286, 1998.

130. Caritis, S., Sibai, B., Hauth, J., Lindheimer, M. D., Klebanoff, M., Thom, E., Van Dorsten, P., Landon, M., Paul, R., Miodovnik, M., Meis, P., Thurnau, G., Low-dose aspirin to prevent preeclampsia in women at high risk, *N. Engl. J. Med.*, 338, 701, 1998.

131. Roderick, P. J., Wilkes, H. C., Meade, T. W., The gastrointestinal toxicity of aspirin: An overview of randomised controlled trials, *Br. J. Clin. Pharmacol.*, 35, 219, 1993.

132. Diener, H. C., Cunha, L., Forbes, C., Sivenius, J., Smets, P., Lowenthal, A., European stroke prevention study: II. Dipyridamole and acetylsalicylic acid in the secondary prevention of stroke, *J. Neurol. Sci.*, 143, 1, 1996.

133. Kelly, J. P., Kaufman, D. W., Jurgelon, J. M., Sheehan, J., Koff, R. S., Shapiro, S., Risk of aspirin-associated major upper-gastrointestinal bleeding with enteric-coated or buffered product, *Lancet*, 348, 1413, 1996.

134. Yeh, S. P., Hsueh, E. J., Wu, H., Wang, Y. C., Ticlopidine-associated aplastic anemia: a case report and review of literature, *Ann. Haematol.*, 76, 87, 1998.

135. Bennett, C. L., Weinberg, P. D., Rozenberg-Ben-Dror, K., Yarnold, P. R., Kwaan, H. C., Green, D., Thrombotic thrombocytopenic purpura associated with ticlopidine: a review of 60 cases, *Ann. Intern. Med.*, 128, 541, 1998.

136. Tcheng, J. E., Clinical challenges of platelet glycoprotein IIb/IIIa receptor inhibitor therapy, bleeding, reversal, thrombocytopenia, and retreatment, *Am. Heart J.*, 139, 38, 2000.

137. Cairns, J. A., Chair, J., Kennedy, W., Fuster, V., Coronary thrombolysis, *Chest*, 114, 634S, 1998.

138. Hyers, T. M., Hull, R. D., Weg, J. G., Antithrombotic therapy for venous thromboembolic disease, *Chest*, 102, 408S, 1992.

139. Arcasoy, S. M., Kreit, J. W., Thrombolytic therapy of pulmonary embolism. A comprehensive review of current evidence, *Chest*, 115, 1695, 1999.

140. Gulba, D. C., Bode, C., Runge, M. S., Huber, K., Thrombolytic agents: an overview, *Ann. Haematol.*, 73, S9, 1996.

141. Kohnert, U., Rudolph, R., Verheijen, J. H., Weening-Verhoeff, E. J., Stern, A., Opitz, U., Martin, U., Lill, H., Prinz, H., Lechner, M., Biochemical properties of the kringle 2 and protease domains are maintained in the refolded t-PA deletion variant BM 06.022, *Prot. Engineer.*, 5, 93, 1992.

142. Keyt, B. A., Paoni, N. F., Refino, C. J., Berleau, L., Nguyen, H., Chow, A., Lai, J., Pena, L., Pater, C., Ogez, J., Etcheverry, T., Botstein, D., Bennett, W. F., A faster-acting and more potent form of tissue plasminogen activator, *Proc. Natl. Acad. Sci. U.S.A.*, 91, 3670, 1994.

143. Gurewich, V., Pannell, R., A comparative study of the efficacy and specificity of tissue plasminogen activator and prourokinase: demonstration of synergism and of different threshold of non-selectivity, *Thromb. Res.*, 44, 217, 1986.

144. Monk, J. P., Heel, R. C., Anisoylated plasminogen streptokinase activator complex (APSAC): a review of its mechanism of action, clinical pharmacology, and therapeutic use in myocardial infarction, *Drugs*, 34, 25, 1987.

145. Collen, D., Linjen, H. R., Basic and clinical aspects of fibrinolysis and thrombolysis, *Blood*, 78, 3114, 1991.

146. Collen, D., Fibrin-selective thrombolytic therapy for acute myocardial infarction, *Circulation*, 93, 857, 1996.

147. Agnelli, G., Rationale for bolus t-PA therapy to improve efficacy and safety, *Chest*, 97(Suppl.), 161S, 1990.

148. Collen, D., Staphylokinase: a potent, uniquely fibrin-selective thrombolytic agent, *Nature Med.*, 4, 279, 1998.

149. Yusuf, S., Collins, R., Peto, R., Furberg, G., Stampler, M. J., Goldhaber, S. Z., Hennekens, C. H., Intravenous and intracoronary fibrinolytic therapy in acute myocardial infarction: overview of results on mortality, reinfarction and side effects from 33 randomized controlled trials, *Eur. Heart J.*, 6, 556, 1985.

150. Gruppo italiano per lo studio della streptokinase nell' infarto miocardico (GISSI). Effecctiveness of intravenous thrombolytic treatment in acute myocardial infarction, *Lancet*, 1, 397, 1986.

151. Fibrinolytic therapy trialists' (FTT) collaborative group. Indications for fibrinolytic therapy in suspected acute myocardial infarction: collaborative overview of early mortality and major morbidity results from all randomized trials of more than 1,000 patients, *Lancet*, 343, 311, 1994.

152. AIMS trial study group. Effect of intravenous APSAC on mortality after acute myocardial infarction: preliminary report of a placebo-controlled clinical trial, *Lancet*, 1, 545, 1988.

153. Wilcox, R. G., Van der Lippe, G., Olsson, C. G., Jensen, G., Skene, A. M., Hampton, J. R., Effects of alteplase in acute myocardial infarction: 6-months results from the ASSET study, *Lancet*, 335, 1175, 1990.

154. ISIS-3 collaborative group. ISIS-3: a randomized comparison of streptokinase vs. tissue plasminogen activator vs. anistreplase and of aspirin plus heparin vs. aspirin alone among 41,299 cases of suspected acute myocardial infarction, *Lancet*, 339, 753, 1992.

155. Gruppo italiano per lo studio della sopravvivenza nell'infarto miocardico. GISSI-2: a factorial randomized trial of alteplase and heparin versus no heparin among 12,490 patients with acute myocardial infarction, *Lancet*, 336, 65, 1990.

156. The GUSTO investigators. An international randomized trial comparing four thrombolytic strategies for acute myocardial infarction, *N. Engl. J. Med.*, 329, 673, 1993.

157. The global use of strategies to open coronary arteries (GUSTO III) investigators. A comparison of reteplase with alteplase for acute myocardial infarction, *N. Engl. J. Med.*, 337, 1118, 1997.

158. International joint efficacy comparison of thrombolytics. Randomized, double-blind comparison of reteplase double-bolus administration with streptokinase in acute myocardial infarction (INJECT): trial to investigate equivalence, *Lancet*, 346, 329, 1995.

159. The continuous infusion versus double-bolus administration of alteplase (COBALT) investigators. A comparison of continuous infusion of alteplase with double-bolus administration for acute myocardial infarction, *N. Engl. J. Med.*, 337, 1124, 1997.

160. Coller, B. S., Platelets and thrombolytic therapy, *N. Engl. J. Med.*, 322, 32, 1990.

161. Lew, A. S., Laramee, P., Cercek, B., Shah, P. K., Ganz, W., The hypotensive effect of intravenous streptokinase in patients with acute myocardial infarction, *Circulation*, 72, 1321, 1985.

162. Smith, W. L., Prostanoid biosynthesis and mechanism of action, *Am. J. Physiol.*, 268, F181, 1992.

163. Prescott, S. M., Majerus, P. W., Characterization of 1,2-diacylglycerol hydrolysis in human platelets. Demonstration of an arachidonyl-monoacylglycerol intermediate, *J. Biol. Chem.*, 258, 764, 1983.

164. Sigal, E., The molecular biology of mammalian arachidonic acid metabolism, *Am. J. Physiol.*, 260, L113, 1991.

165. Coleman, R. A., Smith, W. L., Narumiya, S., International Union of Pharmacology Classification of Prostanoid Receptors: properties, distribution and structure of the receptors and their subtypes, *Pharmacol. Rev.*, 46, 205, 1994.

166. Moncada, S., Gryglewski, R., Bunting, S., Vane, J. R., An enzyme isolated from arteries transforms prostaglandin endoperoxides to an unstable substance that inhibits platelet aggregation, *Nature*, 263, 663, 1976.

167. Zachariae, H., Halkier-Sorensen, L., Bjerring, P., Heickendorff, L., Treatment of ischaemic digital ulcers and prevention of gangrene with intravenous iloprost in systemic sclerosis, *Acta Derm. Venereol.*, 76, 236, 1996.

168. Wigley, F. M., Wise, R. A., Seibold, J. R., McCloskey, D. A., Kujala, G., Medsger, T. A. Jr., Steen, V. D., Varga, J., Jimenez, S., Mayes, M., Clements, P. J., Weiner, S. R., Porter, J., Ellman, M., Wise, C., Kaufman, L. D., Williams, J., Dole, W., Intravenous iloprost infusion in patients with Raynaud's phenomenon secondary to systemic sclerosis, *Ann. Intern. Med.*, 120, 199, 1994.

169. Black, C. M., Halkier-Sorensen, L., Belch, J. J., Ullman, S., Madhok, R., Smit, A. J., Banga, J. D., Watson, H. R., Oral iloprost in Raynaud's phenomenon secondary to Systemic Sclerosis: a multicentre, placebo-controlled, dose-comparison study, *Br. J. Rheumatol.*, 37, 952, 1998.

170. Hiida, M., Hushiyama, O., Suzuki, N., Ohta, A., Nagasawa, K., Yamaguchi, M., The effect of beraprost sodium on the Raynaud's phenomenon, *Nippon Rinsho Meneki Gakkai Kaishi*, 19, 193, 1996.

171. Vayssarait, M., and the French Microcirculation Society Multicenter Group for the Study of Vascular Acrosyndromes, Controlled multicenter double blind trial of an analog oral of prostacyclin in the treatment of primary Raynaud's phenomenon, *J. Rheumatol.*, 23, 1917, 1996.

172. Lau, C. S., Belch, J. J., Madhok, R., A randomised, double-blind study of cicaprost, an oral prostacyclin analogue, in the treatment of Raynaud's phenomenon secondary to systemic sclerosis, *Clin. Exp. Rheumatol.*, 11, 35, 1993.

173. Rubin, L. J., Mendoza, J., Hood, M., McGoon, M., Barst, R., Williams, W. B., Diehl, J. H., Crow, J., Long, W., Treatment of primary pulmonary hypertension with continuous intravenous prostacyclin (esoprostenol), *Ann. Med. Int.*, 112, 485, 1990.

174. Ignaszewski, A. P., Percy, J. S., Humen, D. P., Successful treatment of pulmonary hypertension, *J. Rheumatol.*, 2, 367, 1993.

175. Mok, M. Y., Tse, H. F., Lau, C. S., Pulmonary hypertension secondary to systemic lupus erythematosus: prolonged survival following treatment with intermittent low dose of iloprost, *Lupus*, 8, 328, 1999.

176. Humbert, M., Sanchez, O., Fartoukh, M., Jagot, J. L., Sitbon, O., Simmoneau, G., Treatment of severe pulmonary hypertension secondary to connective tissue diseases with continuous IV epoprostenol (prostacyclin), *Chest*, 114 (Suppl.), 80S, 1998.

177. Humbert, M., Sanchez, O., Fartoukh, M., Jagot, J. L., Le Gall, C., Sitbon, O., Parent, F., Simmoneau, G., Short-term and long-term epoprostenol (prostacyclin) therapy in pulmonary hypertension secondary to connective tissue diseases: results of a pilot study, *Eur. Respir. J.*, 13, 1351, 1999.

32 Hormone Replacement Therapy for "At Risk" Patients with Connective Tissue Diseases

Anne Gompel

CONTENTS

0-8493-1335-X/01/$0.00+$.50
© 2001 by CRC Press LLC

I. INTRODUCTION

Autoimmune and connective tissue diseases often increase the risk in cardiovascular diseases and osteoporosis, directly or by means of corticosteroids (CS) treatments. Thus, postmenopausal patients with connective tissue diseases theoretically could have even greater benefits from Hormone Replacement Therapy (HRT) than normal women. But the CS together with the connective disease also increase the risk of thrombo-embolic diseases, so that the choice in estrogen and progestin have to be cautious in this aspect.

The benefits of HRT are established for the treatment of hypoestrogenic symptoms with improvement in well-being, hot flashes, libido, depression, and urogenital symptoms. Another major benefit is osteoporosis prevention. However, prevention of cardio-vascular diseases, and in particular heart diseases, remains discussed in its importance since many biases may have led to the very favorable scope given by observational studies. Indeed, women treated with estrogen appear to be more healthy, more compliant, have a higher socio-economic status, and are at lower risk for cardio-vascular diseases since, until recently, hypertension, diabetes, and heart diseases were considered as contraindications for HRT.[1] Moreover, no benefit seems to be recorded on stroke,[2-4] and the overall benefit described on total mortality[5-9] could only reflect the better risk of "more healthy" women under estrogens.[1]

Most of the studies also reported that the protective effect was of short duration after discontinuation of therapy.[9] However, a study has shown a greater benefit in women with higher risk (Table 32.1). A more recent possible, but not definitely proven, benefit is an improvement in Alzheimer's disease,[10,11] but additional data will come from a large randomized intervention study, the Women's Health Initiative. In balance to the demonstrated benefits, some side-effects are also well demonstrated, such as a 2- to 3-fold increase in deep vein thrombosis (DVT).[12] Data on increase in breast cancer risk are more conflicting, but an increase to a level of 1.3 is generally admitted after 5 to 10 years of use.[1,13] In addition to these classical side-effects described in normal women, some additional effects may be observed in women with autoimmune diseases since estrogens are well-known enhancers of autoimmunity.

Not all connective tissue diseases display the same pathogenesis and some patients may be particularly at risk of worsening with HRT, whereas some other patients could improve from such treatments. Indeed, systemic lupus erythematosus (SLE), a disease linked to excess in Th2 cytokine (IL-4, IL-10) production, predominantly affects women in reproductive years, whereas rheumatoid arthritis (RA), characterized by deficient Th2 cytokine production, is also more common in women, but its highest incidence is at menopause as well as some other connectivite diseases such as systemic sclerosis. SLE and RA are undoubtedly oppositely influenced by pregnancy (and oral

TABLE 32.1
HRT and Cardiovascular Diseases

		RR (CI95%)
Grodstein et al. 1996	CHD	CE:0.60 (0.43–0.83)
		E+P:0.39 (0.19–0.78)
Falkeborn et al. 1992	MI	CE,E2:0.9 (0.7–1.2)
		E+P:0.53(0.3–0.87)
Rosenberg et al. 1993	MI	CE: 0.9 (0.6–1.2)
		E+P:1.2 (0.6–2.4)
Grodstein et al. 1997	CV high-risk women	0.52 (0.45–0.57)
	CV low-risk women	0.89 (0.62–1.28)
Sourander et al. 1998	C-V mortality (current-users)	0.21 (0.08–0.59)
	C-V morbidity (current-users)	1.07 (0.86–1.32)

contraceptives), and these observations can be explained by the shift during pregnancy between Th1 and Th2 cytokine production.[14]

II. PHARMACOLOGY AND PRINCIPLES OF TREATMENT

The aim of HRT is to alleviate the postmenopausal consequences of estradiol deficiency. It thus consists of an administration of estrogen combined with progestin.

A. ESTROGEN/PROGESTIN TREATMENT

1. Estrogens

Different estrogens are marketed in the world. The more physiological product is estradiol (E2), which is the main potent natural estrogen secreted from the ovary. E2 seems now to be predominantly used in European countries. Also used is an E2 ester, estradiol valerate, which is administered orally and is very close to E2. In the United States, conjugated estrogens (CE) remain the dominant prescription. These estrogens are extracted from the urine of pregnant mares and represent a mixture of human (E2, E1, E1 sulfate) and equine estrogens (equiline, equiniline, dihydroequiniline, dihydroequiline). They thus appear to have a relatively stronger estrogenic potency than E2 and are composed of various derivatives, the effects of which have not being systematically studied. Estriol, a very weak estrogen, is also used orally as a systemic treatment of estrogen deficiency, but it has no proven effect regarding bone protection.

Estradiol (E2) can be administrated orally, transdermally, or percutaneously. It is differentially metabolized according to the route of administration. After an oral administration there is a rapid intestinal metabolism into estrone (E1), which is thereafter even enhanced at the hepatic level. Thus the ratio between E2 and E1 is less than 1, whereas in case of extra-digestive administration the ratio is the inverse and thus more physiologic.[15,16] The main difference between these routes of administration is the hepatic first-pass effect with the oral route, which modifies more significantly some markers of the vascular risk at the hepatic level: HDL-cholesterol is higher and LDL-cholesterol lower using digestive pathway. As a correlation, triglycerides are increased as well as some of the clotting factors, and some anticoagulants are decreased.[15-20] In general, extradigestive administration very minimally alters the hepatic proteins involved in coagulation and fibrinolysis.[19-22] Oral estradiol displays some moderate modifications which are, however, maximal with CE.[23] Some of these hepatic alterations may appear as the biological basis of the CHD protective effect, but others are also linked to the increase in risk of DVT. Considered as beneficial biological alterations are the modifications in the lipid profile (which is considered to be responsible for about 25% of the protective effect) and lowering of fibrinogen[24] and plasminogen activator inhibitor type 1 (an antagonist of fibrinolysis). Concerning these fibrinolytic variables, oral estrogens are more potent than extradigestive estrogens.[20,25] E2, however, seems to also operate at the vascular level where it has a strong vasodilatation effect via different mechanisms.[26-30] It has calcium antagonist properties[26] and controls the NO synthesis[32] as well as some vasculotrope proteins (endothelin-1, prostacycline, thromboxane)[27,28] acting at the endothelial level and indirectly on smooth muscles of the arterial wall. It also acts as an antioxidant, decreasing the oxidation of LDL-cholesterol. These direct vascular actions are observed with E2 independently of its route of administration.[32] These estrogen actions can give a biological plausibility for the reported protective effect in observational studies on HRT and CHD. Indeed, the average ratio for diminishing the incidence of myocardial infarction is 35 to 50% (Table 32.1). A very recent meta-analysis reported a risk of coronary heart diseases (CHD) of 0.70 (CI, 0.65 to 0.75) in women upon estrogen use compared to nontreated women.[1] The RR of mortality is 0.8 (0.55 to 0.97) according to another meta-analysis, without any effect on stroke.[3] Most of the studies have been done with patients who used CE, and no epidemiological data are available for E2 extradigestive administration. Concerning stroke, the

TABLE 32.2
HRT and DVT

HRT and DVT Risk Meta-Analysis Studies	Douketis et al. RR (CI95%)	Oger and Scarabin RR (CI95%)	
Case-control	2.4 (1.7–3.5)	2.2 (1.4–3.2)	
Prospective cohort	1.7(1.0–2.9)	2.1 (1.2–3.8)	
Randomized	0.7(0.3–1.6)		

HRT and DVT Duration	Gutthan et al. OR(CI95%)	Daly et al. RR(CI95%)	Jick et al. RR(CI95%)
6 months	4.6 (2.5–8.4)		
6–12 months or <1 year	3 (1.4–6.5)	6.7 (2.1–21.3)	6.7 (1.5–30.8)
>1 year	1.1 (0.6–2.1)		
Total	2.1 (1.4–2.2)	3.5 (1.8–7.0)	3.6 (1.6–7.8)
Estrogen Dose			
Low (0.625 mg EC, 25–50 μg E2TTS)	2.1 (1.2–3.4)	3.7 (1.3–10.2)	3.3 (1.4–7.8)
High (1.25 mg, 100 μg E2TTS)	2.4 (1–5.6)	6.6 (2.2–19.6)	6.9 (1.5–33.0)
Route			
Oral	2.1 (1.3–3.6)	4.6 (2.1–10.1)	
TTS	2.1 (0.9–4.6)	2.0 (0.1–7.6)	

results are more conflicting. Some studies reported a beneficial effect,[5,6] whereas the Nurses' Health Study gave an RR of 1.3 (1 to 1.7) for users of estrogen alone, and 1.1 (0.7 to 1.8) for E+P.[2] A prospective cohort in Finland[9] gave the RR of 1.08 (0.55 to 2.10) for former users and 0.86 (0.42 to 1.75) for current users. However, no information is available concerning the risk for the different routes of administration.

At the opposite, efficiency of the different routes of administration has been demonstrated in alleviating the postmenopausal symptoms and on bone protection. Osteoporosis prevention and reduction of the risk of fractures is the best established benefit of E2 therapy[33] without considering the route of administration.[34]

Concerning the increase in thrombo-embolism risk, it was recently demonstrated with the oral route.[12,35-41] A significant increase has been reported by a few studies related to estrogen oral dose and was maximal during the first year of use (Table 32.2). Most of these studies do not find any significant risk after one year (maybe because women at high risk have stopped it within the first year) (Table 32.2). The addition of progestins did not modify the range of the risk. Two studies also found an increased risk with transdermal E2, but it was not significant[36,39] (Table 32.2). Thus we still do not know if there is a real increase in DVT with extradigestive E2, despite the absence of any modification of proteins involved in coagulation and fibrinolysis with these treatments.

2. Progestins

Progesterone or progestins have to be combined with E2 in order to avoid endometrial hyperplasia. There are different types of progestins that have no equivalence between them.

a. Progesterone

It is the natural hormone. It can be delivered orally in a micronized preparation, or vaginally. It has no effect by itself or when combined with E2 on the hepatic proteins taken as risk markers for cardiovascular effects. There are some conflicting data on its effect on the vascular tone.[41-45] One author has reported that after P treatment a drop in hand blood flow increased due to E2,[45] whereas others have not observed any modification of the vasodilator effect of E2 combined with P.[42-44] In addition, it is as efficient as the other progestins in endometrial safety.[46] It thus seems to be the best candidate to treat patients at risk for cardiovascular diseases. However, progesterone, as well as all the synthetic progestins, has a relaxation effect on smooth muscles which can be responsible for leg cramps in patients with histories of DVT.

b. Normethyltestosterone Derivatives

They are mainly used for contraceptive purposes. They have some androgenic properties and can exert some estrogenic properties,[47] which may explain the modifications on lipid fractions and hemostasis. They decrease HDL-cholesterol and triglycerides, increase moderately LDL-cholesterol, antagonize the E2 effects on vitamin K-dependent factors, and decrease fibrinogen and plasminogen. They seem to be able to antagonize the vasodilatory effect of E2. However, these effects are dose-dependent and more pronounced at concentrations used for contraception. At 10 mg/day, there is no doubt that they can be thrombo-embolic, but no proof has been obtained for such an effect at 1 mg/day, the usual dose of norethisterone in HRT. However, since other progestins devoid of any influence on the vascular markers are marketed, we do not recommand these products in HRT, especially in women with thrombo-embolic risk.

c. Pregnane and 19 Norprogesterone Derivatives

The most often used derivative in the U.S. is medroxyprogesterone acetate (MPA). It has some mild androgenic and glucocorticoid properties, which can explain its mild effects on lipid fractions and hemostasis. The PEPI trial demonstrated that it was able to reverse the beneficial effects of CE on HDL-cholesterol, whereas progesterone was less active.[48] A cross-sectional analysis of some hemostasis parameters demonstrated that MPA could reverse the CE increase in factor VII and protein C, and it had an inverse effect on antithrombin III.[18] However, in the PEPI trial, all of the treatment regimens (MPA cyclic or daily, or cyclic progesterone combined with CE) prevented the rise in fibrinogen observed in women with placebo, a marker of increased risk in cardiovascular diseases.[24] In a nonhuman primate model, MPA was shown to be a vasoconstrictor on coronary arteries, whereas progesterone did not prevent the beneficial effect of E2.[49] Thus, it appears that MPA can alter some of the beneficial effects of E2 on the markers of cardiovascular risk.[50] However, the epidemiologic studies, which have been done mainly with CE and MPA, have shown the same magnitude of protective effect on CHD by the association than with CE alone; indeed, a recent meta-analysis reported an RR for CHD of 0.66 (CI, 0.53 to 0.84) with the CE+MPA treatments,[1] which is similar to the value for CE alone. No such data are available with other kinds of pregnane derivatives or with progesterone. We can only speculate that a higher beneficial effect could be obtained using more physiologic compounds. Indeed, other pregnane derivatives are marketed and largely used in France since studies of the metabolic and vascular markers have shown the absence of any alterations with these molecules when used alone in contraception[51-53] or associated with E2 in HRT.[54]

One of the most widespread compounds is chlormadinone acetate. We used it routinely in the contraception of women with high risk in thrombosis and metabolic diseases, as well as in women with SLE and antiphospholipids.[52] Its use in HRT is also recommended to the same extent as natural progesterone. It also has a good safety record at the endometrial level.

Other compounds are used in HRT such as medrogestone (a methylpregnane); dydrogestone, a weak progestin; promegestone (a 19norprogesterone); and nomegestrol acetate (a 19norprogesterone) with stronger progestin properties. These compounds have also been demonstrated to be neutral with respect to the proteins involved in the risk for vascular diseases.[51,53-55] None of the pregnane derivatives can reverse the bone protection effect of E2.[56,57] They have an additional interest, which is to be able to cure hot flashes, as shown in add-back studies in women treated with GnRH analogues.[58] In addition, some studies suggest that they could have, by themselves, a beneficial effect on bone.[59] Thus, in women with contraindication to estrogen therapy, the use of progesterone or pregnane derivatives can help to alleviate hot flashes and night sweats, and may be beneficial for osteoporosis, even if these results are still contradictory. There is no information, however, on the association of CS and progesterone on bone, since CS acts through osteoblasts and osteocytes apoptosis, and progesterone on osteoblasts differentiation and proliferation, increasing bone formation rate.[60-64]

3. Principles of Treatment

a. Types

The treatment by E2 and progestin can be sequential, cyclic, or continuous. The sequential treatment was the first to be proposed. It generally consists of an administration of estrogen for 21 to 25 days a month, associated with progestin for at least 10 days for 21 days of estrogen, or 12 days for 25 days of estrogen. This duration for progestins has been shown to prevent, with the greatest efficiency, endometrial hyperplasia.[65] This sequence of treatment is associated with menstruation so that most women now prefer to get "nonbleeding" treatments. Continuous treatments are provided associating estrogen and progestins every day. However, about 40% of breakthrough bleeding occurs during the first year of treatment[66] so that some cyclic schemes are now proposed with a lower rate of bleeding. Different sequences are proposed. In our own experience, the best combination is E2 and progesterone or a pregnane during 25 days per month. Breast tolerance (mastalgia) might also be improved (personal data). Some studies have shown differential efffects on HDL-cholesterol between cyclic or daily MPA administration,[48] but there is no certainty of a differential effect at the cardiovascular end-point.

b. Estrogen Dose

Concerning the estrogen dose, studies have well defined the minimal dose for bone protection: CE has to be administered at 0.625 mg/day, and E2 at 2 or 1 mg/day orally, E2 to 50 mg/patch and to 3 mg/day percutaneously in order to get an E2 plasmatic concentration about 60 pg/ml.[67] The necessary dose to alleviate postmenopausal symptoms is usually considered to be of the same magnitude or even lower. However, no data have precisely evaluated the dose-range effects for cardiovascular protection. Most of the epidemiological studies reporting a protective effect on CHD have concerned populations treated with 1.2 mg and 0.625 mg/day CE. Concerning the thrombo-embolic risk, it appears that the magnitude of the risk is strongly correlated to the estrogen dose (Table 32.2) according to studies with CE and, in particular, the Coronary Drug Project, which demonstrated a high risk of DVT and arterial thrombosis in men treated with CE at higher dosage than now used in HRT.[35] These observations have also been raised from studies with ethinyl-estradiol (a more potent estrogen) showing a dose-relationship between the rate of DVT and the ethinyl-estradiol dose.[68]

For endometrial safety, there is also a dose-relationship between estrogen and hyperplasia and endometrial cancer risk.[65] However, the estrogen-progestin ratio is the most important factor for endometrial protection, and an increase in estrogens can be compensated by an increase in the progestin dose.

c. Progestin Dose

The dosage for progestin has been well studied concerning endometrial eutrophy.[46] The aim in HRT is to get a hypoplastic endometrium which is best provided by a sufficient dosage in progestin. For sequential treatments, the usual doses for micronized progesterone are 200 mg/day, 10 mg for chlormadonine acetate and medrogestone, 500 mg of promegestone, and 20 mg of dydrogesterone. For cyclic or continuous treatments, half of these dosages are usually sufficient.

d. Duration of HRT

This is an unsolved point. However, in the Nurse Health Study, ten or more years of current use was associated with a reduction in the benefit of treatment with an RR of mortality of 0.80 (0.67

to 0.96), mainly due to an increase in breast cancer risk, compared to RR = 0.63 (0.56 to 0.70) of mortality in the cohort for current users.[9]

Concerning bone protection, the Rancho Bernardo Study has shown no differences in BMD levels between women who had a 20 years' use of estrogen, beginning at menopause, and those who have a 9 years' use corresponding to a beginning after 60 years.[69,70] A ten-year treatment, initially recommended to prevent osteoporosis, to be started as soon as menopause is confirmed, has shown to be insufficient in older persons (more than 75 years).

The incidence in breast cancer increases with duration of treatment, after a 5 to 10 years duration, at least in the published American studies which concern mainly women who used unopposed CE. The same methodological bias reported for CHD risk may also have been raised for breast cancer; women with a higher socio-economic level, for example, are known to be at risk for breast cancer.

Another increase in risk related with long-time treatment has been reported concerning endometrial cancer.[72] However, this is the only report of an increase in risk in estrogen-progestin-treated women, RR 2.5% (CI, 1.1 to 5.5) for progestins associated to estrogens, more than 10 days each month, after an HRT use of five or more years. This increase could be either due to a real increase in risk, the emergence of nonhormone-dependent cancer, or a lower compliance in progestins with treatment time increasing. Thus, taking together these different benefits and side-effects, it is still not clear which guidelines can be provided for the duration of HRT.

B. ALTERNATIVES TO THE ESTROGEN/PROGESTIN TREATMENTS

1. Steroid Estradiol Modulators (SERMs)

These products are synthetic compounds which develop some of the beneficial effects of estrogen, in particular at the bone level, theoretically without any proliferative effects on the endometrium, and with a possible beneficial effect on breast cancer since they are antiestrogens. The first compound to be used was tamoxifen. It is efficient on fractures but increases the risk of endometrial cancer and DVT to the same extent as HRT.[72,73] More recently, raloxifene was proposed in the prevention of osteoporosis in patients with contraindication to estrogens. This product has a demonstrated efficiency on vertebral fracture prevention and not on cortical fracture, but increases the rate of hot flashes, has no proven effect on urogenital symptoms, and increases the risk of DVT to the same extent as estrogen or tamoxifen.[47] It is thus doubtful that it can offer any advantages in women with a high risk of thrombosis. It could be of interest in other patients, in the case of intolerance of estrogen and increased risk in osteoporosis. However, the discussion in these indications has to include the possibility of prescription of biphosphonates. They do not provide any thrombo-embolic risk and their effects are more efficient than raloxifene on bone, at least at short term since no long-term studies are available.[74] An additional benefit for raloxifene or tamoxifen could be the decrease in breast cancer incidence. It was reported in two large series that raloxifene decreases the occurrence of estradiol receptor positive breast cancers after two to three years of use.[75] However, there is no information on the recommended duration of treatment, nor on the long-term effect of raloxifen on breast cancer risk. Concerning tamoxifen, it was shown, at least in breast cancer patients, that its beneficial effects were observed after five years of treatment, but not after a longer exposure.[72]

2. Tibolone

It is a 19 nortestosterone derivative with progestogenic, androgenic, and estrogenic properties. It is proposed as an HRT in postmenopausal women and has been shown to be protective on bone and efficient on menopause symptoms, without any effect at the endometrial level.[76,77] Biological studies have shown that it decreases HDL-cholesterol, triglycerides, fibrinogen, does not significantly modify the coagulation markers, and may have beneficial effects on the arterial wall.[78] There are no data on its tolerance in patients with a thromboembolic risk, so it can be used at the moment only in women devoid of this risk; its pharmacological profile (with a mild androgenic effect) suggests that it could be interesting in autoimmune diseases, but this has yet to be evaluated.

III. INDICATIONS FOR CONNECTIVE TISSUE DISEASES

Immunity is involved in most of the connective tissue diseases. However, different mechanisms are underlying the various diseases. HRT can be deleterious in these diseases for two dominant reasons: exacerbation of autoimmunity and an increase in the risk of thrombo-embolic diseases. Estradiol receptors have been localized on the cells involved in the immune response, such as epithelial cells in the thymic medulla, macrophages, and endothelial cells.[14,79-81] It has been shown in various models that E2 enhances the T-helpers and suppresses some cell-mediated immunity and natural killer cell functions; increases B-cell differentiation; increases the production of some autoantibodies, and in particular antiphospholipids autoantibodies, at least in animal model;[82] decreases apoptosis of peripheral blood mononuclear cells with reduced tumour-necrosis-factor-alpha production in patients with SLE;[83,84] and is able to modulate the production of certain interleukins. E2 appears to skew T-cell activation from a Th1 to a Th2 phenotype, and downregulates proinflammatory cytokine production.[80] However, if there is strong evidence that SLE can be worsened by estrogen and rheumatoid arthritis may be improved, the figure is less clear for most of the other connective tissue diseases, even if some have a female predominance (Table 32.3). Indeed, in sclerodermia, Sjögren's syndrome, and various forms of vasculitis (Wegener's syndrome, Churg-Strauss, polyarteritis nodosa, and Takayasu's disease) the role of hormonal factors has not been proven.

A. Systemic and Cutaneous Lupus

SLE is the autoimmune disease where the deleterious effect of estrogen has been the best studied in experimental animal models. Hormonal manipulations have shown in NZB/NZW F1 mice that females have a spontaneous earlier mortality compared with their male counterparts, and that estrogen or androgen treatments can worsen or ameliorate the course of the disease after castration. The most suggestive evidence for estrogen's deleterious effect in women is the female-to-male ratio and its variation with hormonal status (Table 32.3). Moreover, the risk of worsening is generally admitted during oral contraceptives and pregnancy. The deleterious effects of estrogen are still uncompletely understood. However, as mentionned above, estrogens are known to have many implications in the regulation of autoimmunity and, in particular, on cytokine production. SLE patients have been reported to have an increase in the Th2 cytokines, particularly an increase

TABLE 32.3
Sex Ratio of Connectivite Diseases

	Female/Male
SLE: before puberty	3:1
after puberty	9:1
RA	2–4:1
Scleroderma	3–4:1
Sjögren's syndrome	9:1
Myasthenia gravis	2:1
Vasculitis	
PAN	1:2–3
Churg-Strauss	1:2–3
Wegener granulomatosis	1:2–3
Takayasu's arteritis	9:1

TABLE 32.4
Estradiol and Cytokine Production

Bone marrow/bone	IL1	Increase (low doses) or decrease (high doses)
	IL6	Increase (low doses) or decrease (high doses)
	IL7	Decrease
	TNFa	Increase (low doses) or decrease (high doses)
Th1 cytokine		Decrease ?
	IFNγ	
	IL2	
Th2 cytokine		Increase ?
	IL4	
	IL10	Increase
	IL13	

in the IL10:IFNγ ratio compared with controls, and estrogens are reported to enhance Th2 cytokine production (Table 32.4).[14,80,85-90] However, the increased risk of arterial diseases in patients with SLE, as well as of osteoporosis in relation to CS used for long years, and the relative frequency of premature ovarian failure, raise questions about the use of HRT in these patients. The frequency and severity of SLE usually decrease after menopause, and one can speculate an increased risk by prolonging the life-time of estrogen exposition. In addition, if indicated, HRT in SLE seems to have to be of long-term use in these women with particular high risk of CHD and osteoporosis.

Some studies have begun to address the question of the risk or benefit in women with SLE. Two prospective studies have reported a significant increase in the incidence of new disease in patients receiving HRT (Table 32.5).[91,92] Moreover, both of these studies pointed out the increase of risk with duration of HRT. Interestingly, the study from Meier[92] reported a lower risk in patients treated with estrogen and progestin than with unopposed estrogen (Table 32.5), and an increase in the magnitude of the risk with increasing the estrogen dose. This study showed the same increase in risk for SLE and for discoid lupus with HRT. On the contrary, some retrospective studies have found no evidence for a significant increase in clinical flares or SLEDAI.[93-95] However, in the study by Arden et al., the magnitude of change in disease activity was not mentioned. In the study from Kreidstein et al., menopausal status between cases and controls was not equivalent. In the study from Mok et al., the maximum follow-up was three years. No significant increase in the various indexes of disease activity was observed. However, none of these studies was randomized, and it cannot be precluded that the absence of deleterious effect is due to a bias of selection in patients receiving HRT, the weak number of patients, and, at least in two studies, the short duration of treatment. If the benefit of the treatment was demonstrated on well-being, and no major increase in DVT appeared, their short-term was not allowed to show beneficial cardiovascular effect and none of them, curiously, analyzed the possible beneficial effect on BMD (maybe because they were retrospective studies).

Moreover, one may be concerned by a theoretical increased risk in breast cancer in patients treated with immunosuppressive agents, a risk which may be increased by a promoting effect of long-term treatment by E2. Concerning the risk of malignancy in SLE, some studies have reported an increase in non-Hodgkin's lymphoma,[96-98] but only one study has shown an increased risk of breast cancer in these women without HRT (RR:2.9 (1.4 to 6.4)).[99]

Most of the studies on HRT in women with SLE are partially reassuring. However, they are not entirely convincing since bias may have a role. It is necessary to wait for the results of the prospective SELENA (Safety of Estrogens Erythematosus National Assessment), an assay conducted in the U.S. to better determine which patients may benefit from HRT.

TABLE 32.5
HRT and SLE

RR of SLE during HRT	OR(IC95%)
Sanchez-Guerrero	2.1 (1.1–4) ever users
Nurse health study: cohort	2.5 (1–2.5) current users
1 to 4 years	1.8 (0.9–3.8)
5 to 10 years	2.7 (1.2–6.4)
>11 years	3.5 (1.2–10.9)
Meier et al. case-control (UK, GPs)	
Long term-users (>2 years)	2.8 (1.3–5.8)
Short term-users	2.8 (0.9–9.0)
Estrogen users	5.3 (1.5–18.6)
E+P users	2 (0.8–5.0)

RR of flares in SLE	RR(IC95%)
Arden et al.	30 users vs. 30 nonusers
Mean follow-up: 12 months	No differences
Kreidstein et al.	16 users vs. 32 nonusers
Mean follow-up: 12 months	No differences
Mok et al.	11 users vs. 23 nonusers
Mean follow-up: 36 months	No differences

Because of the immunomodulatory effects of androgens, some assays have been conducted in women with SLE with a weak androgen, DHEA. There was an apparent benefit on the course of the disease,[100] but with some androgenic side-effects and no demonstrated protective effect on osteopenia.

In the meantime, what can be suggested is, if a woman has serious complaints from hypoestrogenic symptoms, treatments other than estrogens can be used as first-line treatments, bearing in mind that progesterone, which can have some immunosuppressive properties, at least in animal models, can alleviate hot flashes and may be beneficial at the bone level. Vaginal estrogens can be prescribed at low dose and frequency; twice a week is usually sufficient to cure vaginal dryness, and this topical administration of estrogens can also help urogenital symptoms. Concerning osteoporosis, treatment by biphosphonates have been studied in CS osteoporosis and can be recommended in association with sequential treatment with calcium, vitamin D, and exercise.[101-105]

Estradiol could be prescribed in patients with quiescent diseases for a few years. The choice would be to prefer E2 by extradigestive administration, and natural progesterone or close pregnane derivatives, since these compounds provide the lowest risk DVT with the same efficiency at the bone level. However, a stringent clinical and biological follow-up appears necessary. The existence of antiphospholipids (aPL) constitutes, in our opinion, until more data are obtained, a strict contraindication for HRT.

B. MIXED CONNECTIVE TISSUE DISEASE

It is an autoimmune connective tissue disease defined by the presence of high titers of U1-RNP autoantibodies with clinical features commonly seen in SLE, scleroderma, polymyositis, or RA.[106] A Raynaud's phenomenon can be frequently present. The clinical pattern can be genetically determined.[107] It is usually less severe than SLE, in particular during pregnancy.[108] However, since some patients can evolve to SLE, HRT may be prescribed with careful assessment of the clinical and biological status. Any indication for an SLE evolution may lead to discussion of the indication of the treatment. At the opposite, a rheumatoid arthritis-like disease can help to prescribe HRT in these patients.

C. Primary Antiphospholipid Syndrome

The aPL syndrome is characterized by a variety of clinical manifestations in relation to arterial and venous thrombosis. It is, thus, whether it is primary or associated with SLE, a disease with a very high risk of thrombosis. Moreover, it is an autoimmune disease and estrogens have been shown, in animal models, to stimulate the production of antibodies with anticardiolipine specificity.[82]

There are different clinical situations. Patients with a history of thrombosis are usually treated with anticoagulant, and one can discuss the remaining risk of thrombo-embolic events in such patients. However, the possible triggering in autoantibodies raises concern for the use of estrogens in such patients. The figure may be different in patients without any history of thrombosis despite pregnancy or surgery during their lives, and with an occasional positivity in aPL. In the study by Arden et al.[93] there were five patients with aPL under HRT. One had a DVT during the course of the treatment, but no systematic worsening was reported. However, no detail were given on the clinical and biological characteristics of these patients (history of thrombosis in particular) or on the associated treatments. Thus, at the moment it is not possible to recommend an estrogen treatment in these patients. Progesterone alone can be used to help allieviate hot flashes. Controlled studies are necessary to evaluate the risk and benefits of HRT in patients with aPL.

D. Rheumatoid Arthritis

Some studies have reported the influence of adjuvant therapy with estrogens in RA because of the first report from the GPs showing a protective effect of oral contraception on RA, and because of the improvement of RA during pregnancy.[110] However, the beneficial effect of exogenous estrogens has not been confirmed.[111] Indeed, during pregnancy, the level of estradiol is very high, and other steroids are secreted in excess such as progesterone and glucocorticoid, which may be involved in the improvement of inflammation in these patients. One cohort prospective study has not shown an increase in the incidence of RA in women under HRT (Table 32.6).[112] Case-control studies reported conflicting results on the incidence of RA under HRT (Table 32.6).[113-116]

One of the major interests of HRT in RA is its action on osteoporosis, which is multifactorial and especially a risk for women with RA.[117] Indeed, three studies have confirmed a beneficial effect of HRT on osteoporosis in women with RA.[117-119] The risk of breast cancer has not been found to be increased in RA patients.[120,121] There is a decrease of intestinal cancer and a reported increase

TABLE 32.6
HRT and RA

Prospective Study	OR(IC95%)
Hernandez-Avila et al.	
Nurse health study: cohort	
Current users	1.3 (0.9–2)
Past users	0.7 (0.5–1.2)
Ever users	1 (0.7–1.4)
Cases-Controls Studies	**RR(IC95%)**
Linos et al.	2.2 (1–5.2)
Vandenbroucke et al.	0.32 (0.16–0.64)
Carette et al.	0.9 (0.56–1.44)

in leukemia.[120,121] The effect of testosterone has also been evaluated in RA with a benefit on disease activity and well-being.[122] However, it seems difficult to recommend the use of androgens in women because of the side-effects of these compounds. Tibolone could be of interest in these patients, but has not been evaluated.

E. SYSTEMIC SCLEROSIS

Systemic sclerosis (ss) is a systemic disorder of the connective tissue characterized by vascular lesions, fibrosis, and degenerative changes in the skin and some organs. These lesions are due to paracrine interactions between different cells: activated cells of the immune system, endothelial cells, and fibroblasts. These cells produce various cytokines and growth factors such as IL-1, IL-6, IL-8, IGF-1, PDGF, TGF-β, and ET-1 for the endothelial cells; IL-1, TNF, IL-2,-4,-6,-8, and bFGF for the immune or inflammatory cells; and TNF, IL-1,-6, TGF-β, IGF-1, and DGF for the sclerodermal fibroblasts.[123] Since estrogens can alter the secretion of some of these proteins (decreasing IL-1, TNF, and TGF-β, for example) but maybe act differently on some of them, the resultant action of hormones in this disease is still far from clear. Furthermore, some autoantibodies have been associated with the disease and may be enhanced by estrogens.

Some studies have reported a benefit with weak estrogens in the treatment of ss.[123,124] A recent study reported a particular benefit at the vascular level in patients with Raynaud's phenomenon secondary to ss. The endothelial function of these patients is altered and the administration of quite high doses of CE (1.25 mg) over four weeks led to vasodilatation, but no clinical evaluation was reported in this study.[125] However, the vasodilation action of E2 is well demonstrated in normal women, and since it seems from this study also present in patients with Raynaud's phenomenon, this action is an additional benefit from HRT. Furthermore, osteopenia is a frequent phenomenon in patients with ss who statistically also have an earlier menopause.[126] This osteopenia can be partially linked to calcium malabsorption and renal failure, but is also present in patients devoid of these complications.[126] There is a reported increased risk in the lung and skin, but not especially of gynecological malignacies in these patients.[127] Thus, HRT may be recommended in these patients, but the choice may also be extradigestive E2 combined with progesterone, the more physiologic way to administer HRT, even if clinical studies have to be conducted to confirm the benefit of the treatments, in particular at the vascular end-point.

F. SJÖGREN SYNDROME

It is characterized by alterations in the production of saliva and tears, with perivascular lymphoid infiltration of submucosal glands. This syndrome can be isolated or associated with SLE or RA. It seems to be a predominant Th1 disease with an increase in T CD4+ lymphocytes and T-helpers, increased production in IL-2 and IL-10, and INFγ in the salivary glands. Some autoantibodies are associated with the disease (anti-Rho/SSA, anti-La/SCA). An animal study reported a beneficial effect of estrogen on T-cell-mediated vasculitis and sialadenitis in MRL Ipr/Ipr mice.[128] Thus, very few data are available on the use of hormones in this disease. From actual knowledge, however, only benefits can be predicted from the use of HRT in these patients, in particular if vaginal dryness is a concern.

G. VASCULITIS

It is characterized by leucocytic infiltration of the vessels which can be large (Takayasu's), medium (periarteritis nodosa), or small (Wegener's granulomatosis, Churg-Strauss).[130] The disease has different clinical presentations according to the localization of vasculitis. The pathogenesis is not entirely known. In PAN, viruses have been implicated, but most of the pathogenesis remains to be understood in these disorders despite the recent discovery of ANCA in Wegener's granulomatosis, which can also be found in other forms of vasulitis.

There is no female predominance in these diseases except for Takayasu's arteritis (Table 32.3). They mainly occur at the perimenopausal period, except for Takayasu's arteritis, which is a disease of young women. The main risk of HRT in these patients is exacerbation of thrombosis which has been reported during pregnancy.[12,31]

Some of the forms of vasculitis are severe but usually of short duration under treatment (CS and immunosuppressive agents), such as PAN. In these cases, it seems wiser to wait to the end of the flare before beginning the treatment and, in any case, to prefer a combination neutral on the markers of vascular risk since hypertension is a nonexceptional feature. In chronic diseases, no scientific answer can be given at the moment concerning the use of HRT in these patients; it appears, from the sparse data in the literature, that estrogen may improve vasculitis, at least in some models.[129]

We thus recommend the use also of HRT, which was the lowest risk of thrombosis in patients who are subjected to long courses of CS treatments.

H. DERMATOMYOSITIS AND POLYMYOSITIS

These are idiopathic inflammatory myopathies. There is a female-to-male predominance of about 2:1, and they occur predominantly in the fifth decade. Dermatomyositis is associated with immune complex deposition in the vessels, whereas polymyositis is linked to direct T-cell-mediated muscle injury. Dermatomyositis is considered to be a humorally-mediated disorder with an inflammatory infiltrate of B-cells and a predominance of CD4+ over CD8+ T-cells. Polymyositis is associated with an increase in CD8+ T-cells in the muscle. There is one report of worsening of polymyositis during pregnancy,[131] but no data are available on HRT. Since the rate of malignancies has been reported to be increased in dermatomyositis,[134] a special screening might be proposed for breast and endometrial cancers in these patients. Since they are often treated by CS, they indeed can benefit from HRT for the cardiovascular and the bone end-points.

III. CONCLUSIONS

HRT may be beneficial in patients with connective diseases, especially those who take CS. However, the use of HRT is limited in these patients by the risk of DVT and by the exacerbation of autoimmunity. It is thus necessary to better estimate the risk linked to exogenous estrogens in autoimmune diseases, or to develop other molecules. Alternative treatments such as biphosphonates may be useful in osteopenia, but they do not act on postmenopausal symptoms. SERMs are less efficient than HRT on menopausal symptoms, have no proven beneficial effects at the cardiovascular level, and increase DVT frequency to the same extent as HRT.

REFERENCES

1. Barrett-Connor, E., Grady D., Hormone replacement therapy, heart disease, and other considerations, *Ann. Rev. Public Health*, 19, 55, 1998.
2. Grodstein, F., Stampfer, M.J., Manson, J.E., Colditz, G.A., Willett, W.C., Rosner, B., Speizer, F.E., Hennekens, C.H., Speizer, F.E., Postmenopausal estrogen and progestin use and the risk of cardiovascular disease, *New. Engl. J. Med.*, 335, 453, 1996.
3. Scarabin, P.Y., Plu-Bureau, G., Quantitative evaluation of the cardiovascular risk associated with hormone substitution therapy during menopause, *Arch. Mal. Coeur. Vaiss.*, 86, 243, 1993.
4. Paganini-Hill, A., Estrogen replacement therapy and stroke, *Progr. Cardio. Vasc. Dis.*, 38, 223, 1995.
5. Henderson, B.E., Paganini-Hill, A., Ross, R.K., Decreased mortality in users of estrogen replacement therapy, *Arch. Intern. Med.*, 151, 75, 1990.
6. Hunt, K., Vessey, M., Mc Pherson, K., Mortality in a cohort of long-term users of hormone replacement therapy: an updated analysis, *Br. J. Obstet. Gynaecol.*, 97, 1080, 1990.
7. Ettinger, B., Friedman, G.D., Bush, T., Quesenberry, C.P. Jr., Reduced mortality associated with long-term post menopausal estrogen therapy, *Obstet. Gynecol.*, 87, 6, 1996.

8. Sourander, L., Rajala, T., Räihä, I., Mäkinen, J., Erkkola, R., Helenius, H., Cardiovascular and cancer morbidity and mortality and sudden cardiac death in postmenopausal women on oestrogen replacement therapy (ERT), *Lancet*, 352, 1965, 1998.

9. Grodstein, F., Stampfer, Graham, A., J.E., Colditz, G.A., Walter, C., Willett, W.C., Manson, J.E., Joffe, M., Rosner, B., Fuchs, C., Hankinson, S.E., Hunter, D.J., F.E., Hennekens, C.H., Postmenopausal hormone therapy and mortality, *New Engl. J. Med.*, 336, 1769, 1997.

10. Henderson, V.W., Paganini-Hill, A., Emanuel C.K., Dunn, M.E., Buckwalter, J.G., Estrogen replacement therapy in older women: comparisons between Alzheimer's disease cases and nondemented control subjects, *Arch. Neurol.*, 51, 896, 1994.

11. Paganini-Hill, A., Oestrogen replacement therapy and Alzheimer's disease, *Br. J. Obstet. Gynaecol.*, 103, (suppl.13), 80, 1996.

12. Oger, E., Scarabin, P.Y., Assessment of the risk for venous thromboembolism among users of hormone replacement therapy, *Drugs & Aging*, 14, 55, 1999.

13. Colditz, G.A., Hamkinson, S.E., Hunter, D.J. Willett, W.C., Manson, J.E., The use of estrogens and progestins and the risk of breast cancer in postmenopausal women, *N. Engl. J. Med.*, 332, 1589, 1995.

14. Wilder, R.L., Hormones, pregnancy, and autoimmune diseases, *Ann. N.Y. Acad. Sci.*, 840, 45, 1998.

15. Elkik F., Gompel A., Mercier-Bodard C., Kuttenn F., Guyenne P.N., Corvol P., Mauvais-Jarvis P. Effects of percutaneous estradiol and conjugated estrogens on the level of plasma proteins and triglycerides in post-menopausal women, *Am. J. Obstet. Gynecol.*, 143, 888, 1982.

16. De Lignières, B., Basdevant, A., Thomas, G., Thalabard, J.C., Mercier-Bodard, C., Conard J., Guyenne, T.T., Mairon, N., Corvol P., Guy-Grand, B., Mauvais-Jarvis, P., Biological effects of estradiol-17-b in postmenopausal women: oral versus percutaneous administration, *J. Clin. Endocrinol. Metab.*, 62, 536, 1986.

17. Faguer de Moustier, B., Conard, J., Guyenne, T.T., Sitt, Y., Denys, I., Arnoux-Rouveyre, M., Pelissier, C., Comparative metabolic study of percutaneous versus oral micronized 17-beta-estradiol in replacement therapy, *Maturitas*, 11, 275, 1989.

18. Nabulsi, A.A., Folsom, A.R., White, A., Patsch, W., Heiss, G., Wu, K.K., Szlo, M., Association of hormone-replacement therapy with various cardiovascular risk factors in postmenopausal women, *N. Engl. J. Med.*, 328, 1069, 1993.

19. Conard, J., Samama, M., Basdevant, A. et al., Differential ATIII response to oral and parenteral administration of 17-b estradiol (letter), *Thromb. Haemost.*, 49, 245, 1983.

20. Scarabin, P.Y., Alhenc-Gelas, M., Plu-Bureau, G., Taisne, P., Agher, R., Aiach, M., Effects of oral and transdermal estrogen/progesterone regimens on blood coagulation and fibrinolysis in postmenopausal women: a randomized controlled trial, *Arterioslcer. Thromb. Vasc. Biol.*, 17, 3071, 1997.

21. Scarabin, P.Y., Plu-Bureau, G., Bara, L., Bonithon-Kopp, C., Guize, L., Samama, M.M., Haemostatic variables and menopausal status: influence of hormone replacement therapy, *Thromb. Haemost.*, 70, 584, 1993.

22. The Writing Group for the Estradiol Clotting Factors Study, Effects on haemostasis of hormone replacement therapy with transdermal estradiol and oral sequential medroxyprogesterone acetate: a 1-year, double blind, placebo-controlled study, *Thromb. Haemost.*, 75, 476, 1996.

23. Caine, Y.G., Bauer, K.A., Barzegar, S., Coagulation activation following estrogen administration in postmenopausal women, *Thromb. Haemost.*, 68, 392, 1992.

24. Kannel, W.B., Wolf, P.A., Castelli, W.P., d'Agostino, R.B., Fibrinogen and risk of cardiovascular disease. The Framingham study, *JAMA*, 258, 1183, 1987.

25. Koh, K.K., Mincemoyer, R., Bui, M.N., Csako, G., Pucino, F., Guetta, V., Waclawiw, M., Cannon, R.O., Effects of hormone replacement therapy on fibrinolysis in postmenopausal women, *N. Engl. J. Med.*, 336, 683, 1997.

26. Skafar, D.F., Xu, R., Morales, J., Ram, J., Sowers, J.R., Female sex hormones and cardiovascular disease in women, *J. Clin. Edocrinol. Metab.*, 82, 3913, 1997.

27. Farhat, M.Y., Lavigne, M.C., Ramwell, P.W., The vascular protective effects of estrogen, *FASEB J.*, 10, 615, 1996.

28. White, M.M., Zamudio, S., Stevens, T., Tyler, R., Lindenfeld, J., Leslie, K., Moore L.G., Estrogen, progesterone, and vascular reactivity: potential cellular mechanisms, *Endocrine Reviews*, 16, 739, 1995.

29. Gilligan, D.M., Badar, D.M., Panza, J.A., Guyyumi A.A., Cannon, R.O. III, Acute vascular effects of estrogens in post menopausal women, *Circulation*, 90, 786, 1994.

30. Giraud, G.D., Morton, M.J., Wilson, R.A., Burry, K.A., Speroff, L., Effects of estrogen and progestin on aortic size and compliance in post menopausal women, *Am. J. Obstet. Gynecol.*, 174, 1708, 1996.

31. Collins, P., Rosano, G.M., Jiang, C., Lindsay, D., Sarrel, P.M., Poole-Wilwon, P.A., Cardiovascular protection by oestrogen-a calcium antagonist effect? *Lancet*, 341, 1264, 1993.

32. Cicinelli E., Ignarro, L.J., Lograno, M., Matteo, G., Falco, N., Schonauer, L.M., Acute effects of transdermal estradiol administration on plasma levels of nitric oxide in post menopausal women, *Fertil. Steril.*, 67, 63, 1997.

33. Weiss, N.S., Ure, C.L., Ballard, J.H., Decreased risk of fractures of the hip and lower forearm with postmenopausal use of estrogen, *N. Engl. J. Med.*, 303, 1195, 1980.

34. Lufkin, E.G., Wahner, H.W., O'Fallon, W.M., Hodgson, S.F., Kotowicz, M.A., et al., Treatment of postmenopausal osteoporosis with transdermal estrogen, *Ann. Intern. Med.*, 117, 1, 1992.

35. Coronary Drug Project Research Group, Findings leading to discontinuation of the 2.5 mg/day estrogen group, *JAMA*, 226, 652, 1973.

36. Daly, E., Vessey, M., Hawkins, M., Carson, J., Gough, P., Marsh S., Risk of venous thromboembolism in users of hormone replacement therapy, *Lancet*, 348, 977, 1996.

37. Grady, D., Hulley, S.B., Fuberg, C., Venous thromboembolic events associated with hormone replacement therapy, *JAMA*, 278, 477, 1997.

38. Grodstein, F., Stampfer, M., Goldhaber, S., Manson, J., Colditz, G., Speizer, F.E., Willett, W.C., Hennekens, C.H., Prospective study of exogenous hormones and risk of pulmonary embolism in women, *Lancet*, 348, 983, 1996.

39. Gutthann, S.P., Rodriguez, L.A.B., Castellsague, J., Oliart, A.D., Hormone replacement therapy and risk of venous thromboembolism: population based case-control study, *Br. Med. J.*, 314, 796, 1997.

40. Jick, H., Derby, L., Myers, M., Vasilakis, C., Newton, K., Risk of hospital admission for idiopathic venous thromboembolism among users of postmenopausal oestrogens, *Lancet*, 348, 981, 1996.

41. Douketis, J.D., Ginsberg, J., Holbrook, A., Crowther, M., Duku, E.K., Burrows, R.F., A reevaluation of the risk for venous thromboembolism with the use of oral contraceptives and hormone replacement therapy, *Arch. Intern. Med.*, 157, 1522, 1997.

42. Adams, M.R., Kaplan, J.R., Manuck, S.B., Koritnik, D.R., Praks, J.S. et al., Inhibition of coronary artery atherosclerosis by 17-beta estradiol in ovariectomized monkeys. Lack of an effect of added progesterone, *Arteriosclerosis*, 10, 1051, 1990.

43. Morey, A.K., Pedram, A., Razandi, M., Prins, B.A., Hu, R.M., Biesiaba, E., Levin, E.R., Estrogen and progesterone inhibit vascular smooth muscle proliferation, *Endocrinology*, 138, 3330, 1997.

44. Belfort, M.A., Saade, G.R., Suresh, M., Vedernikov, Y.P., Effects of estradiol-17β and progesterone on isolated human omental artery from premenopausal nonpregnant women and from normotensive and preeclamptic pregnant women, *Am. J. Obstet. Gynecol.*, 174, 246, 1996.

45. Sarrel, P., Effects of ovarian steroids on the cardiovascular system, in *The Circulation in the Female*, Ginsberg, J., Ed., Carnoth, UK: Parthenon, 1989, 117.

46. Whitehead, M., Fraser, D., The effects of estrogens and progestogens on the endometrium, *Obstet. Gynecol. Clin. North Am.*, 14, 299, 1987.

47. Kuhl, H., Effects of progestogens on haemostasis, *Maturitas*, 24, 1, 1996.

48. Writing Group for the PEPI Trial, Effects of estrogen or estrogen/progestin regimens on heart disease risk factors in postmenopausal women, *JAMA*, 273, 199, 1995.

49. Adams, M.R., Register, T.C., Golden, D.L., Wagner, J.D., Williams, J.K., Medroxyprogesterone acetate antagonizes inhibitory effects of conjugated equine estrogens on coronary artery artherosclerosis, *Arterioscler. Thromb. Vasc. Biol.*, 17, 217, 1997.

50. Miyagawa, K., Rösch, J., Stanczyk, F., Hersmeyer, K., Medoxyprogesterone interferes with ovarian steroid against coronary vasospasm, *Nature Med.*, 3, 324, 1997.

51. Basdevant, A., Pelissier, C., Conard, J., Degrelle, H., Guyenne, T.T., Thomas, J.L., Effects of nomegestrol acetate (5mg/d) on hormonal, metabolic and hemostatic parameters in premenopausal women, *Contraception*, 44, 599, 1991.

52. Chabbert-Buffet, N., Blétry, O., Clauvel, J.P., Frances, C., Guillevin, L., Wechsler, B., Piette, J.C., Gompel, A., Pregnane progestin is a safe contraception in systemic lupus erythematosus., *Lupus*, 7 (Suppl. 1), 111, 1998.

53. Basdevant, A., Conard, J., Denis, C., Guyenne, T.T., Egloff, H., Denys, T., Effets métaboliques et hormonaux de l'administration de 1 mg/24 h de Promegestone (R5020). *Gynécologie*, 40, 17, 1989.

54. De Ziegler, O., Effect of progestins on vascular tone? *Fertil. Steril.*, 60, 590, 1993.

55. Tremollieres, F.A., Pouilles, J.M., Ribot, C.A., A prospective two-year study of progestin given alone in postmenopausal women: effect on lipid and metabolic parameters. *Am. J. Obstet. Gynecol.*, 173, 85, 1995.

56. The writing groupe for the PEPI, Effects of hormone therapy on bone mineral density: results from the postmenopausal estrogen/progestin interventions (PEPI) trial, *JAMA*, 276, 1389, 1996.

57. Gibaldi, M., Prevention and treatment of oesteoporosis: does the future belong to hormone replacement therapy? *J. Clin. Pharmacol.*, 37, 1087, 1997.

58. Cedars, M.I., Lu, J.K., Meldrum, D.R., Judd, H.L., Treatment of endometriosis with a long-acting gonadotropin-releasing hormone agonist plus medroxyprogesterone acetate, *Obstet. Gynecol.*, 75, 641, 1990.

59. Tremollieres, F., Pouilles, J.M., Ribot, C., Effect of long-term administration of progestogen on post-menopausal bone loss: result of a two-year, controlled randomized study. *Clin. Endocrinol.* (Oxf), 38, 627, 1993.

60. Manolagas, S.C., Cellular and molecular mechanisms of osteoporosis, *Aging*, 10, 182, 1998.

61. Ishida, Y., Bellows, C.G., Tertinegg, I., Heeersche, J.N., Progesterone-mediated stimulation of osteoprogenitor proliferation and differentiation in cell populations derived from adult or fetal rat bone tissue depends on the serum component of the culture media. *Otseoporos Int.*, 7, 323, 1997.

62. Barengolts, E.I., Koutznestova, T., Segalene, A., Odvina, C., Kukreja, S.C., Unterman, T.G., Effects of progesterone on serum levels of IGF-1 and on femur IGF-1 mRNA in ovariectomized rats. *J. Bone Miner. Res.*, 11, 1406, 1996.

63. Scheven, B.A., Damen, C.A., Hamilton, N.J., Verhaar, H.J., Duursma, S.A., Stimulatory effects of estrogen and progesterone on proliferation and differentiation of normal human osteoblast-like cells *in vitro*, *BBRC*, 186, 54, 1992.

64. Yamamoto, Y., Kurubayashi, T., Tojo, Y., Yahata, T., Honda, A., Tomita, M., Tanaka, K., Effects of progestins on the metabolism of cancellous bone in aged oophorectomized rats, *Bone*, 22, 533, 1998.

65. Paterson, M.E.L., Wade-Evans, T., Sturdee, D.W., Thom, M.H., Studd, J.W.W., Endometrial disease after treatment with estrogens and progestogens in the climacteric, *B. Med. J.*, 822, 1980.

66. Magos, A.L., Brincat, M., Studd, J.W.W., Wardle, P., Schlesinger, P., O'Dowd, T., Amenorrhea and endometrial atrophy with continuous oral estrogen and progestogen therapy in postmenopausal women, *Obstet. Gynecol.*, 65, 496, 1985.

67. Lindsay, R., Hart, D.M., Clark, B.M., The minimum effective dose of estrogen for prevention of postmenopausal bone loss, *Obstet. Gynecol.*, 63, 759, 1984.

68. Gerstman, B.B., Piper, J.M., Tomita, D.K., Ferguson, W.J., Stadel, B.V., Lundin, F.E., Oral contraceptive estrogen dose and the risk of deep venous thromboembolic disease, *Am. J. Epidemiol.*, 133, 32, 1991.

69. Lindsay, R., Hart, D.M., Aitken, J.M., Mac Donald, E.B., Anderson, J.B., Clarke, A.C., Long-term prevention of postmenopausal osteoporosis by estrogen:evidence for an increased bone mass after delayed onset of estrogen treatment, *Lancet*, 1, 1038, 1976.

70. Schneider, K. L., Barrett-Connor, E.L., Morton, M.A., Timing of postmenopausal estrogen for optimal bone mineral density, *JAMA*, 277, 543, 1997.

71. Voight, L.F., Weiss, N.S., Chu, J., Daling, J.R., Mc Knight, B., van Belle, G., Progestagen supplementation of exogenous oestrogens and risk of endometrial cancer, *Lancet*, 338, 274, 1991.

72. Early breast cancer trialists'collaborative group Tamoxifen for early breast cancer: an overview of the randomized trials, *Lancet*, 351, 1451, 1998.

73. Fisher, B., Costantino, J.P., Wickerham, D.L., Tamoxifen for prevention of breast cancer: report of the National Early breast cancer trialists'collaborative group. Surgical Adjuvant Breast and Bowel Project P-1 Study, *J. Natl. Cancer Inst.*, 90, 1371, 1998.

74. Meunier, P.J., Evidence-based medicine and osteoporosis: a comparison of fracture risk reduction data from osteoporosis randomised clinical trials, *Int. J. Clin. Pract.*, 53, 122, 1999.

75. Cummings, S.R., Eckert, S., Krueger, K.A., Grady, D., Powles, T.J., Cauley, J.A., Norton Nickelsen, T., Bjarnason, N.H., Morrow, M., Lippman, M.E., Black, D., Glusman, J.E., Costa, A., Jordan, V.C., The effect of raloxifene on risk of breast cancer in postmenopausal women: results from the MORE randomized trial. Multiple Outcomes of Raloxifene Evaluation. *JAMA*, 281, 2189, 1999.

76. Hammar, M., Christau, S., Nathorst-Böös, J., Rud, T., Garre, K.A., Double-blind randomised trial comparing the effects of tibolone and continuous combined hormone replacement therapy in post-menopausal women with menopausal symptoms. *Br. Med. J.*, 105, 904, 1998.

77. Bjarnason, W.H., Bjarnason, K., Haarbo, J., Rosenquist, C., Christiansen, C., Tibolone: prevention of bone loss in late postmenopausal women, *J. Clin. Endocrinol. Metab.*, 1, 2419, 1996.

78. Llyod, G.W.L., Patel, N.R., McGing, E.A., Coper, A.F., Kamavand, K., Jackson, G., Acute effects of hormone replacement with tibolone on myochardial ischaemia in women with angina, *IJCP*, 52, 155, 1998.

79. Ahmed, S.A., Penhale, W.J., Talal, N., Sex hormones, immune responses and autoimmune diseases, *Am. J. Pathol.*, 121, 531, 1985.

80. Jansson, L., Holmadhl, R., Estrogen-mediated immunosuppression in auto-immune diseases, *Inflamm. Res.*, 47, 290, 1998.

81. Lahita, R.G., The connectivite tissue diseases and the overall influence of gender, *Int. J. Fertil.*, 41, 156, 1996.

82. Ansar Ahmed, S., Vertelyi, D., Antibodies to cardiolipin in normal C57BL/6J mice. Induction by estrogen but not dihydrotestosterone, *J. Autoimmun.*, 6, 265, 1993.

83. Grossman, C.J., Regulation of the immune system by sex steroids, *Endocr. Rev.*, 5, 435, 1984.

84. Evans, M.J., MacLaughlin, S., Marvin R.D., Abdou, N.I., Estrogen decreases *in vitro* apoptosis of peripheral blood mononuclear cells from women with normal menstrual cycles and decreases TNF-alpha production in SLE but not in normal cultures, *Clin. Immunol. Immunopathol.*, 82, 258, 1997.

85. Cutolo, M., Sulli, A., Villaggio, B., Seriolo, B., Accardo, S., Relations between steroid hormones and cytokines in rheumatoid arthritis and systemic lupus erythematosus, *Ann. Rheum. Dis.*, 57, 573, 1998.

86. Lahita, R.G., The importance of estrogens in systemic lupus erythematosus, *Clin. Immunol. Immunopathol.*, 63, 17, 1992.

87. Masi, A.T., Kaslow, R.A., Sex effects in systemic lupus erythematosus: a clue to pathogenesis, *Arthritis Rheum.*, 21, 480, 1978.

88. Munoz, J.A., Gil, A., Lopez-Dupla, J.M., Vasquez, J.J., Gonzalez-Gancedo, P., Sex hormones in chronic systemic lupus erythematosus, *Ann. Med. Intern.*, 145, 459, 1994.

89. Richard-Patin, Y., Alcocer-Varela, J., Llorente, L., High levels of Th2 cytokine gene expression in systemic lupus erythematosus, *Rev. Invest. Clin.*, 47, 267, 1995.

90. Houssiau, F.A., Lefebre, C., Van den Berghe, M., Lambert, M., Devogelear, J.P., Renuald, J.J., Serum interleukin-10 titers in systemic lupus erythematosus reflect disease activity, *Lupus*, 4, 393, 1995.

91. Sanchez-Guerrero, J., Liang, M.H., Karlson E.W., Hunter, D.J., Colditz, G.A., Postmenopausal estrogen therapy and the risk of developing systemic lupus erythematosus, *Ann. Inter. Med.*, 122, 430, 1995.

92. Meier, C.R., Sturkenboom, M.C.J.M., Cohen, A.S., Hershel, J., Postmenopausal estrogen replacement therapy and the risk of developing systemic lupus erythematosus or discoid lupus, *J. Rheumatol.*, 25, 8, 1998.

93. Arden, N.K., Lloyd, M.E., Spector, T.D., Hughes, G.R., Safety of hormone replacement therapy (HRT) in systemic lupus erythematosus (SLE), *Lupus*, 3, 11, 1994.

94. Mok, C.C., Lau, C.S., Ho, C.T.K., Lee, K.W., Mok, M.Y., Wong, R.W.S., Safety of hormonal replacement therapy in postmenopausal patients with systemic lupus erythematosus, *Scand. J. Rheumatol.*, 27, 342, 1998.

95. Kreidstein, S., Urowitz, M.B., Gladman, D.D., Gough, J., Hormone replacement therapy in systemic lupus erythematosus, *J. Rheumatol.*, 24, 2149, 1997.

96. Pettersson, T., Pukkala, E., Teppo, L., Friman, C., Increased risk of cancer in patients with systemic lupus erythematosus, *Ann. Rheum. Dis.*, 51, 437, 1992.

97. Abu-Shakra, M., Gladman, D.D., Urowitz, M.B., Malignancy in systemic lupus erythematosus, *Arthritis Rheum.*, 39, 1050, 1996.

98. Mellemkjaer, L., Andersen, V., Linet, M.S., Gridley, G., Hoover, R., Olsen, J.H., Non-Hodgkin's lymphoma and other cancers among a cohort of patients with systemic lupus erythematosus, *Arthritis Rheum.*, 40, 761, 1997.

99. Ramsey-Goldman, R., Mattai, S.A., Schilling, E., Chiu, Y.L., Alo, C.J., Howe, H.L., Manzi, S., Increased risk of malignancy in patients with systemic lupus erythematosus, *J. Investig. Med.*, 46, 217, 1998.

100. Van Vollenhoven, R.F., Morabito, L.M., Engleman, E.G., Mcuire, J.L., Treatment of SLE with DHEA: 50 patients treated up to 12 months, *J. Rheumatol.*, 25, 285, 1998.

101. Karpf, D., Shapiro, D.R., Seeman, E., Ensrud, K.E., Johnston, C.C., Admai, S., Prevention of non-vertebral fractures by alendronate: a meta-analysis, *JAMA*, 277, 1159, 1997.

102. Aloia, J.F., Vaswani, A., Yeh, J.K., Ross, P.L., Flaster, E., Dilmanian, F.A., Calcium supplementation with and without hormone replacement therapy to prevent postmenopausal bone loss, *Ann. Intern. Med.*, 120, 97, 1994.

103. Reid, I.A., Therapy of oesteoporosis: calcium, vitamin D, and exercise, *Am. J. Med.*, 312, 278, 1996.

104. Luckert, B.P., Johnson, B.E., Robinson, R.G., Estrogen and progesterone replacement therapy reduces corticoid-induced bone loss, *J. Bone Miner. Res.*, 7, 1063, 1992.

105. Stevenson J.C., Management of corticosteroid-induced osteoporosis, *Lancet*, 352, 132, 1998.

106. De Clerck, L.S., Meijers, K.A., Cats, A., Is MCTD a distinct entity? Comparison of clinical and laboratory findings in MCTD, SLE, PSS, and RA patients, *Clin. Rheumatol.*, 8, 29, 1989.

107. Gendi, N.S., Welsh, K.I., van Venrooij, W.J., Vanchees Waran, R., Gilroy, J., Black, C.M., HLA type as a predictor of mixed connective tissue disease differentiation. Ten-year clinical and immunogenetic followup of 46 patients, *Arthritis Rheum.*, 38, 259, 1995.

108. Kaufman, R.L., Kitridou, R.C., Pregnancy in mixed connective tissue disease comparison with systemic lupus erythematosus, *J. Rheumatol.*, 9, 549, 1982.

109. Wingrave, S.J., Kay, C.R., Royal College of General Practiioners study, Reduction in incidence of rheumatoid arthritis associated with oral contraceptives, *Lancet*, 34, 1, 1978.

110. Ostensen, M., Aune, B., Husby, G., Effects of pregnancy and hormonal changes on the activity of rheumatoid arthritis, *Scan. J. Rheumatol.*, 12, 69, 1983.

111. Hammerford, P.C., Kay, C.R., Hirsch, S., Oral contraceptives and rheumatoid arthritis: new data from the Royal College of General Practioners' oral contraception study, *Ann. Rheum. Dis.*, 49, 744, 1990.

112. Hernandez-Avila, Liang, M.H., Willett, W.C., Stampfer, M.J., Colditz, G.A., Rosner, B., Chang, R.W., Hennekens, C.H., Speizer, F.E., Exogenous sex hormones and the risk of rheumatoid arthritis, *Arthritis Rheumatism*, 33, 947, 1990.

113. Linos, A., Worthington, J.W., O'Fallon, W.M., Kurland, L.T., The epidemiology of rheumatoid arthritis in Rochester, Minnesota: A study of its incidence, prevalence and mortality, *Am. J. Epidemiol.*, 111, 87, 1980.

114. Koespsell, T.D., Dugowson, C.E., Nelson, J.L., Voigt, L.F., Daling, J.R., Non-contraceptive hormones and the risk of rheumatoid arthritis in menopausal women, *Int. J. Epidemiol.*, 23, 1248, 1994.

115. Van Den Broucke, J.P., Witteman, J.C., Valkenburg, H.A., Boersma, J.W., Cats, A., Festen, J., Hartman, A.P., Huber-Bruning, O., Rasker, J.J., Weber, J., Non contraceptive hormones and rheumatoid arthritis in perimenopausal women, *JAMA*, 255, 1299, 1986.

116. Carette, S., Marcous, S., Gingras, S., Postmenopausal hormones and the incidence of rheumatoid arthritis, *J. Rheumatol.*, 16, 911, 1986.

117. Van Den Brink, H.R., Lems, W.F., Van Everdingen, A.A., Bijlsma, J.W.J., Adjuvant oestrogen treatment increases bone mineral density in postmenopausal women with rheumatoid arthritis, *Ann. Rheum. Dis.*, 52, 302, 1993.

118. Hall, G.M., Daniels, M., Doyle, D.V., Spector, T.D., Effect of hormone replacement therapy on bone mass in rheumatoid arthritis patients treated with and without steroids, *Arthritis Rheum.*, 37, 1499, 1994.

119. Sambrook, P., Birmingham, J., Champion, D., Kelly, P., Kempler, S., Freund, J., Eisman, J., Post-menopausal bone loss in rheumatoid arthritis: Effect of estrogens and androgens, *J. Rheumatol.*, 19, 3, 1992.

120. Cibere, J., Sibley, J, Haga, M., Rheumatoid arthritis and the risk of malignancy, *Arthritis Rheum.*, 40, 1580, 1997.

121. Gridley, G., McLaughlin, J.K., Ekbom, A., Klareskog, L., Adami, H.O., Hacker, D.G., Hoover, R., Fraumeni, J.F., Incidence of cancer among patients with rheumatoid arthritis, *J. Natl. Cancer Inst.*, 85, 307, 1993.

122. Booij, A., Biewenga-Booij, C.M., Huber-Bruning, O., Cornelis, C., Jacobs, J.W.G., Bijlsma, J.W.J., Androgens as adjuvant treatment in postmenopausal female patients with rheumatoid arthritis, *Ann. Rheum. Dis.*, 55, 811, 1996.

123. Denton, C.M., Black, C.M., Korn, J.H., De Combrugghe, B., Systemic slerosis: current pathogenetic concepts and future prospects for targeted therapy, *Lancet*, 347, 1453, 1996.

124. Herbai, G., Treatment of progressive systemic sclerosis with a synthetic weak estrogen:cyclofenil (Sexovid-R). Report of a case, *Acta Med. Scand.*, 6, 537, 1974.

125. Katayama, H., Ohsawa, K., Yaoita, H., Improvement of progressive systemic sclerosis (PSS) with estriol treatment, *Acta Derm. Venereol.*, 64, 168, 1984.

126. Lekakis, J., Papamichael, C., Mavrikakis, M., Voutsas, A., Stamatelopoulos, S., Effect of long-term estrogen therapy on brachial arterial endothelium-dependent vasodilation in women with Raynaud's phenomenon secondary to systemic sclerosis, *Am. J. Cardiol.*, 82, 1555, 1998.

127. La Montagna, G., Vatti, M., Valentini, G., Tirri, G., Osteopenia in systemic sclerosis. Evidence of a participating role of earlier menopause, *Clin. Rheum.*, 10, 18, 1991.

128. Rosenthal, A.K., Mc Laughlin, J.K., Gridley, G., Nyren, O., Incidence of cancer among patients with systemic sclerosis, *Cancer*, 76, 910, 1995.

129. Carlsten, H., Nilsson, N., Jonsson, R., Bâckman, K., Holmdahl, R., Tarkowski, A., Estrogen accelerates immune complex glomerulonephritis but ameliorates T cell-mediated vasculitis and sialadenitis in autoimmune MRL Ipr/Ipr Mice, *Cell. Immunol.*, 144, 190, 1992.

130. American College of Rheumatology 1990 criteria for the classification of vasculitis, Introduction. *Arthritis Rheum.*, 33, 1065, 1990.

131. Hunder, G.G., Arend, W.P., Block, D.A., Calabrese, L.H., Fauci, A.S., Fries, J.F., Leavitt, Ishikawa, K., Matsuura, S., Occlusive thromboaortopathy (Takayasu's disease) and pregnancy, *Am. J. Cardiol.*, 50, 1293, 1982.

132. Gutierrez, G., Dagnino, R., Mintz, G., Polymyositis/dermatomyositis and pregnancy, *Arthritis Rheum.*, 27, 291, 1984.

133. Risk of cancer in patients with dermatomyositis and polymyositis A population based-study, *N. Eng. J. Med.*, 326, 363, 1992.

33 Surgical Treatments

Matthew Waltham and Kevin G. Burnand

CONTENTS

I. INTRODUCTION

Surgical biopsy of muscle or selected vessels is often valuable in the diagnosis of vascular manifestations of systemic autoimmune diseases. Operative surgery is, however, rarely indicated in the treatment of many "vasculitides" and should only be utilized in carefully selected patients.

II. OCCLUSIVE VASCULITIC DISEASES

Systemic autoimmune diseases commonly cause transmural inflammation of the wall of small vessels, and may progress to cause arterial occlusion and distal limb ischemia in some patients. This may present as pain, ulceration, or gangrene in the affected limb. Individual crural vessels, pedal arch vessels, and the metatarsal and digital arteries can all be affected. The more distal the occlusion, the less the prospect of collateral pathways developing and the greater the likelihood of critical ischemia. Many of the vasculitides present with severe Raynaud's phenomenon (digital pallor followed by cyanosis, then reactive hyperaemia) in response to cold exposure. This is often intractable and may progress to digital ulceration and even frank gangrene.

0-8493-1335-X/01/$0.00+$.50
© 2001 by CRC Press LLC

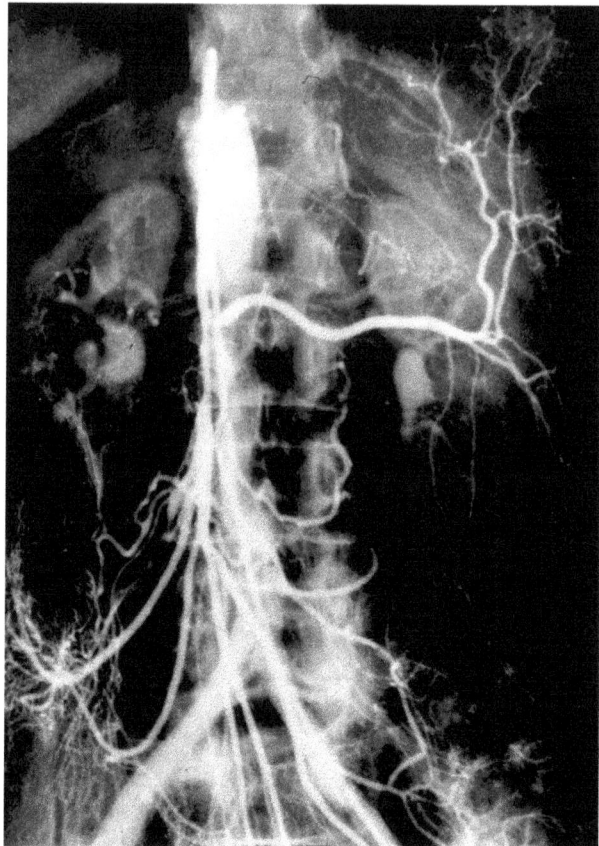

FIGURE 33.1 Mesenteric angiogram of a patient with symptoms of mesenteric ischaemia. The angiogram shows vasculitic stenosis of the mesenteric arteries.

Affected limbs feel cool, distal pulses are impalpable, and ischemic paronychia are common around the nails. Doppler pressures are reduced in the pedal vessels and duplex scanning shows normal blood flow to the popliteal arteries. Unfortunately, the distal nature of most of the vasculitides means that surgical options are limited and often have poor outcomes. Surgery should only be considered for intractable pain or in cases where there is ulceration or frank gangrene. In those patients in whom surgery is indicated, the distal extent of the disease should first be assessed by arteriography to define its nature and plan appropriate treatment. Duplex scanning is less valuable, as it rarely defines disease in the distal vasculature.

Occasionally, vasculitis can affect the mesenteric vessels and present with symptoms of pain following eating ("mesenteric angina"). This should be considered when other causes of the symptoms have been excluded by abdominal ultrasonography and esophagogastroduodenoscopy. The diagnosis can be confirmed by selective mesenteric arteriography (Figure 33.1). The vasculitides can also involve the coronary, subclavian, carotid, cerebral, and renal arteries where they can cause angina, infarction, transient ischemic attacks, strokes, and hypertension. The basic surgical options for treating occlusive inflammatory arterial disease are sympathectomy, bypass procedures, and amputation.

A. Sympathectomy

The arteries to the skin and muscles of the limbs are innervated by the sympathetic nervous system. The nerves to the skin are mainly vasoconstrictor, whereas those to muscles have both vasoconstrictor and vasodilator fibers. At rest, vasoconstrictor tone predominates. Following sympathetic vasomotor blockade there is a marked increase in skin blood flow which can be at the expense of a reduced muscle flow. Although this may reduce the claudication distance, the increased skin blood flow will often allow ischemic nail folds and ulceration to heal, and the blockage of pseudomotor activity dries up ischemic and infected ulcers. Dividing the sympathetic chain also reduces the afferent pain fiber pathways and reduces or abolishes pain. Sympathectomy is, however, ineffective in reversing or improving frank gangrene and, if this is present, it must be combined with ablation. Although the effects are often short-lived, the healing of ischemic areas combined with the cessation of smoking may provide long-term benefit.

Sympathectomy can be achieved by either surgical excision of part of the sympathetic chain or by chemical ablation of the chain. Chemical sympathectomy is performed by injection of phenol around the chain using local anesthetic and radiographic control. Surgical excision is preferable in patients with vasculitides because recurrence following chemical sympathectomy can occur, and salvage surgical sympathectomy following a failed chemical sympathectomy is a very difficult procedure.

The most successful application of sympathectomy is in the treatment of thromboangiitis obliterans (Buerger's disease). In this condition the distal vessels of the upper and lower limbs become progressively obliterated. Luminal thrombosis is common, and the accompanying veins may also become inflamed, which may lead to superficial and deep vein thrombosis. Patients usually present with poorly healing ulcers or digital gangrene, which may be preceded by a history of intermittent claudication. Patients are usually young, cigarette-smoking males, although cannabis smoking has also recently been implicated,[1] and the disease also occurs in women. Arteriography shows a characteristic pattern of normal proximal vessels and distal occlusions with many "corkscrew" collaterals (Figure 33.2). Progressive ischemia leads first to digital gangrene, and then to more major amputations of the limbs if cigarette smoking continues.[2,3] Sympathectomy may be particularly effective in Buerger's disease, perhaps because the condition is characterized by a significant component of vasospasm. Sympathectomy often relieves rest pain, and may allow small areas of gangrene to heal.[4,5]

Sympathectomy is rarely if ever indicated for Raynaud's phenomenon, and many patients can achieve satisfactory symptom control by simply avoiding cold, abstaining from tobacco, and wearing warm or heated gloves in the winter. Vasodilator drugs should be used cautiously during attacks, and the use of in-hospital courses of systemic prostacyclin by infusion may be very valuable in severely affected patients. Sympathectomy often produces a dramatic early benefit,[6] but this is only short-lived and, after a year or two, the benefits are marginal.[7,8]

1. Cervical Sympathectomy

The sympathetic fibers to the arm synapse in the second to fifth thoracic ganglia, with the first thoracic ganglion fusing with the inferior cervical ganglion to form the stellate ganglion. Inadvertent injury to this will result in a permanent Horner's syndrome. Cervical sympathectomy may be performed by cervical (anterior),[9] transaxillary,[10] or thoracoscopic[11] approach depending on surgical preference.

a. Thoracoscopic Cervical Sympathectomy

The thoracoscopic approach is now well established and has become the standard procedure, although complications are not uncommon. Damage to the first cervical ganglion is most easily avoidable using this approach, as it is not usually possible to get any higher than the second rib from the pleural space. The procedure is performed under general anesthesia, preferably using a double lumen tube, with the patient supine and with the arms abducted. The ipsilateral lung is deflated and an artificial pneumothorax established. A 5-mm laparoscope is inserted through the third intercostal space and advanced across the pleural cavity to identify the sympathetic ganglia and chain passing over the necks of the ribs. The appropriate ganglia and interconnecting rami are

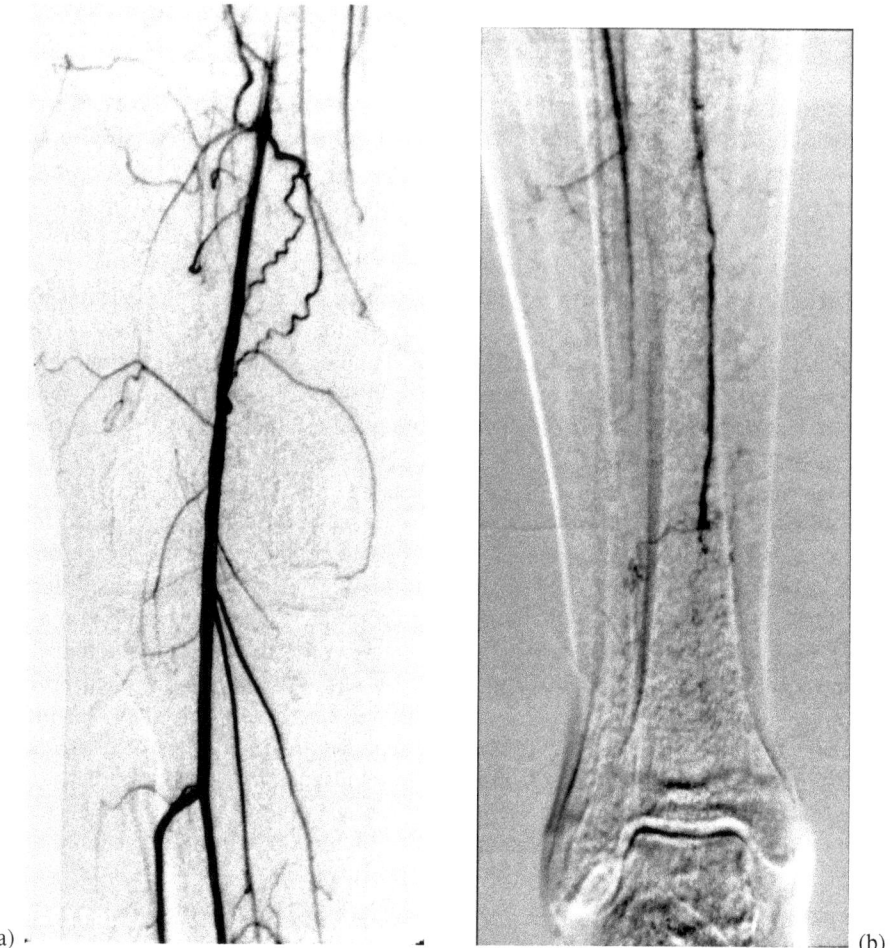

(a) (b)

FIGURE 33.2 (a) Arteriogram showing typical corkscrew collaterals in Buerger's disease. (b) Arteriogram shows predominantly distal disease, with occluded crural vessels.

coagulated using a diathermy probe inserted through a separate incision. This blunderbuss technique fails to remove the sympathetic chain for histology and can, if poorly performed, fail to interrupt the chain. For this reason a two-port technique with careful excision of the chain is preferable. Care must be taken not to damage the first thoracic ganglion. The lung is reinflated at the end of the procedure, the laparoscope is removed, and the wounds closed. A postoperative chest radiograph is performed to identify any residual pneumothorax.

b. Transaxillary Cervical Sympathectomy

This operation has largely been replaced by the laparoscopic procedure. The patient is placed in a lateral position with the operated side uppermost and the axilla widely displayed by abducting the arm and flexing the forearm. An 8-cm oblique incision is made from latissimus dorsi, running forward and down across the third rib as far as the posterior border of pectoralis major. The periosteum of the rib is exposed, divided with diathermy, and reflected from the superior surface to expose the costal pleura. This is divided along the upper border of the rib, and a rib retractor is inserted and opened widely. The apex of the lung is displaced downward and the ganglia and interconnecting chain identified running beneath the costal pleura over the necks of the ribs. The overlying pleura is opened and the chain and rami lifted and divided above the T2 and below the T5 ganglia. The wound is closed and the lung re-expanded. A postoperative chest radiograph is performed.

c. Anterior Cervical Sympathectomy

The traditional access to the sympathetic chain is through the cervical approach. The patient is placed feet-down supine with a sandbag under the shoulders and the head turned to the opposite side. A 5-cm incision is placed 1 cm above the clavicle with the medial end just overlying the sternomastoid. The platysma, lateral fibers of sternomastoid, and any intervening veins are divided to expose the scalenus anterior. This is divided low down, preserving the phrenic nerve on its surface by reflecting it medially. This exposes the subclavian artery, which is retracted upward or downward by dividing its branches to expose the costopleural membrane, which, in turn, is incised to expose the apex of the lung. The sympathetic chain is exposed by carefully stripping the lung downward with a finger. The chain is excised between the stellate and fourth cervical ganglia.

2. Lumbar Sympathectomy

This may be performed either by an open operation or by injecting phenol around the lumbar chain using radiological guidance. The latter has a very low morbidity and so has gained popularity. It may be particularly appropriate for treating some elderly patients with ischemic rest pain. For younger patients, surgical sympathectomy should be performed to ensure complete removal of the sympathetic chain. At operation the second and third lumbar ganglia are removed. In males, the first lumbar ganglion on at least one side must be retained in order to preserve normal ejaculation.

Patients with distal vessel occlusive disease, and therefore not suitable for reconstructive procedures, may be suitable for lumbar sympathectomy to relieve rest pain and sometimes rescue critically ischemic tissue. The major benefit is in the treatment of rest pain, but only 60% of cases may be relieved for up to three years. The amputation rate is not affected.[12] Surgical lumbar sympathectomy can either be performed by an open procedure or laparoscopically.

a. Open Lumbar Sympathectomy

The lumbar sympathetic chain is approached through a transverse incision lateral to, but at the level of, the umbilicus on the side to be denervated. The oblique muscles of the abdominal wall are divided to expose the peritoneum. This is freed by blunt dissection from the deep surface of the transversus abduminus muscle and retracted medially to expose the retroperitoneal space. The psoas is found on the posterior wall and the groove between the medial border of this muscle, the lumbar vertebrae and the aorta on the left, and the inferior vena cava on the right are defined. The lumbar sympathetic chain can usually be palpated as a firm cord punctuated by a number of swellings lying in this groove on the front of the vertebrae. The chain is picked up with a nerve hook and dissected up to the diaphragmatic crura, and down to the pelvic brim. All of the rami that join the ganglia are divided and the first, second, and third ganglia are excised. The wound is closed in layers with suction drainage.

b. Endoscopic Lumbar Sympathectomy

The technique of laparoscopic lumbar sympathectomy has been described as an alternative to the traditional open approach. This may be performed using transperitoneal[13] or retroperitoneal (balloon-assisted)[14] approaches. The benefits of this method have yet to be demonstrated, but may combine the advantages of a minimally invasive approach with the certainty of surgical excision of the sympathetic chain.

B. Arterial Bypass Procedures

1. Bypass Procedures in Patients with Vasculitides

Bypass procedures for patients with lower limb ischemia have been performed for many years. Autologous vein grafts, usually using the long saphenous vein, or artificial materials (such as polytetrafluoroethylene) are used to bypass from patent proximal vessels to distal vessels (Figure

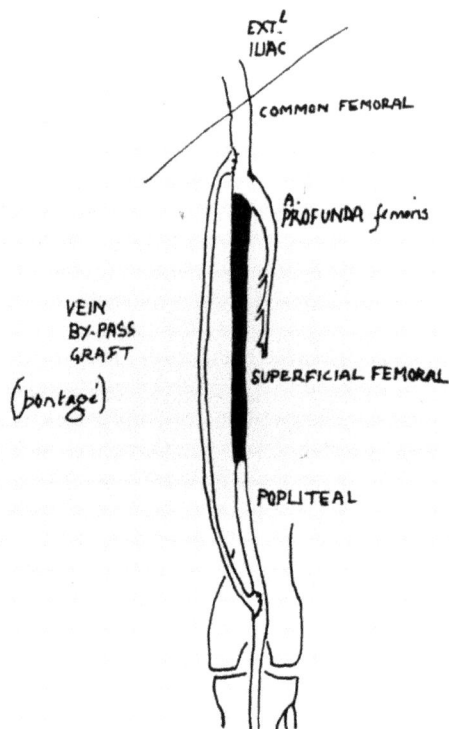

FIGURE 33.3 Diagram of above-knee femoro-popliteal bypass with occluded superficial femoral artery.

33.3). Whereas bypass surgery is modestly successful in atheromatous occlusion, it is much less successful in patients with Buerger's disease. This is largely because the secondary periarteritis is often very severe and makes dissection of the vessels very difficult. Unfortunately, autoimmune vasculitis also tends to affect distal vessels, and distal bypass procedures have a much lower flow rate and patency rate than proximal procedures. Results are therefore poor, and these procedures should only be considered in exceptional cases. In many cases of Buerger's disease, bypass surgery is impossible as a consequence of the distal nature of the disease, although there are some reports of successful results.[15] Even in cases where the graft only remains patent for a short time, this may allow ulceration to heal. The ulcers often do not recur if the graft then fails, provided the patient stops smoking. Intestinal ischemia secondary to Buerger's disease has been described, and this may also need to be treated by vascular bypass.[16]

2. Bypass Procedures in Patients with Takayasu's Disease

Takayasu's disease and the middle aortic syndrome are diseases which are very amenable to surgical bypass. Takayasu's disease most commonly affects the subclavian and innominate arteries and aortic arch, followed by the descending aorta and aorto-iliac region. The presenting symptoms depend upon which vessels are affected, but transient ischemic attacks, visual problems, and arm and leg claudication can all occur.[17] The aortic arch and its branches, the descending, thoracic, and the abdominal aorta, can also be affected, and the disease may be either stenotic or aneurysmal. Arteriography must be performed to assess the disease and plan surgery; this often demonstrates either a smooth tapering stenosis of the affected vessel or total occlusion (Figure 33.4). Surgical bypass to normal vessels beyond the limits of the disease is indicated for patients with ischemic symptoms, aneurysms, or significant renal artery disease.[18-20] Using standard operative techniques, good results can be achieved.[21-23] Surgery may take the form of carotid artery reconstruction,

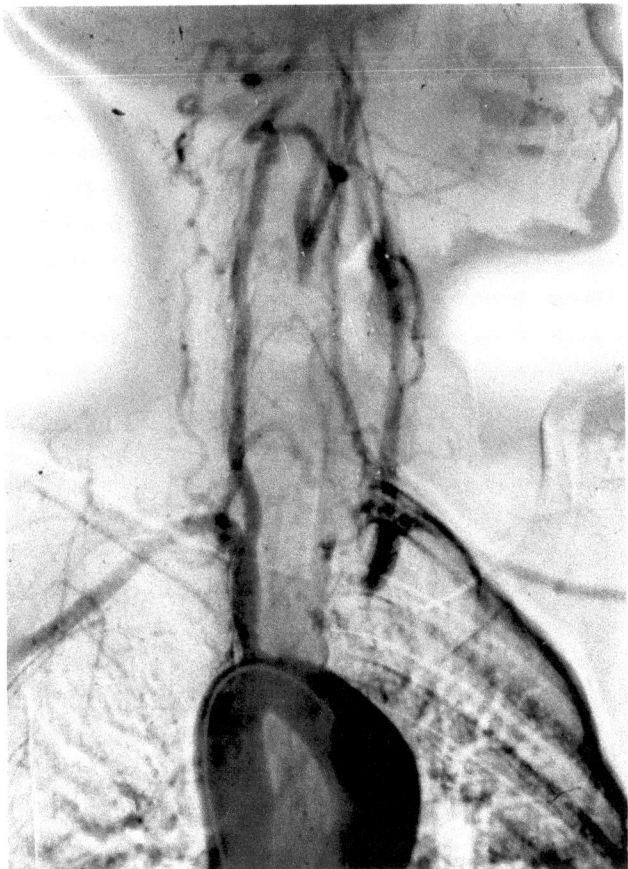

FIGURE 33.4 Arch aortogram showing brachiocephalic artery occlusion in a patient with Takayasu's disease.

thoraco-abdominal aortic bypass, renal artery reconstruction, or aneurysm repair.[24,25] If possible, the surgery should be performed in one stage to correct all affected vessels, with multiple reconstructions if necessary. It is also important to ensure that the disease is not active at the time of bypass. Patients should be treated with steroids and cytotoxic agents until their erythrocyte sedimentation rate is low.[26]

C. AMPUTATION

When the above procedures are not indicated or fail, then there is often no alternative but to amputate critically ischemic or gangrenous tissue (Figure 33.5). Amputation should be as conservative as possible while ensuring that satisfactory healing is achieved. Dead or devitalized tissue or bone must be completely removed.

D. OTHER PROCEDURES

1. Implantable Spinal Cord Stimulators

Implantable spinal cord stimulators have been used in some patients to treat ischemic pain. A temporary lead is placed percutaneously in the dorsal aspect of the epidural space related to the symptomatic dermatomes. If this is effective, then it can be replaced with a permanent lead with a pulse generator. It is relatively simple, minimally invasive and reversible, but unfortunately expensive. Doubts have been cast on the value of this procedure, especially once gangrene is present.

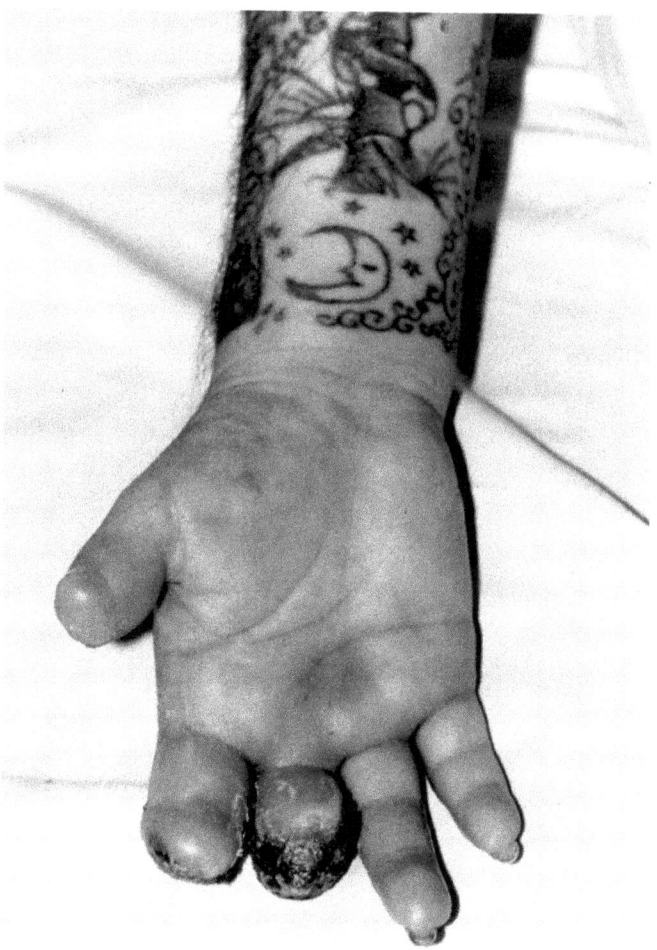

FIGURE 33.5 (a) Ischemia of the digits and amputation in a patient with Buerger's disease.

2. Omentopexy

This experimental technique has been used to attempt to improve the perfusion of ischemic legs in patients with nonreconstructable arterial disease. The greater omentum is mobilized on a vascular pedicle and transposed to the ischamic leg, where it is anastomosed to the femoral vessels. It is then passed down through a subfascial tunnel to the ankle. The omentum has angiogenic properties and promotes new vessel formation. The long-term results of the procedure are not known.[27]

3. Injection of Angiogenic Growth Factors

Preliminary trials suggest that intramuscular injection of angiogenic growth factors such as vascular endothelial growth factor may improve ulcer healing in patients with advanced Buerger's disease in whom other medical and surgical treatment has failed.[28]

III. DIAGNOSIS OF GIANT-CELL ARTERITIS

The diagnosis of giant-cell arteritis can be confirmed surgically by taking a segment of the superficial temporal artery under local anaesthetic. The incision is placed directly over the vessel. Histology

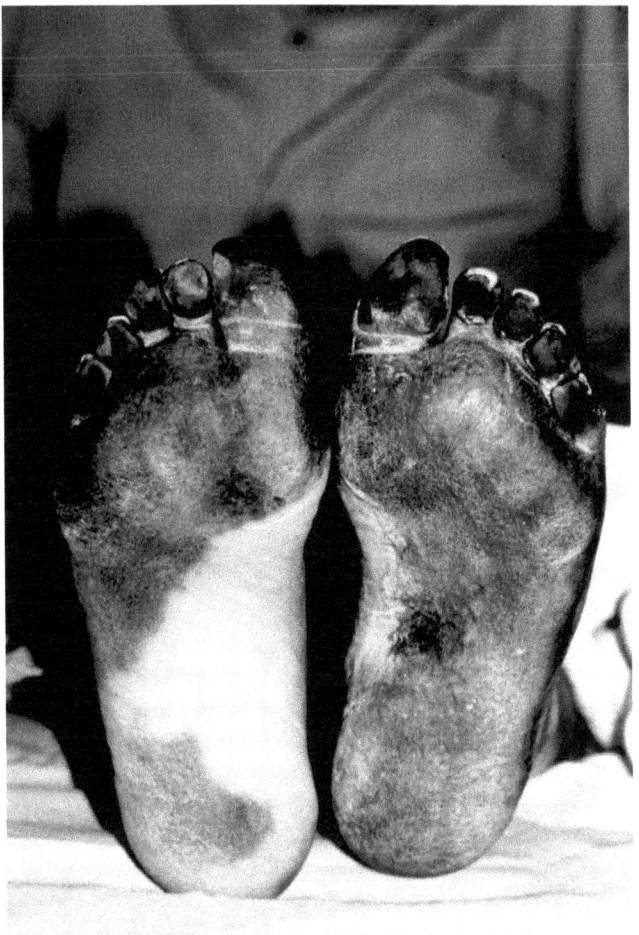

FIGURE 33.5 (b) Gangrene of the feet.

shows a pronounced intimal thickening, a round cell infiltration through all layers of the arterial wall with destruction of the internal elastic lamina, and the presence of a few giant cells.

IV. BEHÇET'S DISEASE

This disease is managed primarily by medical therapy, but has a wide variety of manifestations that sometimes require surgical treatment.[29] It may present with gastrointestinal ulceration, mesenteric ischemia and infarction, occlusive and aneurysmal arterial disease (including intracranial and pulmonary disease), cardiac valve disease, and urological complications. Patients with Behçet's disease have an abnormal response to the trauma of surgery, which leads to poor wound healing and, thus, complications are more frequent.

V. CONCLUSION

Surgery has a limited role in treating patients with vasculitides. Sympathectomy is the most commonly performed operation. Bypass procedures are most effective in patients with Takayasu's disease and the midaortic syndrome. Amputation may be necessary in patients with gangrene.

REFERENCES

1. Schneider, H. J., Jha, S., and Burnand, K. G., Progressive arteritis associated with cannabis use, *Eur. J. Vasc. Endovasc. Surg.*, 18, 366, 1999.
2. McPherson, J. R., Juergens, J. L., and Gifford, R.W., Thromboangiitis obliterans and arteriosclerosis obliterans: clinical and prognostic differences, *Ann. Intern. Med.*, 59, 288, 1963.
3. Kinmonth, J. B., Thromboangiitis obliterans. Results of sympathectomy and prognosis, *Lancet*, 2, 717, 1948.
4. Ohta, T., and Shionoya, S., Fate of the ischaemic limb in Buerger's disease, *Br. J. Surg.*, 75, 259, 1988.
5. Kunlin, J., Lengua, F., Testart, J., and Pajot, A., Thromboangiosis or thromboangeitis treated by adrenalectomy and sympathectomy from 1942 to 1962. A follow-up study of 110 cases, *Journal of Cardiovascular Surgery*, 14, 21, 1973.
6. Baddeley, R. M., The place of upper dorsal sympathectomy in the treatment of primary Raynaud's disease, *Br. J. Surg.*, 52, 426, 1965.
7. Gifford, R. W., Hines, E. A., and Craig, W. M., Sympathectomy for Raynaud's phenomenon, *Circulation*, 17, 5, 1958.
8. Johnson, E. N. M., Summerly, R. and Birnstingl, M., Prognosis in Raynaud's phenomenon after sympathectomy, *Br. Med. J.*, 962, 1965.
9. Telford, E. D., The technique of sympathectomy, *Br J Surg*, 23, 448, 1935.
10. Atkins, H. J. B., Peraxillary approach to the stellate and upper thoracic ganglia, *Lancet*, 2, 1152, 1949.
11. Hederman, W. P., Sympathectomy by thoracoscopy, in *Vascular and Endovascular Surgical Techniques*, Greenhalgh, R. M., Ed., W. B. Saunders, London, 1994, 281.
12. Cotton, L. T., and Cross, F. W., Lumbar sympathectomy for arterial disease, *Br. J. Surg.*, 72, 678, 1985.
13. Wattanasirichaigoon, S., Ngaorungsri, U., Wanishayathanakorn, A., Hutachoke, T., and Chulakamontri, T., Laparoscopic transperitoneal lumbar sympathectomy: a new approach, *J. Med. Assoc. Thailand*, 80, 275, 1997.
14. Elliott, T. B., and Royle, J. P., Laparoscopic extraperitoneal lumbar sympathectomy: technique and early results, *Aus. N. Z. J. Surg.*, 66, 400, 1996.
15. Shionoya, S., Ban, I., Nakata, Y., Matsubara, J., and Hirai, M., Vascular reconstruction in Buerger's disease, *British Journal of Surgery*, 63, 841, 1976.
16. Kempczinski, R. F., Clark, S. M., Belbea, J., Koelliker, D. D., and Fenoglio-Preiser, C., Intestinal ischaemia secondary to thromboangiitis obliterans, *Ann. Vasc. Surg.*, 7, 354, 1993.
17. Lupi-Herrera, E., Sanchez-Torres, G., Marcushamer, J., Mispireta, J., Horwitz, S., and Vela, J. E., Takayasu's arteritis. Clinical study of 107 cases, *Am. Heart. J.*, 93, 94, 1977.
18. Crawford, E. S., De Bakey, M. E., Morris, G. C., and Cooley, D. A., Thrombo-obliterative disease of the great vessels arising from the aortic arch, *J. Thorac Cardiovasc. Surg.*, 43, 38, 1962.
19. Crawford, E. S., Snyder, D. M., Cho, G. C., and Roehm, J. O., Jr., Progress in treatment of thoraco-abdominal and abdominal aortic aneurysms involving celiac superior mesenteric and renal arteries, *Ann. Surg.*, 188, 404, 1978.
20. Thompson, B. W., Read, R. C., and Campbell, G. S., Aortic arch syndrome, *Archives of Surgery*, 98, 607, 1969.
21. Robbs, J. V., Human, R. R., and Rajaruthnam, P., Operative treatment of nonspecific aortoarteritis (Takayasu's arteritis), *J. Vasc. Surg.*, 3, 605, 1986.
22. Fraga, A., Mintz, G., Valle, L., and Flores-Izquierdo, G., Takayasu's arteritis: frequency of systemic manifestations (study of 22 patients) and favorable response to maintenance steroid therapy with corticosteroids (12 patients), *Arthritis Rheum.*, 15, 617, 1972.
23. Weaver, F. A., Yellin, A. E., Campen, D. H., Oberg, J., Foran, J., Kitridou, R. C., Lee, S. E., and Kohl, R. D., Surgical procedures in the management of Takayasu's arteritis, *J. Vasc. Surg.*, 12, 429, 1990.
24. Lande, A., Abdominal Takayasu's aortitis, the middle aortic syndrome and atherosclerosis: A critical review, *Int. Angiol.*, 17, 1, 1998.
25. Takagi, A., Tada, Y., Sato, O., and Miyata, T., Surgical treatment for Takayasu's arteritis, *J. Cardiovasc. Surg.*, 30, 553, 1989.
26. Pokrovsky, A. V., Nonspecific aortoarteritis, in *Vascular Surgery,* 3rd Ed., Rutherford, R. B., W. B. Saunders Co., Philadelphia, 1989.

27. Khazanchi, R.K., Nanda, V., Kumar, R., Garg, P., Guleria, S., and Bal, S., Omentum autotransplantation in thromboangiitis obliterans: a report of three cases, *Surgery Today*, 29, 86, 1999.

28. Isner, J. M., Baumgartner, I., Rauh, G., Schainfeld, R., Blair, R., Manor, O., Ravzi, S., and Symes, J. F., Treatment of thromboangiitis obliterans (Buerger's disease) by intramuscular gene transfer of vascular endothelial growth factor: Preliminary clinical results, *J. Vasc. Surg.*, 28, 964, 1998.

29. Bradbury, A. W., Milne, A. A., and Murie, J. A., Surgical aspects of Behçet's disease, *Brit. J. Surg.*, 81, 1712, 1994.

34 Therapy of Systemic Vasculitis

*David M. Carruthers, Karim Raza,
and Paul A. Bacon*

CONTENTS

0-8493-1335-X/01/$0.00+$.50
© 2001 by CRC Press LLC

I. INTRODUCTION

The primary systemic necrotizing vasculitides (1°SNV) is a rare group of diseases[1] characterized by recurrent episodes of disease activity, during which time irreversible organ damage or even death can occur. These may require urgent treatment to control the disease before organ failure develops — and there is good evidence that the longer the treatment is delayed, the worse the general prognosis. Appropriate treatment can induce long periods of remission (complete or partial) which then require less aggressive therapy to avoid drug toxicity. At this stage it is important to move from the concept of one drug for vasculitis to that of more complex regimes which apply different combinations of therapy at different stages of the disease. The oncological model is relevant here — an aggressive induction phase followed by a consolidation regime followed by long-term mild maintenance regime, unless there is a relapse requiring a return to more aggressive therapy. In this way treatment is aimed at the patient and not at the diagnosis. In particular, it is aimed at the current state of the patient at different phases of the disease. There are now good clinical tools for detailed assessment, allowing much better definition of the current disease state. Thus, drugs can be tailored to the individual patient at different stages of disease, which will improve the overall therapy.

No current regime is perfect, so it is important to monitor the benefit each patient derives so that future treatment can be based on better evidence. Large-scale, randomized, controlled trials have always been seen as the mainstay of evidence-based medicine, but they are not always possible with rare diseases, particularly when these have wide variability in individual disease manifestations, as does vasculitis. In this case, objective measures of improvement, for example in individual organ function, can provide important evidence for therapeutic benefit of any particular agent from even a small number of patients. Future improvements in treatment need to be based both on broad principles of approach and such detailed evidence in order to move therapy from the empirical and, thus, provide real advances in future treatment.

The success of current therapy has transformed the prognosis of 1°SNV from high early mortality to a group of chronic disease with high morbidity. A considerable portion of that morbidity relates to scars from previous episodes of disease activity, as well as the toxicity of long-term noncurative immunosuppressive therapy. The accumulation of items of damage, or irreversible scars, contributes to the morbidity, quality of life, and late mortality. Patients with fatal systemic vasculitis have more active disease prior to death,[2] and have also sustained more organ damage during the course of the disease.[3] In addition to the damage due to disease activity, there is increasing evidence of long-term toxicity from drug therapy.[4] Thus, the general aims of therapy in this group of diseases must include:

1. To turn off disease activity early, thus limiting disease-related damage and minimizing the duration or total dose of drug needed to induce remission. An initial, very aggressive phase followed by a less toxic consolidation phase may be the best approach to this.
2. To maintain long-term remission with relatively mild agents, thus reducing the high relapse rate that is another main cause of current morbidity. To achieve this, a diagnosis of vasculitis is not sufficient, and the key to successful management in 1°SNV rests in accurate patient assessment for early recognition of disease activity, spectrum of organ involvement, and the severity of overall disease.

A. ASSESSMENT

1. Activity

At acute presentation of 1°SNV, or during flares of disease activity, the diagnosis of active vasculitis involving critical organ systems may be obvious and may prompt the institution of therapy prior to the results of diagnostic tests being available. This is particularly important in the presence of a mononeuritis multiplex, where acute foot drop, for instance, may respond to early therapy. If left untreated until confirmatory tests are available, the opportunity to reverse the lesion may be lost, leading to permanent damage and disability.

In other instances more evidence of disease activity may be necessary before embarking upon potentially toxic therapy. In these cases information provided by laboratory, radiology, and histopathology tests may be valuable to support the clinical picture. The Birmingham Vasculitis Activity Score (BVAS) was developed as a clinical tool to help differentiate clinical features due to disease activity from those due to damage from earlier activity.[2] BVAS provides a numerical score, which is weighted depending on the organ involved and the severity of that involvement, with more severe disease generating a higher score. This clinical tool has been validated and shown to correlate with serological markers of inflammation (CRP). A high score, reflecting critical organ involvement (e.g., kidney, lung) or multisystem disease, indicates that a more aggressive and urgent approach to therapy may be required. In addition to disease activity, the damage that occurs during the course of the illness also contributes to morbidity.

2. Damage

The Vasculitis Damage Index (VDI) was developed to record items of organ damage that have been present for a period of three months since the onset of the disease and are attributable to the disease, therapy, or any undefined causes.[5] By definition, the VDI score is cumulative and cannot reduce with time. It has been validated and compares well with other scoring systems for multisystem disease. A high damage score, reflecting multiple organ involvement, identifies a subgroup of patients with more severe or fatal disease.[6]

3. Prognosis

Clinical assessment is also useful for prognostic reasons. The anatomical distribution, severity of involvement, and degree of disease activity in polyarteritis nodosa (PAN) can be used to identify a group of patients with a poor prognosis. A prospective study of 342 patients with PAN and Churg-Strauss syndrome (CSS) identified the following factors as being associated with a poor outcome: cardiomyopathy, gastrointestinal or central nervous system involvement, age over 50, and proteinuria > 1g and creatinine > 140 μmol/l.[7] Patients with two or more of these risk factors who were treated with cyclophosphamide (CP) and corticosteroid (CS) for one year had a 46% mortality, in contrast to a 96% five-year survival in those with good prognosis PAN. Other studies support the poor outcome associated with renal and cardiac disease in this group of patients.[8] These studies also demonstrate that accurate assessment can be used to direct therapy. In patients with CSS and absence of any of the preceding poor prognostic factors, CP appears unnecessary for initial therapy, but should be considered for second-line therapy in case of treatment failure or relapse. In patients with microscopic polyangiitis (MPA) poor prognosis factors have also been identified and include age > 50 and renal failure.[9] The five-year follow-up in another study of patients with MPA showed a 65% survival with 2 of the 3 deaths related to active renal or pulmonary vasculitis.[10] The five-year survival of a cohort of patients with Wegener's granulomatosis (WG) from specialist referral centers in the U.S. illustrates that there is still a high mortality associated with this disease.[11] A slightly longer study by the British Thoracic Society, including all patients seen by the membership, showed over half the patients died, with a mean survival of 8.5 years.[12] The overall conclusion is that life expectancy is still seriously reduced.

4. Laboratory Tests

Laboratory tests can support the clinical impression of disease activity but are nonspecific (anemia, neutrophilia, esinophilia, thrombocytosis, high CRP, and ESR). Infection, which may present with a similar clinical picture to active vasculitis, or may actually precipitate relapse, often needs excluding before administration of immunosuppressive therapy. However, in the presence of active 1°SNV, once infection is under control or excluded, therapy should not be delayed. Immunological tests may help if applied in the right clinical context. Since the identification of antineutrophil cytoplasmic antibodies (ANCA) there has been an apparent increase in incidence of 1°SNV,[13] which probably relates to increased awareness of these conditions. However, they are not diagnostic and may occur in a variety of other conditions (e.g., inflammatory bowel disease, chronic infection). A rising ANCA titer can be useful in predicting relapse in patients with a known diagnosis of WG,[14] but should not be used as the sole indicator to institute changes in therapy. Biopsy of involved tissue is the gold standard for diagnosis in 1°SNV, but tissue samples can also be used to direct therapy where evidence of ongoing activity is necessary. For example, we have reported five cases of WG where transthoracic needle biopsy of isolated pulmonary lesions confirmed the presence of ongoing disease activity histologically, thus allowing an informed decision to be made on future immunosuppressive therapy.[15]

5. Localized or Systemic Disease

Thorough assessment can be used to distinguish localized from systemic disease. We have taken an expectant approach to the management of some patients where a diagnosis of 1°SNV was made after resection of ischemic bowel, but thorough clinical, laboratory, and radiological investigation revealed no evidence of disease activity elsewhere.[16] In contrast, detailed assessment has identified other patients with clinically unexpected extensive organ involvement, leading to a much more aggressive approach to therapy.

II. PRIMARY SYSTEMIC NECROTIZING VASCULITIS

A. Standard Therapy for Remission Induction

After thorough assessment, therapy for 1°SNV should be considered in several stages (Table 34.1). With current therapy the prognosis for patients with 1°SNV has improved considerably. The five-year survival of PAN prior to the introduction of immunosuppressive therapy was 4%,[17] and the mean survival of untreated WG was five months, with a one-year mortality of 85%.[18] Corticosteroids, introduced in the 1950s, reduced disease activity and improved survival at five-year follow-up to 48%, though the prognosis was worse in those with renal disease.[19] The first studies of

TABLE 34.1
Stages of Therapy for Patients with SNV

Phase of Therapy	Main Therapeutic Options
Remission induction	Cyclophosphamide (continuous oral or intermittent pulse) + corticosteroids
Escalation/enhanced therapy	Pulse methylprednisolone
	Plasma exchange
	IVIg
	High dose cyclophosphamide
Consolidation therapy	Cyclophosphamide
	Methotrexate
	Azathioprine
	Cyclosporin A
Maintenance therapy	Methotrexate
	Azathioprine
	Trimethoprim/sulphamethoxazole
Relapse therapy	Short course cyclophosphamide
	Methotrexate
Rescue therapy	Monoclonal antibody therapy
	Stem cell rescue
Surgery (for damage repair)	Sinus drainage
	Tracheostomy
	Renal transplant
	Cosmetic

immunosuppressives in combination with CS for 1°SNV were generally retrospective but demonstrated a considerable improvement in five-year survival (80% compared to 50% for steroids alone and 15% for untreated patients).[20] Fauci et al.[21] showed a considerable reduction in mortality with CP, but the mean duration of steroid therapy prior to the introduction of CP was 22 months, suggesting that this group of patients probably had good prognosis disease, as patients with severe uncontrolled vasculitis were likely to have died already. Despite the methodological problems with these early studies, daily oral CP became the standard therapy for severe 1°SNV, and the debate now focuses not on whether, but how best to administer it.

1. Cyclophosphamide

The introduction of CP for the therapy of 1°SNV has improved survival, but long-term morbidity from disease-related damage and drug-related toxicity is now becoming an increasingly important issue for survivors.[4] The aims of therapy must be to induce remission as rapidly as possible, with minimum short-term drug toxicity, and thus limit disease-related organ damage. Less toxic long-term therapy is then necessary to maintain remission and prevent relapses of disease activity, thus reducing the damage that can occur after chronic CP administration. On this basis, we and several other groups now favor short induction courses of CP followed by consolidation and then maintenance therapy with agents such as methotrexate or azathioprine in combination with low doses of oral steroids.

CP may be administered as continuous oral therapy or by intermittent high-dose pulses given either intravenously or orally. There is much debate about the preferred dosing schedule, but we favor an intermittent pulse regime, which gives a more rapid clinical response but may allow a higher relapse rate later on.[22] However, continuous oral therapy has been successfully introduced when pulse CP has failed or relapse has occurred within the first six months of therapy.[23] It is standard therapy at the onset of therapy in many units. The largest cohort of patients treated with continuous oral CP therapy (2 mg/kg/day) comes from the NIH, where complete or partial remission was induced in 90% of WG patients, of which 75% were in complete remission.[24] CP was given in conjunction with daily oral prednisolone (1 mg/kg/day) which was reduced after about one month, aiming for a dose of 60 mg prednisolone on alternate days. The dose of steroid was then further tapered and withdrawn depending on the patient's response. However, remission induction was often slow (up to two years in some patients), increasing the need for prolonged CP therapy (which was reduced by 25 mg decrements every two to three months one year after disease remission was achieved). Relapses still occurred and morbidity was high due to both the disease process (86% of patients) and its therapy (42%). Infertility, serious infections, and nonglomerular hematuria (50% of patients, with macroscopic changes compatible with hemorrhagic cystitis in 57% of these) were the most common side-effects. The worrying incidence of late bladder carcinoma in these patients (5%) has recently been reported,[4] with an estimated incidence of bladder cancer of 16% at 15 years after first exposure to CP. Intermittent pulses of CP, possibly due to a lower cumulative dose of drug, may represent a safer approach to therapy.

The interval between pulses is an important and frequently ignored issue. Monthly pulses of CP in an uncontrolled study of 14 patients with WG induced remission in only 50%, all of whom relapsed after one or two years.[25] A similar poor rate of remission induction (42%) was seen in a study of 43 WG patients also treated with monthly pulse CP.[26] However, a third study showed that monthly pulses were as effective at inducing and maintaining remission as daily oral CP.[27] In patients with good prognosis PAN or CSS, monthly pulses of CP (0.6 g/m^2) were found to be as effective as continuous oral CP in inducing remission, but were possibly associated with less toxicity.[28]

A more recent study comparing pulses of CP at three weekly intervals to continuous oral CP (2 mg/kg/day) in patients with WG found similar remission induction rates at six months (88.9% vs. 78.3%, respectively).[22] Although relapse rates were higher in the pulse group (59% vs. 13% for continuous oral CP), five-year survival was equal (66.7 vs. 56.5%, respectively). Infectious complications were more frequent with continuous oral CP (69.6% vs. 40.7% for pulse CP) and contributed more often to death in this group (60% vs. 33.3%). The high mortality in both groups highlights the need for new and better approaches to therapy for 1°SNV. Other units have used smaller-dose pulses (500 mg) at weekly intervals with complete or partial remission achieved in 74% of patients with 1°SNV.[29]

Our standard regimen for remission induction in 1°SNV involves pulse CP (15 mg/kg) initially every two weeks, with a dose interval that increases with time.[30] After one year of therapy a lower total dose of CP is given compared to standard continuous oral CP regimes. This two-weekly-pulse regime was compared with continuous oral CP in a study of 54 patients with 1°SNV where both groups received the same total dose of CP (12 months pulse therapy or 3 to 6 months of continuous oral CP followed by azathioprine).[30] Clinical response was similar in the two groups (mortality, treatment failure, relapse, and dialysis requirements) but toxicity was less in the pulse group (less marrow suppression and infection). The better response rate to pulse therapy in these studies compared to the earlier pulse CP studies may reflect the shorter interval between pulses during the induction phase. Our standard pulse CP regime, which we use for patients with medium- and small-vessel necrotizing vasculitis,[30] is shown below.

2. Standard Pulse Cyclophosphamide Regime

a. Induction Period

Intravenous pulses of CP 15 mg/kg immediately preceded by methylprednisolone 10 mg/kg at weeks 0, 2, and 4 followed by oral pulses of CP 5 mg/kg/day plus prednisolone 3.3 mg/kg/day for 3 days each at weeks 7, 10, and 13.

b. Consolidation Period

Induction therapy is then followed by a consolidation regime of: 8 oral pulses of CP 5 mg/kg/day plus prednisolone 3.3 mg/kg/day for 3 days each at weeks 17, 21, 25, 30, 35, 40, 46, and 52. Daily

TABLE 34.2
Dose Reduction for Pulse Cyclophosphamide in Renal Impairment

Creatinine (μmol/l)	Cyclophosphamide Pulse (mg/kg)	Methylprednisolone Pulse (mg/kg)
<150	15	10
150–250	10	10
251–500	7.5	10
>500	5	7

oral steroid is given to most patients (starting dose 20 to 40 mg/day depending on clinical condition), and the dose is reduced after the first three CP pulses, aiming for 10 mg/day by three months.

c. Caveats

The maximum dose per pulse of CP was originally arbitrarily limited at 1000 mg. However, recent experience shows us that higher doses are often well tolerated. In the absence of indications for dose reductions (see below), the final dose from the mg/kg calculation shown above may be required, at least for the induction doses. Some patients do not tolerate oral pulses well due to side-effects, such as nausea, and it is sometimes necessary to continue with intravenous pulses throughout.

Dose reductions are made for each pulse for the following indications:

1. renal impairment: (see Table 34.2)
2. marrow toxicity: after the first pulse a white cell count (wcc) is checked at days 7, 10, and 14 to ensure that the wcc nadir has passed before the second pulse is given. Prior to each subsequent pulse the neutrophil count is checked, and if <2.5 × 10^9/l, pulse therapy is delayed until it returns to the normal range. The dose of subsequent CP may then be reduced by 25% to avoid subsequent neutropenia.
3. age: if greater than 70 years old, CP dose is reduced to 10 mg/kg
4. infection: CP is not given in the presence of untreated infection, but is delayed for at least one or two days depending on the patients' disease activity and the seriousness of the infection.

d. Additional Therapy

The drugs in Table 34.3 are started on the day of each pulse.

3. Alternative Immunosuppressants for Remission Induction

Another alkylating agent, chlorambucil, might be equally as effective as CP for remission induction in 1°SNV, but its long-term use is limited by the high incidence of cutaneous and hematological

TABLE 34.3
Additional Therapies Given during Pulse Therapy

Drug	Dose	Duration	Indication
Amphoteracin lozenges	10 mg qds	10 days	Candidiasis prophylaxis
Ranitidine	150 mg bd	10 days	Gastroprotection
Granisetron or maxolon	1 mg bd 10 mg tds	2–3 days	Nausea prophylaxis
Mesna	20–40% of CP dose qds	1 day	Bladder protection

malignancies seen in patients treated with this drug.[31] The use of azathioprine for initial therapy for PAN has now been superseded by CP, but studies of methotrexate (MTX) therapy are showing promise for therapy of 1°SNV. An open-label study of 42 patients without immediately life-threatening WG (15 new disease, 27 relapsing disease) treated with weekly oral MTX (plus prednisolone at an initial dose of 1 mg/kg/day) induced remission in 71%, with a median time to remission of 4.2 months.[32] A total of 36% of those in whom remission was induced relapsed after a median time of 29 months, while either on MTX alone or after MTX had been discontinued. This drug, therefore, has promise in remission induction as a less toxic, if less active, alternative to CP in certain categories of ANCA-associated vasculitis. The results of a comparative study of 12 months of MTX vs. 3 months of continuous oral CP followed by azathioprine for remission induction in nonrenal ANCA-associated vasculitis are awaited from EUVAS (European Vasculitis Group). At present we view the place of MTX as consolidation and longer-term maintenance rather than primarily induction therapy.

4. Supportive Therapy

During episodes of disease activity general supportive measures must not be ignored. Expert management of renal impairment is essential, but there are other important aspects. This includes parenteral or enteral nutrition, prophylaxis for opportunistic infection (e.g., low-dose septrin for *Pneumocystis carinii* pneumonia where this is locally prevalent[33]), pain control, pressure sore prevention, blood pressure control, physiotherapy, and patient education.

B. ESCALATION THERAPY AND ENHANCED REGIMENS

Patients with progressive disease activity despite CP therapy, or those who have suffered dose-limiting toxicity from previous CP, may need alternative therapeutic approaches to their management.

1. Pulse Methyl Prednisolone

Empirical therapy with 1000-mg boluses of methylprednisolone on three consecutive days for uncontrolled 1°SNV is sometimes used in conjunction with supportive therapy, particularly for rapidly progressive glomerulonephritis or the pulmonary renal syndrome. However, the administration of CP must not be delayed in this group of patients who often have severe uncontrolled disease.

2. Plasma Exchange

Plasma exchange (PE) removes soluble mediators of inflammation, such as immune complexes, from the circulation and enhances the ability of the reticuloendothelial system to clear remaining immune complexes.[34] There is evidence of better recovery of renal function (from rapidly progressive glomerulonephritis) with PE in combination with prednisolone and CP, but the mortality (chiefly from infection) is high in this group.[35] However, PE may be considered in patients with ANCA-associated vasculitis with rapidly deteriorating renal function, particularly when the serum creatinine is >500 μmol/l at presentation; those who are dialysis-dependent;[36] and those with lung hemorrhage. Other studies have found that PE provided no additional benefit in the initial treatment of CSS or MPA presenting with glomerulonephritis.[37] However, PE in combination with antiviral agents (vidarabine or interferon-alpha 2b) is the treatment of choice in PAN associated with hepatitis B infection,[38] suppressing viral replication and giving a ten-year survival of 83%. There may also be a role for PE in non-hep B PAN, where relapse has occurred despite CP and CS therapy, but it has no place in the initial therapy of non-hep B PAN or in CSS.[39]

3. Intravenous Immunoglobulin

Intravenous immunoglobulin (IVIg) successfully prevents the development of coronary aneurysms in Kawasaki disease if given early[40] and has been used, with mixed results, in ANCA-associated vasculitis. In patients who had active disease despite conventional therapy, a substantial benefit was seen with a reduction in the need for other immunosuppressive therapy in 11 of 12 patients treated with IVIg (400 mg/kg/day for 5 days) at a mean follow-up of 12 months.[41] Another study found a lower response rate (40%) with ENT, skin and joint disease improving more than renal, lung, or eye disease.[42] The likely mechanisms of action of this therapy are wide,[43] but side-effects are rare (risk of renal deterioration and hyperviscosity). We use this as adjuvant therapy in patients with severe active disease and life-threatening complications while induction therapy is starting to work.

4. High-Dose Cyclophosphamide

In an attempt to induce early remission in patients with severe flares of 1°SNV, thereby limiting disease-related damage, we have given a high-dose CP pulse (up to 2.5 gm/m^2) to 15 patients. This dose of CP resulted in severe but self-limited neutropenia. It achieved the initial aim to induce remission more rapidly than with standard therapy (no new disease activity after three pulses of CP in eight patients with 1°SNV).[44] However, early relapse occurred in four patients with ANCA-associated vasculitis, possibly precipitated by infection associated with the severe myelosuppression. We are currently exploring alternative regimes (of 1.2 to 1.4 gm/m^2 CP) to improve outcome and limit early drug toxicity. However, since neutrophils are part of the cellular infiltrate in the vessel wall in active vasculitis, inhibition of their function may be an important part of an induction regime.

One approach to induction therapy may be to use a decremental dose with the initial pulse the highest. This may be followed by an earlier switchover to a milder consolidation regime, e.g., MTX. In this case it is important to avoid any gap between the two therapies by starting the consolidation agent during the induction phase. For example, we normally commence MTX after the first four CP pulses and build it up to a clinically effective dose of at least 15 mg/week by the end of the six-pulse regime. In this way a short course of high individual pulse dose (but low total dose) CP can be given to induce rapid remission with an early change to a consolidation regime to avoid relapse or CP toxicity. The precise details of the regimes needed to achieve this aim may vary according to disease activity and severity.

C. CONSOLIDATION AND MAINTENANCE THERAPY

The need for longer-term therapy depends on the natural history of the particular syndrome. In comparison to PAN, which has a low relapse rate but high morbidity (peripheral neuropathy, renal insufficiency, and hypertension), MPA and CSS have a high frequency of relapse which often occurs when treatment is reduced or stopped altogether.[9] Initial CP therapy in this latter group does not seem to reduce the risk of relapse once remission is achieved, but several groups believe that consolidation therapy prolonged for $1^1/_2$ to 2 years may do so. Relapse rates are also high in patients with WG, occurring in a cumulative fashion over long-term observation. This highlights the need for a mild, long-term maintenance therapy in ANCA-associated vasculitis once remission has been induced and consolidated with immunosuppressive therapy. There is a trend toward shorter courses of CP for remission induction (three to six months of pulse or continuous oral CP) before switching to less toxic consolidation immunosuppressive therapy. The benefits of continuing low doses of azathioprine vs. alternative approaches to preventing relapse are just beginning to be explored. The latter includes control of nasal infection or mild anti-TNF agents such as pentoxifylline, but new approaches are urgently needed.

1. Azathioprine and Methotrexate

Azathioprine (2 mg/kg/day) has been the mainstay of therapy after remission induction by CP, but MTX and cyclosporin A (CyA) are alternative agents for consolidation and maintenance therapy. In a study, 69% of WG patients with persistent or relapsing disease activity, who had previously been treated with CP or azathioprine, were induced into remission with MTX (0.15 to 0.3

mg/kg/week).[45] In a large cohort of WG patients (50% who had renal involvement), 71% achieved remission while on MTX, though relapse rates were still reasonably high (36%).[32] When compared to trimethoprim/sulphamethoxazole, weekly MTX was found to be safe and effective at maintaining remission.[46] MTX, therefore, seems a reasonable option as consolidation therapy for patients who have grumbling disease activity or for those who relapse without major organ involvement (e.g., renal or pulmonary hemorrhage), and may be continued as prolonged maintenance therapy in 1°SNV as in rheumatoid arthritis.

2. Cyclosporin A

CyA and FK506, used to prevent transplant rejection without myelosuppression, may have a role in consolidation therapy. Uncontrolled studies on its use in active WG that did not respond to CP suggest that high doses (5 mg/kg/day) are needed to control disease activity at an increased risk of nephrotoxicity, while low doses (1 to 2 mg/kg/day) were not effective at maintaining remission.[47] Others, in a preliminary report of seven patients in remission with ANCA-associated vasculitis, found that after a mean follow-up of 24 months none had relapsed while on CyA (mean dose 2.9 mg/kg/day). The role of these agents is still unclear but may best be reserved for those patients without severe renal involvement or where myelotoxicity has been a problem. Their effectiveness as maintenance agents may be improved where the induction regime has produced a complete remission of disease activity rather than when they are used to consolidate as well as maintain.

3. Trimethoprim/Sulphamethoxazole

Antimicrobial therapy has been studied in WG in view of the persistent infection with *Staphylococcus aureus* that is seen in the paranasal sinuses of patients with WG.[48] The subgroup of WG patients with nasal carriage of *S. aureus* (found in 63% of 57 patients) was identified as being at increased risk of relapse (relative risk of relapse 7.16).[49] In a controlled, two-year prospective trial, trimethoprim/sulphamethoxazole (T/S) (160/800 mg twice daily) maintained remission better than placebo in WG patients (7 of 41 relapsed with T/S, 16 of 40 relapsed with placebo).[50] Another study has shown that the T/S combination is not as effective at maintaining remission in generalized WG, though it was found to be successful when used to induce and maintain remission in >50% of patients with limited disease.[51,52] Due to combined inhibition of folic acid metabolism there is an increased risk of toxicity in patients on MTX and T/S, and this combination should therefore be avoided.

It is entirely possible that the effect of T/S relates to actions other than its antimicrobial role (e.g., an effect on white cell function). In view of the problems of *S. aureus* carriage, it is our practice to screen all patients with WG for nasal carriage of *S. aureus* and, if present, we try and eradicate it with cyclical topical bactroban ointment. Controlled trials of the efficacy of local nasal antibiotics in preventing late relapse are in progress.

D. RELAPSE

Disease activity at relapse is often recognized earlier by the patient and family doctor, highlighting the importance of patient education in these rare diseases. Fewer items of damage accumulate after relapse than at first disease flare,[6] however, patients who relapse once are more likely to relapse again and are therefore more likely to be exposed to recurrent courses of CP, increasing the long-term toxicity risks. For major relapses we tend to use shorter courses of pulse CP (six pulses of standard 15 mg/kg or higher dose over a three-month period) with early transfer to maintenance MTX, azathioprine, or, rarely, cyclosporin A. These drugs, except azathioprine, are started before completion of the CP pulses (after pulse 4) so that their therapeutic benefit is not delayed until after completion of the CP pulses. This avoids the gap often seen between induction/relapse and consolidation regimes, which may predispose to early relapse. MTX may be used as an alternative to CP at relapse if the use of further CP is limited by previous toxicity or there is no evidence of significant renal or major organ involvement. Relapse also offers the opportunity for experimental therapy, which may range from IVIg to monoclonal antibody treatment.

E. Rescue Therapy

Several approaches have been tried in selected centers for patients with increasing disease activity or relapses despite all conventional therapy. These have included anti-T-cell antibodies, antithymocyte globulin,[53] and bone marrow transplantation. Studies with depleting (Campath-1H) and nondepleting (anti-CD4) anti-T-cell monoclonal antibody therapy have been carried out in patients with T-cell-associated vasculitis and ANCA-associated disease[54] with some success. A rapid reduction in ANCA titer was seen without undue toxicity. The place of anti-T-cell monoclonals and anti-TNFα therapy in systemic vasculitis remains to be defined. Successful autologous stem cell rescue after intensive immunosuppressive therapy in two patients with severe WG[55] suggests a potential role for this approach to the therapy of 1°SNV in the future. The overall message from these small studies is that in patients with disease activity in the absence of crippling fixed damage, further attempts at less conventional therapy are often rewarding.

F. Surgery

For patients with grumbling disease activity or accumulating damage, surgery may also be required, particularly in WG. Drainage for chronic sinusitis or otitis media may be necessary, as may ocular surgery to relieve nasoloacrimal duct obstruction or relief of proptosis secondary to retro-orbital granulation tissue. Subglottic stenosis can occur secondary to active disease or scarring and may need temporary or permanent tracheostomy. Dilatation of noninflamed lesions or intralesional steroids may also be contemplated.[56] When disease is inactive, cosmetic surgery for nasal bridge reconstruction can be considered important by patients, and if in sustained remission, kidney transplantation is generally successful.[24]

III. OTHER PRIMARY VASCULITIC SYNDROMES

The vasculitic syndromes may be classified according to the size of vessel involved,[57,58] and important management issues not covered in the preceding sections will be discussed below for some of these vasculitides.

A. Large-Vessel Vasculitis

1. Giant-Cell Arteritis

Where possible, we try to obtain tissue confirmation of the diagnosis of giant-cell arteritis (GCA), but do not delay therapy while awaiting the result. Not only does a positive biopsy confirm the diagnosis, but it provides evidence that the diagnosis was correct should there be future complications of therapy or difficulty withdrawing steroids. The aims of therapy are to reduce pain and disability as well as to prevent damage, particularly visual loss. Treatment is generally tailored to the individual patient. Corticosteroids are the treatment of choice, and for patients with moderate symptoms without visual disturbance, a starting dose of 40 mg is often sufficient. In those with more severe pain or visual symptoms, 60 mg should be used. Some have advocated the use of pulse intravenous CS if visual impairment occurs, but there are no controlled trials to support this. Once symptoms are controlled and a fall in the ESR is observed, the prednisolone dose should be reduced by 5 to 10 mg every 2 to 4 weeks until 15 mg is reached, when the dose reduction should be slower (1 mg every month). A too-rapid reduction in steroid dose may result in relapse, which is also more likely within one year of steroid withdrawal.[59] Although the aim is to stop steroid therapy by two years, studies have shown that 42% of patients require steroids for more than five years,[60] and the median duration of therapy is longer in women (5.5 years) than in men (2.3 years).[61] Several case reports and small studies illustrate the potential steroid-sparing effect of immunosuppressives late in the disease,[62] but the role of these drugs given in conjunction with CS at the time of diagnosis is still unclear.[63] There may be a role for anti-T-cell therapy such as CyA at disease onset in view of recent evidence supporting GCA as an antigen-driven, T-cell-dependent disease.[64]

2. Takayasu's Arteritis

Assessment of disease activity in this group of patients can be difficult, and no single factor should be used. A combination of clinical, laboratory, and imaging investigations should be used to provide a global picture. CS have been the mainstay of therapy, but no randomized studies have been performed. The time to remission induction can be long (median 22 months),[65] and recurrent courses of high-dose steroid are necessary because of the risk of relapse. Reports of treatment success with steroids vary from 20 to 100%.[66] The addition of MTX (mean dose 17.1 mg/week), in an open study of 18 patients with steroid-resistant disease, induced remission in 81% of the 16 patients who completed the study.[67] Relapses occurred in 44% of patients as their steroids were withdrawn, and three patients had disease progression despite therapy. CP has also been used in patients with steroid-resistant disease and is the therapy preferred by some groups. Our own practice in patients with active disease would be to consider a short course of CP (6 pulses) followed by maintenance MTX at 15 to 20 mg/week. The ability of such regimes to prevent complications requires detailed objective evidence in individuals as well as controlled trials.

The most common complication is hypertension due to renal artery stenosis. This may be surgically correctable if the stenosis is greater than 70%, when angioplasty can be considered.[68] Alternatively, management should be medical with β-blockers and ACE-inhibition (care with bilateral renal artery stenosis). One of the problems with assessment of hypertension in these patients is the difference that may exist between peripheral and central blood pressure if significant subclavian or brachial disease exists. Blood pressure needs to be measured in all four limbs and the presence of carotid stenosis actively looked for. Aspirin or even full anticoagulation needs to be considered in patients with TIAs, and smokers must be firmly encouraged to stop.

B. MEDIUM-VESSEL VASCULITIS

1. Kawasaki Disease

The introduction of IVIg as therapy for Kawasaki disease has improved the prognosis considerably.[40] The diagnosis is often delayed while infection as a cause for symptoms is excluded, and during this period general support, hydration, and antibiotics are important. When the diagnosis is suspected, coronary aneurysms should be looked for by 2-D echocardiography, and IVIg should be commenced (2 gm/kg over 12 to 18 hours or 400 mg/kg/day for 5 days).[40,69] Regression of aneurysms can occur, either spontaneously or more frequently after IVIg therapy. Aspirin is useful to reduce fever and also for its antiplatelet effect, but warfarin should be considered if aneurysms are present. Plasma exchange and prostacyclin have been suggested as possible additional therapy in the presence of large coronary artery aneurysms.[70] CS may be useful in those patients who do not respond to IVIg, but are not generally advocated as routine use and may actually worsen the prognosis.[71] Long-term follow-up is advisable due to the future potential risk of atherosclerosis.

C. SMALL-VESSEL VASCULITIS

1. Henoch-Schonlein Purpura

Steroids are often used, if only to make the patient feel better, but have no proven efficacy in Henoch-Schonlein purpura (HSP). They do not seem to improve the purpura but do bring about an earlier resolution of abdominal pain (24 hours instead of 72 hours).[72] Nonsteroidal antiinflammatory drugs (NSAIDs) can be used for arthralgia and do not exacerbate the purpura, but in the presence of renal disease it is probably best to avoid them altogether. When nephritis is present a combination of CS pulses (30 mg/kg/day) in addition to CP (2 mg/kg/day) and prednisolone (2 mg/kg/day) improves prognosis.[73] Dipyramidole (5 mg/kg/day) for six months may also be added. Combinations of steroids with azathioprine, CyA, or IVIg have been tried without convincing benefit.

2. Cutaneous Leucocytoclastic Vasculitis

Exclusion of an associated systemic disease or the identification of an underlying causative stimulus is important. In their absence, symptomatic therapy with antihistamines (H1 and H2 blockers) may be useful for the pruritis and burning pain that can be present, especially with urticarial vasculitis. Colchicine (0.5 mg twice daily), by reducing neutrophil chemotaxis and degranulation, can help with up to 80%, responding within two weeks.[74] Corticosteroids are also used, sometimes with the addition of MTX, allowing the withdrawal of the steroids in conditions such as cutaneous PAN.[75] Azathioprine may also be useful in some patients with resistant disease. Dapsone has been used, but hemolytic anemia is often dose limiting. Dapsone reduces neutrophil chemotaxis, lysosomal activity, and adherence, thus reducing neutrophil activity at inflammatory sites. More effective, less toxic alternatives to immunosuppression are needed for recurrent or severe cases.

3. Cogan's Syndrome

This rare vasculitic illness presents with interstitial keratitis, which may be managed by topical therapy alone,[76] and vestibuloauditory symptoms which require systemic therapy. Prednisolone is regarded as the mainstay of treatment, and if given early after the onset of hearing loss can lead to some improvement. Additional immunosuppressive therapy is sometimes needed to control disease activity and CP, azathioprine, MTX, and CyA have been reported to be helpful in some cases.[77-79]

4. Cerebral Vasculitis

Primary angiitis of the CNS (PACNS), like the CNS vasculitis associated with Behcet's, often needs prolonged therapy with CP and CS for up to one year after remission is induced.[80] A more benign form of cerebral vasculitis (BACNS) may exist which generally has a better prognosis and may not require more than a short course of CS therapy.[81,82]

IV. SECONDARY VASCULITIS

Vasculitis can occur in association with another underlying systemic illness, when it is referred to as secondary vasculitis. The approach to management is not very different from that described for 1°SNV, but evidence for the underlying condition needs to be sought and may need to be treated independently.

A. Vasculitis Associated with Connective Tissue Diseases

The onset of systemic rheumatoid vasculitis (SRV) has been linked with the initiation of, or a sudden change in, the dose of steroid in patients with RA.[83] High doses of CS are often used to treat rheumatoid vasculitis, but usually at the cost of significant toxicity. Azathioprine has been used in conjunction with steroids to control severe disease, but we prefer to immunosuppress with CP, using daily oral prednisolone in as low a dose as possible. In a similar approach to that outlined for 1°SNV, we use pulse CP for remission induction.[84] Although the pulse interval (initially twice weekly) and the duration of therapy (three to six months depending on response) is similar, we have found that this group of patients may be more sensitive to myelosuppression from CP and the dose may have to be adjusted down for age, low wcc, or renal function. This shortened course of CP therapy reduces drug-induced toxicity, but the high frequency of relapses dictates the requirement for maintenance therapy, for which we use either azathioprine or MTX.

Untreated, SRV has a high mortality (both early and late in disease) and significant morbidity.[83] At the onset of vasculitis, arthritis is often inactive; however, immunosuppressive therapy may push patients from active vasculitis to active synovitis.

Vasculitis is rarely associated with Sjögren's syndrome, dermatomyositis, systemic sclerosis, and mixed connective tissue disease.[85] Depending on the spectrum of disease (organ involvement and severity), immunosuppressive therapy with CP may be required.

Mild lupus vasculitis may respond to CS with or without the addition of azathioprine. In more severe disease where there is renal, pulmonary, nervous, or gastrointestinal involvement with clear evidence of arteritis, pulse CP is used as in 1°SNV. A less aggressive regime of 10 mg/kg is used at monthly intervals for six months with proven benefit in lupus renal disease.[86] Differentiation from the antiphospholipid antibody syndrome is important, but the two can coexist, requiring dual therapy.[87,88]

B. Mixed Essential Cryoglobulinemic Vasculitis

Steroids are useful to treat the purpura and arthralgias of a mixed cryoglobulinemia (0.1 to 0.2 mg/kg/day). The natural history is often of a mild but very chronic illness, so it is important to avoid or minimize drug toxicity. When motor neuropathy, widespread vasculitis, or glomerulonephritis are present, then higher doses of CS, CP, and plasma exchange are used to control the flare.[89] In the presence of hepatitis C infection, additional treatment with alpha-interferon should be considered to eliminate the virus.[90]

C. Urticarial Vasculitis

A variety of therapies have been found to have some therapeutic benefit in these patients, however, only a few respond to combined antihistamines (H1 and H2 blockade). Short courses of prednisolone (15 to 30 mg/day) may be useful, though NSAIDs can also help. Gold and colchicine have some effect, as does dapsone at a dose of 100 mg/day.

V. OTHER VASCULITIC SYNDROMES

A. Behçet's Syndrome

This disease is characterized by exacerbations and remissions. Flares in disease activity may be mild, in the form of genital or oral ulceration, or severe with sight threatening disease or cerebral involvement. Oral ulceration may require little more than local application of hydrocortisone tablets allowed to dissolve in the mouth in close proximity to the ulcer. Tetracycline mouthwash may help, but complications from oral thrush may result from a combined approach with topical steroids. Severe exacerbations of oral/genital ulceration may respond to a short course of thalidomide (doses up to 300 mg daily for 3 to 5 days), which can also be used to maintain remission at a lower dose (50 mg three times a week). Side-effects are common, and peripheral neuropathy may require discontinuation of the drug.[91] In patients to be maintained on thalidomide long term, we obtain baseline nerve conduction studies and repeat them after six months to detect early, subclinical disease that may require cessation of thalidomide therapy. The teratogenic effects of this drug are well known, but the risk must be reinforced in female patients, who must be using adequate contraception. Azathioprine (2 mg/kg) may also be used for maintenance therapy as can colchicine, though the latter drug is generally more effective for arthralgias and cutaneous lesions (erythema nodosum). NSAIDs and sulphasalazine may be effective for the joint disease associated with Behçet's.

Rapid control of Behçet's eye disease can be achieved with CyA, though the effect tends to decrease with time.[92] In contrast, azathioprine has more benefit in the maintenance of visual acuity and prevention of development of disease in the other eye.[93] Azathioprine may thus be useful once remission has been induced by CyA. Short pulses of CS can also be used to induce remission when flares in eye disease occur that cannot be controlled by local application of steroids. Though CNS vasculitis is rare in association with Behçet's, it does require immunosuppression with CP when it occurs. Our experience with pulse CP in neuro-Behçet's suggests that protracted courses of therapy (12 months at pulse interval of 2 to 3 weeks) are required to halt disease progression and prevent relapses. Severe skin disease may also require pulse CP therapy.

Behçet's is also associated with a prothrombotic tendency (venous, portal vein, and cerebral venous sinus thrombosis), and lifelong anticoagulation may be required if these complications arise.

B. Pseudo Vasculitis

This heterogeneous group of disorders needs to be considered when a clear clinical diagnosis of a specific vasculitis cannot be made. Embolism from cardiac sources (atrial myxoma, valvular lesions, SBE) or cholesterol emboli from atherosclerotic plaques may present as a digital vasculopathy.[94,95] This diagnosis is often missed. Biopsy evidence of cholesterol crystals within target organs (skin and muscle, usually) is often required for a definite diagnosis of cholesterol atheroembolism. Antiphospholipid syndromes may present in a similar fashion. Treatment of the underlying disorder may be sufficient to prevent further events, but during the acute stages there may be significant inflammation requiring antiinflammatory therapy with short courses of CS, but not the prolonged immunosuppression needed for 1°SNV.

VI. FUTURE DIRECTIONS FOR THERAPY

A. New Drugs

There are several new immunosuppressants which are currently undergoing trials in transplant rejection (mycophenolate mofetil and rapamycin) or are being introduced as second-line drug therapy in rheumatoid arthritis (leflunomide). The experience with these agents in vasculitis is limited at present, but they may offer less toxic alternatives for maintenance, and possibly remission induction therapy in the future. Leflunomide has been used successfully to maintain remission in 13 patients with WG over a period of 11 months,[96] and reports have suggested that mycophenolate may also be of use as a maintenance therapy in vasculitis[97] or in patients with Takayasu's arteritis who are resistant to conventional therapy.[98]

B. New Targets for Therapy

An increase in understanding of the molecular mechanisms that lead to cell recruitment to sites of inflammation and their survival in these tissues may present attractive targets for therapy. The expression of specific adhesion molecules may allow selective recruitment of inflammatory cells to inflamed endothelium. Other signals involved in transmigration and selective retention of leucocytes at sites of inflammation are as yet not clearly defined. Targeting these processes (with monoclonal antibodies) may lead to new avenues for therapy. Cell survival within inflammatory sites may also perpetuate inflammation, and the signals that contribute to this survival are becoming increasingly recognized in inflammatory joint disease.[99] The induction of apoptosis in tissue infiltrating leucocytes is an attractive proposition for turning off inflammation.

TABLE 34.4
Mechanism of Action of Immunosuppressants

Drug	Mechanism of Action	Effect on Cellular Processes
Prednisolone	Binds to intracellular receptor, enters nucleus, binding to DNA promoter region: - inhibits DNA coding for several molecules - ↓ synthesis of lipocortin, inhibiting PLA$_2$ - inhibits inflammatory response Pulse CS redistribute lymphocytes to L/N and inhibit IL2 production	↓ synthesis and release of inflammatory mediators from macrophages (e.g. TNFα, IL1, and IL6) ↓ expression MHCII. ↓ expression of adhesion molecules ↓ eicosanoids ↓ exudation and inhibits ↑ in vascular permeability Inhibit macrophage migration and division ↓ protease release Stabilizes lysosomal membranes ↓ circulating lymphocytes for hours Esinophils ↓, neutrophils ↑
Cyclophosphamide	Alkylates and cross-links DNA Has anti-inflammatory properties	B and T-cell lymphopenia ↓ Ig synthesis ↓ number of activated T-cells Suppresses cell-mediated/humoral responses.
Methotrexate	Anti-metabolite: - inhibits dihydrofolate reductase and thymidylate synthetase - antagonizes folic acid metabolism and function (folate depletion not responsible for therapeutic effect in inflammatory disease) Increased adenosine release from fibroblasts and endothelial cells	↓ purine synthesis ↓ neutrophil chemotaxis and LTB4 production ↓ IL1 and IL2 production ↓ IL6 production Inhibition of neutrophil adhesion to endothelium
Azathioprine	Intereferes with adenine and guanine ribonucleosides	↓ circulating B and T-cells (CD8 > CD4) ↓ IgG, IgM and IL2 synthesis
Cyclosporin A	Binds to cytosolic isomerases, inhibiting calcineurin activation by Ca^{2+}-calmodulin	IL2 gene activation in T-cells inhibited ↓ T-cell response and interaction
Trimethoprim/ sulphamethoxazole	Clears *S aureus* infection and/or acts as a free-radical scavenger	Toxin from *S. aureus* may act as a superantigen Cell wall components of *S. aureus* are effective B-cell mitogens (may ↑ ANCA production) ↓ stimulation of neutrophils by *S. aureus* ↓ α1 antitrypsn
IVIg	Blocks Fc receptors on phagocytic cells Direct NK or T-cell inhibition Anti-idiotypic antibodies	Interferes with complement system, prevents complement mediated immune damage Inhibits cytokine production, ↓ Ab synthesis Bind to idiotypic determinants in pathogenic autoantibodies, down regulate B-cell receptors or bind to T-cell receptors Anti-idiotypic activity against ANCA

TABLE 34.5
Toxicity of SNV Therapies

Drug	Short Term	Long Term
Prednisolone	Glucose & electrolyte imbalance	Osteoporosis, osteonecrosis, tendon rupture myopathy,
	Infection risk	Cataract, glaucoma
	Peptic ulceration	Brusing, alopecia, obesity
	Psychosis, depression	Hypertension, infection
Cyclophosphamide	Neutropenia	Myelodysplasia
	Thrombocytopenia	Infertility — in women risk increases with increasing age (total
	Infection	dose CP age >40 — 5.2 g, 30-39 ,9.3 g and 20-29 years -20g)
	Alopecia	— in men doses >18 g
	Nausea	Hemorrhagic cystsitis (caused by acrolein — breakdown
	Oligo or amenorrhea	product of CP), bladder fibrosis or carcinoma — risk of these
		significantly greater with long term continuous oral CP
Methotrexate	Stomatitis	Teratogenecity common
	Dyspepsia	Oncogenicity rare
	Leucopenia	Liver fibrosis or cirrhosis (rare)
	Pulmonary hypersensitivity	Pulmonary fibrosis
	Transaminitis	
Azathioprine	Bone marrow suppression	Increased risk malignant disease (particularly non-Hodgkins
	Gastrointestinal disturbances	lymphoma)
	Hepatitis	
Cyclosporin A	Dose related	Renal interstitial fibrosis and tubular atrophy
	- hypertension,	
	- increase in creatinine	
	Hepatotoxicity, nausea	
	Hypertrichosis, gum hyperplasia	
	Hyperkalemia, hyperuricemia	

TABLE 34.6
Mechanism of Action and Toxicity of Other SNV Therapies

Therapy	Mechanism	Toxicity
Plasma exchange	Clears soluble mediators of inflammation and enhances activity of reticuloendothelial system	Hypotension Increased infection risk
Leflunomide	Inhibits pyrimidine synthesis by inhibition of dihydroorotate dehydrogenase and tyrosine kinases Arrest of stimulated cells at the G1 phase	Uncommon Rash, allergic reactions Gastrointestinal disturbances Reversible alopecia
Mycophenolate	Inhibits *de novo* purine synthesis by inhibition of inosine monophosphate dehydrogenase. DNA synthesis and cell proliferation reduced	Leucopenia/neutropenia (rare) Gastrointestinal disturbances Headache, dizziness, rash, insomnia
Rapamycin	Binds to immunophilin FK506BP. Inhibition of signalling through IL2 receptor on T-cells. Cell cycle progression halted between G1 and S phase. Decreased activation of T and B cells	

REFERENCES

1. Watts, R.A., Carruthers, D.M., Scott, D.G.I. Epidemiology of systemic vasculitis — changing incidence or definition, *Seminars in Arthritis and Rheumatism,* 25, 28, 1995.
2. Luqmani, R.A., Bacon, P.A., Moots, R.J., Janssen, B.A., Pall, A., Emery, P., Savage, C., Adu, D. Birmingham Vasculitis Activity Score (BVAS) in systemic necrotizing vasculitis, *Quarterly Journal of Medicine,* 87, 671, 1994.
3. Exley, A.R., Bacon, P.A., Luqmani, R.A., Kitas, G.D., Carruthers, D.M., Moots, R. Examination of disease severity in systemic vasculitis from the novel perspective of damage using the vasculitis damage index (VDI), *Brit. J. Rheum.,* 37, 57, 1998.
4. Talar-Williams, C., Hijazi, Y.M., Walther, M.M., Lineham, W.M., Hallahan, C.W., Lubensky, I., Kerr, G.S., Hoffman, G.S., Fauci, A.S., Sneller, M.C. Cyclophosphamide-induced cystitis and bladder cancer in patients with Wegener granulomatosis, *Annals of Internal Medicine,* 124, 477, 1996.
5. Exley, A.R., Bacon, P.A., Luqmani, R.A., Kitas, G.D., Gordon, C., Savage, C.O.S., Adu, D. Development and initial validation of the vasculitis damage index for the standardized clinical assessment of damage in the systemic vasculitides, *Arthritis and Rheumatism,* 40, 371, 1997.
6. Exley, A.R., Carruthers, D.M., Luqmani, R.A., Kitas, G.D., Gordon, C., Janssen, B.A., Savage, C.O.S., Bacon, P.A. Damage occurs early in systemic vasculitis and is an index of outcome, *Qjm-Monthly Journal of the Association of Physicians,* 90, 391, 1997.
7. Guillevin, L., Lhote, F., Gayraud, M., Cohen, P., Jarrousse, B., Lortholary, O., Thibult, N., Casassus, P. Prognostic factors in polyarteritis nodosa and Churg-Strauss syndrome. A prospective study in 342 patients, *Medicine* (Baltimore), 75, 17, 1996.
8. Fortin, P.R., Larson, M.G., Watters, A.K., Yeadon, A.K., Choquette, C.A., Esdaile, J.M. Prognosis factors in systemic necrotizing vasculitis of the polyarteritis nodosa group. A review of 45 cases, *Journal of Rheumatology,* 22, 78, 1995.
9. Gordon, M., Luqmani, R.A., Adu, D., Greaves, I., Richards, N., Michael, J., Emery, P., Howie, A.J., Bacon, P.A. Relapses in patients with a systemic vasculitis, *Quarterly Journal of Medicine,* 86, 779, 1993.
10. Savage, C.O.S., Winearls, C.G., Evans, D.G., Rees, A.J., Lockwood, C.M. Microscopic polyarteritis: Presentation, pathology and prognosis, *Quarterly Journal of Medicine,* 56, 467, 1985.
11. Matteson, E.L., Gold, K.N., Bloch, D.A., Hunder, G.G. Long-term survival of patients with Wegener's granulomatosis from the American College of Rheumatology Wegener's Granulomatosis Classification Criteria Cohort, *American Journal of Medicine,* 101, 129, 1996.
12. Anderson, G., Coles, E.T., Crane, M., Douglas, A.C., Gibbs, A.R., Geddes, D.M., Peel, E.T., Wood, J.B. Wegener granuloma — a series of 265 British cases seen between 1975 and 1985 — a report by a sub-committee of the British Thoracic Society Research Committee, *Quarterly Journal of Medicine,* 83, 427, 1992.
13. Andrews, M., Edmunds, M., Campbell, A., Walls, J., Feehally, J. Systemic vasculitis in the 1980s — is there an increasing incidence of Wegeners granulomatosis and microscopic polyarteritis, *Journal of the Royal College of Physicians of London,* 24, 284, 1990.
14. Gaskin, G., Savage, C.O.S., Ryan, J.J. Anti-neutrophil cytoplasmic antibodies and disease activity during long-term follow-up of 70 patients with systemic vasculitis, *Nephrol. Dial. Transplant.,* 6, 689, 1991.
15. Carruthers, D.M., Guest, P., Howie, A.J., Exley, A.R., Buckley, C.D., Raza, K., Bacon, P.A. Percutaneous X-Ray guided lung biopsy in ANCA positive Wegener's Granulomatosis, *Clin. Exp. Immunol.,*112:(S1), 31, 1998.
16. Raza, K., Exley, A.R., Carruthers, D.M., Buckley, C., Hammond, L.A., Bacon, P.A. Localized bowel vasculitis — postoperative cyclophosphamide or not? *Arthritis and Rheumatism,* 42, 182, 1999.
17. Rose, G.A., Spencer, H. Polyarteritis nodosa, *Quarterly Journal of Medicine,* 26, 43, 1957.
18. Walton, E.W. Giant cell granuloma of the respiratory tract (Wegener's Granulomatosis), *British Medical Journal,* 2, 265, 1957.
19. Frohnert, P.P., Sheps, S.G. Long-term follow-up study of periarteritis nodosa, *American Journal of Medicine,* 43, 8, 1967.
20. Lieb, E.S., Restivo, C., Paulus, H.E. Immunosuppressive and corticosteroid therapy of polyarteritis nodosa, *American Journal of Medicine,* 67, 941, 1979.

21. Fauci, A.S., Katz, P., Haynes, B.F., Wolff, S.M. Cyclophosphamide therapy of severe systemic necrotising vasculitis, *New England Journal of Medicine*, 301, 235, 1979.
22. Guillevin, L., Cordier, J.F., Lhote, F., Cohen, P., Jarrousse, B., Royer, I., Lesavre, P., Jacquot, C., Bindi, P., Bielefeld, P., Desson, J.F., Detree, F., Dubois, A., Hachulla, E., Hoen, B., Jacomy, D., Seigneuric, C., Lauque, D., Stern, M., Longy-Boursier, M. A prospective, multicenter, randomized trial comparing steroids and pulse cyclophosphamide versus steroids and oral cyclophosphamide in the treatment of generalized Wegener's granulomatosis, *Arth. Rheum.*, 40, 2187, 1997.
23. Genereau, T., Lortholary, O., Le Clerc, P. Treatment of systemic vasculitis with cyclophosphamide and steroids: daily oral low dose cyclophosphamide after failure of pulse IV high dose regimen in 4 patients, *Brit. J. Rheum.*, 33, 959, 1994.
24. Hoffman, G.S., Kerr, G.S., Leavitt, R.Y., Hallahan, C.W., Lebovics, R.S., Travis, W.D., Rottem, M., Fauci, A.S. Wegener granulomatosis — an analysis of 158 patients, *Annals of Internal Medicine*, 116, 488, 1992.
25. Hoffman, G.S., Leavitt, R.Y., Fleisher, T.A., Minor, J.R., Fauci, A.S. Treatment of Wegener's granulomatosis with intermittent high-dose intravenous cyclophosphamide, *American Journal of Medicine*, 89, 403, 1990.
26. Reinhold-Keller, E., Kekow, J., Schnabel, A. Effectiveness of cyclophosphamide pulse-treatment in Wegener's granulomatosis. *Adv. Exp. Med. Biol.*, 336, 483, 1993.
27. Haubitz, M., Schellong, S., Gobel, U., Schurek, H.J., Schaumann, D., Koch, K.M., Brunkhorst, R. Intravenous pulse administration of cyclophosphamide versus daily oral treatment in patients with antineutrophil cytoplasmic antibody-associated vasculitis and renal involvement: a prospective, randomized study, *Arthritis and Rheumatism*, 41, 1835, 1998.
28. Gayraud, M., Guillevin, L., Cohen, P., Lhote, F., Cacoub, P., Deblois, P., Godeau, B., Ruel, M., Vidal, E., Piontud, M., Ducroix, J.P., Lassoued, S., Christoforov, B., Babinet, P. Treatment of good prognosis polyarteritis nodosa and Churg-Strauss syndrome: comparison of steroids and oral or pulse cyclophosphamide in 25 patients. French cooperative study group for vasculitides, *Brit. J. Rheum.*, 36, 1290, 1997.
29. Martin-Suarez, I., D'Cruz, D., Mansoor, M., Fernandes, A.P., Khamashta, M.A., Hughes, G.R. Immunosuppressive treatment in severe connective tissue diseases: effects of low dose intravenous cyclophosphamide, *Ann. Rheum. Dis.*, 56, 481, 1997.
30. Adu, D., Pall, A., Luqmani, R.A., Richards, N.T., Howie, A.J., Emery, P., Michael, J., Savage, C.O., Bacon, P.A. Controlled trial of pulse versus continuous prednisolone and cyclophosphamide in the treatment of systemic vasculitis, *Quarterly Journal of Medicine*, 90, 401, 1997.
31. Patapanian, H., Graham, S., Sambrook, P.N., Browne, C.D., Champion, G.D., Cohen, M.L., Day, R.O. The oncogenicity of chlorambucil in rheumatoid arthritis, *Brit. J. Rheum.*, 27, 44, 1988.
32. Sneller, M.C., Hoffman, G.S., Talar-Williams, C., Kerr, G.S., Hallahan, C.W., Fauci, A.S. An analysis of forty-two Wegener's granulomatosis patients treated with methotrexate and prednisone, *Arthritis and Rheumatism*, 38, 608, 1995.
33. Godeau, B., Mainardi, J.L., Roudot-Thoraval, F., Hachulla, E., Guillevin, L., Huong Du, L.T., Jarrousse, B., Remy, P., Schaeffer, A., Piette, J.C. Factors associated with pneumocystis carinii pneumonia in Wegener's granulomatosis, *Ann. Rheum. Dis.*, 54, 991, 1995.
34. Lockwood, C.M. Reversal of impaired splenic function of patients with nephritis or vasculitis (or both), *New England Journal of Medicine*, 300, 524, 1979.
35. Hind, C.R.K., Lockwood, C.M., Peters, D.K., Paraskevakou, H., Evans, D.J., Rees, A.J. Prognosis after immunosuppression of patients with crescentric nephritis requiring dialysis, *Lancet*, 1, 263, 1983.
36. Pusey, C.D., Rees, A.J., Evans, D.J., Peters, D.K., Lockwood, C.M. Plasma exchange in focal necrotising glomerulonephritis without anti-GBM antibodies, *Kidney Int.*, 40, 757, 1991.
37. Guillevin, L., Cevallos, R., Durand-Gasselin, B., Lhote, F., Jarrousse, B., Callard, P. Treatment of glomerulonephritis in microscopic polyangiitis and Churg-Strauss syndrome. Indications of plasma exchanges, meta-analysis of 2 randomized studies on 140 patients, 32 with glomerulonephritis, *Ann. Med. Interne* (Paris), 148, 198, 1997.
38. Guillevin, L., Lhote, F., Cohen, P., Sauvaget, F., Jarrousse, B., Lortholary, O., Noel, L.H., Trepo, C. Polyarteritis nodosa related to hepatitis B virus. A prospective study with long-term observation of 41 patients, *Medicine* (Baltimore), 74, 238, 1995.

39. Guillevin, L., Lhote, F., Cohen, P., Jarrousse, B., Lortholary, O., Genereau, T., Leon, A., Bussel, A. Corticosteroids plus pulse cyclophosphamide and plasma exchanges versus corticosteroids plus pulse cyclophosphamide alone in the treatment of polyarteritis nodosa and Churg-Strauss syndrome patients with factors predicting poor prognosis. A prospective, randomized trial in sixty-two patients, *Arthritis and Rheumatism*, 38, 1638, 1995.

40. Newburger, J.W., Takahashi, M., Burns, J.C., Beiser, A.S., Chung, K.J., Duffy, C.E., Glode, M.P., Mason, W.H., Reddy, V., Sanders, S.P., Shulman, S.T., Wigins, J.W., Hicks, R.V., Fulton, D.R., Lewis, A.B., Leung, D.Y.M., Colton, T., Rosen, F.S., Melish, M.E. The treatment of Kawasaki syndrome with intravenous gamma globulin, *New England Journal of Medicine*, 315, 341, 1986.

41. Jayne, D.R.W. Intravenous immunoglobulin in the therapy of systemic vasculitis, *Transfusion Science*, 13, 317, 1992.

42. Richter, C., Schnabel, A., Csernok, E., deGroot, K., Reinhold-Kkeller, E., Gross, W.L. Treatment of antineutrophil cytoplasmic antibody (ANCA)-associated systemic vasculitis with high-dose intravenous immunoglobulin, *Clin. Exp. Immunol.*, 101, 2, 1995.

43. Jordan, S.C., Toyoda, M. Treatment of autoimmune-diseases and systemic vasculitis with pooled human intravenous immune globulin, *Clin. Exp. Immunol.*, 97, 31, 1994.

44. Carruthers, D.M., Exley, A.R., Williams, R., Buckley, C.D., Amft, N., Raza, K., Rowe, I., Bacon, P.A. Intensive pulse cyclophosphamide for remission induction in systemic necrotising vasculitis, *Arthritis and Rheumatism*, 41, 545, 1998.

45. Hoffman, G.S., Leavitt, R.Y., Kerr, G.S., Fauci, A.S. The treatment of Wegener's granulomatosis with glucocorticosteroids and methotrexate, *Arthritis and Rheumatism*, 35, 1322, 1992.

46. de Groot, K., Reinhold-Keller, E., Tatsis, E., Paulsen, J., Heller, M., Nolle, B., Gross, W.L. Therapy for the maintenance of remission in sixty-five patients with generalized Wegener's granulomatosis. Methotrexate versus trimethoprim/sulfamethoxazole, *Arthritis and Rheumatism*, 39, 2052, 1996.

47. Allen, M.B., Caldwell, D.S., Rice, J.R. Cyclosporin A therapy for Wegener's granulomatosis, *Adv. Exp. Med. Biol.*, 336, 473, 1993.

48. Fauci, A.S., Haynes, B.F., Katz, P., Wolff, S.M. Wegeners granulomatosis — prospective clinical and therapeutic experience with 85 patients for 21 years, *Annals of Internal Medicine*, 98, 76, 1983.

49. Stegeman, C.A., Tervaert, J.W.C., Sluiter, W.J., Manson, W.L., deJong, P.E., Kallenberg, C.G.M. Association of chronic nasal carriage of staphylococcus aureus and higher relapse rates in Wegener granulomatosis, *Annals of Internal Medicine*, 120, 12, 1994.

50. Stegeman, C.A., Cohen Tervaert, J.W., de Jong, P.E., Kallenberg, C.G. Trimethoprim-sulfamethoxazole (co-trimoxazole) for the prevention of relapses of Wegener's granulomatosis. Dutch Co-Trimoxazole Wegener Study Group, *New England Journal of Medicine*, 335, 16, 1996.

51. de Groot, K., Reinhold-Keller, E., Tatsis, E., Paulsen, J., Heller, M., Nolle, B., Gross, W.L. Therapy for the maintenance of remission in sixty-five patients with generalized Wegener's granulomatosis — methotrexate versus trimethoprim/sulfamethoxazole, *Arthritis and Rheumatism*, 39, 2052, 1996.

52. Reinhold-Keller, E., de Groot, K., Rudert, H., Nolle, B., Heller, M., Gross, W.L. Response to trimethoprim sulfamethoxazole in Wegener's granulomatosis depends on the phase of disease, *Qjm-Monthly Journal of the Association of Physicians*, 89, 15, 1996.

53. Jayne, D.R.W. Immunotherapy for ANCA-associated systemic vasculitis, *Clin. Exp. Immunol.*, 112, 12, 1998.

54. Lockwood, C.M., Thiru, S., Stewart, S., Hale, G., Isaacs, J., Wraight, P., Elliott, J., Waldmann, H. Treatment of refractory Wegener's granulomatosis with humanized monoclonal antibodies, *Qjm-Monthly Journal of the Association of Physicians*, 89, 903, 1996.

55. Bacon, P., Exley, A., Carruthers, D., Russell, N., McColl, G., Rentsch, J., Grigg, A., Szer, J. Immune ablation with stem cell rescue for Wegeners, *Arthritis and Rheumatism*, 41, 499, 1998.

56. Lebovics, R.S., Hoffman, G.S., Leavitt, R.Y., Kerr, G.S., Travis, W.D., Kammerer, W., Hallahan, C., Rottem, M., Fauci, A.S. The management of subglottic stenosis in patients with Wegeners granulomatosis, *Laryngoscope*, 102, 1341, 1992.

57. Jennette, J.C., Falk, R.J., Andrassy, K., Bacon, P.A., Churg, J., Gross, W.L., Hagen, E.C., Hoffman, G.S., Hunder, G.G., Kallenberg, C.G.M., Mccluskey, R.T., Sinico, R.A., Rees, A.J., Vanes, L.A., Waldherr, R., Wiik, A. Nomenclature of systemic vasculitides — proposal of an international consensus conference, *Arthritis and Rheumatism*, 37, 187, 1994.

58. Fries, J.F., Hunder, G.G., Bloch, D.A., Michel, B.A., Arend, W.P., Calabrese, L.H., Fauci, A.S., Leavitt, R.Y., Lie, J.T., Lightfoot, R.W., Masi, A.T., Mcshane, D.J., Mills, J.A., Stevens, M.B., Wallace, S.L., Zvaifler, N.J. The American College of Rheumatology 1990 criteria for the classification of vasculitis — summary, *Arthritis and Rheumatism,* 33, 1135, 1990.
59. Nordborg, E., Bengtsson, B.A. Death rates and causes of death in 284 consecutive patients with giant-cell arteritis confirmed by biopsy, *British Medical Journal,* 299, 549, 1989.
60. Healey, L.A. Relation of giant-cell arteritis to polymyalgia rheumatica, *Baillieres Clinical Rheumatology,* 5, 371, 1991.
61. Nordborg, E., Nordborg, C., Malmvall, B.E., Andersson, R., Bengtsson, B.A. Giant cell arteritis, *Rheum. Dis. Clin. North Am.,* 21, 1013, 1995.
62. Wilke, W.S., Hoffman, G.S. Treatment of corticosteroid resistant giant cell arteritis, *Rheum. Dis. Clin. North Am.,* 21, 59, 1995.
63. van der Veen, M.J., Dinant, H.J., van Booma-Frankfort, C., van Albada-Kuipers, G.A., Bijlsma, J.W. Can methotrexate be used as a steroid sparing agent in the treatment of polymyalgia rheumatica and giant cell arteritis?, *Ann. Rheum. Dis.,* 55, 218, 1996.
64. Weyand, C.M., Goronzy, J.J. Giant-cell arteritis as an antigen-driven disease, *Rheum. Dis. Clin. North Am.,* 21, 1027, 1995.
65. Kerr, G.S., Hallahan, C.W., Giordano, J., Leavitt, R.Y., Fauci, A.S., Rottem, M., Hoffman, G.S. Takayasu arteritis, *Annals of Internal Medicine,* 120, 919, 1994.
66. Fraga, A., Mintz, G., Valle, L., Flores-Izquierdo, G. Takayasu's arteritis: frequency of systemic manifestations (study of 22 patients) and favorable response to maintenance steroid therapy with adrenocorticosteroids (12 patients), *Arthritis and Rheumatism,* 15, 617, 1972.
67. Hoffman, G.S., Leavitt, R.Y., Kerr, G.S., Rottem, M., Sneller, M.C., Fauci, A.S. Treatment of glucocorticoid-resistant or relapsing Takayasu arteritis with methotrexate, *Arthritis and Rheumatism,* 37, 578, 1994.
68. Sharma, S., Saxena, A., Talwar, K.K., Kaul, U., Mehta, S.N., Rajani, M. Renal artery stenosis caused by nonspecific arteritis (Takayasu disease) — results of treatment with percutaneous transluminal angioplasty, *American Journal of Roentgenology,* 158, 417, 1992.
69. Newburger, J.W., Takahashi, M., Beiser, A.S., Burns, J.C., Bastian, J., Chung, K.J., Colan, S.D., Duffy, C.E., Fulton, D.R., Glode, M.P., Mason, W.H., Meissner, H.C., Rowley, A.H., Shulman, S.T., Reddy, V., Sundel, R.P., Wiggins, J.W., Colton, T., Melish, M.E., Rosen, F.S. A single intravenous-infusion of gamma-globulin as compared with 4 infusions in the treatment of acute Kawasaki syndrome, *New England Journal of Medicine,* 324, 1633, 1991.
70. Tizard, E.J., Suzuki, A., Levin, M., Dillon, M.J. Clinical aspects of 100 patients with Kawasaki disease, *Archives of Disease in Childhood,* 66, 185, 1991.
71. Dillon, M.J., Ansell, B.M. Vasculitis in children and adolescents, *Rheum. Dis. Clin. North Am.,* 21, 1115, 1995.
72. Rosenblum, N.D., Winter, H.S. Steroid effects on the course of abdominal pain in children with Henoch-Schonlein purpura, *Pediatrics,* 79, 1018, 1987.
73. Oner, A., Tinaztepe, K., Erdogan, O. The effect of triple therapy on rapidly progressive type of Henoch-Schonlein nephritis, *Pediatric Nephrology,* 9, 6, 1995.
74. Callen, J.P. Colchicine is effective in controlling chronic cutaneous leukocytoclastic vasculitis, *Journal of the American Academy of Dermatology,* 13, 193, 1985.
75. Jorizzo, J.L., White, W.L., Wise, C.M., Zanolli, M.D., Sherertz, E.F. Low-dose weekly methotrexate for unusual neutrophilic vascular reactions — cutaneous polyarteritis nodosa and Behçet's disease, *Journal of the American Academy of Dermatology,* 24, 973, 1991.
76. Chynn, E.W., Jakobiec, F.A. Cogan's syndrome: ophthalmic, audiovestibular, and systemic manifestations and therapy, *International Ophthalmology Clinics,* 36, 61, 1996.
77. Raza, K., Karokis, D., Kitas, G.D. Cogan's syndrome with Takayasu's arteritis, *Brit. J. Rheum.,* 37, 369, 1998.
78. Vollertsen, R.S., Mcdonald, T.J., Younge, B.R., Banks, P.M., Stanson, A.W., Ilstrup, D.M. Cogan's-syndrome — 18 cases and a review of the literature, *Mayo Clinic Proceedings,* 61, 344, 1986.
79. Allen, N.B., Cox, C.C., Cobo, M., Kisslo, J., Jacobs, M.R., Mccallum, R.M., Haynes, B.F. Use of immunosuppressive agents in the treatment of severe ocular and vascular manifestations of Cogan's syndrome, *American Journal of Medicine,* 88, 296, 1990.

80. Calabrese, L.H., Duna, G.F. Evaluation and treatment of central nervous system vasculitis, *Curr. Opin. Rheumatol.*, 7, 37, 1995.

81. Calabrese, L.H., Gragg, L.A., Furlan, A.J. Benigh angiopathy: A distinct subset of angiographically defined primary angiitis of the central nervous system, *Journal of Rheumatology*, 20, 2046, 1993.

82. Calabrese, L.H., Duna, G.F., Lie, J.T. Vasculitis in the central nervous system, *Arthritis and Rheumatism*, 40, 1189, 1997.

83. Vollertsen, R.S., Conn, D.L., Ballard, D.J., Ilstrup, D.M., Kazmar, R.E., Silverfield, J.C. Rheumatoid vasculitis — survival and associated risk-factors, *Medicine*, 65, 365, 1986.

84. Scott, D.G.I., Bacon, P.A. Intravenous cyclophosphamide plus methylprednisolone in treatment of systemic rheumatoid vasculitis, *American Journal of Medicine*, 76, 377, 1984.

85. Bacon, P.A., Carruthers, D.M. Vasculitis associated with connective-tissue disorders, *Rheum. Dis. Clin. North Am.*, 21, 1077, 1995.

86. Boumpas, D.T., Austin, H.A., Vaughn, E.M., Klippel, J.H., Steinberg, A.D., Yarboro, C.H., Balow, J.E. Controlled trial of pulse methylprednisolone versus 2 regimens of pulse cyclophosphamide in severe lupus nephritis, *Lancet*, 340, 741, 1992.

87. Ames, P.R.J., Cianciaruso, B., Bellizzi, V., Balletta, M., Lubrano, E., Scarpa, R., Brancaccio, V. Bilateral renal-artery occlusion in a patient with primary antiphospholipid antibody syndrome — thrombosis, vasculitis or both, *Journal of Rheumatology*, 19, 1802, 1992.

88. Goldberger, E., Elder, R.C., Schwartz, R.A., Phillips, P.E. Vasculitis in the antiphospholipid syndrome — a cause of ischemia responding to corticosteroids, *Arthritis and Rheumatism*, 35, 569, 1992.

89. Ferri, C., Moriconi, L., Gremignai, G., Migliorini, P., Paleologo, G., Fosella, P.V., Bombardieri, S. Treatment of the renal involvement in mixed cryoglobulinemia with prolonged plasma-exchange, *Nephron*, 43, 246, 1986.

90. Ferri, C., Marzo, E., Longombardo, G., Lombardini, F., Lacivita, L., Vanacore, R., Liberati, A.M., Gerli, R., Greco, F., Moretti, A., Monti, M., Gentilini, P., Bombardieri, S., Zignego, A.L. Interferon-alpha in mixed cryoglobulinemia patients — a randomized, crossover-controlled trial, *Blood*, 81, 1132, 1993.

91. Gardner-Medwin, J.M.M., Smith, N.J., Powell, R.J. Clinical-experience with thalidomide in the management of severe oral and genital ulceration in conditions such as Behçet's-disease — use of neurophysiological studies to detect thalidomide neuropathy, *Ann. Rheum. Dis.*, 53, 828, 1994.

92. Masuda, K., Urayama, A., Kogure, M., Nakajima, A., Nakae, K., Inaba, G. Double-masked trial of cyclosporine versus colchicine and long-term open study of cyclosporine in Behçet's-disease, *Lancet*, 1, 1093, 1989.

93. Yazici, H., Pazarli, H., Barnes, C.G., Tuzun, Y., Ozyazgan, Y., Silman, A., Serdaroglu, S., Oguz, V., Yurdakul, S., Lovatt, G.E., Yazici, B., Somani, S., Muftuoglu, A. A controlled trial of azathioprine in Behçet's syndrome, *New England Journal of Medicine*, 322, 281, 1990.

94. Lie, J.T. Cholesterol atheromatous embolism — the great masquerader revisited, *Pathology Annual*, 27, 17, 1992.

95. Cappiello, R.A., Espinoza, L.R., Adelman, H., Aguilar, J., Vasey, F.B., Germain, B.F. Cholesterol embolism — a pseudovasculitic syndrome, *Seminars in Arthritis and Rheumatism*, 18, 240, 1989.

96. Metzler, C., Reinhold-Keller, E., Schmitt, W., Gross, W.L. Maintenance of remission with leflunomide in 11 patients with Wegener's granulomatosis, *Arthritis and Rheumatism*, 40, 808, 1997.

97. Nowack, R., Birck, R., VanderWoude, F.J. Mycophenolate mofetil for systemic vasculitis and iga nephropathy, *Lancet*, 349, 774, 1997.

98. Daina, E., Schieppati, A., Remuzzi, G. Mycophenolate mofetil for the treatment of Takayasu arteritis: report of three cases, *Annals of Internal Medicine*, 130, 422, 1999.

99. Salmon, M., Scheel-Toellner, D., Huissoon, A.P., Pilling, D., Shamsadeen, N., Hyde, H., Dangeac, A.D., Bacon, P.A., Emery, P., Akbar, A.N. Inhibition of t-cell apoptosis in the rheumatoid synovium, *J. Clin. Invest.*, 99, 439, 1997.

35 Anticoagulation Therapy for the Antiphospholipid Syndrome

Scott Goodnight

CONTENTS

I. INTRODUCTION

The optimal treatment of vascular thrombosis in patients who have antiphospholipid antibodies has proven to be a challenge. The diversity of the thromboses — venous, arterial, and microvascular — suggests that multiple pathogenic mechanisms are involved.[1] However, anticoagulants (heparin, low-molecular-weight heparin, and oral anticoagulants) have generally proven effective for the prevention of thrombotic recurrences regardless of their vascular origin. Prospective randomized clinical trials of anticoagulants are urgently needed to refine treatment indications, as well as the intensity and duration of therapy. This chapter will discuss the use of anticoagulants for the treatment of venous and arterial thromboembolism in patients with antiphospholipid antibodies. In addition, complications of anticoagulant therapy and the special problems associated with monitoring anticoagulant treatment in patients with the lupus anticoagulant will be covered.

II. TREATMENT OF VENOUS THROMBOSIS

Venous thromboembolism is a common clinical problem in patients with antiphospholipid antibodies.[2] In addition to classic deep venous thrombosis and pulmonary embolism, patients may develop superficial thrombophlebitis as well as thrombi in unusual sites, such as the central abdominal veins or the cerebral dural sinuses. In many instances additional risk factors are present which include physical (inactivity, trauma, surgery), hormonal (oral contraceptives, pregnancy), or plasma disorders (homocysteinenia,[3] protein S deficiency,[4] activated protein C resistance[5]). Thrombotic recurrences following a first venous thromboembolism also tend to be venous in location in up to 90% of patients.[6,7]

Acute venous thrombosis or pulmonary embolism in patients with antiphospholipid antibodies is treated with a standard approach using therapeutic doses of unfractionated or low-molecular-weight heparin as soon as the diagnosis is established.[8] Oral anticoagulants are begun in the first 24 to 48 hrs of heparin treatment.[9] The heparin or low-molecular-weight heparin should be continued

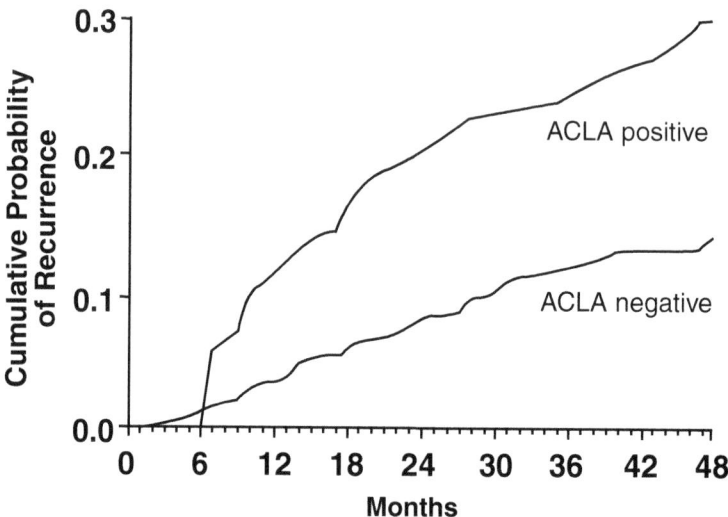

FIGURE 35.1 Cumulative probability of a recurrent venous thromboembolism in patients after a first episode who were anticoagulated for six months. ACLA refers to IgG anticardiolipin antibodies. From Schulman et al.[12]

until the INR has reached a therapeutic range (usually an INR of 2 to 3) for at least 24 hrs. and preferably longer to allow prothrombin and other clotting factor concentrations to fall to a protective range.[10] This may be particularly relevant for patients with antiphospholipid antibodies in whom the likelihood of a recurrence is quite high. Importantly, pretreatment laboratory studies including a prothrombin time (PT), activated partial thromboplastin time (aPTT), and platelet count should be obtained to detect any influence of a lupus anticoagulant on screening coagulation tests, or the presence of severe thrombocytopenia, which could increase the risk of bleeding with anticoagulant treatment. If the pretreatment PT or aPTT are elevated, then alternative methods to monitor anticoagulant therapy must be used.

In the absence of adequate oral anticoagulant treatment, thrombotic recurrence rates in patients with antiphospholipid antibodies are very high. Early studies in selected patient populations suggested that at least 50% of patients would have a recurrent thromboembolism in the next two years.[11] In the large retrospective studies of Rosove[6] and Khamashta,[7] thrombosis recurrence rates were as high as 20% per year in the absence of treatment, although the recurrences were not separated by these investigators into arterial or venous events. More recently, prospective studies have documented high rates of recurrent venous thrombosis in patients with IgG anticardiolipin antibodies (see Figure 35.1)[12] or the lupus anticoagulant.[13] Based on this data, oral anticoagulant treatment is clearly warranted for the prevention of recurrent thrombosis in patients with antiphospholipid antibodies.[14]

A therapeutic range for the INR of 2 to 3 appears to be sufficient for the treatment of most patients with antiphospholipid antibody-associated venous thromboembolism. Evidence for this recommendation includes the retrospective study of Rosove in which venous thrombosis did not recur if the INR was maintained between 2 and 3.[6] More recently, a Swedish study of patients with a first or second episode of venous thrombosis and IgG anticardiolipin antibodies showed that oral anticoagulant treatment with an INR of 2 to 2.85 eliminated recurrences in the on-treatment group.[12] Similarly, a study by Kearon et al. of patients with carefully defined idiopathic venous thrombosis showed that warfarin treatment (INR 2 to 3) also eliminated recurrences in their group, which included individuals with lupus anticoagulants and anticardiolipin antibodies.[13] The presence of a lupus anticoagulant (but not anticardiolipin antibodies) predicted recurrent thromboembolism (Hazard Ratio 6.8 (p=0.03)). Low or absent recurrences of venous thrombosis at INRs of 2 to 3 have been reported by other investigators as well.[14,15]

The optimal duration of oral anticoagulant treatment for patients with antiphospholipid anti-body-associated venous thromboembolism remains uncertain. However, the reported high rates of recurrence suggest that, in general, longer treatment is justified in many patients if they do not have excessive risks of bleeding. Long-term therapy in this context may be defined as treatment durations of >6 months, and in some instances treatment should be continued indefinitely. Patients who may benefit from long-term anticoagulation include those with a history of recurrent throm-boses, massive venous thrombosis, or life-threatening pulmonary emboli. Longer term treatment should also be strongly considered in patients with antiphospholipid antibodies who have a first major idiopathic (unprovoked) thrombosis.[13]

Shorter treatment durations may be sufficient (e.g., 3 to 6 months) in subjects who have a first provoked thrombosis in which the additional risk factors are not persistent or can be eliminated (e.g., surgery, pregnancy, or oral contraceptives). However, such patients remain at an increased likelihood of recurrent thrombosis and should be counseled on the signs and symptoms of new venous thromboses or pulmonary emboli, and arrangements should be made for prompt diagnostic testing should symptoms occur. Intensive antithrombotic prophylaxis (e.g., low-molecular-weight heparin) should be administered for periods of high risk such as surgery, trauma, pregnancy, inflammatory states, or even prolonged immobility.[16] Antithrombotic therapy is not indicated for patients with antiphospholipid antibodies who lack a history of thrombosis, since the risk of a first thrombosis is sufficiently low (at the most, 2.5% per year) that the risks of long-term anticoagulant therapy are not warranted.[2]

III. TREATMENT OF ARTERIAL THROMBOEMBOLISM

Antiphospholipid antibodies have long been linked to cerebral ischemic events, acute myocardial infarction, and other arterial thrombotic disorders.[2] Optimal treatment of these patients poses a major clinical dilemma because of the variable nature of the disease and the lack of prospective trials of antithrombotic therapy. For example, neurologic symptoms due to cerebral ischemia are common in patients with antiphospholipid antibodies, but the signs and symptoms can be due to a multitude of causes, not all of which should be treated with anticoagulants. For example, patients may have:

- A major thromboembolic stroke in conjunction with high titer antiphospholipid antibod-ies, or a potent lupus anticoagulant in the absence of atherosclerosis.[17,18] These patients may also have livido reticularis and thrombocytopenia.[19]
- A dural sinus thrombosis (more properly a venous thrombosis).[20]
- Recurrent, relatively minor cerebral ischemic events often associated with cardiac abnor-malities on transesophageal echocardiography.[21]
- Multiple risk factors for atherosclerotic arterial disease and relatively low titer antiphos-pholipid antibodies.[22] In this instance, the antiphospholipid antibodies may be markers for the underlying vascular disease.
- Striking "unidentified bright objects" (hyperintense foci on T_2-weighted MRI brain scans) which may be associated with symptoms suggestive of multiple sclerosis.[23] These lesions may represent local *in situ* small vessel disease (but not necessarily thrombosis) in the brain.
- Systemic lupus erythematosus (SLE) with cerebral vasculitis which happens to be asso-ciated with the lupus anticoagulant or solid-phase antiphospholipid antibodies.

Clearly, the most appropriate therapy for each of the above conditions may be quite different, and could include anticoagulants in some instances; but in others, anticoagulant treatment could pose major risks of bleeding along with little benefit. Unfortunately, controlled prospective studies in well-defined cohorts of patients with these clinical syndromes are not yet available. The diagnostic approach to patients with cerebral ischemia should include a thorough neurologic clinical evaluation including magnetic resonance scanning, in some instances cerebral angiography, carotid and other vascular studies, and transesophageal echocardiography to evaluate cardiac valves and potential right-to-left cardiac shunts.[24]

Patients with major thromboembolic stroke, particularly in the absence of extensive atherosclerosis, who have high titer antiphospholipid antibodies and/or a lupus anticoagulant are likely to benefit from long-term oral anticoagulant therapy, based on large but uncontrolled retrospective studies.[6,7] The optimal intensity of anticoagulant treatment is not clear, but the above studies suggest that an INR range of 2.5 to 3.5 may be needed to prevent recurrences. Many of these patients had lupus anticoagulants which potentially could have excessively prolonged the prothrombin times that were used to monitor the anticoagulant therapy. This effect could give a false impression that higher INR's are necessary for adequate therapy, although this effect seems unlikely to account for all of their results. At this time, then, it remains unclear whether oral anticoagulant treatment at INR ranges of 2 to 3 or the higher range of 2.5 to 3.5 will provide optimal protection with the lowest risks. Low-dose aspirin can be added to oral anticoagulants if patients have recurrent central nervous system events while treated with anticoagulants alone, although the risk of hemorrhage, particularly gastrointestinal bleeding, will often be increased.

Many patients have relatively minor but recurrent cerebral ischemic events that occur despite antithrombotic therapy with warfarin and/or aspirin.[17,18,21] The optimal treatment of these individuals is uncertain, at best. However, if MR scans show clear evidence of cerebral infarction, then oral anticoagulant therapy with INR's in the 2.5 to 3.5 range seems reasonable. Anticoagulant treatment is probably not necessary for many patients with antiphospholipid antibodies and recurrent neurologic symptoms, but in whom brain scans are entirely normal and who show no evidence of cerebral infarction.

Therapeutic decisions are even more difficult for those patients with multiple risk factors for cerebral or coronary vascular disease (e.g., smoking, diabetes, hypertension) who are discovered (often incidentally) to have low titer solid-phase antibodies (e.g., IgG or IgM anticardiolipin antibodies).[22] In many of these patients, the antiphospholipid antibodies may reflect the underlying arterial vascular disease. In such patients a standard treatment regimen that includes antiplatelet agents may pose less risk than oral anticoagulant therapy.

Finally, a group of patients with antiphospholipid antibodies has been described that have headache, unidentified bright objects on brain scan, and slowly progressive symptoms reminiscent of multiple sclerosis (but often lacking the oligoclonal bands in the spinal fluid).[23] It is not known whether thrombosis plays a role in the genesis or progression of these lesions or whether antithrombotic therapy would provide benefit. However, if the hyperintense foci are associated with frank infarcts, then anticoagulant treatment should be considered.

IV. BLEEDING COMPLICATIONS ASSOCIATED WITH ANTICOAGULANT TREATMENT

The risks of anticoagulant-induced bleeding in patients with thrombosis and antiphospholipid antibodies could be somewhat higher than in subjects without this immune disorder. Factors that could well increase the risks of bleeding include:

- Coexisting active SLE or other collagen vascular disorder
- Antiphospholipid antibody-associated immune thrombocytopenia [25]
- Possible platelet function defect in patients with the lupus anticoagulant[26]
- Concomitant administration of antiplatelet and anticoagulant therapy[27]
- Coexisting acquired prothrombin deficiency[28]

Unfortunately, no data on the direct comparison of bleeding risks in antiphospholipid antibody versus nonantiphospholipid antibody patients has been published, particularly in subjects with truly comparable INRs. Two retrospective studies of antiphospholipid antibody patients suggested that the risk of major life-threatening bleeding with oral anticoagulant treatment was 2 to 3% per year.[6,7] In studies of bleeding risk in other groups of patients who were not selected for antiphospholipid antibodies, the annual incidence of major bleeding, life-threatening bleeding, and fatal bleeding was approximately 2%, 1%, and 0.25%, respectively.[29] A very recent prospective controlled study of warfarin treatment for patients with idiopathic venous thromboembolism found a somewhat higher major bleeding rate of 3.8% per year.[13] Therefore, the available data do not support a greatly increased risk of bleeding in anticoagulated antiphospholipid antibody patients, but individual patients with severe thrombocytopenia, prothrombin deficiencies, or those treated with higher INRs may constitute a particularly high-risk subgroup.

Patients with mild or moderate immune thrombocytopenia in concert with antiphospholipid antibodies can often be safely treated with oral anticoagulants.[25] Those individuals with more severe reductions in platelet count (e.g., <50,000/cmm) pose a larger problem. Therapeutic measures such as corticosteroids, intravenous IgG, Rh immune globulin, or splenectomy may be necessary to raise platelet counts to a level that allows the safe administration of anticoagulant therapy. Acquired prothrombin deficiency due to circulating prothrombin-antiprothrombin immune complexes poses a similar and is sometimes a more difficult problem in management.[28,30] Very low levels of prothrombin activity greatly increase the risk of bleeding with both heparin and coumarin anticoagulants. In some patients, corticosteroids or other immunosuppressive treatment may increase prothrombin levels sufficiently to allow adequate oral anticoagulant treatment.[31,32]

V. MONITORING ANTICOAGULANTS IN THE PRESENCE OF A LUPUS ANTICOAGULANT

The lupus anticoagulant can occasionally prolong the results of the coagulation tests used to monitor heparin or oral anticoagulant therapy.[33] Lupus anticoagulant-induced prolongation of the PT and aPTT depends in part on the characteristics of the inhibitor in individual patients, but also on the reagents and the instruments used for the laboratory assays.[34-37] For example, Innovin®, a recombinant tissue factor PT reagent, may be particularly sensitive, giving higher INR results in the presence of a lupus anticoagulant than other thromboplastins.[35,38,39] Screening PT and aPTT tests should be obtained prior to starting anticoagulant treatment with the reagent-instrument combination to be used for future monitoring of anticoagulant therapy.

Heparin monitoring in the presence of a lupus anticoagulant is best performed using an anti-factor Xa heparin assay rather than depending on the aPTT to guide therapy.[40] The anti-Xa heparin assay does not require phospholipid and therefore is not affected by the inhibitor. Alternatively, the patient can be treated with low-molecular-weight heparin, which does not usually need laboratory monitoring.[8] Low-molecular-weight heparin levels (again by an anti-Xa method) can be helpful if patients are at high risk of bleeding or recurrent thrombosis, have extremes of body weight, suffer renal insufficiency, are pregnant, or are younger than 10 years of age.[41]

Patients with prolonged PTs prior to anticoagulation with the coumarins, or those who appear to be unduly sensitive to oral anticoagulant therapy, require alternative monitoring strategies. Options include the selection of a thromboplastin reagent known to be insensitive to the patient's lupus inhibitor, the use of the prothrombin and proconvertin (P-and-P) time test, or measuring clotting factor X levels using a chromogenic factor X assay.[33] The P-and-P test is unlikely to be influenced by a lupus anticoagulant because the patient's plasma is diluted prior to performing the test, reducing the effect of the inhibitor in the test system. Unfortunately, the reagents for the P-and-P test may be difficult to obtain. Generally speaking, P-and-P levels of 45 to 15% correlate with an INR of 2 to 3.[33,39] The chromogenic factor X assay (factor X is a vitamin K-dependent clotting factor and is reduced by coumarin treatment) is effective in the presence of the lupus anticoagulant because phospholipid is not used in the test. Factor X levels of 10 to 40% have been shown to correlate with INRs of 3 to 2 (i.e., the lower factor X activity level correlates with higher INR values and indicates a greater degree of anticoagulation).

REFERENCES

1. Greaves, M., Antiphospholipid antibodies and thrombosis, *Lancet*, 353, 1348, 1999.
2. Finazzi, G., Brancaccio, V., Moia, M., Ciavarella, N., Mazzucconi, M. G., Schinco, P., Ruggeri, M., Pogliani, E. M., Gamba, G., Rossi, E., Baudo, F., Manotti, C., D'Angelo, A., Palareti, G., De Stefano, V., Berrettini, M. and Barbui, T., Natural history and risk factors for thrombosis in 360 patients with antiphospholipid antibodies: A four-year prospective study from the Italian Registry, *Am. J. Med.*,100, 530, 1996.
3. Petri, M., Roubenoff, R., Dallal, G. E., Nadeau, M. R., Selhub, J. and Rosenberg, I. R., Plasma homocysteine as a risk factor for atherothrombotic events in systemic lupus erythematosus, *Lancet*, 348, 1120, 1996.
4. Ginsberg, J. S., Demers, C., Brill-Edwards, P., Bona, R., Johnston, M., Wong, A. and Denburg, J. A., Acquired free protein S deficiency is associated with antiphospholipid antibodies and increased thrombin generation in patients with systemic lupus erythematosus, *Am. J. Med.*, 98, 379, 1995.
5. Galli, M., Ruggeri, L. and Barbui, T., Differential effects of anti-β_2-glycoprotein I and antiprothrombin antibodies on the anticoagulant activity of activated protein C, *Blood*, 91, 1999, 1998.
6. Rosove, M. H. and Brewer, P. M. C., Antiphospholipid thrombosis: Clinical course after the first thrombotic event in 70 patients, *Ann. Intern. Med.*, 117, 303, 1992.
7. Khamashta, M. A., Cuadrado, M. J., Mujic, F., Taub, N. A., Hunt, B. J. and Hughes, G. R. V., The management of thrombosis in the antiphospholipid-antibody syndrome, *N. Engl. J. Med.*, 332, 993, 1995.
8. Hyers, T. M., Agnelli, G., Hull, R. D., Weg, J. G., Morris, T. A., Samama, M. and Tapson, V., Antithrombotic therapy for venous thromboembolic disease, *Chest*, 114, 561S, 1998.
9. Hirsh, J., Dalen, J. E., Anderson, D. R., Poller, L., Bussey, H., Ansell, J., Deykin, D. and Brandt, J. T., Mechanism of action, clinical effectiveness, and optimal therapeutic range, *Chest*, 114, 445S, 1998.
10. Zivelin, A., Rao, L. V. and Rapaport, S. I., Mechanism of the anticoagulant effect of warfarin as evaluated in rabbits by selective depression of individual procoagulant vitamin K-dependent clotting factors, *J. Clin. Invest.*, 92, 2131, 1993.
11. Derksen, R. H. W. M., de Groot, P. G., Kater, L. and Nieuwenhuis, H. K., Patients with antiphospho-lipid antibodies and venous thrombosis should receive long term anticoagulant treatment, *Ann. Rheum. Dis.*, 52, 689, 1993.
12. Schulman, S., Svenungsson, E., Granqvist, S., and Duration Anticoagulation Study Group, Anticar-diolipin antibodies predict early recurrence of thromboembolism and death among patients with venous thromboembolism following anticoagulant therapy, *Am. J. Med.*, 104, 332, 1998.
13. Kearon, C., Gent, M., Hirsh, J., Weitz, J., Kovacs, M. J., Anderson, D. R., Turpie, A. G., Green, D., Ginsberg, J. S., Wells, P., MacKinnon, B. and Julian, J. A., A comparison of three months of anticoagulation with extended anticoagulation for a first episode of idiopathic venous thromboembo-lism, *N. Engl. J. Med.*, 340, 901, 1999.
14. Prandoni, P., Simioni, P. and Girolami, A., Antiphospholipid antibodies, recurrent thromboembolism, and intensity of warfarin anticoagulation, *Thromb. Haemost.*, 75, 859, 1996.
15. Ginsberg, J. S., Wells, P. S., Brill-Edwards, P., Donovan, D., Moffatt, K., Johnston, M., Stevens, P. and Hirsh, J., Antiphospholipid antibodies and venous thromboembolism, *Blood*, 86, 3685, 1995.
16. Clagett, G. P., Anderson, F. A., Jr., Geerts, W., Heit, J. A., Knudson, M., Lieberman, J. R., Merli, G. J. and Wheeler, H. B., Prevention of venous thromboembolism, *Chest*, 114, 531S, 1998.
17. Levine, S. R., Brey, R. L., Sawaya, K. L., Salowich-Palm, L., Kokkinos, J., Kostrzema, B., Perry, M., Havstad, S. and Carey, J., Recurrent stroke and thrombo-occlusive events in the antiphospholipid syndrome, *Ann. Neurol.*, 38, 119, 1995.
18. Levine, S. R., Salowich-Palm, L., Sawaya, K. L., Perry, M., Spencer, H. J., Winkler, H. J., Alam, Z. and Carey, J. L., IgG anticardiolipin antibody titer >40 GPL and the risk of subsequent thrombo-occlusive events and death — A prospective cohort study, *Stroke*, 28, 1660, 1997.

19. Tourbah, A., Piette, J. C., Iba-Zizen, M. T., Lyon-Caen, O., Godeau, P. and Frances, C., The natural course of cerebral lesions in Sneddon syndrome, *Arch. Neurol.*, 54, 53, 1997.

20. Carhuapoma, J. R., Mitsias, P. and Levine, S. R., Cerebral venous thrombosis and anticardiolipin antibodies, *Stroke*, 28, 2363, 1997.

21. Verro, P., Levine, S. R. and Tietjen, G. E., Cerebrovascular ischemic events with high positive anticardiolipin antibodies, *Stroke*, 29, 2245, 1998.

22. Tanne, D., D'Olhaberriague, L., Schultz, L. R., Salowich-Palm, L., Sawaya, K. L. and Levine, S. R., Anticardiolipin antibodies and their associations with cerebrovascular risk factors, *Neurology*, 52, 1368, 1999.

23. Karussis, D., Leker, R. R., Ashkenazi, A. and Abramsky, O., A subgroup of multiple sclerosis patients with anticardiolipin antibodies and unusual clinical manifestations: Do they represent a new nosological entity?, *Ann. Neurol.*, 44, 629, 1998.

24. DeRook, F. A., Comess, K. A., Albers, G. W. and Popp, R. L., Transesophageal echocardiography in the evaluation of stroke, *Ann. Intern. Med.*, 117, 922, 1992.

25. Galli, M., Finazzi, G. and Barbui, T., Thrombocytopenia in the antiphospholipid syndrome, *Br. J. Haematol.*, 93, 1, 1996.

26. Orlando, E., Cortelazzo, S., Marchetti, M., Sanfratello, R. and Barbui, T., Prolonged bleeding time in patients with lupus anticoagulant, *Thromb. Haemost.*, 68, 495, 1992.

27. Turpie, A. G. G., Gent, M., Laupacis, A., Latour, Y., Gunstensen, J., Basile, F., Klimek, M. and Hirsh, J., A comparison of aspirin with placebo in patients treated with warfarin after heart-valve replacement, *N. Engl. J. Med.*, 329, 524, 1993.

28. Bajaj, S. P., Rapaport, S. I., Fierer, D. S., Herbst, K. D. and Schwartz, D. B., A mechanism for the hypoprothrombinemia of the acquired hypoprothrombinemia-lupus anticoagulant syndrome, *Blood*, 61, 684, 1983.

29. Hirsh, J., Kearon, C. and Ginsberg, J., Duration of anticoagulant therapy after first episode of venous thrombosis in patients with inherited thrombophilia, *Arch. Intern. Med.*, 157, 2174, 1997.

30. Galli, M. and Barbui, T., Antiprothrombin antibodies: Detection and clinical significance in the antiphospholipid syndrome, *Blood*, 93, 2149, 1999.

31. Bajaj, S. P., Rapaport, S. I., Barclay, S. and Herbst, K. D., Acquired hypoprothrombinemia due to non-neutralizing antibodies to prothrombin: mechanism and management, *Blood*, 65, 1538, 1985.

32. Simel, D. L., St.Clair, E. W., Adams, J. and Greenberg, C. S., Correction of hypoprothrombinemia by immunosuppressive treatment of the lupus anticoagulant-hypoprothrombinemia syndrome, *Am. J. Med.*, 83, 563, 1987.

33. Moll, S. and Ortel, T. L., Monitoring warfarin therapy in patients with lupus anticoagulants, *Ann. Intern. Med.*, 127, 177, 1997.

34. Arnout, J. and Vermylen, J., Lupus anticoagulant: Influence on the international normalized ratio, *Thromb. Haemost.*, 81, 847, 1999.

35. Arnout, J., Meijer, P. and Vermylen, J., Lupus anticoagulant testing in Europe: An analysis of results from the first European Concerted Action on Thrombophilia (ECAT) survey using plasmas spiked with monoclonal antibodies against human β_2-glycoprotein 1, *Thromb. Haemost.*, 81, 929, 1999.

36. Lawrie, A. S., Purdy, G., Mackie, I. J. and Machin, S. J., Monitoring of oral anticoagulant therapy in lupus anticoagulant positive patients with the anti-phospholipid syndrome, *Br. J. Haematol.*, 98, 887, 1997.

37. Lawrie, A. S., Mackie, I. J., Purdy, G. and Machin, S. J., The sensitivity and specificity of commercial reagents for the detection of lupus anticoagulant show marked differences in performance between photo-optical and mechanical coagulometers, *Thromb. Haemost.*, 81, 758, 1999.

38. Arnout, J., Vanrusselt, M., Huybrechts, E. and Vermylen, J., Optimization of the dilute prothrombin time for the detection of the lupus anticoagulant by use of a recombinant tissue thromboplastin, *Br. J. Haematol.*, 87, 94, 1994.

39. Robert, A., Le Querrec, A., Delahousse, B., Caron, C., Houbouyan, L., Boutière, B., Horellou, M. H., Reber, G., Sié, P. and Group Methodol Hemostase Group Etud Hem, Control of oral anticoagulation in patients with the antiphospholipid syndrome — Influence of the lupus anticoagulant on international normalized ratio, *Thromb. Haemost.*, 80, 99, 1998.

40. Hirsh, J., Warkentin, T. E., Raschke, R., Granger, C., Ohman, E. M. and Dalen, J. E., Heparin and low-molecular-weight heparin — Mechanisms of action, pharmacokinetics, dosing considerations, monitoring, efficacy, and safety, *Chest*, 114, 489S, 1998.

41. Laposata, M., Green, D., Van Cott, E. M., Barrowcliffe, T. W., Goodnight, S. H. and Sosolik, R. C., College of American Pathologists Conference XXXI on Laboratory Monitoring of Anticoagulant Therapy — The clinical use and laboratory monitoring of low-molecular-weight heparin, danaparoid, hirudin and related compounds, and argatroban, *Arch. Pathol. Lab. Med.*, 122, 799, 1998.

36 The Treatment of Raynaud's Phenomenon

Marco Matucci-Cerinic, Sergio Generini, and James R. Seibold

CONTENTS

I. THE BASAL APPROACH TO RAYNAUD'S PHENOMENON

Raynaud's phenomenon (RP) occurs in a remarkably diverse clinical setting ranging from a nuisance manifestation of normal health[1] to the disabling ischemic injury of systemic sclerosis. Consideration of mechanism has been covered elsewhere in this text but should include recognition of the roles of thermoregulatory homeostasis, vasospasm, structural abnormalities, disturbances of hemorheology, and the role of locally-generated vasoconstrictors. It should come as no surprise that there is a diverse number of pharmacologic agents, with both an underlying rationales and supportive clinical experience, employed in the clinical management of RP.

To a large extent, choice of management is influenced by the dominant pathophysiology in the individual patient. However, there are general measures and nonspecific medications useful in virtually all subjects. We propose that therapy of RP must define the goals of treatment (OUTCOME), but that choice of therapy is strongly dependent on pathophysiologic reasoning (PROCESS).

A. The Goals

After a diagnostic algorithm and the possible identification of the cause of RP, it is mandatory to identify clearly the goals of the therapy, which should be tailored to the patient's characteristics. The goals may be observed from two points of view, one clinical and the other pathophysiological.

Independently from the nature of RP, the main clinical goals may be identified in the reduction of the frequency and severity of the attacks of early RP, the maintenance of blood flow, and the healing of ulcers in advanced RP. The strategy is thus to lessen the continuous episodes of vasoconstriction and reperfusion that are detrimental to the microcirculatory environment. In more advanced cases, when the vascular structural modifications and critical finger ischemia are already in action, the strategy is to keep a satisfactory vasodilation in order to maintain blood flow, prevent flow breakdown, and avoid the evolution to gangrene and digital loss.

The pathophysiological goals consider the endothelium and the peripheral nervous system as intermediate targets and the smooth muscle cells as ultimate targets for the design of the treatment of RP. The main purpose is to protect the endothelium and restore a balanced control of vascular tone. The reduction of the episodes of vasoconstriction, reperfusion and injury, and, consequently, the reduction of oxygen radicals formation, may not only be achieved by reducing the number of RP attacks, but also by reducing the impact on the endothelial wall of reactive oxygen species and polymorphonuclear cells. In some cases of RP, the loss of capillaries may need a vigorous therapeutic strategy for the restoration of the angiogenic potential. Another aim is also to control the function of the peripheral nervous system, keep its vasodilating capacity, and modulate its vaso-constricting capacity. Ultimately, the target is represented by the smooth muscle cells that are the effectors of any message coming from the endothelium and/or the peripheral nervous system. The drug regimen may be thus aimed directly at the smooth muscle cell, or it may use the endothelium and the peripheral nervous system as intermediate producers of vascular tone-controlling substances.

B. The General Measures

All patients with RP benefit from patient education and simple modifications in lifestyle. Recognition of the role of reflex vasoconstriction as a principal mechanism of thermoregulation is an example of helpful information. All patients with RP benefit from measures to minimize core body heat loss. This would include the wearing of hats and dressing the trunk in layered clothing in addition to attention to appropriate hand and footwear. Patients should be encouraged to look for daily circumstances associated with predictable occurrences of Raynaud episodes. Common sense advice can be offered in their planning of activities of daily living. Nicotine delivery systems, most notably smoking, must be avoided. Many patients benefit to the point of not requiring pharmaceuticals if smoking cessation is made the main goal of therapy. Occasional patients may seem unduly intolerant of minor stimulants, including caffeine. Stress reduction techniques (yoga, biofeed-back, relaxation) can be encouraged in those patients, typically primary Raynaud, in whom both emotional stress and cold are precipitants of attacks.

II. THE DRUGS

A. Vasodilators

1. Calcium Channel Blockers

Calcium channel blockers extrude the calcium from smooth muscle cells, inducing vasodilatation. Depending on the binding site, they are divided into four classes, but the main difference is between dihydropyridine and nondihydropyridine.[2] The former has a selective tropism for peripheral smooth muscle cells, while the latter has a tropism for cardiac muscle cells. This difference is clear in clinics because the former vasodilates and affects the cardiac function, indirectly increasing the heart rate, while the latter has a potent negative effect on heart function.

Calcium channel blockers are still considered the first-line drug for RP.[2] Several dihydro and non-dihydro pyrimidines may be useful for the treatment of RP (see Table 36.1). Usually, nifedipine is the reference calcium antagonist[3] that is not only a vasodilator, but also exerts an inhibition of an *in vivo* platelet activation and antithrombotic effect.[4] Nifedipine may reach significant vasodilation, but also has several side-effects (edema, gastrointestinal symptoms, headache, dizziness) that may jeopardize its use in RP. However, many other calcium antagonists (Table 36.1) can be employed according to personal experience and the patient's tolerability. The effect of nicardipine, felodipine, and diltiazem in RP is still controversial.[2,5] A beneficial effect of novel calcium antagonists, isradipine and amlodipine,[2,6,7] has been reported on vasospastic episodes in RP. The drugs had favorable effect reducing the frequency, severity, and disability due to RP. Isradipine seems to significantly lower the circulating endothelin-1 levels, thus explaining the improvement of tissue perfusion.[6] Amlodipine has a slower onset of action and results in a reduction of the frequency and severity of RP attacks with a lower incidence of side-effects.[2,7] Our experience with nitrendipine shows that the drug is very potent and rapid on RP frequency and severity, but sometimes the tolerance of the patient to the rapid vasodilatition is limited and suggests the use of lower dosages. Verapamil is not effective in most patients with severe RP.[8]

2. Nitrates and L-Arginine

Sustained release transdermal glyceryl trinitrate patches are reported to effect a reduction in the number of and severity of RP attacks,[9,10] but without any improvement in thermography.[10] The use of the drug seems to be limited by the high incidence of headache (80%).[10]

L-arginine is one of the main components of the NO pathway and it has shown the capacity to inhibit platelet aggregation and human monocyte adhesion to vascular endothelium. However, despite initial encouraging results,[11] L-arginine did not result in an increase of endothelium-dependent relaxation in RP.[12]

3. Prostanoids

Prostacyclin and Prostaglandin E$_1$ (PGE$_1$) have been employed in the treatment of RP.[13,14] Both drugs have side-effects related to vasodilation, but their efficacy is short-lived and frequent repetition of the treatment is needed.[15,16] Recently, PGE$_1$ has shown a significant effect on chronic critical limb ischemia[16] and in the healing of digital ulcers in RP,[17] while prostacyclin has been used to fight severe pulmonary hypertension in scleroderma patients.[18] In the last decade, a stable prostacyclin analogue, iloprost, has shown a potent vasodilating and platelet antiaggregating effect, and it has been used in the treatment of RP[19] and pulmonary hypertension.[20] Iloprost has a long-lived effect on the frequency and severity of RP that can reach at least eight weeks. The infusion of iloprost for five consecutive days is surely effective, but its repetition every month is a heavy procedure. Interesting is the recent proposal for a single-day infusion every four weeks after the inducing infusion of five days.[21] Iloprost may also be useful in healing ulcers[22] and in blocking imminent gangrene.[23] The frequency of side-effects such as headache, flushing, nausea, vomiting, and diarrhea may frequently limit the use of the drug.

Oral preparations of iloprost showed poor efficacy,[24,25] while limaprost, an oral preparation of PGE$_1$, showed a significant efficacy in only a limited number of patients with RP.[26] More controversial results emerged with a prostacyclin oral analog, beraprost: on one side a significant reduction of the duration and incidence of RP was found,[27] while on the other a 37% improvement of RP attacks but with a lack of statistical significance was detected.[28] Prostanoids are very interesting molecules for the management of RP. In particular, iloprost is now considered the gold standard

TABLE 36.1
Clinical Trials for Raynaud's Phenomenon

Medication	Category	Dose	Response	Adverse Events	Entity of Adverse Effects
Amlodipine[7]	CCA	5-10 mg/day	↓ frequency, severity and disability	Flushing and headache	+
Beraprost[27,28]	PG	60 µg/day	Lack of statistical significance vs placebo[27]. ↓ duration and incidence of RP with significant increase of the skin temperature.[28]	No severe side effects but headache	+
Diltiazem[2]	CCA		↓ frequency and duration of attacks	None	+
Enalapril[36]	ACEi	20 mg/day	no significant changes in number and severity of RP attacks, no subjective benefit (VAS, 5 point rating scales, skin temperature response to cold challenge)	No major side effects	+
Felodipine[5]	CCA	10 mg/day	Dose-dependent improvement in RP symptomatology	Edema	+
Glyceryl trinitrate[10]	ND	patches 0.2 mg/h	↓ number and severity of attacks	Headache	+++
I.V. Iloprost[19]	PG	0.6-2 ng/kg/min IV over 6 hrs daily for 5 days	Improvement in patient rated overall severity; weekly attack frequency; MD overall severity digital ulcers healing, response to cold challenge improved	Facial and peripheral flushing; diarrhea, headache, jaw pain, vomiting, myalgia, injection site pain and local reactions, hypotension and mild tachycardia	++
Oral Iloprost[24,25]	PG	50-100 µg x 2/day[24] 50 µg x 2/day[25]	Reduced total daily duration and severity but not frequency of attacks[24] no significant difference with placebo[25]	Headache, dizziness, nausea, vomiting, jaw or tight pain, chest pain; 27 and 51% of treatment discontinuation for adverse events with 50 and 100 µg x 2/day respectively[24]	+++
Isradipine[6]	CCA	5 mg/day	reduction of frequency, severity and disability	Flushing and headache	++
Limaprost[26]	PG		Improvement in peak blood flow velocity in SLE and MCTD patients but not in SSc patients	Headache, dizziness, flushing, dhiarrea, abdominal pain	+++
Losartan[38]	ATIIrA	12.5 mg/day	Improvement in number and severity of attacks	No significant side effects	-
Nicardipine[2]	CCA		Moderate effect on clinical activity	Palpitations, flushing, nausea, edema, headache	++
Nifedipine[3,4]	CCA		Decreased frequency and severity of attacks; improved digital ulcer healing	Dizziness, headaches, constipation, edema, GI symptoms	+++
Nisoldipine[2]	CCA		↓ frequency of attacks	None	
Nitrendipine[2]	CCA	5-20 mg/day	Rapid improvement in number and severity of RP. Improvement of fingertips ulcers.	Headache, ephygastralgy	++
Prazosin[41-44]	αBl		Subjective improvement; increased digital vessel potency with cold challenge	Dizziness, dyspnea, edema, headache, rash, orthostatic hypotension	+
Terazosin[45]	αBl	5 mg/day	↓ number, intensity and duration of attacks		
Verapamil[8]	CCA	80-120 mg/day	Subjective improvement, not statistically significant, in RP frequency		++

Note: CCA: calcium channel antagonist, ACEi: Angiotensin converting enzyme inhibitor, αBl: alpha blocking, PG: prostanoid; ND: nitroderivatives; ATIIrA: angiotensin II receptor antagonist.

for any new vasodilating therapy, but more work is needed to identify the real usefulness of oral analogs in RP.

B. Other Kinds of Drugs and Approaches

1. Fibrinolytic Enhancers

In RP, fibrinolysis has been frequently reported impaired, and for this reason drugs restoring deficient fibrinolysis have been employed.[29] Low-weight-molecular dextran and stanozolol, an anabolic steroid which increases fibrinolysis, have been proposed for the treatment of RP but have never found confirmation. Recently, fibrinolytic activators seem to have more success in the treatment of RP: tissue plasminogen activator was effective in healing finger ulcers in severe RP,[30] and urokinase improved skin sclerosis (ultrasound evaluation) and took to the resolution of ulcers and the improvement of microcirculatory conditions.[31]

2. Estrogens

In the last year, interesting reports addressed the potential efficacy of estrogens in the improvement of endothelial dependent and independent function in RP.[32,33] Indeed, infused estrogens were able to reverse cold-induced coronary RP, leading to the normalization of the cold-induced Thallium-201 defect.[34] Estrogen potentiates endothelium-dependent vasodilation, upregulates the transcription of NO synthase, enhances its activity in nonvascular tissue, and has a potent antioxidant effect due to its phenolic ring. The development of new estrogen derivatives, such as raloxifene, might provide new potential vasoactive drugs devoid of detrimental side-effects, and of pivotal interest in the management of RP.

3. ACE Inhibitors

ACE inhibitors are currently used in the treatment of kidney involvement and lung hypertension in SSc. After an initial enthusiasm,[35] ACE inhibitors did not prove effective in controlling RP.[36,37] Instead, inhibitors of type I receptor for angiotensin II seem highly effective in the reduction of vasospastic attacks in RP.[38] However, this whole group of drugs, ACE and ATII receptor inhibitors, need large, controlled studies for the definition of their real utility in RP treatment.

4. Serotonin Antagonists

Local release of serotonin, presumably of platelet origin, has been hypothesized to be of importance in both primary and secondary RP. Ketanserin, a selective antagonist of serotonin-2 receptors, was found to improve digital artery perfusion across a broad range of finger temperatures[39] in patients with systemic sclerosis. In contrast, this highly selective agent reversed, but did not prevent, cold-induced vasoconstriction in subjects with primary RP.[40] Unfortunately, the mechanism-based toxicity of all serotonin-2 receptors or prolongation of the rate-corrected Qt interval has limited their development.

5. Sympatholytics and Sympathectomy

A large number of sympatholytic drugs (guanethidine, methyldopa, phentolamine, prazosin, reserpine, tolazoline, and others) may be useful in RP, but their use is limited by side-effects. Contradicting results have been obtained with α_1-adrenergic blockers. Prazosin was shown to be effective in reducing both the frequency and the severity of vasospasm in both primary and secondary RP patients,[41,42] but it is not able to induce complete relief from cold-induced attacks.[43] Other experiences suggest that it has a poor effect in RP secondary to SSc.[44] Therazosin determines a decrease in number, intensity, and duration of vasospastic attacks to the hands as well as an improvement of telethermographic and ultrasonographic findings.[45] Yohimbine, a selective alpha$_2$ antagonist, is limited by unpredictable bioavailability after oral administration.[46]

It has been recently reported that, in both normal and Raynaud's subjects, selective antagonism of alpha 1- or alpha 2-adrenergic receptors does not abolish local cold-induced vasoconstriction,[47] although several reports indicate that increased activation of α_2-adrenergic receptors, with a shift in the balance of alpha 1- and alpha 2-adrenoceptors on the vascular smooth muscle and in endothelium-derived relaxing and contracting factors, may be responsible for the vasospastic attacks in RP.[48] Flavahan and colleagues have demonstrated a profound increase (approximately 300-fold) to alpha$_2$-adrenoceptor-mediated vasoconstriction in both endothelium-containing and endothelium-denuded arterioles obtained from patients with systemic sclerosis.[49] This finding may be of particular importance because a nonselective treatment aimed at α_1 receptors might result in a deleterious effect. Thus, the use of specific α_2 receptor antagonists in the effort to control vasospastic attacks in RP might prove useful in the treatment of RP.[50] Sympathectomy has been reported to be effective in the management of RP:[51] the surgical approach, such as digital, thoracoscopic, or percutaneous thoracic sympathectomy, is strictly reserved for severe cases of RP refractory to medical treatments. Sympathectomy should be considered only in those subjects who manifest appropriate clinical responses to short-term sympathetic blockade, e.g., bipuvicaine stellate block. Recently, adventitial stripping of digital arteries was found extremely useful in refractory RP because of its sympathetic denervation, but also for its decompression of the ischemic vessel through removal of a fibrotic and noncompliant adventitia.[52] In order to avoid nerve section, a simpler approach might be the block of the digital, cervical, or stellate ganglion for the temporary control of severe RP.[53] However, the section of the nerve is very gross and deprives the patient of the role that the sympathetic system exerts on vascular tone. The application of this invasive approach to RP patients should be carefully revised.

6. Neuropeptides

Calcitonin gene-related peptide is one of the most potent endothelial-independent vasodilators that acts directly on the smooth muscle cells. The infusion of the drug in a randomized single-blind, controlled study obtained a significant vascular dilation in severe Raynaud's phenomenon.[54]

III. THE THERAPEUTIC STRATEGY

The large number of drugs available may sometimes be a confusing factor in making the choice of the right drug for the case to be treated. First of all, the physician must consider and treat appropriately the disease that causes RP. It is clear that the specific treatment for RP may vary according to the main clinical and laboratory features of the disease.

It is important to determine the severity of RP. If RP is mild, only general measures and the use of calcium antagonists may be suggested. If RP is severe, with the presence of ulcers and gangrene, it is mandatory to act rapidly in order to avoid the breakdown of the blood flow evolving to gangrene.[55] The therapy must be aggressive; in these cases the continuous infusion of iloprost may be helpful with the potential combination of different vasodilators and with the cooperation also of thrombolytic, anticoagulant, and profibrinolytic therapy.

IV. FUTURE THERAPIES

The scavenging strategy may become the leading therapeutic strategy in the future. Antioxidant drugs have already shown their efficacy in favoring vasodilation in RP,[56] and new drugs potentiating the expression of scavenging enzymes and the reduction of the adhesion of polymorphonuclear cells in order to block their homing to tissues may be interesting options.

More likely, the knowledge of the function of the peripheral nervous system may lead to identification of new agents, such as calcitonin gene-related peptide, that may be of benefit to achieve the control of the vascular tone. Capsaicin might be a potential drug inducing the selective release of substance P and CGRP from sensory motor nerves, but its use is limited by the risk of depleting the nerve fiber. Unfortunately, no drugs are known to act on and modulate the peripheral nerve terminals. The future development of such drugs will probably allow the control of vascular tone by manipulating the peripheral terminals.

REFERENCES

1. Hadler, NM: "Primary Raynaud's" is not a disease or even a disorder: It's a trait. *J. Rheumatol.*, 1998; 25: 2291-2294.
2. Sturgill, MG, Seibold, JR: Rational use of calcium-channel antagonists in Raynaud's phenomenon. *Curr. Opinion. Rheumatol.*, 1998;10: 584-588.
3. Rodeeheffer, RJ, Rommer, JA, Wigley, F, Smith, CR: Controlled double blind trial on nifedipine in the treatment of Raynaud's phenomenon. *N. Engl. J. Med.*, 1983; 308: 880-883.
4. Rademaker, M, Meyrick, Thomas, RH, Kirby, JD, Kovacs, IB: The anti-platelet of nifedipine in patients with systemic sclerosis. *Clin. Exp. Rheumatol.*, 1992;10: 57-62.
5. Gradman, AH: Treatment of hypertension with felodipine in patients with concomitant diseases. *Clin. Cardiol.*, 1993; 16: 294-301.
6. La Civita, L, Giuggioli, D, Del Chicca, G, Longombardo, G, Pasero, GP, Ferri, C: Effect of isradipine on endothelin 1 plasma concentrations in patients with Raynaud's phenomenon. *Ann. Rheum. Dis.*, 1996; 55: 331-334.
7. La Civita, L, Pitaro, N, Rossi, M: Amylodipine in the treatment of Raynaud's phenomenon: A double blind placebo controlled crossover study. *Clin. Drug Invest.*, 1996; 11 (suppl): 126-131.
8. Kinney, EL, Nicholas, GG, Gallo, J, Pontoriero, C, Zelis, R: The treatment of severe Raynaud's phenomenon with verapamil. *J. Clin. Pharmacol.*, 1982; 22: 74-76.
9. Franks, AG: Topical glyceryl trinitrate as adjunctive treatment of Raynaud's phenomenon. *Lancet*, 1982; 1: 76-77.
10. Teh, LS, Manning, J, Moore, T, Tully, MP, O'Reilly, D, Jayson, MIV: Sustained release transdermal glyceryl trinitrate patches as a treatment for primary and secondary Raynaud's phenomenon. *Br. J. Rheum.*, 1995, 34: 636-641.
11. Agostoni, A, Marasini, B, Biondi, ML, Bassani, C, Cazzaniga, A, Bottasso, B, Cugno, M: L-Arginine therapy in Raynaud's phenomenon? *Int. J. Clin. Lab. Res.*, 1991; 21: 202-203.
12. Khan, F, Litchfield, SJ, McLaren, M, Veale, DJ, Littleford, RC, Belch, JJ: Oral L-arginine supplementation and cutaneous vascular responses in patients with primary Raynaud's phenomenon. *Arth. Rheum.*, 1997; 40: 352-357.
13. Belch, JJF, Newman, P, Drury, JK, et al.: Intermittent epoprosteronol (Prostacyclin) infusion in patients with Raynaud's disease. *Lancet*, 1981; i: 313-315.
14. Langevitz, P, Buskila, D, Lee, P, Urowitz, MB: Treatment of refractory ischemic skin ulcers in patients with Raynaud's phenomenon with PGE1 infusion. *J. Rheumatol.*, 1989; 16: 1433-1435.
15. Kingma, K, Wollersheim, H, Thien, T: Double blind placebo controlled study of intravenous prostacyclin on hemodynamics in severe Raynaud's phenomenon: the acute vasodilatory effect is not sustained. *J. Cardiovasc. Pharmacol.*, 1995; 26: 388-393.
16. The ICAI study group: Prostanoids for chronic critical leg ischemia. A randomized, controlled, open label trial with PGE1. *Ann. Int. Med.*, 1999; 130:142: 412-421.
17. Lamprecht, P, Schnabel, A, Gross, WL: Efficacy of alprostadil and iloprost in digital necrosis due to secondary Raynaud's phenomenon. *Br. J. Rheumatol.*, 1998; 37: 703-704.
18. Olschewski, H, Walmrath, D, Schermuly, R, Ghofrani, Grimminger, F, Seeger, W: Aerosolized prostacyclin and iloprost in severe pulmonary hypertension. *Ann. Int. Med.*, 1996; 124: 820-824.
19. Wigley, FM, Wise, RA, Seibold, JR, et al.: Intravenous iloprost infusion in patients with Raynaud's phenomenon secondary to systemic sclerosis: a multicenter placebo controlled double blind study. *Ann. Int. Med.*, 1994; 120: 199-206.

20. Bartosik, I, Eskilsson, J, Scheja, A, Akesson, A: Intermittent iloprost infusion therapy of pulmonary hypertension in scleroderma — a pilot study. *Br. J. Rheumatol.,* 1996; 35:1187-1188.

21. Ceru, S, Pancera, S, Sansone, S, Sfondrini, G, Codella, O, De Sandre, G, Lechi, A, Lunardi, C: Effects of five days versus one day infusion of iloprost on the peripheral microcirculation in patients with systemic sclerosis. *Clin. Exp. Rheumatol.,* 1997; 15: 381-385.

22. Wigley, FM, Seibold, JR, Wise, RA, et al.: Intravenous iloprost treatment of Raynaud's phenomenon and ischemic ulcers secondary to systemic sclerosis. *J. Rheumatol.,* 1992; 19: 1407-1414.

23. Zachariae, H, Halkier-Sorensen, L, Bjerring, P, Heickendorff, L: Treatment of ischaemic digital ulcers and prevention of gangrene with intravenous iloprost in systemic sclerosis. *Acta Derm. Venereol.,* 1996, 76: 236-238.

24. Black, CM, Halkier-Sorensen, L, Belch, JJ, Ullman, S, Madhok, R, Smit, AJ, Banga, JD, Watson, HR: Oral iloprost in Raynaud's phenomenon secondary to systemic sclerosis: a multicentre, placebo-controlled, dose-comparison study. *Br. J. Rheumatol.,* 1998; 37: 952-960.

25. Wigley, FM, Korn, JH, Csuka, ME, et al.: Oral iloprost in patients with Raynaud's phenomenon secondary to systemic sclerosis: a multicenter placebo controlled double blind study. *Arth. Rheum.,* 1998; 41: 670-677.

26. Tsukamoto, H, Nagasawa, K: Successful treatment of Raynaud's phenomenon with limaprost, an orla prostaglandin E1 analogue. *Br. J. Rheumatol.,* 1991; 30: 317.

27. Hiida, M, Hushiyama, O, Suzuki, N, Ohta, A, Nagasawa, K, Yamaguchi, M: The effect of beraprost sodium on the Raynaud's phenomenon. *Nihon Rinsho Meneki Gakkai Kaishi,* 1996; 19: 193-200.

28. Vayssairat, M: Controlled multicenter double blind trial of an oral analog of prostacyclin in the treatment of primary Raynaud's phenomenon, French microcirculation society multicenter group for the study of vascular acrosyndromes. *J. Rheumatol.,* 1996; 23: 1917-1920.

29. Cimminiello, C: Clinical trials with defibrotide in vascular disorders. *Semin. Thromb. Hemost.,* 1996; 22 (suppl 1):29-34.

30. Maestrello, SJ, Vazquez-Abad, D, Waterman, JR: Tissue plasminogen activator treatment of severe Raynaud's phenomenon and associated ischemic ulcerations. *Arth. Rheum.,* 1995; 38 (s336): 1095.

31. Ciompi, ML, Bazzichi, L, Melchiorre, D, De Giorgio, F, Bondi, F, Puccetti, L: A placebo controlled study on urokinase therapy in systemic sclerosis. *Biomed. Pharmacother.,* 1996; 50: 363-368.

32. Lekakis, J, Papamichael, C, Mavrikakis, M, Voutsas, A, Stamateloupolos, S: Effect of long-term estrogen therapy on brachial arterial endothelium dependent vasodilation in women with Raynaud's phenomenon secondary to systemic sclerosis. *Am. J. Cardiol.,* 1998; 82: 1555-1557.

33. Lekakis, J, Mavrikakis, M, Papamichael, C, et al.: Short-term estrogen administration improves anormal endothelial function in women with systemic sclerosis and Raynaud's phenomenon. *Am. Heart J.,* 1998; 136: 905-912.

34. Lekakis, J, Mavrikakis, M, Emmanuel, M, Prassopoulos, V, Papamichael, C, Moulopoulou, D, Ziaga, A, Kostamis, P, Moulopoulos, S: Acute estrogen administration can reverse cold-induced coronary Raynaud's phenomenon in systemic sclerosis. *Clin. Exp. Rheumatol.,* 1996; 14: 421-424.

35. Miyazaki, S, Miura, K, Kasia, Y, Abe, K, Yoshinga, K: Relief from digital vasospasm by treatment with captopril and its complete inhibition by serine proteinase inhibitors in Raynaud's phenomenon. *BMJ,* 1982; 284: 310-311.

36. Challenor, VF, Waller, DG, Hayward, RA, Griffin, MJ, Roath, OS: Subjective and objective assessment of enalapril in primary Raynaud's phenomenon. *Br. J. Clin. Pharmacol.,* 1991; 31: 477-480.

37. Challenor, VF: Angiotensin converting enzyme inhibitors in Raynaud's phenomenon. *Drugs,* 1994; 48: 864-867.

38. Pancera, P, Sansone, S, Secchi, S, Covi, G, Lechi, A: The effects of thromboxane A_2 inhibition (picotamide) and angiotensin II receptor blockade (losartan) in primary Rayanud's phenomenon. *J. Int. Med.,* 1997; 242: 373-376.

39. Seibold, JR, Jageneau, AHM: Treatment of Raynaud's phenomenon with ketanserin, a selective antagonist of the serotonin-2 (5-HT-2) receptor. *Arth. Rheum.,* 1984; 27: 139-146.

40. Seibold, JR, Terregino, CA: Selective antagonism of serotonin-2 receptors relieves but not prevent cold-induced vasoconstriction in idiopathic Raynaud's phenomenon. *J. Rheumatol.,* 1986; 13: 337-340.

41. Surwit, RS, Gilgor, RS, Allen, LM, Duvic, M: A double-blind study of prazosin in the treatment of Raynaud's phenomenon in scleroderma. *Arch. Dermatol.,* 1984; 120: 329-31.

42. Wollersheim, H, Thien, T, Fennis, J, van Elteren, P, van 't Laar, A: Double-blind, placebo-controlled study of prazosin in Raynaud's phenomenon. *Clin. Pharmacol. Ther.,* 1986; 40: 219-25.

43. Nielsen, SL, Vitting, K, Rasmussen, K: Prazosin treatment of primary Raynaud's phenomenon. *Eur. J. Clin. Pharmacol.,* 1983; 24: 421-3.

44. Russell, IJ, Lessard, JA: Prazosin treatment of Raynaud's phenomenon: a double blind single crossover study. *J. Rheumatol.,* 1985 Feb;12(1):94-8.

45. Paterna, S, Pinto, A, Arrostuto, A, Cannavo, MG, Di Pasquale, P, Cottone, C, Licata, G: Raynaud's phenomenon: effects of terazosin. *Minerva Cardioangiol.,* 1997; 45: 215-21.

46. Grasing, K, Sturgill, MG, Rosen, RC, et al.: Individual AUC values determine yohimbine effects on autonomic measures. *J. Clin. Pharmacol.,* 1996; 36: 814-82.

47. Cooke, JP, Creager, SJ, Scales, KM, Ren, C, Tsapatsaris, NP, Beetham, WP, Jr, Creager, MA: Role of digital artery adrenoceptors in Raynaud's disease. *Vasc. Med.,* 1997; 2: 1-7.

48. Shepherd, RF, Shepherd, JT: Raynaud's phenomenon. *Int. Angiol.,* 1992; 11: 41-5.

49. Wigley, FM, Flavahan, NA: Raynaud's phenomenon. *Rheumatic Clin. N. Amer.,* 1996; 22: 765-781.

50. Freedman, RR, Baer, RP, Mayes, MD: Blockade of vasospastic attacks by α_2 adrenergic but not $\alpha1$ adrenergic antagonists in idiopathic Raynaud's disease. *Circulation,* 1995; 92: 1448-1451.

51. Wazieres, BD, Bartholomot, B, Fest, T, Combes, J, Kastler, B, Dupond, JL: Percutaneous thoracic sympathectomy under x-ray computed tomographic control in hyperhidrosis and refractory ischemia. Apropos of 17 cases. *Ann. Med. Int. Paris,* 1996; 147: 299-303.

52. Yee, AM, Hotchkiss, RN, Paget, SA: Adventitial stripping: a digit saving procedure in refractory Raynaud's phenomenon. *J. Rheumatol.,* 1998; 25: 269-76.

53. Klyscz, Th, Juenger, M, Meyer, H, Rassner, G: Improvement of acral circulation in a patient with systemic sclerosis with stellate blocks. *Vasa,* 1998; 27: 39-42.

54. Bunker, CB, Reavley, C, O'Shaughnessy, DJ, Dowd, PM: Calcitonin gene related peptide in the treatment of severe peipheral vascular insufficiency in Raynaud's phenomenon. *Lancet,* 1993; 342: 80-83.

55. Wigley, FM: Management of severe Raynaud's phenomenon. *J. Clin. Rheumatol.,* 1996; 2: 103-111.

56. Denton, CP, Bunce, T, Wilson, H, Howell, K, Bruckdorfer, KR, Black, CM: Anti-oxidant therapy for Raynaud's phenomenon — a controlled trial comparing probucol with nifedipine. *Arth. Rheum.,* 1995; 38: S152.

37 Treatment of Pulmonary Hypertension

Simon P. Wharton and Tim W. Higenbottam

CONTENTS

I. INTRODUCTION

The treatment of pulmonary hypertension (PH) in the setting of autoimmune disease draws from the experience gained in treating both the connective tissue diseases and the primary form of the disease. Early approaches to the treatment of PH focused largely on the use of anticoagulants, supplemental oxygen, and oral vasodilators. Calcium channel blockers seemed particularly useful. With these treatments, increased survival was seen (in patients with no evidence of right ventricular failure and an ability to vasodilate on acute testing).[1]

Prognosis for the untreated is dismal. Furthermore, as patients may relapse after responding to initial therapy, there is an urgent need for new treatments to improve the prognosis of patients with all forms of pulmonary hypertension.

The newest therapies are nitric oxide (NO) and continuous intravenous prostacyclin (epoprostenol, PGI_2). These are endogenously-produced substances and their therapeutic efficacy is not limited to vasodilation; only 30% of primary pulmonary hypertension (PPH) patients show acute vasodilation in response to these agents.[2] Their efficacy probably lies in their capacity to regulate the processes of endothelial remodeling that occurs in PH. They were initially used to treat primary pulmonary hypertension with some success, and their use is being extended to the secondary form of the disease.

Immunosuppressants have been used in the treatment of connective tissue disease, and their role in the treatment of pulmonary hypertension has been evaluated with some evidence of benefit. In particular, attention has focused on the use of cyclophosphamide in systemic sclerosis (SSc).

II. IMMUNOSUPPRESSANT THERAPY

Pulmonary hypertension secondary to interstitial lung disease and primary PH are two of the most serious complications of connective tissue disease. They have been described in rheumatoid arthritis,[3] systemic lupus erythematosus,[9] and mixed connective tissue disease,[10] but are particularly associated with systemic sclerosis. Prednisolone, azathioprine, and methotrexate have all been used, but cyclophosphamide seems to be the most effective. These treatments are all potentially toxic.

The use of cyclophosphamide in systemic sclerosis was introduced in 1981.[4] There is evidence that it has beneficial effects on both cutaneous and interstitial manifestations as measured by spirometry and transfer factors. Cyclophosphamide therapy improves FVC, DLCO, and static lung compliance.[4-8] It may be most effective in those patients with raised acute-phase reactants.[5] Case reports describe PH in SLE and mixed connective tissue disease responding to cyclophosphamide, with improvement in pulmonary function and pulmonary artery pressure (PAP).[9,10] Unpublished data may describe similar findings in SSc.[11]

Cyclophosphamide therapy is associated with serious side-effects such as sepsis, hemorrhagic cystitis, and an increased incidence of malignancy, especially carcinoma of the bladder, although the frequency of this last complication has been disputed.[11] It is not known at what point treatment should be started. The onset of interstitial lung disease and pulmonary hypertension are often silent. Given that the early use of cyclophosphamide may modify disease progression, markers of extent and onset would be useful. The extent of alveolitis on thin-section CT slices is reflected by DLCO. Both this and the estimated PAP by transthoracic echocardiography are noninvasive methods of evaluating patients. They may provide a basis upon which to make decisions about commencing potentially toxic treatment.

III. NITRIC OXIDE THERAPY

Endothelium-derived NO is a potent vasodilator and inhibitor of vascular smooth muscle cell proliferation and platelet aggregation.[12] A lack of NO-mediated vasorelaxation may be important in the pathogenesis of PH.[13,14] Inhaled NO (iNO) can be used to substitute for the deficiency of endogenously-produced NO. This may protect against the development of PH.

iNO is a selective pulmonary vasodilator[15] that acts on the precapillary pulmonary arteries.[16] The absence of a systemic effect is a result of NO that enters the alveoli, being rapidly taken up by the capillaries.[17] It is thought to bind to hemoglobin, limiting its vasodilatory effects to the pulmonary circulation. iNO activates smooth muscle soluble guanylate cyclase to increase cGMP, so causing vasorelaxation.[18] The iNO distributes to ventilated areas of the lung and, in Adult Respiratory Distress Syndrome (ARDS), it can improve arterial oxygenation.[19] In a recent study of PPH patients receiving vasodilatory therapy prior to transplantation, NO therapy in combination with O_2 successfully reduced pulmonary artery resistance in 74% (20 of 27) of patients compared with 11% of those receiving either O_2 or O_2 and prostacyclin.[20] Even when there is no change in pulmonary artery pressure following NO administration, transesophageal echocardiography has demonstrated that global myocardial function may improve.[21] However, in PH associated with chronic hypoxic lung disease, gas exchange is worsened by iNO,[22] and it is in neonatal PH that iNO is most effective.[23] There remains a need to develop an ambulatory delivery system for iNO. Currently, only patients on a mechanical ventilator can safely receive long-term iNO. Delivering NO as a "spike" at the start of each inhalation may limit the dose required and facilitate the development of a portable system for the delivery of inhaled NO.[24]

IV. PROSTACYCLIN THERAPY

Prostacyclin (PGI_2) is a metabolite of arachidonic acid. It is a potent, short-acting vasodilator. It is also a potent inhibitor of platelet aggregation, vascular smooth muscle proliferation, and leucocyte adherence to the vascular wall, maintaining vascular tone and vessel patency. The decreased expression of prostacyclin synthase in lung tissue of both primary and secondary PH patients is taken as representing reduced endothelial cell PGI_2 synthesis. Lack of PGI_2 has been implicated in pulmonary vascular remodeling, a key pathogenic feature of chronic PH. PGI_2 has a short half-life and must be delivered by continuous intravenous infusion. It activates specific PGI_2 receptors on vascular smooth muscle cells coupled to the adenylate cyclase systems. Vasodilation follows the rise of cAMP levels in the vascular smooth muscle cells.[25] PGI_2, or stable analogues such as iloprost, can be administered intravenously, as intermittent or continuous infusion, or as aerosols.

A. CONTINUOUS INFUSION IN THE TREATMENT OF PULMONARY HYPERTENSION

PGI_2 is given by continuous intravenous infusion because of its short plasma half-life. The drug is delivered via a portable infusion pump attached to a permanent indwelling central venous catheter. Ambulatory intravenous prostacyclin, which began as a bridging therapy to transplantation, now has a recognized place in the management of PH. It even produces sustained hemodynamic responses in patients who have no demonstrable acute response to infusion. These benefits may accrue through modulating vascular growth, ameliorating vascular remodeling, and preventing pulmonary thrombosis. However, there are drawbacks to this approach. Indwelling catheters are associated with sepsis, there is a small risk of pump malfunction, and treatment is expensive.

The clinical effectiveness of intravenous PGI_2 in PH was demonstrated by Higenbottam et al.[26] PGI_2 therapy can improve hemodynamic factors and increase exercise capacity in PPH refractory to conventional oral vasodilators,[27] and long-term treatment improves both survival and quality of life. Intravenous PGI_2 therapy improves the survival of patients with severe PH awaiting heart-lung transplantation, and doubles the chance of successful transplantation compared to untreated controls.[28]

The effect of treatment can also be assessed by changes in exercise capacity; compared with conventional therapy alone, treatment with PGI_2 significantly improves exercise capacity.[29] Quality of life (QoL) measures have been assessed using the Nottingham Health Profile (NHP) and Congestive Heart Failure Questionnaire (CHFQ). Compared with baseline, patients who received PGI_2 therapy over the 12-week period had a significant improvement in all four domains of the CHFQ, and two of the six domains of the NHP. Patients receiving conventional therapy alone experienced either no improvement or a worsening of their conditions.

B. INHALATION OF PROSTANOIDS

Intravenous prostanoid therapy represents a major advance in the treatment of PH. However, continuous infusion is accompanied by diminished hypoxic pulmonary vasoconstriction, reduced arterial oxygenation, and systemic vasodilation.[30] This, together with the complex delivery system and the risk of catheter-related infections and thrombosis, has driven the search for alternative routes of administration.

Inhaled or nebulized iloprost may provide a future way forward for the treatment of PH. Studies of inhaled aerolized PGI_2 indicate that iloprost induces pulmonary vasodilation and reduces pulmonary vascular resistance (PVR) without affecting systemic circulation.[31] Inhaled nitric oxide (a selective pulmonary vasodilator) and inhaled iloprost are equally effective in producing selective pulmonary vasodilation in patients with perioperative PH during cardiac surgery.[32] In mechanically ventilated patients with ARDS and pneumonia, inhaled prostacyclin and inhaled NO were equally effective in improving V/Q matching.[33] Anecdotal evidence from patients with PH treated with prostanoids suggests that optimum effects are achieved with six to nine inhalations per day, separated by short intervals in the morning and longer intervals in the evening. Inhaled iloprost has no effect on systemic artery pressure (Olschewski, H., personal communication). In patients with interstitial lung disease, inhaled iloprost also produced a greater reduction in PVR compared with calcium antagonists, intravenous PGI_2, and inhaled NO. It appears to be well tolerated, producing mild to moderate adverse effects, of which irritation of the upper respiratory tract is the most common (Olschewski, H., personal communication). Drug-related systemic side-effects are relatively rare, consistent with the drug's selective pulmonary action.

Current clinical evidence suggests inhaled iloprost is a good candidate for achieving selective pulmonary vasodilation with a decreased risk of complications. Its selectivity decreases the risk of systemic side-effects and allows treatment of patients with preexisting ventilation/perfusion (V/Q) mismatch, such as in fibrosis and pneumonia. Administration by inhalation avoids the need for implantation of an intravenous catheter, and only mild and transient irritation of the upper respiratory tract has been reported with inhaled iloprost. Inhaled therapy also offers the prospect of considerable cost savings compared with continuous intravenous infusions, and may make prostanoid therapy available for more patients. In contrast to intravenous prostanoid therapy and inhaled NO, there is no risk of rebound PH with inhaled iloprost.

C. Prostanoids for Pulmonary Hypertension in Patients with Systemic Sclerosis

Conventional therapies for the treatment of PH have generally proved ineffective in cases of isolated pulmonary hypertension, a frequent complication of limited systemic sclerosis (lcSSc) and PH secondary to fibrosis in patients with the diffuse form of the disease (dcSSc). Calcium channel blockers, such as nifedipine, have been used in patients with systemic sclerosis (SSc), but with limited success.[64] Although nifedipine has been used to treat Raynaud's syndrome in patients with lcSSc for many years, some 15 to 18% still go on to develop PH. Little is known about the efficacy of angiotensin conversor enzyme (ACE) inhibitors in the treatment of PH associated with SSc. Captopril has been investigated, however, in patients with connective tissue diseases and has been found to reduce pulmonary artery pressure during both acute and chronic administration.[34] Current opinion remains divided on the potential benefits of using anticoagulant therapy with warfarin or heparin in patients with SSc. The antiproliferative properties of these drugs have yet to be explored in such patients.

Similarities between PPH and PH associated with SSc have led to considerable interest in the use of some of the newer therapies for PPH. Iloprost has recently been investigated with encouraging results in patients with SSc. Intravenous iloprost was initially administered as a 6 to 8 hour infusion over 5 days, at doses up to the maximum tolerated of 2 ng/kg/min, to treat peripheral vascular disease associated with scleroderma.[35] A subsequent long-term study, in which intravenous iloprost was administered by infusion every 4 to 6 weeks over a 6-month period to 12 patients, 9 with lcSSc, showed it produced significant reductions in pulmonary artery pressure without any evidence of rebound effects.[36]

The success of these early studies led to a larger study of patients receiving intermittent iloprost therapy on a 3-month basis. Results of a 7-year follow-up of 42 patients with lcSSc, and 11 patients with dcSSc, who had received serial iloprost infusions suggested that patients with moderately raised pulmonary artery pressure (30 to 60 mmHg) had a better response to pulsed therapy over a period of years than those with severe disease (>60 mmHg) (Black, C., personal communication). Interestingly, patients with dcSSc and secondary PH due to interstitial lung disease, who also responded well to iloprost, appeared to have a milder form of disease than the lcSSc patients with PHT.

In addition to encouraging results obtained with intermittent iloprost therapy, there is also evidence to suggest that 24-hour ambulatory iloprost produces acute improvements in cardiac output, pulmonary artery O_2 saturation, and pulmonary artery resistance in patients with connective tissue diseases.[30] Over 32 weeks, ambulatory iloprost led to improvements in both exercise tolerance and quality of life, even though the hemodynamic response was more variable.

While intravenous iloprost is clearly beneficial in delaying the progression of PH in patients with SSc, its use tends to be limited to patients with severe established disease. Since PH progresses rapidly once established, and is difficult to reverse by current therapeutic measures, there is a need both to treat the disease in its earliest phases and to use alternatives to intravenous infusion. The oral form of iloprost represents an attractive formulation for the treatment of PH associated with SSc, and studies to evaluate its effectiveness in comparison with standard oral vasodilators are in progress.

V. CONCLUSION

Pulmonary hypertension is a relatively rare, but usually fatal, lung disorder. The endothelium of the pulmonary vasculature is central to the maintenance of normal vascular structure and function, providing a nonthrombogenic surface and barrier to cell cytotoxic effects. There is growing evidence to suggest that endothelial cells undergo a phenotypic change, which promotes vasoconstriction and enhanced thrombus formation. The pulmonary resistance vessels of patients with PH have a markedly decreased expression of prostacyclin synthase, a critical enzyme in the conversion of arachidonic acid to PGI_2. This finding, together with evidence that overexpression of prostacyclin synthase may protect against the development of PH, confirms the importance of reduced PGI_2 activity in PH. Decreased PGI_2 activity not only promotes vasoconstriction of the pulmonary artery, but also leads to increased proliferation of smooth muscle cells and activation of platelets, contributing to pulmonary vascular remodeling. This suggests that readjusting the level of prostacyclin within the pulmonary circulation may be beneficial in patients with PH. This provides the rationale for using continuous infusions of prostacyclin in the treatment of this disease. Cyclophosphamide therapy appears to have a role in modifying the disease progress in systemic sclerosis, including interstitial lung disease and pulmonary hypertension. Recent evidence of decreased prostacyclin synthase expression in plexiform lesions of the lungs of patients with PH has underlined the importance of diminished synthesis of PGI_2 in the pathogenesis of this disorder. It has reinforced the view that prostanoid therapy is a logical approach to the treatment of PH.

REFERENCES

1. Rich, S, Kaufman, E, Levy, PS. The effect of high doses of calcium-channel blockers on survival in primary pulmonary hypertension. *N. Engl. J. Med.,* 1992; 327: 76–81.
2. Rubin, LJ, Rich, S. Medical management. In: Rubin, LJ, Rich, S. (Eds). *Primary Pulmonary Hypertension.* New York: Marcel Dekker, 1997: pp 271–288.
3. Asherson, RA, Morgan, SH, Hackett, D, et al. Rheumatiod arthritis and pulmonary hypertension. A report of three cases. *J. Rheumatol.,* 1985; 12(1): 154-9.
4. Dau, PC, Kakaleh, MB, Sagebiel, RW. Plasmapheresis and immunosuppresive therapy in scleroderma. *Arthritis Rheum.,* 1981; 24: 1128-36.
5. Åkesson, A, Scheja, J, Lundin, A, et al. Improved pulmonary function in systemic sclerosis after treatment with cyclophosphamide. *Arth. Rheum.,* 1994; 37: 729-35.
6. Silver, RM, Warrick, JH, Kinsella, MB, et al. Cyclophosphamide and low dose prednisolone therapy in patients with systemic sclerosis (scleroderma) and interstitial lung disease. *J. Rheumatol.,* 1993; 20: 838-44.
7. Steen, VD, Lanz, JK, Conte, C, et al. Therapy for severe interstitial lung disease in systemic sclerosis. *Arth. Rheum.,* 1994; 37: 1290-96.
8. Behr, J, Vogelmeir, C, Beinert, T, et al. Bronchoalveolar lavage for evaluation and management of scleroderma disease of the lung. *Am. J. Respir. Crit. Care Med.,* 1997; 40(suppl): 555.
9. Groen, H, Bootsma, H, Potsma, DS, et al. Primary pulmonary hypertension in a patient with systemic lupus erythematosus: partial improvement with cyclophosphamide. *J. Rheumatol.,* 1993; 20: 1055-57.
10. Dahl, M, Chalmers, A, Wade, J, et al. Ten year survival of a patient with advanced pulmonary hypertension and mixed connective tissue disease treated with immunosuppressive therapy. *J. Rheumatol.,* 1992; 19: 1807-9.
11. Åkesson, A. Cyclophosphamide therapy for scleroderma. *Curr. Opin. Rheumatol.,* 1998; 10(6): 579-83.
12. Moncada, S, Palmer, R, Higgs, E. Nitric oxide: Physiology, pathophysiology and pharmacology. *Pharmacol. Rev.,* 1991; 43: 109–142.
13. Dinh-Xuan, AT, Higenbottam, TW, Clelland, CA, et al. Impairment of endothelium-dependent pulmonary-artery relaxation in chronic obstructive lung disease. *N. Engl. J. Med.,* 1991; 324: 1539–1547.
14. Giaid, A, Saleh, D. Reduced expression of endothelial nitric oxide synthase in the lungs of patients with pulmonary hypertension. *N. Engl. J. Med.,* 1995; 333: 214–221.

15. Pepke Zaba, J, Higenbottam, TW, Dinhxuan, AT, et al. Inhaled nitric-oxide as a cause of selective pulmonary vasodilatation in pulmonary-hypertension. *Lancet*, 1991; 338: 1173-1174.

16. Cremona, G, Takao, M, Hall, LW, Bower, EA, Higenbottam, HW. Route and site of action of inhaled nitric oxide in the vasculature of the isolated pig lung. *Journal of Applied Physiology*, 1997; 82: 23-31.

17. Borland, CDR, Higenbottam, TW. A simultaneous single breath measurement of pulmonary diffusing capacity with nitric oxide and carbon monoxide. *European Respiratory Journal*, 1989; 2: 56-63.

18. Zapol, W, Rimar, S, Gillis, N, et al. Nitric oxide and the lung. *Am. J. Respir. Crit. Care Med.*, 1994; 149: 1375–1380.

19. Rossaint, R, Falke, KJ, Lopez, F, et al. (1993). Inhaled nitric-oxide for the adult respiratory-distress syndrome. *New England Journal of Medicine*, 328, 399-405.

20. Turanlahti, MI, Laitinen, PO, Sarna, SJ, Pesonen, E. Nitric oxide, oxygen and prostacyclin in children with pulmonary hypertension. *Heart*, 1998; 79: 169–174.

21. Schulze-Neick, I, Uhlmann, F, Nurnberg, JH, et al. Aerosolized prostacyclin for preoperative evaluation and post-cardiosurgical treatment of patients with pulmonary hypertension. *Z. Kardiol.*, 1997b; 86: 71–80.

22. Barbera, JA, Roger, N, Roca, J, Rovira, I, Higenbottam, TW, Rodrifuez-Roisin, R. Worsening of pulmonary gas exchange with nitric oxide inhalation in chronic obstructive pulmonary disease. *Lancet*, 1996; (347): 436-440

23. Kinsella, JP, Neish, SR, Shaffer, E, et al. (1992). Low-dose inhalational nitric-oxide in persistent pulmonary-hypertension of the newborn. *Lancet*, 340, 819-820.

24. Katayama, Y, Higenbottam, TW, Cremona, G, et al. Minimizing the dose of NO with breath-by-breath delivery of spikes of concentrated gas. *Circulation*, 1998 Dec; 98(22):2429-32.

25. Nootens, M, Schrader, B, Kaufmann, E, et al. Comparative acute effects of adenosine and prostacyclin in primary pulmonary hypertension. *Chest*, 1995; 107: 54–57.

26. Higenbottam, TW, Wheeldon, D, Wells, F, et al. Long-term treatment of primary pulmonary hypertension with continuous intravenous epoprostenol (prostacyclin). *Lancet*, 1984; 1: 1046–1047.

27. Rubin, LJ, Mendoza, J, Hood, M, et al. Treatment of primary pulmonary hypertension with continuous intravenous prostacyclin (epoprostenol). *Ann. Intern. Med.*, 1990; 112: 485–491.

28. Higenbottam, TW, Spiegelhalter, D, Scott, JP, et al. The value of prostacyclin (epoprostenol) and heart-lung transplantation for severe pulmonary hypertension. *Br. Heart J.*, 1993; 70: 366–370.

29. Guyatt, GH, Sullivan, MJ, Thompson, PJ. The six-minute walk: A new measure of exercise capacity in patients with chronic heart failure. *Can. Med. Ass. J.*, 1985; 132: 919–923.

30. Booke, M, Hinder, F, Meyer, J. Limitations of inhaled vasodilators. *Anaesthetist*, 1996; 45: 1097–1107.

31. Haraldsson, A, Kieler-Jensen, N, Ricksten, SE. Inhaled prostacyclin for treatment of pulmonary hypertension after cardiac surgery or heart transplantation: a pharmacodynamic study. *J. Cardiothorac. Vasc. Anesth.*, 1996; 10: 864–868.

32. Schulze-Neick, I, Bultmann, M, Werner, H, et al. Right ventricular function in patients treated with inhaled nitric oxide after cardiac surgery for congenital heart disease in newborns and children. *Am. J. Cardiol.*, 1997a; 80: 360–363.

33. Walmrath, D, Schneider, T, Schermuly, R, et al. Direct comparison of inhaled nitric oxide and aerosolised prostacyclin in acute respiratory distress syndrome. *Am. J. Respir. Crit. Care Med.*, 1996; 153: 991–996.

34. Alpert, MA, Pressly, TA, Mukerji, V, et al. Short- and long-term hemodynamic effects of captopril in patients with pulmonary hypertension and selected connective tissue disease. *Chest*, 1992; 102: 1407–1412.

35. Bartram, SA, Denton, CP, du Bois, RM, et al. Sustained improvement in scleroderma associated pulmonary hypertension following pulsed intravenous prostacyclin therapy. *Arthritis Rheum.*, 1995; 38 (Suppl): S307, 927.

36. Bartosik, I, Eskilsson, J, Scheja, A, et al. Intermittent iloprost infusion therapy of pulmonary hypertension in scleroderma — a pilot study (Letter). *Br. J. Rheumatol.*, 1996; 35: 1187–1188.

Index

A